(Courtesy of Michael Vollan Photography, Inc.)

EDITOR

SUZANN K. CAMPBELL, PT, PhD, FAPTA

Professor
Department of Physical Therapy
College of Associated Health Professions
University of Illinois at Chicago
Chicago, Illinois

ASSOCIATE EDITORS

DARL W. VANDER LINDEN, PT, PhD

Assistant Professor
Department of Physical Therapy
Eastern Washington University
Spokane, Washington

ROBERT J. PALISANO, PT, ScD

Associate Professor
School of Occupational Therapy and Physiotherapy
Faculty of Health Sciences
McMaster University
Hamilton, Ontario, Canada

Physical Therapy for Children

W.B. SAUNDERS COMPANY
A Division of Harcourt Brace & Company
Philadelphia London Toronto Montreal Sydney Tokyo

W.B. SAUNDERS COMPANY
A Division of
Harcourt Brace & Company

The Curtis Center
Independence Square West
Philadelphia, PA 19106

Library of Congress Cataloging-in-Publication Data

Physical therapy for children /
[edited by] Suzann K. Campbell, Robert J. Palisano, Darl W. Vander Linden.
p.   cm.
ISBN 0–7216–6503–9
1. Physical therapy for children.   I. Campbell, Suzann K.
  II. Palisano, Robert J.   III. Vander Linden, Darl W.
    [DNLM: 1. Physical Therapy—in infancy & childhood.   2. Physical
Therapy—methods.   WB 460 P578 1994]
RJ53.P5P52   1994
615.8'2'083—dc20
DNLM/DLC   95-10990

Physical Therapy for Children   ISBN 0–7216–6503–9

Printed in the United States of America.

Last digit is the print number: 9   8   7   6   5   4

This book is dedicated to all the children who have enriched
our personal and professional lives, but especially to

DIANNE AND DEBBIE,
ABBY AND MITCHELL,
AND
CHRISTINA, JOEY, AND MICHAEL

Contributors

JENNIFER L. AGNEW-COUGHLIN, BScPT, BHK
Guest Lecturer, Department of Physical Therapy, University of Toronto; Physiotherapist, Chest Program, Hospital for Sick Children, Toronto, Ontario, Canada

JO A. ASHWELL, BScPT
Physiotherapist, Hospital for Sick Children, Toronto, Ontario, Canada

DONNA BERNHARDT-BAINBRIDGE, PT, ATC, EdD
Clinical Faculty Affiliate, Department of Physical Therapy, The University of Montana; Director, Northern Rockies Sports Rehabilitation, Missoula, Montana

DEBRA ANN BLEAKNEY, PT
Chief Clinical Therapist, Alfred I. DuPont Institute, Wilmington, Delaware

STEPHANIE BOYD, BScPT
Physiotherapist, Kitchener-Waterloo Hospital, Kitchener, Ontario, Canada

NINA S. BRADLEY, PT, PhD
Assistant Professor, Department of Biokinesiology and Physical Therapy, University of Southern California, Los Angeles, California

DINA BROOKS, BScPT, MSc
Lecturer and Course Coordinator, Department of Physical Therapy, University of Toronto; Physiotherapist, Hospital for Sick Children, Toronto, Ontario, Canada

SUZANN K. CAMPBELL, PT, PhD, FAPTA
Professor, Department of Physical Therapy, College of Associated Health Professions, University of Illinois at Chicago, Chicago, Illinois

SHIRLEY J. CARLSON, PT, PCS, MS
Assistant Director and Physical Therapy Consultant, Reaching Out—The Family and Child Inclusion Project; Physical Therapist, Spokane Guilds' School and Neuromuscular Center, Spokane, Washington

KATHRYN STEYER DAVID, PT, PCS, MS
Physical Therapist, Heartland Area Education Agency, Johnston, Iowa; Consultant for Physical Therapy Services, Bureau of Special Education, Iowa Department of Education, Des Moines, Iowa

MAUREEN DONOHOE, PT
Clinical Specialist, Alfred I. DuPont Institute, Wilmington, Delaware

SUSAN K. EFFGEN, PT, PhD
Associate Professor, Department of Orthopedic Surgery and Rehabilitation, Hahnemann University; Director, Pediatric Physical Therapy, Hahnemann University Hospital, Philadelphia, Pennsylvania

LINDA EZZELLE, PT, MS
Physical Therapist, Montgomery Public Schools, Montgomery, Alabama

CARRIE G. GAJDOSIK, PT, MS
Associate Professor, Physical Therapy Department, School of Pharmacy and Allied Health Sciences, The University of Montana, Missoula, Montana

RICHARD L. GAJDOSIK, PT, PhD
Professor, Physical Therapy Department, School of Pharmacy and Allied Health Sciences, The University of Montana, Missoula, Montana

SUSAN R. HARRIS, PT, PhD, FAPTA
Professor and Head, Division of Graduate Studies, School of Rehabilitation Sciences, University of British Columbia; Faculty Clinical Associate, Sunny Hill Health Centre for Children, Vancouver, British Columbia, Canada

KATHLEEN A. HINDERER, PT, MS, MPT
Doctoral Student, Department of Kinesiology, Division of Movement Science, University of Michigan, Ann Arbor, Michigan

STEVEN R. HINDERER, PT, MD, MS
Assistant Professor, Department of Physical Medicine and Rehabilitation, Wayne State University School of Medicine; Medical Director of Research and the Clinical Rehabilitation Research Unit, Rehabilitation Institute of Michigan; Medical Director of Rehabilitation Services, Harper Hospital, Detroit, Michigan

BETSY A. HOWELL, PT, MS
Clinical Specialist, Pediatric Cardiopulmonary Physical Therapist, University of Michigan Medical Center, Ann Arbor, Michigan

LINDA KAHN-D'ANGELO, PT, ScD
Professor of Physical Therapy, University of Massachusetts, Lowell, Massachusetts

M. KATHLEEN KELLY, PT, MS
Instructor, Department of Physical Therapy, Rangos School of Health Sciences, Duquesne University; Senior Physical Therapist, Children's Hospital of Pittsburgh, Pittsburgh, Pennsylvania

THUBI H. A. KOLOBE, PT, PhD
MCH Clinical Coordinator and Lecturer, Department of Physical Therapy, College of Associated Health Professions, University of Illinois at Chicago, Chicago, Illinois

HÉLÈNE M. LARIN, PT, PhD
Assistant Professor, Faculty of Health Sciences, School of Occupational Therapy and Physiotherapy, McMaster University, Hamilton, Ontario, Canada

JUDY LEACH, PT
Clinical and Research Coordinator, Pediatric Orthopedic and Scoliosis Medical Group; Staff, Physical Therapy Department, Children's Hospital, San Diego, California

BENJAMIN R. LOVELACE-CHANDLER, PT, PCS, PhD
President, Kids' SPOT, Little Rock, Arkansas

VENITA S. LOVELACE-CHANDLER, PT, PCS, PhD
Professor and Chairperson, Department of Physical Therapy, University of Central Arkansas, Little Rock, Arkansas

CYNTHIA L. MAGEE, PT, MS
Medford, New Jersey

TERESA L. MASSAGLI, MD
Assistant Professor, Departments of Rehabilitation Medicine and Pediatrics, University of Washington; Attending Physician, Children's Hospital and Medical Center; Consulting Physician, University of Washington Medical Center, Harborview Medical Center, Overlake Hospital Medical Center, Veterans Administration Hospital, Seattle, Washington

IRENE McEWEN, PT, PCS, PhD
Associate Professor, University of Oklahoma Health Sciences Center, Oklahoma City, Oklahoma

SANDRA M. McGEE, PT
Assistant Director of Physical Therapy, Children's Seashore House; Consultant, Comprehensive Hemophilia Clinic, Children's Hospital of Philadelphia, Philadelphia, Pennsylvania

MERILYN L. MOORE, PT
Guest Lecturer, University of Puget Sound, Tacoma, Washington, and University of Washington, Seattle, Washington; Physical Therapy Supervisor, Harborview Medical Center, Seattle, Washington

SANDRA J. OLNEY, BSc(P&OT), MEd, PhD
Professor, School of Rehabilitation Therapy, Queen's University, Kingston, Ontario, Canada

ROBERT J. PALISANO, PT, ScD
Associate Professor, Department of Physical Therapy, Allegheny University of The Health Sciences, Philadelphia, Pennsylvania; Co-Investigator, Neurodevelopmental Clinical Research Unit, McMaster University, Hamilton, Ontario, Canada

CHERYL PATRICK, PT
Senior Physical Therapist, Children's Memorial Hospital, Chicago, Illinois

WENDY E. PHILLIPS, PT, PCS, MA, MS
Senior Physical Therapist, Egleston Children's Hospital at Emory University, Atlanta, Georgia

CAROLE RAMSEY, OTR/L
Senior Occupational Therapist, Division of Developmental Disabilities, University Hospital School, University of Iowa, Iowa City, Iowa

SHIRLEY A. SCULL, PT, MS
Adjunct Assistant Professor, Philadelphia College of Pharmacy and Science; Clinical Assistant Professor, Hahnemann University; Director, Department of Physical Therapy, Children's Seashore House, Philadelphia, Pennsylvania

DAVID B. SHURTLEFF, MD
Professor, Department of Pediatrics, and Chief, Birth Defects Clinic, University of Washington; Co-Chairman, Quality Improvement/Peer Review Committee, Children's Hospital and Medical Center; Staff, University Hospital, Seattle, Washington

TERESA L. SOUTHARD, PT
Staff, The Puget Sound Physical Therapy Registry, Seattle, Washington

JOYCE W. SPARLING, PT, OT, PhD
Assistant Professor, Division of Physical Therapy, University of North Carolina at Chapel Hill, Chapel Hill, North Carolina

MICHAEL L. SPOTTS, JD
Assistant District Attorney, Fulton County, Atlanta, Georgia

MEG STANGER, PT, PCS, MS
Director of Program Services, Easter Seal Society of Lancaster County, Lancaster, Pennsylvania

JEAN L. STOUT, PT, MS
Research Physical Therapist, Motion Analysis Laboratory, Gillette Children's Hospital, St. Paul, Minnesota

WAYNE A. STUBERG, PT, PCS, PhD
Associate Professor and Director of Physical Therapy, Meyer Rehabilitation Institute; Associate Professor of Physical Therapy, Assistant Professor of Anatomy, University of Nebraska Medical Center; Adjunct Assistant Professor of Physical Therapy and Occupational Therapy, Creighton University, Omaha, Nebraska

DARL W. VANDER LINDEN, PT, PhD
Assistant Professor, Department of Physical Therapy, Eastern Washington University, Spokane, Washington

MARILYN J. WRIGHT, BScPT, MEd
Physiotherapist, Chedoke McMaster Hospitals, Hamilton, Ontario, Canada

Preface

As Cherry[1] said in a description of philosophy and science in pediatric physical therapy, specialty practice in pediatrics derives from the general philosophy of physical therapy but must address additional concerns that are different from those of physical therapy for adults. For example, clinical decision making must be guided by the knowledge that the natural development of children interacts with disability. As a result, physical therapists must anticipate and provide for children's changing needs. In addition, treatment must be adapted to children's attention to the here and now and to their dependence on adult caregivers. These significant adults must be intimately involved in both the planning of needed care and its implementation in natural settings for children—the home, school, and playground.

Another conceptual basis for the clinical practice of pediatric physical therapy is the model of the disabling process developed at the National Center for Medical Rehabilitation Research (NCMRR)[2] of the U.S. National Institutes of Health. This model defines a variety of dimensions of disablement, including (1) *impairments* of organ systems, such as deformities and limited strength, (2) *functional limitations* in whole body or body segment activity, such as locomotion or manipulation, and (3) *disabilities* in performing age-appropriate roles or activities, such as community mobility and play with peers, or independence in activities of daily living. The editors believe that all interventions that physi-

cal therapists provide should have as their ultimate goal the reduction of disability as defined in the NCMRR model. Use of this model is helpful in directing attention toward the real purpose of providing therapy for children; therefore, a focus is maintained in this book on prevention of disability throughout childhood and during the transition to living successfully as an adult.

The NCMRR model and the special needs of pediatric clients form the basis for this first comprehensive reference book for the practice of pediatric physical therapy. In the design of *Physical Therapy for Children*, the Associate Editors and I attempted to meet these needs through inclusion of (1) comprehensive coverage of the most common conditions seen in pediatric practice, (2) current information on the characteristics of best practice both from the research literature and from the experiences of the scientific practitioners who wrote each chapter, (3) delineation of critical issues during successive stages of living well with a disability from infancy to adulthood, and (4) a focus on the process of disablement from the organ systems level to functional capacities of the whole child and to disability in participating in role functions typical of children's daily interactions in natural settings.

To meet our goal of providing a comprehensive reference for pediatric practice, we believed that it was necessary to begin the book by addressing essential foundational knowledge in development, motor control, motor learning, and clinical decision making. Section One therefore begins the book with seven chapters on understanding motor performance in children. These chapters provide information on the development of *functional motor skills, gait, and the musculoskeletal structures; motor control; health-related physical fitness; and motor learn-*

[1]Cherry, DB. Pediatric physical therapy: Philosophy, science, and techniques. Pediatric Physical Therapy, 3:70–75, 1991.

[2]National Institutes of Health. Research Plan for the National Center for Medical Rehabilitation Research. NIH Pub. No. 93-3509. Bethesda, MD: National Institutes of Health, 1993.

ing. The final chapter on *clinical decision making* presents the model of the disabling process that was used as the conceptual basis for subsequent chapters on specific pediatric conditions. Although the reader will find each chapter to be self-contained, an early reading of this chapter will facilitate understanding of the structure of the material that follows.

Sections Two through Four of the book describe the pathophysiology and physical therapy management of common pediatric *musculoskeletal, neurologic*, and *cardiopulmonary* conditions, respectively. Application of the content is illustrated with case histories from the authors' practice. Physical therapy concerns are presented in each chapter in a way that makes explicit the relationships and the differences among treatment goals aimed at impairments, functional limitations, and disabilities. The Editors of this book believe that a clear delineation of each of the dimensions of the disabling process will lead to improved patient care, development of measurement tools with a strong underlying conceptual basis, and clinical research that clarifies the linkages among the various dimensions to improve the effectiveness and efficiency of clinical practice.

Finally, Section Five of *Physical Therapy for Children* addresses *special settings and special considerations*, including the *burn unit, the special care nursery, family-centered early intervention, the educational environment, private practice*, and *medicolegal issues*, such as child abuse and neglect and public laws addressing disabilities in childhood.

Just as children's health and development depend on the presence of a supportive environment, the completion of a project like this would not be possible without a variety of supports. I would like to thank my outstanding Associate Editors, Darl Vander Linden and Robert Palisano; the Senior Editor for Health-Related Professions at W.B. Saunders, Margaret Biblis, who pursued the initiation of this project until I could no longer say no and continued her support for making the book the best it could be; my husband, Richard Campbell, who has always encouraged me to do more than I thought I could do (and been right); and my Department Head at the University of Illinois at Chicago, Jules Rothstein, for allowing the time commitment this work involved. Partial support was also provided by the Maternal and Child Health Bureau of the U.S. Department of Health and Human Services, which has funded my work and that of my former graduate students (including the Associate Editors) over two decades of partnership in building the science and practice of pediatric physical therapy. Finally, I would like to thank my colleagues and mentors in pediatric physical therapy who have given me the knowledge and support to empower children with disabilities and their families to be all that they can be: Leila Green, Georgia Shambes, Margaret Moore, Mary Clyde Singleton, Marc Hansen, Ernest Kraybill, Earl Siegel, Irma Wilhelm, Carolyn Heriza, Janet Wilson, Gay Girolami, Hélène Larin, and Thubi Kolobe.

SKC

Contents

Section One

Understanding Motor Performance in Children

SUZANN K. CAMPBELL, PT, PHD, FAPTA

Section Editor

Chapter 1

The Child's Development of Functional Movement

SUZANN K. CAMPBELL, PT, PhD, FAPTA

Working knowledge of motor development is the very basis of the practice of pediatric physical therapy. It provides the norms for functioning of children at various ages that guide treatment planning through emphasis on selection of age-appropriate skills as goals. Effective program planning for children also requires knowledge of the milestones of cognitive development that must be recognized to provide treatment in a stimulating and motivating environment and to take advantage of interactions between cognitive and motor development. Developing such an environment for the provision of treatment typically involves use of play activities at a cognitive level appropriate for an individual child, regardless of the level of the child's motor development. The challenge is perhaps greatest when motor and cognitive levels in a particular child are exceedingly different.

Movement, on the other hand, also promotes cognitive and perceptual development (Bertenthal & Campos, 1987). The two go hand in hand to foster the development of functional performance. Therapists must consider in their treatment planning how to structure therapy to facilitate best all

aspects of their clients' development and to take advantage of the interactive nature of developmental subsystems, especially when functional limitations are present and likely to be lifelong. When to emphasize treatment of physical impairments and functional limitations through exercise and other therapeutic modalities, when to concentrate on finding compensatory means to prevent or limit disability in a variety of developmental areas, and when to combine the two are important components of an ongoing debate among practitioners.

In order to contribute to this debate, the specific purpose of this chapter is to describe the important milestones in the development of functional movement in children and to introduce a discussion of the processes by which development occurs, which will be elaborated on by Bradley in Chapter 2 on motor control. It seems appropriate first to define what is meant by functional movement. Fisher (1992) has reviewed the various meanings of the term function that rehabilitation professionals have used in the design and evaluation of assessment measures. Function is variously described as having a definite end or purpose and as being goal-directed as well as meaningful. A functional limitation represents a failure of the individual's performance to meet a standard expectation. When permanent, functional limitations result in a reduction in behavioral skills, task accomplishment, or fulfillment of appropriate social roles. This chronic effect of functional limitations on behavior or social roles is defined for the purposes of this volume as constituting a disability (see Chapter 7 on clinical decision making for further elaboration of definitions). In rehabilitation, impaired functional performance resulting in disabilities is frequently evaluated by assessing the degree of assistance the client needs to perform activities of daily living (ADLs). The use of technology to compensate for functional limitations, however, means that disability in performing age-appropriate social roles can be avoided through alternative means for achieving independence in daily life functions (Butler, 1991).

Certainly all therapists would agree that ADLs should be considered under the rubric of "functional." But children engage in many meaningful movement activities that appear to lack a well-defined goal. Spinning, bouncing, and endless repetition of newly learned movements, such as going up and down steps and putting things into containers and taking them out, are just a few examples (Shirley, 1931). We would probably call this "play" or "practice," but regardless of terminology, therapists surely see these activities as important aspects of motor development, motor learning, and environmental mastery. In other words, they are functional behaviors for the child's stage of development despite their lacking apparent goals. Certainly, children demonstrate a remarkable intensity of purpose when practicing emerging skills. Vander Linden (personal communication, 1993) provides several examples of his daughter Abby's development. Abby played almost compulsively with nesting cups for about 2 weeks, and when she could nest all 10, she was no longer interested in them. Similarly, she repeatedly went up and down a 4-inch step onto a screened porch in their home, insisting that her parents open the porch door for her to access the porch and resisting enticements to play with toys instead.

Based on many observations such as these, the definition provided by Fisher (1992) that I prefer is that function, or occupation, in the framework of occupational therapy theory and practice, is "what people do" (p. 184). These words imply that functional movements are self-chosen, self-directed, and, therefore, meaningful in the life of the individual at his or her particular place in the life cycle (Fisher, 1992; Oppenheim, 1981). Given this definition, our descriptive presentation will review information regarding how children develop, what they do, and the general order in which they do it, beginning with infants' spontaneously generated, that is, self-directed, movements and gradually incorporating information on tasks that are easier for adults to identify as purposeful and goal-directed.

In keeping with the importance to pediatric physical therapists of knowledge of functional motor development, the main objectives of this chapter are to 1) briefly review the historical development of theories of motor development, 2) describe current information and hypotheses regarding general principles of motor development, and 3) provide an overview of the developmental stages of acquisition of upright posture and mobility and of object manipulation—the two most basic functions that underlie meaningful activity. Brief attention will be paid to issues in cognitive development and the interaction of motor skill acquisition and perceptual-cognitive development. Finally, the chapter concludes with an abbreviated review of tests of motor development and functional motor behavior of use to physical therapists from the point of view of the theoretic perspectives provided in earlier parts of the chapter.

MOTOR DEVELOPMENT THEORIES

Throughout the history of physical therapy, theories of child development have changed dramatically, eliciting successive revisions of intervention approaches to maximizing motor development and functional performance in children. Underlying the changes in developmental theory are differing conceptualizations of the respective roles of changing structure and function within the individual and of the influence of the environment on the developmental course. Thelen and colleagues (1987) summarized the major theoretic approaches as encompassing three theories: 1) neural-maturationist, 2) cognitive, and 3) dynamical systems. Each has an interesting history that in itself makes fascinating reading because of the strong role that changing biases and accumulation of new knowledge play in how research efforts are designed and how their results are interpreted and judged (Bergenn et al., 1992; Thelen & Adolph, 1992). These theories will be reviewed briefly in this chapter; further elaboration can be found in Chapter 2 on motor control.

Neural-Maturationist Theories

The neural-maturationist point of view was pioneered by Gesell (1928a,b, 1945; Gesell et al., 1934, 1940, 1975), Shirley (1931), and others. This view proposed that the ontogeny of behavior is "an intrinsic property of the organism, with maturation leading to an unfolding of predetermined patterns, supported, but not fundamentally altered by the environment" (Thelen et al., 1987, p. 40). According to this approach, functional behaviors appear as the nervous system matures, with more complex behaviors being based on the activity of progressively higher levels of the nervous system. This theory, therefore, depends on the assumption of hierarchic maturation of neural control structures.

Gesell's point of view and research findings resulted in the development of important tests of motor milestones and other adaptive behaviors that have had, and continue to have, a monumental influence on practice in the area of diagnosis of developmental delay or deviance (Thelen & Adolph, 1992). Virtually all subsequent tests of development contained items derived from Gesell's work and ideas. Gesell emphatically believed in stages of development as biologic imperatives. Although he recognized that there are individual differences among children and was a strong believer in freedom of human action, he never resolved the paradox between these beliefs and his insistence on maturation as the predominant force driving development.

Thelen and Adolph (1992) pointed out, however, that among Gesell's less remembered contributions is the idea that the nature of development forms a spiraling function, with alternations between extremes in a variety of behavioral realms, including alternating dominance between flexor and extensor muscle activity. He believed in a principle of functional asymmetry in which the child needs to break free of symmetric movement patterns to achieve functional goals such as manipulation.

Pediatric physical therapy developed according to this theoretic model and, consequently, emphasized the assessment of stages of reflex development and motor milestones as reflections of increasingly higher levels of neural maturation (Horak, 1991). Treatment of the child with central nervous system (CNS) dysfunction was organized around inhibition of primary reflexes that were believed to persist and produce functional limitations, and it emphasized facilitation of righting and equilibrium reactions that were supposedly the underlying coordinative structures for development of skilled voluntary motor behavior.

Cognitive Theories

BEHAVIORAL THEORY

Cognitive theories of motor skill development are of two types. Skinner (1972; Bijou, 1989; Catania & Harnad, 1988) developed a behavioral approach to development that emphasizes the importance of contingent learning and posits reinforcement from the environment as the motivator and shaper of both motor and cognitive development. In this theoretic approach, the environment is the site of developmental control.

In more contemporary developmental psychology, behavioral analysis theory has been based on Skinner's later radical behaviorism and on the interbehaviorism of Kantor, in which the developing individual is conceived of as a pattern of psychologic responses in interaction with the functional environment (Bijou, 1989). Progressions in development depend on opportunities and circumstances inherent in the individual's makeup and in his or her past and present physical and social environments. Developmental progress occurs through Pavlovian responses to previous stimulation and by operant processes in which responses are controlled by consequences. Operant responses are acquired and maintained by contingent stimuli with acquired or primary reinforcing functions, and the strength of these interactions is affected by conditions such as timing and frequency of reinforcements. Although sometimes misused, behavior modification approaches have greatly aided the training of specific skills for children with mental retardation (Bijou, 1989), and the knowledge base of the behavioral approach helped therapists to break down skills into component parts for easier learning by children with impaired neural control mechanisms. Clinical problems are approached based on the beliefs that each problem has its unique history and that the treatment program should be individually tailored to the specific problem behavior.

A frequently misunderstood aspect of behavioral analysis theory is the role of individuals in their own development. The individual is not perceived of as passive and responding only when stimulated. Rather, the individual is considered to be adjusting in continual interaction with the environment. The critical feature of this theory is that it is a psychology of the individual in interaction with the environment. Stages of development are considered to be merely empirical descriptions and not in any sense causal explanations of behavior. The research methodology of behavioral analysis is, therefore, one of single-subject designs or within-subject comparisons designed to demonstrate functional relationships rather than to test theories. The elaboration of such designs has been a significant contribution to clinical research science in physical therapy and other helping professions.

PIAGETIAN THEORY

A second cognitive theory based primarily on the work of Piaget (1952) emphasizes an interaction between maturation of cognitive-neural structures and environmental opportunities to promote action (Beilin, 1989; Flavell, 1963). Control functions are found in the development of higher level plans based in biologic structures, termed schemata in Piagetian theory, or motor programs or subroutines in motor control theory (Bruner, 1970; Connolly, 1970). Cognitive mechanisms of all types are believed to derive from knowledge gained through action based at first on innate hereditary reflexes and instinctual capacities and later on experience forming concrete intelligent operations. Cognitive development culminates in abstract intelligence based on coordination of fundamental cognitive operations.

Piagetian theory had little effect on pediatric physical therapy from the perspective of planning the motor aspects of therapeutic programming because it was primarily a cognitive theory and because it continued to emphasize the evolution of functional behaviors from reflexive movements. These movements were believed to be practiced and coordinated with developing mental structures. Adaptive responses were thought to develop through psychologic processes interacting with maturation of neural structures. In this view, the most important processes are successive equilibration, disequilibrium, re-equilibration, resulting from the interaction of maturation and experience. An important aspect of Piagetian theory is the view of the individual as possessing a self-regulating system of psychologic processes that provides balance between assimilation of environmental experiences and accommodation of existing cognitive structures to that experience. The individual is a homeorrhetic system that, by virtue of its self-regulating characteristics, constantly adjusts itself to maintain equilibrium despite disturbances from the environment, thus driving developmental progress.

Viewing the operation of these psychologic processes in children who were observed while solving interesting problems led to theories of the mental structures constructed by children as a result of their activity. Neo-Piagetian work has emphasized research on the functioning of these psychologic processes (Beilin, 1989).

The concept of stages played a major role in early Piagetian theory, although in his later conceptions of development, when faced with evidence contradicting some of his hypotheses, he realized that stage theory tended to lead one to think in terms of periods of rest or equilibrium, whereas development was, in fact, never static (Beilin, 1989). In later years, Piaget, like Gesell, tended to see development as a spiraling process, an important principle that we will return to later. Description of stages, nonetheless, forms the framework for discussions of development of cognitive systems in Piagetian theory.

Four main stages were posited, each with multiple substages. The first is the stage of sensorimotor intelligence from birth to about 18 to 24 months (Beilin, 1989). Repetition in action is a major factor in this stage, culminating in the major achievement of symbolic functioning. The second period of representational thought, from 1.5 to 2 through 6 years of age, involves the development of language and of one-way mappings of logical thought that allow classifications to be developed.[1] Much work on experiments detailing the errors of logical thought in this period was influential in revealing the lack of sophistication in children's mental constructions that was not previously obvious. In the third period of concrete operations, thought processes become reversible, allowing conservation of number, weight, and volume under transformation conditions. In the final period of cognitive development, formal operations beginning at about age 11 permit logical thinking in a hypotheticodeductive mode.

The impact of Piagetian theory on pediatric physical therapy was primarily on the inclusion of interesting spectacles and problem-solving activities in therapeutic programs to assist in the cognitive-motivational aspects of facilitating motor development. Therapists used problems such as the search for hidden objects (object permanence) and problems involving means-ends relationships and container-contained ideas as therapeutic media to

---

[1]Current work on classifications suggests that they can be performed perceptually much earlier than Piaget projected, probably as early as 3 months of age in a primitive form (Hayne et al., 1987).

motivate children to move and to assess and promote the perceptual-cognitive aspects of development and motor learning (Campbell & Wilson, 1976; Fetters, 1981).

Dynamical Systems Theory

Thelen and colleagues (1987, 1989, 1993; Thelen & Ulrich, 1991; Ulrich, 1989) have proposed a dynamical functional perspective on motor development that emphasizes process rather than product or hierarchically structured plans and places neural maturation on an equal plane with other structures and processes that interact to promote motor development. These "control structures become progressively integrated with the self-organized properties of the system" (Thelen et al., 1987, p. 41) to gradually optimize skilled function. Cooperating systems include musculoskeletal components, sensory systems, central sensorimotor integrative mechanisms, and arousal and motivation and are discussed by Bradley in Chapter 2 (Heriza, 1991; Horak, 1991; Shumway-Cook & Woollacott, 1985, 1993; Thelen et al., 1987). In this theoretic approach, both these internal components of the organism and the external context of the task are equivalent in determining the outcome of behavior because behavior is task-specific. In this model of infant motor development, therefore, the environment is as important as the organism. Because the infant's cooperating systems, such as those leading to strength and postural control, do not develop at the same rate, however, certain components are seen as rate-limiting or constraining to the performance of any specific behavior.

In a seminal paper in the physical therapy literature, Heriza (1991) described the basic concepts of dynamical systems theory and suggested various approaches to testing its utility in planning and assessing therapeutic interventions. For example, eight subsystems are postulated to be involved in the development of infant locomotion. They are

1. Pattern generation of the coordinative structure leading to reciprocal lower extremity activity, consisting primarily of alternating flexor muscle activation
2. Development of reciprocal muscle activity of flexor and extensor muscles
3. Strength of extensor muscles needed for opposing the force of gravity
4. Changes in body size and composition
5. Antigravity control of upright posture of the head and trunk
6. Appropriate decoupling of the tight synchron-

ization characteristic of early reciprocal lower extremity movements, such that the knee moves out of phase with the hip and ankle
7. Visual flow sensitivity required to maintain posture while moving through the environment
8. Ability to recognize the requirements of the task and be motivated to move toward a goal

This listing makes it clear that the development of a particular motor pattern depends on a combination of mechanical, neurologic, cognitive, and perceptual factors in addition to environmental contributions specific to both the task and the context of the infant's action. Each of the subsystems develops at its own rate but is constrained or supported by physical and environmental factors, such as opportunities to practice standing upright and stepping. The movements of locomotion are conceived not as derived from a set of instructions from the nervous system nor as built from chains of reflexes but as self-organizing and emergent as a result of the interaction of the subsystems described. The locus of control for function shifts over time, depending on the dominance or constraints of various subsystems. Transitional periods, when movement patterns appear more variable, are conceived of as sensitive periods in development when intervention might be particularly effective. Future research is likely to identify these sensitive periods in the development of specific functional behaviors, thereby providing new knowledge to guide intervention by therapists.

Although use of dynamical systems theory to drive therapeutic theory and practice in physical therapy is still in its infancy, it is already clear that this model focuses the attention of the therapist on a number of important aspects of the therapeutic process of facilitating functional motor development. They include 1) search for the constraints in subsystems, such as contractures, that limit motor behavior; 2) creation of an environment that supports or compensates for weaker or less mature (rate-limiting) components of the systems that contribute to development of motor control; 3) attention to setting up a therapeutic environment that affords opportunities to practice tasks in a meaningful and functional context; and 4) search for control parameters, such as speed of movement, that can be manipulated in therapy to facilitate the attainment of therapeutic goals, especially during sensitive periods of development during which behavior is less stable (Fetters, 1991a,b; Heriza, 1991). Chapter 2 on motor control and Chapter 6 on motor learning explore these concepts as therapeutic guides in more detail.

Myrtle McGraw, although generally considered a

member of the maturationist school, developed a theory of motor development in the 1930s that contained the rudiments of many of the components of the modern dynamical systems approach to understanding the development of motor skills (Bergenn et al., 1992; McGraw, 1935). McGraw was a psychologist who studied the effects of intensive intervention, beginning at 20 days of age, with Johnny, the weaker of twin boys named Johnny and Jimmy. Her research was conducted at the height of the nature-nurture controversy between maturationists and behaviorists. In summary, her work showed that providing up to 7 hours a day of exercise of newly emerging developmental skills in the first year of life did not increase the rate of motor development. Her anecdotal comments, however, indicated that the exercised twin had more relaxed muscle tone and better coordination of movement than the twin whose movements and exploration had been restricted to a crib for much of the day, with no interaction with people other than for needed care.

McGraw's work was interpreted at the time as supporting the maturationist theory that the environment had little effect on child development. In the second year of his life, however, McGraw provided Johnny with a stimulating environment and extensive practice opportunities (3 h/d) for developing motor skills that were not otherwise likely to develop in a child younger than 2 years, such as roller skating, climbing inclines of 70°, and jumping off high pedestals. Under these conditions, Johnny excelled in physical growth, problem-solving of difficult motor control situations, and attainment of skills that Jimmy refused even to try during the periodic testing sessions that occurred. McGraw also noted the remarkable persistence in tasks demonstrated by Johnny as well as his extensive visual review of the situation before embarking on a task. Films of the twins at the age of 40 years, moreover, demonstrated that the twin who exercised intensively during the first 2 years had an impressive physique and elegantly coordinated movement compared with those of his twin.

Although the results of an analysis of 2 individual cases cannot be accepted as providing fundamental laws of motor development, McGraw's study makes it clear that we have little idea of the possibilities inherent in the very young child who is seldom stimulated to achieve the full potential of early motor skill development. By analogy, we can assume that we have barely scratched the surface in our understanding of how therapeutic intervention might be used to mitigate the effects of CNS dysfunction. In recounting her life's work and its interpretation by herself and others, McGraw also illus-

trated how the biases of the times are reflected in the design of research efforts and how their results are interpreted and received.

DEVELOPMENTAL PRINCIPLES

Based on her study of Johnny and Jimmy as well as 68 other babies studied longitudinally without special intervention, McGraw constructed a set of developmental principles, many of which remain current (or are once again current) today. She conceived of movements as behaviors within an action system in which objects in the environment are as important a part of the action system as the movements themselves. "Any activity is composed of many ingredients, some of which may for convenience be considered as external and others as internal with respect to the organism, but none of these factors can be considered as external to the behavior" (McGraw, 1935, p. 303). McGraw also recognized that multiple components are interwoven in the development of behavior patterns:

The growing of a behavior-pattern is likened to a design in the process of being woven, composed as it is of various colored threads. All of the threads do not move forward at the same time nor at the same rate. The weaver picks up the gold thread and weaves it back and forth, though at the same time steadily forward. Then he drops it in order to bring the blue thread forward a distance, until finally the two become united to make the pattern complete. The design is contingent upon the interrelation of the various threads. It is not the summation of the blue and gold threads but their position with respect to each other and to the piece as a whole which determines the design.

(MCGRAW, 1935, PP. 302–303.)

McGraw also described the uneven nature of development, in which a given behavior pattern has a period of "inception, incubation, consummation, and decline" (1935, p. 305). The results of her longitudinal studies on the intratask course of development of important motor patterns were published in 1945 (McGraw, 1963) and remain highly informative today (although her description of brain development itself has long been out of date). Because of her daily observations, she often saw a movement pattern appear only once or twice (examples of beginner's luck) and then disappear before becoming a stable part of the infant's repertoire. When first becoming stable, the activity seems overworked and exaggerated. Further, she noted that "as the child begins to get control over a pattern or an aspect of a pattern, the activity itself becomes the incentive for repetition" (McGraw, 1935, p. 307). Thus, early in life, movement for the sake of movement is a functional activity. Therapists who perceive these evanescent periods of self-driven motivation to practice emerging movements and who follow the lead of children in the flow of therapy are likely to be among those whose clients are both happy and productive in intervention sessions.

McGraw suggested that a stable movement pattern may seem to disappear as a part of the child's repertoire, becoming superseded by some rapidly developing new behavior, but ultimately the movement is restricted to its most specific and economic form. She was among the first to note the presence of normal regressions in motor behavior and has been credited as one of the first developmental psychologists to recognize the bidirectionality of neural and behavioral development (Bergenn et al., 1992; Bevor, 1982; Oppenheim, 1981; Provost, 1981). A behavior may also become integrated with other behaviors to form a complex activity; thus, McGraw noted that the developmental course of a behavior may look quite different during different stages of its maturation. A "second wind" for a behavioral pattern in decline as a part of the movement repertoire was also noted.

Because McGraw noted these various characteristics across many developing movement patterns, she believed that fits and starts, spurts and regressions, and overlapping of patterns undergoing emergence, development, and decline were firm developmental principles and that snapshots of development, such as motor milestone tests, could not adequately reflect the underlying processes of development (Bergenn et al., 1992). McGraw firmly believed that there were sensitive periods (she actually used the term "critical period" but later regretted it because of its "use it or lose it permanently" interpretation in biology) in which interventions could produce the most influence on developing behavioral patterns. The period of greatest susceptibility to exercise was believed to be one in which the pattern was entering its most rapid phase of development. Delay did not mean that intervention could no longer affect the behavior pattern (the concept of critical period), but rather that the interference of other ongoing developmental programs, including changes in anthropometric configuration of the body with growth, can decrease effectiveness. Unfortunately, we still have little idea of how these developmental principles might be systematically applied in a therapeutic milieu, but dynamical systems theory has brought them back to the forefront of scientific thinking about the processes of motor

development. When research provides prescriptions for most effectively structuring therapy based on a child's current repertoire, readiness level for learning new skills, and environmental characteristics that will be influential in evoking developmental progress, we are likely to make great strides in the efficient packaging of therapeutic programs (Bower & McLellan, 1992). Perhaps even more important will be knowledge that helps therapists to coach children more effectively in their own self-initiated attempts to drive developmental progress.

McGraw ended her monumental study of human development by foreseeing the development and potential of dynamical systems–based motion analysis! "Perhaps the time will come when the movements of growth can be expressed in mathematical formulas as precisely as the movements of celestial bodies, but until that time arrives we shall have to be content with cumbersome descriptive analyses" (McGraw, 1935, p. 312). Although both McGraw and Gesell believed that neural maturation was the primary force driving development, the observations and theories of each pointed up the dynamic nature of motor development. The approach of dynamical systems analysis has added knowledge gained from many kinds of physical systems, including nonbiologic systems. In decades to come, we shall see how this new approach contributes to explaining the observations of the theorists who pioneered the study of motor development.

Contemporary Issues in Understanding Principles of Motor Development

Despite a new theoretic perspective that models development as encompassing multiple organismic components in the creation of coordinative structures for posture and movement and emphasizing the crucial role of the environment and task characteristics in organizing emergent movements, certain principles of motor development have rather consistently appeared in the concepts of various students of motor development. These include the notions that development of motor skills generally proceeds in a cephalocaudal and proximodistal direction, that neural maturation is an important component of unfolding skill development, and that motor development appears, at least on the surface, to be more stage-like than continuous, having a spiralling nature in which regressions, consolidations, and reappearances of underlying fundamental processes occur (Bevor, 1982).

What is becoming clear is that these long-standing theoretic concepts must be expanded to incorporate a new understanding of the underlying developmental processes. For example, new research on developmental processes discussed in Chapter 2 on motor control has revealed that certain factors are rate-limiting to motor development, with postural control and perceptual analysis capabilities being among the most important. When compensations are provided experimentally to eliminate the effects of these rate-limiting factors, the developing motor system may display previously unrecognized potential. Patterns of movement appear that seem precocious because they were previously denied expression owing to immaturity of other cooperating systems.

Dynamical systems theory has also demonstrated that stage-like external behavior can emerge from continuously changing underlying processes. Here a new stage seems to appear de novo only because the continuous developments of a number of cooperating systems finally merge in a way that allows the new behavior to appear. The behavior appears to reflect an entirely novel stage of development when, in fact, the underlying processes in multiple systems were developing continuously in a gradually accretive fashion. We will use new information about the development of eye-hand coordination to illustrate these points.

CEPHALOCAUDAL AND PROXIMODISTAL DEVELOPMENTAL DIRECTION

The processes involved in functional reaching include 1) visual fixation to localize the object and choose a hand transport program, 2) foveal analysis for perceptual identification of the object needed for anticipatory adaptation of the action to fit the characteristics of the object, 3) manual capture, and 4) object manipulation (Hay, 1990). By the time of birth, a primitive body scheme has already developed that provides the infant with a hand transport program. Infants have been observed in utero during real-time ultrasound imaging to perform hand-to-mouth activities, touch other parts of their own bodies, and explore the uterine walls—all, of course, without visual guidance (Sparling, 1993). Shortly after birth, they are able to launch the hand toward a visualized object, preferring one that is moving (von Hofsten, 1982).[2] The hand, although

open, does not engage in actual grasping in most cases, and the coordination of the movement does not include corrections of direction or hand-shaping for the object's properties during the course of the reach (Vinter, 1990). In fact, the entire arm is launched as a single unit in a pattern that can best be described as a swipe, a coordinative strategy that is quite unlike the lift-project strategy typical of more mature reaching.

Because we know that further development will include gradual refinement of hand use as part of reaching and grasping, this sequence of development would appear to follow the proximodistal developmental rule. The course of development, however, is much more complicated. First, reaching at 1 to 2 months is typically done with a fisted hand, rather than the open hand of the newborn, and reaching under visual control with an open hand begins anew at 4 to 5 months (Vinter, 1990). Furthermore, successful reach-and-grasp under visual control can often occur in the period from 1 to 2 months if the head is supported to eliminate a major problem in developing a successful coordinative strategy. Thus, when external controls are provided for the posturally incompetent head, the infant may be able to coordinate a reach-and-grasp successfully.

These and other observations have led to the suggestions that postural control is a rate-limiting factor in early motor development (Shumway-Cook & Woollacott, 1993) and that distal competence may be masked by deficiencies in postural control of the head and neck. Although it seems readily apparent that the ability to control the head to maintain stability of visual perception is an important early competence in a general sequence of cephalocaudal progression of development, many aspects of proximal and distal control of the extremities are undergoing contemporaneous development that may not be overtly observable under normal conditions (see Fetters et al., 1989; Heriza, 1991; and Loria, 1980, for further examples).

An important consequence of understanding these new findings from research is that therapists should not conceive of individual body parts as developing independently, sequentially, or purely as a result of nervous system maturation when planning therapeutic intervention. Although various segments of the body may develop their patterns of control for any given task at different rates, any movement pattern is a composite, involving coordination of all of the body subsystems. Furthermore, the apparent directionality of development does not appear to be inherent only in the genetic direction of nervous system development, but rather is a result of the interactive functioning

---

[2]This competence fits well with the known characteristics of early development of the retina, which is more mature in the movement-sensitive periphery than in the foveal area (Abramov et al., 1982).

of the multiple systems children bring to exploration of the problems and possibilities inherent in a particular task at a particular point in their development (Thelen, 1990). The characteristics and demands of the task are critical in organizing the response of the subsystems, but each child's response is unique in its kinematics and time of appearance (Thelen et al., 1993). In early infancy, for example, the enormous mass of the child's head relative to the size of the rest of the body places constraints on the functions that are possible. Lifting the head and sustaining its upright position while the body is prone, therefore, entail coordinating the trunk and extremities to create a stable base for head movement. The role of the neck extensor muscles may be comparatively minor, yet until the head can be adequately stabilized in space, other movement functions of the body in the prone position cannot be fully expressed. In attempts to lift the head while prone to look at an interesting object, each child produces a unique and specific pattern of movement that depends on individual anthropometric characteristics, muscle strength and limb compliance, visual acuity, previous experience, and interest in the object.

In summary, what seems to play a major role in the general observation of cephalocaudal progression of development is the infant's anthropometric characteristics, that is, the large mass of the head relative to the rest of the body and the high center of mass. Cephalocaudal progression is a notion that continues to hold as an overall generalization regarding the postural control of the whole body, but its basis is probably not in the sequence of development of the nervous system. This notion should not be assumed to imply that one part of the body is functioning alone, because most movements used by infants entail the coordination of multiple body parts to be effective. Finally, many exceptions to a proximodistal progression of development have been found (Heriza, 1991).

The examples given earlier illustrate the potential power of the dynamical systems perspective by pointing out that multiple systems and processes are developing at any given time, each at its own rate and instantaneous level of competence. What then appears to be a newly appearing stage may merely be the time at which one or more rate-limiting factors finally achieve a level of development in a continuous trajectory that supports the appearance of a new behavior. The new behavior appears discontinuous with what went before only because the underlying processes were not visible. Further research to identify these critical processes and systems should be productive in refining intervention strategies to promote motor development.

NERVOUS SYSTEM MATURATION AS ONE DRIVING FORCE FOR DEVELOPMENT

Although McGraw (1963), Gesell (1928a,b), and Shirley (1931) emphasized brain maturation as being the major force driving development (despite their own contrary evidence for the important role of external factors), dynamical systems theory has sometimes seemed to view neural maturation with less credence than I believe it deserves. The nervous system in dynamical systems theory is described as merely another system in its developmental contribution, no more important than any other system. In many children with mental retardation or cerebral motor dysfunction, however, therapists are well aware of the limitations in adapting movement to functional purposes imposed by a compromised CNS.

Research suggests that about 30% of the entire genome is expressed only in the brain (Nowakowski, 1987). Although it is true that we now know that experience drives brain development in just as important a way as do genetic programs (Greenough et al., 1987), the notion that no hierarchy of important functions or no unique function of structures exists is simply not true, especially in the human brain, with its highly encephalized processes. What is true is that lower levels of the nervous system, such as the midbrain and the spinal cord, have been recognized to be capable of controlling many finely coordinated movements, not only simple reflexes, and that vast amounts of the CNS are involved in the production and control of even the most basic movements. For example, animal research described by Bradley in Chapter 2 has revealed that well-coordinated stepping movements can be evoked from activation of spinal cord circuits. Involvement of higher levels of the nervous system, however, is necessary to control the body's overall equilibrium during gait and to express the intentionality of functional movements. The locus of control for a given movement within the CNS varies, however, depending on task requirements and previous experience with similar tasks. Thus, environmental demands become a part of the neural ensemble for producing movement.

To return to the example of development of eye-hand coordination, humans display a major shift from subcortically directed movement in the first 3 to 4 months to increasing involvement of cortical circuits at 4 to 5 months (Paillard, 1990). Infants with later evidence of cortical blindness, for example, may be able to track an object visually in the newborn period, using brain stem processing mechanisms reflecting genetically constructed neural networks. Although the organism's own activity is influential in directing the course of neural plasticity during development (Greenough et al., 1987), this example of deviant development reinforces the concept that the higher levels of the CNS are necessary (but not sufficient) for normal human development to occur.

Reaching, too, differs fundamentally in the newborn and the 6-month-old (Paillard, 1990). Reaching is a unitary action in the young infant; a differentiation among reach, grasp, manipulation, and release will later result from maturation of cortical systems in conjunction with learning gained from experiences in the world of objects (Fentress, 1990). As seen in patients with a stroke that affects fine hand function, cortical activity is necessary for the more delicate aspects of motor control of the hand, and it cannot develop adequately unless the encephalic structures are intact. No examples have been reported in the literature of a capability of higher primates to develop or regain fine finger control in the absence of primary motor cortex. In humans, individual finger movements cannot be evoked by electrical stimulation of the motor cortex before 3 months of age (Fentress, 1990).

Establishment of monosynaptic connections between the motor cortex and spinal cord motoneurons is associated with the appearance of selective control of digital movements in primates (Schoen, 1969); these connections are not present in neonatal monkeys and develop gradually during the first 8 months after birth. Improvement in monkeys' abilities to retrieve small pieces of food from indentations is seen when a wide range of rapid, small movements involving the forearm or shoulder joint appear to assist more efficient distal performance of the digits. This description is remarkably similar to descriptions of the development of fidgety movements in human infants at 2 to 3 months of age (Hadders-Algra & Prechtl, 1992). These movements herald the development of goal-directed movements, including the emergence of consistently effective reaching and grasping. These small synergistic movements in monkeys do not survive pyramidotomy, nor do selective digital movements.

According to Paillard (1990), four features characterize the evolution of the primate nervous system, culminating in the human brain, that promote use of the hand as an elaborate tool for manipulating the environment. These features are 1) extension of the precentral cortex developed principally for fine sensory-guided steering and control of the hand and digits; 2) enlargement of the lateral cerebellum, again relating to control of forelimb segments and to timing and smoothing of movements; 3) specialization of the parietal association cortex

for precise visual guidance of goal-directed arm and hand movements; and 4) prominent development of the frontal association areas that funnel information to motor control regions, mainly through basal ganglia loops.

The frontal areas process information related to goal-directed behavior and anticipated consequences of intended acts involving the basic capacity to guide response choice by stored information (Goldman-Rakic, 1987; Paillard, 1990). Major developments in this area in the human infant begin at about 8 months and reach a maximum at 2 years of age. Activity in frontal areas cooperates in motor functions through basal ganglia circuits (Hoover & Strick, 1993). The basal ganglia are involved in the internal generation of automatic movements, the predictive monitoring of head and arm activities (Fentress, 1990), and the acquisition and learning of motor skills through their five parallel pallidal-thalamocortical loops, including projections to primary motor cortex, where the dynamics of movement patterns are developed (Georgopoulos et al., 1992).

Eye-head-body orientation activities and target-reaching activities have been shown in lower vertebrates to be coordinated primarily by brain stem centers, prominently involving the superior colliculus (Paillard, 1990). In keeping with identification of these behaviors in very young infants, arm projection at that age is possible without cerebral cortical control. Functional manipulation, such as the fine digital control involved in food taking in experimental primates, however, depends on the additional coordinated action of cortical pathways from higher centers (Fentress, 1990). Elegant hand-grasping and manipulation movements of the primate are dependent on inputs from cerebral cortical levels that are coordinated with lower level eye-hand-head programming. Overall, however, the primary role of higher level structures is to tune, guide, learn, and adapt or inhibit execution of basic programs located at the brain stem level. The therapist views this as increasing ability to control movements selectively and adapt them to functional purposes.

Motor control functions are not assumed at successively higher hierarchic levels, leaving behind previously used primitive behaviors and control centers; rather, many levels of the nervous system cooperate in the production of movement behaviors. Typically, no single control site for any particular behavior can be identified; behavior is, rather, an emergent property of the cooperation of various subsystems, with task characteristics organizing the response (Thelen et al., 1993). This statement should not, however, be construed to suggest that any area of the nervous system can substitute for any other. The next section of this chapter elaborates on a theory of nervous system function that provides an appropriate explanatory model for how the developing organism actively constructs its own operating system for functional behavior.

The Theory of Neuronal Group Selection

According to a popular summary by Edelman (1992) of current theories of nervous system functioning, previous psychologic theories have failed spectacularly in shedding light on how the human mind originates in the functioning of the physical brain because they have neglected the biology of the system. Popular models describing the brain as analogous to a computer with hardware (neurons) and software (motor programs) bear only superficial resemblance to the actual operation of the brain. Edelman's theory is based instead on facts that are garnered from biologic research but are consistent with behavioral observations. Called the neuronal group selection theory, it has three basic tenets. These tenets describe how the anatomy of the brain is produced during development, how experience selects for strengthening certain patterns of responses from the anatomic structures, and how the resulting maps of the brain give rise to uniquely individual behavioral functions through a process called reentry.

The first tenet of Edelman's theory (1992) is concerned with developmental selection by which the characteristic neuroanatomy of a species is formed. The genetic code of the species does not specify the wiring diagram but instead describes the constraints of the process of formation of neural networks, resulting in a primary repertoire of species-specific behavior. In humans, for example, these behaviors appear to include rhythmic movements of the lower extremities, expressed in kicking and neonatal stepping (Thelen, 1990), mouth-to-hand behaviors, and visual following and projection of the arm toward moving objects (von Hofsten, 1982). An overproduction of early synaptic connections formed by activity and cell death or retraction of unexercised connections may explain why individual wiring diagrams vary somewhat while still maintaining the same general form across members of the species.

The second tenet of Edelman's (1992) neuronal group selection theory involves the development of a secondary repertoire of functional circuits from the basic neuroanatomic network through a process of selective activation that strengthens or weakens synaptic connections based on individual experience. The secondary repertoire includes mechanisms underlying skilled motor behavior, memory, and other important functions and is unique to the individual.

Edelman's third tenet describes how the first two selectional processes interact to connect biology with psychology. The primary and secondary repertoires of species-typical and uniquely individual functional neural circuits must form maps connected by massively parallel and reciprocal connections. Edelman gives the example that the visual system of the monkey consists of more than 30 different maps, each with a unique degree of functional segregation for orientation, color, movement, and other functions and each linked to the others by parallel and reciprocal connections that can be accessed by the reentry process.

Selection occurs over neuronal groups from various maps throughout the region and the nervous system as a whole to produce a particular behavior. The behavior is unique to the individual in whom it occurs because of variations in maps caused by the effects of individual experience on their development. The combination of neuronal groups from selected multiple maps of an area's function (for example, the hand motor area of primary cerebral motor cortex combined with selections from maps that are concerned with receipt of visual and tactile information and ones concerned with postural function of the neck and shoulder) allows the production of a movement that is precisely tuned to the environmental demands for functional performance yet unique to the individual's capacity for receiving sensory inputs and for combining selections of neuronal groups from his or her individual regional maps.

Such a model is consistent with the research of Keshner and colleagues (1989), demonstrating that when overtly similar movements are studied in a group of individuals, each person performs the movement with his or her own unique combination of synergistic muscle activation patterns. Thelen and colleagues (1993) have demonstrated similar findings in infants learning to reach. Although a group of infants tended to use a similar strategy of coactivating muscular antagonists when first learning to reach, each infant came at the task in a unique way based on preferred posture, movement, and energy level. Two quiet infants, for example, organized their reaches by lifting their arms and extending them slowly forward. Two other infants, who were highly active and frequently engaged in bilateral arm flapping, needed to damp down their oscillations to reach successfully. These infants used high-velocity swipes to orient their arms toward the toy.

In keeping with each individual's march to a personal internal drum, each phenotypic neuronal group has a combination of excitatory and inhibitory connections, allowing the final motor output to be assembled selectively based on current demands and past experience with the task that has strengthened or weakened the tendencies to select particular groups from particular maps (Edelman, 1992; Thelen, 1990). Resulting from these selections, higher order dynamic structures called global maps are formed that link sensory and motor maps. These global maps are able to interact with memory processes and other unmapped functions such as those of the basal ganglia and cerebellum. Global maps allow the connection between local maps and motor behavior, new sensory inputs, and further neural processing as important aspects of development and learning.

Neuronal group selection theory does not hold that programs are executed by the nervous system; rather, dynamic loops are created that continually match movements and postures to task-related sensory signals of multiple kinds. Functioning is based on statistical probabilities of signals, not coded signals or preformed programs. Georgopoulos and colleagues (1993), for example, have demonstrated that the precise directionality of a reaching movement can be specified by vectors calculated from the neural activity of large populations of cells in the motor cortex, each of which individually has a preferred directionality but also fires in relation to movements in multiple directions. Edelman (1992) further theorized that the system has biologic "values" that are species-specific and drive the selective strengthening of synaptic activities based on experience. These values influence adaptive processes by linkage between the global mappings and activity in hedonic centers and the limbic system of the brain in a way that fulfills homeostatic needs of the organism that have been set through evolution.

In a computer model of a visual system with a set "value" (similar to that produced in humans by evolution) that prefers light to no-light conditions in the center of a "visual" field, initially nondirected movements of an "arm" have been shaped to target an object (Edelman, 1992). If one appreciates that newborn infants possess a primary repertoire that includes moving the mouth to the hand, seeking light, and producing head turns or arm projections in response to moving objects in the visual field, it is not difficult to perceive of the theory of neuronal group selection as an explanation for the gradual process of learning to reach successfully to grasp an object and put it into the mouth.

With repeated experience in reaching and grasping as an "individual problem-solver working each day" (Thelen et al., 1993), infants modulate their intrinsic dynamics, discovering the most stable trajectory, joint coordination, and patterns of muscle activation (Thelen et al., 1993), and thereby creating their own personal maps. For example, Strick and Preston (1982a,b) have suggested that separate representations of hand motor patterns at cerebral cortical levels may reflect the modular organization of sensorimotor units underlying the distinctive uses of the hand for power gripping or as a palpatory sensory surface.

Experience-Expectant and Experience-Dependent Neural Maturation

Greenough and colleagues (1987) have also discussed the importance of environmental experience in driving development of the brain, and their work provides further elaboration on Edelman's theory of neuronal group selection in a maturational context. Although no scientific evidence exists to suggest that training or an enriched environment leads to development of new neurons, extensive evidence documents the effect of training and environment on numbers and properties of synaptic connections among neural cells. Greenough and colleagues (1987) suggested that genetically specified directions lead to initial synaptic connectivities through a process of overproduction of populations of cells that are pruned by exposure to experiences common to all members of a species, such as the array of visual inputs to which infants are typically exposed. The result is species-typical behaviors akin to the primary repertoire described by Edelman (1992).

Greenough and colleagues (1987) called this process experience-expectant development and suggested that it occurs through the death of cells that do not establish productive connections. It has been discovered, however, that the genetic code may actually program cell death (Barinaga, 1993). If neurons have access to particular nerve growth factors, they may be able to escape their programmed fate. By such genetic-environmental interactions, development occurs by a size-matching process whereby the appropriate number of neurons survives to serve peripheral needs. By one's own developmental processes, therefore, each individual obtains a personal, unique structure and functional movement.

A second process, akin to Edelman's secondary repertoire and called experience-dependent neural maturation, is proposed to be the process by which each individual achieves further uniqueness in structure and function through exposure to an individualized set of experiences that establishes strong connectivities among cells based on strengthening of neural synapses that are "exercised" through both sensory and motor experiences (Greenough et al., 1987). The specific structure and function of a person, therefore, depend on both species-typical connectivities and the amount and strength of other connections resulting from personal experiences specific to each individual and his or her life history. Of most importance, in both aspects of neural plasticity, synaptic connectivity is linked to the individual's own activity in conjunction with genetic programs and environmental opportunities. Thus, the individual in a very real sense is the creator of his or her own unique brain and, by extension, functional motor behavior (Thelen, 1990).

Bertenthal and Campos, in a 1987 commentary on Greenough and colleagues' theory, summarized research that may support the theory that experience-expectant and experience-dependent maturation of neural systems could be the basis of sensitive periods in development. They stressed that experience-dependent plasticity of the nervous system can initiate the generation of new synaptic connections and is available throughout the life span. The effects of experiences during a sensitive period, however, are expected to be qualitatively different from those at other points in the life span. The theory also predicts that sensitive periods in experience-expectant development can be extended by various means, including deprivation of sensory inputs that allow synaptic competition for connections to persist longer than is usual.

Most of the animal research on the influence of environmental stimuli on neural plasticity has been on cerebral cortical areas, especially those devoted to visual function, but some evidence also exists to suggest effects on the motor cortex and the cerebellum (Greenough et al., 1987). Research has documented the existence of sensitive, and in some cases, critical, periods for development of visual-perceptual skills, once again suggesting the superior benefits of intervention earlier, rather than later, in life.

Several sensitive periods in cognitive development have been demonstrated to occur during infancy (Fischer, 1987). At 2 to 4 months, infants demonstrate the ability to vary activity within a single action sequence to reach a simple goal, such as grasping a toy within reach. At 7 to 8 months, several actions can be related in a single functional unit, such as a delayed response task, using vision to guide a manual manipulation or compare multiple objects, and using a string to activate a toy. By 12 to 13 months, a number of actions can be coordinated to perform a function such as putting a ball into a small hole in a toy box. At 18 to 21 months,

symbolic representation is achieved in which a memory of an object can activate an action without the object's being present. Various types of evidence, such as changes in rates of synaptogenesis and electroencephalographic changes, show discontinuities at related time periods. Whether these demonstrated discontinuities in developmental rates at the level of neuronal groups and behavioral stages are compatible with the dynamical systems view of continuity in subsystem development remains to be demonstrated. Much of the confusion regarding whether development is continuous or discontinuous may reflect disagreement among researchers working at different levels of analysis.

Unfortunately, only few data are available on the subject of sensitive periods as they affect motor skill development, particularly in children with acquired or congenital disabilities. Zelazo and colleagues (1972, 1983), however, demonstrated the effect of early stepping experience in human infants on maintenance of stepping behavior and earlier age of walking. Heriza (1991) has proposed that sensitive periods exist in the development of locomotor behavior that can be identified through kinematic analysis of rhythmic alternating movements of the legs based on dynamical systems theory and hypothesized that these transitional periods are important points for intervention in children at risk for developmental disabilities. Kanda and colleagues (1984) have also shown the superior benefits on quality of movement and walking in children with cerebral palsy of early, as opposed to later, exposure to Vojta therapy, and Scherzer and colleagues (1976) suggested that children with cerebral palsy who were treated at an earlier age than others also demonstrated greater benefits. These preliminary suggestions that intervention to promote motor development may vary in effectiveness based on timing of therapy are tantalizing, and further research on this topic is direly needed for improving the scheduling of intervention for maximizing outcomes. To be successful, however, research designs must be tailored specifically to the search for answers to the sensitive period question.

PERIODIC EQUILIBRATION IN A SPIRALING PATTERN OF DEVELOPMENT

Piaget suggested that the experience of acting on the world (assimilation) with whatever sensorimotor schema is currently dominant was frequently met with resistance because the objects of interest were not easily adapted to the current schema (e.g., handling a soft cookie when the motor activity of crumpling or shaking was currently popular). This misfit between the child's current sensorimotor functioning and the response of handled objects leads to disequilibrium, which drives developmental progress through the child's persistence in gradually accommodating to the properties of objects eliciting interest. In so doing, the child eventually develops a different approach to handling the cookie and thereby alters the cognitive structure as well.

Ames and colleagues (1979), following from Gesell's earlier observations, posited a similar process of alternating equilibrium and disequilibrium in behavioral characteristics that they believed cycled periodically. For example, toddlers at 18 months[3] are likely to be trying to their parents because they have definite wants but few words with which to express them and communicate with crying and tantrums instead. At 2 years, the child has developed more language and coordination and is emotionally on an even keel. Disequilibrium returns again at about 2.5 years, when this little person becomes more difficult to live with — bossy, rigid, and oppositional. Cooperation and sharing in play have not yet appeared, and the 2.5-year-old wants to hold onto any toy "he is playing with, has played with, or might in the future want to play with" (Ames et al., 1979, p. 28). The age of 3 years is again an easy time emotionally, whereas at 3.5 years children are insecure and anxious, yet determined and self-willed. At 3, children need their security blankets and thumbs a great deal. The 4-year-old is described as wild and wonderful. This child loves humor and is secure and self-confident, although going overboard in either enthusiasm or anger, even threatening to run away when upset. Five-year-olds are more inwardly directed, prefer to stay within known boundaries, and have less interest in novel experiences. These children are careful to attempt only what can most definitely be achieved but are, nonetheless, expansive intellectually, loving to talk and learn about things. "Why?" is the word of choice. By 5.5 years, however, another period of disequilibrium seems to occur, but it is one characterized by extremes — shy at one moment, extremely bold the next. The child may seem to be in a constant state of tension, chewing on pencils and fidgeting. By 6.5 years, however, a calmer, more even-tempered child again emerges, moving toward the inner-directed 7-year-old.

Gesell (Heriza, 1991), Rood (Stengel et al., 1984), Bly (1983), and others have suggested that motor development also consists of an alternation and recombination of patterns of flexion, extension, and symmetry versus asymmetry, leading ever onward toward improved mobility and stability in posture and movement in opposition to the force of gravity. At different times, various patterns predominate, but an alternation between stability and instability of functioning characterized also by switches between symmetry and asymmetry is thought to be characteristic of normal developmental progression. Heriza has summarized these principles based on Gesell's early work as viewing growth "not as a linear process but a spiral one where structure and function jointly mature leading to regression, asymmetries, and reorganization. Although Gesell is best known for his principles of direction of development and individuating maturation, his principle of reciprocal interweaving . . . foreshadows [a] contemporary systems view of motor development" (Heriza, 1991, p. 102). As we have seen, McGraw (1935) held a similar view, but she and other early developmental researchers lacked the contemporary ability to reveal the underlying systems changes that produce these overtly observed patterns of development.

To summarize, studies have suggested that development proceeds in a continuous spiral characterized by "paired-but-opposed types of responses that occur in repeated alternation" (Ames et al., 1979, p. 4) and with relative periods of stability and instability (Heriza, 1991) that may or may not reflect underlying developmental continuity within subsystems involved in maturation. Regressions are also normal aspects of developmental processes (Bevor, 1982; Oppenheim, 1981; Provost, 1981). The ages of 2, 5, 10, and 16 years are considered to be periods of emotional equilibrium; 3.5, 7, and 13 as periods of relative inwardness and withdrawal; and ages 4, 8, and 14 as periods of expansive behavior (Ames et al., 1979). More recent research has suggested that periods of rapid behavioral changes of many kinds occur at approximately 4, 6 to 7, 10 to 12, and 14 to 16 years (Fischer, 1987). Similarly, Shumway-Cook and Woollacott (1985) have suggested that motor patterns in the development of postural stability undergo a period of disequilibrium between 4 and 6 years, when a physical growth spurt occurs. Changes in perceptual functions during this period offer an alternative, or possibly an additional, explanation.

Whether these findings can be correlated with specific periods of brain growth is an interesting question. Epstein (1979) has found that there are major periods of accelerated brain growth (relative to body growth) in the periods from 3 to 10 months, and from 2 to 4, 6 to 8, 10 to 12+, and 14

---

[3]The reader should note that in this and other sections of the chapter, ages given are normative or average times of appearance of described behaviors; individual developmental rates may, of course, differ to some extent.

to 16+ years. Between 3 and 12 months, a major area of myelinization in the human is the inferior parietal cortex, a cross-modal association area. The cerebellum also shows its major, and virtually final, growth during this period, demonstrating an approximately 3-fold increase in DNA compared with the cerebrum. Except for the first period in infancy, however, growth is not accompanied by a net increase in brain DNA, so growth after about 1.5 years is assumed to be composed primarily of elaboration of networks of axons and dendrites and of axon myelinization. The latter is primarily associated with enhanced speed of neural processing.

Overall brain growth stages have been correlated with mind growth, a process called "phrenoblysis" (Epstein, 1979). Although Greenough and colleagues (1987) cautioned that spurts in growth of the whole brain or in head circumference may not be reflective of relative differences in timing of growth rates in the various regions of the brain, Goldman-Rakic (1987) has shown that concurrent spurts of synaptogenesis take place in many regions of the cerebral cortex of rhesus monkeys during the period of rapid behavioral growth in ability to perform delayed-response tasks. In humans, this stage occurs beginning at about 8 months, with rapid developments in understanding of object permanence, and can be correlated with rapid synaptogenesis in the visual cortex (Fischer, 1987; Goldman-Rakic, 1987). In humans, however, the prefrontal cortex, the area of the brain that has been related to delayed-response tasks, has an extensive period of synaptogenic development, peaking at 1 to 2 years and remaining high until about 7 years.

During the second postnatal brain growth stage (2–4 yr), there are striking developments in sensory function, including binocularity, hearing, and language. Evidence suggests that earlier occurring defects in these functions can be remedied only during the growth stage. For example, the fact that children with strabismus leading to amblyopia will never have normal binocularity if the strabismus is not corrected during the first 3 years of life is important evidence of a critical period in development (Banks, et al., 1975; Hohmann & Creutzfeldt, 1975).

For cognitive function also, Epstein (1979) contended that mental age shows developmental stages that generally agree with those of brain growth. He suggested that the reason for successful enhancement of the cognitive development of children who begin attending the federally funded Head Start programs by age 2 versus those who do not begin until 4 to 6 years was that minimal brain growth occurs during the later period. Physical therapists,

of course, have long suggested that treatment of developmental motor dysfunction, such as that found in cerebral palsy, is more successful when begun during the first year of life, a period in which the cerebellum shows massive growth. As previously noted, however, only a small amount of suggestive evidence to support this conjecture is currently available (Kanda et al., 1984; Scherzer et al., 1976).

In summary, significant principles of motor development include 1) overall cephalocaudal progression, 2) spiraling development characterized by periods of relative stability and instability and sensitive periods in which development is especially responsive to environmental influences and therapeutic intervention, and 3) self-regulating active construction of developmental progress on the part of the child. Developmental milestones that appear to reflect discontinuous stages may actually reflect underlying continuity of development in subsystems maturing at different rates. The finding of punctuated periods of rapid synaptogenesis in the brain may contradict this view at the cellular level, but they are likely to provide the means by which genetic programs provide a general framework for development of the individual. Each human brain is uniquely inscribed through active creation of functional networks of neuronal groups selected by species-typical values shaping selective processes driving development and learning. Most developmentalists would now agree that the individual is formed through interaction between genetically determined processes, individual history, and environmental opportunities at least partially created by the organism itself.

"STAGES" OF MOTOR DEVELOPMENT

The next section will elaborate on the observable "stages" of gross and fine motor development that represent milestones of developmental progress toward achieving the goals of upright posture, mobility, and manipulation—essential elements of environmental mastery and control. As infants attain and perfect these major developmental motor skills, they are incorporated into functional ADLs such as self-care, feeding, and play. Important milestones of motor development in later years of childhood will also be briefly addressed.

The major gross motor milestones of the first 12 to 18 months include achieving an indefinitely maintained upright head posture, attaining prone-on-elbows position, rolling from supine to prone, independent sitting, attaining hands-and-knees position, moving from sitting to four-point position and prone, creeping on hands and knees, pulling to a stand, standing independently, and walking independently (van Blankenstein et al., 1962). As each position or skill is attained, further development will entail the perfecting of postural control in these positions and the ability to make rapid, effortless transitions from one position to another. These developments are discussed by Bradley in Chapter 2.

Despite the greater complexity of our more recent view of the development of any motor behavior, including the idea of underlying continuity of development in multiple systems, it is possible to summarize the perfection of use of various parts of the body in an overall schema of cephalocaudal direction. During the first quarter of the first year of life, infants develop the ability to control their heads in virtually all positions in space, although control will continue to be fine-tuned during successive months. The second quarter reveals major advances in control of the arms and upper trunk, although once again continued refinements occur later. During the third quarter, initial stages involving mastery of control of the lower trunk and pelvis in the upright position occur, and the final quarter of the first year reveals the development of milestones in mobility and control of the lower parts of the legs in conjunction with upright stance and overall postural control.

Infancy

FUNCTIONAL HEAD CONTROL

At birth, infants already have the capacity to right the head from either full flexion or full extension when they are supported in an upright position. A stable vertical head position, however, cannot usually be sustained for more than a second or two, if at all. Supine, or with the head supported in a reclining position, head-turning to either side of midline can usually be elicited by attracting the infant's visual orientation to a moving object. At about 2 months, the infant can sustain the head in midline in the frontal plane during supported sitting but often appears to be looking down at his or her feet, so that the eyes are oriented about 30° below the horizontal plane as in Figure 1–1 (Campbell, SK, Kolobe, TH, Osten, E, Girolami, G, & Lenke, M, unpublished research, 1992). Turning of the unsupported head in the upright position is not usually possible. If the child can be enticed to lift the head to the vertical position, oscillations are typically seen with inability to maintain a stable upright posture. Finer synergistic

FIGURE 1–1. Early head control in space is characterized by ability to stabilize the head in midline but with eyes angled downward from the vertical. (From van Blankenstein, M, Welbergen, UR, & de Haas, JH. le développement du nourrisson: sa première année en 130 photographies. Paris: Presses Universitaires de France, 1962, p. 26.)

control of neck flexor and extensor muscles typically appears in the third month, when the head is indefinitely stable in a vertical position and can be freely turned to follow visual stimulation, although sometimes with brief oscillations and loss of control.

When stabilizing control of the head in the upright position has been attained, the infant can typically organize head and trunk activity so that when placed prone with the arms extended along the sides of the body, the prone-on-elbows position is rapidly assumed by lifting the head and extending the thoracic spine while simultaneously bringing both arms up to rest on the elbows (Fig. 1–2). Given the large weight of the head relative to the rest of the body at this age, presumably a stabilizing postural function of the legs and pelvis provides a stable base of support for simultaneous neck and trunk extension with arm movement. Turning the head to either side while prone on the elbows may still be difficult to coordinate at this stage, and lateral head-righting also remains imperfect. Nevertheless, by the end of the third or fourth postnatal

FIGURE 1–2. Early stage of prone-on-elbows posture with stable neck extension, elbows close to trunk, and flexed hips and knees. (From van Blankenstein, M, Welbergen, UR, & de Haas, JH. le développement du nourrisson: sa première année en 130 photographies. Paris: Presses Universitaires de France, 1962, p. 25.)

month, the head, in conjunction with organized trunk and lower extremity extension, has largely perfected the maintenance of stable positioning in space appropriate for the further development of eye-head-hand control and of independent sitting to come (Fig. 1–3).

Commensurate with acquisition of functional control of head positioning are important developments in control of the arms. During the second and third months, generalized movements of the arms and body have altered their earlier writhing quality (Cioni & Prechtl, 1990). Small fidgety movements appear throughout the body, the arms and legs may show oscillations during movement, and ballistic swipes and swats with legs or arms appear for the first time (Hadders-Algra & Prechtl,

1992). For example, if the legs are flexed up to the chest and then released while the infant is supine, the legs may extend so that the heels pound the supporting surface, or when excited, the infant may make large arm-swiping movements in the air. Hadders-Algra et al. (1992) have demonstrated that the first evidence of reciprocal activity of muscular antagonists about the shoulder underlies the ability to perform these ballistic movements. Ferrari and colleagues (1990) suggested the importance of these developing qualitative changes in spontaneous movement by demonstrating that they herald the appearance of goal-directed reaching and by indicating that they do not appear in children destined to be diagnosed as having cerebral palsy. Children with CNS dysfunction tend to move in tight ranges characterized by simultaneity of activity in multiple limbs, referred to as cramped synchrony.

UPRIGHT TRUNK CONTROL

Midway through the first year, the average child has achieved the ability to sit alone (Fig. 1–4) and can successfully manipulate objects with one hand while the other hand holds it although sitting and

FIGURE 1–4 Early stage of independent sitting with arms used for balance. (From van Blankenstein, M, Welbergen, UR, & de Haas, JH. le développement du nourrisson: sa première année en 130 photographies. Paris: Presses Universitaires de France, 1962, p. 39.)

FIGURE 1–3. Advanced stage of prone-on-elbows posture, with free movement of head and arms and extended lower extremities. (From van Blankenstein, M, Welbergen, UR, & de Haas, JH. le développement du nourrisson: sa première année en 130 photographies. Paris: Presses Universitaires de France, 1962, p. 34.)

manipulating at once may still be a challenge. Poking fingers explore crevices and crumbs and herald the fine selective digital control that characterizes the human organism. Strong extension throughout the body in the prone position allows significant freedom of action for the arms and head (Fig. 1–5). While sitting, however, the child lacks the fine pelvic and lower extremity control needed for moving into and out of the position or for turning the trunk freely on a stable base. Pelvic control functions begin to be developed at this time, however, in rolling from supine to prone (Fig. 1–6), pivoting while prone, and playing with the legs and feet while supine.

LOWER TRUNK CONTROL IN THE UPRIGHT POSITION

During the third quarter of the first year, functional movements free the child from a spot on which she or he is placed by others. Control of lower trunk and pelvis, combined with previously achieved upper body skills, provides new mobility when prone (Fig. 1–7), crawling and creeping (Fig.

FIGURE 1–5. In the most advanced stage of the prone posture, arms and legs move freely from a stable trunk. (From van Blankenstein, M, Welbergen, UR, & de Haas, JH. le développement du nourrisson: sa première année en 130 photographies. Paris: Presses Universitaires de France, 1962, p. 37.)

FIGURE 1–6. Rolling from supine to prone with head-righting. (From van Blankenstein, M, Welbergen, UR, & de Haas, JH. le développement du nourrisson: sa première année en 130 photographies. Paris: Presses Universitaires de France, 1962, p. 36.)

1–8), pulling to a stand, moving from supine to four-point and sitting positions, and moving down to hand and knees or prone from sitting (Fig. 1–9). Inherent in each activity are freedom from a strong midline symmetry that previously characterized postural control and the continued refinement of rotational abilities within the axis of the trunk.

The presence of oscillations also continues to

FIGURE 1–7. Dynamic play in prone includes push-ups on extended arms and "flying" with strong trunk extension and scapular retraction. (From van Blankenstein, M, Welbergen, UR, & de Haas, JH. le développement du nourrisson: sa première année en 130 photographies. Paris: Presses Universitaires de France, 1962, p. 47.)

herald new developments. Rocking on four points before launching into creeping, and bouncing while standing before beginning to cruise along furniture, are examples of self-induced actions that appear to be important precursors of functional skills.

FINE LOWER EXTREMITY CONTROL IN THE UPRIGHT POSITION

Once the child has attained competence at standing and cruising along furniture, the legs and feet move toward perfection of selective control since the trunk and pelvis are increasingly reliable supports that permit freedom of lower extremity activities. In creeping, pelvic swiveling motions give way to reciprocal hip flexion and extension activity, and creeping velocity increases as an arm and leg on the same side of the body can be placed in simultaneous flight. The child can lower himself or herself from standing (Fig. 1–10); bear-walk with dorsiflexed ankles, flexed hips, and partially extended

knees (Fig. 1–11); and finally stand and walk independently at 9 to 15 months of age (Fig. 1–12).

The gradual refinement of gait is described by Stout in Chapter 3. During the next several months of walking experience, creeping is gradually abandoned and heel-strike in gait develops, allowing faster walking with longer strides. Roberton and Halverson (1984) hypothesized the following temporal sequence of development of foot locomotion patterns: walking; running; single leap, jumping down or bounce-jumping, and galloping (in uncertain order, but generally at about 2–2.5 y); hopping on dominant foot (seldom before age 3) then nondominant foot; and skipping and sideways galloping or sliding. Although some children may manage a skip by age 4, many reach an early level of proficiency only by age 7. A rhythmic step-and-hop movement is even more difficult and does not appear until well into the primary school years, when it may be used in many dance forms. Before describing the further development of gross motor skills in preschoolers, however, the sequence of development of functional hand use in infancy will be described.

FIGURE 1–8. Creeping on hands and knees. (From van Blankenstein, M, Welbergen, UR, & de Haas, JH. le développement du nourrisson: sa première année en 130 photographies. Paris: Presses Universitaires de France, 1962, p. 53.)

FIGURE 1–9. The infant moves from sitting to the four-point position over one leg. (From van Blankenstein, M, Welbergen, UR, & de Haas, JH. le développement du nourrisson: sa première année en 130 photographies. Paris: Presses Universitaires de France, 1962, p. 57.)

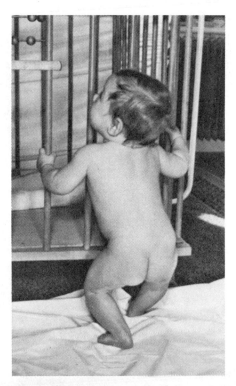

FIGURE 1–10. Lowering from standing to the floor with control. (From van Blankenstein, M, Welbergen, UR, & de Haas, JH. le développement du nourrisson: sa première année en 130 photographies. Paris: Presses Universitaires de France, 1962, p. 57.)

FIGURE 1–11. "Bear-walking" on hands and feet. (From van Blankenstein, M, Welbergen, UR, & de Haas, JH le développement du nourrisson: sa première année en 130 photographies. Paris: Presses Universitaires de France, 1962, p. 54.)

OBJECT MANIPULATION

Development of fine motor function entails two major features: control of the hand as a terminal device for reaching and grasping and object manipulation and release. Postural control for reaching and grasping will be detailed in Chapter 2; an excellent volume devoted to development of all aspects of the capacity to reach, grasp, and release as well as the functional use of the hands has been edited by Bard and colleagues (1990). This chapter will emphasize development of the manipulative functions of the hand.

Karniol (1989) has documented the stages of object manipulation in the first year of life. These stages of spontaneous behaviors observed in daily life occur in a hierarchic form that progresses from rotation (angular displacement) to translation (movement parallel to the object itself) to vibration (rapid periodic movements of either translation or rotation). Later stages involve combinations of these actions and bimanual activities. The invariant sequence of spontaneous behaviors documented by Karniol (1989) includes

Stage 1, Rotation of Held Objects—By 2 Months: With vision, holding objects becomes an intentional act. Objects are first held when they come directly into the infant's reach and are later (by 3–4 mo) twisted while being held. Karniol (1989) indicated that through this action, infants learn that objects can be held and transformed by rotation

Stage 2, Translation of Grasped Objects—By 3 Months: Typical of this stage is reaching for an object while in the prone position and bringing it to the mouth. The object may also be rotated. What the infant learns through these types of action is that he or she can translate objects in order to look at, or mouth, them and that it is not possible to reach objects further distant than the length of the arm.

Stage 3, Vibration (Shaking) of Held Objects—By 4 Months: In this stage infants learn that they can make interesting noises by rapidly flexing and extending their arms and can make the noise stop by holding still. If the object does not produce a noise, it may be translated or rotated and examined before being dropped, but visual attention is not a dominant part of this activity.

Stage 4, Bilateral Hold of Two Objects—By 4.5 Months: The infant may hold an object in one hand and shake an object held in the other, thereby learning that it is possible to do more than one thing at a time (Fig. 1–13).

Stage 5, Two-Handed Hold of a Single Object—By 4.5 Months: First use of bimanual holding is to hold an object, such as a bottle, steady, but it rapidly advances to holding (and often rotating) large objects that require the use of two hands. These actions allow the child to learn that two hands can steady and rotate objects better than can one hand as well as permit the holding of large objects.

Stage 6, Hand-to-Hand Transfer of an Object—At 4.5–6 Months: Transfer is usually followed by repeated actions on the object with the second hand, thereby learning that whatever can be done with the right hand can also be done with the left.

Stage 7, Coordinated Action with a Single Object in which One Hand Holds the Object While the Other Manipulates or Bangs It—At 5–6.5 Months: A quintessential example of this type of activity is holding a toy in one hand while picking at it with the other (Fig. 1–14). Displacements of the object caused by handling are followed by rotational readjustments of the hand that holds it. These activities teach the infant that two hands can do more than can one alone and that noise can be produced from striking objects that do not respond to vibrating

Stage 8, Coordinated Action with Two Objects, Such As Striking Two Blocks Together—At 6–8.5 Months: Through these actions, the infant learns to produce interesting effects by moving one object toward another.

FIGURE 1–12. The infant walks and carries a toy, with wide-based gait and hands in "guard" position. (From van Blankenstein, M, Welbergen, UR, & de Haas, JH. le développement du nourrisson: sa première année en 130 photographies. Paris: Presses Universitaires de France, 1962, pp. 64–65.)

Stage 9, Deformation of Objects—At 7–8.5 Months: At this stage, the infant learns that it is possible to alter the way things look or sound by ripping, bending, squeezing, or pulling them apart.

Stage 10, Instrumental Sequential Actions—At 7.5–9.5 Months: These activities involve the sequential use of two hands for goal-oriented functions, so that the infant learns that coordinated use of the hands leads to desired outcomes. The infant may, for example, open a box with one hand and take out its contents with the other.

The achievement of these stages completes the development of the essentials of manual manipulation. More complex actions follow that are related to the functional characteristics of objects or to imaginary play in which an object can be whatever one pretends it to be (Karniol, 1989). Manual ma-

nipulations become automatized, leaving attention to be more directed toward the functional use of objects.

Based on the previously discussed research of Edelman (1922), Thelen and colleagues (1993; Thelen, 1990), and Keshner and colleagues (1989), we can hypothesize that, although functional hand use develops in a regular, invariant sequence, it is likely that each infant uses unique coordinative patterns and kinetics to achieve manipulative goals that are circumscribed by individual variations in body structure, experiences, and rate of neural and physical maturation. If, as Thelen and colleagues believe, the task characteristics also structure the infant's unique response, parents play an important role in providing opportunities that support development.

Karniol (1989) suggested that parents and others who choose toys for infants have two important functions: helping infants to master the abilities of each stage by providing objects that are appropriate

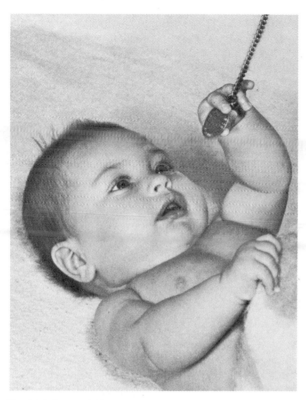

FIGURE 1–13. Bilateral hold of two objects: One hand holds the blanket, the other reaches for a keychain (stage 4 of Karniol, 1989). (From van Blankenstein, M, Welbergen, UR, & de Haas, JH. le développement du nourrisson: sa première année en 130 photographies. Paris: Presses Universitaires de France, 1962, p. 91.)

for emerging skills and facilitating infants' developing sense of capability to control their world by providing objects that are responsive to current ma-

FIGURE 1–14. Coordinated action with a single object: holding a toy with one hand while poking at it with another (stage 7 of Karniol, 1989). (From van Blankenstein, M, Welbergen, UR, & de Haas, JH. le développement du nourrisson: sa première année en 130 photographies. Paris: Presses Universitaires de France, 1962, p. 93.)

nipulative abilities. Thus, Karniol and others believed that mastery of controlling objects in the environment is influential in development of the infant's general sense of competence as well as in providing initial sensorimotor knowledge of the permanence of objects and of cause-effect relationships. Karniol reviewed research demonstrating the influence on persistence at tasks and IQ at age 3 of play with objects that provide contingent feedback and are appropriate for the infant's manual manipulative competencies.

As each stage is attained, the presentation of any object results in action appropriate to the motor stage, whether or not the object lends itself well to that action. Thus, in stage 3, all objects are considered shakeable whether or not they make noise when shaken. This fact is not well explained by developmental theories that suggest that children perceive the affordances of the environment and act on them (Fetters, 1991a,b; Pick, 1992; Thelen, 1990); this type of function was recognized by Piaget (Flavel, 1963) and included in his principle of assimilation. This principle states that when cognitive structures develop a particular schema, it is applied indiscriminately to objects in the environment, assimilating them to the existing cognitive structure. Piaget also posited that repeated experiences with attempted assimilations of inappropriate objects results in gradual accommodation to their properties and the appearance of both new behaviors and new cognitive structures.

The Preschool and Early School Years

FUNCTIONAL MOTOR SKILLS IN PRESCHOOLERS

We return now to a description of the functional skills of preschool children, combining information on both gross and fine motor function in practical use. In the second year, children walk well (although steps are still quite short and rather constrained) and enjoy the sheer pleasure of movement through running, climbing up and down stairs independently, and jumping off the bottom step (Ames et al., 1979). The 2-year-old child can kick a ball and steer a push-toy, and by 2.5 years the child can walk on tiptoes, jump with both feet, stand on one foot, and throw and catch a ball using arms and body together. Galloping may appear, but only leading with the preferred foot (Roberton & Halverson, 1984). The more practical pleasures of dressing independently (pulling on a simple garment at 2 years and pulling off pants and socks by 2.5 years) and eating with a spoon with little spilling also develop (Ames et al., 1979). Food preferences can become a touchy subject by around 2.5 years, however!

The 3-year-old child can alternate feet easily when ascending stairs, can control speed of movement well, and takes pleasure in riding a tricycle (Ames et al., 1979). Hopping may emerge, although it is often a momentary, single hop on the preferred foot (Roberton & Halverson, 1984). Surprisingly, however, by 3.5 years, the child may seem less secure and physically coordinated, stumbling frequently and showing a fear of falling (Ames et al., 1979). Hands may show excessive dysmetria during block stacking. Nevertheless, typical 3-year-olds feed themselves well and can hold a glass with only one hand. At 3.5 years, mealtime may again become trying because the food must be put on the plate in a certain way and the sandwich has to be cut just so. The same may be true of the dressing process, with special objection being expressed against clothing that goes over the head. The typical 3-year-old can put on pants, socks, and shoes, but buttoning may be difficult. Nearly all 3-year-olds are consistently dry during the daytime, and bowel training is well established.

Four-year-olds have been described by Ames and colleagues (1979) as typically out-of-bounds in their exuberance. Behavior in all spheres is frequently wild, and self-confidence and bragging seem endless. The 4-year-old can walk downstairs with one foot per step, catch with hands only, and learn to use roller skates or a small bicycle. (But remember McGraw's experiments demonstrating that learning these skills is possible much earlier!) Athletic activities are particularly enjoyed, especially running, jumping, and climbing. Four-year-olds can button large buttons and lace shoelaces, feed themselves independently except for cutting, and talk and eat at the same time. Most can take responsibility for washing hands and face and brushing teeth as well as dressing and undressing without help except for tying their shoes or differentiating front from back of some garments.

Five-years-olds tend to be more conforming than the exuberant 4-year-old (Ames et al., 1979). During the fifth year the child can skip, long jump about 2 feet, climb with sureness, jump rope, and do acrobatic tricks. Children begin to learn to dodge well at 5 years (Roberton & Halverson, 1984). Handedness is well established,[4] and overhand throwing is accomplished (Ames et al., 1979). The 5-year-old likes to help with household tasks, play with blocks, and build houses. Eating is independent, including using a knife except for cutting

meat, although dawdling and wriggling in the chair may be trying to parents. The challenge of dressing oneself is past, so children of 5 may ask for more help than they need (usually only for tying shoes or buttoning difficult buttons), and overall, undressing is generally easier than dressing.

At age 6, children are constantly on the go, "lugging, tugging, digging, dancing, climbing, pushing, pulling" (Ames et al., 1979, p. 49). Six-year-olds seem to be consciously practicing body balance in climbing, crawling over and under things, and dancing about the room. They swing too high, build too tall, and try activities exceeding their ability. Indoors, awkwardness may cause accidents, and the child seems less coordinated than during the fifth year. Despite excellent eating skills, falling out of the chair or knocking over full glasses is not uncommon.

STEPS IN MOTOR SKILL DEVELOPMENT

In the various motor skills developed in the preschool and elementary school years, each body segment has its own developmental trajectory within the overall coordinative structure; one part can be at a different level of skill than another, although all parts tend to be at a primitive level early or at an advanced level when skills are well learned (Roberton & Halverson, 1984). Furthermore, when demands of the task change (increased height, distance, or accuracy requirements), or when fatigue sets in, one body component may regress in its action while another continues to perform at an advanced level of skill. Thus, task requirements are once again seen to be influential in determining the characteristics of motor response. For hopping and other skills, such as catching, throwing, and jumping, Roberton and Halverson provided detailed analyses and photographs of the intratask developmental steps for each critical body component, instruction in how to make detailed observations to categorize the level of skill of body segments, and advice for guiding the learning of these childhood skills.

Physical therapists would find this information useful in planning intervention for children with mild physical disabilities or clumsiness. For example, as children learn to throw, the trunk goes through similar stages of development as those found in early developmental motor activities. The trunk is initially passive, then increasingly a stabilizer for the function of the extremities, and finally a participant in actively imparting force to the flight of the ball. Jumping changes from a functional activity characterized best as falling and catching to one of projection, flight, and landing, each with

---

[4]Current research suggests that hand preference is already stable by 12 to 13 months in most children (Fagard, 1990).

components that add force and speed or shock absorption to lend elegance and style to the activity.

Although many tests of motor development include assessment of hopping skills, most therapists probably would not view this as a particularly functional activity because children seldom hop spontaneously (Roberton & Halverson, 1984). Physical educators, however, believe that hopping is an important developmental skill because a hop is often required in situations such as controlling momentum during sudden stops and in handling unexpected perturbations to balance as well as for pleasurable play activities such as skipping. Hopping is also an excellent activity for describing the development of various strategies leading, finally, to skillful action.

Skillful hopping requires projected flight off the supporting leg and a pumping action of the swinging leg that assists in force production. Initial prehop attempts involve extension of the supporting leg as the child tries to lift off with the nonsupporting leg raised high. The first successful strategy, however, is usually a quick hip-and-knee flexion that pulls the supporting leg off the floor and into momentary flight (actually falling off-balance and flexing the leg) while the swing leg remains inactive. At the next level of skill, the supporting leg again extends but with limited range and early timing relative to point of takeoff. In skillful hopping, the swinging leg leads the takeoff, and extension of the supporting leg occurs late; thus the action becomes one of "land, ride, and extend" (Roberton & Halverson, 1984, p. 62).

Sports and playground games become increasingly important parts of children's motor activities when they enter school and when complex feats of coordination become possible. Children have, however, individual rates of development of the components of motor skill, some undoubtedly innate, some based on cultural characteristics and family interest in development of physical skills. McGraw's (1935) work demonstrates, for example, that toddlers can develop motor skills that are usually considered inappropriate, primarily because of safety issues. Furthermore, research has generally supported the belief that African-American children have superior motor skills, especially those involving speed and agility, relative to white children (Cintas, 1988; Lee, 1980; Plimpton & Rigimbal, 1992). Although most authors have explained these differences on the basis of socioeconomic status and differences in permissiveness of child rearing (Williams & Scott, 1953), we found differences among ethnic groups that approached statistical significance on test scores of the Test of Infant Motor Performance (TIMP) in 142 infants younger than 3.5 months (Campbell, SK, Girolami, GL,

Kolobe, THA, Lenke, M, & Osten, E, unpublished data 1993). Both African-American and Latino infants scored slightly better on the TIMP than did white infants.

Interactions between Perceptual-Cognitive Development and Motor Development

The work of Bertenthal and Campos (1987) is significant in demonstrating that experience, not maturation alone, drives perceptual-cognitive development and that self-induced movement is critical in evoking advancements in a number of important cognitive processes. Through ingenious studies that varied locomotor experience levels by studying natural differences, such as length of time infants had been creeping, and unusual childhood events, such as being confined to a cast for a long period or being given a walker to induce locomotion before it occurred independently, Bertenthal and Campos have shown that self-induced locomotion is a critical ingredient in the development of depth perception that mediates avoidance of heights when a child is placed on a visual cliff. This behavior normally develops between 7 and 9 months of age but is related more to degree of locomotor experience than to age at locomotion. Bertenthal and Campos also reviewed other evidence that self-produced locomotion promotes developmental progress in functions such as memory for locations and ability to localize objects objectively with reference to external landmarks rather than egocentrically. Children who did not creep have also been demonstrated to be cognitively delayed when compared with children with creeping experience (McEwan et al., 1991). These findings call into question the previous assumption that varying patterns of development of locomotion are merely that, variations without developmental significance.

In general, therapists must take into account in treatment planning the long period of development of spatial-cognitive and other perceptual functions. For example, infants can adapt their reaching to the actual distance of an object at 3.5 to 5.5 months (Vinter, 1990). Depth perception is based on kinetic information at 3 months, binocular information at 5 months, and pictorial information at 7 to 9 months. Children preform the hand for the anticipated shape of an object at about 9 to 10 months and can adapt for anticipated weight by 14 to 16 months (Corbetta & Mounoud, 1990). Children under the approximate age of 6 are not able to conserve the amount of a substance when the shape of its container is altered (Beilin, 1989). By 7 or 8 years of age, however, they recognize that pouring water from a wide container to one that is narrower has not increased the amount of water (Roberton & Halverson, 1984). Weight, however, is not conserved until 9 or 10 years, and volume not until 11 or 12.

Gibson used the term differentiation to describe the improvements that occur in perception over the course of development (Pick, 1992). According to Pick, Gibson stated that "Progressive differentiation occurs with respect to information specifying the meaningful properties of the world" (Pick, 1992, p. 789). Gibson believed that perception involves an active effort to make sense of the world, but the action is exploratory, not executive in the sense of using physical manipulation. Perception improves because we detect more of the aspects, features, and nuances that convey the meaning of objects and events. It seems likely that the alternations in apparent self-confidence, coordination, and other characteristics of children reported by Ames and colleagues (1979) are related to their best attempts to make sense of the world as physical characteristics, neural maturation, perceptual abilities, and other developmental subsystems change with growth and learning.

Although the importance of motor experience in development of many of the perceptual functions described earlier has not, to my knowledge, been explored, the finding that self-directed activity is influential in other spatial-cognitive functions suggests the need to pay attention to providing compensations for functional limitations that may hinder children's development when physical disabilities are present. Bertenthal and Campos (1987), for example, have shown that use of a walker before endogenously produced locomotion was present positively affected performance on the visual cliff problem. Thus, maneuvering under self-control appears to be more important than does locomotor movement per se. Perhaps therapists need to reconsider prohibitions regarding the use of walkers for children with developmental disabilities.

Using Developmental Sequences As a Therapeutic Framework

Most of our contemporary clinical approaches to developing intervention plans for children with disabilities were originally based on use of the developmental sequence as the primary framework for planning intervention. New theoretic models for understanding the achievement of functional motor skills suggest that this framework, as a rigid

structure for approaching intervention, is inadequate. Atwater (1991), for example, suggested that a number of issues must be considered when deciding whether to follow a normal developmental sequence in planning treatment. These issues include the knowledge that 1) multiple underlying processes involving both distal and proximal function develop contemporaneously; 2) motor milestones and their components develop in overlapping sequences, with spurts and regressions being common; 3) many variations in the development of motor milestones occur in perfectly normal children, and thus motor milestones cannot be considered to be an invariant sequence leading to skill; 4) development in multiple domains must be considered; 5) the age of the child and the extent and type of disability are important considerations in determining which skills will be most functional for a child at any given time; and 6) child and family involvement in decisions regarding the goals of therapy must be considered. The discussion earlier in the chapter regarding contemporary theories of development and neural plasticity provide an additional basis in support of Atwater's suggestion (1991). She aptly quotes Bobath and Bobath in stating that

Treatment should not attempt to follow the sequence of development . . . regardless of the age and physical condition of the individual child. Rather, it should be decided what each child needs most urgently at any one stage or age, and what is absolutely necessary for him to participate for future functional skills, or for improving the skills he has but performs abnormally.

(ATWATER, 1991, P. 91.)

I would add the suggestion that an emphasis on processes underlying developmental progress, such as the role of self-induced movement in both motor learning and cognitive development, and the motivation on the part of children to engage in repetitive, apparently goal-less, practice of activities during sensitive periods of development, should be considered in treatment planning. Further information on sensitive periods of development for basic motor functions will be needed to target times appropriately for most effective intervention, especially for children with disabilities.

Also of great importance is identification of the most effective strategies for promoting the attainment of functional goals involving motor activity. Based on research on facilitation of cognitive development in disadvantaged children, early learning environments, and basic learning strategies, Ramey and Ramey (1992) have identified the following essential daily ingredients to promote intellectual development in children: 1) encouragement of exploration; 2) mentoring in basic skills such as labeling, sequencing, and noting means-ends relations; 3) celebration of developmental advances; 4) guided rehearsal and extension of new skills; 5) protection from inappropriate disapproval, teasing, or punishment; and 6) provision of a rich and responsive language environment. Many of these ingredients are likely to be equally important in promoting motor development in children with physically challenging conditions; research on the design of specific teaching and learning strategies for such children is direly needed. Chapter 6 on motor learning by Larin reviews what is known.

Atwater (1991) recommended that treatment planning should focus on encouragement of functional independence to prevent cognitive retardation and learned helplessness that will be highly disabling in adolescence and adulthood, even when this means giving up goals for improving movement quality. Fetters (1991c) and Harris (1990) agree, suggesting that ecologically valid treatment programs have as their goals the movements that are necessary and useful to humans as they move about in their environment. Fetters (1991c), however, emphasized that there may be tradeoffs inherent in working for function of which therapists should be cognizant. Independence in ambulation may be accomplished only with high physiologic cost; the achievement of faster reaching may result in poorer trunk control.

Although I agree wholeheartedly with the recommendations and observations of these three thoughtful scientific practitioners, I have also argued that therapists must choose wisely when making decisions regarding use of compensatory patterns or assistive devices to facilitate functioning of children with CNS dysfunction. Wise decision making involves giving due consideration to whether use of compensatory patterns may lead to later secondary impairments of a musculoskeletal nature that could also be severely disabling in the future (Campbell, 1991). It is not acceptable to include in a treatment plan a goal for functional movement that does not also meet a requirement that working toward such an objective will not be likely to contribute to potential future deformity, skin breakdown, osteoporosis, or other preventable secondary impairment. A focus on health promotion and disease prevention, in addition to a focus on functional improvement for current and future needs, is required.

To accomplish these objectives, we need both our extensive knowledge of biomechanics and more information on the natural history of conditions we treat. Indeed, I believe that the combination of attention to assisting persons with disabilities to improve their functional capabilities through promoting achievement of useful, meaningful activities performed as efficiently as possible, along with prevention of musculoskeletal and other complications, constitutes the unique features of physical therapy. In Chapter 7 and throughout this book, we therefore recommend that therapists use a framework for describing the disabling process developed by the National Center for Medical Rehabilitation Research that approaches disability from the perspective of the multiple, interacting dimensions of the human organism, from the cellular to the societal (National Advisory Board on Medical Rehabilitation Research, 1993).

Such a comprehensive approach to clinical decision making requires the use of appropriate assessments on which to base treatment planning and outcome assessment. Tests of motor development and functional skills that meet appropriate psychometric standards and are useful in clinical settings are discussed in the next section.

TESTS OF MOTOR DEVELOPMENT AND FUNCTIONAL PERFORMANCE

Physical therapists use motor milestone and functional performance tests to document children's developmental level in relation to age norms and to observe the functional limitations that may be present. Tests of specific functional skills, such as dressing and feeding, are also used to assess current levels of functioning and to document developmental progress and achievement of treatment goals. In conjunction with family interviews and sometimes home observations, therapists can assess competencies in fulfilling age-appropriate roles and identify areas of disability that should be addressed with a therapeutic program in consultation with other professionals and the family.

Although all tests to be described in this chapter are standardized scales with acceptable psychometric properties according to the American Physical Therapy Association's Standards for Tests and Measurements in Physical Therapy (Task Force on Standards for Measurement in Physical Therapy, 1991), some tests remain under development, so complete information is not available. Those selected for brief discussion include the Test of Infant Motor Performance, Alberta Infant Motor Scale, the Denver II, the Miller First Step, the Miller Toddler and Infant Motor Evaluation, Bayley Infant Neurodevelopmental Screen, Bayley Scales of Infant Development, Gesell Revised Developmental Schedules, Peabody Developmental Motor scales, Bruininks-Oseretsky Test of Motor Proficiency, Gross Motor Function Measure, Pediatric Evaluation of Disability Inventory, and the Functional Independence Measure for Children. The reader may consult Palisano (1993) or Stengel (1991) for more information on these and other tests.

Although the tests described are at various stages of development, none are tests of disability in daily life in which observations take place in an ecologically valid setting. Those that purport to assess disability do so through report of a knowledgeable informant, such as the parent, guardian, or teacher. Some tests assess spontaneously generated or self-chosen movements; others involve specifying the tasks a child is to perform in a particular way. Some are more useful for individual treatment planning, others for comparing global performance to age norms for diagnostic and classification purposes or for programmatic assessment of overall rehabilitation outcomes. Use of a combination of the tests would provide comprehensive assessment of functional skills in children with physical disabilities, although better tests and well thought out comprehensive protocols are still needed (Campbell, 1989; Fetters, 1991c; Haley et al., 1993).

Screening Tests

The Alberta Infant Motor Scale (AIMS) is an observational scale for assessing gross motor milestones in infants from birth through the stage of independent walking (Piper & Darrah, 1994; Piper et al., 1992). Function in this test is defined as spontaneously engendered motor behaviors performed with a specified level of postural control. Gross motor maturation is assessed by 58 items in four physical positions: supine, prone, sitting, and standing. Items are scored dichotomously based on descriptors that specify demonstration of weight bearing, posture, and antigravity movement appropriate for each skill. Both inter-rater and test-retest reliability are reported with intraclass correlation coefficients of 0.99, and concurrent validity with the Bayley motor scale is 0.98 and with the Peabody Motor Developmental Scale is 0.97. The test was normed on 506 infants in the Canadian province of Alberta, and the discriminative validity for identifying abnormal infants as abnormal was 89%. The test takes 15 minutes to administer and is noninvasive because only observation is involved.

The Miller First Step (Screening Test for Evaluating Preschoolers; Miller, 1992) is a screening test to identify children at risk for developmental delays. The test is appropriate for assessing cognitive, communicative, physical, social-emotional, and adap-

tive function in children from 2 years 9 months to 6 years 2 months of age. Function is defined as performance on games using toys that are entertaining and exciting for children in this age group. The test was normed on a U.S. national sample of 100 boys and 100 girls in each 6-month age grouping. It takes 17 minutes to administer and score performance on the 18 games.

The Denver II is a revision of the Denver Developmental Screening Test (DDST) that was re-normed on 2096 children from 1 week to 6 years of age in the Denver area (Frankenburg et al., 1990, 1992). The test has no single underlying construct, but was designed to include items that could be precisely identified as occurring in 90% of children at one of the 12 specific ages corresponding with American Academy of Pediatrics–recommended schedules for pediatric health maintenance. According to the selection criterion, 125 items were included in the four domains of the scale: personal-social, fine motor–adaptive, language, and gross motor. Differences from the DDST include increased numbers of language items, two articulation items, a new age scale, a category of item interpretation to identify milder delays, a behavior rating scale, and the availability of new training materials. The test requires about 15 minutes to administer. All items included in the scale had kappa statistics of 0.75 or better (mean = 0.99) for inter-rater agreement, but 23% of the items had 7- to 10-day test-retest kappa values of less than 0.75 (mean = 0.90). Glascoe and colleagues (1992), however, reported that in screening 104 children between 3 and 72 weeks of age for developmental delay, the Denver II had an 83% sensitivity but only 43% specificity and a high over-referral rate. The authors did not recommend its use for developmental screening until more research on test validity is completed.

The Bayley Infant Neurodevelopmental Screen (BINS; Aylward, 1992, in press) was originally published as the Early Neuropsychologic Optimality Rating Scales (ENORS) and actually has no direct relationship to the Bayley Scales of Infant Development (Bayley, 1969). The purpose of the test is to assess brain-behavior relationships in the context of developmental change and maturation, expressed in tests for use at 3, 6, 9, 12, 18, and 24 months (± 1 month). Functions are assessed in five neuropsychologic areas: basic neurologic function or intactness (tone, reflexes, signs), receptive functions (visual, auditory, verbal), expressive functions (fine motor and oral motor, gross motor), processing of higher order functions (memory, problem solving, object permanence), and mental activity (goal-directed behavior, attention). The test at each age contains 16 to 22 items. Scoring is based on the optimality concept, and percentage scores (the number optimal divided by the sum of the number optimal and the number nonoptimal) are used as cutoff values for delay-nondelay. Although age equivalents have not yet been developed, the test identifies specific functional areas needing additional assessment. Correlations with the Bayley Scales range from 0.55 at 3 months to 0.82 at 24 months. Sensitivity is highest at 24 months (92%, with 76% specificity) when compared with Bayley scores, and specificity values peak at 12 months (94%, with sensitivity only 68%). The time required to complete a test at any age is about 15 minutes.

Comprehensive Diagnostic Developmental Assessments

The Bayley Scales of Infant Development (BSID) (Bayley, 1969) contain norm-referenced motor and mental scales for children from birth to 30 months of age. Functions on the mental scale include object permanence, memory, manipulation, problem solving, and verbal communication and comprehension assessed with a subset for any particular aged child taken from 163 items scored pass-fail. The motor scale assesses both fine and gross motor function, including 81 items assessing hand function, posture, and locomotion. All items after the 9-month age level are gross motor only. The BSID have just undergone revision and renorming on 1700 able-bodied U.S. children and several hundred children with developmental disabilities of various types; the revised motor scale includes fine motor items across the ages for which the test is appropriate, and the age range of the test has been increased to 42 months (Bayley, 1993).

The older version of the BSID was normed prior to 1969 on over 1200 infants from 2 to 30 months of age from across the United States. Approximately 90% agreement on items is achieved on inter-rater reliability assessments, and the Bayley mental scale is correlated at 0.57 with the Stanford-Binet Intelligence Scale for children older than 2 years. Scores of infants tested longitudinally in the first year have not been demonstrated to be stable (Coryell et al., 1989), and Bayley herself recommended that three consecutive tests should be used to estimate performance during the first 15 months of life (Rosenblith, 1992). Also problematic is the fact that the 1969 age norms overestimate ability of 12-month-old infants by an average of about 0.6 standard deviation (SD) (Campbell et al., 1986). Scores at other ages during infancy are probably

inflated also, particularly at 4 months, when many clinics first perform developmental follow-up on high-risk infants (Coryell et al., 1989; Palisano, 1993). Therapists are advised to be conservative in assuming normality from scores on the old BSID. The BSID take about 45 to 60 minutes to administer.

The Gesell Revised Developmental Schedules (Knobloch et al., 1980) are comprehensive scales for assessing adaptive, gross and fine motor, language, and personal-social development in children from birth to 36 months of age. Function in these scales is assumed to capture neurologic maturation. The adaptive domain contains 145 items reflecting perception and problem solving. The gross (98 items) and fine (56 items) motor domains assess locomotion and postural control and reach, grasp, and manipulation, respectively. The personal-social domain consists of 81 items reflecting ADLs and social skills. The test was normed on 927 children living in the area of Albany, NY. Inter-rater reliability averages about 90% agreement on items, and results are correlated with BSID performance. Both scales, however, appear to result in higher age equivalents than does the Peabody Developmental Motor Scales (Campbell et al., 1988). The test takes about 45 minutes to administer because only a few items in each domain are administered at any given age level.

Motor Assessments

The Test of Infant Motor Performance (TIMP; Campbell et al., 1993) is a test under development for infants younger than age 4 months, including prematurely born infants as young as 32 weeks postconceptional age. Function on this scale is defined as the postural and selective control needed for functional movements in early infancy, including head and trunk control in prone, supine, and upright positions. The test has 27 items scored pass-fail on the basis of observations of spontaneous activity and 26 scaled items administered by the examiner according to a standardized format. Elicited items present the infant with problems to solve that require organization of head and trunk posture in space to orient to interesting spectacles, interact with the tester, or regain a preferred positional configuration. Items are internally consistent (0.97), correlate with age at 0.80, and are sensitive to degree of medical complications experienced in the newborn period ($R^2 = 0.71$, $p < 0.0001$, when age and risk are used to predict test performance). The test has not yet been normed. Intra- and inter-rater reliabilities are high, as demonstrated by

Rasch model assessment of 5% or fewer misfitting ratings by each of five experienced examiners on 14 videotaped tests (Osten, unpublished master's thesis, University of Illinois at Chicago, 1992). The test takes 25 to 45 minutes to administer.

The Peabody Developmental Motor Scales (PDMS; Folio & Fewell, 1983; Hinderer et al., 1989) contains separate scales for gross and fine motor assessment for children from birth to 42 months of age. Functions assessed by the gross motor scale include reflexes, balance, nonlocomotor and locomotor activities, and receipt and propulsion of objects. The fine motor scale contains items for assessing grasp, hand functions, eye-hand coordination, and manual dexterity. The PDMS was normed on 617 children from across the United States, and relatively small numbers of children were assessed at any given age level. The test takes 45 to 60 minutes to administer. Inter-rater reliabilities of 0.97 for the gross motor scale and 0.94 for the fine motor scale were reported by the test developers; others have found the fine motor ratings to be more reliable for children with delays (0.96) than for those without delays (0.76), but these results were related more to the statistical effect created by the greater variability of the delayed group than to actual disagreements between raters (Stokes et al., 1990). Age-equivalent scores on the PDMS are generally lower than on the Gesell or BSID, perhaps reflecting the more current national norms on the PDMS (Campbell et al., 1988). The PDMS will need to be again compared with the Bayley II now that revision is complete. Although correlations among these three tests are high, they cannot be considered to give exactly comparable results in terms of normative scores or age equivalents. These issues are discussed more thoroughly by Palisano (1993).

The Toddler and Infant Motor Evaluation (TIME; Miller, in press) is a comprehensive qualitative motor assessment for children from birth to 42 months with suspected motor delay or dysfunction. In addition to seven subtests of mobility, stability, motor organization, atypical positions, quality, component analysis, and behavior during testing, a 15-minute parent interview assesses functional performance in dressing and other activities. The test is intended for use in treatment planning and in research on treatment efficacy. Testing is based on parent-elicited play and naturalistic observations of movement. A national study involving 1400 subjects is under way.

The Bruininks-Oseretsky Test of Motor Proficiency is a test of gross and fine motor function for children from 4.5 to 14.5 years of age (Bruininks, 1978). The 46-item test takes 45 to 60 minutes to administer (a 15- to 20-minute short form is available) and has subscales for running speed and agility, balance, bilateral coordination, strength, upper limb coordination, response speed, visual-motor control, and upper limb speed and dexterity. Although the test is largely one of coordination and balance (Krus et al., 1981), several subtests have items that are clearly related to functional demands for school-aged children, such as cutting within lines and ball activities and physical education skills such as sit-ups, shuttle-runs, and long jumping. The test was normed on 765 subjects reflective of the U. S. population. Inter-rater reliability has been reported to be 0.90 or greater; test-retest reliability for total scores was reported to be 0.89 for second graders and 0.86 for sixth graders.

Assessments Designed for Children with Disabilities

The Gross Motor Function Measure (GMFM; Rosenbaum et al., 1990; Russell et al., 1989) is a test specifically designed and validated for measuring change over time in gross motor function in children with cerebral palsy. Function in this test is defined as the child's degree of achievement of a motor behavior (regardless of quality) when instructed to perform or placed in a particular position. Spontaneously chosen movements are not assessed. The test contains 88 items of gross motor function distributed over five dimensions to measure how much children can do, not the quality with which they do it. These dimensions include lying and rolling; sitting; crawling and kneeling; standing; and walking, running, and jumping. All items are achievable by 5-year-olds with normal motor function. Intraclass correlation coefficients for intrarater and inter-rater reliability of 0.99 have been reported. The test was validated for sensitivity to change over a 6-month period in children with cerebral palsy from 5 months to 16 years of age. Correlations between test scores and judgments of change were 0.54 if made by parents and 0.65 if made by therapists. Change judged from blind evaluation of videotapes was correlated with GMFM test scores at 0.82. The test requires 45 to 60 minutes to administer. The test has not been normed on a sample of able-bodied children, and little research has yet been published on its value for use in clinical practice and decision making. One study suggests, however, that scores on the total test and on the subsections using predominantly the legs are correlated with independently obtained assessments of leg strength, accounting for 55 to 65% of the common variance, but are not correlated with aerobic power or with arm strength (Parker et al., 1993). The Gross Motor Performance Measure, a companion test of postural control in items from the GMFM, will be described in the next chapter.

The Pediatric Evaluation of Disability Inventory (PEDI) is a discriminative device for detecting functional limitations and disability in age-appropriate independence and a tool for program evaluation in tracking progress in individual children with disabilities (Feldman et al., 1990; Haley et al., 1991, 1992). Function in this scale is defined as ability to perform ADLs with or without modifications or assistance as reported by a knowledgeable informant. On the PEDI, 197 items measure functional skills in self-care, and mobility and social function, and 20 items assess the extent of caregiver assistance and modifications needed to reduce or eliminate disabilities in each domain. Inter-rater and inter-respondent reliabilities greater than 0.90 have been reported, and concurrent validity with the Battelle and the Functional Independence Measure for Children ranges from 0.70 to 0.90. The test was normed on 412 nondisabled children, and initial validity for discriminating function and assistance needed was derived from a clinical sample of 102 children with various disabilities (Feldman et al., 1990). Both normative standard scores and scaled scores are provided for each of its three domains. The test takes 20 to 30 minutes to complete by therapists or teachers and 45 to 60 minutes by structured parent interview. Hey and colleagues at Boston Children's Hospital have developed a parent self-administered version of the PEDI that took an average of 35 minutes to complete in a sample of 110 parents (Hey, LA, Kasser, J, Rosenthal, R, Ramsing, N, & Katz, J, unpublished data, 1992). Scoring software to obtain Rasch logit measures is available. Direct testing of children's performance in an ecologically valid setting is not specified but could be done.

The Functional Independence Measure for Children (WeeFIM) is a discipline-free tool of disability for assessing functions in self-care, sphincter control, mobility, locomotion, and communication and social cognition (Granger et al., 1989; Msall et al., 1992a). Function in this scale is defined as caregiver assistance needed to accomplish daily tasks. The WeeFIM is descriptive of caretaker and special resources required because of functional limitations and is useful in tracking outcomes over time across health, developmental, and community settings. Although insufficient detail is provided to be useful in making treatment decisions, it is an excellent tool for description of overall rehabilitation outcomes, for use in program evaluation, and for cross-disciplinary communication. The test has 18 items measured on a seven-point ordinal scale for use with children with developmental disabilities from 6 months to 12 years of age. Test-retest and inter-rater reliabilities have been reported to be greater than 0.90, and pilot normative work on a sample of 222 children demonstrated significant correlations between total WeeFIM scores and age ($r = .80$) (Msall et al., 1992b). The test has been used with children with extreme prematurity, cerebral palsy, Down syndrome, congenital limb disorders, myelodysplasia, and traumatic brain injury (Msall, ME, personal communication, 1992). The test requires 20 to 30 minutes to complete.

In summary, a number of well-designed tests are available for screening and assessing mental and motor development in children, and several new tests assess specific motor constructs or functional limitations of children with disabilities. Many of these new tests remain to be validated in clinical practice, but early results are promising. No standardized tests have yet emerged from the new interest in contemporary theories of motor development and motor control.

Analysis of the results of tests of function and disability gives the therapist knowledge of what the child can do, with or without assistance from technology or caregivers. These results are important in diagnosis of developmental delay or deviance and for providing basic information regarding the child's motor competencies for accomplishing the important tasks of childhood play and for experiencing the joy of movement used for pleasure and for purposeful exploration of the world. More information, however, is needed for planning intervention when functional limitations are identified. Roberton and Halverson (1984) have described, in a beautifully succinct way, the process of developing a plan for helping a child to learn movement. Once having observed in what way and how the child responds to a movement task believed to be developmentally appropriate, the prospective teacher needs both to consider what the environment demands for the child to succeed at the task and to interpret the child's response. "What is the meaning of a child's solution to a particular movement problem? Does it indicate a more advanced form of movement? Does it suggest improved perceptual functioning? Is the solution a cognitive attempt to avoid a balance-threatening position? Does the child's response suggest that the task is too stressful, too complex at that particular moment—that the child is not 'ready' for it?" (Roberton & Halverson, 1984, p. 3) Based on task analysis and an interpretation of the child's solution, the teacher must decide whether to intervene or to leave the child and the environment alone. If the decision is to intervene, then the teacher must decide whether to redesign the physical environment, verbally or physically coach the child, or show the child a possible solution. After implementing the decision, reassessment is used to evaluate the effectiveness of the intervention. The chapters that follow in this section will provide further information to aid the physical therapist with these basic processes of clinical instruction and decision making. These chapters include information on the development of gait, motor control and motor learning processes and principles, and physical growth and fitness and suggestions for structuring clinical decision making using a scientific approach. The information provided in these chapters will enable pediatric physical therapists to apply current concepts and research for the benefit of our clients—children with disabilities and their families.

Acknowledgments

I would like to express my appreciation to Darl Vander Linden, Robert Palisano, and Carolyn Heriza for their critical review of and excellent suggestions for improving this chapter. They bear no responsibility for misinterpretations of the literature I may have made. Partial support for work described in this paper was provided by the Foundation for Physical Therapy.

References

Abramov, I, Gordon, J, Hendrickson, A, Hainline, L, Dobson, V, & LaBossiere, E. The retina of the human infant. Science, *217*:265–267, 1982.

Ames, LB, Gillespie, C, Haines, J, & Ilg, FL. The Gesell Institute's Child from One to Six: Evaluating the Behavior of the Preschool Child. New York: Harper & Row, 1979.

Atwater, SW. Should the normal motor developmental sequence be used as a theoretical model in pediatric physical therapy? In Lister, MJ (Ed.), Contemporary Management of Motor Control Problems: Proceedings of the II STEP Conference. Alexandria, VA: Foundation for Physical Therapy, 1991, pp. 89–93.

Aylward, GP. Bayley Infant Neurodevelopmental Screen Manual. San Antonio, TX: Psychological Corporation, 1992.

Aylward, GP. Update on early developmental neuropsychological assessment: The Early Neuropsychologic Optimality Scales. In Tramontana, MG, & Hooper, SR (Eds.), Advances in Child Neuropsychology, Vol. 2. New York: Springer-Verlag, in press.

Banks, M, Aslin, R, & Letson, R. Sensitive period for the development of human binocular vision. Science, *190*:675–677, 1975.

Bard, C, Fleury, M, & Hay, L (Eds.). Development of Eye-Hand Coordination across the Life Span. Columbia, SC: University of South Carolina Press, 1990.

Barinaga, M. Death gives birth to the nervous system. But how? Science, *259*:762–763, 1993.

Bayley, N. Bayley II. San Antonio: Psychological Corporation, 1993.

Bayley, N. Manual for the Bayley Scales of Infant Development. New York: Psychological Corporation, 1969.

Beilin, H. Piagetian theory. In Vasta, R (Ed.), Annals of Child Development, Vol. 6. Greenwich, CT: JAI Press, 1989, pp. 85–131.

Bergenn, VW, Dalton, TC, & Lipsitt, LP. Myrtle B. McGraw: A growth scientist. Developmental Psychology, *28*:381–395, 1992.

Bertenthal, BI, & Campos, JJ. New directions in the study of early experience. Child Development, *58*:560–567, 1987.

Bevor, TG. Regressions in Mental Development: Basic Phenomena and Theories. Hillsdale, NJ: Lawrence Erlbaum Associates, 1982.

Bijou, SW. Behavior analysis. In Vasta, R (Ed.), Annals of Child Development, Vol. 6. Greenwich, CT: JAI Press, 1989, pp. 61–83.

Bly, L. The Components of Normal Movement during the First Year of Life and Abnormal Motor Development. Oak Park, IL: Neuro-Developmental Treatment Association, 1983.

Bobath, B, & Bobath, K. The neuro-developmental treatment. In Scrutton, D (Ed.), Management of the Motor Disorders of Children with Cerebral Palsy. London: Spastics International Medical Publications, 1984, pp. 6–18.

Bower, E, & McLellan, DL. Effect of increased exposure to physiotherapy on skill acquisition of children with cerebral palsy. Developmental Medicine and Child Neurology, *34*:25–39, 1992.

Bruininks, RH. Bruininks-Oseretsky Test of Motor Proficiency: Examiner's Manual. Circle Pines, MN: American Guidance Service, 1978.

Bruner, JS. The growth and structure of skill. In Connolly, K (Ed.), Mechanisms of Motor Skill Development. New York: Academic Press, 1970, pp. 63–94.

Butler, C. Augmentative mobility: Why do it? Physical Medicine and Rehabilitation Clinics of North America, *2*(4):801–815, 1991.

Campbell, SK. Measurement in developmental therapy: Past, present, and future. In Miller, LJ (Ed.), Developing Norm-Reference Standardized Tests. Binghamton, NY: Haworth Press, 1989, pp. 1–13.

Campbell, SK. Framework for the measurement of neurologic impairment and disability. In Lister, MJ (Ed.), Contemporary Management of Motor Control Problems: Proceedings of the II STEP Conference. Alexandria, VA: Foundation for Physical Therapy, 1991, pp. 143–153.

Campbell, SK, Osten, ET, Kolobe, THA, & Fisher, AG. Development of the Test of Infant Motor Performance. In Granger, CV, & Gresham, GE (Eds.), New Developments in Functional Assessment. Philadelphia: WB Saunders, 1993, pp. 541–550.

Campbell, SK, Siegel, E, Parr, CA, & Ramey, CT. Evidence for the need to renorm the Bayley Scales of Infant Development based on the performance of a population-based sample of twelve-month-old infants. Topics in Early Childhood Special Education, *6*(2):83–96, 1986.

Campbell, SK, Wilhelm, IJ, Phillips, W, & Slaton, DS. Comparative performance of infants on three tests of gross motor development (Abstract). Physical Therapy, *68*:818, 1988.

Campbell, SK, & Wilson, JM. Planning infant learning programs. Physical Therapy, *56*:1347–1357, 1976.

Catania, A, & Harnad, S (Eds.). The Selection of Behavior—The Operant Behaviorism of B.F. Skinner: Comments and Consequences. New York: Cambridge University Press, 1988.

Cintas, HM. Cross-cultural variation in infant motor development. Physical and Occupational Therapy in Pediatrics, *8*(4):1–20, 1988.

Cioni, G, & Prechtl, HFR. Preterm and early postterm behaviour in low-risk premature infants. Early Human Development, *23*:159–191, 1990.

Connolly, K. Skill development: Problems and plans. In Connolly, K (Ed.), Mechanisms of Motor Skill Development. New York: Academic Press, 1970, pp. 3–21.

Corbetta, D், & Mounoud, P. Early development of grasping and manipulation. In Bard, C, Fleury, M, & Hay, L (Eds.), Development of Eye-Hand Coordination across the Life Span. Columbia, SC: University of South Carolina Press, 1990, pp. 188–213.

Coryell, J, Provost, BM, Wilhelm, IJ, & Campbell, SK. Stability of Bayley Motor Scale scores in the first two years. Physical Therapy, 69:834–841, 1989.

Edelman, GM. Bright Air, Brilliant Fire: On the Matter of the Mind. New York: Basic Books, 1992.

Epstein, HT. Correlated brain and intelligence development in humans. In Hahn, ME, Jensen, C, & Dudek, BC (Eds.), Development and Evolution of Brain Size: Behavioral Implications. New York: Academic Press, 1979, pp. 111–131.

Fagard, J. The development of bimanual coordination. In Bard, C, Fleury, M, & Hay, L (Eds.), Development of Eye-Hand Coordination across the Life Span. Columbia, SC: University of South Carolina Press, 1990, pp. 262–282.

Feldman, AB, Haley, SM, & Coryell, J. Concurrent and construct validity of the Pediatric Evaluation of Disability Inventory. Physical Therapy, 70:602–610, 1990.

Fentress, JC. Animal and human models of coordination development. In Bard, C, Fleury, M, & Hay, L (Eds.), Development of Eye-Hand Coordination across the Life Span. Columbia, SC: University of South Carolina Press, 1990, pp. 3–25.

Ferrari, F, Cioni, G, & Prechtl, HRF. Qualitative changes of general movements in preterm infants with brain lesions. Early Human Development, 23:193–231, 1990.

Fetters, L. Object permanence development in infants with motor handicaps. Physical Therapy, 61:327–333, 1981.

Fetters, L. Foundations for therapeutic intervention. In Campbell, SK (Ed.), Pediatric Neurologic Physical Therapy. New York: Churchill Livingstone, 1991a, pp. 19–32.

Fetters, L. Cerebral palsy: Contemporary treatment concepts. In Lister, MJ (Ed.), Contemporary Management of Motor Control Problems: Proceedings of the II STEP Conference. Alexandria, VA: Foundation for Physical Therapy, 1991b, pp. 219–224.

Fetters, L. Measurement and treatment in cerebral palsy: An argument for a new approach. Physical Therapy, 71:244–247, 1991c.

Fetters, L, Fernandez, B, & Cermak, S. The relationship of proximal and distal components in the development of reaching. Journal of Human Movement Studies, 17:283–297, 1989.

Fischer, KW. Relations between brain and cognitive development. Child Development, 58:623–632, 1987.

Fisher, AG. Functional measures, Part 1: What is function, what should we measure, and how should we measure it? American Journal of Occupational Therapy, 46:183–185, 1992.

Flavell, JH. The Developmental Psychology of Jean Piaget. Princeton, NJ: Van Nostrand, 1963.

Folio, M, & Fewell, R. Peabody Developmental Motor Scales and Activity Cards. Allen, TX: DLM Teaching Resources, 1983.

Frankenberg, WK, Dodds, J, Archer, P, Bresnick, B, Maschka, P, Edelman, N, & Shapiro, H. Denver II. Denver: Denver Developmental Materials, 1990.

Frankenburg, WK, Dodds, J, Archer, P, Shapiro, H, & Bresnick, B. The Denver II. A major revision and restandardization of the DDST. Pediatrics, 89:91–97, 1992.

Georgopoulos, AP, Ashe, J, Smyrnis, N, & Taira, M. The motor cortex and the coding of force. Science, 256:1692–1695, 1992.

Georgopoulos, AP, Taira, M, & Lukashin, A. Cognitive neurophysiology of the motor cortex. Science, 260:47–52, 1993.

Gesell, A. Infancy and Human Growth. New York: Macmillan, 1928a.

Gesell, A. The Mental Growth of the Pre-school Child: A Psychological Outline of Normal Development from Birth to the Sixth Year, Including a System of Developmental Diagnosis. New York: Macmillan, 1928b.

Gesell, A. The Embryology of Behavior. New York: Harper & Row, 1945.

Gesell, A, Amatruda, CS, Castner, BM, & Thompson, H. Biographies of Child Development: The Mental Growth Careers of Eighty-four Infants and Children. New York: Arno Press, 1975.

Gesell, A, Halverson, HM, Thompson, H, Ilg, FL, Castner, BM, Ames, LB, & Amatruda, CS. The First Five Years of Life. New York: Harper & Row, 1940.

Gesell, A, Thompson, H, & Amatruda, CS. Infant Behavior: Its Genesis and Growth. New York: McGraw-Hill, 1934.

Glascoe, FP, Byrne, KE, Ashford, LG, Johnson, KL, Chang, B, & Strickland, B. Accuracy of the Denver-II in developmental screening. Pediatrics, 89:1221–1225, 1992.

Goldman-Rakic, PS. Development of cortical circuitry and cognitive function. Child Development, 58:601–622, 1987.

Granger, CV, Hamilton, BB, & Kayton, R. Guide for the Use of the Functional Independence Measure (WeeFIM) of the Uniform Data Set for Medical Rehabilitation. Buffalo, NY: Research Foundation, State University of New York, 1989.

Greenough, WT, Black, JE, & Wallace, CS. Experience and brain development. Child Development, 58:539–559, 1987.

Hadders-Algra, M, & Prechtl, HFR. Developmental course of general movements in early infancy. I. Descriptive analysis of change in form. Early Human Development, 28:201–213, 1992.

Hadders-Algra, M, Van Eykern, LA, Klip–van den Nieuwendijk, AWJ, & Prechtl, HFR. Developmental course of general movements in early infancy. II. EMG correlates. Early Human Development, 28:231–253, 1992.

Haley, SM, Baryza, MJ, & Blanchard, Y. Functional and naturalistic frameworks in assessing physical and motor disablement. In Wilhelm, IJ (Ed.), Physical Therapy Assessment in Early Infancy. New York: Churchill Livingstone, 1993, pp. 225–256.

Haley, SM, Coster, WJ, & Faas, RM. A content validity study of the Pediatric Evaluation of Disability Inventory. Pediatric Physical Therapy, 3:177–184, 1991.

Haley, SM, Coster, WJ, Ludlow, LH, Haltiwanger, JT, & Andrellos, PJ. The Pediatric Evaluation of Disability Inventory: Development Standardization and Administration Manual. Boston: New England Medical Center Publications, 1992.

Harris, SR. Efficacy of physical therapy in promoting family functioning and functional independence for children with cerebral palsy. Pediatric Physical Therapy, 2:160–164, 1990.

Hay, L. Developmental changes in eye-hand coordination behaviors: Preprogramming versus feedback control. In Bard, C, Fleury, M, & Hay, L (Eds.), Development of Eye-Hand Coordination across the Life Span. Columbia, SC: University of South Carolina Press, 1990, pp. 217–244.

Hayne, H, Rovee-Collier, C, & Perris, EE. Categorization and memory retrieval by three-month-olds. Child Development, 58:750–767, 1987.

Horak, C. Motor development: Traditional and contemporary theories. In Lister, MJ (Ed.), Contemporary Management of Motor Control Problems: Proceedings of the II STEP Conference. Alexandria, VA: Foundation for Physical Therapy, 1991, pp. 99–126.

Hinderer, KA, Richardson, PK, & Atwater, SW. Clinical implications of the Peabody Developmental Motor Scales: A constructive review. Physical and Occupational Therapy in Pediatrics, 9(2):81–106, 1989.

Hohmann, A, & Creutzfeldt, OD. Squint and the development of binocularity in humans. Nature, 254:613–614, 1975.

Hoover, JE, & Strick, PL. Multiple output channels in the basal ganglia. Science, 259:819–821, 1993.

Horak, FB. Assumptions underlying motor control for neurologic rehabilitation. In Lister, MJ (Ed.), Contemporary Management of Motor Control Problems: Proceedings of the II STEP Conference. Alexandria, VA: Foundation for Physical Therapy, 1991, pp. 11–27.

Kanda, T, Yuge, M, Yamori, Y, Suzuki, J, & Fukase, H. Early physiotherapy in the treatment of spastic diplegia. Developmental Medicine and Child Neurology, 26:438–444, 1984.

Karniol, R. The role of manual manipulative stages in the infant's acquisition of perceived control over objects. Developmental Review, 9:205–233, 1989.

Keshner, EA, Campbell, D, Katz, R, & Peterson, BW. Neck muscle activation patterns in humans during isometric head stabilization. Experimental Brain Research, 75:335–364, 1989.

Knobloch, H, Stevens, F, & Malone, AF. Manual of Developmental Diagnosis (rev. ed.). New York: Harper & Row, 1980.

Krus, PH, Bruininks, RH, & Robertson, G. Structure of motor abilities in children. Perceptual and Motor Skills, 52:119–129, 1981.

Lee, AM. Child-rearing practices and motor performance of black and white children. Research Quarterly for Exercise and Sport, 51:494–500, 1980.

Loria, C. Relationship of proximal and distal function in motor development. Physical Therapy, 60:167–172, 1980.

McEwan, MH, Dihoff, RE, & Brosvic, GM. Early infant crawling experience is reflected in later motor skill development. Perceptual and Motor Skills, 72:75–79, 1991.

McGraw, MB. Growth: A Study of Johnny and Jimmy. New York: Appleton-Century, 1935.

McGraw, MB. The Neuromuscular Maturation of the Human Infant. New York: Hafner, 1963. (Original work published by Columbia University Press, 1945.)

Miller, LJ. The Miller First Step (Screening Test for Evaluating Preschoolers). New York: Psychological Corporation, 1992.

Miller, LJ. The Toddler and Infant Motor Evaluation. Tucson, AZ: Communication Skill Builders, in press.

Msall, ME, Braun, S, Duffy, L, DiGaudio, K, LaForest, S, & Granger, C. Normative sample of the Pediatric Functional Independence Measure: A uniform data set for tracking disability (Abstract). Developmental Medicine and Child Neurology, 34(suppl 66):19, 1992a.

Msall, ME, Braun, S, Granger, C, DiGaudio, K, & Duffy, L. The Functional Independence Measure for Children (WeeFIM), Developmental Edition (Version 1.5). Buffalo, NY: Uniform Data Set for Medical Rehabilitation, 1992b.

National Advisory Board on Medical Rehabilitation Research. Research Plan for the National Center for Medical Rehabilitation Research. NIH Publication No. 93-3509. Bethesda, MD: National Institutes of Health, 1993.

Nowakowski, RS. Basic concepts of CNS development. Child Development, 58:568–595, 1987.

Oppenheim, RW. Ontogenetic adaptations and retrogressive processes in the development of the nervous system and behavior: A neuroembryological perspective. In Connolly, K, & Prechtl, HFR (Eds.), Maturation and Development: Biological and Psychological Perspectives. Philadelphia: JB Lippincott, 1981, pp. 73–109.

Paillard, J. Basic neurophysiological structures of eye-hand coordination. In Bard, C, Fleury, M, & Hay, L (Eds.), Development of Eye-Hand Coordination across the Life Span. Columbia, SC: University of South Carolina Press, 1990, pp. 26–74.

Palisano, RJ. Neuromotor and developmental assessment. In Wilhelm, IJ (Ed.), Physical Therapy Assessment in Early Infancy. New York: Churchill Livingstone, 1993, pp. 173–224.

Parker, DF, Carriere, L, Hebestreit, H, Salsberg, A, & Bar-Or, O.

Muscle performance and gross motor function of children with spastic cerebral palsy. Developmental Medicine and Child Neurology, 35:17–23, 1993.

Piaget, J. The Origins of Intelligence in Children. New York: International Universities Press, 1952.

Pick, HL, Jr. Eleanor J. Gibson. Learning to perceive and perceiving to learn. Developmental Psychology, 28:787–794, 1992.

Piper, MC, Darrah, J. Motor Assessment of the Developing Infant. Philadelphia: WB Saunders, 1994.

Piper, MC, Pinnell, LE, Darrah, J, Maguire, T, & Byrne, PJ. Construction and validation of the Alberta Infant Motor Scale (AIMS). Canadian Journal of Public Health, 83(suppl 2):S46–S50, 1992.

Plimpton, CE, & Regimbal, C. Differences in motor proficiency according to gender and race. Perceptual and Motor Skills, 74, 399–402, 1992.

Provost B. Normal development from birth to 4 months: Extended use of the NBAS-K. Part II. Physical and Occupational Therapy in Pediatrics, 1(3):19–34, 1981.

Ramey, CT, & Ramey, SL. Effective early intervention. Mental Retardation, 30(6):337–345, 1992.

Roberton, MA, & Halverson, LE. Developing Children — Their Changing Movement. A Guide for Teachers. Philadelphia: Lea & Febiger, 1984.

Rosenbaum, P, Russell, D, Cadman, D, Gowland, C, Jarvis, S, & Hardy, S. Issues in measuring change in motor function in children with cerebral palsy: A special communication. Physical Therapy, 70:125–131, 1990.

Rosenblith, JF. A singular career: Nancy Bayley. Developmental Psychology, 28:747–758, 1992.

Russell, D, Rosenbaum, P, Cadman, D, Gowland, C, Hardy, S, & Jarvis, S. The Gross Motor Function Measure: A means to evaluate the effects of physical therapy. Developmental Medicine and Child Neurology, 31:341–352, 1989.

Scherzer, AL, Mike, V, & Ilson, J. Physical therapy as a determinant of change in the cerebral palsied infant. Pediatrics, 58:47–52, 1976.

Schoen, JHR. The corticofugal projection to the brain stem and spinal cord in man. Psychiatry, Neurology and Neurosurgery, 72:121–128, 1969.

Shirley, MM. The First Two Years: A Study of Twenty-five Babies. Vol. I. Postural and Locomotor Development. Minneapolis, MN: University of Minnesota Press, 1931.

Shumway-Cook, A, & Woollacott, M. The growth of stability: Postural control from a developmental perspective. Journal of Motor Behavior, 17:131–147, 1985.

Shumway-Cook, A, & Woollacott, M. Theoretical issues in assessing postural control. In Wilhelm, IJ (Ed.), Physical Therapy Assessment in Early Infancy. New York: Churchill Livingstone, 1993, pp. 161–171.

Skinner, BF. Cumulative Record: A Selection of Papers (3rd ed.). New York: Meredith, 1972.

Sparling, JW (Ed.). Concepts in Fetal Movement Research. New York: Haworth Press, 1993.

Stengel, TJ. Assessing motor development in children. In Campbell, SK (Ed.), Pediatric Neurologic Physical Therapy (2nd Ed.). New York: Churchill Livingstone, 1991, pp. 33–65.

Stengel, TJ, Attermeier, SM, Bly, L, & Heriza, CB. Evaluation of sensorimotor dysfunction. In Campbell, SK (Ed.), Pediatric Neurologic Physical Therapy. New York: Churchill Livingstone, 1984, pp. 13–87.

Stokes, NA, Deitz, JL, & Crowe, TK. The Peabody Developmental Fine Motor Scale: An interrater reliability study. American Journal of Occupational Therapy, 44:334–340, 1990.

Strick, PL, & Preston, JB. Two representations of the hand in area 4 of a primate. I. Motor output organization. Journal of Neurophysiology, 48:139–149, 1982a.

Strick, PL, & Preston, JB. Two representations of the hand in area 4 of a primate. II. Somatosensory input organization. Journal of Neurophysiology, 48:150–159, 1982b.

Task Force on Standards for Measurement in Physical Therapy. Standards for tests and measurements in physical therapy practice. Physical Therapy, 71:589–622, 1991.

Thelen, E. Coupling perception and action in the development of skill: A dynamic approach. In Bloch, H, & Bertenthal, BI (Eds.), Sensory-Motor Organization and Development in Infancy and Early Childhood. Dordrecht, Netherlands: Kluwer Academic, 1990, pp. 39–56.

Thelen, E, & Adolph, KE. Arnold L. Gesell: The paradox of nature and nurture. Developmental Psychology, 28:368–380, 1992.

Thelen, E, Corbetta, D, Kamm, K, Spencer, JP, Schneider, K, & Zernicke, R. The transition to reaching: Mapping intention and intrinsic dynamics. Child Development, 64:1058–1098, 1993.

Thelen, E, Kelso, JAS, & Fogel, A. Self-organizing systems and infant motor development. Developmental Review, 7:39–65, 1987.

Thelen, E, & Ulrich, BD. Hidden skills: A dynamic systems analysis of treadmill stepping during the first year. Monographs of the Society for Research in Child Development. Serial No. 223, Vol. 56, No. 1. Chicago: University of Chicago Press, 1991.

Thelen, E, Ulrich, BD, & Jensen, JL. The developmental origins of locomotion. In Woollacott, MH, & Shumway-Cook, A (Eds.), Development of Posture and Gait across the Life Span. Columbia, SC: University of South Carolina Press, 1989, pp. 23–47.

Ulrich, BD. Development of stepping patterns in human infants: A dynamical systems perspective. Journal of Motor Behavior, 21:329–408, 1989.

van Blankenstein, M, Welbergen, UR, & de Haas, JH. le développement du nourrisson: sa première année en 130 photographies. Paris: Presses Universitaires de France, 1962.

Vinter, A. Manual imitations and reaching behaviors: An illustration of action control in infancy. In Bard, C, Fleury, M, & Hay, L (Eds.), Development of Eye-Hand Coordination across the Life Span. Columbia, SC: University of South Carolina Press, 1990, pp. 157–187.

von Hofsten, C. Eye-hand coordination in the newborn. Developmental Psychology, 18:450–461, 1982.

Williams, JR, & Scott, RB. Growth and development of Negro infants: Motor development and its relationship to child-rearing practices in two groups of Negro infants. Child Development, 24:103–121, 1953.

Zelazo, PR. The development of walking: New findings and old assumptions. Journal of Motor Behavior, 15:99–137, 1983.

Zelazo, PR, Zelazo, NA, & Kolb, S. "Walking" in the newborn. Science, 176:314–315, 1972.

Chapter 2

Motor Control: Developmental Aspects of Motor Control in Skill Acquisition

NINA S. BRADLEY, PT, PhD

What does it mean to say, "I use a motor control approach" in my clinical practice? The term "motor control" is appearing with increasing frequency in physical therapy literature (e.g., Barnes et al., 1990; Giuliani, 1991; Horak, 1992; Ostrosky, 1990), but the reader may feel uncertain as to what the term means, given the variety of ways it is applied. This chapter seeks to familiarize the clinician with the field of motor control and, more specifically, with how motor control applies to issues of development. For this purpose, four objectives are set forth. Because the field of motor control emerged from the scholarly and research activities of scientists interested in motor behavior, the first objective of this chapter is to provide a brief discussion of some theories and hypotheses that have shaped the direction of research and views on motor control. Results of research testing theories and hypotheses of motor control, in turn, have led scientists to suggest that physiologic, psychologic, and mechanical processes or mechanisms play specific roles in the control of movement that can be studied under conditions of controlled observation. Thus, the second objective of this chapter is to describe some of the processes that may control movement initiation or execution. The third objective of this chapter, and its primary emphasis, is to present the work of researchers that both describes motor skill acquisition and attempts to reveal the processes that drive or permit acquisition of skills such as posture, gait, reaching, and grasping. The fourth objective is to explore how a physical therapist might assess a child's movement problems in light of our current knowledge of motor control.

THEORIES, HYPOTHESES, AND MODELS

Defining the term "motor control" and describing many of the theoretic constructs common to the field are no easy tasks, in part due to the fact that motor control is a multidisciplinary field of study that draws from a broad range of disciplines, including anatomy, physiology, psychology, kinesiology, engineering, and increasingly, physical therapy. Historically, theories of motor control emerged from either anatomy or psychology, whereas hypotheses and models have tended to emerge from the integration of ideas across fields. One consequence of this cross-pollination is that theoretic constructs and terminology may take on slightly different definitions from one disciplinary view to the next, often leaving resolution of the discrepancy in definitions to the interested student. In this section, we will briefly review some of the better known theories, hypotheses, and models of motor control, both to gain an understanding of the ideas commonly embraced or challenged and to discuss some of the differences in terminology one may encounter in the literature.

Theories of motor control attempt to unite various observations and laws that emerge from scientific study to explain why they exist and how they relate to one another. Theories also provide the foundation for development of hypotheses, models, and new theories. Three distinctly different theoretic perspectives are currently encountered in motor control literature: maturational, learning, and dynamical-based views. In the discussion to follow, we will briefly consider each view. Hypotheses, by contrast, attempt to predict the relationship between observations and defined (or experimental) conditions. For example, the maturational-based theory of motor control proposes that emergence of behavior is attributable to maturational changes in the nervous system. Thus, one might hypothesize in accordance with this theory that the capacity for independent finger movements emerges at 7 months of age because of specific physiologic changes that occur in the primary motor cortex just before 7 months. When experiments by a large number of scientists test hypotheses and obtain consistent findings, hypotheses become laws. Thus, laws define highly predictable relationships between variables, and in some instances these relationships can be mathematically defined. Fitts' Law, for example, states that accuracy requirements and the distance over which a movement occurs can be used to predict movement time (Fitts, 1954). Models, on the other hand, are idealized constructs that typically incorporate a number of variables and are used by scientists both to visualize and to test theories. A basic understanding of hypotheses and models is useful because it provides the underpinnings for many of the research designs and views currently found in motor control literature. For further elaboration on these points, the reader is referred to the discussion by Schmidt (1988).

A Historical Perspective

Near the turn of the twentieth century, the neurologist Ramón y Cajal discovered that the Golgi silver stain could selectively label individual nerve cells—an advance that set the course for neurobiologic research and thinking throughout the century (Hamburger, 1980), including those of the maturational-based theory of motor control. Using the silver stain, anatomists could for the first time see individual neurons, distinguish differences among populations of neurons, and distinguish morphologic changes related to development. Such findings eventually led to the view that all behavioral functions are the consequence of how the nervous system is structurally (i.e., anatomically) organized, a relation referred to as "structure-function" organization. Equipped with the ability to define distinct neuroanatomic networks visually, physiologists discovered the means for isolating portions of the nervous system (also referred to as reduced preparations) capable of producing stereotypic movements such as the stretch reflex, the brisk contraction of a muscle in response to a quick elongation of the muscle and its proprioceptors. Many studies of reflex function in the spinal cord of cats, dogs, and monkeys led Sherrington (1947) to propose a hierarchic view of neural function based on the integrative action of many reflexes. In the classic treatise, *Integrative Action of the Nervous System,* first published in 1906, Sherrington put forth the notion that the simple reflex (composed of a receptor, conductor, and effector organ) is the fundamental unit of neural integration. Integrative action of the nervous system, he proposed, is the composite coordination of simple reflexes, called reflex-chaining, that results from the summation of excitatory and inhibitory actions at the synapse.

MATURATIONAL-BASED THEORIES

The Sherringtonian notion of reflex-chaining so dominated the study of physiology in the first half of this century that physiologists gave little attention to other views of motor control in their attempts to explain behavior (Gallistel, 1980). During much of this century, concepts of structure-function organization and reflex-chaining were routinely enlisted in studies of motor development. Experimental designs were often based on temporal correlations between emerging stimulus-evoked behavior and anatomic changes in neural pathways (e.g., Humphrey, 1964; Langworthy, 1933). Typically, such studies assumed that behavioral change was due to a change in anatomy. Thus, early studies sought to identify what anatomic changes occurred about the time a new behavior emerged without considering whether other variables contributed to the behavioral change. Based on numerous studies in many different species employing similar temporal correlations, scientists proposed that certain predictable changes during neural maturation are the primary determinants of motor development (Hooker, 1958; McGraw, 1945), forming the basis for a maturational theory. Concurrent with these views, the Sherringtonian notion of reflex-chaining evolved into the view that reflexes are arranged in a hierarchic order and reflect an animal's phylogenetic origins (Humphrey, 1970). Such views merged into the notions that an animal's earliest movements are primitive behaviors controlled by phylogenetically older neural structures and that they eventually disappear as the older neural structures are inhibited by later, differentiating neural structures that are phylogenetically more recent (Touwen, 1984). Little or no scientific evidence challenged these neuromaturational views, perhaps because little attention was given by students of development to other directions in neurobiologic research that were emerging at the time (Gallistel, 1980).

LEARNING-BASED THEORIES

During this same period, psychologists were also attempting to form theories of development. Behaviorism looked to the role of the environment in shaping behavior and sought to determine what attributes of the environment trigger or shape behavior. The theory of response-chaining, for example, proposed that feedback becomes more strongly associated with action over practice, such that it automates sequences of actions executed by the nervous system (Rosenbaum, 1991). According to the theory of response-chaining, the environment is the controller of the automating process. With response-chaining, as with Sherrington's reflex-chaining, the ordering of movements is explained as the consequence of feedback from one movement that in turn activates the next movement. Thorndike extended the notion of response-chaining specifically to the question of how motor skills are learned, and in the Law of Effect, he proposed that skills emerge as we repeat actions that are rewarded, an idea that was enlisted and popularized by BF Skinner in techniques of behavior modification (Schmidt, 1988).

The Law of Effect and the emphasis on feedback can also be identified in contemporary theories and models of motor learning such as Adams's closed-loop theory (Adams, 1971). This theory proposed that we develop a perceptual memory trace for what a correct movement should feel like (expected sensory consequences) based on intrinsic feedback generated during movement implementation. The perceptual trace evaluates the actual sensory consequences (feedback) of a movement each time it is executed and selects the movement attributes that are compatible with the perceptual memory trace to establish a memory trace for movement execution parameters. As developed in Adams's learning-based theory, feedback during movement is required to learn a movement, but subsequently obtained evidence indicated that we do not need to monitor ongoing movements in order to reinforce desirable movement parameters (Taub & Berman, 1968). This inconsistency between experimental results and theoretic prediction was subsequently addressed by Schmidt's Schema Theory, to be discussed later (Schmidt, 1975).

As theories are tested, the outcomes reveal their shortcomings, clarify the boundaries of our understanding, and raise a new generation of questions. For example, tests of response-chaining theories raised such questions as how do we learn or execute movements when we cannot constantly monitor movement-dependent feedback and how do we manage to execute an apparently endless variety of new and varied movements, usually with minimal difficulty. Cognitive and developmental psychologists, much interested in these questions, sought to explain the development of new skills as either the determinants or the consequences of increasing cognitive abilities. For example, Piaget proposed that early motor skill acquisition is the outcome of preverbal learning processes that incorporate sensorimotor experience to form early notions of causation and that these notions are stored to serve later as an internal reference during the development of language and concrete cognitive operations. According to Piagetian theory, preverbal learning and motor skill acquisition are developmental (maturational) processes that permit concrete and abstract learning to take place (Bower, 1979; Keogh & Sugden, 1985). In contrast to maturational-based theories, learning-based theories suggest that development of motor skill is the consequence of learning by trial and error to master and sequence units of action that in their rudimentary form are genetically determined. Connolly (1977) proposed, for example, that the infant is genetically endowed with the equivalent of computer hardware (neurologic and biomechanical features) and that the infant's cognitive activities, comparable to computer software, function to modify and adapt rudimentary units of movement into skilled action.

Perhaps the most widely embraced of the learning theories, Schema Theory, proposed that motor development is a function of learning rules to evaluate, correct, and update memory traces for a given class of movements (Connolly, 1977; Keogh & Sugden, 1985; Schmidt, 1988). Schema Theory assumes the presence of three constructs: general motor programs and two types of memory traces, namely, recall schema and recognition schema. In Schema Theory, general motor programs are loosely defined as sets of instructions that are responsible for organizing the invariant or fundamental components of a movement. Recall schema are defined as memories of relationships between past movement parameters and past initial conditions and the movement outcomes they produced. Recognition schema are defined as memories of relationships between past movement parameters and past initial conditions and the sensory consequences they produced. In theory, recall schema function to establish rules regarding the relationship between movement parameters of a general motor program, such as force or velocity, and movement outcome for a given set of initial conditions that can be used to plan similar movements under anticipated conditions. Recognition schema, in turn, are proposed to compare sensory consequences with movement outcome in light of initial conditions to form a second set of rules that can be used to predict the expected sensory consequences for similar movement outcomes during anticipated initial conditions. The expected sensory consequences are hypothesized to serve as a perceptual memory trace for evaluating new movements. When movements are generated too quickly, ballistically, to be corrected by feedback as they are executed (i.e., open loop), it is theorized that intrinsic feedback, an efferent copy of the motor command, can be compared with the expected sensory consequences to evaluate the movements during execution or after they are completed. In theory, the schema are established and refined as a function of practice. See Chapter 6 by Larin for further discussion of motor-learning theories.

Schema Theory does not attempt to explain the establishment of motor programs, nor does it attempt to ascribe them to specific neural structures; because motor programs are frequently invoked to explain aspects of motor control, however, a few comments about them are warranted. The term "motor programs" is employed in a variety of ways by researchers from different disciplinary backgrounds, as demonstrated in a collection of papers (Jeannerod, 1990), which may help to explain why there is no consensus as to what constitutes a motor program (Rosenbaum, 1991). In general, motor programs are called upon to account for behavioral phenomena that appear to document their existence. In motor-learning literature, motor programs are commonly invoked to explain the stereotypic attributes of a complex movement pattern that persists as movement parameters or context is altered. For example, it has been suggested that we have a general motor program for writing our names and its instructions are recognized in the features common to signing our names under different conditions with different tools, different parameters of movement, and even different sets of muscles (Raibert, 1977). Motor-learning literature also ascribes to motor programs the ability to generate complex movements without benefit of concurrent feedback. This includes movements executed under deafferented conditions, such as reaching for a target after administration of a local anesthetic or tourniquet, as well as ballistic movements that may be completed before feedback can contribute to the movement (Schmidt, 1988). In each of these instances, motor programs are viewed as learned sets of instructions. In neurobiology, however, motor programs, also called pattern generators, are viewed as genetically inherited sets of instructions that control the stereotypic features of innate behaviors such as mating, defense, and locomotion (Kupfermann, 1991). It has also been suggested that motor programs control human gait (Shapiro et al., 1981). These applications of the term appear to suggest that motor programs are in some way related to central pattern generators, a term we will discuss within the topic of locomotion. Some of the strongest evidences for the existence of general motor programs are the many examples of an animal's ability to execute functional movements in the absence of feedback (Lashley, 1917; Polit & Bizzi, 1979; Taub & Berman, 1968). Where the movement instructions are stored is yet to be determined, but some investigators implicate the sensorimotor cortex (Asanuma & Keller, 1991) or the cerebellum (Sanes et al., 1990) in motor learning, and the prefrontal association cortex in motor memory and planning (Kupfermann, 1991).

DYNAMICAL-BASED THEORY

One theory put forth to explain the development of motor control is the Dynamical Systems Theory proposed by Thelen and colleagues (Thelen & Ulrich, 1991). The Dynamical Systems Theory springs from a fundamental hypothesis that multiple identifiable variables, such as muscle power, body mass, arousal, neural networks, motivation, and environmental forces (e.g., gravity and friction), establish a context for movement initiation and execution. A second hypothesis fundamental to the theory is that the relationship between such variables is in constant flux and therefore shapes the features of a movement as it unfolds (Ulrich, 1989). In a comprehensive presentation of Dynamical Systems Theory, Thelen and Ulrich (1991) formalized the problems of motor development they wished to address that had not been handled satisfactorily by previous theories and assumptions about what drives skill acquisition. For example, why do we typically describe development as a sequence of stages and how does a child move from one stage to another? Lacking an explanation for transitions between stages, progressions may appear to be quantum leaps, suggesting something more miraculous than mechanistic. The Dynamical Systems Theory proposes, by contrast, that changes in motor behavior and skill performance can be explained in terms of dynamics common to physical, biologic, and computational systems. Transitions in behavior may occur as the consequence of changes in one or more variables that add to or subtract from expression of an action. In some instances, the variable may be present or absent, whereas in other instances, the variable might be scaled differently. For example, in the absence of sufficient postural control, coordinated limb movements may not be apparent until postural control requirements are addressed (Bradley, 1992). Or the pattern of limb movements may vary abruptly with changes in movement parameters such as velocity (Scholz, 1990). The beauty of theories like Dynamical Systems and Schema is that they readily afford hypothesis development and testing, and unlike maturational views, they imply that there are variables that may be readily manipulated to produce significant changes in motor behavior. The last-mentioned property suggests that research based on these theories may offer important new or refined concepts of therapeutic intervention for children with disabilities.

Current Hypotheses of Motor Control

Rather than propose some unifying theory, most current hypotheses of motor control attempt to identify controlling variables for specific types of movement. Central pattern generators are proposed to account for the basic neural organization and function required to execute coordinated, rhythmic movements such as locomotion (Grillner, 1981), chewing (Luschei & Goldberg, 1981), and respiration (von Euler, 1980). In most instances, central pattern generators are defined as interneuronal networks located in either the spinal cord or brain stem that order the selection and sequencing of motoneurons independent of descending or peripheral afferent neural input. It is generally held that descending neural input activates central pattern generators (Jordan, 1986), and that descending input (Armstrong, 1986) and peripheral afferent

input (Loeb, 1986) modify the output of central pattern generators to make the resulting behavior adaptive to the movement context. Central pattern generators can also modify the inputs they receive, gating potentially disruptive reflex actions such as nociceptive activation of flexor withdrawal when a limb is fully loaded during the stance phase of locomotion (Rossignol & Drew, 1986). A considerable body of evidence suggests that central pattern generators, including that for locomotion, are established during initial differentiation of the nervous system and are potentially capable of producing orderly or coordinated motor patterns with the onset of embryonic movement (Bradley & Bekoff, 1989, 1990). There has been some suggestion that central pattern generators may be one class of general motor programs (Shapiro et al., 1981), but central pattern generators are hypothesized only to control repetitive, stereotypic movements and are typically modeled as discrete populations of neurons (Grillner, 1981; Pearson, 1976). General motor programs, by contrast, are hypothesized to control classes of related movements, including discrete movements (e.g., reaching for a toy), and may or may not be defined by discrete neural structures.

A number of hypotheses of motor control specifically attempt to explain how we control discrete arm movements. According to the equilibrium-point hypothesis, also called the mass-spring hypothesis, the nervous system strives to control joint position in space, and every position can be defined by a unique combination of agonist and antagonist muscle forces that result in a net stiffness (Feldman, 1986). It is argued that muscles function like springs, and once a motor program is sufficiently established, it activates the appropriate muscles to contract and move a limb segment until the segment reaches the point in space where all active and passive muscle forces are in equilibrium. One version of this hypothesis proposes that the equilibrium points composing a trajectory endpoint of movement are achieved as a function of neural commands that regulate coactivation of alpha and gamma motoneurons (Feldman, 1986). Another version of the hypothesis proposes that these equilibria may be achieved as a consequence of neural commands to alpha motoneurons alone. This later version of the hypothesis was proposed because it was found that, after partially deafferented monkeys (by dorsal root transection of brachial nerves) were able to point to a target within viewing their arms, even when the arm was moved unknowingly before the onset of the movement (Polit & Bizzi, 1978). Other hypotheses attempt to distinguish whether we learn to control movement with respect to intrinsic body coordinates of joint position, referred to as joint-space, or with respect to extrinsic coordinates, referred to as hand-space in the case of reaching (Abend et al., 1982). Finally, some hypotheses attempt to determine which parameters, such as time, distance, or force, are controlled during movement initiation and prior to correction. Most notable among these, the impulse-timing hypothesis proposes that the nervous system controls movement by planning the phasing and duration of muscle contractions (Schmidt et al., 1979). For further discussions on hypotheses of motor control, the reader is referred to reviews (Rosenbaum, 1991; Schmidt, 1988) and a collection of several excellent papers (Jeannerod, 1990).

Researchers have also begun to investigate the use of models for motor control by looking to the fields of robotics and neural networks. Both approaches seek to incorporate perception and action to explain control of movement. Robotic models are based on the physics of perception and movement, assigning mathematic values to known neural and biomechanical relationships to explain movement outcome. Neural network models are based on the assumption that no simple, predictable relationship exists between nerve cells that can explain movement, but rather that the phenomenon of their complex interactions explains the movement outcome. An introductory overview of these topics is provided by Rosenbaum (1991), and a collection of papers presents a wide range of specific examples currently under study (Jeannerod, 1990). Models of motor control are in a sense an endpoint, the assimilation of data from experiments testing hypotheses derived from theories. Models can then, in turn, be used to determine the extent to which we can generalize the findings of studies testing hypotheses and theories. As these ideas withstand the test of challenge, we can become more confident in estimating how they may be effectively applied in addressing practical and clinical problems of motor control.

▌ MOTOR CONTROL VARIABLES

Characteristic of contemporary motor control research is the notion that multiple variables contribute to the initiation and execution of a movement. Thus, it is generally assumed that to understand how movements are controlled one must be able to identify which variables are important and to determine how these variables interact during movement. In this section, we will identify some possible variables and consider how investigators currently think these variables contribute to motor control. Borrowing from the ideas of Bernstein (1967), a Soviet physiologist, some investigators speak of motor control variables as systems or subsystems of control composed of many intra- and extrapersonal variables (Thelen & Ulrich, 1991). In more eclectic terms, variables may be anything, whether physical, physiologic, or psychologic, that has an impact on movement planning or execution. Thus, to identify the underlying processes that determine skill acquisition during development, one needs to know not only which variables are important at a given age but also how each variable changes during development and the impact of that change on all the other variables involved. To accomplish such a task successfully requires an experimental approach that controls as many variables as possible while methodically manipulating the one in question—a task that is rarely feasible in human studies. Nonetheless, researchers are attempting to identify variables that are critical to skill acquisition. By nature, these variables are interactive, but for convenience we will refer to them here as being sensorimotor variables, mechanical variables, cognitive variables, and task requirements.

Sensorimotor Variables

Sensorimotor variables are those physiologic mechanisms or processes that reside within the nervous system. Central pattern generators, discussed in the previous section, are an example of a sensorimotor contribution. By selecting and timing the activity of motoneurons, central pattern generators play a key role in determining the pattern of muscle activity during movement (Grillner, 1981). For example, in the case of locomotion, central pattern generators determine which muscles are active in the stance phase of gait and which are active in swing. Experiments have demonstrated that central pattern generators can produce motor patterns similar to those produced during normal behavior even when deprived of afferent (sensory) information. Some investigators refer to the muscle activity produced by central pattern generators as synergies, with each rhythmic movement having its own synergy (Smith et al., 1986), but these pattern generators are not the only determinants of the synergies that characterize rhythmic movements. When a cat rapidly shakes a paw to dislodge an irritant, for example, a novel combination of flexor and extensor activity is produced, referred to as a mixed synergy. The mixed synergy is partially determined by spinal neural circuits (a central pattern generator) and partially determined by motion-dependent feedback from the leg (Koshland & Smith, 1989).

Movement synergies and neural mechanisms that alter or regulate them can also be viewed as sensorimotor variables controlling movement. A common view is that the formation of synergies for movement is the nervous system's solution to the problem of controlling the multiple degrees of freedom inherent in coordinating a multisegmented body (Bernstein, 1967). Although synergies have long been viewed as the stereotypic motoneuron patterns inherent in spinal neural circuitry, such as flexor and extensor synergies, current views suggest that movement synergies not only are context-specific and highly individualistic (Keshner, 1990) but also may include any pattern of motoneuron activity characterizing a given form of movement (Lee, WA, 1984). Supporting this view, anatomic and physiologic data from cats have suggested that motoneuron pools for biarticular muscles of the leg are actually a collection of smaller pools that can be separately recruited in a task-specific manner (Pratt & Loeb, 1991). For example, portions or all of these pools may be recruited depending on movement parameters such as velocity or acceleration (Smith & Zernicke, 1987). Other studies suggest that muscle synergies characterizing voluntary movement, particularly of the upper extremities, may be controlled by premotor cortical areas because specific patterns of corticoneuronal activity in these areas are initiated prior to the onset of practiced movements (Georgopolous, 1990; Ghez, 1991). Sensorimotor variables that may contribute to regulation of muscle synergies to enhance performance include mechanisms controlling joint stiffness (Hasan, 1986) and visuomotor and visuospatial processes (Lee, DN, et al., 1990; Schmidt, 1988) and, in essence, all other perceptuomotor processes tuned to participate in planning or executing a movement. Developmental aspects of sensorimotor variables also include processes of change such as differentiation and refinement of neural networks, changes in sensory perception, neural conduction characteristics, changing motor unit properties, and force-producing capabilities. The two topics last named will be considered more fully with respect to musculoskeletal development in Chapter 4 of this text.

Mechanical Variables

Mechanical contributions to motor control have enjoyed renewed attention. Changes in total body mass and relative distribution of mass during development are accompanied by changes in length and center of mass per body segment. These changes, in turn, alter inertial forces due to gravity and to friction during movement. In some instances, these inertial forces may assist movement. In other instances, they may oppose movement. Together with other variables, they help shape movement (Smith & Zernicke, 1987). Several studies in animals and humans have demonstrated that motor skills are greatly affected by inertial forces (Hoy et al., 1985; Schneider et al., 1990) and that part of learning to perfect a skill is learning to anticipate and use these forces to execute a movement more efficiently (Schneider et al., 1989; see also section on Locomotion, this chapter). The viscoelastic properties of musculoskeletal tissues are also an important mechanical variable in the control of movement (Hoy & Zernicke, 1985; Siegler et al., 1984; Tardieu et al., 1989). The passive elastic attributes of these tissues contribute to action by absorbing and releasing energy and have been thought to reduce neural programming requirements for movement execution (Schneider et al., 1989; Smith & Zernicke, 1987).

Cognitive Variables

Cognitive variables may include variables that are dependent on both conscious and subconscious processes such as reasoning, memory, or judgment to optimize performance. Such variables might include arousal, motivation, anticipatory strategies, and the selective use of feedback, practice, and memory. Variations in arousal can probably modify any other control variable, such as pattern generation (Thelen et al., 1982), or may even determine whether a behavior is demonstrated (Bradley & Smith, 1988a,b). Motivation may make multiple contributions to the control of movement. In some instances, it may serve primarily to trigger activity, and in other instances motivation may determine the form of the consequent movement. For example, it has been suggested that an infant's hand-path is straighter during reaches for a moving target than for a stationary one because the infant is more motivated to reach and make contact with a moving target (Hofsten, 1991).

Anticipatory strategies, also called feedforward strategies, are movement adjustments time locked to voluntary movements (Massion, 1992). In the control of posture, anticipatory strategies minimize equilibrium disturbance, and in other acts, they minimize the amount of attention dedicated to monitoring feedback and making corrections after initial movement execution. Although anticipatory strategies are not usually conscious cognitive processes, it can be argued that they involve subconscious forecasting processes (Massion, 1992), as is suggested for the control of perceptuomotor tasks (Viviani & Mounoud, 1990) and by the considerable training required for anticipatory postural adjustments observed in dancers (Mouchnino et al., 1990). Indeed, it is argued that anticipatory strategies are learned and relatively fixed under stable conditions but are adapted in less fixed situations only by learning from past movement experiences (Massion, 1992). Anticipatory strategies are observed in postural adjustments before the onset of whole body movements (Nashner & Forssberg, 1986), in postural adjustments before the onset of arm movements (Horak et al., 1984; Lee, WA, 1980), in shaping and orientation of the hand before contact with an object to be grasped (Jeannerod, 1984), and in strategies to time body movements with timing demands of the environment (Viviani & Mounoud, 1990). Children, like adults, demonstrate anticipatory postural adjustments in trunk and leg muscles before lifting their arms (Riach & Hayes, 1990) or rising onto tiptoe (Haas et al., 1989) as early as 4 years of age. Anticipatory strategies during preparation to grasp, however, can be observed as early as 9 months of age (Forssberg et al., 1991; Hofsten & Rönnqvist, 1988), and appear to be present by 3 to 4 postnatal months, as evidenced by the postural adjustments in neck and trunk musculature when infants are about to be pulled to a sitting position or picked up when supine (Bayley, 1969).

Whether all these anticipatory strategies share some fundamental means of regulation has not to this author's knowledge been addressed experimentally, but it is speculated that similarities may exist between feedforward strategies in postural and arm trajectory control (Massion, 1992). In addition, there is no clear locus of control for any of the identified anticipatory strategies. To date, it is generally thought that anticipatory postural adjustments are controlled by local spinal cord and brain stem networks as well as by transcortical loops, including the motor and premotor cortices (Massion, 1992). Models of feedforward control hypothesize that the controller is likely to be a network that receives and compares afferent feedback with a copy of the motor commands for the desired movement (also called an efferent copy) to set gain adjustments for modifying movement commands as they are executed (Massion, 1992). Feedforward strategies may also function to reprogram postural responses (Horak & Nashner, 1986) or delay initiation of the voluntary command (Massion, 1992) when the command is destabilizing. Limited evidence to date suggests that feedforward strategies emerge subsequent to feedback strategies during development of a skill such as postural control in stance (Haas et al., 1989) and that these strategies are disrupted in children with cerebral palsy

(Nashner et al., 1983) and delayed or inadequate in children with Down syndrome (Sugden & Keogh, 1990).

The amount of attention dedicated to monitoring a movement is also viewed as a variable that can be modified to perfect a motor skill. It has been suggested that during development, children initially execute new movements in a ballistic manner, ignoring feedback, then swing to the opposite extreme, attempting to process excessive amounts of feedback, before finally learning to attend to feedback selectively. An example of this transition proposed by Hay (1979) is described in the section in this chapter on reaching. It is generally thought that once the child (or adult) learns to attend selectively to feedback, more attention (or mental processing) can be assigned to reading the environment and predicting the environmental changes and movement outcome as the movement is executed. For further information on these issues, see discussions by Keogh and Sugden (1985). Other cognitive variables related to learning, such as form and quantity of practice and the role of memory, will be addressed within the context of motor learning in Chapter 6 of this text.

Task Requirements

Finally, task requirements can also be considered to be distinct motor control variables. Task requirements may include any variable that can contribute to, or in some way alter, movement, including biomechanical requirements, meaningfulness, predictability, and any other variable associated with a given movement context. Because task requirements are also identified as variables in studies of motor control, we will consider them briefly. Physiologic recordings from several sensorimotor centers of the brain indicate that their participation in a task is context-specific (Crutcher & Alexander, 1990; Ghez, 1991; Lemon, 1988). Task requirements shape such motor strategies as the response selection to postural perturbations, for example, to recover a posture, step into a new posture, or execute protective extension of the arms (Horak & Nashner, 1986). Task requirements can also result in the gating of reflexes, as when a noxious stimulus applied to the foot produces a flexor withdrawal response if the leg is in the swing phase of a gait, but produces an extensor "contact" response if the leg is in the stance phase (Rossignol & Gauthier, 1980). Similarly, task requirements may alter the strategy a child uses to reach for an object (Hofsten, 1991), and research suggests that the meaningfulness of the task may enhance or mask performance (van der Weel et al., 1991). The role of meaningfulness is demonstrated by comparing performance when a child is asked to perform a relatively abstract task (e.g., verbally instructed to pronate then supinate as far as possible) versus a concrete task (e.g., verbally instructed to hit a tambourine, a task requiring pronation and supination). Children with cerebral palsy generate larger movement excursions following the concrete instructions than following the abstract instructions (van der Weel et al., 1991). Task requirements, like all other variables we have considered, appear to play a crucial role in the control of movement. Control variables may add to or subtract from movement in such a way that there may be multiple possible behavioral outcomes for a given set of centrally generated movement instructions. Thus, learning more about how control variables shape movement may lead us to a better understanding of how to help our clients improve their motor skills.

MOTOR SKILL ACQUISITION IN CHILDREN

This section will examine specific areas of motor development in children and the variables currently viewed as critical to the process of skill acquisition. As will be demonstrated, many of the apparently key sensorimotor variables for control of a skill are already present in the earliest phases of postnatal development, suggesting that the basic neural substrate for orderly generation of skilled movement is likely to be in place months or years before the maturation of the nervous system is complete and adult behaviors are observed. Although neural maturation of sensorimotor variables for motor control is necessary to attain adult levels of skill, it is not sufficient to account fully for how or when skilled movement is achieved. We will consider some of the variables identified by researchers and how these variables may contribute to the control of four specific skill areas, postural control, locomotion, reaching, and grasping, during development.

Postural Control

Postural control is thought to be achieved via the cooperative interaction of multiple neural systems, most notably the visual, vestibular, and somatosensory systems (Horak et al., 1990, Nashner et al., 1982). Although each of these systems is considered essential to optimal control of both static and dy-namic posture, each system can compensate to some extent for the functions of the other two (Horak et al., 1990), and the relative importance of each system appears to vary with contextual demands (Horak & Nashner, 1986; Horak et al., 1989). As we will see, acquiring skill to process this ensemble of sensory information to select a motor strategy may more fully account for the postnatal development of postural control than do indices of physiologic maturation of any given sensory system. The functioning of these systems to achieve postural control is often described in terms that emphasize the closed-loop, or feedback, aspects of balance correction; adaptive postural control, however, also employs open-loop or feedforward, strategies. These anticipatory strategies function to minimize potential postural perturbations arising with movement initiation. Thus, the process of establishing effective anticipatory strategies may also more fully account for the development of postural control than do indices of postnatal changes in the closed-loop attributes of any given sensory system or its impairment during development (Horak et al., 1988). In this section we will consider the contribution of sensorimotor variables, most notably in the visual, vestibular, and somatosensory systems, and other variables contributing to the acquisition of postural control.

VISUAL SYSTEM

Vision is perhaps the most powerful sensory system functioning to regulate posture, both for feedback correction and for selection of anticipatory postural strategies (Butterworth & Hicks, 1977; Lee, DN, & Aronson, 1974). The first to ascribe a proprioceptive function to vision, Gibson (1966) suggested that as light from the visual field strikes the retina, changes in light associated with movement create "optical flow patterns" interpreted by the brain to determine the position of our head and body with respect to the surrounding environment. It is argued that the large-amplitude postural sway observed in blind individuals is due to the absence of this optical flow information (Lee, DN, 1980). Optical flow patterns can evoke dramatic postural responses in both children and adults. In a now classic set of studies, DN Lee and Lishman (1975) demonstrated that when an adult stands inside a closed space formed by three walls and a ceiling, a forward or backward movement of the wall facing the person (center wall, Fig 2–1) triggers a larger sway amplitude than occurs under static visual conditions; the effect is greater if the postural task is made more difficult, as by standing on one leg. The effect of this visual stimulus is greatest if the visual

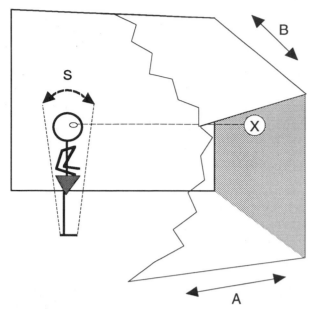

FIGURE 2–1. The subject is placed in the center of a partial room, formed by three walls and a ceiling, that can be slid along in direction A or B. When the subject is facing wall X, room motion in direction A creates a looming or receding visual stimulus and triggers an increase in the magnitude of the subject's sway (S) in the anteroposterior plane. Younger children are likely to sway closer to their limits of stability (noted by the dashed lines forming an inverted cone) when presented with a looming visual stimulus but not when the visual stimulus moves side to side (direction B). (Adapted from Lee, DN, & Aronson, E. Visual proprioceptive control of standing in human infants. Perception and Psychophysics, *15*:529–532, 1974. Reprinted by permission of Psychonomic Society, Inc.)

stimulus moves along the anterior-posterior axis of vision (referred to as a looming visual stimulus, Fig. 2–1*A*) and least if it moves tangentially (side to side, Fig. 2–1*B*) to the visual axis. In the latter case, extraocular muscle activity during visual tracking is thought to provide proprioceptive information used to discriminate between environment and body movements (Butterworth & Hicks, 1977; Lee, DN, & Lishman, 1975). For example, if facing the center wall as it is slowly moved closer, the subject sways backward; if the wall is moved away, the subject leans forward. If the entire enclosure is moved sideways from the subject's left to right (or vice versa), however, little or no change in posture is detected.

Children begin to demonstrate distinct postural responses to optical flow patterns early in development (Butterworth & Hicks, 1977; Lee, DN, & Aronson, 1974). When placed in the moving room, children from 13 to 17 months old with 0.5 to 6.5 months of walking experience sway excessively and

are likely to fall in response to a looming visual stimulus (Butterworth & Hicks, 1977). Forward and backward sway responses to looming visual stimuli are also observed during independent sitting in infants at 11 to 16 months (Butterworth & Hicks, 1977). The potential for such responses appears to be functional by the age of 2 postnatal months and perhaps as early as by 6 postnatal days. For example, when a looming visual stimulus is presented to an infant supported in an infant seat, directionally appropriate neck muscle activity is observed; namely, approaching stimuli trigger neck extensor activity, whereas withdrawing stimuli trigger neck flexor activity (Ball & Tronick, 1971; Bower et al., 1970; Yonas et al., 1977). Visual proprioception appears to play a dominant role in postural control during early childhood, for if the eyes are closed during postural displacements in the anterior-posterior plane on a movable platform under conditions of normal vestibular and somatosensory information, the magnitude of sway for children 4 to 6 years of age is significantly greater than for children 7 to 10 years of age (Shumway-Cook & Woollacott, 1985a). By 7 to 10 years of age, with eyes closed, children demonstrate responses similar to those of adults with eyes closed (Shumway-Cook & Woollacott 1985a).

VESTIBULAR AND SOMATOSENSORY SYSTEMS

Evidence also suggests that the vestibular and somatosensory systems actively participate in the control of posture early in the postnatal period. When infants are supported in a seated position and experience anterior-posterior displacements administered via horizontal movement of a computer-controlled platform, neck flexor and extensor muscle activity is paired with the direction of displacement (Woollacott et al., 1987). Namely, anterior platform movements produce backward displacement of the head and subsequent activation of neck flexors to realign the head over the shoulders. The role of the vestibular and somatosensory systems combined as a single unit is underscored here by the finding that the directionally appropriate responses are more consistent (occurring in as much as 100% of trials) when vision is occluded (Woollacott et al., 1987).

Vestibular and somatosensory systems are also capable of generating directionally-appropriate responses in the trunk and legs to anterior-posterior displacements during the earliest phases of independent sitting and standing (Forssberg & Nashner, 1982; Haas et al., 1989; Woollacott et al., 1987). Commonly used testing methods and leg responses

FIGURE 2–2. When a child is placed standing on a movable platform that is then displaced at a fixed rate and duration by a computer-driven mechanism in the posterior direction, the child sways forward and the posterior synergy is activated in a distal to proximal sequence over time to realign the head and trunk over the base of support *(A₁)*. Conversely, displacement of the platform in the anterior direction produces a posterior sway that is corrected by activation of the anterior muscle synergy, also in a distal to proximal sequence *(A₂)*. In both conditions illustrated, normal visual, vestibular, and somatosensory inputs are available. If the platform is rapidly rotated to produce ankle dorsiflexion *(B)* or plantar flexion (not shown), visual and vestibular input remains relatively stable throughout the perturbation, whereas somatosensory receptors register displacement. If, however, the platform is rapidly rotated in the same direction synchronously with normal sway *(C)*, somatosensory input remains relatively stable, because the ankle angle changes little during the perturbation, whereas vestibular and visual receptors register the postural sway. Visual information regarding sway can be altered during testing by having the subject close the eyes or by placing a dome around the subject's head to provide a stable visual field *(D)*. If vision is stabilized during platform *translations*, as in *A*, visual input will be in conflict with normal vestibular and somatosensory information. If vision is stabilized during platform *rotations*, as in *B*, both visual and vestibular inputs will be in conflict with somatosensory information. Finally, if vision is stabilized during platform rotations synchronized to normal sway, visual and somatosensory inputs will be in conflict with normal vestibular information. Vertical arrows in A_1 and A_2 indicate onset of first muscle responses. For additional discussion on methods and development of postural control, the reader is referred to a review and discussion by Woollacott et al. (1989) Abd = abdominal muscle, Gast = gastrocnemius, Ham = hamstring muscles, Para = paraspinal muscles, Quad = quadriceps muscles, Tib = tibialis anterior. *(A,* Adapted from Nashner, LM, Shumway-Cook, A, & Marin, O. Stance posture control in select groups of children with cerebral palsy: Deficits in sensory organization and muscular coordination. Experimental Brain Research, *49:*393–409, 1983. *B,* Adapted from Horak, FB, & Nashner, LM. Central programming of postural movements: Adaptation to altered support surface configurations. Journal of Neurophysiology, *55:*1369–1381, 1986.)

are illustrated in Figure 2–2. By 7 to 10 months of age, children occasionally demonstrate directionally appropriate leg muscle responses after the onset of mechanically induced sway. By 14 to 15 months of age, infants can regain upright posture independently, and some can consistently demonstrate directionally appropriate responses (Forssberg & Nashner, 1982; Haas et al., 1989; Shumway-Cook & Woollacott, 1985a; Woollacott et al., 1987). Leg muscle responses have thus far not been observed in children younger than 7 to 10 months of age who require postural assistance. Failure to obtain leg responses before the onset of independent stance may be due to the presence of an external support removing the need for a postural response, or there may be insufficient stretch-induced proprioceptive input at the ankle to trigger leg responses as a consequence of the external support (Woollacott et al., 1987, 1989).

As may be expected, muscle onset latencies and consistency of response to tests of postural skill gradually approach adult levels of performance during childhood. In the earliest phases of skill acquisition in stance, activation of leg responses tends to be slower and more variable (Forssberg & Nashner, 1982; Shumway-Cook & Woollacott, 1985a). These findings, however, may be due in part to the fact that vision is typically available in such studies. For, when vision is occluded, infants produce more reliable vestibular- and somatosensory-evoked neck responses after anterior-posterior displacements while sitting (Woollacott et al., 1987). In tests of standing posture, if the platform is rotated to produce dorsiflexion rather than translated horizontally, visual and vestibular inputs remain generally stable (see Fig. 2–2). Under these conditions, somatosensory-induced leg responses undergo progressive refinement with age. Adult-like muscle onset latencies for postural responses are not attained until approximately 10 to 15 years of age (Haas et al., 1989), but one need only consider the early acquisition of skills in world-class gymnasts to realize that the maturation of these closed sensorimotor loops is not sufficient to account for the acquisition of common postural skills in childhood.

INTERSENSORY CONFLICTS

Perhaps a more powerful account of initial limitations in postural control and progressive skill acquisition is set forth in studies that test a child's ability to manage intersensory conflict situations. Younger children find it nearly impossible to ignore visual information, even when it is grossly incorrect, as underscored by the tendency of children to sway and fall when confronted by a looming visual stimulus (Butterworth & Hicks, 1977; Lee, DN, & Aronson, 1974). The looming stimulus actually presents a sensory conflict for the child. That is, visual proprioception indicates that the relationship between posture and environment has changed, while vestibular information regarding the relationship between posture and gravity and somatosensory information regarding the relationship between posture and support surface have not

changed. If, during a postural displacement while standing on a movable platform, children are presented with conflicting sensory information and are posturally displaced, the magnitude of sway is increased. This observation holds particularly for children 4 to 6 years of age, the youngest found to be cooperative under these testing conditions (Shumway-Cook & Woollacott, 1985a). Even in instances when visual and vestibular sensory information is reliable, conflicting somatosensory input, induced by rotation of the platform (see Fig. 2–2), results in excessive sway or falls in 4- to 6-year-old children (Shumway-Cook & Woollacott, 1985a).

MUSCLE RESPONSE LATENCIES

During stance perturbations, children 4 to 6 years of age often have muscle response latencies that are greater and more variable than do children younger than 4 years (Shumway-Cook & Woollacott, 1985a). For example, when displaced in an anterior direction, children as young as 15 months of age demonstrate distinct muscular responses characterized by the initial activation of the gastrocnemius followed by the activation of the hamstring muscles, a combination of responses referred to as posterior synergy (Forssberg & Nashner, 1982; Shumway-Cook & Woollacott, 1985a). Even at 15 months of age, onset latency of the gastrocnemius and temporal delay in onset of the hamstring muscles may fall within the ranges for 7- to 10-year-old children and adults, whereas the average and range in temporal values for these parameters are considerably greater in 4- to 6-year-olds. It has been suggested that the greater variability observed in children 4 to 6 years old may reflect a period of transition as vision becomes less important and somatosensory information becomes more important in the control of posture (Shumway-Cook & Woollacott, 1985a). During this transition, children may be trying to process excessive amounts of information rather than selectively attending to the most pertinent sensory information, as has been suggested for other types of motor skill acquisition (Hay, 1979). Children may attempt to process excessive amounts of information as a strategy for coping with limited ability to anticipate change in the environment. (For an extensive discussion of this topic, the reader is referred to an excellent chapter on information processing in children by Keogh & Sugden, 1985.)

ANTICIPATORY STRATEGIES

Learning to predict postural requirements and to select anticipatory strategies for movement in a given environment may be rate-limiting variables in postural control development. Typically, as we become expert in a movement task, we learn to recognize those sensory cues most reliable for predicting how the environment may change during movement execution, and we can learn to ignore less useful cues. Simultaneously, we learn to predict how our movements will change our relationship with respect to this more or less predictable environment and, therefore, determine the postural requirements for the task. For example, when an adult is asked to rise onto tiptoes (from a plantigrade to digitigrade posture), ankle dorsiflexors are activated nearly 200 milliseconds before ankle plantar flexors, apparently to shift the center of pressure at the interface between foot and floor a sufficient amount forward before onset of postural elevation (Haas et al., 1989). Similar responses can be observed in some children as young as 4 years of age, the youngest children thus far cooperative in such laboratory recordings, whereas some children are unable to achieve digitigrade stance even by 10 years of age. The latter children exhibit insufficient anticipatory forward shifts in center of pressure before onset of postural elevation with dorsiflexor to plantar flexor muscle onset latencies of less than 60 ms (Haas et al., 1989). Similar anterior shifts in center of pressure are present before raising an arm while standing by 4 years of age, the youngest age tested (Riach & Hayes, 1990), and activation of directionally appropriate leg muscle synergies is initiated before voluntary arm push-pull tasks at 7 to 9 years of age, the youngest age tested (Nashner et al., 1983). The overlap in refinements of feedback (perturbation-triggered corrections) and feedforward postural control in children between 4 and 10 years of age suggests that they are two distinct processes that emerge in parallel during development. Further, it is suggested that children begin to learn anticipatory postural strategies to coordinate posture and locomotion with the onset of voluntary movements to sit and crawl (Haas et al., 1989), but much work remains to be done to determine how such strategies are learned and modified with skill acquisition.

BIOMECHANICAL CONSTRAINTS

In children younger than 4 years of age, it appears that some key rate-limiting variables are biomechanical in nature (Forssberg & Nasher, 1982; Shumway-Cook & Woollacott, 1985a). Most notably, in the first postnatal year, the center of mass is proportionately higher than at any other age due to the combination of a large head and short limbs, requiring large force generation and regulation by

neck and upper trunk musculature to counter the inertial forces created by displacements of the head. Secondly, in young walkers, the actual distance between floor contact and the center of mass is very small and results in much higher frequencies of postural sway with relatively larger arcs of motion than occur at later ages (Forssberg & Nashner, 1982; Shumway-Cook & Woollacott, 1985a). Consequently, younger children sway faster and closer to their limits of stability than do older children and adults. Although younger children can produce adult-like muscle synergies for postural correction at latencies similar to adult values, given the biomechanical constraints described, adult-like responses may be too slow for regaining upright posture.

POSTURAL RESPONSE STRATEGIES

Some mention should be made regarding the failure of researchers to find distinct sequences of development in postural responses (Perham et al., 1987). This failure likely reflects the fact that complex neuromuscular responses are available very early in development, but a child's ability to select the most favorable strategy and the immediate context in question are critical determinants. Children with Down syndrome can produce correct neuromuscular patterns (i.e., posterior synergy with a distal to proximal activation of leg and thigh muscles) in response to postural perturbations in stance, but the patterns are initiated at a greater latency than in other children of similar chronologic age (Shumway-Cook & Woollacott, 1985b). Thus, in children with Down syndrome, motor patterns for postural control appear to be available and similar to those in normal children but may not be adequately timed to regain upright posture in an efficient manner before reaching the boundaries of stability in stance. Protective responses, however, appear to emerge before righting and equilibrium responses in children with Down syndrome (Haley, 1987), providing a highly effective strategy for limiting injury and a reasonably adaptive strategy if one cannot rely on other postural strategies.

Collectively, these findings and previous points of discussion suggest at least one possible hypothesis regarding the emergence of postural skill; namely, children may possess the potential to produce a particular postural response despite the inability to evoke it under given testing conditions, but the postural response may be masked or overridden by more reliable strategies for a given context. The context specificity of a response is further underscored by the gradual changes in strategy observed during repeated trials when the postural perturbation is modified (Forssberg & Nashner, 1982). When children 4 to 6 years of age are subjected to repeated mechanical rotations of the ankle (into dorsiflexion) in stance, after earlier trials of anterior or posterior horizontal platform displacement, the posterior synergy is gradually suppressed because, under these conditions, activation of the posterior synergy (although appropriate for reactions to horizontal displacements) is now potentially destabilizing (Shumway-Cook & Woollacott, 1985a). It is argued that these changes occur as a function of reweighting each of the sensory cues in light of the postural context (Forssberg & Nashner, 1982). Clearly, more work is needed in this area to understand the development and refinement of postural control in children as they acquire the adaptive characteristics of mature postural skills (Horak & Nashner, 1986; Horak et al., 1989). The availability of such information could enhance the ability of therapists to devise effective interventions for children with motor control deficiencies.

Locomotion

The locomotor capabilities of the neonate and young infant have been vigorously explored since the early 1980s. Many of the advances in our knowledge of locomotor control in humans have been due to important physiologic studies in animals. With the advent of locomotor studies in animals in the 1970s (Grillner, 1981), there developed a rapid expansion of interest in rhythmic behaviors more generally. This new interest was important because it helped to move investigations of motor control from a focus on classic reflex paradigms to the broader domain of natural, spontaneous motor behavior and the development of new research methods to study both naturally occurring behavior and corresponding physiologic systems under behaviorally restricted conditions (Bradley & Bekoff, 1989). In particular, because locomotion is a rhythmic behavior with many kinematic and electromyographic (EMG) features that are repeated across cycles in predictable patterns under stable conditions, studies typically focus on the production of these features to test specific hypotheses of locomotor control and theories of motor control more generally. Animal models of locomotor control continue to assist in refining research methods and in interpreting data from human studies; thus findings from both human and non-human animal studies applicable to our discussion will be addressed in this section as we explore the emergence of locomotor control. Detailed discussion on the refinement of locomotion during childhood is presented in Chapter 3 on gait.

DEVELOPMENT OF LOCOMOTION IN ANIMALS

All animals studied thus far demonstrate the potential to produce either locomotion or related forms of rhythmic limb movements early in development (Bradley & Bekoff, 1989). Newborn kittens, when separated from their mothers during feeding, take a few hypermetric and awkward steps to return to their mother's teats, often falling in the process (Bradley & Smith, 1988a). During these efforts, steps are occasionally characterized by the stereotypic features of reciprocal flexor and extensor EMG patterns similar to those occurring during adult locomotion. Adult-like muscle patterns are most readily apparent, however, when kittens are posturally supported while stepping on the moving belt of a treadmill or making stepping motions in midair (air stepping). Typically, steps over ground are accompanied by extensive coactivation of antagonists at the ankle, suggesting that coactivation of ankle antagonists may be a functional strategy for increasing joint stiffness to compensate for limitations in postural control and muscle force production (Bradley & Smith, 1988a). The appearance of adult features for locomotion in muscle activity of newborns suggests that the neural networks for locomotion are established in the prenatal period. Studies of embryonic motility in chicks support this view, for repetitive limb movements are characterized by orderly patterns of alternating flexor and extensor muscle activity (Bradley & Bekoff, 1990) and limb kinematics (Bradley, 1992; Chambers & Bradley, 1991). Since extensive evidence indicates that many of these stereotypic features of locomotion are mediated by spinal circuitry (Grillner, 1981), it appears that the circuitry is established with differentiation of the embryonic spinal cord (Bradley & Bekoff, 1989, 1990).

PARALLELS BETWEEN DEVELOPING ANIMALS AND HUMANS

Several parallels can be drawn between the studies previously mentioned and studies on locomotion or rhythmic leg movements in infants. When supported on the treadmill, infants perform repetitive leg movements that are characterized by several kinematic features similar to adult locomotor behavior (Forssberg 1985; Thelen, 1986; Thelen & Ulrich, 1991). Although infants of 6 to 12 months of age become more reliable in producing a sustained pattern of alternating steps that is timed to the treadmill belt speed, even infants at the youngest ages tested (1 and 2 months) occasionally demonstrated these features (Thelen & Ulrich, 1991). Neonatal infant stepping shares many features with early treadmill stepping. Most notably, hip, knee, and ankle joints are synchronously flexed during the swing phase and synchronously extended during the extensor phase; the excursions are accompanied by nonspecific EMG patterns; and there is an absence of both heel-strike and push-off at the transitions between swing and stance (Forssberg 1985; Thelen, 1986). These features are also characteristic of infant kicking (Thelen, 1986; Thelen & Fisher, 1982; Thelen et al., 1981) suggesting that some of the mechanisms controlling treadmill stepping, and therefore locomotion, are already functional at birth. These findings also suggest that infant stepping need not be inhibited for normal gait to emerge during the first year of life, a point of view now held by a number of investigators (Forssberg 1985; Thelen et al., 1984; Zelazo, 1983).

The presence of some potential for locomotion at birth raises the question of whether that potential is established early in fetal development. Ultrasound studies of human fetal movement indicate that isolated kicks are initiated during the ninth embryonic week, and alternating leg movements, reported to resemble neonatal stepping, are initiated with postural changes (backward somersaults) in utero during the fourteenth embryonic week (de Vries et al., 1982). Thus, human fetuses appear to exhibit stepping motions during the first half of the gestational period, at about the same portion of the embryonic period that chicks exhibit organized EMG and kinematic features during spontaneous motility (Bradley, 1992; Bradley & Bekoff, 1990; Chambers & Bradley, 1991). Given that low-risk preterm infants born at 34 weeks gestational age demonstrate orderly kinematic patterns similar to those of full-term newborns and that those features differing from full-term infants appear to be attributable to dynamic interactions emerging during movement (Heriza, 1988), the parallel between human fetuses and chick embryos appears reasonable (Fig. 2-3). The neural foundations for locomotion may be assembled during initial differentiation of spinal neural networks in humans, as they appear to be in other animals (Bradley & Bekoff, 1989).

DEVELOPMENT OF LOCOMOTOR MUSCLE PATTERNS IN HUMANS

Thus far, the adult features of EMG recordings have not been observed during locomotor efforts in infants (Forssberg & Wallenberg, 1980) until approximately 2 years of age, when ankle muscles

FIGURE 2-3. Kinematic analyses indicate that lower extremity movements are organized very early in development. When preterm infants initiate a sequence of several kicks at 40 weeks of gestational age, the alternation of flexion and extension at the hip is synchronous with motions of the knee and ankle in the same direction *(A)* and is similar to kicking movements during spontaneous motility in chick embryos in ovo at 9 embryonic days of age *(B)*. *(A*, Adapted from Heriza, CB. Comparison of leg movement in preterm infants at term with healthy full-term infants. Physical Therapy, *68*:1687–1693, 1988. Reprinted from *Physical Therapy* with the permission of the American Physical Therapy Association.)

finally demonstrate stable reciprocal patterns (Sutherland et al., 1988). Failure to observe adult-like EMG patterns is often attributed to late myelinization of descending paths at caudal spinal levels (Sutherland et al., 1980; however, see Sutherland et al., 1988), late dendritic arborization of caudal spinal motoneurons (Scheibel & Scheibel, 1971), maturation of cortical structures (Forssberg, 1985, 1992; Leonard et al., 1988), or late myelinization of peripheral nerves (Sutherland et al., 1988). The failure to observe adult-like EMG patterns during locomotion or stepping efforts in prewalkers and early walkers may also be attributable to adaptive strategies that mask this potential. For example, infants may coactivate antagonist muscles to increase joint stiffness and stabilize limb posture as a compensation for insufficient control of posture or force generation (timing or magnitude of force or both) to support and transport body mass (Bradley & Smith, 1988a). Testing conditions may also mask the potential to generate adult-like locomotor EMG patterns, in that support in stance or movement against gravity while supine alters the task requirements, necessitating a different EMG pattern. Conversely, the testing conditions may lack key features to support expression of EMG patterns. For instance, in cats, the velocity of limb movements contributes to the generation of certain EMG patterns (Smith & Zernike, 1987), a finding that also appears to apply to locomotion and other rhythmic movements in young kittens (Bradley & Smith, 1988b).

Although there is wide support for the view that basic features of locomotion are spinally mediated, some argue that uniquely human features of gait emerge as spinal neural networks are transformed with maturation of higher neural centers (Forssberg, 1985, 1992; Forssberg & Wallberg, 1980; Leonard et al., 1988). Specifically, it is argued that the basic patterns of alternating flexion and extension observed during neonatal stepping persist with development of locomotion but that maturing sensorimotor input suppresses activation of ankle extensor motoneurons to permit heel contact at the onset of stance (Forssberg and Wallberg, 1980). As further support for this view, it is argued that the absence of heel-strike in children with cerebral palsy is because cerebral injury impairs development of higher center control over spinal neural networks for locomotion (Forssberg, 1985; Leonard et al., 1988). Similarly, it is argued that absence of heel-strike in adults after a cerebrovascular accident is because the lesion results in a loss of higher center control (Forssberg, 1985).

Conversely, some researchers speculate that attributes of gait, such as heel-strike, need not be specifically dictated by higher neural centers, for they may emerge from the inertial interactions and associated feedback between body segments during movement (Smith & Zernicke, 1987; Thelen & Cooke, 1987; Thelen & Ulrich, 1991). For example, when cats walk at relatively fast walking speeds, the sartorius muscle produces a two-burst pattern, one during late stance and one during late swing, but the second burst does not consistently occur at slower walking speeds. Kinematic and kinetic analyses suggest that the burst in late swing functions to counteract extensor forces at the knee during faster walking speeds but is not required, and therefore not recruited, at slower speeds because viscoelastic properties of knee flexors are sufficient to counter these forces. Whether the muscle activity associated with heel-strike is due to centrally organized commands or the result of motion-dependent feedback or both has yet to be tested. Thus, to explore neural versus cortical control of heel-strike further, one may experimentally test whether ankle angles during gait are velocity dependent. For example, do controlled increases in walking velocity produce larger dorsiflexion angles during swing? Perhaps the maximum velocity typically achieved during early locomotion is insufficient to express adult-like ankle control in the step cycle, or perhaps the changes in velocity are insufficient.

BIOMECHANICAL VARIABLES

The emergence of locomotion during development is also determined by the interactive aspects of anatomy and environment during movement. Morphologic features of the infant appear to play a critical role in determining whether the infant expresses stepping behaviors (Thelen & Fisher, 1983). Typically, infant stepping cannot be elicited beyond the first to second postnatal month under standard testing conditions, and it has long been argued that the behavior disappears as a consequence of encephalization processes (the taking over of control) by maturing higher motor centers (McGraw, 1940). The postnatal decreases in rate of stepping, however, temporally correlate with rapid weight gain, suggesting that morphologic changes in body mass contribute to the disappearance of infant stepping. Two lines of evidence support this hypothesis. One, when infants are submerged in water up to chest level, both stepping rate and amplitude increase in comparison with these values during stepping out of water (Thelen et al., 1984). Two, if weights equivalent to the weight gains at 5 and 6 postnatal weeks of age are added to the ankles of infants at 4 postnatal weeks of age, both stepping rate and amplitude decrease in comparison with the rate and amplitude for stepping without ankle weights (Thelen et al., 1984). Thus, buoyancy appears to diminish the dampening effect of body mass and gravitational interactions, whereas added weight appears to augment the effect of these interactions.

Animal studies help to underscore the notion that morphologic features of the organism interact with the environment either to express or to mask potential abilities. Fetal rat pups, for example, exhibit interlimb coordination during spontaneous movements under buoyant conditions before they do under nonbuoyant conditions (Bekoff & Lau, 1980; Bekoff & Trainer, 1979). Frog tadpoles exhibit coordinated leg movements several stages earlier in development if they can push off from a mesh surface placed in an aquatic tank (Stehouwer & Farel, 1984). The last-mentioned point invites redress of the previous discussion regarding heel contact in gait: heel-strike may not be observed until independent walking is established, owing to immature morphologic characteristics of the infant's foot. Given the considerable structural change the foot undergoes during the first postnatal year or more, it is conceivable that initial biomechanical features of the foot do not readily afford initiation of heel strike or push-off in the young infant.

VARIABLES UNDER INVESTIGATION

Several new lines of investigation into locomotor control are now being established and will no doubt add greatly to our understanding of normal and abnormal locomotor development in the near future. Application of kinematic and kinetic analysis methods to the study of intersegmental dynamics of leg movement in 3-month-old infants while kicking when supine demonstrates that young infants may use motion-dependent forces (torques) to coordinate limb movements (Schneider et al., 1990). In some instances, for example, the flexor phase of kicking appears attributable to active flexor (muscle) forces, whereas the extensor phase is attributable to passive (inertial) forces and active flexor (muscle) forces (Fig. 2–4). The presence of active flexor forces during the extensor phase suggests that lengthening flexor muscle contractions are used to control the lowering of the leg, and this may be one explanation for why reciprocal EMG patterns have not been observed during kicking or stepping movements in studies thus far. Application of perceptual research methods to the study of locomotion in adults demonstrates that vision contributes importantly to the kinematics of movement (Patla, 1991). Also, new information is emerging on how secondary movements are accommodated during locomotion (Patla, 1986) and how segmental reflexes are gated during locomotion (Bolanger & Patla, 1987; Crenna & Frigo, 1984; Yang & Stein, 1990). Many of these studies, like ones previously discussed, are based on earlier animal studies of locomotion (Carter & Smith, 1985; Forssberg et al., 1975) and demonstrate the important contribution animal studies are likely to continue to make in expanding our understanding of motor control in humans. Similar questions have yet to be considered in studies of locomotion development, but one may surmise that they will be in the near future.

FIGURE 2–4. Motions of adjacent limb segments during kicking may arise from active forces due to muscle activity and passive forces due to gravity and inertia of the limb segments. For example, in the data presented here, an infant initiates a kick cycle starting from a semiextended position of 125° and achieves a peak flexion of 80° at 0.32 second (vertical dashed line in *A* and *B*) before the hip returns to the extended position. The motion into flexion is attributable primarily to an initial hip (Hip) flexor force or torque that is maximal at the outset (0.0 s) and begins to decrease as the hip moves into flexion *(A)*. The hip flexor force is due to active muscle force (MUS) during the first 0.2 second *(B)*. An extensor force develops between 0.2 and 0.3 second *(A)* as active hip flexor force decreases to 0 newton-meter *(B)* and serves to slow and reverse the hip motion into extension (0.32 s). Throughout the extension of the hip, there are small passive extensor forces due to gravity (GRA) and inertia (MDT) and a growing active hip flexor force (MUS) to lower the leg. (Adapted from Schneider, K, Zernicke, RF, Ulrich, BD, Jensen, JL, & Thelen, E. Understanding movement control in infants through the analysis of limb intersegmental dynamics. Journal of Motor Behavior, 22:493–520, 1990. Reprinted with permission of the Helen Dwight Reid Educational Foundation. Published by Heldref Publications, Washington, D.C. Copyright 1990.)

Reaching

Since the late 1970s, studies have produced dramatic demonstrations and reappraisals of the reaching abilities of newborn and young infants. In commonly employed static testing situations, with the infant placed supine, reaching for a dangling, stationary target, such as a red ring, is initiated at a mean age of 3.8 postnatal months, as tested by item 46 in the mental scale of the Bayley Scales of Infant Development (Bayley, 1969). Investigators have demonstrated, however, that if newborns are adequately supported in an inclining posture and presented with a moving target, rudimentary eye-hand coordination can be distinguished from random hand movements within days of birth. By 4 months of age, infants are adept at contacting a moving object, and by 9 months they demonstrate adult-like reaching patterns as they catch a moving object. In this section, features characterizing the development of reaching and tracking skills will be described. For additional discussion on the control of reaching, the reader may wish to refer to chapters on reaching, grasping, and visual proprioception by Keogh and Sugden (1985) and by Rosenbaum (1991).

RUDIMENTARY REACHING SKILLS

Arm movements of the neonate, like kicking movements, may be rudimentary expressions of skilled reaching actions that emerge during the first postnatal year (Trevarthen, 1974). It has been suggested by a number of investigators that the arm movements of newborns are not strictly random events, but rather intentional actions (McDonnell, 1979) or practice of subroutines for movement of the arms against gravity that are aroused by a visual stimulus (Bruner, 1973) and are directionally oriented (Hofsten, 1982). These views are supported by observation of a variety of spontaneous behaviors, such as concurrent midline hand activity and mouth movements, upon presentation of a visual stimulus (Bruner, 1973) and the increased probability that the mouth will be open throughout a reach when the hand actually ends up in the mouth (Butterworth, 1986). Further, when newborn infants 6 to 20 days of age are presented with an approaching visual stimulus, responses include widening of the eyes, extension of the neck, and raising of the hands between the face and object in an apparent avoidance response (Bower et al., 1970).

It is generally held that reaching in the neonatal period is visually triggered and that hand-trajectories reveal directed actions. For example, the number of arm movements is significantly greater when 3-day-old infants visually fixate on an object than when they do not (Hofsten, 1982). Similarly, when presented with a ball or a picture of a ball, infants 8 to 16 days old make more directed arm movements (defined as lateral arm extensions, arcing movements of the arm toward midline, or flexion of the arm toward upper half of chest) than they do when presented with a blank card (Rader & Stern, 1982). The directness of neonatal reaches was quantified in a study of 3-day-old newborns who were supported in a reclining infant seat and presented with a stimulus moving in an arc 12 cm from the eyes (Hofsten, 1982). Measurements for every hand movement exceeding 5 cm indicated that forward extending arm movements are aimed much closer to the target (32° off-target) when infants visually fixate on a target than when they look elsewhere (52° off-target) or close their eyes (54° off-target). A study of newborns also suggests that presentation of an object in the visual field elicits longer horizontal and vertical hand-paths during arm movements than when no stimulus is present (Bergmeier, 1992). These observations may indicate that a genetically established neural coordinate system links the trajectories of the hand with the face and visually fixated objects within reach (Hofsten, 1982; Trevarthen, 1974). This does not appear to be an unrealistic hypothesis, because ultrasound study of human fetuses indicates that infants make hand-to-face contact by 10 weeks of gestation (de Vries et al., 1982), suggesting the presence of a functional neural network that relates hand-space to body-space (see Chapter 4, Directional Coding of Reaching, in Jeannerod, 1988) by the end of the first trimester of fetal development. Further study is required to test such hypotheses, however, because an early hand-trajectory could be the product of biomechanical variables that shape arm movements rather than the product of detailed neural commands (Fetters & Todd, 1987).

Infants 1 to 19 weeks of age, when presented with a slowly moving object, continue to display interest in the object, but during the weeks that neonatal reaching is transformed into functional reaching, the role of vision appears to change somewhat and there are periods when reaching is less readily observed. Age-dependent declines in reaching responses are reported to occur between 8 and 16 postnatal days (Rader & Stern, 1982) and in the seventh postnatal week (Hofsten, 1984). Because neonatal reaching was initially viewed as a primitive, reflex-like behavior, the age-dependent decline was attributed to maturation of descending neural inputs, an argument similar to that for the disappearance of infant stepping (Connolly, 1977; Humphrey, 1969; McGraw, 1945). It has also been suggested that the decline in reaching may occur because object contact, and therefore behavioral reinforcement, is rare or because the infant does not have sufficient optimal opportunities (e.g., postural context) to practice during this time (Bower, 1979). Alternatively, as infants become much more interested in looking at objects, visual attendance may function to extinguish neonatal reaching efforts (Bergmeier, 1992; Hofsten, 1984). In the neonatal period, the hand is typically open during forward extension of the arm (Hofsten, 1982), but around the seventh postnatal week, when the rate of reaching briefly decreases, infants seem more interested in looking at the object and the hand posture is more likely to be fisted (Hofsten, 1984). Around 12 postnatal weeks, however, the frequency of reaching increases, and the hand resumes an open posture during reaches (Hofsten, 1984). During this time, infants appear to acquire some visual ability to determine realistic reaching distances because they rarely initiate effort to contact objects out of reach (Field, 1977). Between 12 and 16 weeks of age, infants acquire considerable skill in aiming their reaches (Hofsten & Rönnqvist, 1988; Lockman & Ashmead, 1983). By 15 weeks, infants can contact a moving object in 90% of trials, and between 15 and 18 weeks, contact shifts from merely touching to catching the moving object (Hofsten, 1979). Vision functions to elicit reaching throughout the transition from neonatal to functional reaching, but it is not used to guide hand-trajectory (Lasky, 1977; Wishart et al., 1978) or to orient the hand toward the object before initial contact (Lockman et al., 1984). These findings seem to suggest that younger infants initiate reaching using a ballistic strategy to aim the hand toward the target and then switch to a feedback strategy to make corrective movements for grasping after the hand pauses near the object. At 5 months of age, reaches are as good with vision available during the reach as when vision is removed after onset of the reach (Wishart et al., 1978).

INFANT REACHING STRATEGIES

During the period from 12 to 36 postnatal weeks, several major changes occur in the form of reaching that suggest the development of a new control strategy (Hofsten, 1979, 1991). To determine how reaching is performed and to investigate strategies used to control reaching during development, the velocity and distance of hand transport are measured from video records of infant performances. In accordance with research methods standard in studies of adult behavior, trajectories are dissected into movement units, each containing one acceler-

ation phase and one deceleration phase (Jeannerod, 1981). Adult reaches are characterized by 1 or 2 movement units; the first unit functions to transport the hand 70 to 80% of the distance to the target and is relatively long in duration, whereas the second unit functions to home in on the object and is relatively short in duration (Jeannerod, 1981). Between 19 and 31 postnatal weeks, infants progressively restructure reaches for a moving object from an average of 4 movement units per reach to 2 movement units (Hofsten, 1991), yet even at 19 weeks of age, 22% of reaches contain only 1 or 2 movement units. The sequencing of movement units is also modified; the transport unit is the first movement unit in half of the reaches at 19 weeks, extending an average distance of 80 cm, whereas at 31 weeks, it is the first unit in 84% of reaches and extends 137 cm. Finally, the hand-path straightens with age (Fig. 2–5), suggesting that by 31 weeks of age, improved spatial planning contributes to advances in aiming skill since the hand is now transported closer to the target in a more efficient manner during the first movement unit, requiring fewer subsequent units to correct for errors (Hofsten, 1991).

This pattern of control does not appear to apply, however, when infants 5 to 9 months of age reach to grasp a stationary object placed on a horizontal surface such as a table (Fetters & Todd, 1987). Under these conditions, movement units tend to be similar in duration (200 ms) for all ages, reaching distances, and positions (or order) within a reach (Fig. 2–6). Furthermore, there may not be a decrease in the number of movement units within the path or a change in the straightness of the hand-path under these conditions between 5 and 9 months of age. Both hand-path distance (equivalent to twice the shortest possible distance) and mean reaching duration (800 ms) also appear to be stable across ages and within adult limits, but they are more variable. These findings suggest that the movement speed and curvature of early functional reaching observed under stationary reaching conditions may be fundamental properties of both skilled and unskilled reaching controlled by biologic and physical constraints emerging from body-environment interactions (Fetters & Todd, 1987). These findings also point to the effect of task context on measurements used to explore control variables and to the likelihood that control strategies vary with context (Hofsten, 1991). For example, hand-path may be straighter when reaching for a moving object than when reaching for a stationary one (Hofsten, 1979).

During the period from 5 to 9 months of age, infants begin to use visual information at the end of

FIGURE 2–5. Hand-paths become straighter and contain fewer movement units during the first postnatal year when the infant is reaching for a moving target. During a reach at 19 weeks of age *(A)*, 5 movement units are identified (by smaller arrows) in views from the front *(A₁)* and the side *(A₂)*. Note that these movement units are similar in length. During a reach at 31 weeks of age in the same infant *(B)*, only 4 movement units are identified from the front *(B₁)* and side *(B₂)*. Note that most of the reaching distance is covered in the first movement unit. S↑ = start of motion. (Adapted from Hofsten, C von. Structuring of early reaching movements: A longitudinal study. Journal of Motor Behavior, *32*:280–292, 1991. Reprinted with permission of the Helen Dwight Reid Educational Foundation. Published by Heldref Publications, Washington, D.C. Copyright 1991.)

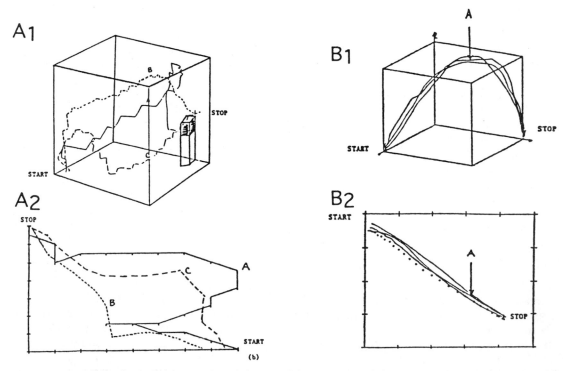

FIGURE 2–6. When reaching for a stationary object, infants exhibit reaches containing multiple movement units of a similar duration. Three reaches (A, B, & C) are shown for a 9-month-old infant from a side view *(A₁)* and overhead view *(A₂)*. Note the irregularities both within and between reaches as compared with adult performance from a side view *(B₁)* and overhead view *(B₂)*. (Adapted from Fetters, L, & Todd, J. Quantitative assessment of infant reaching movements. Journal of Motor Behavior, *19*:147–166, 1987. Reprinted with permission of the Helen Dwight Reid Educational Foundation. Published by Heldref Publications, Washington, D.C. Copyright 1987.)

the reach as the hand approaches the target to correct for errors in trajectory (Hofsten, 1977; McDonnell, 1975). Before 5 months of age, they take little notice of the hand during flight, but thereafter, if vision of the hand is blocked, as when infants reach for a virtual (mirror image) object, performance is frequently disrupted (Lasky, 1977). Although infants continue to use a ballistic reaching strategy well into childhood, withdrawal of visual feedback begins to impair their reaching skill at 6 to 7 months of age (Lasky, 1977; Wishart et al., 1978). To determine how reaching movements are controlled, investigators have explored parameters that characterize the straightness of the hand-trajectory. In adults, the curve of the hand-path during reaching is composed of straight line segments linked sequentially (Abend et al., 1982). The end of one segment and the beginning of the next corresponds to a "speed valley" (deceleration and reacceleration) and a change in direction of the hand (Jeannerod, 1981). Each movement segment may be ballistically generated and corrections may be made at these junctions between movement segments (Brooks, 1974). To test whether path corrections are necessarily restricted to these speed valleys, Mathew and Cook (1990) examined the curved hand-path in reaching trials of infants between 4 and 8 months old presented with a suspended object having some motion. Three-dimensional analyses of hand-trajectories indicated that the initial movement segment is directed toward the object at all ages tested and that changes in the path after onset of reaching tend to curve the hand toward the target to correct for error (Fig. 2–7). Also, measures of hand speed within a movement segment correlate with veering of the hand toward the target within the movement segment, suggesting that error correction occurs continuously rather than only at discrete intervals in hand transport. The relationship between veering within a movement unit and target location may indicate that when vision is available, reaching is not executed using a ballistic strategy. By contrast, continuous veering within a movement unit may be the biomechanical consequence of projecting the arm through space, a notion that is consistent with the equilibrium-point hypothesis for joint position in the mass spring model of arm control (Hofsten, 1991; Polit & Bizzi, 1979)

REACHING STRATEGIES IN SCHOOL-AGE CHILDREN

Studies in older children suggest that reaching strategies change very little from 9 months until approximately 7 years of age, at which time there

FIGURE 2–7. Analyses of hand-path trajectories indicate that corrective movements occur throughout the reach even in young infants. Measurements of veering within a movement unit *(A)* indicate that initial hand trajectory is oriented toward the target and that correction in hand-path is not limited exclusively to speed valleys (troughs indicated by arrows in B_2 and C_2) adjoining consecutive movement units. Speed valleys, characteristic of adult reaching *(C₂)*, are also characteristic of infant reaching at as early as 6 postnatal months *(B₂)* but are more numerous and greater in relative magnitude due to the greater number of irregularities in hand-path *(B₁ vs C₁)*. (Adapted from Mathew, A, & Cook, M. The control of reaching movements by young infants. Child Development, *61*:1238–1258, 1990.)

appears to be a transitional period leading to an adult reaching strategy. When the visual field is displaced by a prism, children 5 years of age reach out to the apparent target location in 1 or 2 movement units before making corrective movements to move the hand to the actual target location (Hay, 1979). By contrast, 7-year-olds execute multiple small movement units (referred to as early braking), producing hand-paths that begin to veer toward the actual target location early in the trajectory, whereas 9- to 11-year-olds execute an initial movement unit that approaches the virtual target location but is then followed by a second, corrective unit (referred to as smooth braking) that alters the

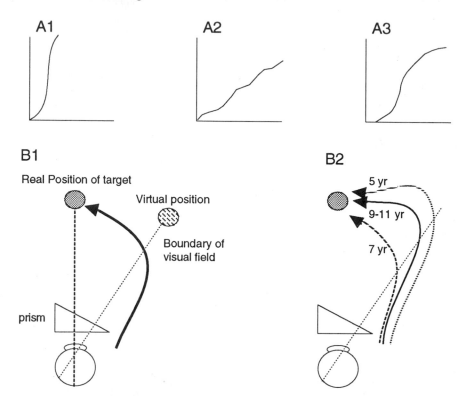

FIGURE 2–8. Hand-paths during reaching toward a stationary target correspond to the use of visual information to plan and control reaching. Ballistic reaches exhibit smooth trajectories with no distinct points of path correction, suggesting that they are preplanned and executed open-loop *(A₁)*, whereas early braking reaches are executed closed-loop, using vision to continuously monitor and correct error *(A₂)*. Late braking reaches, by contrast, combine open- and closed-loop strategies to maximize reaching efficiency by preplanning 70 to 80% of the trajectory and then correcting trajectory error in the final approach to the target *(A₃)*. The use of these three strategies can be demonstrated by using a prism to displace the visual field *(B₁)*. Under these conditions, it is apparent that children 5 years of age use a ballistic reaching strategy, for they correct their hand-paths only after they have reached or surpassed the target's virtual position *(B₂)*. By contrast, 7-year-olds, using an early braking strategy, identify the discrepancy between real and virtual target position as soon as the hand enters the visual field, and 9- to 11-year-olds, using a late braking strategy, almost reach the virtual target position before detecting the discrepancy. (Adapted from Hay, L. Spatial-temporal analysis of movements in children: Motor programs versus feedback in the development of reaching. Journal of Motor Behavior, *11*:188–200, 1979. Reprinted with permission of the Helen Dwight Reid Educational Foundation. Published by Heldref Publications, Washington, D.C. Copyright 1979.)

trajectory before the hand reaches the virtual target location (Fig. 2–8). These findings suggest that 5-year-olds continue to use ballistic strategies much like those of older infants, whereas 7-year-olds constantly monitor their movements in a closed-loop strategy to control their reaches. Finally, between 9 and 11 years of age, children begin to combine these strategies to increase the efficiency of their movements and to reduce the amount of attention required (Hay, 1979; Keogh & Sugden, 1985), which is a likely explanation for why many of the reach parameters in 9-month-old infants appear similar to those of adults. Similar examples of visual guidance at these ages were also reported by McDonnell (1975) and McCracken (1983).

In a related vein, one current view of the clumsi-

ness seen in children with mild to moderate movement dysfunction is that a sensory or attentional problem hinders their ability to identify or attend selectively to the most pertinent information during a reach (Schellekens et al., 1983). For example, study of hand-paths during movement between two buttons in a repetitive tapping task in 8- to 10-year-olds with minimal neurologic dysfunction suggests that they must constantly monitor and correct their actions. It is believed that using this closed-loop strategy leaves them with little opportunity to attend to information that might enable them to execute anticipatory adjustments and minimize the amount of error correction during movement. In comparison with age-matched controls, children with minimal neurologic dysfunction appear to execute more movement units per reach (4 units vs 2 units), the first movement unit is less likely to be the longest unit or to achieve the greatest acceleration, and each unit tends to contain more subpeak accelerations or irregularities (Schellekens et al., 1983). Not surprisingly, these children tend to have more difficulty in maintaining task orientation. It is generally thought that children with these types of movement dysfunction tend to rely heavily on vision, for when it is available to assist manual tracking of a continuously moving stimulus (a coincident-timing task) with a predictable path, clumsy children (ages 6 and 11) are slower than age-matched controls (van der Meulen et al., 1991a). Their movement distance during an acceleration phase is more variable than is that of control children, their tracking motions are more delayed (e.g., time to peak excursion), and they perform more trials with apparently suboptimal attention. When these children are presented with an unpredictable tracking task, they have greater difficulty in attending to the task than do age-matched controls, perhaps because they cannot identify a compensatory strategy (van der Meulen et al., 1991b). When presented with a predictable tracking task, however, 7-year-olds with minimal brain dysfunction give themselves more time to cope with less efficient reaching skills by planning a hand-trajectory that will intercept a moving target further along its trajectory (Forsström & Hofsten, 1982). For discussion on the establishment of coincident-timing strategies, the reader is referred to a review by Goodgold-Edwards (1991).

In summary, the variables and processes that contribute to an emerging control of reaching skills during infancy and childhood are similar to those contributing to control of posture and locomotion. In each instance, rudimentary aspects of control can be observed in very young infants if optimal conditions are provided, suggesting that some neural contributions to control of these skills are established in the fetal or neonatal period of development. In each instance, early skills appear to be more or less automatic in that they appear to be activated by relevant stimuli and shaped by contextual variables, such as the biomechanical interactions of moving body segments in space. Feedback does not appear to play an important role in controlling these early skills. Each of these early skills, however, undergoes important transformations as children learn to monitor their movements, predict the potential consequences of their actions for a given context, and develop anticipatory strategies for efficient movement execution. As will be shown in the section to follow, these variables also contribute to the development of grasp control.

Grasping

Hand function has traditionally been viewed as one of the key responsibilities of the motor cortex. Classic studies linked onset of fine motor milestones with myelinization of the lateral precentral gyrus (Lawrence & Hopkins, 1976). Pyramidal lesion studies in monkeys (Lawrence & Kuypers, 1968) led to a general acceptance that reaching and grasping are controlled by separate subcortical neural systems. After lesion of the lateral brain stem, monkeys cannot control hand movements independently of arm movements, yet they can use their limbs for walking and climbing. With a lesion of the ventrolateral path, by contrast, monkeys can no longer control the posture of the limb but they can pick up food with their hands. Studies suggest that the potential for coordinated hand movements may be present earlier than previously appreciated and that anatomic changes in descending neural paths, while necessary, may not be sufficient to account for development of hand control. For example, ultrasound recordings indicate that human fetuses begin extending their fingers during isolated arm movements by 12 weeks of gestation (de Vries et al., 1982), long before myelinization processes can account for these rudimentary actions. Furthermore, observation of spontaneous hand movements in neonates indicates that the hand is not always in a stereotypic posture of flexion (closed fist) or extension (open). The hands continuously move between these extremes, and in so doing, they exhibit considerable variability, suggesting that the potential for independent finger control is present at birth. If there is sufficient neural substrate to produce motor commands for independent finger actions at birth, why do fine motor milestones typically emerge several months later? In this section, the acquisition of grasp control and studies identifying variables that may help to account for its acquisition are reviewed.

RUDIMENTARY PERCEPTUAL CONTROL OF GRASPING

Although reaching and grasping skills are intimately related in a functional sense, control of grasping is distinguished from control of reaching by the different roles ascribed to the anatomic structures previously discussed and by the apparent differences in perceptuomotor control of these two skills (Hofsten, 1990). The initial trajectory of reaching (phase 1 reaching) is based on visual definition of the object's location in space and executed using a ballistic or open-loop strategy, processes that do not appear to be linked with control of grasping. During execution of the reach (phase 2 reaching), visual feedback (Jeannerod, 1981) or proprioceptive feedback (Prablanc & Pélisson, 1990) or both may be used to define arm position as part of a closed-loop strategy to correct for initial errors in trajectory. At the onset of phase 2 reaching, the hand is open maximally and then begins to close immediately before target contact, suggesting that anticipatory preparation for grasping is integrated with phase 2 reaching (Jeannerod, 1981).

Currently available data indicate that during neonatal reaching, only the ballistic phase is executed and activity of the hand is not controlled separately from that of the limb to attempt grasping. Thus, the prevailing view is that during reaching in the neonatal period, the arm and hand are synergistically coupled (Hofsten, 1990). In support of this view, one study of neonatal reaches indicated that the hand is typically open during reaching, but hand posture does not vary during the trajectory, nor does it vary with or without visual fixation of the target (Hofsten, 1984). This synergistic link between arm and hand is said to be functionally disconnected at approximately 2 postnatal months, for the hand is more frequently fisted during arm movements into extension, and by 3 months of age, the hand begins to open once again during reaching but only when the infant visually fixates on the target (Hofsten, 1984). Such gains are typically attributed to anatomic changes in corticomotoneuronal connections (Lawrence & Hopkins, 1976), but another variable to consider at this age is the development of binocular vision (Hofsten, 1990). Acquisition of grasp control at this particular period of development may be primarily attributable to the emergence of adequate visual processing, so that the infant can begin learning how to implement closed-loop (visually dominated) control of hand movements. By 4 months of age, infants can use vision to correct their reaching trajectory when it is displaced by a prism (McDonnell, 1975), and by 5 to 6 months, infants expect to see their hand during a reach, but if vision of the hand is blocked, their performance is disturbed (Lasky, 1977). Around 6 postnatal months, infants can occasionally execute an adult-like movement pattern when reaching to grasp, and by 9 months, they can execute the pattern reliably (Hofsten, 1979). To return briefly to an earlier question regarding control of independent finger movements, we might also hypothesize that independent finger movements and grasping skills emerge in the middle of the first year because the visual system is then sufficiently operational to employ and sculpture available corticomotoneuronal networks or because infants require a sufficient amount of initial visual experience of the hand to master control of the fingers. In the latter case, postural requirements, that is, stability of both head and hand positions to visualize the effects of self-initiated finger actions, may be another rate-limiting variable in acquisition of independent finger movements. Establishment of visual and visuomotor processes may be the rate-limiting variables that normally determine when potential motor abilities are expressed.

EMERGENCE OF ANTICIPATORY CONTROL

With the onset of functional reaching, reaching behaviors indicate that infants begin to develop perceptual abilities to read the environment in such a way as to shape reaching and grasping skills. At the onset of functional reaching, they are less inclined to reach for objects that are placed at the perimeter of their reach (Fetters & Todd, 1987), and at 5 months of age, they begin to orient the hand toward the object, either just before or at the beginning of the reach (Hofsten & Fazel-Zandy, 1984). At this age, infants primarily rely on contact with the object to orient and grasp the object successfully, but during the next 3 months, infants begin to use visual information both to anticipate contact and to orient the hand with respect to the object (Lockman et al., 1984). When adults reach to grasp an object, the distance between index finger and thumb is set with respect to object size at the onset of reaching (Jakobson & Goodale, 1991; Jeannerod, 1981). Anticipation of object size is similarly observed in the hand posture of 9- to 13-month-old infants during reaching (Hofsten & Rönnqvist, 1988), suggesting that young infants quickly learn to preprogram reaches for object size, location, and distance on the basis of visual information. The grasp of infants older than 9 months continues to exhibit some immature features, one being the relatively constrained range in hand opening when infants are presented with an assortment of objects varying in size. The hand may open in exaggerated postures, often considered residual retention of more primitive or yet undifferentiated manual behaviors due to corticomotoneuronal immaturity (Twitchell, 1970). As an alternative hypothesis, however, infants may open the hand wide as a strategy to compensate for limited ability to estimate the task requirements for grasping an object (Hofsten, 1990); adults exhibit similar exaggerated hand postures when visual feedback is either withdrawn or its availability is unpredictable (Jakobson & Goodale, 1991).

MATURATION OF GRIP FORCE CONTROL

Once contact is initiated, the infant must coordinate normal (grip) and frictional (load) forces to grasp and lift an object (Johansson & Westling, 1988). Adults coordinate these forces synchronously, whereas infants and young children coordinate them sequentially (Forssberg et al., 1991). For quantitative examination of grip control, infants are encouraged to pick up an object such as a toy that is equipped with force transducers to measure the grip forces of the opposing thumb and index finger and the load force necessary to lift the object off a table (Fig. 2–9). Under these conditions, infants as young as 8 months of age, the youngest age tested, coordinate their grip and load forces sequentially to lift the object. During the preload phase (initial contact with the object), young infants contact the object with one finger before the other, creating a latency to onset of grip force that is significantly greater than it is in infants 18 months of age or older. Infants and young children also tend to press down on the object, creating a negative load force, before reversing the direction of

force to lift the object off the table successfully. Infants and young children generate a significant portion of the total grip force (often twice the magnitude of adult grasps) for grasping before initiating the load force, and during the load phase, they typically exhibit multiple peaks in records for both these forces. Adults, by contrast, scale the increases in grip and load forces in an economic, synchronous, and nearly linear manner, with only a single peak near the middle of the load phase (Forssberg et al., 1991; Johansson & Westling, 1988). These findings suggest that the smooth execution of an adult grasp is the consequence of anticipating the object's weight so as to select an appropriate target force magnitude and scaling of magnitude over time (Forssberg et al., 1991; Johansson & Westling, 1988).

Several points can be made with respect to the work on grasp. First, it is apparent that by 8 months of age infants can produce each of the actions re-

FIGURE 2–9. One method to quantitatively describe grasping skills and examine aspects of motor control is to measure the combination of grip and load forces over time. Precision grip force is the net normal force exerted by the index finger (Grip force 1) and thumb (Grip force 2), and load force is the tangential or frictional force exerted when lifting the object against gravity (positive force values) or pushing the object down into the table (negative force values). The mass of the object can be varied by exchanging weights (C), and displacement of the object can be detected by infrared diodes (B) and a sensor (D). By 8 months of age, infants first press down on the object (negative x values), then increase grip force (positive y values) before initiating a load force (positive x values) to lift the object. By 2 years of age, positive load and grip forces are scaled in a synchronous and more linear fashion similar to that seen in adults, and negative load force is less apparent than at younger ages. (Adapted from Forssberg, H, Eliasson, AC, Kinoshita, H, Johansson RS & Westling, G. Development of human precision grip. I. Basic coordination of force. Experimental Brain Research, 85:451–457, 1991.)

quired for a precision grip, and by 12 months of age, infants can occasionally assemble all the components of action needed to produce adult-like force patterns but they demonstrate considerable variability across trials (Forssberg et al., 1991). Here again, it appears that infants possess the neural substrate necessary to execute skilled motor patterns early in development, but demonstration of this potential is unreliable. Second, infants and young children use far more force than is required. In general, this is a common finding in studies of motor development (Keogh & Sugden, 1985). On the one hand, the variability and the excessive forces used in their strategies may be the consequence of as yet immature corticospinal pathways or motor units (Forssberg et al., 1991). On the other hand, the variability and excessive forces may be compensatory strategies to cope with limited experience and one or more limited perceptuomotor abilities, such as the ability to extract sufficient information from visual input and the ability to estimate the potential consequences of a motor action. In other words, do infants fail to exhibit independent finger actions and complex grasp patterns earlier than 8 postnatal months because they lack sufficient corticomotoneuronal command pathways to execute these actions (Muir & Lemon, 1983)? Or do they begin to demonstrate precision grip at 8 postnatal months because visual acuity, biomechanics, context, experience, and other learning-related requirements typically reach some minimal threshold to support successful performance?

In a similar vein, developmental literature frequently implies that reflexes exert control over early behaviors such as grasping and that their influence subsides as the motor cortex and corticospinal tract develop (Humphrey, 1960, 1969; McGraw, 1945). Because it was assumed that the nervous system is hierarchically organized, it has long been believed that reflexes determine when certain behaviors emerge or disappear by either dominating action or failing to support actions owing to immaturity in neural transmission (Twitchell, 1970). Reflexes are also commonly identified as the mechanisms responsible for the aberrant grasping behavior observed in children with movement dysfunction. Such assumptions do not appear to be compatible, however, with current electrophysiologic studies of the motor cortex. Although motor cortex and corticospinal inputs function to recruit hand muscles (Lemon & Mantel, 1989), motor cortex activity does not exhibit a consistent relationship with respect to either a movement or a movement-related activity in other areas of the brain, leading investigators to support a heterarchic rather than a hierarchic view of motor control (Kalaska & Crammond, 1992).

Studies on the control of the precision grasp in children with cerebral palsy underscore a point raised repeatedly in this chapter, that maturation of the motor cortex and corticomotoneuronal pathways, although necessary, is not sufficient to account for the development of normal or abnormal control of movement. Many other issues, such as anticipatory control and effective use of feedback information, must also be considered if control of movements is to be more fully understood. When normal children 6 to 8 years of age are asked to grasp and lift a 200-gram object repeatedly, they initiate nearly synchronous, linear increases in grip and load forces with a single peak in magnitude, as do adults. Children with cerebral palsy (diplegia or hemiplegia), by contrast, tend to initiate the forces sequentially, as do younger normal children (Eliasson et al., 1991). At least some children with cerebral palsy can produce the requisite forces, but they have difficulty in selecting and executing efficient grasp strategies. Available data indicate that these children have difficulty in regulating the timing and magnitude of force during both dynamic and static phases and they tend to bear down on the object before lifting it (Fig. 2–10). When these children are asked in blocked and randomized trials to grasp and lift objects of two different weights, they also have difficulty in scaling forces with respect to object weight during both random and nonrandom presentation of the two weights (Eliasson et al., 1992). Thus, it appears that in the population studied to date, children with cerebral palsy, unlike their peers without motor disabilities, have difficulty in using feedback to regulate their movements effectively, yet they are especially dependent on feedback to modify their actions because they have difficulty in establishing feedforward or anticipatory strategies based on previous experience. Children with cerebral palsy may also have difficulty in stabilizing their gaze so that they can effectively use the available visual information (Lee, DN, et al., 1990). Given that the normal acquisition of grasp control has a protracted period of development (Forssberg et al., 1991, 1992), it is also reasonable to hypothesize that these children do not experience sufficient amounts and variety of practice to use available information for developing efficient strategies, an issue previously raised by Goodgold-Edwards (1991).

Refinements in the control of grasping continue to occur well into late childhood. Young children execute grasps characterized by multipeaked variations in grip and load forces and do not execute the smooth, coincident increases and decreases in these forces characteristic of adult grasping until approximately 8 years of age (Forssberg et al., 1991). These developmental changes may be in part due to grad-

FIGURE 2-10. Children with cerebral palsy demonstrate some of the same force patterns during grasping to lift as do younger normal children. Although age-matched (6-8) normal children *(A₁)* exhibit synchronous scaling of grip and load forces, some children with diplegia *(A₃)* and hemiplegia *(A₄)* exhibit marked negative load force at the onset of a grasp, serial ordering of grip and positive load forces, and grip force magnitudes twice those of normal children. Children with less severely disabling cerebral palsy, however, as one child with mild diplegia *(A₂)*, may exhibit more normal, age-appropriate grasp patterns. In addition to difficulty in coordinating grip and load forces, children with hemiplegia *(B₂)* and diplegia *(B₃)* have greater difficulty in scaling grip force with respect to object weight than do normal children *(B₁)*. During lifts of a 400-gram weight *(dashed lines)*, normal children apply larger grip forces than for a 200-gram weight *(solid lines)*, and grip force quickly peaks then drops to a stable level. Grip forces in children with cerebral palsy, by contrast, are slow to reach peak magnitude, are unstable during the static phase of the lift, and are not scaled reliably with respect to object weight. (*A*, adapted from Eliasson, AC, Gordon, AM, & Forssberg, H. Basic co-ordination of manipulative forces of children with cerebral palsy. Developmental Medicine and Child Neurology, *33*:661–670, 1991. *B*, Adapted from Eliasson, AC, Gordon, AM, & Forssberg, H. Impaired anticipatory control of isometric forces during grasping by children with cerebral palsy. Developmental Medicine and Child Neurology, *34*:216–225, 1992.)

ual improvements in anticipatory strategies. To test the use of anticipatory strategies, one study examined the grip and load forces produced as children of 1 to 15 years of age lifted each of two different weights over 6 consecutive trials and then presented randomly over 25 trials (Forssberg et al., 1992). Under these conditions, children as young as 1 to 2 years of age can scale grip and load force magnitude to adjust for lifting each weight based on information from the preceding lift of the object, and by 2 to 3 years of age, they can use this information to adjust the rate of increase in grip and load force for

each weight. It appears that the scaling of grip and load force rates continues to change until approximately 8 to 15 years, depending on the order of presentation of the weights, suggesting that anticipatory skills do not achieve adult levels until this age range. Children begin to use visual information (size of object to estimate its weight) to anticipate task requirements and to scale grip and load forces by 3 to 4 years of age (Gordon et al., 1992), but how vision and other perceptual processes contribute to the refinement of grasp control, or to anticipatory strategies more generally, remains to be explored.

Collectively, the studies described in this section demonstrate that grasping is a complex skill involving many different aspects of sensorimotor control. Innate or rudimentary skills, biomechanics, and other context-dependent variables contribute to setting the stage for rapid changes in motor control during the first year of life. Already in these earliest exercises of skill, infants are probably building a database of information they will begin to use to transform their skills as they become increasingly intent on shaping their own experiences. Probably one of the views enjoying the greatest consensus among researchers in the field of motor control today is the view that all aspects of movement execution, including the basic physiology, biomechanics, perceptual processing, and development of strategies, must be closely examined under varying movement conditions to provide a better understanding of the acquisition of motor control during normal development. The potential implications of this view when development goes awry will be the focus of the final portion of this chapter.

MOTOR CONTROL RESEARCH: CLINICAL IMPLICATIONS

The implied assumption of motor control research is that it can, and will, advance clinical interventions to improve or restore motor function limited as a consequence of disease or injury. This is indeed an exciting time for those researchers and clinicians interested in building links between movement science and clinical rehabilitation practice to improve assessment and treatment of movement problems. New ideas and approaches are emerging as scientists and clinicians begin to test the generality of theory-driven findings applied to various patient populations. It will take well-designed studies addressing specific links between science and practice, however, to reveal more precisely the implications of motor control studies for specific problems encountered in rehabilitation practice. In this last section, some possible implications of movement science for clinical practice are briefly discussed with respect to assessment and treatment of motor control problems.

Clinical Assessments

The vast majority of currently available tools for assessment of motor control are based on neural maturational or learning theories, but some newly developed tools appear to reflect changing views of development, such as that espoused by Thelen and Ulrich (1991) in the Dynamical Systems Theory. Maturational-based tools can be readily identified by their emphasis on reflex testing (Palisano, 1993). Such tools focus on reflex, or evoked, behaviors because it is assumed that expression of these behaviors indicates the level of neural integration and function achieved (Touwen, 1984). In many of these tests, little or no consideration is given to other variables that may enhance, depress, or otherwise alter expression of the evoked behaviors. Even some maturational-based tools are beginning to encompass broader views of motor development, however, since variables such as state behavior (e.g., level of arousal) are included in testing protocols or grading of responses. In many cases, the theoretic underpinnings of a given assessment are not clear. For instance, some motor assessments are composed of tests to determine milestone achievements and may be viewed as indicators of the extent of neural maturation and corticospinal control, as proposed by McGraw (1940, 1945), or as behavioral indicators of cognitive maturation, as originally proposed by Piaget (Keogh & Sugden, 1985). In other instances, assessments are composed of milestones solely because they appear to display statistical or diagnostic significance (Hopkins & Prechtl, 1984). Although no tool has yet been developed to reflect a dynamical-based view of development, interest in spontaneous, self-produced movements under naturalistic conditions reflects both a departure from earlier assessment approaches and the possibility of recognizing contributions to movement of multiple variables (Hadders-Algra & Prechtl, 1992). In this section, the following tools for assessment of motor skill acquisition will be briefly reviewed with respect to some of the motor control issues discussed in this chapter: General Movement (GM) assessment, Dubowitz Neurological Assessment, Movement Assessment of Infants (MAI), Gross Motor Performance Measure (GMPM), Miller Assessment for Preschoolers (MAP), Sensory Integration and Praxis Tests (SIPT), and Assessment of Motor and Process Skills (AMPS).

GENERAL MOVEMENT ASSESSMENT

A quality of GM assessment, developed by researchers at the University of Groningen in The Netherlands, is a relatively new tool developed to assess the spontaneous movements of newborn and young infants (Hopkins & Prechtl, 1984). To date, the GM assessment tool has been used for full-term and preterm infants from 2 to 18 postnatal weeks (Cioni & Prechtl, 1990; Hadders-Algra & Prechtl, 1992). The assessment consists of observation and classification of spontaneous movements while the infant lies in the supine position. Duration of observation has not been standardized; reports are based on periods varying from 15 minutes to more than 2 hours. Only movements generated while the infant is in an awake, noncrying state are analyzed and identified as belonging to one of five possible classifications of movement quality: writhing, fidgeting, wiggling-oscillating, saccadic, and ballistic. Classification definitions distinguish the frequency, amplitude, power, speed, flow, irregularity, and abruptness of onset. Thus far, studies have focused primarily on identifying age-related trends in the occurrence of each movement quality (Cioni & Prechtl, 1990; Hadders-Algra & Prechtl, 1992). A finding of cramped, synchronous movement quality, however, has been related to the outcome of spastic cerebral palsy in a small sample of high-risk infants (Ferrari et al., 1990) and suggests that larger scale outcome studies are needed to determine the predictability of this outcome when using the GM assessment tool.

The GM assessment is based on ethologic methods for studying behavior, describing the form of movement and its consequences on physical and social dimensions of the environment. The design of the GM assessment reflects a theoretic view that maturation is not a fixed sequence of differentiation, but rather a continuous transformation of behavior (Hopkins & Prechtl, 1984). The GM assessment also views general spontaneous movements as distinct, coordinated patterns of activity in the healthy newborn, but when such movements become totally disorganized, excessively monotonous, or stereotypic, they may be indicative of neural malformations or severe brain lesions (Prechtl, 1983, 1990). Interestingly, one study compared the age-related trends in movement quality classifications with a neurologic assessment consisting of commonly elicited reflexes and behaviors and found no correlation between the two measures (Hadders-Algra & Prechtl, 1992). The lack of correlation between these measures may indicate that the GM assessment captures behaviors controlled by processes different from the processes underlying behaviors assessed by traditional neurologic tests. Developers of the GM assessment acknowledge the possibility that self-organizing processes of neural networks and extrinsic factors as well as endogenous maturational processes are likely contributors to the emergence of these movement qualities and raise the possibility that different movements emerge with changes within different brain regions (Hadders-Algra & Prechtl, 1992). Future studies using the GM assessment may help to identify specific neural and extraneural variables and the roles they play in the control of movements in young infants.

DUBOWITZ NEUROLOGICAL ASSESSMENT

The Dubowitz Neurological Assessment is an example of a tool based on traditional, neuromaturational views of development and designed to assess preterm and full-term infants soon after birth and during the neonatal period for the purpose of detecting deviations and resolutions of neurologic problems (Dubowitz & Dubowitz, 1981). It consists of 32 items selected to evaluate 4 areas: habituation to stimuli, movement and tone, reflexes, and behavior. Using a 5-point scale, scoring of each item is criterion-referenced and criteria are ordered according to expected changes with increasing gestational age. The infant's state of arousal is considered in the interpretation of findings. Selection and design of the test items for the Dubowitz Neurological Assessment were based on the following criteria: to reflect expected findings for full-term infants at 3 days of age; to achieve good agreement between observers; to include some measure of higher neurologic function; and to be useful for assessing ill infants. Nearly all items are examiner-evoked responses, with the exception of one item for describing the quality of spontaneous body movements and another for identifying the presence of specific abnormal movement or posture. The authors reported that a cluster of abnormal scores, the presence of asymmetries or increased tone, and diminished leg mobility, in particular, may indicate that an intraventricular hemorrhage has occurred (Dubowitz & Dubowitz, 1981) and that motor abnormalities may eventually emerge (Dubowitz et al., 1984). They also suggested that an abnormal test score during initial assessment may be of less prognostic significance than milder but more persisting clinical signs. From the findings it may be suggested that these examiner-evoked movements provide little information on the control of movement or its development except when viewed collectively, and even then the primary information seems to be an indication of general neural intactness, not of the specific motor pathologic processes likely to unfold. The lack of sensitivity to specific motor function or dysfunction in these types of assessments may occur because the test procedures only superficially screen brain function, whereas reasons for dysfunction can be varied and even multifactorial (Prechtl, 1983)

MOVEMENT ASSESSMENT OF INFANTS

The MAI is a tool designed for the purposes of identifying motor dysfunction and changes in the status of motor dysfunction and of establishing an intervention program for infants from birth to 1 year of age (Chandler et al., 1980). The MAI is a criterion-referenced examination composed of 65 items selected to evaluate four areas: muscle tone, reflexes, automatic reactions, and volitional movement. Each item is scored on a scale of 0–4 or 0–6 points and checked for asymmetric or rostrocaudal variations to obtain an "at-risk score" for motor dysfunction. Like other maturational-based assessments, the current version of the MAI contains many examiner-evoked test procedures, and it does not attempt to control for contextual variables such as state of arousal. It does include, however, items to assess spontaneous motor features such as self-initiated postures and behaviors commonly identified in milestone schedules of development that are scored for quality and level of proficiency. Theoretic justification for items of the MAI has not been specified, but it would appear that each item is included for its statistical potential to discriminate abnormal deviations in motor development.

Unlike many assessments currently available, the testing properties of the MAI have been studied by several investigators and the findings reviewed (Palisano, 1993). Studies on the predictive value of the MAI have focused primarily on the reliability of scores for infants at 4 months of age or on the sensitivity and specificity of the 4-month scores with respect to outcomes at later ages. In general, studies seem to indicate that reliability is poor to fair for items requiring handling of the infant by the examiner and fair to good for those not requiring handling (Haley et al., 1986). Studies appear to indicate also that the MAI is sensitive, readily identifying deviations in motor development that may predict motor dysfunction at later ages, but that it exhibits poor specificity because it also identifies some normal infants as being at risk for later motor dysfunction (Harris, 1987; Swanson et al., 1992). It appears that the most consistently reliable and predictive portion of the MAI is the section on volitional movement, because it was the only section to exhibit a strong relationship with outcome (at 18 months) at both the 4-month and 8-month assessments (Swanson et al., 1992). To date, no data suggest that the MAI can predict the types of motor dysfunction likely to emerge during development, nor to this author's knowledge have studies yet tested the ability of the MAI to address the tasks (treatment and change in status) for which it was also designed. Revised versions of the MAI are under development by Chandler (1986, 1990) and by Harris (1991).

GROSS MOTOR PERFORMANCE MEASURE

The Gross Motor Function Measure (GMFM, see Chapter 1 by Campbell) and its companion, the GMPM, were specifically designed to assess the status and change in status of motor proficiency due to therapeutic interventions in children with cerebral palsy (Boyce et al., 1991; Russell et al., 1989). The GMPM consists of qualitative rating on 60 items, based on GMFM motor skills commonly performed by normal children younger than 5 years of age, to measure proficiency in eight categories of motor function in activities carried out in the supine, prone, four-point, sitting, kneeling, and standing positions and during walking and climbing. Performance quality is scored on a 5-point scale to indicate the postural alignment, selective control, coordination, stabilization, and weight shift characteristic of the task. Most items involve either movements requiring a change in posture, such as during locomotion (crawling or walking), or movements while maintaining a posture (extending an arm while sitting or in four-point position). The theoretic basis for design of the GMFM was the measurement of responsiveness, that is, the ability to show change in motor function, in children from 5 months to 12 years of age who had cerebral palsy. Preliminary study of the assessment by its authors suggested that the GMFM is a responsive tool for measurement of change in young children with cerebral palsy (Russell et al., 1989). The GMPM was designed to assess qualities of movement believed by therapists to be problematic in children with cerebral palsy but amenable to intervention. Research findings on the measurement properties of the GMPM are not yet available. The use of physical aids or orthoses is noted on the score sheet, but use of these devices is not reflected in scoring and no other possible variables affecting motor control are considered. Further, the GMPM does not assess qualities of performance such as speed, effort, or efficiency.

MILLER ASSESSMENT FOR PRESCHOOLERS

The MAP was designed as a screening tool to identify mild or moderate delays in the development of children between approximately 3 and 6 years of age at risk for future school-related problems and to refer them for more in-depth assessments (Miller, 1982). The current version of the MAP consists of 27 core items to address sensory, motor, cognitive, and combined abilities that are drawn from previously existing tools based on statistical support, time required to execute an item, and extent of equipment required. To date, there are few readily available publications of MAP measurement properties, but a review of such studies is provided by King-Thomas and Hacker (1987). Sensorimotor items include tests of position and movement sense, stereognosis, postural stability, mobility, and coordination (fine motor, gross motor, oral). Unlike most available motor assessments, the MAP treats some sensorimotor items as cognitive-dependent, as, for example, the ability to sequence or imitate movements. The assessment also considers the role of behavior (e.g., concentration, need for reward, and social interaction) in assessment of performance. Thus, design of the MAP suggests it has the potential for reflecting dynamical-based views of development, but this remains to be explored.

SENSORY INTEGRATION AND PRAXIS TESTS

The SIPT, formerly known as the Southern California Sensory Integration Tests, is a sensorimotor assessment for children between the ages of 4 and 9 years having mild to moderate learning impairment in the absence of frank organic disease, mental retardation, or primary sensory deficit (Ayres, 1989). Unlike many assessments, the SIPT has a theoretic basis for design, Sensory Integration Theory, that is precise; it is composed of three primary postulates: 1) learning is dependent upon the intake and processing of sensory experiences from movement and the environment; 2) deficits in sensory processing can lead to deficits in motor planning and execution; 3) active participation in meaningful tasks can improve sensory integrative processes and motor learning (Fisher & Bundy, 1992). The assessment is composed of 17 tests. Initial SIPT examining balance, proprioceptive and tactile sensation, and control of specific movements are used to identify whether there is a sensory processing disorder in one of three areas — vestibular proprioception, tactile discrimination, or sensory modulation — that may be indicative of integrative dysfunction. If a cluster of scores suggests dysfunction in one of these areas, subsequent SIPT are used to identify a disorder in bilateral integration and sequencing praxis, somatodyspraxia, or sensory modulation. Although the SIPT seek to identify only sensory processing problems, they do look at motor performance across a broad range of tasks and include tests for tactile discrimination, movement planning, tactile defensiveness, perception of form and space, and visuomotor coordination. Like most formalized assessments of sensorimotor abilities, the SIPT are standardized, but unlike most such assessments, the SIPT are scored by computer (at Western Psychological Services in Los Angeles, CA).

ASSESSMENT OF MOTOR AND PROCESS SKILLS

The AMPS is a new tool developed to evaluate motor skills and series of actions (called process skills) leading to completion of a task (Fisher, in press). Design of the AMPS is based on Sensory Integration Theory for the purpose of evaluating the behavioral manifestation of sensory integrative dysfunction in children (Bundy & Fisher, 1992) and adults (Fisher, in press). Selection of specific items in the AMPS is based on the assumption that collectively they represent the abilities underlying performance of common tasks and therefore can be used to estimate overall function as well as to identify specific deficits limiting function for use in planning therapeutic intervention. The AMPS contains 15 motor skills items to assess strength, posture, mobility, fine motor and subtle postural adjustment capabilities, and 20 process skills to measure attentional, conceptual, organizational, and adaptive capabilities. To evaluate these skills, the subject selects a common activity, such as fixing a meal, from a range of 30 possible activities listed in the AMPS manual. Each of the skills is then scored on a 4-point scale describing levels of competence displayed while the subject completes the activity. Scores for each of the motor skills are then adjusted for the level of task difficulty, so that performance can be related to a continuum of performance capacity to compare and predict performance for tasks of lesser or greater difficulty. Findings for a preliminary study of some AMPS test properties are available (Fisher, in press). Although the AMPS was specifically designed with reference to Sensory Integration Theory, the inclusion of contextual sensitivity suggests that it has the potential for being adapted to any naturalistic setting as well as multiple settings so as to be interpreted also with respect to a dynamical-based theory.

In summary, there are a number of motor assessments currently available, and only a small representative sample is reviewed here. As efforts are made to extend research in motor control to issues of assessment, greater attention to theoretic framework and purpose of test design is required to scrutinize whether an assessment tool not only exhibits good measurement properties but also yields measures consistent with current knowledge of the processes and mechanisms of motor control. Many assessments commonly used in rehabilitation are based primarily on maturational-based theories (Palisano, 1993) and possess few, if any, properties reflecting current views of motor control. It is likely that as rehabilitation specialists take more interest in research supporting dynamical-based theories, a new generation of assessment tools will reflect this view as well. By way of example, study in young children with hemiplegia due to cerebral palsy nicely demonstrated how one variable alone, task specificity, can alter the results of a simple measurement such as joint angle (van der Weel et al., 1991). How many more variables are yet to be identified that affect assessment and interpretation of motor performance?

Implications for Treatment

As one attempts to relate contemporary research in motor control to potential implications for treatment in clinical practice, one finds that the issues are similar to those considered for assessment. Conceptualization begins with understanding the theoretic basis for why a certain action is taken and specifying the expected consequences predicted by the theory enlisted. Excellent reviews of the theoretic bases and expected consequences enlisted by physical therapists during much of this century are available (Gordon, 1987; Horak, 1991, 1992) and will only be highlighted here. Some examples of possible implications for treatment drawn from motor control research will complete this section and chapter.

EVOLVING BASES FOR TREATMENT

Most neurotherapeutic approaches used in physical therapy were originally based on reflex and hierarchic models of motor control (Gordon, 1987; Horak, 1991). Treatment approaches based on maturational theory typically subscribed to a hierarchic model of motor skill acquisition and enlisted a facilitation model of treatment. In practical terms, it was assumed that motor development in the child progressed in a specific sequence of reflexes, movement patterns, and milestones, and that a child had to experience each facet of this sequence to acquire normal, age-appropriate motor control. Based on the facilitation model of treatment, it was assumed that externally driven sensory experience of these sequences, such as the passive and guided movements generated by a therapist or caregiver, could alter the damaged nervous system in such a way that the child with motor impairment might acquire more normally functioning motor pathways. The facilitation model also assumed that abnormal or undesirable movement experiences could reinforce pathologic pathways, severely limiting ultimate gains in motor control. Such logic can be found in various forms of treatment adapted from theoretic neurorehabilitation models developed by (but not limited to) Bobath and Bobath (1984), Brunnstrom (1970), Knott (1966), and Vojta (Aufschnaiter, 1992). Typically, maturational-based treatment approaches have emphasized inhibiting abnormal postural muscle tone and primitive reflexes, breaking up abnormal move-

ment patterns, and providing movement experiences in prescribed sequences to acquire motor skills (e.g., proximal to distal progression of body control and hierarchically ordered motor milestones). Documented dissatisfactions with this approach include poor carryover to functional activities, insufficient active movement by the patient, lack of attention to movement-related variables that are extrinsic to the nervous system, and failure to produce normal movement patterns once abnormal muscle tone or primitive reflexes were inhibited (Horak, 1991).

As dissatisfaction with maturational-based approaches to treatment and other related therapies has grown, aspects of each have been combined and modified to incorporate the later findings of motor control research. One approach, developed by Carr and Shepherd (1987), is organized around goal-directed, functional behaviors and takes into account the importance of both peripheral and central neural function and the environment in learning to accomplish specific functional goals. The goal-oriented approach is based on the systems model of motor control first proposed by Bernstein (1967). According to this model, function of each contributing system and interaction among systems are dictated by the demands of task goals during a given movement (Fig. 2–11A). Thus, unlike other approaches, the goal-directed approach assumes that movement patterns vary according to the goal and the systems contributing to a given movement. Similarly, the goal-directed approach assumes that there may be multiple satisfactory movement pattern solutions for achieving a goal; a patient is therefore encouraged to find multiple strategies for accomplishing a goal. Active, self-initiated movement is encouraged, and principles of motor learning are used to enhance practice and learning of new movement strategies. Because it is relatively new, this approach includes aspects that are yet undeveloped, such as concise methods for more precisely specifying the quality of movement and methods for enhancing motor learning processes implied in the approach (Horak, 1991). Thus far, the approach also fails to address whether the learner has limited or vast movement experience (i.e., a young child vs an adult), and it is not coupled with a specified assessment methodology. Thus far, too, this goal-directed treatment approach is the closest approximation to a dynamical theory–based (or systems) model of rehabilitation found in clinical practice.

In relation to the goal-directed approach, Horak (1992) has proposed the development of an approach that more precisely reflects the systems model of Bernstein. In this model of rehabilitation,

FIGURE 2–11. The Systems Model of Motor Control *(A)* and Systems Model of Rehabilitation *(B)* specify a collection of systems that contribute to the control of movement. The organization of these systems is heterarchic rather than hierarchic, suggesting that control shifts among the contributing systems as a function of the goal for a given task. (*A* adapted and reprinted with permission from Horak, FB. Assumptions underlying motor control for neurologic rehabilitation. In Lister, MJ [Ed.], Contemporary Management of Motor Control Problems, Proceedings of the II Step Conference. Alexandria, VA: Foundation for Physical Therapy, Inc., 1991, pp. 11–28. Reprinted with permission from the Foundation for Physical Therapy, Inc. *B* adapted from Horak, FB. Motor control models underlying neurologic rehabilitation. In Forssberg, H, & Hirschfeld, H [Eds.], Movement Disorders in Children; Medicine and Sport Science, Vol. 36. Basel: Karger, 1992, pp. 21–30.)

Horak draws together each of the systems identified in motor control research as contributors to a class of goals, such as postural stability (Fig. 2–11*B*). Starting from the upper right corner of Figure 2–11*B*, the *Musculoskeletal System* contributes the net biomechanical forces for postural control resulting from active contractile forces, passive elastic forces, and displacements of multilinked body segments. *Central Set* provides anticipatory strategies based on past experience to minimize the potential for postural instability as it emerges during movement. *Environmental Adaptation* provides a means for using both feedforward and feedback control to adapt postural strategies to a particular task or environment. Using somatosensory, vestibular, and visual information, *Perception of Orientation* deter-

mines the postural orientation goal for the task at hand. *Sensory Interaction* provides a means for adjusting the relative dominance of all sensory inputs based on current postural context, previous postural experience, and postural expectations. Finally, *Sensorimotor Strategies* provide a collection of innate and learned movement strategies that can be adapted by the actions of all other systems to simplify planning of an action and effectively meet the postural goal.

HYPOTHETIC APPLICATIONS

With the close of this chapter, a few hypothetic examples of how the systems model for rehabilitation might be used are provided for the reader to ponder. First, consider a new walker eagerly attempting to reach for a bright, shiny toy with one hand while standing and holding on to a small piece of furniture with the other hand. Moving about the model illustrated by Figure 2–11*B*, the infant's stability goal is to remain standing while reaching for the toy. The *Musculoskeletal System* generates biomechanical variables such as a relatively high center of gravity (e.g., high sway frequency) and produces responses limited by a small and relatively undeveloped lever system formed by the leg, ankle, and foot for generating force against the floor. Because the infant is a new walker and has little experience, *Central Set* has few predictive abilities and anticipatory strategies from which to generate a plan for minimizing a shift in center of gravity as the reach is initiated. Thus, *Central Set* may be viewed as a limiting system in this task. Given limited predictive skills, *Environmental Adaptation* may be limited to dependence on feedback strategies to correct postural perturbations. Because the infant has several months of experience in a gravitational environment, *Perception of Orientation* is not likely to be a limiting system in this task. The infant will likely rely almost exclusively on vision to control posture, since *Sensory Interaction*, also a limiting system, has not yet determined how to adjust the relative dominance of each contributing sensory system. Owing to biomechanical variables (faster sway and shorter distance to the limits of stability) and a dependence on feedback, rather than feedforward, correction strategies, the timing and sequencing of ankle (sensorimotor) strategies may not be sufficiently effective or reliable to correct posture before the infant sways to the limits of stability. In which case, *Sensorimotor Strategies* may favor either generating cocontraction of antagonist muscles to provide stiffness about the ankle as a way to stabilize posture (Bradley & Smith, 1988a) or selecting a protective extension response.

In contrast to the hypothetic interpretations mentioned earlier, immature motor skills or actions have typically been viewed as indicative of a nervous system not yet able to execute adaptive, coordinated motor commands. If one embraces multifactorial assumptions of motor control, however, immature motor actions may also be viewed as adaptive strategies to cope with inherent immaturity in one or more contributing systems. The failure to see a motor pattern associated with more mature responses need not mean that it cannot be produced by *Sensorimotor Strategies;* rather, the pattern may be potentially available but not seen because other member systems cannot support it (Bradley, 1992). Immature motor actions may also be the emergent consequences of biomechanical or other environmental constraints and affordances that contribute forces or cues and shape the movement differently as it is executed through a physical space or movement context. Studies by Thelen and colleagues provide a wide range of examples describing how infant kicking is altered with changes in biomechanics and environment (for review, see Thelen & Ulrich, 1991; also see Heriza, 1991).

If a neural lesion is added to the systems model, consideration must also be given to the various direct and indirect effects of the lesion, including disuse, on each contributing system. Because each system is viewed as being organized around a specific task, even abnormal or atypic motor behaviors can be interpreted as being the patient's current solution for attempting to achieve a goal. Returning to the new walker's attempt to reach, consider the presence of mild spastic diplegia. Attempting to reach for the toy, the infant rises up on the toes, the heels seldom in contact with the ground. In this instance, in addition to the contributions of normal rate-limiting systems, weakness of leg muscles further diminishes the effectiveness of the postural lever system. Given the state of other systems, *Sensorimotor Strategies* may select to activate extensors excessively in an effort to control posture for a number of possible reasons. For example, the extensor activity may keep the center of mass forward within a new cone of stability that is biomechanically more effective than if the center of mass were shifted posteriorly; for if the center of mass shifts posteriorly, the anterior postural synergy may not be sufficient, due to weakness, to make a correcting anterior adjustment in posture. Another possible reason for selection of the extensor synergy may be to reduce the number of degrees of freedom in the leg to enhance stiffness where phasing or force generation of muscle is insufficient. According to the systems model, each contributing system is also influenced by the function of all other systems.

Thus, another implication of the model is that if function of one or more systems is altered by a pathologic process, other systems will be altered as well. Similarly, if these systems have not fully matured at the time a pathologic process occurs, maturational processes of any or all systems may be seriously altered. Thus, another implication for rehabilitation is the need to anticipate both the direct and the indirect effects of a pathologic process on each contributing system. For example, a lesion affecting the *Musculoskeletal System* may result in a significantly reduced level of activity, practice, and variety of experiences necessary for maturation of the *Central Set* and any other contributing systems. The reader is similarly encouraged to try to develop examples that may be more meaningful to a clinical problem at hand.

As one becomes discontent with the current state of knowledge, experience, or practice, it is difficult not to be overly frustrated and critical. Criticism of accepted practices may take on a life of its own, creating the impression that the current state of affairs, in this case clinical practice, is in a sorry state. Such is not necessarily the case or necessarily the view of those generating the criticism. As discussed previously in this chapter, maturational-based views and approaches to practice have undergone considerable criticism of late. As research in motor control began to take hold, however, maturational-based approaches to treatment were also undergoing modification by their creators (Bobath & Bobath, 1984), a point not always appreciated by either the practitioners or the critics of maturational-based views (Mayston, 1992). Future research and efforts to link science and practice may even lead to preservation of many facets of current treatment approaches (Ostrosky, 1990), but advances in knowledge may also suggest reasons or expected outcomes different from those previously ascribed to established approaches. The challenge is to identify and test the motor control assumptions underlying practice and critique the results thoughtfully.

References

Abend, W, Bizzi, E, & Morasso, P. Human arm trajectory formation. Brain, *105*:331–348, 1982.

Adams, JA. A closed-loop theory of motor learning. Journal of Motor Behavior, *3*:111–149, 1971.

Armstrong, DM. The motor cortex and locomotion in the cat. In Grillner, S, Stein, PSG, Stuart, DG, Forssberg, H, & Herman, RM (Eds.), Neurobiology of Vertebrate Locomotion. London: Macmillan Press, 1986, pp. 121–137.

Asanuma, H, & Keller, A. Neuronal mechanisms of motor learning in mammals. Neuroreport, *2*:217–224, 1991.

Aufschnaiter, D von. Vojta: A neurophysiological treatment. In

Forssberg, H, & Hirschfeld, H (Eds.), Movement Disorders in Children; Medicine and Sport Science, Vol. 36. Basel: Karger, 1992, pp. 7–15.

Ayres, AJ. Sensory Integration and Praxis Tests. Los Angeles: Western Psychological Services, 1989.

Ball, WA, & Tronick, E. Infant responses to impending collision, optical and real. Science, 171:818–820, 1971.

Barnes, MR, Crutchfield, CA, Heriza, CB, & Herman, SJ. Reflex and Vestibular Aspects of Motor Control, Motor Development and Motor Learning. Atlanta, GA: Stokesville, 1990.

Bayley, N. Bayley Scales of Infant Development. New York: Psychological Corporation, 1969.

Bekoff, A, & Lau, B. Interlimb coordination in 20 day-rat fetuses. Journal of Experimental Zoology, 214:173–175, 1980.

Bekoff, A, & Trainer, W. The development of interlimb coordination during swimming in postnatal rats. Journal of Experimental Zoology, 83:1–11, 1979.

Belanger, M, & Patla, AE. Phase-dependent compensatory responses to perturbation applied during walking in humans. Journal of Motor Behavior, 19:434–453, 1987.

Bergmeier, SA. An investigation of reaching in the neonate. Pediatric Physical Therapy, 4:3–11, 1992.

Bernstein, N. The Coordination and Regulation of Movements. London: Pergamon Press, 1967.

Bobath, K, & Bobath, B. The neuro-developmental treatment. Clinics in Developmental Medicine, 90:6–18, 1984.

Bower, TGR. Human Development. San Francisco: Freeman, 1979.

Bower, TGR, Broughton, JM, & Moore, MK. Infant responses to approaching objects: An indicator of response to distal variables. Perception and Psychophysics, 19:193–196, 1970.

Boyce, W, Gowland, C, Hardy, S, Rosenbaum, P, Lane, M, Plews, N, Goldsmith, C, & Russell, D. Development of a quality of movement measure for children with cerebral palsy. Physical Therapy, 71:820–832, 1991.

Bradley, NS. What are the principles of motor development? In Forssberg, H & Hirschfeld, H (Eds.), Movement Disorders in Children; Medicine and Sport Science, Vol. 36. Basel: Karger, 1992, pp. 41–49.

Bradley, NS, & Bekoff, A. Development of locomotion: Animal models. In Woollacott, MH, & Shumway-Cook, A (Eds.), Development of Posture and Gait across the Lifespan. Columbia, SC: University of South Carolina Press, 1989, pp. 48–73.

Bradley, NS, & Bekoff, A. Development of coordinated movement in chicks: I. Temporal analysis of hindlimb muscle synergies at embryonic days 9 and 10. Developmental Psychobiology, 23:763–782, 1990.

Bradley, NS, & Smith, JL. Neuromuscular patterns of stereotypic hindlimb behaviors in the first two postnatal months. I. Stepping in normal kittens. Developmental Brain Research, 38:37–52, 1988a.

Bradley, NS, & Smith, JL. Neuromuscular patterns of stereotypic hindlimb behaviors in the first two postnatal months. III. Scratching and the paw-shake response in kittens. Developmental Brain Research, 38:69–82, 1988b.

Brooks, VB. Some examples of programmed limb movements. Brain Research, 71:299–308, 1974.

Bruner, JS. Organization of early skilled action. Child Development 44:1–11, 1973.

Brunnstrom, S. Movement Therapy in Hemiplegia. New York: Harper & Row, 1970.

Bundy, AC, & Fisher, AG. Evaluation of sensory integration dysfunction. In Forssberg, H, & Hirschfeld, H (Eds.), Movement Disorders in Children: Medicine and Sport Science, Vol. 36. Basel: Karger, 1992, pp. 272–277.

Butterworth, G. Some problems in explaining the origins of

movement control. In Wade, MG, & Whiting, HTA (Eds.), Motor Development in Children: Problems of Coordination and Control. Dordrecht, Netherlands: Martinus Nijhoff, 1986, pp. 23–32.

Butterworth, G, & Hicks, L. Visual proprioception and postural stability in infancy. A developmental study. Perception, 6:255–262, 1977.

Carr, JH, & Shepherd, RB. Assumptions underlying physical therapy intervention: Theoretical and historical perspectives. In Carr, JH, & Shepherd, RB (Eds.), Movement Science Foundations for Physical Therapy in Rehabilitation. Rockville, MD: Aspen Publishers, 1987, pp. 31–92.

Carter, M, & Smith, JL. Simultaneous control of two rhythmical behaviors. I. Locomotion and the paw-shake response in normal cat. Journal of Neurophysiology, 56:171–183, 1985.

Chambers, SH, & Bradley, NS. Intra- and interlimb coordination during motility in chick embryos (Abstract). Society for Neuroscience, 17:937, 1991.

Chandler, LS. Screening for movement dysfunction in infancy. Physical and Occupational Therapy in Pediatrics, 6(3):171–190, 1986.

Chandler, LS. Neuromotor assessment. In Gibbs, ED, & Teti, DM (Eds.), Interdisciplinary Assessment of Infants: A Guide for Early Intervention Professionals. Baltimore: Brookes, 1990, pp. 45–61.

Chandler, LS, Andrews, MS, & Swanson, MW. Movement Assessment of Infants. Rolling Bay, WA: Chandler, Andrews, and Swanson, 1980.

Cioni, G, & Prechtl, HFR. Preterm and early postterm motor behaviour in low-risk premature infants. Early Human Development, 23:159–191, 1990.

Connolly, K. The nature of motor skill development. Journal of Human Movement Studies, 3:128–143, 1977.

Crenna, PF, & Frigo, C. Evidence of phase-dependent nociceptive reflexes during locomotion in man. Experimental Neurology, 85:336–345, 1984.

Crutcher, MD, & Alexander, GE. Movement-related neuronal activity selectively coding either direction or muscle pattern in 3 motor areas of the monkey. Journal of Neurophysiology, 64:151–163, 1990.

de Vries, JIP, Visser, GHA, & Prechtl, HFR. The emergence of fetal behavior: I. Qualitative aspects. Early Human Development, 7:301–322, 1982.

Dubowitz, L, & Dubowitz, V. The neurological assessment of the preterm and full-term newborn infant. Clinics in Developmental Medicine, 79:1–103, 1981.

Dubowitz, LMS, Dubowitz, V, Palmer, PG, Miller, G, Fawer, C-L, & Levine, MI. Correlation of neurologic assessment in the preterm newborn infant with outcome at 1 year. Journal of Pediatrics, 105:452–456, 1984.

Eliasson, AC, Gordon, AM, & Forssberg, H. Basic co-ordination of manipulative forces of children with cerebral palsy. Developmental Medicine and Child Neurology, 33:661–670, 1991.

Eliasson, AC, Gordon, AM, & Forssberg, H. Impaired anticipatory control of isometric forces during grasping by children with cerebral palsy. Developmental Medicine and Child Neurology, 34:216–225, 1992.

Feldman, AG. Once more on the Equilibrium Point Hypothesis (λ model) for motor control. Journal of Motor Behavior, 18:17–54, 1986.

Ferrari, F, Cioni, G, & Prechtl, HFR. Qualitative changes of general movements in preterm infants with brain lesions. Early Human Development, 23:193–231, 1990.

Fetters, L, & Todd, J. Quantitative assessment of infant reaching movements. Journal of Motor Behavior, 19:147–166, 1987.

Field, J. Coordination of vision and prehension in young infants. Child Development, 48:97–103, 1977.

Fisher, AG. Development of a functional assessment that adjusts ability measures for task simplicity and rater leniency. In Wilson, M (Ed.), Objective Measurement: Theory into Practice, Vol. 2. Norwood, NJ: Ablex, in press.

Fisher, AG, & Bundy, AC. Sensory integration theory. In Forssberg, H, & Hirschfeld, H (Eds.), Movement Disorders in Children; Medicine and Sport Science, Vol. 36. Basel: Karger, 1992, pp. 16–20.

Fitts, PM. The information capacity of the human motor system in controlling the amplitude of movement. Journal of Experimental Psychology, 47:381–391, 1954.

Forssberg, H. Ontogeny of human locomotor control. I. Infant stepping, supported locomotion and transition to independent locomotion. Experimental Brain Research, 57:480–493, 1985.

Forssberg, H. Evolution of plantigrade gait: Is there a neuronal correlate? Developmental Medicine and Child Neurology, 34:920–925, 1992.

Forssberg, H, Eliasson, AC, Kinoshita, H, Johansson, RS, & Westling, G. Development of human precision grip. I. Basic coordination of force. Experimental Brain Research, 85:451–457, 1991.

Forssberg, H, Grillner, S, & Rossignol, S. Phase dependent reflex reversal during walking in chronic spinal cats. Brain Research, 85:103–107, 1975.

Forssberg, H, Kinoshita, H, Eliasson, AC, Johansson, RS, Westling, G, & Gordon, AM. Development of human precision grip. II. Anticipatory control of isometric forces targeted for object's weight. Experimental Brain Research 90:393–398, 1992.

Forssberg, H, & Nashner, LM. Ontogenetic development of postural control in man: Adaptation to altered support and visual conditions during stance. Journal of Neuroscience, 2:545–552, 1982.

Forssberg, H, & Wallberg, H. Infant locomotion: A preliminary movement and electromyographic study. In Berg, K, & Eriksson, BO (Eds.), Children and Exercise IX. Baltimore: University Park Press, 1980, pp. 32–40.

Forsström, A, & Hofsten, C von. Visually directed reaching of children with motor impairments. Developmental Medicine and Child Neurology, 24:653–661, 1982.

Gallistel, CR. The Organization of Action: A New Synthesis. Hillsdale, NJ: Lawrence Erlbaum Associates, 1980.

Georgopolous, AP. Neurophysiology of reaching. In Jeannerod, M (Ed.), Attention and Performance XIII. Hillsdale, NJ: Lawrence Erlbaum Associates, 1990, pp. 227–263.

Ghez, C. Voluntary movements. In Kandel, ER, Schwartz, JH, & Jessell, TM (Eds.), Principles of Neuroscience (3rd ed.). New York: Elsevier, 1991, pp. 609–625.

Gibson, JJ. The Senses Considered As Perceptual Systems. Boston: Houghton Mifflin, 1966.

Giuliani, CA. Dorsal rhizotomy for children with cerebral palsy: Support for concepts of motor control. Physical Therapy, 71:248–259, 1991.

Goodgold-Edwards, SA. Cognitive strategies during coincident timing tasks. Physical Therapy, 71:236–243, 1991.

Gordon, AM, Forssberg, H, Johansson, RS, Eliasson, AC, & Westling, G. Development of human precision grip. III Integration of visual cues during the programming of isometric forces. Experimental Brain Research, 90:399–403, 1992.

Gordon, J. Assumptions underlying physical therapy intervention: Theoretical and historical perspectives. In Carr, JH, & Shepherd, RB (Eds.), Movement Science Foundations for Physical Therapy in Rehabilitation. Rockville, MD: Aspen Publishers, 1987, pp. 1–30.

Grillner, S. Control of locomotion in bipeds, tetrapods, and fish. In Brookhart, JM, & Mountcastle, VB (Eds.), Handbook of Physiology, Vol. 2, Part 2. Bethesda, MD: American Physiological Society, 1981, pp. 1179–1236.

Haas, G, Diener, HC, Rapp, H, & Dichgans, J. Development of feedback and feedforward control of upright stance. Developmental Medicine and Child Neurology, 31:481–488, 1989.

Hadders-Algra, M, & Prechtl, HFR. Developmental course of general movements in early infancy. I. Descriptive analysis of change in form. Early Human Development, 28:201–213, 1992.

Haley, SM. Sequence of development of postural reactions by infants with Down syndrome. Developmental Medicine and Child Neurology, 29:674–679, 1987.

Haley, SM, Harris, SR, Tada, WL, & Swanson, MW. Item reliability of the Movement Assessment of Infants. Physical and Occupational Therapy in Pediatrics, 6(1):21–39, 1986.

Hamburger, VS. Ramón y Cajal, R.G. Harrison, and the beginnings of neuroembryology. Perspectives in Biology and Medicine, 23:600–616, 1980.

Harris, SR. Early detection of cerebral palsy: Sensitivity and specificity of two motor assessment tools. Journal of Perinatology, 7:11–15, 1987.

Harris, SR. Development of an Infant Neuromotor Test. Final Report. Washington, DC: National Institute on Disability and Rehabilitation Research, U.S. Department of Education, 1991.

Hasan, Z. Optimized movement trajectories and joint stiffness in unperturbed, inertially loaded movements. Biological Cybernetics, 53:373–382, 1986.

Hay, L. Spatial-temporal analysis of movements in children: Motor programs versus feedback in the development of reaching. Journal of Motor Behavior, 11:188–200, 1979.

Heriza, CB. Comparison of leg movements in preterm infants at term with healthy full-term infants. Physical Therapy, 68:1687–1693, 1988.

Heriza, CB. Motor development: Traditional and contemporary theories. In Lister, MJ (Ed.), Contemporary Management of Motor Control Problems, Proceedings of the II Step Conference. Alexandria, VA: Foundation for Physical Therapy, 1991, pp. 99–126.

Hofsten, C von. Binocular convergence as a determinant of reaching behavior in infancy. Perception, 6:139–144, 1977.

Hofsten, C von. Development of visually guided reaching: The approach phase. Journal of Human Movement Studies, 5:160–178, 1979.

Hofsten, C von. Eye-hand coordination in the newborn. Developmental Psychology, 18:450–461, 1982.

Hofsten, C von. Developmental changes in the organization of prereaching movements. Developmental Psychology, 20:378–388, 1984.

Hofsten, C von. A perception-action perspective on the development of manual movements. In Jeannerod, M (Ed.), Attention and Performance XIII. Hillsdale, NJ: Lawrence Erlbaum Associates, 1990, pp. 739–762.

Hofsten, C von. Structuring of early reaching movements: A longitudinal study. Journal of Motor Behavior, 23:280–292, 1991.

Hofsten, C von, & Fazel-Zandy, S. Development of visually guided hand orientation in reaching. Journal of Experimental Child Psychology, 38:208–219, 1984.

Hofsten, C von, & Rönnqvist, L. Preparation for grasping an object: A developmental study. Journal of Experimental Psychology: Human Perception and Performance, 14:610–621, 1988.

Hooker, D. Evidence of Prenatal Function of the Central Nervous System in Man. New York: American Museum of Natural History, 1958.

Hopkins, B, & Prechtl, HFR. A quantitative approach to the development of movements during early infancy. Clinics in Developmental Medicine, 94:179–197, 1984.

Horak, FB. Assumptions underlying motor control for neurologic rehabilitation. In Lister, MJ (Ed.), Contemporary Management of Motor Control Problems, Proceedings of the II

Step Conference. Alexandria, VA: Foundation for Physical Therapy, 1991, pp. 11–28.

Horak, FB. Motor control models underlying neurologic rehabilitation. In Forssberg, H, & Hirschfeld, H (Eds.), Movement Disorders in Children; Medicine and Sport Science, Vol. 36. Basel: Karger, 1992, pp. 21–30.

Horak, FB, Diener, HC, & Nashner, LM. Influence of central set on human postural responses. Journal of Neurophysiology, 62:841–853, 1989.

Horak, FB, Esselman, P, Anderson, ME, & Lynch, MK. The effects of movement velocity, mass displaced, and task certainty on associated postural adjustments made by normal and hemiplegic individuals. Journal of Neurology, Neurosurgery and Psychiatry, 47:1020–1028, 1984.

Horak, FB, & Nashner, LM. Central programming of postural movements: Adaptation to altered support-surface configurations. Journal of Neurophysiology, 55:1369–1381, 1986.

Horak, FB, Nashner, LM, & Diener, HC. Postural strategies associated with somatosensory and vestibular loss. Experimental Brain Research, 82:167–177, 1990.

Horak, FB, Shumway-Cook, A, Crowe, TK, & Black, FO. Vestibular function and motor proficiency of children with impaired hearing, or with learning disability and motor impairments. Developmental Medicine and Child Neurology, 30:64–79, 1988.

Hoy, MG, & Zernicke, RF. Modulation of limb dynamics in the swing phase of locomotion. Journal of Biomechanics. 18:49–60, 1985.

Hoy, MG, Zernicke, RF, & Smith, JL. Contrasting roles of inertial and muscle moments at the knee and ankle during paw-shake response. Journal of Neurophysiology, 54:1282–1294, 1985.

Humphrey, T. The development of the pyramidal tracts in human fetuses, correlated with cortical differentiation. In Tower, DB, & Schadé, JP (Eds.), Structure and Function of the Cerebral Cortex. Amsterdam: Elsevier, 1960, pp. 94–103.

Humphrey, T. Some correlations between the appearance of human reflexes and the development of the nervous system. Progress in Brain Research, 4:93–135, 1964.

Humphrey, T. Postnatal repetition of human prenatal activity sequences with some suggestions of their neuroanatomical basis. In Robinson, RJ (Ed.), Brain and Early Behavior. London: Academic Press, 1969, pp. 43–84.

Humphrey, T. The development of human fetal activity and its relation to postnatal behavior. Advances in Child Development and Behavior, 5:1–57, 1970.

Jakobson, LS, & Goodale, MA. Factors affecting higher order movement planning—A kinematic analysis of human prehension. Experimental Brain Research, 86:199–208, 1991.

Jeannerod, M. Intersegmental coordination during reaching at natural visual objects in infancy. In Long, J, & Baddeley, A (Eds.), Attention and Performance IX. Hillsdale, NJ: Lawrence Erlbaum Associates, 1981, pp. 153–168.

Jeannerod, M. The timing of natural prehension movement. Journal of Motor Behavior, 26:235–254, 1984.

Jeannerod, M. The Neural and Behavioral Organization of Goal-Directed Movements. Oxford: Clarendon Press, 1988.

Jeannerod, M (Ed.). Attention and Performance XIII. Hillsdale NJ: Lawrence Erlbaum Associates, 1990.

Johansson, RS, & Westling, G. Coordinated isometric muscle commands adequately and erroneously programmed for the weight during lifting task with precision grip. Experimental Brain Research, 71:59–71, 1988.

Jordan, LM. Initiation of locomotion from the mammalian brainstem. In Grillner, S, Stein, PSG, Stuart, DG, Forssberg, H, & Herman, RM (Eds.), Neurobiology of Vertebrate Locomotion. London: Macmillan Press, 1986, pp. 21–37.

Kalaska, JF, & Crammond, DJ. Cerebral cortical mechanisms of reaching movements. Science, 255:1517–1523, 1992.

Keogh, J, & Sugden, D. Movement Skill Development. New York: Macmillan, 1985.

Keshner, EA. Equilibrium and automatic postural reactions as indicators and facilitators in the treatment of balance disorders. In: In Touch: Topics in Pediatrics (Lesson 4). Alexandria, VA: American Physical Therapy Association, 1990, pp. 1–17.

King-Thomas, L, & Hacker, BJ (Eds.). A Therapist's Guide to Pediatric Assessment. Boston: Little, Brown and Company, 1987.

Knott, M. Neuromuscular facilitation in the child with central nervous system deficit. Journal of the American Physical Therapy Association, 41:741, 1966.

Koshland, GF, & Smith, JL. Paw-shake responses with joint immobilization—EMG changes with atypical feedback. Experimental Brain Research, 77:361–373, 1989.

Kupfermann, I. Localization of higher cognitive and affective functions: The association cortices. In Kandel, ER, Schwartz, JH, & Jessell, TM (Eds.), Principles of Neuroscience (3rd ed.). New York: Elsevier, 1991, pp. 823–838.

Langworthy, OR. Development of behavior patterns and myelinization of the nervous system in the human fetus and infant. Contributions to Embryology, Carnegie Institute, 24: 1–57, 1933.

Lashley, KS. The accuracy of movement in the absence of excitation from the moving organ. American Journal of Physiology, 43:169–194, 1917.

Lasky, RE. The effect of visual feedback of the hand on the reaching and retrieval behavior of young infants. Child Development, 48:112–117, 1977.

Lawrence, DG, & Hopkins, DA. The development of the motor control in the rhesus monkey: Evidence concerning the role of corticomotoneuronal connections. Brain, 99:235–254, 1976.

Lawrence, DG, & Kuypers, HGJ. The functional organization of the motor system in the monkey: I. The effects of bilateral pyramidal lesions. Brain, 91:1–14, 1968.

Lee, DN. The optic flow-field: The foundation of vision. Philosophical Transactions of the Royal Society of London. (Series B): Biological Sciences, 290:169–179, 1980.

Lee, DN, & Aronson, E. Visual proprioceptive control of standing in human infants. Perception and Psychophysics, 15:529–532, 1974.

Lee, DN, Daniel, BM, Turnbull, J, & Cook, ML. Basic perceptuo-motor dysfunctions in cerebral palsy. In Jeannerod M (Ed.), Attention and Performance XIII. Hillsdale, NJ: Lawrence Erlbaum Associates, 1990, pp. 583–603.

Lee, DN, & Lishman, JR. Visual proprioceptive control of stance. Journal of Human Movement Studies, 1:87–95, 1975.

Lee, WA. Anticipatory control of postural and task muscles during rapid arm flexion. Journal of Motor Behavior, 12:185–196, 1980.

Lee, WA. Neuromotor synergies as a basis for coordinated intentional action. Journal of Motor Behavior, 16:135–170, 1984.

Lemon, R. The output map of the primate motor cortex. Trends in Neurosciences, 11:501–506, 1988.

Lemon, R, & Mantel, GWH. The influence of changes in discharge frequency of corticospinal neurones on hand muscles in the monkey. Journal of Physiology, 413:351–378, 1989.

Leonard, CT, Hirschfeld, H, & Forssberg, H. Gait acquisition and reflex abnormalities in normal children and children with cerebral palsy. In Amblard, B (Ed.), Development Adaptation and Modulation of Posture and Gait. Amsterdam: Elsevier, 1988, pp. 33–45.

Lockman, JJ, & Ashmead, DH. Asynchronies in the development of manual behavior. In Lipsitt, LP, & Rovee-Collier, CK (Eds.), Advances in Infant Research, Vol. 2. Norwood, NJ: Ablex, 1983, pp. 114–136.

Lockman, JJ, Ashmead, DH, & Bushnell, EW. The development of anticipatory hand orientation during infancy. Journal of Experimental Child Psychology, 37:176–186, 1984.

Loeb, GE. Kinematic factors in the generation and role of sensory feedback during locomotion. In Grillner, S, Stein, PSG, Stuart, DG, Forssberg, H, & Herman, RM (Eds.), Neurobiology of Vertebrate Locomotion. London: Macmillan Press, 1986, pp. 547–561.

Luschei, ES, & Goldberg, LJ. Neural mechanisms of mandibular control: Mastication and voluntary biting. In Brooks, VB (Ed.), Handbook of Physiology, Vol. 2. Bethesda, MD: American Physiological Society, 1981, pp. 1237–1274.

Massion, J. Movement, posture and equilibrium—Interaction and coordination. Progress in Neurobiology, 38:35–56, 1992.

Mathew, A, & Cook, M. The control of reaching movements by young infants. Child Development, 61:1238–1258, 1990.

Mayston, MJ. The Bobath concept—Evolution and application. In Forssberg, H, & Hirschfeld, H (Eds.), Movement Disorders in Children; Medicine and Sport Science, Vol. 36. Basel: Karger, 1992, pp. 1–6.

McCracken, HD. Movement control in a reciprocal tapping task: A developmental study. Journal of Motor Behavior, 15:262–279, 1983.

McDonnell, P. The development of visually guided reaching. Perception and Psychophysics, 18:181–185, 1975.

McDonnell, P. Patterns of eye-hand coordination in the first year of life. Canadian Journal of Psychology, 33:253–267, 1979.

McGraw, MB. Neuromuscular development of the human infant as exemplified in the achievement of erect locomotion. Journal of Pediatrics, 17:747–771, 1940.

McGraw, MB. The Neuromuscular Maturation of the Human Infant. New York: Hafner Press, 1945.

Miller, LJ. Miller Assessment of Preschoolers. Littleton, CO: Foundation for Knowledge in Development, 1982.

Mouchnino, L. Aurenty, R, Massion, J, & Pedotti, A. Coordinated control of posture and equilibrium during leg movement. In Brandt, T, Paulus, W, Bles, W, Dieterich, M, Krafczyk, S, & Straube, A (Eds.), Disorders of Posture and Gait. Stuttgart: Georg Thieme, 1990, pp. 68–71.

Muir, RB, & Lemon, RN. Corticospinal neurons with a special role in precision grip. Brain Research, 261:312–316, 1983.

Nashner, LM, Black, FO, & Wall, C. Adaptation to altered support and visual conditions during stance: Patients with vestibular deficits. Journal of Neuroscience, 2:536–544, 1982.

Nashner, LM, & Forssberg, H. Phase-dependent organization of postural adjustments associated with arm movements while walking. Journal of Neurophysiology, 55:1382–1394, 1986.

Nashner, LM, Shumway-Cook, A, & Marin, O. Stance posture control in select groups of children with cerebral palsy: Deficits in sensory organization and muscular coordination. Experimental Brain Research, 49:393–409, 1983.

Ostrosky, KM. Facilitation vs motor control. Clinical Management, 10:34–40, 1990.

Palisano, RJ. Neuromotor and developmental assessment. In Wilhelm, IJ (Ed.), Physical Therapy Assessment in Early Infancy. New York: Churchill Livingstone, 1993, pp. 173–224.

Patla, AE. Adaptation of postural responses to voluntary arm raises during locomotion in humans. Neuroscience Letters, 68:334–338, 1986.

Patla, AE. Visual control of human locomotion. In Patla, AE (Ed.), Adaptability of Human Gait. Amsterdam: Elsevier, 1991, pp. 55–97.

Pearson, K. The control of walking. Scientific American, 235:72–86, 1976.

Perham, H, Smick, JE, Hallum, A, & Nordstrom, T. Development of the lateral equilibrium reaction in stance. Developmental Medicine and Child Neurology, 29:758–765, 1987.

Polit, A, & Bizzi, E. Processes controlling arm movements in monkeys. Science, 201:1235–1237, 1978.

Polit, A. & Bizzi, E. Characteristics of motor programs underlying arm movements in monkeys. Journal of Neurophysiology, 42:183–194, 1979.

Prablanc, C, & Pélisson, D. Gaze saccade orienting and hand pointing are locked to their goal by quick internal loops. In Jeannerod, M (Ed.), Attention and Performance XIII. Hillsdale, NJ: Lawrence Erlbaum Associates, 1990, pp. 653–676.

Pratt, CA, & Loeb, GE. Functionally complex muscles of the cat hindlimb. 1. Patterns of activation across sartorius. Experimental Brain Research, 85:243–256, 1991.

Prechtl, HFR. Risk factors and the significance of early neurological assessment. In Brazelton, TB, & Lester, BM (Eds.), New Approaches to Developmental Screening of Infants. Amsterdam: Elsevier, 1983, pp. 125–135.

Prechtl, HFR. Qualitative changes of spontaneous movements in fetus and preterm infant are a marker of neurological dysfunction. Early Human Development, 23:151–158, 1990.

Rader, N, & Stern, JD. Visually elicited reaching in neonates. Child Development, 53:1004–1007, 1982.

Raibert, MH. Motor control and learning by the state-space. Cambridge, MA: Massachusetts Institute of Technology, Artificial Intelligence Laboratory Technical Report AI-TR-439, 1977.

Riach, CL, & Hayes, KC. Anticipatory postural control in children. Journal of Motor Behavior, 22:250–266, 1990.

Rosenbaum, DA. Human Motor Control. San Diego: Academic Press, 1991.

Rossignol, S, & Drew, T. Phasic modulation of reflexes during rhythmic activity. In Grillner, S, Stein, PSG, Stuart, DG, Forssberg, H, & Herman, RM (Eds.), Neurobiology of Vertebrate Locomotion. London: Macmillan Press, 1986, pp. 517–534.

Rossignol, S, & Gauthier, L. An analysis of mechanisms controlling the reversal of crossed spinal reflexes. Brain Research, 182:31–45, 1980.

Russell, DJ, Rosenbaum, PL, Cadman, DT, Gowland, C, Hardy, S, & Jarvis, S. The Gross Motor Function Measure: A means to evaluate the effects of physical therapy. Developmental Medicine and Child Neurology, 31:341–353, 1989.

Sanes, JN, Dimitrov, B, & Hallett, M. Motor learning in patients with cerebellar dysfunction. Brain, 113:103–120, 1990.

Scheibel, ME, & Scheibel, AB. Developmental relationship between spinal motoneuron dendrite bundles and patterned activity in the forelimb of cats. Experimental Neurology, 30:367–373, 1971.

Schellekens, JMH, Scholten, CA, & Kalverboer, AF. Visually guided hand movements in children with minor neurological dysfunction: Response time and movement organization. Journal of Child Psychology and Psychiatry and Allied Disciplines, 24:89–102, 1983.

Schmidt, RA. A schema theory of discrete motor skill learning. Psychological Review, 82:225–260, 1975.

Schmidt, RA. Motor Control and Learning, a Behavioral Emphasis (2nd ed.). Champaign, IL: Human Kinetics, 1988.

Schmidt, RA, Zelaznik, HN, Hawkins, B, Frank, JS, & Guinn, JT. Motor output variability: A theory for the accuracy of rapid motor acts. Psychological Review, 86:415–451, 1979.

Schneider, K, Zernicke, RF, Schmidt, RA, & Hart, TJ. Changes in limb dynamics during the practice of rapid arm movements. Journal of Biomechanics, 22:805–817, 1989.

Schneider, K, Zernicke, RF, Ulrich, BD, Jensen, JL, & Thelen, E. Understanding movement control in infants through the analysis of limb intersegmental dynamics. Journal of Motor Behavior, 22:493–520, 1990.

Scholz, JP. Dynamic pattern theory—Some implications for therapeutics. Physical Therapy, 70:827–843, 1990.

Shapiro, DC, Zernicke, RF, Gregor, RJ, & Diestel, JD. Evidence for generalized motor programs using gait pattern analysis. Journal of Motor Behavior, 13:33–47, 1981.

Sherrington, CS. The integrative action of the nervous system. New Haven: Yale University Press, 1947. (Original work published 1906).

Shumway-Cook, A, & Woollacott, M. The growth of stability: Postural control from a development perspective. Journal of Motor Behavior, 17:131–147, 1985a.

Shumway-Cook, A, & Woollacott, M. Dynamics of postural control in the child with Down syndrome. Physical Therapy, 9:1315–1322, 1985b.

Siegler, S, Moskowitz, GD, & Freedman, W. Passive and active components of the internal moment developed about the ankle joint during human ambulation. Journal of Biomechanics, 17:647–652, 1984.

Smith, JL, Bradley, NS, Carter, MC, Giuliani, CA, Hoy, MG, Koshland, GF, & Zernicke, RF. Rhythmical movements of the hindlimbs in spinal cat: Considerations for a controlling network. In Goldberger, ME, Gorio, A, & Murray, M (Eds.), Development and Plasticity of the Mammalian Spinal Cord. New York: Springer-Verlag, 1986, pp. 347–362.

Smith, JL, & Zernicke, RF. Predictions for neural control based on limb dynamics. Trends in Neurosciences, 10:123–128, 1987.

Stehouwer, DJ, & Farel, PB. Development of hindlimb locomotor behavior in the frog. Developmental Psychobiology, 17: 217–232, 1984.

Sugden, DA, & Keogh, JF. Problems in Movement Skill Development. Columbia, SC: University of South Carolina Press, 1990.

Sutherland, DH, Olshen, RA, Biden, EN, & Wyatt, MP. The development of mature walking. Clinics in Developmental Medicine, 104/105:1–227, 1988.

Sutherland, DH, Olshen, R, Cooper, L, & Woo, SL. The development of mature gait. Journal of Bone and Joint Surgery (British), 62:336–353, 1980.

Swanson, MW, Bennet, FC, Shy, KK, & Whitfield, MF. Identification of neurodevelopmental abnormality at four and eight months by the Movement Assessment of Infants. Developmental Medicine and Child Neurology, 34:321–337, 1992.

Tardieu, C. Laspargot, A, Tabary, C, & Bret, M. Toe-walking in children with cerebral palsy: Contributions of contracture and excessive contraction of triceps surae muscle. Physical Therapy, 69:656–662, 1989.

Taub, E, & Berman, AJ. Movement and learning in the absence of sensory feedback. In Freedman, SJ (Ed.), The Neuropsychology of Spatially Oriented Behavior. Homewood, IL: Dorsey Press, 1968.

Thelen, E. Treadmill-elicited stepping in seven-month-old infants. Child Development, 57:1498–1506, 1986.

Thelen, E, Bradshaw, G, & Ward, JA. Spontaneous kicking in month-old infants: Manifestation of a human central locomotor program. Behavioral and Neural Biology, 32:45–53, 1981.

Thelen, E, & Cooke, DW. Relationship between newborn stepping and later walking. A new interpretation. Developmental Medicine and Child Neurology, 29:380–393, 1987.

Thelen, E, & Fisher, DM. Newborn stepping: An explanation for a "disappearing" reflex. Developmental Psychology, 18:760–775, 1982.

Thelen, E, & Fisher, DM. The organization of spontaneous leg movements in newborn infants. Journal of Motor Behavior, 15:353–377, 1983.

Thelen, E, Fisher, DM, & Ridley-Johnson, R. The relationship between physical growth and a newborn reflex. Infant Behavior and Development, 7:479–493, 1984.

Thelen, E, Fisher, DM, Ridley-Johnson, R, & Griffin, NJ. Effects of body build and arousal on newborn infant stepping. Developmental Psychobiology, 15:447–453, 1982.

Thelen, E, & Ulrich, BD. Hidden skills: A dynamic systems analysis of treadmill stepping during the first year. Society for Research in Child Development, 56:1–98, 1991.

Touwen, BCL. Primitive reflexes—Conceptional or semantic problem? Clinics in Developmental Medicine, 94:113–125, 1984.

Trevarthen, C. The psychobiology of speech development. Neurosciences Research Program Bulletin, 12:570–585, 1974.

Twitchell, TE. Reflex mechanisms and the development of prehension. In Connolly, K (Ed.), Mechanisms of Motor Skill Development. London: Academic Press, 1970, pp. 25–37.

Ulrich, BD. Development of stepping patterns in human infants: A dynamic systems perspective. Journal of Motor Behavior, 21:392–408, 1989.

van der Meulen, JHP, Vandergon, JJD, Gielen, CCA, Gooskens, RHJ, & Willemse, J. Visuomotor performance of normal and clumsy children. 1. Fast goal-directed arm-movements with and without visual feedback. Developmental Medicine and Child Neurology, 33:40–54, 1991a.

van der Meulen, JHP, Vandergon, JJD, Gielen, CCA, Gooskens, RHJ, & Willemse, J. Visuomotor performance of normal and clumsy children. 2. Arm-tracking with and without visual feedback. Developmental Medicine and Child Neurology, 33:118–129, 1991b.

van der Weel, FR, van der Meer, ALH, & Lee, DH. Effect of task on movement control in cerebral palsy: Implications for assessment and therapy. Developmental Medicine and Child Neurology, 33:419–426, 1991.

Viviani, P, & Mounoud, P. Perceptuomotor compatibility in pursuit tracking of two-dimensional movements. Journal of Motor Behavior, 22:407–443, 1990.

von Euler, C. Central pattern generation during breathing. Trends in Neurosciences, 3:275–277, 1980.

Wishart, JG, Bower, TGR, & Dunkeld, J. Reaching in the dark. Perception, 7:507–512, 1978.

Woollacott, M, Debu, B, & Mowatt, M. Neuromuscular control of posture in the infant and child. Journal of Motor Behavior, 19:167–186, 1987.

Woollacott, MH, Shumway-Cook, A, & Williams, HG. The development of posture and balance control in children. In Woollacott, MH, & Shumway-Cook, A (Eds.), Development of Posture and Gait across the Life Span. Columbia, SC: South Carolina Press, 1989, pp. 77–96.

Yang, JF, & Stein, RB. Phase-dependent reflex reversal in human leg muscles during walking. Journal of Neurophysiology, 63:1109–1117, 1990.

Yonas, A, Bechtold, AG, Frankel, D, Gordon, FR, McRoberts, G, Norcia, A, & Sternfels, S. Development of sensitivity to information for impending collision. Perception and Psychophysics, 21:97–104, 1977.

Zelazo, PR. The development of walking: New findings and old assumptions. Journal of Motor Behavior, 15:99–137, 1983.

Chapter 3

Gait: Development and Analysis

JEAN L. STOUT, PT, MS

One of the first questions asked by many parents whose child has recently been diagnosed as having a motor impairment, or whose child has suffered an injury, is "Will my child walk?" or "Will my child walk again?" The reason for emphasis on the task of walking apart from many other abilities (which are sometimes more functional), I believe, is the measure of independence and social acceptance with which the task of walking is associated. The ultimate goal for families, and sometimes pediatric therapists as well, becomes independent walking for the child or client. Although the variables that contribute to this important ability are numerous and complex, a child is usually able to stand and walk by 9 to 15 months of age (see Chapter 1). Furthermore, the pattern is mature by the age of 3½ (Sutherland et al., 1980), all without instruction. The complexity of the task has been studied extensively since the days of Saunders (1953) and Murray (1964), and study continues today. Improved computerized techniques and new theories of motor control and balance contribute to better understanding of the components of walking. Understanding how we walk was once required only for those in the fields of child development and rehabilitation. Today walking is studied by many disciplines, including engineering. The extent and duration of the research in the area is a statement of its continued importance.

The purpose of this chapter is to provide an overview of the aspects of gait important to physical therapists treating children. These include the development of gait and its refinement in childhood, the normal components of walking as identified by gait analysis, and a description of some of the common abnormalities in gait found in children with physical disabilities. Those interested in more extensive information are referred to a number of excellent resources on the topic (Gage, 1991; Gillette Children's Hospital, 1993; Inman et al., 1981; Ounpuu et al., 1991; Perry, 1992; Rose, SA, et al., 1991; Sutherland, 1984; Sutherland et al., 1980, 1988; Winter, 1979, 1983, 1987, 1990).

DEVELOPMENT OF GAIT

Gage (1991) suggests that normal walking has five major attributes: 1) stability in stance, 2) sufficient foot clearance in swing, 3) appropriate prepositioning of the foot for initial contact, 4) adequate step length, and 5) energy conservation. When independent ambulation begins in the toddler only the prerequisites for these attributes are present. The prerequisites, however, are likely to be more important to the attainment of walking than the attributes themselves, which develop with normal growth, maturation, and refinement of the skill. Loss of the five attributes in pathologic gait occurs because of a loss or failure to achieve the prerequisites. The prerequisites related to the development and skill of locomotion have already been suggested by Campbell in Chapter 1 in her review of the eight subsystems proposed on the basis of the dynamical systems theory (Heriza, 1991). These include adequate motor control and central nervous system maturation (implying an intact neurologic system), adequate range of motion, strength, appropriate bone structure and composition, and intact sensation (proprioception). As suggested by Campbell, the development of a motor pattern (in this case walking) "depends on a combination of mechanical [including structural], neurologic, cognitive, and perceptual factors." A brief description of the biomechanical and neurologic factors that contribute to the development and refinement of walking follows.

Neurologic Factors

Campbell (see Chapter 1) and Bradley (see Chapter 2) have already discussed the primary neurologic factors related to walking and other motor tasks. To briefly review, the basic neural organization and function used to execute locomotion is thought to be controlled by a central pattern generator located either in the spinal cord or in the brain stem (Grillner, 1981). Descending neural input activates the central pattern generator (Jordan, 1986), while descending and peripheral input (Armstrong, 1986; Loeb, 1986) modify the output to adapt the execution. The central pattern generator is believed to organize the activation and firing sequence of muscles during gait. The parallels between developing animals and humans, and the parallels between the sequencing and timing of infant stepping, kicking, and locomotion (Forssberg, 1985; Thelen, 1986; Thelen & Cooke, 1987; Thelen & Ulrich, 1991; Zelazo, 1983), have led individuals to suggest that the neural foundations for locomotion are present at a very early stage in prenatal development (Bradley & Bekoff, 1989). Postnatally, the major periods of accelerated brain growth in relation to body growth occur between 3 and 10 months of age (Epstein, 1979), and the myelination that develops during this time likely contributes to the neural organization required for independent locomotion.

Mechanical Factors

Adequate range of motion, strength, appropriate bone structure and composition, and body composition also affect the emergence of locomotion and its refinement. Gajdosik and Gajdosik present an extensive review of musculoskeletal development and adaptation in Chapter 4. These variables have significant ramifications as mechanical factors in the development of walking. Range of motion, strength, and bony structure of the lower extremities affect the early patterns of walking. In the presence of normal motor control and maturation, constraints in any of these mechanical variables change patterns; as the constraints change so do the movement and the muscle activity depicting motor control. Kugler and colleagues (1982) suggest that changes seen in the development of many skills may be the result of critical dimension changes in the body of the growing child.

Determinants of Walking

Sutherland and colleagues (1980) have identified five important determinants of mature walking. The determinants distinguish walking that is considered "mature" (age 3 years and older) from walking that is "immature" (age 2½ years and younger). The most important of the 13 variables analyzed were the duration of single-limb stance, walking velocity, cadence, step length, and the ratio of pelvic span to ankle spread. The variable with the least discriminating power was the presence or absence of a heel strike at initial contact.

The duration of single-limb stance is, as the name implies, the length of time during which only one foot is on the ground during stance phase. As a child's walking pattern matures the duration of single-limb stance increases, implying a measure of increasing stability and increasing control. The most rapid change occurs between ages 1½ and 3½ years.

Step length is defined as the longitudinal distance between the two feet. It is a parameter closely related to changes in height and leg length. Step length increases throughout childhood until growth is complete. A linear relationship between step length and leg length is present from age 1 to age 7. A linear relationship between step length and age exists from age 1 to age 4.

Walking velocity increases with age from age 1 to age 7, although the rate of change decreases from age 4 to age 7. A child and an adult can often walk at a similar velocity if a child has an increased cadence, or takes more steps per minute than the

TABLE 3–1. **CHANGES IN TIME AND DISTANCE PARAMETERS AT SELECTED AGES FROM THE ONSET OF WALKING THROUGH AGE 7**

Time and Distance Parameters	Age			
	1 YEAR	1½ YEARS	3 YEARS	7 YEARS
Opposite toe-off (% cycle)	17	18	16	12
Opposite foot-strike (% cycle)	49	50	50	50
Single stance (% cycle)	32	32	35	38
Toe-off (% cycle)	67	68	66	62
Step length (cm)	22	25	33	48
Stride length (cm)	43	50	67	97
Cycle time (sec)	0.68	0.70	0.77	0.83
Cadence (steps/min)	176	171	154	144
Walking velocity				
(cm/sec)	64	71	86	114
(m/min)	38.4	42.6	51.6	68.4

Modified from Sutherland, DH, Olshen, RA, Biden, EN, & Wyatt, MP. The Development of Mature Walking. London: Mac Keith Press, 1988.

adult. Cadence gradually decreases with age throughout childhood. The most rapid reduction in cadence occurs between the ages of 1 and 2 years.

The changes with respect to age in these and other determinants are found in Table 3–1. These determinants will be discussed as the refinement of walking is described at various ages.

Refinement of Gait by Age

BIRTH TO AGE 9 MONTHS

The disproportionate contribution of fat content to overall increases in body mass over the first 8 months of postnatal life causes infants to be relatively weak during a time when they are developing the motor control and coordination skills to progress toward independent ambulation (Thelen et al., 1982, 1984). From birth to 6 months of age, body fat of the infant rises from 12% to 25% of body mass (Spady, 1989). Adipose tissue is a major component of weight gain during the first 4 months of postnatal life, with increases in lipids accounting for more than 40% of total weight gain during this time (Fomon, 1967). Between 4 and 12 months of age increased lipid content accounts for approximately 20% of increased weight. With increasing age and mobility, fat content drops and muscle mass increases.

The body structure of infants as they develop the ability to stand upright with support and to cruise independently affects their posture and movement pattern. Flexion contractures are present at the hips, and range of external rotation is slightly greater than range of internal rotation. Range of hip abduction is slightly increased at 8 to 9 months of age but has been slowly decreasing since birth (Coon et al., 1975; Haas et al., 1973; Phelps et al., 1985; Sutherland et al., 1988; Walker, 1991). Femoral anteversion* (a forward or anterior orientation of the head and neck with respect to the frontal plane) and femoral antetorsion (a twist of the bone in its longitudinal axis) of the hips are both present (Bleck, 1982, 1987; Cusick & Stuberg, 1992; Engel & Staheli, 1974; Fabray et al., 1973). The magnitude of the femoral torsion is 30° to 40°.

Structurally, the knees in the frontal plane exhibit genu varum, or bowing in the tibiofemoral angle (Fig. 3–1) (Salenius & Vankka, 1975; Tachdjian, 1990). The tibia and fibula exhibit neutral alignment about the longitudinal axis, which represents slight internal torsion relative to adult values (Staheli & Engel, 1972; Staheli et al., 1985). A medial inclination of the talotibial articulation is present in the infant, producing an everted talocrural mortise (Bernhardt, 1988; Root et al., 1971; Tachdjian, 1985; Valmassy, 1984). The medial inclination of the joint is manifested in an everted heel position in weight bearing. Supported walking at this age is characterized by wide abduction, external rotation, and flexion at the hips (Bly, 1980), bowed legs, and an everted heel position.

The postural control and development of antigravity muscle strength that are gained over the first 9 months of life are important precursors to the development of independent ambulation. Antigravity strength of the hip flexors in the lower extremities is built early on in the developmental process

---

*Femoral anteversion and femoral antetorsion are often used as synonymous terms in orthopaedic literature to refer to the torsion or the medial twist between the axis of the head and neck and the axis of the femoral condyles.

FIGURE 3–1. An 8-month-old infant with physiologic varus in the tibiofemoral angle.

by kicking from the supine position. Hip extensor strength in both concentric and eccentric types of muscle contractions similar to those used in ambulation begins from activities in the prone position but gradually builds as the infant begins creeping and kneeling activities. Bly describes infants of 8 months of age exhibiting the ability to rise from a kneeling to standing position, which requires hip and knee extension. Cruising builds strength of the hip abductors (Bly, 1980).

By 8 months of age, the visual, proprioceptive, and vestibular systems work together to consistently bring the center of mass back to a stable position after perturbation in a seated position (Woollacott et al., 1989). Needed postural corrections in response to visual flow for a particular skill often predate the development of that skill. (Butterworth & Hicks, 1977; Woollacott et al., 1989). For example, Butterworth and Hicks (1977) demonstrated that infants who could sit alone but could not stand independently exhibited the same appropriate postural adjustments to visual information simulating movement as did infants who were able to walk independently.

AGE 9 TO 15 MONTHS

Lower extremity alignment and body structure at the beginning of ambulation are characterized by a standing posture with a wide base of support and the hips in abduction, flexion, and slight external rotation. The tibias display mild internal torsion, and varus is still present in the tibiofemoral angle; and the heel position in weight bearing remains everted because of the inclination of the mortise joint. The child's center of mass is proportionately closer to the head and upper trunk (at the lower thoracic level) than in an older child, whose center of mass is located at midlumbar level, or than an adult, whose center of mass is located at the sacral level (Palmer, 1944). Although differential growth rates are allowing the head to become relatively smaller than the rest of the body, the head is still relatively large. The ratio of body fat to muscle mass is still high, contributing to weakness relative to the demands of upright posture. Coming upright against the force of gravity puts new demands on muscle strength. Muscles (particularly the hip flexors, knee extensors, and ankle dorsiflexors) must now work in new antigravity positions, which further increases functional weakness. Despite the structural limitations, infants exhibit the necessary postural responses to compensate for visual and support-surface perturbations that are inherent in the task of upright locomotion (Berger et al., 1985; Butterworth & Hicks, 1977; Shumway-Cook & Woollacott, 1985; Thelen et al., 1989; Woollacott et al., 1989).

The base of support in an infant at the beginning of ambulation is wide for both structural and stability reasons. Mediolateral (side to side) stability is achieved, but anteroposterior stability is limited. Progression takes place in the sagittal plane; and if the head moves outside the limits of stability at the base of support, balance is lost.

The rate-limiting factors associated with the ability to demonstrate upright locomotion are 1) sufficient extensor muscle strength to support the body's weight on a single-limb base of support and 2) dynamic balance (Thelen et al., 1989). The critical dimension of the body to be controlled is likely to be the head within the limits of stability of that base of support. The pattern displayed by a beginning walker is similar to that of an experienced walker on a slippery surface (i.e., small steps, a widened base of support, and maintenance of the body and limbs very upright in an extended, stiff position). The work of Sutherland and colleagues (1988) characterizes infant ambulation as consisting of a wide base of support, increased hip and knee flexion, full foot initial contact in plantar flexion, a short stride, increased cadence, and a relative footdrop in swing phase.

Motorically, the initial pattern and execution of the first steps are thought to be related to the patterns used in stepping and kicking during early infancy (Thelen & Cooke, 1987) and may be constrained by this pattern. That is, just as the structural makeup of the body drives the initial posture, so may the primitive generator for kicking and stepping drive the muscle activity for early walking. Both kicking and stepping are alternating reciprocal patterns of movement between the limbs. Each has a flexion phase (in gait, analogous to swing) and an extension phase (in gait, analogous to stance). Thelen and colleagues (1989) suggest that the ability to generate step-like patterns is continuous from the newborn period through independent locomotion and that the pattern demonstrated in beginning upright ambulation is a modified, more flexible version of the earlier patterns that has been modified by changes in strength, neurologic maturation, and the mechanics of upright posture.

The electromyographic (EMG) patterns of activity at the onset of independent ambulation demonstrate significant co-contraction across antagonistic muscle groups—the anterior tibialis and gastrocnemius during swing phase and the quadriceps and hamstrings during stance phase, (Kazai et al., 1976; Okamoto & Kumamoto, 1972; Sutherland et al., 1980, 1988; Thelen & Cooke, 1987). Co-activation patterns result from the need for stability.

As stated previously, Thelen and colleagues suggest that it is not the pattern-generating capabilities or motor control postural abilities that constrain the onset of independent locomotion. Development of sufficient extensor strength is believed to be the critical variable (Thelen et al., 1989). This belief is consistent with other views for the requirements of walking, including stance phase stability (Gage, 1991) and the need to maintain a net extensor muscle support moment as described by Winter (1987, 1990).

AGE 18 TO 24 MONTHS

As the child grows, body structure changes, increases in strength, neurologic maturation, and walking experience all likely play a part in altering the walking pattern. By 18 months of age, the varus angulation of the tibiofemoral angle in the frontal plane has resolved and the limb is straight (Fig. 3–2) (Tachdjian, 1990; see also Chapter 4). No change is noted in excessive femoral antetorsion, although limitation in hip extension range of motion is reduced to an average of 4°, indicating that

FIGURE 3–2. Standing posture of an 18-month-old toddler. The varus in the tibiofemoral angle has resolved, and the limb is straight.

remodeling is underway (Fabray et al., 1973; Phelps et al., 1985). Range of hip abduction is no longer excessive. Because of decreased abduction and improved stability, the base of support has decreased. Dynamic balance and strength have also improved. A heel strike has not consistently emerged in the 18-month-old (Sutherland et al., 1980, 1988), but the lessened base of support allows for more anteroposterior movement over the planted foot. Heel position remains everted (Root et al., 1971; Valmassy, 1984). The viscoelastic and inertial properties of the stretched stance limb begin to be exploited to propel the leg in swing (Thelen & Cooke, 1987). A knee flexion wave begins to emerge during initial stance phase as a heel strike develops and knee extensor contraction absorbs some of the impact of floor contact (Sutherland et al., 1980, 1988). The duration of stance phase remains prolonged and cadence is increased relative to mature gait (see Table 3–1).

The efficiency of locomotion slowly improves during the period from 18 to 24 months of age as the center of mass descends from a position high above the lower extremities to one in close proximity to the chief motor power in the legs. Stability of any body is inversely related to the distance of its center of mass from its base of support. Between the first and second years of life, the legs are growing proportionately longer, becoming the most rapidly increasing dimension of the body. These events bring the center of mass closer to the proximal end of the lower limbs (Palmer, 1944).

Controversy exists over whether heel strike develops as a result of neurologic maturation or gradual changes in body structure, base of support, improved strength, and improved stability (Forssberg, 1985, 1992; Thelen & Cooke, 1987; Thelen et al., 1989). It is likely that each variable is important. A consistent heel strike develops by 24 months of age (Sutherland et al., 1980, 1988). Requirements include refined motor control, strength, and dynamic balance to sustain stability on a small area of contact (the heel). Children with impaired walking ability lack a heel strike at initial contact. This may be caused by either lack of motor control or the inherent choice of maintaining stability by use of a larger area of initial contact (Gage, 1991).

The EMG patterns at this age show decreasing co-contraction in antagonistic muscle groups, implying increased control and stability. The primary changes occur in the duration of stance phase activity (Okamoto & Kumamoto, 1972; Sutherland et al., 1980, 1988). The durations of stance phase quadriceps, medial hamstring, and anterior tibialis muscle activity are all decreased in the 18- to 24-month-old as compared with those seen in the 12-month-old. By the age of 2, the late swing phase/early stance phase activity monitored in the gastroc-soleus complex of the 12- to 18-month-old child has disappeared (Sutherland et al., 1980, 1988).

AGE 3 TO 3½ YEARS

Between the ages of 3 and 3½ years, the joint angles associated with walking mature into the adult pattern (Sutherland et al., 1980, 1988). Structurally, the tibiofemoral angle, which was neutral at 18 months of age, now shows maximum valgus alignment (Salenius & Vankka, 1975) (Fig. 3–3). Femoral antetorsion of the hip is decreasing but remains increased in relation to that measured in an adult. The center of mass is closer to the extremities as the rate of lower extremity growth stabilizes (Palmer, 1944). Heel eversion in weight bearing can still be observed but is decreasing. Measurement by motion analysis demonstrates that a heel strike is consistently present in conjunction with a knee

FIGURE 3–3. The tibiofemoral alignment of a 3-year-old showing maximum physiologic valgus.

flexion wave in early stance (Sutherland et al., 1980, 1988). EMG activity has a mature pattern by this age.

AGE 6 TO 7 YEARS

By the age of 7, the gait patterns by standards of movement or motion are fully mature. Minimal changes are noted when compared with the adult pattern, although time and distance variables continue to vary with age and stature (Sutherland et al., 1980, 1988). Balance and postural control have passed to renewed stability after a period of disequilibrium often seen between the ages of 4 and 6 years of age (Shumway-Cook & Woollacott, 1985; Woollacott et al., 1989). Structurally, the tibiofemoral angle has returned to neutral (Tachdjian, 1990), and femoral antetorsion is largely resolved but still slightly higher than measured in the adult (Bleck, 1987; Fabray et al., 1973). The inclination of the talotibial joint is no longer present, and heel position is neutral by age 7 (Valmassy, 1984). A period of disproportionate growth with respect to body dimensions has also passed. The center of mass is still slightly higher than in the adult, at the level of the third lumbar vertebra (Palmer, 1944).

COMPONENTS OF NORMAL GAIT AS MEASURED BY GAIT ANALYSIS

As stated previously, extensive research has been done and continues to be done in the area of gait. Numerous textbooks and basic research articles have been written on the topic (Gage, 1991; Gillette Children's Hospital, 1993; Inman et al., 1981; Ounpuu et al., 1991; Perry, 1992; Rose, SA, et al., 1991; Rose, SA, et al., in press; Sepulveda et al., 1993; Sutherland, 1984; Sutherland et al., 1980, 1988; Winter, 1979, 1983, 1987, 1990; Zajac & Gordon, 1989). This section describes the normal components of mature walking as identified by three-dimensional computerized analysis of movement and forces, electromyography, and energy expenditure in a functional context.

One complete gait cycle refers to a single stride that begins when one foot strikes the ground and ends when the same foot strikes the ground again. The gait cycle is divided into two major phases—stance and swing. Stance phase is associated with the period of time when the foot is on the ground; swing phase is the period of time when the foot is in the air. The stance phase of the gait cycle occupies approximately 60% of the cycle, and the swing phase occupies approximately 40%.

Perry and colleagues (1992) developed a generic terminology for the functional phases of gait that further divided the gait cycle into eight subphases. Each subphase has a functional objective that assists in the accomplishment of one of three basic tasks of the walking cycle: weight acceptance, single-limb support, and limb advancement (Rancho Los Amigos Medical Center, 1989). The basic tasks that Perry's group described are similar to the "attributes" discussed by Gage (1991): weight acceptance and single-limb support (stability in stance and pre-positioning of the foot for initial contact); limb advancement (foot clearance in swing, pre-positioning of the foot for initial contact, and adequate step length).

Stance phase is divided into five subphases or instantaneous events (Fig. 3–4):

1. Initial Contact (0–2% of the cycle)
2. Loading Response (0–10% of the cycle)
3. Midstance (10–30% of the cycle)
4. Terminal Stance (30–50% of the cycle)
5. Preswing (30–60% of the cycle)

Opposite leg toe-off and opposite initial contact occur at 10% and 50% of the gait cycle, respectively.

Thus, there are two periods of double support during the walking cycle when both feet are on the ground. These occur during loading response (just after initial contact) and preswing (just before toe-off). Each occupies approximately 10% of the gait cycle.

Swing phase begins at toe-off and occurs during the period of single support of the stance limb. Three subphases are identified (see Fig. 3–4):

1. Initial Swing (60–73% of the cycle)
2. Midswing (73–87% of the cycle)
3. Terminal Swing (87–100% of the cycle)

Temporal Measurement Definitions and Common Terms

The following definitions will be helpful in the description of walking as used in gait analysis:

Cadence: The frequency of steps taken in a given amount of time, usually measured in steps per minute.

Concentric muscle contraction: A shortening contraction that produces acceleration. Positive work results and power generation occurs.

Eccentric muscle contraction: A lengthening contraction that produces deceleration. Negative work results and power absorption occurs. The efficiency of negative work or power absorption by a muscle is 3 to 9 times higher than that of positive work (Inman et al., 1981).

External load: Ground reaction forces, inertial forces, and gravitational forces that effect joint motion.

Isometric muscle contraction: A stabilizing contraction that produces no net power. Force is produced without length change in the muscle.

Joint moment: A force acting at a distance from an axis causing a rotation about that axis is called a torque or moment (moment = force × perpendicular distance). In the body, moments are produced external to the body by ground reaction forces, forces related to gravity, and inertial forces. Moments internal to the body are produced by muscle forces, ligamentous forces, or forces produced by joint capsules. Joint moments represent the physiologic response of the body generated in response to an external load (Ounpuu et al., 1991).

Joint power: The net rate of energy absorption or generation. Mechanical power is defined as the work performed per unit of time. Joint power is defined as the product of the net joint moment and the joint angular velocity. Muscles are the primary internal power producers in the body.

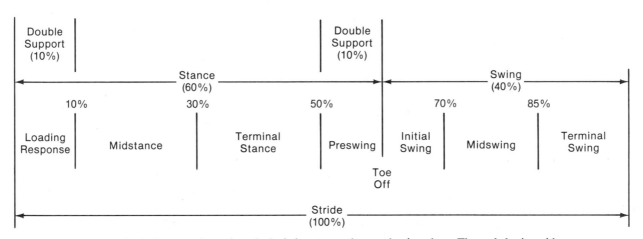

FIGURE 3–4. One complete gait cycle depicting stance phase and swing phase. The cycle begins with initial contact of the right foot. Stance phase has five subphases; swing phase has three subphases. Initial contact and toe-off are instantaneous events. (Adapted from Gage, JR. An overview of normal walking. In Greene, WB (Ed.), Instructional Course Lectures, Vol. 39. Park Ridge, IL: American Academy of Orthopaedic Surgeons, 1990.)

Muscles can also be internal power absorbers. Ligaments usually absorb power.

Kinematics: The parameters used to describe motion without regard to forces. These include linear or angular displacements, velocities, and accelerations.

Kinetics: The parameters that describe the causes of the movement. These include external and internal forces such as gravitational forces, ground reaction forces, inertial forces, muscle or ligament forces, joint moments, and joint powers.

Step length: The longitudinal distance between the two feet. Right step length is measured from the first point of contact of the left foot to the first point of contact of the right foot.

Stride length: The longitudinal distance between the initial contact of one foot and the next initial contact of the same foot. It is the sum of the right

and left step lengths and the distance traversed in one complete gait cycle.

Walking velocity: The rate of walking or the distance traversed in a specified length of time. Velocity can be expressed as stride length divided by cycle time or the product of step length and cadence.

Kinematics

Kinematics in gait analysis can be collected in either two or three dimensions. Common to all types of computerized motion analysis is a reference system such as the use of markers that are placed on the body and aligned with respect to specific anatomic landmarks. Two-dimensional motion systems provide joint angles that are a direct measure of the motion of the marker set placed on the skin. Three-dimensional systems reference the marker coordinate system to an internal coordinate system based on an estimation of the locations of the anatomic joint centers. The outputs, regard-less of two- or three-dimensional technique, are displayed as a series of graphs of a single gait cycle for each joint in a given plane of motion. Figure 3–5 gives an example of three-dimensional motion data from Gillette Children's Hospital.

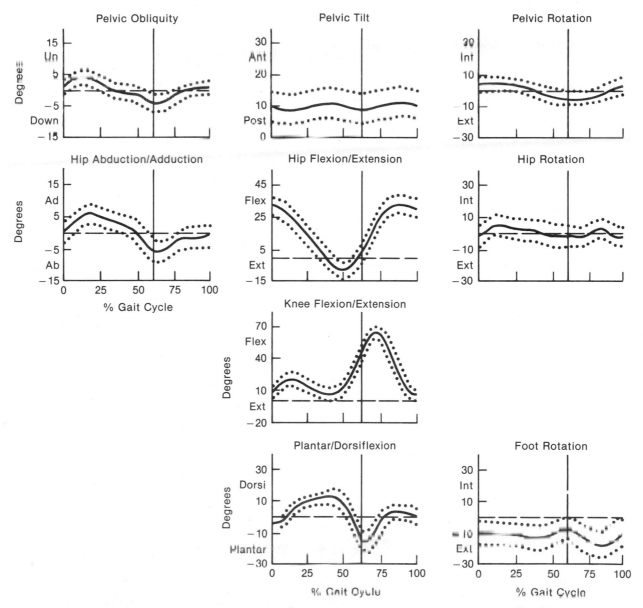

FIGURE 3–5. Representative normal three-dimensional motion data from Gillette Children's Hospital. In this and subsequent normative figures, one complete gait cycle is depicted and is normalized to 100% of the stride. The mean (*solid line*) and one standard deviation (*dotted line*) are displayed of composite data collected from children aged 4 to 19 years of age. Stance phase is separated from swing phase in each graph by the vertical line. Each graph represents the same walking cycle. Each row displays a different joint: from top to bottom are pelvis, hip, knee, and ankle. Each column displays the movements of a different joint in the same plane of motion, from left to right are the coronal plane–front view, sagittal plane–side view, and transverse plane–rotational view. *Note*: The pelvis is measured with respect to laboratory coordinates, the hip with respect to the pelvis, and the knee with respect to the thigh. Foot rotation graph represents foot progression angle, not rotation of the foot with respect to the tibia.

Kinetics

Kinetics represent the parameters that describe the causes of the movement. These include external and internal forces such as gravitational forces, ground reaction forces, inertial forces, muscle or ligament forces, joint moments, and joint powers. Kinetic data as part of two- or three-dimensional analysis are obtained from a combination of force plate and kinematic information and are displayed as joint moments and joint powers. The force plate provides information regarding the ground reaction force, and the kinematics provide information regarding the joint angular velocities. Anthropometric measurements of the body are also required. The method commonly used to calculate joint moments and powers is called *inverse dynamics* and is based on a linked segment model approach (Winter, 1990). A ground reaction force method is another method sometimes used (Winter, 1990).

A moment or torque is a force acting at a distance that causes an object to rotate. A joint moment represents the physiologic response of the body generated in response to an external load (Ounpuu et al., 1991). In my laboratory, what is displayed on the graphs is the net joint moment, which represents the sum of all internal joint moments in a particular plane at a particular joint. The moments refer primarily to the muscle forces that are acting to control segment rotation, but internal joint moments can be generated by ligaments as well. The net joint moment depicts which muscle group is dominant but does not denote the relative contributions of muscle groups on either side of the joint. For example, in the sagittal plane,

a net extensor moment at the hip during stance phase implies that the hip extensors are dominant. Hip flexors may or may not contribute, but the overall moment is an extensor moment. The hip extensor muscles are active to counteract an external moment created by the ground reaction force that is tending to flex the hip (Fig. 3–6). The ground reaction force tends to flex the hip because it is anterior to the joint center.

Power, in mechanical terms, is defined as the rate of doing work. Joint power is defined as the net joint moment multiplied by the joint angular velocity. Muscles are the primary internal power producers in the body. A muscle's ability to produce power is affected by its cross-sectional area. Other factors that affect power include fiber type, the length–tension ratio, and the degree of fatigue (see Chapter 4). Muscles can also be internal power absorbers. Ligaments usually absorb power. The power graphs display whether power is generated (positive work) or absorbed (negative work). Concentric muscle action is associated with power generation, and eccentric muscle action is associated with power absorption. In the previous example of the hip, the hip is extending in the presence of a net extensor moment; therefore, power generation occurs (Fig. 3–7). Normal sagittal plane kinematics and kinetics can be found in Figure 3–8.

Electromyography

The electrical signal associated with the neuromuscular activation of a muscle is measured by electromyography (Basmajian & DeLuca, 1985;

FIGURE 3–6. An example of an internal joint moment produced at the right hip. Because the ground reaction force falls anterior to the hip joint, the joint would flex without internally produced resistance. The joint moment graph demonstrates a net extensor moment at the hip (*shaded*) as the body's internal resistance to the external force. The internal moment is produced by dominant action of the hip extensor muscles. (Adapted in part from Gage, JR. Gait Analysis in Cerebral Palsy. London: Mac Keith Press, 1991.)

FIGURE 3–7 An example of power generation at the right hip. Because the hip is extending and a net extensor moment is present, power generation (*shaded*) occurs. The units for power are watts per kilogram. By convention, power generation is represented by positive deflection on the graph; power absorption is negative. (Adapted in part from Gage, JR. Gait Analysis in Cerebral Palsy. London: Mac Keith Press, 1991.)

Winter, 1990). Electromyographic data can provide information about the timing of muscle activity and, in some cases, about the intensity of muscle contraction. Under some conditions EMG amplitude has been shown to be related to force (Komi, 1973; Vredenbregt & Rau, 1973), but the usefulness of this aspect for assessment of walking is limited because the relationship is valid only under isometric conditions and when no co-activation is occurring. The amplitude of an EMG signal is affected by many factors, including electrode location, type of electrode used, interelectrode distance, skin temperature, and amount of subcutaneous fat (Basmajian & DeLuca, 1985). Comparing EMG amplitudes across muscles, or within or between subjects, should be done with caution and adequate understanding of the complexity involved in interpretation. Current research focuses on understanding the relationship of muscle activity and muscle force with joint kinematics and joint powers using engineering principles (Zajac & Gordon, 1989). Combining engineering principles with neural network representations is advancing the understanding of the effects of EMG activity even further (Sepulveda et al., 1993).

Each muscle has a particular time during the walking cycle when activity is present or absent, and these periods have been documented for both children and adults (Ounpuu et al., 1991; Perry, 1992; Sutherland et al., 1988; Winter & Yack,

1987). An example can be found in Figure 3–9. EMG data can be collected using surface or fine wire (indwelling) electrodes. Reviews on the advantages and disadvantages of each have been published (Kadaba et al., 1985).

KINEMATICS, KINETICS, AND ELECTROMYOGRAPHY IN NORMAL GAIT

A detailed description of activity in the lower extremities during each phase of the gait cycle is now presented, including a summary of hip, knee, and ankle kinematics and kinetics with associated muscle activity. Sagittal plane events are emphasized. The reader should refer to the kinematic and kinetic plots.

Sagittal Plane

At *initial contact* (0% of the gait cycle) the ankle is in a position of neutral dorsiflexion, the knee is in minimal flexion, and the hip is in approximately 35° of flexion. The objective of this event is appropriate pre-positioning of the foot to begin the gait cycle. The ground reaction force at initial contact is passing through the heel and is anterior to both the

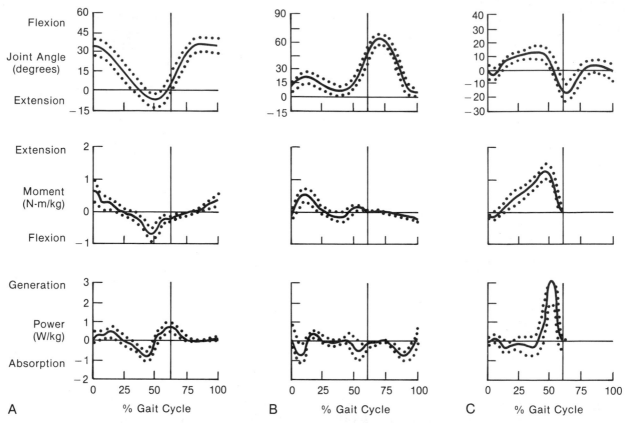

FIGURE 3-8. Sagittal plane kinematics and kinetics of the hip (**A**), knee (**B**), and ankle (**C**). Each graph represents the same walking cycle, with the mean (*solid line*) and ±1 standard deviation (*dashed line*). The top row shows the kinematic graphs; the middle row, the joint moments; and the bottom row, the joint powers. Units for the kinematics are degrees. The units for joint moments (newton-meters/kilogram) and powers (watts/kilogram) are standardized for body weight.

knee and the hip. The gluteus maximus and hamstrings are active to control the external flexor moment at the hip. The hamstrings also assist in preventing knee hyperextension. Anterior tibialis and quadriceps activity initiates the loading response (Fig. 3–10).

Loading response (Fig. 3–11) is a period of acceptance of body weight while maintaining stability and progression. The purpose of loading response is to cushion or absorb the impact of the body's moment of inertia. It is the first period of double support and occurs between 0 and 10% of the gait cycle, beginning after initial contact and ending when the entire foot is in contact with the floor. The ankle is plantar flexing at this time under controlled eccentric contraction of the anterior tibialis muscle. The dominant internal moment at the ankle is a dorsiflexor moment because the dorsiflexor muscles are dominant. The power curve depicts absorption because the anterior tibialis muscle is contracting eccentrically. Gage (1991) refers

to loading response as the first "rocker" of ankle stance phase.

The knee undergoes an initial phase of flexion to approximately 15° (average value). Both hamstring activity and quadriceps muscle activity are present. Because the quadriceps muscles are acting eccentrically to decelerate knee flexion, the power graph depicts absorption. Whenever the joint movement and the joint moment are opposite from each other, power absorption is occurring.

The hip during loading response is extending by concentric action of the hip extensor muscles (gluteus maximus, gluteus minimus, and hamstrings). The hamstrings are able to work as hip extensors because knee motion is stabilized by the single joint muscles of the quadriceps. The internal moment is extensor, and the power graph depicts generation. Because the external ground reaction force falls anterior to the hip joint, without the action of the hip extensors the joint would collapse into flexion.

Midstance (Fig. 3–12) is the beginning of the

Normal Electromyographic Data

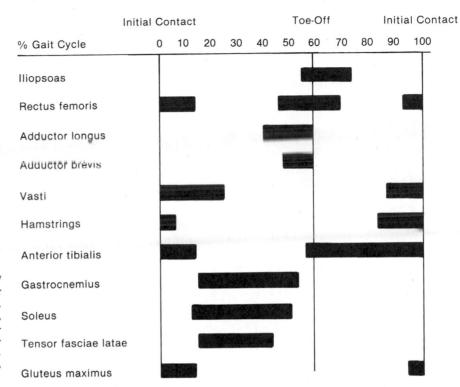

FIGURE 3–9. The phasic (on/off) EMG activity of the major muscles used during walking. (Adapted from Ounpuu, S, Gage, JR, & Davis, RB. Three-dimensional lower extremity joint kinetics in normal pediatric gait. Journal of Pediatric Orthopaedics, *11*:341–349, 1991, p. 344.)

FIGURE 3–10. Initial contact of the gait cycle. (From Gage, JR. Gait Analysis in Cerebral Palsy. London: Mac Keith Press, 1991.)

single-support phase of the gait cycle and extends from the period of 10 to 30% of the cycle. The goal during midstance is to maintain trunk and limb stability and allow smooth progression over a stationary foot when the entire plantar surface is in contact with the floor. The ankle is in a period of increasing dorsiflexion that is controlled by eccentric contraction of the soleus muscle. The moment graph demonstrates a dominant plantar flexor moment and the power graph a period of absorption. The second rocker of ankle stance phase occurs during midstance (Gage, 1991).

The knee extends during midstance. The vastus medialis, vastus intermedius, and vastus lateralis muscles work initially to stabilize the knee until the ground reaction force passes anterior to the knee joint. Once the ground reaction force is anterior to the knee, extension is passive. The joint moment at the knee is an extensor moment. The power graph shows initial decreasing absorption followed by generation. This period of power generation is the only one produced at the knee during the entire gait cycle.

The hip is also extending during midstance. The joint moment is extensor, and power is generated, implicating concentric action of the hip extensor muscles. The internal extension moment, however,

FIGURE 3–11. Loading response (0–10% of the gait cycle). (*A* adapted from Gage, JR. Gait Analysis in Cerebral Palsy. London: Mac Keith Press, 1991.)

is decreasing during this time. When the ground reaction force becomes posterior to the hip joint, a transition occurs from a concentric (power generation) extensor moment to an eccentric (power absorption) flexor moment.

Terminal stance (Fig. 3–13) is the second half of

the single-support phase and occurs from 30 to 50% of the gait cycle. This period begins when the ground reaction force passes anterior to the knee and posterior to the hip and often occurs with heel rise. During this phase of the gait cycle, forward progression of the tibia is arrested and further in-

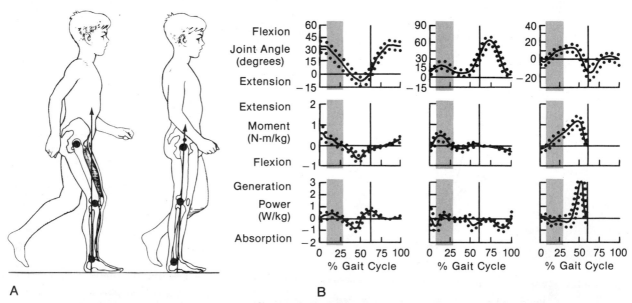

FIGURE 3–12. Midstance (at 10–30% of the gait cycle). (*A* adapted from Gage, JR. An overview of normal walking. In Greene, WB [Ed.], Instructional Course Lectures. Vol. 39. Park Ridge, IL: American Academy of Orthopaedic Surgeons, 1990.)

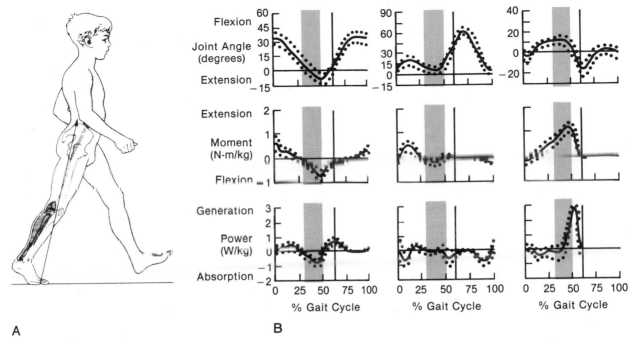

FIGURE 3–13. Terminal stance (at 30–50% of the gait cycle). (*A* adapted from Gage, JR. Gait Analysis in Cerebral Palsy. London: Mac Keith Press, 1991.)

crease in dorsiflexion is limited. The ankle begins a period of decreasing dorsiflexion by concentric contraction of the gastrocnemius and soleus muscles, producing power generation. One of the primary power productions that propels an individual through the walking cycle is generated at the ankle during terminal stance (36% of the total power generation produced during the walking cycle) (Ounpuu et al., 1991; Winter, 1987). Heel rise marks the period of the third rocker of ankle stance phase (Gage, 1991).

The knee moves from relative extension to increasing flexion during terminal stance. An internal flexor moment is dominant because the ground reaction force falls in front of the knee. Power is absorbed. The internal flexor moment is probably produced by a combination of ligamentous resistance and flexor activity of the gastrocnemius muscle.

The hip continues to extend during terminal stance. Because the ground reaction force is posterior to the joint center, extension is resisted by an internal flexor moment. Power is absorbed, suggesting that the flexor moment is produced by tension force of the iliofemoral ligament.

Preswing (Fig. 3–14) is the second period of double support during the walking cycle and occurs at 50 to 60% of the cycle. The function of preswing is to advance the limb into swing; preswing ends at toe-off. The stance phase extremity is unweighted as weight is accepted on the opposite limb. The

ankle is now in true plantar flexion, and the plantar flexor moment remains dominant. The magnitude of the moment is rapidly decreasing, however, and power generation falls rapidly to zero.

The knee joint is flexing during preswing and reaches approximately 45° (average value) at toe-off. The internal muscle moment is extensor, and power is absorbed. Activity of the rectus femoris muscle is probably responsible for this activity and assists the deceleration of the moment of inertia of the shank.

The hip begins to flex in preswing. The dominant moment is a flexor moment, and power is generated. Concentric action of the hip flexor muscles, primarily the iliopsoas, produces the activity. Occasionally the rectus femoris muscle is active to augment hip flexion. This usually occurs at faster walking speeds. Peak flexor power of the hip is generated at toe-off. Hip musculature (both extensors and flexors) is responsible for the majority of positive work performed during the walking cycle (56%), with most being produced during stance phase (Ounpuu et al., 1991).

The objective of *initial swing* (Fig. 3–13) is foot clearance and limb advancement. Initial swing occurs from 60 to 73% of the gait cycle. Maximum plantar flexion occurs at the ankle in initial swing. At the same time, peak knee flexion occurs, uniquely timed for optimal clearance of the foot. The ankle then begins to dorsiflex by activity of the anterior tibialis muscle. The dominant muscle mo-

FIGURE 3–14. Preswing (at 50–60% of the gait cycle). (*A* adapted from Gage, JR. Gait Analysis in Cerebral Palsy. London: Mac Keith Press, 1991.)

FIGURE 3–15. Initial swing (at 60–73% of the gait cycle). (*A* adapted from Gage, JR. An overview of normal walking. In Greene, WB [Ed.], Instructional Course Lectures. Vol. 39. Park Ridge, IL: American Academy of Orthopaedic Surgeons, 1990.)

FIGURE 3-16. Midswing (at 73-87% of the gait cycle). (*A* adapted from Gage, JR. An overview of normal walking. In Greene, WB [Ed.], Instructional Course Lectures. Vol. 39. Park Ridge, IL: American Academy of Orthopaedic Surgeons, 1990.)

ment is a dorsiflexor moment. Power output is negligible.

The hip flexes during initial swing, which also assists foot clearance. A flexor moment remains dominant, and power generation is occurring by concentric activity of the hip flexors.

The goals of *midswing* (Fig. 3-16) remain foot clearance and limb advancement, and it occurs between 73 and 87% of the gait cycle. The ankle is dorsiflexing during this time by concentric action of the anterior tibialis muscle. The knee is extending by inertial forces without muscle activity. The hip is flexing.

The primary purpose of *terminal swing* (Fig. 3-17) is pre-positioning of the limb for weight acceptance. This phase occupies the period between 87 and 100% of the gait cycle. The ankle begins to plantar flex by eccentric action of the anterior tibialis muscle to position the ankle in neutral. A flexor moment is dominant at the knee with power absorption as knee extension is controlled by eccentric action of the hamstrings to decelerate the forward swing of the thigh. The quadriceps muscles also become active to assist with control of the

knee. Minimal movement is noted at the hip at this time.

Coronal Plane

The function of hip and pelvis motion in the coronal plane is to minimize the vertical excursion of the center of mass (Figs. 3-5 and 3-18). At initial contact the pelvis in the coronal plane is level and the hip is in neutral abduction and adduction. The stance side of the pelvis rises 5° at the beginning of loading response in conjunction with adduction of the stance limb. The dropping of the pelvis on the unsupported limb is caused by the ground reaction force on the supported limb, which produces an external adduction moment at hip, knee, and ankle. The external adduction moment is resisted by eccentric control of the hip abductors. This allows the stance side of the pelvis to rise and the unsupported side to drop.

The pelvis and hip motion reverses in midstance as concentric control by the hip abductors of the

A   B

FIGURE 3–17. Terminal swing (at 87–100% of the gait cycle). (*A* adapted from Gage, JR. An overview of normal walking. In Greene, WB [Ed.], Instructional Course Lectures, Vol. 39. Park Ridge, IL: American Academy of Orthopaedic Surgeons, 1990.)

stance limb act to raise the pelvis. This action assists clearance on the swing side. During preswing the hip on the stance side goes into abduction in preparation for toe-off.

Transverse Plane

The end result of transverse plane motion is stride elongation (see Fig. 3–5). This is accomplished by internal pelvis and hip rotation under the control of the adductor magnus muscle. During the first half of stance phase internal rotation occurs at the pelvis and hip that reverses in the last half of stance. The pelvis is at its maximum posterior position at toe-off. The foot is positioned 5 to 10° (average value) external to the line of progression throughout the entire walking cycle.

Energy Expenditure

The purpose of many of the motion events in the walking cycle in all three planes of motion is to minimize energy expenditure or reduce the vertical translation of the center of mass. Gage (1991) includes energy conservation as one of the five attributes of normal gait and states that variation in this attribute encompasses the deviations of the other four attributes.

The mechanisms that the body uses to conserve energy are minimizing the excursion of the center of mass, control of momentum, and active or passive transfer of energy between body segments. The vertical and horizontal displacements of the center of mass are almost sinusoidal and are equal and opposite during typical walking (Winter, 1987). The body accomplishes this through the three pelvic rotations (rotation, tilt, and obliquity) and coordinated knee and ankle motion. Inman and colleagues (1981) demonstrated that without pelvic rotation and with stiff limbs, the center of mass of the body would be lifted approximately 9.5 cm with each step. Normal vertical excursion of the body averages approximately 4.5 cm.

Determination of energy expenditure in gait has been a topic of research since the 1950s (Coates & Meade, 1960; Passmore & Durnin, 1955; Ralston, 1958). Ralston (1958) hypothesized that individuals naturally select a speed of walking that allows a minimum of energy expenditure. If true, this has direct implications for the child with a motor impairment. His research suggested that energy expenditure during walking is directly proportional to the square of velocity.

Research by Waters and associates (1988) includes information on energy expenditure in children. A linear relationship between velocity and rate of oxygen consumption is described, but the data fail to include velocities below 40 m/min or a reference zero velocity data collection. Data collected at my laboratory are consistent with Ralston's research and demonstrate that the rate of oxygen consumption varies with the square of velocity (Koop, SE, & Stout, JL, 1991, unpublished data). These data include standing zero velocity resting values and data collected at walking velocities below 40 m/min (Fig. 3–19A). Preschool children are found to be less efficient than either school-aged children or teenagers (Fig. 3–19B).

An alternative to the use of measuring oxygen consumption to estimate energy expenditure involves calculation of the mechanical work required for walking. Kinematic measurements, anthropometric measurements, and kinetic analyses of internal and external loads are required for use of this method (Olney et al., 1990; Winter, 1990). The advantage of mechanical energy estimation is that the energy requirements of individual joints can be calculated. One of the disadvantages, particularly in the assessment of pathologic gait, is that the use of external loads to judge the work associated with walking does not measure the body's ability to efficiently respond to the external loads. Co-contraction associated with spasticity is unaccounted for (Rose, SA, et al., 1991).

Heart rate is often used as a substitute clinical measure for oxygen uptake and therefore metabolic energy expenditure because of the linear relationship of heart rate to oxygen uptake (Rose, J, et al., 1989, 1990). However, low mechanical efficiency

FIGURE 3–18. Coronal plane hip joint kinetics. (From Gage, JR. Gait Analysis in Cerebral Palsy. London: Mac Keith Press, 1991.)

FIGURE 3–19. (A) Normative values of the rate of metabolic oxygen consumption versus velocity for 150 children 2 to 19 years of age. The units for oxygen consumption are standardized for body weight. The mean and ±2 standard deviations are displayed. (B) Mean values for three age groups: 2–5-year-olds, 6–12-year-olds, and 13–19-year-olds. Unpublished data collected at Gillette Children's Hospital.

creates disproportionately high submaximal heart rates in individuals with cerebral palsy, making submaximal heart rate a poor predictor of aerobic capacity (Bar-Or, 1983). I have observed high and inconsistent heart rate in relation to oxygen uptake in various clinical populations including cerebral palsy. Caution should be taken if consideration is being given to this method of estimation of energy expenditure. See Chapter 5 for more information on aerobic capacity.

USE OF GAIT ANALYSIS IN ASSESSING PATHOLOGY

Gait analysis is a useful tool in assessing walking pathology in children with physical disabilities because it provides objective measurement of the magnitude of deviations. It also allows the interpreter to analyze data from all planes of motion for a single gait cycle. Just as computed tomography has improved on radiography, gait analysis improves on the evaluator's clinical examination and visual observation. Gait analysis data in the hands of a critical evaluator should never be used in isolation. Clinical assessment by a physician, physical therapist, or trained kinesiologist is a vital part of the evaluation. The goals of the family for treatment are important as well.

A gait analysis laboratory should be considered a measurement tool. Information from a gait laboratory can assist in differentiation of primary impairments from secondary compensations. Primary impairments are those abnormalities that are a direct result of the central nervous system injury; secondary compensations refer to the mechanisms used by the individual to circumvent the primary abnormalities. In addition to use in treatment of conditions such as cerebral palsy and myelomeningocele, gait data can also be used to assess the effects on walking of orthotic devices in various populations or of different prosthetic devices in individuals with amputations. Gait analysis at repetitive intervals can assist in the assessment of the progression of a particular deformity or condition or the effects of a particular controlled treatment regimen (including surgery, medication, or physical therapy). With the use of gait laboratory data alone, however, it is often difficult to assist in developing specific physical therapy recommendations. The gait laboratory assessment typically includes only a limited physical evaluation and is not a complete physical therapy assessment. The EMG information from most gait laboratories does not provide information about strength of muscle contraction and cannot be used to determine which muscles are

to be strengthened and how. A thorough knowledge of muscle mechanics and normal gait combined with manual muscle testing allows the therapist to answer these questions. However, EMG activity can determine if muscle activity is present or absent and the timing of that muscle activity, which can be useful to determine if a particular muscle is available for strengthening and what the consequences of that strengthening might be. Kinetic analysis does provide moment and power information that is sometimes useful for this purpose. In summary, the gait laboratory can be an objective measuring tool for the physical therapist.

Returning to the prerequisites for development of any skill, gait pathology can be created by abnormal motor control, spasticity, loss of range of motion, decreased strength, loss of sensation, and bony deformity. Each can result in primary impairments as well as secondary compensatory mechanisms used to produce or to maintain useful function. Gait analysis can be used to distinguish between the two. It can be used to identify areas of bony abnormality and loss of functional range of motion and to document areas of relative weakness or spasticity. The information is always used in conjunction with a clinical evaluation. The use of gait analysis in assessment of impairments in cerebral palsy is discussed here as an example of how information is used and interpreted. Limitations of gait analysis are also discussed. Gait analysis is in no way limited to assessment of cerebral palsy or any one gait pathology.

Common Gait Abnormalities in Cerebral Palsy

BONY DEFORMITIES

Bony deformities are assessed best by clinical examination and radiography. Gait analysis data measure the functional effect of the bony deformity on the child's walking. Bony deformities are examples of secondary impairments because they are not caused directly by the central nervous system lesion. They can result from failure of physiologic bone remodeling as a result of weight bearing, the effects of spasticity and muscle imbalance, disuse, attempts to function, or any combination of these factors. These deformities are often seen in the transverse plane. Once they have occurred they become a primary focus for orthopaedic treatment because they cannot be corrected by conservative management. True bony deformity cannot be corrected by physical therapy. Three common bony abnormalities seen in children with cerebral palsy are femoral anteversion, external tibial torsion, and subtalar joint breakdown.

Excessive Femoral Antetorsion (Internal Femoral Torsion). Visually, excessive femoral antetorsion appears as internal rotation of the femurs during walking and is measured as such on kinematic analysis. Antetorsion is a true structural torsion or twist deformity of the femur. The cause is a combination of lack of resolution of physiologic antetorsion of the infant because of delayed weight bearing or abnormal muscle forces created by spasticity (Bleck, 1987; Gage, 1991). Femoral torsion is not synonymous with valgus angulation of the femoral neck shaft angle, which is a separate hip disorder. Antetorsion can be clinically measured by the degree of internal femoral rotation in the prone position when the greater trochanter is palpated to be most lateral or parallel to the supporting surface. Usually in the presence of internal femoral torsion there is loss of passive external rotation range and the range of internal rotation is excessive; often the

ratio of internal to external rotation is equal to or greater than 3:1 (Fig. 3–20).

External Tibial Torsion. External tibial torsion is an external rotation or torsion of the long axis of the tibia. It is measured most appropriately by physical evaluation of the transmalleolar axis or thigh-foot axis and not by gait analysis, unless the system used measures the rotation of the foot with respect to the tibia. External tibial torsion is a true bony deformity that develops as a compensation to femoral anteversion or limited knee motion and causes repetitive dragging of the foot in an externally rotated posture for clearance. In the presence of femoral anteversion, external tibial torsion is difficult to observe visually because the foot progression angle may not appear abnormal. The knee sometimes has a valgus appearance, but it is not a coronal plane abnormality (Fig. 3–21). The internal torsion of the femur is compensated by external

FIGURE 3–20. An example of kinematic graphs from (**A**) a 10-year-old child with spastic diplegic cerebral palsy compared with (**B**) normative data for pelvic and hip rotation and foot progression. Results of bony deformity are often seen in the transverse or rotational plane. Graphs for the child with cerebral palsy depict the right side (*solid line*) and the left side (*dashed line*) for a representative gait cycle. The normative graphs display the mean (*solid line*) and 1 standard deviation (*dashed line*). The hip rotation graph in the child with cerebral palsy shows bilateral internal hip rotation. The foot rotation graph displays an appropriate external foot progression on the right side (*solid line*) despite internal hip rotation on the right side. This could result from either subtalar joint breakdown or external tibial torsion, or a combination of both. By physical examination this child has bilateral femoral anteversion and a right external tibial torsion.

FIGURE 3–21. A 30-year-old adult with spastic diplegic cerebral palsy. Note the internal hip position on the right side (knee in) and the foot progression angle that is neutral to the line of progression. This individual has an external tibial torsion on the right side.

torsion of the tibia so that the foot remains in the direction of progression (see Fig. 3–20).

Pes Valgus (Subtalar Joint Breakdown). Pes valgus is most common in children with spastic diplegic or spastic quadriplegic types of cerebral palsy and less often occurs in children with spastic hemiplegia. Caused by a relative subluxation of the talus on the os calcis, it usually develops because of abnormal muscle forces with a combination of tightness and weakness. Kinematic data do not identify subtalar joint breakdown. The effect of the deformity is measured in the plantar flexion, dorsiflexion, and foot rotation graphs. Physical and radiographic examination is required.

INADEQUATE RANGE OF MOTION AND SPASTICITY

Gage (1991) often refers to cerebral palsy as a condition that preferentially affects two joint muscles because it is primarily in the two-joint muscles that spasticity contributes to the abnormalities associated with walking. Most two-joint muscles are predominantly fast-twitch muscles used for rapid force production. Loss of range of motion creates static contracture; spasticity imposes loss of range

of motion in dynamic situations because of resistance to stretch (Kruger & Gage, 1986; Rose, SA, et al., in press). The effects of inadequate range of motion and spasticity can be measured in all three planes of motion but are most prevalently seen in the sagittal plane. Examples measured by gait analysis are an abnormal plantar flexion–knee extension couple, crouch gait, and limited swing-phase knee motion.

Abnormal Plantar Flexion–Knee Extension Couple. During normal walking, the plantar flexion–knee extension couple is a force couple whereby the soleus and the gastrocnemius muscles control forward momentum and the forward progression of the ground reaction force by eccentric contraction. Children with cerebral palsy often enter the walking cycle with a footflat initial contact, which rapidly places the gastrocnemius under premature tension at both ends of the muscle. Gage (1991) postulated that in response to the stretch, spasticity is elicited that can restrict tibial advancement, produce knee extension (hyperextension), and reduce the extent of dorsiflexion (plantar flexion). The spastic response is revealed in a bi-phasic pattern during stance phase of increasing dorsiflexion and then decreasing dorsiflexion in the kinematics and by an abnormal plantar flexor power generation coincident in time with the first decrease of dorsiflexion in the cycle in the kinetics. Occasionally, the EMG activity is bi-phasic as well (Fig. 3–22). The functional significance of this abnormal power generation is unclear, but, theoretically, it elevates the body's center of mass.

Crouched Posture. Caused by hip flexion contractures or tightness, knee flexion contractures or tightness, excessive plantar flexor weakness or any combination, increased flexion is seen at all joints in the sagittal plane (Fig. 3–23).

Limited Swing-Phase Knee Motion. Limitation of motion at the knee in swing phase usually begins in preswing, where motion is also inadequate. Momentum for swing phase in normal gait is generated by the acceleration force of the gastrocnemius muscle that drives the ground reaction force behind the knee. When the gastrocnemius force generation is reduced, as is often the case in cerebral palsy, the hip flexors supply the momentum to clear the extremity. The rectus femoris is often recruited as a hip flexor. If this muscle is spastic it maintains its action as a knee extensor. The already diminished knee flexion in preswing is further inhibited by spastic restraint that does not allow further knee flexion (see Fig. 3–23).

WEAKNESS

Weakness cannot be measured directly by gait analysis. The type of electromyography used does

Patient Data

Normal Data

FIGURE 3–22. Kinematics and kinetics at the ankle joint demonstrating **(A)** an abnormal plantar flexion–knee extension couple in a child with cerebral palsy compared with **(B)** normal. The ankle kinematic of the patient displays a bi-phasic pattern in stance phase —increasing dorsiflexion-decreasing dorsiflexion—that repeats itself. This results in a bi-phasic plantar flexor moment as well, and an inappropriate midstance power generation. **(C)** Surface EMG record from the gastrocsoleus complex also exhibits two bursts of activity coinciding with the power generation.

not provide information regarding strength. Kinematic data measure only the effects; it is up to the clinician to interpret whether the pattern is present as the result of weakness or tightness. Kinetic data do provide a limited measure of weakness if full range of motion is available at the joint. Power can be produced only if joint movement is present. The best measure of strength is by physical assessment, although this is complicated by the presence of spasticity.

Abductor Weakness. Weakness of the hip abductor muscles in cerebral palsy, as in any other type of gait disorder, produces pelvic drop on the swing side and lateral trunk shift over the stance limb. The ground reaction force in the coronal plane produces an external adduction moment at all joints of the stance limb. If abductor strength is insufficient, the lateral trunk shift artificially

creates the abduction moment. Hip abductor muscle weakness is frequently (but not necessarily) seen in children with femoral anteversion because the torsion creates an inadequate lever arm over which the gluteus medius muscle is able to act, imposing functional weakness. On kinematic graphs hip abductor weakness is displayed as increased adduction. Differentiation between hip abductor muscle weakness and hip adductor tightness cannot be done solely using kinematic data.

Gastrocnemius Soleus Weakness. Plantar flexor muscle weakness primarily affects terminal stance and preswing phases of the gait cycle, but midstance is also affected. During midstance, the soleus is not able to control the progression of the ground reaction force that is anterior to the ankle, and excessive dorsiflexion results. Heel rise is delayed in terminal stance because gastrocnemius power may

FIGURE 3–23. Example of a crouched posture of increased hip and knee flexion in the sagittal plane of a 10-year-old child with cerebral palsy (**A**) as compared with normal (**B**). Patient data compare the child's right side (*solid line*) with the left (*dashed line*). The posture at the knee is asymmetric, with increased knee flexion during stance phase on the right side. Swing phase knee flexion is also decreased.

also be insufficient. Excessive dorsiflexion can drive the knees into flexion as well. Quadriceps muscle activity is required to maintain an upright posture, resulting in increased energy expense. Clearance is achieved by "pull off" by the proximal hip flexors because the plantar flexor muscles alone are insufficient. This results in an insufficient acceleration force in terminal stance and imposes a slower velocity.

▌ CONCLUSION

The attributes of normal gait are lost in pathologic conditions such as cerebral palsy because of

the primary impairments of loss of selective motor control and balance, abnormal tone, muscle weakness, and loss of sensation and because of secondary impairments such as bony deformity and loss of range of motion. These prerequisites for any motor function, including gait, develop as the central nervous system matures and the body grows, producing physiologic changes in the mechanics and the neurophysiology of the system.

This chapter was designed to provide an overview of the refinement of gait in childhood, the components of normal gait as measured by gait analysis, and a brief introduction to the use of gait analysis in assessment of gait pathology. A gait laboratory is only a measuring tool and is a supplement, not a substitute, for other tools to assess gait pathology.

Research in the area of gait continues to be a topic of great interest. As measurement techniques improve, our knowledge of walking and its development becomes more refined. With a clear understanding of normal gait, we can better understand the mechanisms of pathologic gait. Here the science of physical therapy melds into the art of physical therapy practice for the children we treat.

Acknowledgments

I would like to thank Dr. Jim Gage and Dr. Steven Koop, whose philosophy and understanding of normal gait and treatment of children with gait pathologies are significant contributions to this chapter. I am privileged to work with both of them.

References

Armstrong, DM. The motor cortex and locomotion in the cat. In Grillner, S, Stein, PSG, Stuart, DG, Forssberg H, Herman, RM, & Wallen, P (Eds.), Neurobiology of Vertebrate Locomotion. London: Macmillan, 1986, pp. 121–137.

Bar-Or, O. Neuromuscular diseases. In Bar-Or, O, Pediatric Sports Medicine for the Practitioner. New York: Springer-Verlag, 1983, pp. 227–249.

Basmajian, JV, & DeLuca, CJ. Muscles Alive: Their Functions Revealed by Electromyography (5th ed.). Baltimore: Williams & Wilkins, 1985.

Berger, W, Quintern, J, & Dietz, V. Stance and gait perturbations in children: Developmental aspects of compensatory mechanisms. Electroencephalography and Clinical Neurophysiology, 61:385–395, 1985.

Bernhardt, DB. Prenatal and postnatal growth and development of the foot and ankle. Physical Therapy, 68:1831–1839, 1988.

Bleck, EE. Developmental orthopaedics: III. Toddlers. Developmental Medicine and Child Neurology, 24:533–555, 1982.

Bleck, EE. Orthopaedic Management in Cerebral Palsy. London: Mac Keith Press, 1987, pp. 323–328.

Bly, L. The components of normal movement during the first year of life. In Slaton, DS (Ed.), Development of Movement in Infancy. Chapel Hill, NC: University of North Carolina, 1980, pp. 85–123.

Bradley, NS, & Bekoff, A. Development of locomotion: Animal models. In Woollacott, MH, & Shumway-Cook, A (Eds.), Development of Posture and Gait Across the Lifespan. Columbia, SC: University of South Carolina Press, 1989, pp. 48–73.

Butterworth, G, & Hicks, L. Visual proprioception and postural stability in infancy: A developmental study. Perception, 6:255–262, 1977.

Coates, JE, & Meade, F. The energy demand and mechanical energy demand in walking. Ergonomics, 3:97–119, 1960.

Coon, V, Donato, G, Houser, C, & Bleck, EE. Normal ranges of hip motion in infants six weeks, three months, and six months of age. Clinical Orthopaedics and Related Research, 110: 256–260, 1975.

Cusick, DD, & Stuberg, WA. Assessment of lower-extremity alignment in the transverse plane: Implications for management of children with neuromotor dysfunction. Physical Therapy, 72:3–15, 1992.

Engel, GM, & Staheli, LT. The natural history of torsion and other factors influencing gait in childhood: A study of the angle of gait, tibial torsion, knee angle, hip rotation, and the development of the arch in normal children. Clinical Orthopaedics, 99:12–17, 1974.

Epstein, HT. Correlated brain and intelligence development in humans. In Hahn, ME, Jensen, C, & Dudek, BC (Eds.), Development and Evolution of Brain Size: Behavioral Implications. New York: Academic Press, 1979, pp. 111–131.

Fabray, G, MacEwen, GD, & Shands, AR. Torsion of the femur: A study in normal and pathological conditions. Journal of Bone and Joint Surgery (American), 55:1726–1738, 1973.

Fomon, SJ. Body composition of the male referenced infant during the first year of life. Pediatrics, 40:863–867, 1967.

Forssberg, H. Ontogeny of human locomotor control: I, Infant stepping, supported locomotion and transition to independent locomotion. Experimental Brain Research, 57:480–493, 1985.

Forssberg, H. Evolution of plantigrade gait: Is there a neuronal correlate? Developmental Medicine and Child Neurology, 34:916–925, 1992.

Gage, JR. Gait Analysis in Cerebral Palsy. London: Mac Keith Press, 1991.

Gillette Children's Hospital, Motion Analysis Laboratory, Hagen, BT, & Stout, JL (Producers). Normal Walking: An Overview Based on Gait Analysis. St. Paul, MN: Gillette Children's Hospital Productions, 1993. (Videotape)

Grillner, S. Control of locomotion in bipeds, tetrapods, and fish. In Geiger, SR (Ed.), Handbook of Physiology, Vol. 2. Bethesda, MD: American Physiological Society, 1981, pp. 1179–1236.

Haas, SS, Epps, CH, Jr, & Adams, JP. Normal ranges of hip motion in the newborn. Clinical Orthopaedics, 91:114–118, 1973.

Heriza, C. Motor development: Traditional and contemporary theories. In Lister, MJ (Ed.), Contemporary Management of Motor Control Problems: Proceedings of the II STEP Conference. Alexandria, VA: Foundation for Physical Therapy, 1991, pp. 99–126.

Inman, VT, Ralston, HJ, & Todd, F. Human Walking. Baltimore: Williams & Wilkins, 1981.

Jordan, LM. Initiation of locomotion from the mammalian brainstem. In Grillner, S. Stein, PSG, Stuart, DG, Forssberg, H, Herman, RM, & Wallen, P (Eds.), Neurobiology of Vertebrate Locomotion. London: Macmillan Press, 1986, pp. 21–37.

Kadaba, MP, Wooten, ME, & Gainery, J. Repeatability of phasic muscle activity: Performance of surface and intramuscular electrodes. Journal of Orthopedic Research, 3:350–359, 1985.

Kazai, N, Okamoto, T, & Kumamoto, M. Electromyographic study of supported walking of infants in the initial period of learning to walk. In Komi, PV (Ed.), Biomechanics V: Proceedings of the Fifth International Congress on Biomechanics. Baltimore: University Park Press, 1976, pp. 311–318.

Komi, PV. Relationship between muscle tension, EMG, and velocity of contraction under concentric and eccentric work. In Desmedt, JE (Ed.), New Developments in Electromyography and Clinical Neurophysiology. Basel, Switzerland: S Karger AG, Medical and Scientific Publishers, 1973, pp. 596–606.

Kruger, MP, & Gage, JR. Stance phase foot rocker problems in spastic diplegia. Developmental Medicine and Child Neurology, 28(suppl 53):4, 1986.

Kugler, PN, Kelso, JA, & Turvey, MT. On the control and coordination of naturally developing systems. In Kelso, JAS, & Clark, JE (Eds.), The Development of Movement Control and Coordination. New York: John Wiley & Sons, 1982.

Loeb, GE. Kinematic factors in the generation and role of sensory feedback during locomotion. In Grillner, S, Stein, PSG, Stuart, DG, Forssberg, H, Herman, RM, & Wallen, P (Eds.),

Neurobiology of Vertebrate Locomotion. London: Macmillan Press, 1986, pp. 547–561.

Murray, MP, Drought, AB, & Kory, RC. Walking patterns of normal men. Journal of Bone and Joint Surgery (American), 46:355–360, 1964.

Okamoto, T, & Kumamoto, M. Electromyographic study of the learning process of walking in infants. Electromyography, 12:149–158, 1972.

Olney, SJ, MacPhail, HEA, Hedden, DM, & Boyce, WF. Work and power in hemiplegic cerebral palsy gait. Physical Therapy, 70:431–438, 1990.

Ounpuu, S, Gage, JR, & Davis, RB, III. Three-dimensional lower extremity joint kinetics in normal pediatric gait. Journal of Pediatric Orthopedics, 11:341–349, 1991.

Palmer, CE. Studies of the center of gravity in the human body. Child Development, 15:99–180, 1944.

Passmore, R, & Durnin, GA. Human energy expenditure. Physiological Reviews, 35:801–839, 1955.

Perry, J. Gait Analysis: Normal and Pathological Function. Thorofare, NJ: Slack, 1992.

Phelps, E, Smith, LJ, & Hallum, A. Normal ranges of hip motion of infants between 9 and 24 months of age. Developmental Medicine and Child Neurology, 27:785–793, 1985.

Ralston, HJ. Energy-speed relation and optimal speed during level walking. Internationale Zeitschrift fur Angewandte Physiologie, 17:277–283, 1958.

Rancho Los Amigos Medical Center, Pathokinesiology Department, Physical Therapy Department. Observational Gait Analysis Handbook. Downey, CA: The Professional Staff Association of Rancho Los Amigos Medical Center, 1989.

Root, ML, Orien, WP, Weed, JH, & Hughes, RJ. Biomechanical Examination of the Foot, Vol. 1. Los Angeles: Clinical Biomechanics, 1971.

Rose, J, Gamble, JG, Burgos, A, Medeiros, J, & Haskell, WL. Energy expenditure index of walking for normal children and children with cerebral palsy. Developmental Medicine and Child Neurology, 32:333–340, 1990

Rose, J, Gamble, JG, Medeiros, J, Burgos, A, & Haskell, WL. Energy cost of walking in normal children and in those with cerebral palsy: Comparison of heart rate and oxygen uptake. Pediatric Orthopedics, 9:276–279, 1989.

Rose, SA, DeLuca, PA, Davis, RB, III, Ounpuu, S, & Gage, JR. Kinematic and kinetic evaluation of the ankle following lengthening of the gastrocnemius fascia in children with cerebral palsy. Journal of Pediatric Orthopedics. In press.

Rose, SA, Ounpuu, S, & DeLuca, PA. Strategies for the assessment of pediatric gait in the clinical setting. Physical Therapy, 71:961–980, 1991.

Salenius, P, & Vankka, E. The development of the tibiofemoral angle in children. Journal of Bone and Joint Surgery (American), 57:259–261, 1975.

Saunders, JB, Inman, VT, & Eberhart, HD. The major determinants in normal and pathological gait. Journal of Bone and Joint Surgery (American), 35:543–559, 1953.

Sepulveda, F, Wells, DM, & Vaughan, CL. A neural network representation of electromyography and joint dynamics in human gait. Journal of Biomechanics, 26:101–109, 1993.

Shumway-Cook, A, & Woollacott, MH. The growth of stability: Postural control from a developmental perspective. Journal of Motor Behavior, 17:131–147, 1985.

Spady, DW. Normal body composition of infants and children. Ross Conference on Pediatric Research, Ross Laboratories, Columbus, Ohio, 98:67–73, 1989.

Staheli, LT, Corbett, M, Wyss, C, & King, H. Lower extremity rotational problems in children. Journal of Bone and Joint Surgery (American), 67:39–47, 1985.

Staheli, LT, & Engel, GM. Tibial torsion: A method of assessment and a survey of normal children. Clinical Orthopaedics, 86:183–186, 1972.

Sutherland, DH. Gait Disorders in Childhood and Adolescence. Baltimore: Williams & Wilkins, 1984.

Sutherland, DH, Olshen, RA, Biden, EN, & Wyatt, MP. The Development of Mature Walking. London: Mac Keith Press, 1988.

Sutherland, DH, Olshen, RA, Cooper, L, & Woo, S. The development of mature gait. Journal of Bone and Joint Surgery (American): 62:336–353, 1980.

Tachdjian, MO. The Child's Foot. Philadelphia: WB Saunders, 1985.

Tachdjian, MO. Pediatric Orthopaedics (2nd ed.), Vol. 4. Philadelphia: WB Saunders, 1990, pp. 2820–2835.

Thelen, E. Treadmill elicited stepping in seven-month-old infants. Child Development, 57:1498–1506, 1986.

Thelen, E, & Cooke, DW. Relationship between newborn stepping and later walking: A new interpretation. Developmental Medicine and Child Neurology, 29:380–393, 1987.

Thelen, E, Fisher, DM, & Ridley-Johnson, R. The relationship between physical growth and a newborn reflex. Infant Behavior and Development, 7:479–493.

Thelen, E, Fisher, DM, Ridley-Johnson, R, & Griffin, NJ. Effects of body build and arousal on newborn infant stepping. Developmental Psychobiology, 15:447–453, 1982.

Thelen, E, & Ulrich, BD. Hidden skills: A dynamic systems analysis of treadmill stepping during the first year. Monographs of the Society for Research in Child Development, 56:1–98, 1991.

Thelen, E, Ulrich, BD, & Jensen, JL. The developmental origins of locomotion. In Woollacott, MH, & Shumway-Cook, A (Eds.), Development of Posture and Gait Across the Lifespan. Columbia, SC: University of South Carolina Press, 1989, pp. 25–47.

Valmassy, RL. Biomechanical evaluation of child. In Ganley, JV (Ed.), Symposium on Podopediatrics. Philadelphia: WB Saunders, 1984, pp. 563–579.

Vredenbregt, J, & Rau, G. Surface electromyography in relation to force, muscle length, and endurance. In Desmedt, JE (Ed.), New Developments in Electromyography and Clinical Neurophysiology. Basel, Switzerland: S Karger AG, Medical and Scientific Publishers, 1973, pp. 607–622.

Walker, JM. Musculoskeletal development: A review. Physical Therapy, 71:878–889, 1991.

Waters, RL, Lunsford, BR, Perry, J, & Byrd, R. Energy-speed relationship of walking: Standard tables. Journal of Orthopaedic Research, 6:215–222, 1988.

Winter, DA. The Biomechanics of Human Movement. New York: John Wiley & Sons, 1979.

Winter, DA. Biomechanical motor patterns in normal walking. Journal of Motor Behavior, 15:302–330, 1983.

Winter, DA. The Biomechanics of Motor Control and Human Gait. Waterloo, Ontario: University of Waterloo Press, 1987.

Winter, DA. Biomechanics and Motor Control of Normal Human Movement (2nd ed.) New York: John Wiley & Sons, 1990.

Winter, DA, & Yack, HJ. EMG profiles during normal human walking: Stride to stride and intersubject variability. Electroencephalography and Clinical Neurophysiology, 67:402–411, 1987.

Woollacott, MH, Shumway-Cook, A, & Williams, HG. The development of posture and balance control in children. In Woollacott, MH, & Shumway-Cook, A (Eds.), Development of Posture and Gait Across the Lifespan. Columbia, SC: University of South Carolina Press, 1989, pp. 77–96.

Zajac, FE, & Gordon, ME. Determining muscle's force and action in multiarticular movement. Exercise Science and Sports Sciences Reviews, 17:187–231, 1989.

Zelazo, PR. The development of walking: New findings and old assumptions. Journal of Motor Behavior, 15:99–137, 1983.

Chapter 4

Musculoskeletal Development and Adaptation

CARRIE G. GAJDOSIK, PT, MS
RICHARD L. GAJDOSIK, PT, PhD

Pediatric physical therapists routinely address clinical conditions that influence the growth and development of the musculoskeletal system, either directly or indirectly. Therapeutic interventions are frequently designed to promote musculoskeletal adaptations in an effort to prevent or correct physical impairments with the hope of enhancing functional outcomes. Accordingly, knowledge of normal growth and development and of the principles of adaptation of the musculoskeletal system is essential for understanding the efficacy of interventions. The purposes of this chapter are to 1) describe the growth and development of muscle and bone and 2) describe the adaptation of muscle and bone, including the effects of various interventions designed to promote desired adaptations.

MUSCULOSKELETAL DEVELOPMENT

Muscle Tissue

The embryologic development of muscle has been well described in many texts and articles, and few controversies exist regarding the sequence of gross anatomic changes during the embryologic period (Davis & Dobbings, 1974; Moore, KL, 1988; Owen et al., 1980). Embryonic myoblasts arise from mesodermal cells and eventually differentiate to form myotubes. These immature, multinucleate tubular structures, which develop from two distinct lineages, are labeled either "primary" or "secondary" (Grove, 1989; Mastaglia, 1974; Sanes, 1987). The primary myotubes are first observed at approximately 5 weeks of gestational age and are known to develop and differentiate without neural influence (Butler et al., 1982; Grove, 1989; Thompson et al., 1990). The secondary myotubes are seen several weeks later. The growth and development of these myotubes are more heavily dependent on neural input, without which they are smaller and fewer in number (Grove, 1989; Thompson et al., 1990). By 20 weeks of gestational age, most myotubes have fused to form muscle fibers and many of the fibers have a microscopic content similar to that of adult fibers.

The motor unit, which consists of a motoneuron and the muscle fibers it innervates, begins its formation with the development of the neuromuscular junction. At a defined localized area, acetylcholine receptors develop in the myotubular membrane during the tenth or eleventh week of gestation (Kamieniecka, 1968). At the same time, the muscle spindle, with small intrafusal fibers and a thin connective tissue capsule, is seen (Kamieniecka, 1968). Motor activity, observed by 12 weeks of gestation, indicates that a viable connection between the neuromuscular junction and the motor axon has occurred. Several motor axons originating from different somites innervate the newly formed end plates. This polyneuronal innervation results in motor units that are much larger than those found in adults. During the prenatal and early neonatal periods, synaptic elimination results in each neuromuscular junction receiving innervation by only one axon. This adult pattern of one nerve per muscle fiber permits a reproducible and predictable increase of force during performance of a task (Purves & Lichtman, 1980; Thompson, 1986). Why fetal muscles are innervated initially by several axons and later undergo the elimination of all but one axon is not well established. It does not appear that the reason is to ensure that every muscle fiber is innervated. In partially denervated muscles of animals, the few remaining motoneurons still undergo synaptic elimination, thus reducing the size of the motor unit (Brown et al., 1976; Thompson & Jansen, 1977). During the last half of gestational growth, the number and size of muscle fibers increase rapidly so that most of the skeletal muscle has developed by birth. Through the first year of life, muscle fibers continue to increase in number from either the process of splitting existing cells or the differentiation of myoblasts to secondary myotubes (Mastaglia, 1974). During the growing years, muscle fibers increase in length and cross-sectional area by the addition of sarcomeres (Kitiyakara & Angevine, 1963). Their final size is dependent on many factors, including blood supply, innervation, nutrition, genetics, and exercise.

During fetal development, the myotubes differentiate into the two basic types of muscle fibers, type I (slow twitch) and type II (fast twitch) (Slaton, 1981). Two basic theories of how fetal muscle fiber differentiates into two types have been proposed. From the 1960s to the early 1980s, the widely accepted concept was that the fiber type of developing undifferentiated myotubes was determined by the innervating motoneurons (Buller et al., 1960; Kamieniecka, 1968). Later studies, however, supported a second concept that fetal muscle fibers can differentiate without neuronal input (Butler et al., 1982; Sanes, 1987; Thompson et al., 1990). Both theories may be correct since myotubes are now known to develop from two distinct lineages. Mus-

cle tissue derived from primary myotubes expresses the two basic fiber types without the influence of the motoneuron, whereas muscle tissue derived from the secondary myotubes is dependent on innervation for differentiation into muscle fiber types (Butler et al., 1982; Grove, 1989). In adults, the expression of muscle fiber types depends on neuronal input, regardless of whether the muscle was derived from primary or secondary myotubes. Fiber type preference is also strongly influenced by disease and by the function of the muscle.

Skeletal and Articular Structures

Like muscle tissue, both the skeletal and articular tissues arise from the mesodermal layer of the embryo. Mesenchymal cells condense to form templates of the skeleton. From this point, two distinct processes of bone formation take place: 1) endochondral ossification and 2) intramembranous ossification. All bones, with the exception of the clavicle, mandible, and skull, are formed by endochondral ossification (also called intracartilaginous ossification) (Moore, KL, 1988; Royer, 1974; Walker, 1991). During the early embryonic period, collagenous and elastic fibers are deposited on the mesenchymal models and form cartilaginous models. Bone minerals are deposited on these new models and gradually replace the cartilage in the process of ossification. Intramembranous ossification occurs directly in the mesenchymal model. Mesenchymal cells differentiate into osteoblasts that deposit a matrix called osteoid tissue. This tissue is organized into bone as calcium phosphate is deposited (Moore, KL, 1988).

Ossification at the primary ossification centers, typically in the center of the diaphyses or body of the bone (Royer, 1974), commences at the end of the embryonic period (eighth fetal week). By the time of birth, the diaphyses are almost ossified, whereas the epiphyses, or distal ends of the bone, remain cartilaginous. During early childhood, the secondary ossification centers appear in the epiphyses, and ossification proceeds in this section of the bone. The timing of complete ossification varies with each particular bone. Most bones are fully ossified by 20 years of age, but for a few bones the process can continue into adulthood (Moore, KL, 1988). After birth, long bones grow in length at the epiphyseal plate, which is between the diaphysis and the epiphysis. This cartilaginous plate rapidly proliferates on the diaphyseal side of the bone. The resultant chondrocytes, arranged in parallel columns, become enlarged and are then converted into bone by endochondral ossification (McKibbin,

1980; Rodriguez et al., 1992). Eventually the epiphyseal plate is ossified, the diaphyses and epiphyses are joined, and the growth of the bone in length is considered complete.

Bone also increases in size through appositional growth, which is the accumulation of new bone on the bone surfaces. This results in an increase in thickness and density of the diaphyses. The most rapid period of bone growth is prenatal. A marked decrease in the rate of growth is noted at birth, but throughout childhood the decline is more gradual. A midgrowth spurt occurs at age 7 and again at puberty (Gasser et al., 1991).

Joint formation begins about the time that the cartilaginous models are formed (Moore, KL, 1988; Walker, 1991). In a specialized area between these models, the interzonal mesenchyma differentiates to form the joint. The basic structures of the joint are formed during the sixth to eighth week of gestation, but the final shape develops throughout early childhood under the influence of the forces of movement and compression (Drachman & Sokoloff, 1966). The hip is a good example of how a joint changes shape during the fetal period. At 11.5 weeks of gestational age, the acetabulum is extremely deep and the head of the femur, which is quite round, is well covered (Ralis & McKibbin, 1973). As the fetus increases in age, the relative depth of the acetabulum decreases as the head of the femur becomes more hemispheric. At birth, the acetabulum is so shallow that it covers less than one half of the femoral head to result in an unstable hip. This is thought to allow for easier passage through the vaginal canal. During postnatal growth, the forces of compression and movement contribute to an increase in the depth of the acetabulum. The head of the femur becomes rounder, but it never achieves the roundness it had during the early fetal period.

ADAPTATIONS OF MUSCLE AND BONE

The musculoskeletal system demonstrates a remarkable ability to adapt to the physical demands, or lack of physical demands, placed on the system. The presence of a pathologic condition may adversely influence the structure and function of any component of the system, and this process may result in secondary impairments. For example, congenital deformities, disease processes, or abnormal growth of bone may lead to strength and length adaptations of the muscle-tendon unit (MTU). Congenital or acquired central nervous system deficits, for example, cerebral palsy (CP), bring about sensorimotor impairments that may promote unwanted adaptations of the MTU and ultimately compromise the structural and functional integrity of the joints and bone. Pathologic conditions of the MTU itself, for example, muscular dystrophies, may also lead to secondary, unwanted adaptations of the joints and bone. Normal adaptations can either enhance function or lead to impairment, functional limitations, and disability.

Changes in Muscle Fiber Types

Muscle fiber types are susceptible to both internal and external influences. In normal muscle, fiber types are randomly distributed to form a mosaic pattern and there is little variation in fiber size. In the presence of disease or dysfunction, this pattern is altered. One fiber type can predominate, size can change, or the mosaic pattern can be lost when similar fiber types clump together. These changes have been useful in diagnosis of certain pathologic conditions of muscle. Less information is available on changes in fiber types for children with disabilities than for adults, and there may be some differences between the two age groups (Brooke & Engel, 1969; Tanabe & Nonaka, 1987). Selective atrophy of type II fibers is commonly seen in individuals with muscle disease, especially when muscle strength is compromised by disuse or impairment. Adults with steroid-induced weakness have selective type II atrophy (Rothstein & Rose, 1982). This same pattern may be seen in children who receive steroids to treat such diseases as juvenile rheumatoid arthritis. Children with spastic CP show atrophy of type II fibers in muscles that are spastic (Brooke & Engel, 1969; Slaton, 1984). Denervated muscles show atrophy of both major types of fibers, but type II fibers have more atrophy than do type I fibers. This pattern is probably true for children with myelodysplasia, although it has not been documented. Malnourished children are at risk for a loss of type II fibers, which are thought to be converted to type I fibers (Ward & Strickland, 1991). Selective atrophy of type I fibers is less common but is seen in children with hypotonia (Brooke & Engel, 1969) and in children with congenital myotonic dystrophy (Farkas-Bargeton et al., 1988). An immobilized limb has been reported to show a greater atrophy of type I fibers than of type II fibers, although this change appears to be variable and dependent on the presence or absence of pain, the length of time the limb was immobilized, or the particular muscle that was immobilized (Rose & Rothstein, 1982).

Predominance of either fiber type may occur in the presence of disease. Type I predominance is typically seen in myopathic conditions such as Duchenne's muscular dystrophy (Brooke & Engel, 1969), whereas type II predominance is associated with motoneuron diseases such as spinal muscular atrophy type 3 (Kugelberg-Welander disease) (Brooke, 1986).

Why do pediatric physical therapists need to know about muscle fiber types and their responses to outside influences? This question is difficult to answer because the clinical significance is unknown. Speculation has been put forth about whether the predominant fiber type in athletes influences performance, but athletes are not part of the patient population of the vast majority of pediatric therapists. Rose and Rothstein (1982) speculated that the loss of fast-twitch fibers could affect the muscle's ability to protect joints during periods of sudden weight loading, whereas the person with a small number of slow-twitch fibers may not be able to preserve the joint integrity when endurance is required. Over time, either of these scenarios could lead to degenerative joint changes.

Although it is known that children with CP have atrophy of type II fibers and have difficulty with ballistic movement, whether a causal relationship exists is unknown. How does the disorganization of movement affect atrophy of fibers? Working on ballistic exercises may increase the size of the type II fibers, but the important issue is whether this type of exercise influences function. Further studies of changes in fiber types and the effect of the changes on function are needed. In the meantime, physical therapists should be aware that the two basic types of muscle fibers are influenced by exercise differently, that is, the effects of exercise on muscle fibers are training-specific. Endurance training enhances the performance of type I fibers, whereas strength training enhances performance of type II fibers.

Structure and Function of the Normal Muscle-Tendon Unit

The normal MTU comprises skeletal muscle tissue proper (muscle fibers with actin and myosin protein filaments); the supportive connective tissues within and around the muscle belly (endomysium, perimysium, and epimysium); and the dense regular connective tissues of the tendons that secure the MTU to bone. The total muscle force production is influenced by many factors, including the size of the muscle fibers, the firing rate of motor unit action potentials, the recruitment and derecruitment patterns, the muscle's architecture, the angle of pull, the lever arm, and the changes in the muscle's length.

The two basic components of the total muscle force are produced by the active and passive components of the MTU (Fig. 4–1), both of which are influenced by its length. To determine the active force produced by the MTU, the passive force is subtracted from the total force (see Fig. 4–1). The force produced by the active component depends primarily on the amount of overlap of the actin and myosin filaments. The maximum isometric force is produced near the resting length of an isolated muscle, and the isometric force decreases as the muscle is either lengthened or shortened relative to the resting length. The change in force in relation to the change in length forms the basis of the sliding filament theory of muscle contraction (Gordon et al., 1966; Huxley & Peachey, 1961). The isometric force is nearly maximal at the resting length because the actin and myosin filaments are in a position of optimal overlap (Figs. 4–2, 4–3). The force generated by the active component of the MTU depends on the integrity of the central and peripheral nervous systems, the excitation-contraction coupling mechanism, and the cross-sectional area of the skeletal muscle tissues. In a completely re-

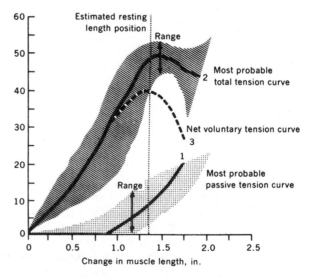

FIGURE 4–1. Classic length-tension curves for skeletal muscle. Net voluntary active tension is predicted by subtracting passive tension from total tension. (With permission from Astrand, P, & Rodahl, K. Textbook of Work Physiology [2nd ed.]. New York: McGraw-Hill, 1977, p. 102.)

FIGURE 4-2. Schematic summary of tension changes in relation to sarcomere length changes. Arrows along the top are placed opposite the striation spacings for critical stages of actin and myosin filament overlap (see Fig. 4-3). (From Gordon, AM, Huxley, AF, & Julian, FJ. The variation in isometric tension with sarcomere length in vertebrate muscle fibers. Journal of Physiology, *184*:185, 1966.)

laxed skeletal muscle (i.e., one in a subject whose central nervous system is not intact or one in which there is no artificial stimulation), no active tension exists.

The force produced by the passive component of the MTU is thought to be brought about by stable cross-links between the actin and myosin filaments (series elastic component), and by deformation of the connective tissues of the muscle (parallel elastic component). The passive component accounts for the resistance felt during passive stretch of a fully relaxed muscle. The results of studies with animals have suggested that in relaxed skeletal muscle, part of the passive tension arises from weak interactions or cross-links between the actin and myosin filaments, the so-called filamentary resting tension hypothesis of passive tension. The stable bonds impart a stiffness because the actin-myosin cross-bridges stretch a short distance from the stable position before the contacts slip and reattach at another bonding site. This stiffness has been reported in whole muscles (Flitney & Hirst, 1978; Hill, 1968,

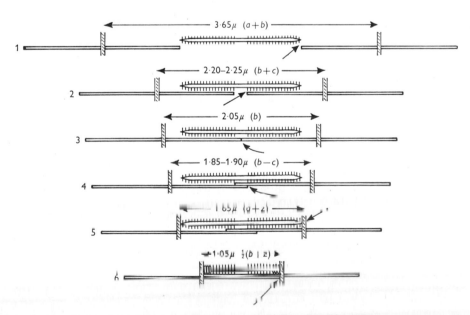

FIGURE 4-3. Critical stages in the increase of overlap between actin and myosin filaments as a sarcomere shortens. Numbers correspond to numbers in Fig. 4-2. (From Gordon, AM, Huxley, AF, & Julian, FJ. The variation in isometric tension with sarcomere length in vertebrate muscle fibers. Journal of Physiology, *184*:186, 1966.)

1970a,b; Huxley & Simmons, 1971; Magid & Law, 1985; Matsubara & Yagi, 1985; Rack & Westury, 1974; Yagi & Matsubara, 1984) and in single muscle fibers (Granzier & Pollack, 1985; Griffiths et al., 1980; Guth et al., 1978). Passive stiffness is the resistance one feels when passively stretching a muscle. Because passive compliance is the reciprocal of stiffness, passive compliance is the "ease" with which the muscle lengthens. Although passive compliance can be represented as the ratio of change in muscle length to change in muscle force (Botelho et al., 1954), to arrive at these measurements normally requires invasive research methods that are usually not possible in humans. Instead, passive compliance in humans is usually measured by the ratio of the change in the size of the angle to the change in the amount of torque (Gajdosik, 1991a; Gajdosik et al., 1990; Tardieu, C, et al., 1982a; Tardieu, G, et al., 1982).

Although some resistance to passive lengthening is probably present at most functional muscle lengths, passive resistance increases as the muscle is lengthened beyond its resting length: passive resistance is the equivalent of resting muscle tone. The increase in passive resistance is influenced by the lengthening of the connective tissues of the endomysium, perimysium, and epimysium of the muscle belly. Tendons are composed of dense regular connective tissues that present very low passive compliance (high stiffness), so the immediate length of tendons can generally be considered constant and noncontributory to the passive length-tension relationships of the stretched MTU (Halar et al., 1978; Stolov & Weilepp, 1966; Tardieu, C, et al., 1982b).

Early studies of whole skeletal muscles indicated that the passive length-tension relationship is linear for length changes associated with small passive tensions (when the muscle is relatively short) but is curvilinear for changes in length at higher tensions (when the muscle approaches maximal length) (Brodie, 1895; Haycraft, 1904; Sichel, 1934), with the concavity toward the tension axis. The length-tension relationship of single skeletal muscle fibers, however, showed a linear relationship when the fibers were passively stretched from 100 to 130% of the resting length (Sichel, 1934). The difference between the results with whole muscles and with single muscle fibers was attributed to variations in the length and orientation of the fibers in whole muscles (i.e., unipenniform, bipenniform, or multipenniform structure), and the orientation of the connective tissues within and around the muscle. During initial loading, the muscle fibers within whole muscles passively resist lengthening, represented by a linear length-tension relationship. The

extent of the linear relationship varies among muscle types. As whole muscles are stretched further, the extracellular connective tissue is uncrimped and brought into alignment, thus increasing the total passive resistance of the MTU and producing a curvilinear relationship at greater lengths and passive tensions (Banus & Zetlin, 1938; Sichel, 1934). Later studies with single muscle fibers found that the passive length-tension curves of fibers stretched beyond 130% of the resting lengths were curvilinear and that the sarcolemma accounted for all of the tension (Casella, 1950; Ramsey & Street, 1940), but that the sarcolemma did not contribute to the passive tension through 100 to 130% of the resting length. These findings suggested that the passive tension of the contractile components probably accounted for the linear length-tension relationship reported earlier for this range of lengthening in single fibers (Sichel, 1934).

Further support for the influence of the connective tissues of skeletal muscles on passive compliance was provided by studies of the normal structure of these tissues. The perimysium has a well-ordered crisscross array of crimped collagen fibers (Rowe, 1974, 1981), and because of this organization, the perimysium is considered tissue that is a major contributor to extracellular passive resistance (Borg & Caulfield, 1980). Examination of the perimysium with light microscopy (Rowe, 1974) and scanning electron microscopy (EM) (Williams & Goldspink, 1984) revealed that the orientation of the crimped collagen changes as the length of the muscle changes. The structure of the perimysium, a system of sheets with a three-dimensional weave surrounding muscle fasciculi, and the structural changes observed during muscle lengthening explain the curvilinear length-tension relationship reported for stretching muscles beyond their resting lengths (Brodie, 1895; Haycraft, 1904; Sichel, 1934). Knowledge of the basic structures contributing to length-tension relationships of muscles is important clinically. The resistance a pediatric therapist feels at the end of the range of a lengthened muscle with spasticity may result from the resistance borne by the passive components (especially the connective tissues) and not from an activation of spasticity.

Force and Length Adaptations in the Muscle-Tendon Unit

ANIMAL STUDIES

Numerous experimental animal models have shown that anatomic and physiologic length adaptations of the MTU can be induced by immobilization, denervation, local contraction by artificial stimulation, or a combination of these methods. Studies have included examination of changes in the active and passive length-tension curves in light of histologic and histochemical changes in the muscles.

When muscles were immobilized in shortened positions they showed a decrease in total force production, resulting from decreases in both the active force and the passive force (Alder et al., 1959; Williams & Goldspink, 1978). Muscle length also decreases (Alder et al., 1959; Ranson & Dixon, 1928; Stolov et al., 1971), a change brought about by a reduction in the number of sarcomeres (Goldspink, G, et al., 1974; Tabary et al., 1972; Williams & Goldspink, 1971, 1973, 1978). The soleus muscles of young mice immobilized in the shortened position demonstrated a decrease in the postnatal addition of sarcomeres (Williams & Goldspink, 1973). Protein synthesis and protein breakdown studies have demonstrated that muscles immobilized in shortened positions showed significant loss of tissue protein because of decreased synthesis and increased degradation (Williams & Goldspink, 1971). The synthesis and degradation occurred primarily at the ends of the muscle fibers. Muscles immobilized in the shortened position presented decreased resting length (Alder et al., 1959; Goldspink, G, et al., 1974; Ranson & Dixon, 1928; Tabary et al., 1972; Tardieu, C, et al., 1982a; Williams & Goldspink, 1978), reduced maximal length, and decreased passive compliance (Tabary et al., 1972; Tardieu, C, et al., 1982b; Williams & Goldspink, 1978). The sarcomeres adapt in length to maintain optimal actin and myosin overlap concomitant with the loss in number of sarcomeres. When the immobilization is discontinued, the muscles readapt to gain their original sarcomere number and length characteristics. Although changes in the resting lengths were attributed to loss of sarcomeres, as already discussed, the changes in passive compliance, demonstrated by changes in the length-tension curves, were attributed to changes in the connective tissues of the muscles (Rowe, 1981; Tabary et al., 1972, Williams & Goldspink, 1978). Muscles immobilized in the shortened position demonstrated a greater abundance (Tabary et al., 1972; Williams & Goldspink, 1984) and remodeling (Williams & Goldspink, 1984) of connective tissues in the early stages of immobilization. Greater abundance of connective tissue has been assessed by determining the relative concentration of hydroxyproline in relation to the total volume of the muscle (Williams & Goldspink, 1984). Muscle fibers, however, atrophy without a decrease in their number (Cardenas et al., 1977); thus, whether the absolute amount of connective tissue increases remains controversial. Evidence for remodeling was provided by scanning EM of the soleus muscles of mice immobilized in the shortened position for 2 weeks (Williams & Goldspink, 1984). The collagen fibers of the perimysium were oriented at more acute angles to the muscle fiber axis than were the collagen fibers of normal muscles fixed in the same position. This collagen fiber arrangement at the immobilized length resembled the arrangement found in normal muscles fixed in lengthened positions (Fig. 4–4). As a result of the remodeling, greater tension per unit of passive elongation, and therefore steeper length-tension curves, produced decreased passive compliance. In addition, both the active and passive length-tension curves shifted to the left, that is, the muscles were shorter and less compliant (stiffer). The length-tension curves for young muscles (Fig. 4–5) and adult muscles were similar.

Immobilization of muscles in lengthened positions caused an increase in muscle length because of increases in the number of sarcomeres (Tabary et al., 1972; Williams & Goldspink, 1973, 1978), particularly at the ends of the muscle fibers. Similar results have been reported during normal postnatal growth of skeletal muscle fibers in young animals (Kitiyakara & Angevine, 1963; Williams & Goldspink, 1971). The addition of sarcomeres is accompanied by weight gain and increased protein synthesis after immobilization (Goldspink, DF, 1977). The increased number of sarcomeres was not so great (19% increase) as the loss of sarcomeres in muscles immobilized in the shortened position (40% loss) (Tabary et al., 1972).

The active and passive length-tension curves for adult muscles were shifted to the right compared with those of adult controls. In young muscles, however, the muscle belly length was decreased, so the curves of the experimental muscles were shifted to the left compared with those of the controls, instead of to the right, as in adult muscle (Williams & Goldspink, 1978) (Fig. 4–6). Evidence suggests that a tendon elongates more readily in young, growing animals than in adult animals. In young mice with muscles immobilized in either the shortened or lengthened position, the overall muscle length was decreased, with a concomitant increase in tendon length (Williams & Goldspink, 1978). Thus, in young animals a shorter muscle belly may result in strength deficits that are independent of the length of the MTU during immobilization. As with muscles immobilized in the shortened position, the sarcomere length adapts to maintain optimal actin and myosin overlap. Also, muscles im-

FIGURE 4-4. Scanning electron micrographs of collagen fibers in the perimysium. *A*, Normal muscle fixed in the lengthened position. *B*, Normal muscle fixed in the shortened position. *C*, Muscle immobilized for 2 weeks in the shortened position and then fixed in the same position. M = muscle fiber, × 1300. (From Williams, PE, & Goldspink, G. Connective tissue changes in immobilized muscle. Journal of Anatomy [London], *138*[2]:347, 1984. Reprinted with the permission of Cambridge University Press.)

mobilized in the lengthened position readapted to their original lengths when the immobilization was discontinued.

Studies of peripheral denervation of skeletal muscles have revealed obvious loss of the ability of the animal to generate voluntary active tension. After denervation, the passive length-tension relationship showed gradual changes over a period of weeks, with steeper length-tension curves and limited extensibility between their resting lengths and

FIGURE 4-5. Length-tension curves for young muscles (*A-D*) immobilized in the shortened position (o) and their controls (●). (From Williams, PE, & Goldspink, G. Changes in sarcomere length and physiological properties in immobilized muscle. Journal of Anatomy [London], *127*[3]:464, 1978. Reprinted with the permission of Cambridge University Press.)

Muscle belly length as % of *in vivo* fully extended length of control

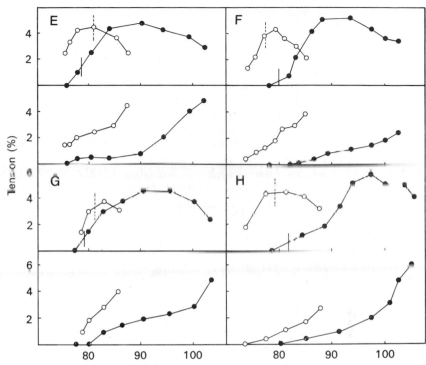

FIGURE 4-6. Length-tension curves for young animals ($E-H$) immobilized in the lengthened position (o) and their controls (●). (From Williams, PE, & Goldspink, G. Changes in sarcomere length and physiological properties in immobilized muscle. Journal of Anatomy [London], *127*[3]:464, 1978. Reprinted with the permission of Cambridge University Press.)

their maximal lengths compared with those of controls (Stolov et al., 1970; Thomson, 1955). These findings support the notion of an influence of the filamentary resting tension on passive resistance in the shorter ranges of muscle lengthening. Studies have also revealed that length adaptations may result from myogenic—but not neurogenic—responses to the length of muscles. Denervated muscles immobilized in shortened positions in adult rats showed muscle belly shortening after 8 weeks (Stolov et al., 1971), and a similar change was seen in adult cats after 4 weeks, with loss of up to 35% of the sarcomeres (Goldspink, G, et al., 1974). The muscle belly shortening and decreased passive compliance were essentially the same as those observed in innervated muscles immobilized in shortened positions.

The reports that muscle length and associated physiologic changes may be independent of neuronal control were supported by studies of muscles stimulated with tetanus toxin (Huet de la Tour et al., 1979a,b; Ranson & Dixon, 1928) and electrical stimulation (Tabary et al., 1981). Local injection of tetanus toxin into the soleus muscles of guinea pigs produced a shift in the passive length-tension curve toward the tension axis (to the left), a decrease in passive compliance, and a 45% decrease in sarcomere number (Huet de la Tour et al., 1979b). The

shortening adaptations were similar to those found after the muscles of cats were immobilized in shortened positions (Tabary et al., 1972). Analysis of the changes in sarcomere numbers in the soleus muscles of guinea pigs after length and tension were varied independently indicated that the length of muscles, not the tension, appeared to be the determining factor in sarcomere regulation (Huet de la Tour et al., 1979a). Contraction of a shortened muscle, however, may hasten sarcomere loss: electric stimulation of the sciatic nerve induced a 25% decrease in sarcomere numbers and decreased passive compliance within 12 hours (Tabary et al., 1981), whereas 5 days of shortening by immobilization in plaster casts alone was required to produce similar changes (Huet de la Tour et al., 1979b).

HUMAN STUDIES AND CLINICAL EVIDENCE

Studies of the length and passive compliance adaptations of the MTU in humans are less common than such studies in animals. Limited attempts to investigate the length and passive compliance responses to imposed changes in muscle length of neurologically impaired children have been reported. Studies of children with CP and hypoextensible triceps surae muscles showed that they have muscle shortening and decreased passive compliance compared with findings in healthy children without CP (Tardieu, C, et al., 1982a).

In another study, 9 children with hypoextensible triceps surae muscles were casted for 3 weeks with these muscles placed in the lengthened position. Four children showed passive length-tension curves that were shifted to the right with decreased slopes, indicating increased passive compliance, whereas 5 children had curves that were shifted to the right without a change in the form of the curve (Tardieu, C, et al., 1979). In the same study, 5 children with hyperextensible triceps surae muscles were casted in a shortened position. The passive length-tension curves shifted to the left with increased slopes, indicating decreased passive compliance, in 4 of the 5 children.

In a follow-up study, children with CP and hypoextensible triceps surae muscles but no evidence of prolonged sustained contractions (group 1) were compared with children with CP and hypoextensible triceps surae muscles caused by an imbalance between triceps surae and dorsiflexion contractions (group 2) (Tardieu, G, et al., 1982). Both groups were treated with progressive casting to lengthen the muscles. Group 1 showed a shift to the right of the passive length-tension curve without a change in the slope of the curve. Group 2 presented curves that were shifted to the right with decreased slopes, showing increased passive compliance (Fig. 4–7).

The authors suggested that the children in group 2 showed normal muscle adaptation because of the passive compliance adaptation. These findings suggest that human muscles undergo adaptations similar to those that have been reported for animals. This is based on the association of the passive compliance curves of animal and of human muscles measured by noninvasive methods, with the histologic and histochemical adaptations in animal muscles. The results of the study also elucidate the variability that can be expected in humans, particularly with regard to the possibility of different pathologic mechanisms underlying the adaptability of hypoextensible muscles in selected patient populations, such as children with CP (Tardieu, G, et al., 1982).

Clinical observations clearly provide evidence that the musculoskeletal system of humans undergoes adaptations in response to immobilization, disuse, postural disturbances, and muscle imbalances in relation to specific pathologic disorders. It is well known that the skeletal muscles of a limb that is immobilized and not used will atrophy as a result of protein degradation (Sargeant et al., 1977). It is equally well known that normal muscle fibers respond to increased force and endurance demands by adaptive responses in structural, physiologic, and biochemical characteristics (Salmons & Hendriksson, 1981). The presence of pathologic conditions that alter skeletal muscles directly (e.g., muscular dystrophy) or indirectly from changes in the neurologic activity to the skeletal muscles (e.g., hypotonia or hypertonia) may lead to postural contractures and deformities from muscle imbalances and chronic positioning (Bunch, 1977; Sharrard, 1967; Tardieu, C, et al., 1982a; Tardieu, G, et al., 1982).

Many of the clinical manifestations of musculoskeletal disorders correlate well with the pathophysiologic conditions of the MTU described from experimental animal models. Children with idiopathic spinal conditions such as scoliosis present shortening adaptations of the MTU on one side of the spine, contralateral MTU lengthening adaptations, and rotational spinal column deformities. Abnormal shape in the structures of the vertebral column (e.g., hemivertebra) presents similar adaptations of the MTU and other soft tissues of the back. If the lower limbs of a child presenting with flaccid paralysis are held in a specific posture for an extended period (e.g., hip flexion, abduction, and lateral rotation), the limbs adopt the characteristic position of the posture (Sharrard, 1967).

Long-term conservative interventions, such as stretching and casting, may facilitate desired adaptations of the MTU and enhance function, but much research is needed to examine these possibilities objectively. By contrast, surgical lengthening of the tendons of the triceps surae muscle group (Reimers, 1990a) and the hamstring muscle group (Damron et al., 1991; Lespargot et al., 1989; Reimers, 1990b) in children with CP has demon-

FIGURE 4–7. Results of successful progressive casting in child from group 2. X = passive torque curve before treatment, ■ = passive torque curve after treatment. The curve shifted to the right with increased passive compliance. (From Tardieu, G, Tardieu, C, Colbeau-Justin, P, & Lespargot, A. Muscle hypoextensibility in children with cerebral palsy: II. Therapeutic implications. Archives of Physical Medicine and Rehabilitation, *63*:106, 1982.)

strated enhanced functional outcomes. Studies that examine the combined influence of both conservative and surgical interventions are clearly needed to determine the most efficacious methods of improving function.

Bone deformities and alterations in the MTU may result from abnormal skeletal growth, or both MTU and bone adaptations may be associated with abnormalities in muscle tonicity and muscle imbalances found with conditions such as spastic diplegia in children with CP. Numerous developmental changes in the musculoskeletal system have been associated with CP, and the changes correlate well with the presence of spasticity and imbalances in muscle force and muscle length. These include changes in the femur and acetabulum resulting in medial femoral torsion and hip disorders (Beals, 1969; Lewis et al., 1964), hip adduction contractures and knee flexion contractures in spastic adductor and hamstring muscles (Reimers, 1974), and severe equinus deformity because of spasticity and shortening adaptations of the calf musculature (Tardieu, G, et al., 1982).

Skeletal Adaptations

The growth and resultant shape of the skeleton are affected by genetic coding, nutrition, and the combination of various mechanical forces that are imposed over time (Carter, 1987). The mass, girth, thickness, curvature, and trabecular arrangement of bone change as the forces of heredity and the environment play their roles. When examining skeletal adaptation, mechanical forces, such as muscle pull and weight bearing, are of interest to the pediatric physical therapist. Martin and McCulloch (1987) reported a case study of a child with congenital absence of a left tibia. At birth the left fibula was larger than the right fibula. This was thought to result from the forces of movement in utero. When the child reached 2 years of age, the fibula was surgically centered in relation to the femur to act as a tibia. Sixteen months later, the fibula looked like a tibia in shape, size, and strength. The authors believed that the mechanical stresses delivered in a functional weight-bearing manner induced the changes in the fibula. Mechanical forces affect the shape of the maturing skeleton, which in turn affects the biomechanical function of the musculoskeletal system. Deformations of the skeletal system can lead to abnormalities in movement and impedance of function (Beals, 1969; Bunch, 1977; King & Staheli, 1984).

EFFECTS OF NORMAL FORCES ON SKELETAL GROWTH

From the time the cartilaginous template is formed, the basic shape of the skeletal system does not change (Bunch, 1977). Each bone grows in length, width, and girth, but its relative form remains unchanged. Natural and atypic angular changes occur from compressive and shear forces at the epiphyseal plate (Arkin & Katz, 1956; LeVeau & Bernhardt, 1984). Compressive forces are perpendicular to the plate. Normal intermittent compressive forces, such as those produced by weight bearing or muscle pull, stimulate lengthening of bone (Arkin & Katz, 1956). If these forces are too great, the rate of growth is diminished.

Asymmetric forces affect the shape of the bone by stimulating growth in noncompressed areas while inhibiting bone development in areas of compression (Arkin & Katz, 1956). Although the bone appears to bend, it is actually growing asymmetrically as the epiphyseal plate realigns to the direction of the force. The clinical use of the effects of compression on the epiphyseal plate is exemplified by surgical stapling of the medial aspect of the epiphyseal plate of the proximal tibia to retard growth on that side to correct a genu valgum deformity (Cozen, 1990). In children with unequal leg lengths, both sides of the plate on the longer leg are stapled to slow its growth until the shorter leg catches up (Edmonson & Crenshaw, 1980). Asymmetric proliferation of one or more epiphyseal growth plates located within a single bone can also lead to bone deformation. The spinal neural arch has six growth centers, three within each half of the arch. Chandraraj and Briggs (1991) speculated that uneven growth of either half of the neural arch may be a significant factor in the later development of idiopathic scoliosis.

Shear forces, which run parallel to the epiphyseal plate, can lead to torsional or twisting changes in the bone. The columns of chondrocytes around the periphery of the plate veer away from the shear forces in a twisting pattern (Arkin & Katz, 1956; Bernhardt, 1988; LeVeau & Bernhardt, 1984). The normal pull of muscles around a joint contributes to the shear forces, resulting in normal torsional changes in the long bones. For example, at birth, the tibia has 5° of medial torsion. By adulthood, the longitudinal orientation of the tibia has changed to 23 to 25° of lateral torsion (Bernhardt, 1988). The combination of atypic shear and compressive forces can lead to skeletal deformities, such as vertebral wedging, femoral anteversion, femoral or tibial-fibular torsion, genu valgum or varum, and pes planovalgus. Abnormalities of the skeletal system can lead to secondary problems of pain and dysfunction.

The normally developing child demonstrates interesting changes in the position of the knee in the frontal plane. Initially, the infant's knees are bowlegged (genu varum), but they undergo progressive straightening until they are completely straight at about 20 months of age. The knee angulation then progresses toward that of genu valgum, reaching its peak when the child is 2.5 years old. After this time, they again undergo gradual realignment until, by the age of 4 to 6 years, they are straight (Fig. 4–8).

The level of compressive forces also affects the thickness and density of the bone shaft (Arkin & Katz, 1956; Martin, 1987; Royer, 1974). The bone thickens via appositional growth with excessive compressive forces, whereas a less than normal amount of compression leads to bone atrophy (Bernhardt, 1988). An increase in bone thickness is found in athletes, who have greater bone density than nonathletes. Nonathletes can, however, increase bone density with regular physical activity

Newborn—Moderate genu varum   6 Months—Minimal genu varum   1 Year, 7 Months—Legs straight

2 Years, 6 Months

a. Physiolgic genu valgum

b. Protective toeing-in

4 to 6 Years— Legs straight

FIGURE 4–8. Physiologic evolution of lower limb alignment at various ages in infancy and childhood. (From Tachdjian, MO. Pediatric Orthopedics [2nd ed.]. Philadelphia: WB Saunders, 1990, p. 2821.)

(Martin, 1987). Children who do not experience normal levels of weight bearing are at risk for osteoporosis, as is observed in children with myelodysplasia (Williamson, 1987) and juvenile rheumatoid arthritis (Hopp et al., 1991).

The formation, growth, and integrity of articular cartilage are stimulated by compressive forces and movement between the bone surfaces (Drachman & Sokoloff, 1966; Ralis & McKibbin, 1973). Intermittent joint loading leads to healthy, thick cartilage, but constant loading interrupts normal nutrition. The cartilage becomes thin and can eventually degenerate, leading to degenerative joint disease (Carter et al., 1987; Trueta, 1974). Adults with CP have reported that pain, in particular joint pain, is a major problem secondary to the CP (Rural Institute on Disabilities, 1989).

The role of movement in the development of joint shape and articular cartilage integrity is not clearly understood. In embryonic chicks, early joint formation occurred in the absence of mobility, but toward the end of the fetal period, cartilaginous bonds between the joint surfaces were present and the articular surfaces were flattened and misshapen (Drachman & Sokoloff, 1966). These changes have not been shown in humans. Movement may play a greater role in joint modeling after the joint is formed.

EFFECTS OF ABNORMAL FORCES ON SKELETAL GROWTH

Skeletal deformities are common in children with muscle imbalances, spasticity, contractures, hypokinesis, and obesity, all of which apply abnormal mechanical forces to the growing skeleton. Although these deformities can occur throughout the growing period, the skeleton is most vulnerable during the first few years of life (prenatal and postnatal) when the rate of growth is greatest (Carter et al., 1987; Curry & Butler, 1975).

Fetal position has been related to various deformities, especially those that occur toward the end of the pregnancy (Katz et al., 1990). The incidence of tibial rotation and metatarsus adductus was reported to increase as the gestational age increased in preterm infants (Katz et al., 1990). Thus, preterm infants born closer to term were more likely to have rotational deformities than were younger preterm infants. Many factors can cause prenatal deformities, including decreased amniotic fluid, the limited space in which the fetus can move in utero, multiple births, and external forces from tightly stretched uterine and abdominal walls. Some associated deformities are congenital torticollis, plagiocephaly (asymmetric head), and pelvic obliquity

(Bernhardt, 1988; Fulford & Brown, 1977; LeVeau & Bernhardt, 1984; Sherk et al., 1981). During the third trimester, the hip is especially vulnerable to dislocating forces because of its shallow acetabulum (Beals, 1969; Ralis & McKibbin, 1973; Sherk et al., 1981). Suzuki and Yamamuro (1986) reported that infants delivered in the single-breech position (hips flexed and knees extended) had a higher incidence of congenital hip dysplasia than did infants born in cephalic, double-breech (i.e., both hips and knees flexed), or footling positions. It was postulated that, with extreme hip flexion combined with knee extension, the hamstrings pulled the head of the femur downward, thus stretching the compliant hip capsule. After birth, the femur was dislocated by the upward pull of the iliopsoas muscle when the infants were diapered and wrapped with the hips extended.

During normal postnatal growth, the depth of the acetabulum increases, progressively covering more of the femoral head until the age of 8 years, when the adult level of head coverage is reached (Beals, 1969). Normal compressive forces through the hip help to form the acetabulum and the femoral head into their appropriate shapes. Atypic pressures, such as those caused by abnormal pull by spastic muscles around the hip, deform the component parts of the hip and leave the child at risk for subluxation or dislocation (Heinrich et al., 1991).

Atypic changes in the shape of the acetabulum and femoral head have been reported in children with unstable or dislocated hips, such as children with congenitally dislocated hips, CP, or myelodysplasia. Buckley and colleagues (1991) examined 33 unstable hips in children with these disabilities and found that all had significantly more shallow acetabulae compared with those of a control group; the hip was most shallow in children with CP. The percentage of coverage of the head of the femur also was less for these children compared with that of control groups of children without disabilities. The children with disabilities had thinly developed articular surfaces and small shallow acetabulae with poorly defined margins. Beals (1969) reported that the acetabulae of children with CP in his study had appeared normal after birth, but that they did not increase in depth as expected by the age of 2 years. Nevertheless, acetabular depth was comparable to that of the normal population when the children were 8 years old. All but 1 of the 40 children included in this study were walking by 8 years of age, suggesting that the dynamic compressive forces of walking contributed to increased depth of the acetabulum. Beals also supported a standing program to increase the depth of the hip joint.

The torsional changes of the bone observed in

children with muscle imbalances or spasticity about the hip joint are good examples of the influence of the muscular system on the skeletal system. Femoral anteversion, or femoral torsion, is a twisting "forward of the head, neck, and trochanteric area of the femur in respect to the transcondylar axis of the knee" (Bleck, 1987, p. 323). At birth, the femoral head, neck, and greater trochanteric area are made of pliable cartilage and attached to the rigid osseus diaphysis. Normal torsional forces about this point of fixation cause a decrease in femoral anteversion as the infant develops. These torques are created by lateral hip rotation and extension (Bleck, 1987). If these movements are lacking, as is frequently observed in children with CP, the infantile femoral anteversion does not decrease as it should (Beals, 1969; Bleck, 1987; Samilson et al., 1972). Excessive femoral anteversion has been associated with the in-toed gait of children with CP (Bleck, 1987). Merchant (1965) explained this association by the decrease in gluteus medius muscle function in the presence of excessive femoral anteversion. The gluteus medius muscle is most effective in stabilizing the pelvis during the stance phase of gait when its insertion on the greater trochanter is in direct alignment with its origin. In excessive femoral anteversion, the greater trochanter is posterior to the midpoint of the ilium. To achieve maximal efficiency, the femur is rotated medially to align the insertion with the origin. The end result is an in-toed posture.

Changes in either the muscular or skeletal system due to internal or external forces often have interactive effects. Understanding the influences of these two systems on the development and final outcome of each system and recognizing the period when these systems are most mutable assist the therapist in designing effective treatment programs as well as in knowing when to discontinue treatment procedures.

ASSESSMENT AND EFFECTS OF INTERVENTION

Fundamental goals of therapeutic intervention for physical disabilities include preventing or correcting the impairments that are secondary to the underlying pathologic condition or to normal physiologic adaptations superimposed upon the pathologic condition. If impairments are prevented or corrected, then presumably function will be enhanced and disability decreased. Impairments of the range of motion (ROM) available about a joint or multiple joints and of the strength of the MTU are generally believed to bring about functional limitations and disability. Achieving maximal ROM by increasing the MTU length and achieving maximal strength are frequently two fundamental goals of therapeutic intervention. Accurate assessments of ROM and strength are, therefore, important components of the physical therapy evaluation.

Range of Motion Assessment

A wide range of methods and instruments has been reported for evaluating the ROM about a joint or multiple joints, including simple visual estimation, use of various protractors and goniometers, measurements made from still photographs, and complex methods using computerized motion analysis systems. To most physical therapists, however, the universal goniometer (i.e., full-circle manual goniometer) remains the most versatile and widely used instrument in clinical practice. The design of the universal goniometer and the procedures for its use have been described in detail in numerous publications. The articles by ML Moore (1949a,b) and the book by Norkin and White (1985) are particularly comprehensive and should be consulted for complete descriptions.

The reliability of goniometry is based on the reproducibility or stability of ROM measurements in relation to 1) the time intervals between comparable measurements or 2) the use of more than one rater. The ROM measurements must be reliable to be considered valid. Many factors influence the reliability and validity of goniometric measurements. These include consistency of the procedures applied, differences among joint actions and among the structure and function of body regions, passive versus active measurements, intrarater measurements (multiple measurements by one examiner) versus inter-rater measurements (multiple measurements by two or more examiners), normal day-to-day variations, and day-to-day variations in different pathologic conditions (Gajdosik & Bohannon, 1987).

Numerous studies have been reported on the ROM characteristics and the reliability of goniometry on adults, but reports on infants and children are more limited in number. Studies have demonstrated that full-term newborns present a limited range of hip and knee extension and greater plantar flexion compared with measurements in adults (Drews et al., 1984; Waugh et al., 1983). These findings were attributed to the effects of intrauterine position and newborn flexor muscle tone. Consequently, clinicians should not use normal adult ROM values for comparisons with limb

ROM measurements of the newborn. Studies with normal healthy children have indicated that ROM can probably be measured reliably (Haley et al., 1986), but studies of children with various pathologic conditions have shown that reliability varies with the number of raters (Pandya et al., 1985; Stuberg et al., 1988) and the pathologic problem (Ashton et al., 1978; Bartlett et al., 1985; Harris et al., 1985). Pandya and colleagues (1985) studied seven upper and lower extremity joint limitations in 150 children with Duchenne's muscular dystrophy and reported that intrarater reliability was high (intraclass correlation coefficient [ICC] range, .81–.91), but inter-rater reliability was lower, with a wide variation from joint to joint (ICC range, .25–.91). Stuberg and colleagues (1988) reported similar findings for children with CP.

Ashton and colleagues (1978) examined the day-to-day inter-rater reliability of measuring ROM of the hip in 4 children with spastic diplegia and found that the reliability tended to be lower for the 2 children with a moderate condition than for children with a mild condition. Harris and colleagues (1985) examined the goniometric reliability for a child with spastic quadriplegic CP and found that intrarater reliability exceeded inter-rater reliability, but both showed wide daily variations. The authors concluded that a difference of $\pm$ 10 to 15° in ROM over time does not signify a meaningful change in a child with spastic quadriplegic CP.

Bartlett and colleagues (1985) compared four methods of measuring hip extension (by prone extension, Thomas's test, Mundale method, and pelvic-femoral angle) in 45 children, of whom 15 had spastic diplegia, 15 had meningomyelocele, and 15 had no known pathologic condition. They reported that the Thomas test was particularly difficult to apply to patients with spastic diplegia and that improved reliability for these children would most likely result by using one of the other methods. The least reliable test in the meningomyelocele group was that of Mundale, probably because of difficulty in identifying bony landmarks in the presence of obesity and deformities.

The results of these few studies clearly indicate that the reliability of ROM measurements is influenced by the specific patient problem. Additional research is needed to clarify the goniometric reliability among the many different types of patients treated by pediatric physical therapists. Moreover, studies are clearly needed to examine the effects of changes in ROM on functional outcomes. In other words, can improved ROM predict improved function? In the meantime, therapists are encouraged to do their own reliability studies to establish confidence intervals for recognizing changes in ROM that are clinically significant. Because intrarater reliability has generally been shown to be acceptable, another alternative would be to have the therapist perform all the goniometric assessments on one child.

Strength Assessment

Accurate assessment of strength is important to identify strength deficits and in documenting changes in strength as a result of interventions. Numerous methods of assessing strength are available, including the traditional procedures of manual muscle testing (Daniels & Worthingham, 1980; Kendall & McCreary, 1983), use of various hand-held force dynamometers (Bohannon, 1987; Bohannon & Andrews, 1987) and computerized isokinetic testing systems (Rothstein et al., 1987). Although manual muscle testing is probably the most versatile and widely used method, recent evidence indicates that hand-held dynamometers may yield more precise measurements. Isokinetic systems are constructed primarily for use with adults, but they can be used with children large enough to fit the various components. The components could be modified, or smaller isokinetic devices could be developed to meet the special size requirements of children. Even so, children must be able to understand the instructions and follow commands to produce accurate and reliable strength measurements. The reliability of the strength measurements may also vary with the time of day, particularly for patients who fatigue by the end of the day. Obtaining reliable strength measurements for children may also depend on the enthusiasm or lack of enthusiasm of the child, the testing environment, and the testing clinician's rapport with the child. As with goniometry, standardization of testing procedures should improve the reliability of strength measurements.

The results of strength testing for children with specific pathologic conditions have been reported. Manual muscle testing was used to examine the force output for 17 upper and lower extremity muscle groups of 21 children with Duchenne's muscular dystrophy (Florence et al., 1984). The investigators examined the intrarater and inter-rater consistency of four physical therapists over a 2 year period and reported good consistency, with improvement in the reliability of the measurements over the period. Fowler and Gardner (1967) used a cable tensiometer and a hand-held dynamometer to assess the stability of measuring the isometric force of 13 muscle groups of 45 healthy boys and 75 children with Duchenne's, limb-girdle, facioscapulohumeral, or myotonic muscular dystrophy. The results showed age-specific force deficits in the children with muscular dystrophy compared with the force of healthy children and demonstrated that the force deficits were related to the type of muscular dystrophy. Similar studies that used hand-held dynamometers (Edwards, 1980; Hosking et al., 1976) and an isokinetic dynamometer (Sockolov et al., 1977) also reported force deficits in children with various types of muscular dystrophy compared with the force of healthy children. Given that strength varies by sex, the increased strength in boys at puberty may enhance their function in certain situations compared with that of girls. This finding may be particularly true for children with impaired lower extremity strength and function but normal upper extremity strength, such as children with meningomyelocele. Sex differences related to specific disorders and pubertal changes are worthy of clarification through controlled research studies.

The validity of strength assessments of muscles with spasticity is disputed. In the past, spastic muscles were not tested because their hypertonicity was believed to confound and compromise objective measurements. Current pediatric assessment procedures usually include evaluating other characteristics of muscle performance, such as reflex responses, movement patterns, movement against gravity, and functional performances. Evidence indicates that the results of strength tests of spastic muscles (tested with a hand-held dynamometer) in patients with adult-onset hemiplegia are related to gait velocity (Bohannon, 1986) and can also be used to show improvement related to the rehabilitation program (Bohannon & Smith, 1987). Similar methods of hand-held dynamometry could be applied to children with hypertonicity (e.g., CP) to yield objective assessments of force production and to document improvements.

The impact of spasticity on the antagonist muscle groups also warrants consideration. The importance of considering strength measurements of antagonists was demonstrated by examination of the strength changes of the dorsiflexor muscles after surgical lengthening of the triceps surae muscle group (Reimers, 1990a) and of the quadriceps muscles after surgical lengthening of the hamstring muscle group (Reimers, 1990b) of children with CP. The strength of the dorsiflexors had increased by 50% 4 weeks postoperatively and by more than 200% 14 months postoperatively (Reimers, 1990a). The strength of the quadriceps muscle group decreased by 70% 4 weeks postoperatively but was regained by 7 months, and by 13 months postoperatively the strength had increased by more than 50% (Reimers, 1990b). Taken together, these studies confirm the idea that antagonist muscle strength improves when the spastic agonist muscle group is lengthened. We encourage clinicians to examine methods of objectively measuring muscle strength in children with CP to study the changes in muscle strength resulting from both conservative and surgical interventions. Moreover, we encourage clinicians to relate strength changes to changes in the functional abilities of the children.

In addition to the possibility of objectively measuring the voluntary force produced in spastic muscles, a combination of technologies may now permit objective assessments of the degree of underlying hypertonicity. Isokinetic passive movements at different velocities, combined with the recording of electromyographic activity of the agonist and antagonist muscles could permit quantification of hypertonicity because muscles with spasticity present an increased velocity-dependent neuromuscular response to passive lengthening (Price et al., 1991). For example, rapid (e.g., 100°/s) passive lengthening of a spastic triceps surae muscle group through a short arc of motion would probably yield a quantifiable increase in the amount of passive resistance and EMG activity compared with a nonspastic triceps surae muscle group. If change in the passive force combined with change in the EMG activity could be assessed, then the effects of therapeutic interventions could be determined and related to functional outcomes. These possibilities are particularly worthy of future study, and clinicians are encouraged to participate in research projects to help examine these possibilities.

Effects of Intervention on the Musculoskeletal System

Objective evidence of the effects of strengthening exercises for particular pediatric patient conditions is limited. In the past, concerns about whether strengthening muscles of children with degenerative disorders would lead to a more rapid progression of the disorders have probably limited the application of strengthening programs. Some of the limited evidence available, however, indicates that "submaximal exercise has no negative effect and may be of limited value in increasing strength in Duchenne muscular dystrophy" (de Lateur & Giaconi, 1979, p. 36). The results of a case study of the effects of a progressive resistive exercise program for an adult with spastic CP suggested that strengthening exercises may improve strength, endurance, and ROM (Horvat, 1987). The development of objective methods of testing strength and the importance of the relationship between strength increases and functional outcomes promise to stimulate vigorous investigations in this area.

Passive and active slow static stretching exercises are used routinely as accepted methods of addressing abnormally short MTUs. Static stretching is believed to promote lengthening adaptations of the MTU, represented clinically by increases in ROM. Given the difficulty of evaluating the direct effects of stretching exercises on muscle and connective tissues in humans, the changes observed in the ROM in humans are based on associated histologic, biochemical, anatomic, and physiologic changes observed directly in animal models. For example, evidence has indicated that static stretching of adult hamstring muscles brings about lengthening and passive resistance adaptations similar to the adaptations reported for animal muscles immobilized in the lengthened position (Gajdosik, 1991b). Even prolonged passive stretching of MTUs in a state of severe contracture from long-term hypertonicity and shortening may promote lengthening adaptations and increased ROM in children with CP (McPherson et al., 1984). Whether changes observed from the stretching regimens are brought about by decreased neurologic excitability (hypertonicity), by adaptations in the muscle and connective tissues of the MTU, or by both remains controversial and worthy of investigation.

Serial casting and inhibitive casting methods have also been used to promote lengthening adaptations of the MTU, especially for children with CP or head injuries. Serial casting employs the principles of lengthening and shortening adaptations within the MTU. As discussed earlier in this chapter, investigators have demonstrated that when hypoextensible, abnormally short muscles of children with CP were serially casted in lengthened positions, length and passive compliance adaptations were enhanced (Tardieu, C, et al., 1979, 1982a; Tardieu, G, et al., 1982). The researchers indicated that the adaptations resulted directly from changes in the MTU; changes in the neurologic excitability of the muscles were not reported. Again, the presumption of an adaptive effect was based on the association of the active force and passive compliance curves of animals and of the human muscles measured by noninvasive methods with the histologic and histochemical adaptations observed in animal muscles.

Given the possibility that connective tissue adaptations (i.e., proliferation and remodeling) may contribute to the adaptations observed in the MTU, soft tissue mobilization procedures could also contribute to the desired adaptations. As a result of increased attention in continuing education offerings, the use of soft tissue mobilization with children is increasing. Case reports and systematic research on this approach are direly needed.

The differences in effect between serial casting and inhibitive casting are difficult to identify. In a review of casting principles and theories, Carlson (1984) indicated that proponents of inhibitive casting suggest that the casting procedures have a neurophysiologic influence on the motoneuron excitability that results in a reduction in spasticity. As stated earlier, the observed lengthening changes in the MTU, as indirectly represented by changes in ROM, may result from changes in the MTU directly or from changes in muscle activation patterns and not necessarily from changes in motoneuron excitability. The finding of enhanced strength and function of the antagonist muscle group after surgical lengthening of the agonist muscle groups (Reimers, 1990a,b) supports the hypothesis that functional changes result from direct changes in muscle length, not from motoneuron excitability. This proposal was also supported by the finding that splinting spastic muscles of patients with brain damage changed ROM without altering the integrated EMG activity of the muscles compared with the activity in muscles that were not splinted (Mills, 1984).

Clearly, a major problem in interpreting the clinical reports of the effects of inhibitory casting centers on the confusing and variable definition of "tone." Is tone caused by central or peripheral influences or by both? Knowledge of the interrelationships among the length, tension, and passive compliance of the MTU and of the neurologic excitability of the muscles of neurologically impaired children and how the interrelationships are influenced by therapeutic interventions remains sparse. Additional research is needed to explore the effects of many therapeutic methods on the active and passive characteristics of the MTU, including such methods as muscle strengthening and stretching and soft tissue mobilization and casting. The application of passive isokinetic movements combined with recording of EMG, as stated earlier in this chapter, could be used to examine the effects of these interventions on spastic muscles. In the meantime, clinicians should maintain objective records of strength and ROM and attempt to correlate these findings with specific therapeutic interventions and functional outcomes.

The shape and size of the skeletal system are most susceptible to alteration during periods of rapid growth; hence, undesirable forces, as well as appropriate corrective forces, are most influential during childhood. Many deformities that occur during the fetal or early postnatal period are more easily corrected in the infant than in the older child. For example, congenitally dislocated hips often readily respond to bracing during the first year of life (Sherk et al., 1981). If, however, the dislocated hip is not diagnosed until after 12 months, surgery is often necessary. Bracing for idiopathic scoliosis is most effective for preventing worsening of the curve during the preteen and teenage years (Cassella & Hall, 1991). Once an individual has stopped growing, the external support is no longer needed.

The influence of orthoses on the growth of children has not been thoroughly investigated. Bleck (1987) reported that full-control hip-knee-ankle orthoses have not been successful in preventing structural deformities in children with CP. These children still developed dislocated hips or hip flexion contractures. In a study of 204 children, Lee (1982) reported that regardless of the type of CP the presence or absence of bracing did not influence the development of deformities. Bracing did not diminish the need for surgery to correct deformities nor did it prevent recurrences of deformities after the surgery. Lee and Bleck (1980) reported a 9% recurrence rate of shortening after Achilles tendon lengthening in children with CP who did not wear night splints to maintain tendon length. This rate, however, was comparable with that reported in other studies of children who did wear night splints (Bleck, 1987). Preventing deformities via bracing may be more difficult in children with abnormal tone than in those with normal tone or paralysis.

Orthoses can also lead to the development of secondary deformities. Lusskin (1966) reported two case studies of children with lower extremity paralysis resulting from polio. Both children had marked tibial-fibular torsion yet were braced in knee-ankle-foot orthoses with the knees and feet facing forward. As a result, a rotational force was placed at the ankle and foot, and these children developed severe metatarsus adductus and heel varus. Children who wear ankle-foot orthoses for most of their growing years may be at risk for stunted growth of the foot and lower limb. The circumferential compressive forces as well as the restriction in active movement can interfere with normal musculoskeletal growth. Pediatric physical therapists have an important responsibility to understand the effects of external devices on the growing child. While trying to solve one problem, the therapist may inadvertently create another.

Weight-bearing activities retard the loss of bone mass as well as help to shape the joint (Beals, 1969; Harrison, 1961; Stuberg, 1992). In a preliminary study, Stuberg found that 60 minutes of standing 4 or 5 times a week increased the bone mineral density of nonambulatory children with severe to profound CP. When the standing program was discontinued, bone mineral density decreased. Standing programs may also help deepen the acetabulum. The contact between the femoral head and the acetabulum in weight bearing helps in the development of the normal shape of the acetabulum, which contributes to a stable hip socket (Beals, 1969; Harrison, 1961).

Movement has been reported to affect the formation and shape of joints in fetal animals (Drachman & Sokoloff, 1966; Murray & Drachman, 1969). Movement allows the compressive forces to be spread throughout the joint surface and not confined to a small area. Combining weight-bearing activities with movement would create more desirable forces for joint formation. Although no research has been reported on the effects on hip formation of stationary standing devices, such as prone boards or standing platforms, it appears reasonable to use caution when using these devices with very young children. Since remodeling of the bone and associated joints takes place most readily during the first few years of life and since the acetabular shape is fairly well defined by the age of 3 years (Ralis & McKibbin, 1973), early intervention with weight-bearing activities may have a substantial influence on the shape and function of the joint. To help shape the joint, chronologic age and not developmental age may be more important when determining when to begin weight-bearing activities. Although standing is important, the length of time the child stands during any one period may need to be controlled.

For the young child with severe delays in motor development in whom independent walking (with or without devices) is unlikely and hip dislocation is a risk, early and prolonged standing may be beneficial in developing a deeper hip joint. The shape of the acetabulum may not be appropriate for walking, but the hip may be more stable. Over time, this early standing may help to prevent or decrease the severity of a dislocated hip. For children with milder delays, less stationary standing time and more weight bearing with movement may help to develop a more normally shaped hip socket. This may contribute to an improved gait and a decrease in the risk of osteoarthritis in adulthood. Certainly, more research in this area would give the pediatric physical therapist valuable information for designing treatment programs with weight-bearing activities.

In summary, this chapter reviewed the normal growth and development of the musculoskeletal system, with emphasis on the adaptations of muscle and bone associated with pathologic conditions encountered by pediatric physical therapists. The microscopic and macroscopic structure and function of the normal MTU and the force and length adaptations to imposed physical changes, such as immobilization and denervation, have been well documented in nonhuman studies using invasive methods of investigation. The results of human studies using noninvasive methods of investigation indicate that the human MTU undergoes adaptations similar to those reported for animals. The clinical evidence for the musculoskeletal adaptations supports these research findings.

In the developing child, atypic changes in the MTU can exert forces on the skeletal system, resulting in bone deformities. Pediatric physical therapists routinely assess physical impairments and develop therapeutic interventions designed to promote musculoskeletal adaptations. To document therapeutic efficacy in relation to specific pediatric disorders, therapists are encouraged to use objective assessments of ROM and strength during specific interventions for correlating changes in musculoskeletal impairments with functional outcomes. Additional research is needed to examine the efficacy of therapeutic strengthening and stretching programs and their interrelation with other interventions, such as surgical procedures. The application of new research technologies, such as isokinetic dynamometry and EMG, may now permit objective assessment of neuromuscular disorders and the effects of interventions designed to influence these disorders. Further controlled studies will enhance the scientific basis for using physical therapy to promote improved functional outcomes.

References

Alder, AB, Crawford, GNC, & Edwards, GR. The effect of limitation of movement on longitudinal muscle growth. Proceedings of the Royal Society of London. Series B: Biological Sciences, 150:554–562, 1959.

Arkin, AM, & Katz, JF. The effects of pressure on epiphyseal growth. Journal of Bone and Joint Surgery (American), 38:1056–1076, 1956.

Ashton, BB, Pickles, B, & Roll, JW. Reliability of goniometric measurements of hip motion in spastic cerebral palsy. Developmental Medicine and Child Neurology, 20:87–94, 1978.

Banus, MG, & Zetlin, AM. The relation of isometric tension to length of skeletal muscle. Journal of Cellular and Comparative Physiology, 12:403–420, 1938.

Bartlett, MD, Wolf, LS, Shurtleff, DB, & Staheli, LT. Hip flexion contractures: A comparison of measurement procedures. Archives of Physical Medicine and Rehabilitation, 66:620–625, 1985.

Beals, RK. Developmental changes in the femur and acetabulum in spastic paraplegia and diplegia. Developmental Medicine and Child Neurology, 11:303–313, 1969.

Bernhardt, DB. Prenatal and postnatal growth and development of the foot and ankle. Physical Therapy, 68:1831–1839, 1988.

Bleck, EE. Orthopedic Management in Cerebral Palsy. Philadelphia, JB Lippincott, 1987.

Bohannon, RW. Strength of lower limb related to gait velocity and cadence in stroke patients. Physiotherapy Canada, 38:204–206, 1986.

Bohannon, RW. Hand-held dynamometry: Stability of muscle strength over multiple measurements. Clinical Biomechanics, 2:74–77, 1987.

Bohannon, RW, & Andrews, AW. Inter-rater reliability of hand-held dynamometer. Physical Therapy, 67:931–933, 1987.

Bohannon, RW, & Smith, MB. Assessment of strength deficits in eight paretic upper extremity muscle groups of stroke patients with hemiplegia. Physical Therapy, 67:522–525, 1987.

Borg, TK, & Caulfield, JB. Morphology of connective tissue in skeletal muscle. Tissue and Cell, 12:197–207, 1980.

Botelho, SY, Cander, L, & Guiti, N. Passive and active tension-length diagrams of intact skeletal muscle in normal women of different ages. Journal of Applied Physiology, 7:93–95, 1954.

Brodie, TG. The extensibility of muscle. Journal of Anatomy and Physiology, 29:367–388, 1895.

Brooke, MH. A Clinician's View of Neuromuscular Disease. Baltimore: Williams & Wilkins, 1986.

Brooke, MH, & Engel, WK. The histographic analyses of human muscle biopsies with regard to fiber types: 4. Children's biopsies. Neurology, 19:591–605, 1969.

Brown, MC, Jansen, JKS, & Van Essen, D. Polyneuronal innervation of skeletal muscle in newborn rats and its elimination during maturation. Journal of Physiology, 261:387–422, 1976.

Buckley, SL, Sponseller, PD, & Maged, D. The acetabulum in congenital and neuromuscular hip instability. Journal of Pediatric Orthopedics, 11:498–501, 1991.

Buller, AJ, Eccles, JC, & Eccles, RM. Differentiation of fast and slow muscles in the cat hind limb. Journal of Physiology, 150:399–416, 1960.

Bunch, W. Origin and mechanism of postnatal deformities. Pediatric Clinics of North America, 24:679–684, 1977.

Butler, J, Cosmos, E, & Brienley, J. Differentiation of muscle fiber types in aneurogenic muscles of the chick embryo. Journal of Experimental Zoology, 224:65–80, 1982.

Cardenas, DD, Stolov, WC, & Hardy, R. Muscle fiber number in immobilization atrophy. Archives of Physical Medicine and Rehabilitation, 58:423–426, 1977.

Carlson, SJ. A neurophysiological analysis of inhibitive casting. Physical and Occupational Therapy in Pediatrics, 4(4):31–42, 1984.

Carter, DR, Orr, TE, Fyhrie, DP, & Schurman, DJ. Influences of mechanical stress on prenatal and postnatal skeletal development. Clinical Orthopedics and Related Research, 219:237–250, 1987.

Casella, C. Tensile force in total striated muscle, isolated fibre and sarcolemma. Acta Physiologica Scandinavica, 21:380–401, 1950.

Cassella, MC, & Hall, JE. Current treatment approaches in the nonoperative and operative management of adolescent idiopathic scoliosis. Physical Therapy, 71:897–909, 1991.

Chandraraj, S, & Briggs, CA. Multiple growth cartilages in the neural arch. Anatomical Record, 230(1):114–120, 1991.

Cozen, L. Knock-knee deformity in children: Congenital and acquired. Clinical Orthopedics and Related Research, 258:191–203, 1990.

Dhanani, S, Brendi, AL, & Hudson, H. Hamstring tenotomies in cerebral palsy: Long-term retrospective analysis. Journal of Pediatric Orthopedics, 11:514–519, 1991.

Daniels, L, & Worthingham, C. Muscle Testing: Techniques of Manual Examination (4th ed.). Philadelphia: WB Saunders, 1980.

Davis, JA, & Dobbing, J (Eds.). Scientific Foundations of Paediatrics. Philadelphia: WB Saunders, 1974.

de Lateur, BJ, & Giaconi, RM. Effect on maximal strength of submaximal exercise in Duchenne muscular dystrophy. American Journal of Physical Medicine, 58:26–36, 1979.

Drachman, DB, & Sokoloff, L. The role of movement in embryonic joint development. Developmental Biology, 14:401–420, 1966.

Drews, JE, Vraciu, JK, & Pellino, G. Range of motion of the joints of the lower extremities of newborns. Physical and Occupational Therapy in Pediatrics, 4(2):49–62, 1984.

Edmonson, AD, & Crenshaw, AH (Eds.). Campbell's Operative Orthopaedics, Vol. 2. St. Louis: CV Mosby, 1980.

Edwards, RHT. Studies of muscular performance in normal and dystrophic subjects. British Medical Bulletin, 36:159–164, 1980.

Farkas-Bargeton, E, Barbet, JP, Dancea, S, Wehrle R, Checouri, A, & Dulac, O. Immaturity of muscle fibers in the congenital form of myotonic dystrophy: Its consequences and its origin. Journal of the Neurological Sciences, 83(2–3):145–159, 1988.

Flitney, FW, & Hirst, DG. Cross-bridge detachment and sarcomere 'give' during stretch of active frog's muscle. Journal of Physiology, 276:449–465, 1978.

Florence, JM, Pandya, S, King, WM, Robison, JD, Signore, LC, Wentzell, M, & Province, MA. Clinical trials in Duchenne dystrophy: Standardization and reliability of evaluation procedures. Physical Therapy, 64:41–45, 1984.

Fowler, WM, & Gardner, GW. Quantitative strength measurements in muscular dystrophy. Archives of Physical Medicine and Rehabilitation, 48:629–644, 1967.

Fulford, G, & Brown, J. Position as a cause of deformity in children with cerebral palsy. Developmental Medicine and Child Neurology, 18:305–314, 1977.

Gajdosik, RL. Passive compliance and length of clinically short hamstring muscles of healthy men. Clinical Biomechanics, 6:239–244, 1991a.

Gajdosik, RL. Effects of static stretching on the maximal length and resistance to passive stretch of short hamstring muscles. Journal of Orthopedic Sports and Physical Therapy, 14:250–255, 1991b.

Gajdosik, RL, & Bohannon, RW. Clinical measurement of range of motion: Review of goniometry emphasizing reliability and validity. Physical Therapy, 67:1867–1872, 1987.

Gajdosik, RL, Guiliani, CA, & Bohannon, RW. Passive compliance of the hamstring muscles of healthy men and women. Clinical Biomechanics, 5:23–29, 1990.

Gasser, T, Kneip, A, Ziegler, P, Largo, R, Molinari, L, & Prader, A. The dynamics of growth of width in distance, velocity and acceleration. Annals of Human Biology, 18(5):449–461, 1991.

Goldspink, DF. The influence of immobilization and stretch on protein turnover of rat skeletal muscle. Journal of Physiology, 64:267–282, 1977.

Goldspink, G, Tabary, C, Tabary, JC, Tardieu, C, & Tardieu, G. Effect of denervation on the adaptation of sarcomere number and muscle extensibility to the functional length of the muscle. Journal of Physiology, 236:733–742, 1974.

Gordon, AM, Huxley, AF, & Julian, FJ. The variation in isometric tension with sarcomere length in vertebrate muscle fibers. Journal of Physiology, 184:170–192, 1966.

Granzier, HLM, & Pollack, GH. Stepwise shortening in unstimulated frog skeletal muscle fibers. Journal of Physiology, 362:173–188, 1985.

Griffiths, PJ, Guth, K, Kuhn, HJ, & Ruegg, JC. Cross bridge slippage in skinned frog muscle fibres. Biophysics of Structure and Mechanism, 7:107–124, 1980.

Grove, BK. Muscle differentiation and the origin of muscle fiber diversity. CRC Critical Reviews of Neurobiology, 4(3):201–234, 1989.

Guth, K, Kuhn, HJ, Herzig, JW, & Ruegg, JC. Evidence for cross bridge slippage in stretched muscle fibre. Experientia, 34:1183–1184, 1978.

Halar, EM, Stolov, WC, Venkatesh, B, Brozovivh, FV, & Harley, JD. Gastrocnemius muscle belly and tendon length in stroke patients and able-bodied persons. Archives of Physical Medicine and Rehabilitation, 59:467–484, 1978.

Haley, SM, Tada, WL, & Carmichael, EM. Spinal mobility in young children: A normative study. Physical Therapy, 66:1697–1703, 1986.

Harris, SR, Smith, LH, & Krukowski, L. Goniometric reliability for a child with spastic quadriplegia. Journal of Pediatric Orthopedics, 5:348–351, 1985.

Harrison, TJ. The influence of the femoral head on pelvic growth and acetabular form in the rat. Journal of Anatomy (British), 95:12–24, 1961.

Haycraft, B. The elasticity of animal tissues. Journal of Physiology, 31:392–409, 1904.

Heinrich, SD, MacEwen, GD, & Zembo, MM. Hip dysplasia, subluxation, and dislocation in cerebral palsy: An arthrographic analysis. Journal of Pediatric Orthopedics, 11:488–493, 1991.

Hill, DK. Tension due to interaction between sliding filaments in resting striated muscle: The effect of stimulation. Journal of Physiology, 199:637–684, 1968.

Hill, DK. The effect of temperature in the range of 0–35°C on the resting tension of frog's muscle. Journal of Physiology, 208:725–739, 1970a.

Hill, DK. The effect of temperature on the resting tension of frog's muscle in hypertonic solutions. Journal of Physiology, 208:741–756, 1970b.

Hopp, R, Degan, J, Gallager, JC, & Cassidy, JT. Estimation of bone mineral density in children with juvenile rheumatoid arthritis. Journal of Rheumatology, 18:1235–1239, 1991.

Horvat, M. Effects of a progressive resistance training program on an individual with spastic cerebral palsy. American Corrective Therapy Journal, 41:7–10, 1987.

Hosking, GP, Bhat, US, Dubowitz, V, & Edwards, HT. Measurements of muscle strength and performance in children with normal and diseased muscle. Archives of Disease in Childhood, 51:957–963, 1976.

Huet de la Tour, E, Tabary, JC, Tabary, C, & Tardieu C. The respective roles of muscle length and muscle tension in sarcomere number adaptation of guinea-pig soleus muscle. Journal de Physiologie, 75:589–592, 1979a.

Huet de la Tour, E, Tardieu, C, Tabary, JC, & Tabary C. Decreased muscle extensibility and reduction of sarcomere number in soleus muscle following local injection of tetanus toxin. Journal of the Neurological Sciences, 40:123–131, 1979b.

Huxley, AF, & Peachey, LD. The maximum length for contraction in vertebrate striated muscle. Journal of Physiology, 156:150–165, 1961.

Huxley, AF, & Simmons, RM. Proposed mechanism of force generation in striated muscle. Nature, 233:533–538, 1971.

Kamieniecka, L. The stages of development of human fetal muscles with reference to some muscular diseases. Journal of the Neurological Sciences, 7:319–329, 1968.

Katz, K, Naor, N, Merlob, P, & Wielunsky, E. Rotational deformities of the tibia and foot in preterm infants. Journal of Pediatric Orthopedics, 10:483–485, 1990.

Kendall, FP, & McCreary, EK. Muscles Testing and Function (3rd ed.). Baltimore: Williams & Wilkins, 1983.

King, HA & Staheli, LT. Torsional problems in cerebral palsy. Foot and Ankle, 4:180–184, 1984.

Kitiyakara, A, & Angevine, DM. A study of the pattern of

post-embryonic growth of M. gracilis in mice. Developmental Biology, 8:322–340, 1963.

Lee, CL. Role of lower extremity bracing in cerebral palsy (Abstract). Developmental Medicine and Child Neurology, 24:250–251, 1982.

Lee, CL, & Bleck, EE. Surgical correction of equinus deformity in cerebral palsy. Developmental Medicine and Child Neurology, 22:287–292, 1980.

Lespargot, A, Tardieu, C, Bret, MD, Tabary, C, & Singh, B. Is tendon surgery for the knee flexors justified in cerebral palsy? French Journal of Orthopedic Surgery, 3(4):446–450, 1989.

LeVeau, BF, & Bernhardt, DB. Effects of forces on the growth, development, and maintenance of the human body. Physical Therapy, 64:1874–1882, 1984.

Lewis, FR, Samilson, RR, & Lucas, DB. Femoral torsion and coxa valga in cerebral palsy: A preliminary report. Developmental Medicine and Child Neurology, 6:591–597, 1964.

Lusskin, R. The influence of errors in bracing upon deformity of the lower extremity. Archives of Physical Medicine and Rehabilitation, 47:520–525, 1966.

Magid, A, & Law, DJ. Myofibrils bear most of the resting tension in frog skeletal muscle. Science, 230:1280–1282, 1985.

Martin, AD, & McCulloch, RG. Bone dynamics: Stress, strain, and fracture. Journal of Sports Sciences, 5:155–163, 1987.

Mastaglia, FL. The growth and development of the skeletal muscles. In Davis, JA, & Dobbing, J (Eds.), Scientific Foundations of Paediatrics. Philadelphia: WB Saunders, 1974, pp. 348–375.

Matsubara, I, & Yagi, N. Movements of cross-bridges during and after slow changes in active frog skeletal muscle. Journal of Physiology, 361:151–163, 1985.

McKibbin, B. The structure of the epiphysis. In Owen, R, Goodfellow, J, & Bullough, P (Eds.), Scientific Foundations of Orthopaedics and Traumatology. Philadelphia: WB Saunders, 1981.

McPherson, JJ, Arends, TG, Michaels, MJ, & Trettin, K. The range of motion of long term knee contractures of four spastic cerebral palsied children: A pilot study. Physical and Occupational Therapy in Pediatrics, 4(1):17–34, 1984.

Merchant, AJ. Hip abduction muscle force. Journal of Bone and Joint Surgery (American), 47:462–475, 1965.

Mills, VM. Electromyographic results of inhibitory splinting. Physical Therapy, 64:190–193, 1984.

Moore, KL. The Developing Human: Clinically Oriented Embryology (4th ed.). Philadelphia: WB Saunders, 1988.

Moore, ML. The measurement of joint motion: Part I. Introductory review of the literature. Physical Therapy Review, 29:195–205, 1949a.

Moore, ML. The measurement of joint motion: Part II. The technique of goniometry. Physical Therapy Review, 29:256–264, 1949b.

Murray, PDF, & Drachman, DB. The role of movement in the development of joints and the related structures: The head and neck in the chick embryo. Journal of Embryology and Experimental Morphology, 22:349–371, 1969.

Norkin, CC, & White, DJ. Measurement of Joint Motion: A Guide to Goniometry. Philadelphia: FA Davis, 1985.

Owen, R, Goodfellow, J, & Bullough, P (Eds.). Scientific Foundations of Orthopaedics and Traumatology. Philadelphia: WB Saunders, 1981.

Pandya, S, Florence, JM, King, WM, Robison, JD, Lyman, M, & Province, MA. Reliability of goniometric measurements in patients with Duchenne muscular dystrophy. Physical Therapy, 65:1339–1342, 1985.

Price, R, Bjornson, KF, Lehmann, JF, McLaughlin, JF, & Hays, RM. Quantitative measurement of spasticity in children with cerebral palsy. Developmental Medicine and Child Neurology, 33:585–595, 1991.

Purves, D, & Lichtman, JW. Elimination of synapses in the developing nervous system. Science, 210:153–157, 1980.

Rack, PMH, & Westbury, DR. The short range stiffness of active mammalian muscle and its effect on mechanical properties. Journal of Physiology, 240:331–350, 1974.

Ralis, Z, & McKibbin, B. Changes in shape of the human hip joint during its development and their relation to stability. Journal of Bone and Joint Surgery (British), 55:780–785, 1973.

Ramsey, RW, & Street, SF. The isometric length-tension diagram of isolated skeletal muscle fibers of the frog. Journal of Cellular and Comparative Physiology, 15:11–34, 1940.

Ranson, SW, & Dixon, HH. The elasticity and ductility of muscle in the myostatic contracture caused by tetanus toxin. American Journal of Physiology, 86:312–319, 1928.

Reimers, J. Contracture of the hamstrings in spastic cerebral palsy: A study of three methods of operative correction. Journal of Bone and Joint Surgery (British), 56:102–109, 1974.

Reimers, J. Functional changes in the antagonists after lengthening the agonists in cerebral palsy: I. Triceps surae lengthening. Clinical Orthopaedics and Related Research, 253:30–34, 1990a.

Reimers, J. Functional changes in the antagonists after lengthening the agonists in cerebral palsy: II. Quadriceps strength before and after distal hamstring lengthening. Clinical Orthopaedics and Related Research, 253:35–37, 1990b.

Rodriguez, TI, Razquin, S, Palacios, T, & Rubio, V. Human growth plate development in the fetal and neonatal period. Journal of Orthopaedic Research, 10(1):62–71, 1992.

Rose, SJ, & Rothstein, JM. Muscle mutability: Part 1. General concepts and adaptation to altered patterns of use. Physical Therapy, 62:1773–1784, 1982.

Rothstein, JM, Lamb, RL, & Mayhew, TP. Clinical uses of isokinetic measurements: Critical issues. Physical Therapy, 67:1840–1844, 1987.

Rothstein, JM, & Rose, SJ. Muscle mutability. Part 2, Adaptation to drugs, metabolic factors, and aging. Physical Therapy, 62:1788–1798, 1982.

Rowe, RWD. Collagen fibre arrangement in intramuscular connective tissue. Changes associated with muscle shortening and their possible relevance to raw meat toughness measurements. Journal of Food Technology, 9:501–508, 1974.

Rowe, RWD. Morphology of perimysial and endomysial connective tissue in skeletal muscle. Tissue and Cell, 13:681–690, 1981.

Royer, P. Growth of bony tissue. In Davis, JA, & Dobbing, J (Eds.), Scientific Foundations of Paediatrics. Philadelphia: WB Saunders, 1974.

Rural Institute on Disabilities. Secondary Disability Surveillance Report for 1989: Cerebral Palsy. Missoula, MT: University of Montana, 1989.

Salmons, S, & Hendriksson, J. The adaptive response of skeletal muscle to increased use. Muscle and Nerve, 4:94–105, 1981.

Samilson, RL, Tsou, P, Aamoth, G, & Green, WM. Dislocation and subluxation of the hip in cerebral palsy. Journal of Bone and Joint Surgery (American), 54:863–873, 1972.

Sanes, JR. Cell lineage and the origin of muscle fiber types. Trends in Neurosciences, 10(6):119–121, 1987.

Sargeant, AJ, Davies, CTM, Edwards, RHT, Maunder, C, & Young, A. Functional and structural changes after disuse of human muscle. Clinical Science and Molecular Medicine, 52:337–342, 1977.

Sharrard, WJW. Paralytic deformity in the lower limb. Journal of Bone and Joint Surgery (British), 49:731–747, 1967.

Sherk, HH, Pasquariello, PS, & Watters, WC. Congenital dislocation of the hip. Clinical Pediatrics, 20(8):513–520, 1981.

Sichel, FJM. The elasticity of isolated resting skeletal muscle fibres. Journal of Cellular and Comparative Physiology, 5:21–42, 1934.

Slaton, D. Muscle fiber types and their development in the human fetus. Physical and Occupational Therapy in Pediatrics, *1*(3):47–57, 1981.

Slaton, D. Mutability of muscle fiber types. Physical and Occupational Therapy in Pediatrics, *4*(1):5–15, 1984.

Sockolov, R, Irwin, B, Dressendorfer, RH, & Bernauer, EM. Exercise performance in 6- to 11-year-old boys with Duchenne muscular dystrophy. Archives of Physical Medicine and Rehabilitation, *58*:195–200, 1977.

Stolov, WC, Riddell, WM, & Shrier, KP. Effect of electrical stimulation on contracture of immobilized, innervated and denervated muscle (Abstract). Archives in Physical Medicine and Rehabilitation, *52*:589, 1971.

Stolov, WC, & Weilepp, TG. Passive length-tension relationship of intact muscle, epimysium, and tendon in normal and denervated gastrocnemius of the rat. Archives in Physical Medicine and Rehabilitation, *47*:612–620, 1966.

Stolov, WC, Weilepp, TB Jr, & Riddell, WM. Passive length-tension relationship and hydroxyproline content of chronically denervated skeletal muscle. Archives in Physical Medicine and Rehabilitation, *51*:517–525, 1970.

Stuberg, WA. Considerations related to weight-bearing programs in children with developmental disabilities. Physical Therapy, *72*:35–40, 1992.

Stuberg, WA, Fuchs, RH, & Miedaner, JA. Reliability of goniometric measurements of children with cerebral palsy. Developmental Medicine and Child Neurology, *30*:657–666, 1988.

Suzuki, S, & Yamamuro, T. Correction of fetal posture and congenital dislocation of hip. Acta Orthopaedica Scandinavica, *57*:81–84, 1986.

Tabary, JC, Tabary, C, Tardieu, C, Tardieu, G, & Goldspink, G. Physiological and structural changes in the cat's soleus muscle due to immobilization at different lengths by plaster casts. Journal of Physiology, *224*:231–244, 1972.

Tabary, JC, Tardieu, C, Tardieu, G, & Tabary, C. Experimental rapid sarcomere loss with concomitant hypoextensibility. Muscle and Nerve, *4*:198–203, 1981.

Tanabe, Y, & Nonaka, I. Congenital myotonic dystrophy. Changes in muscle pathology with ageing. Journal of the Neurological Sciences, *77*:59–68, 1987.

Tardieu, C, Huet de la Tour, E, Bret, MD, & Tardieu, G. Muscle hypoextensibility in children with cerebral palsy: I. Clinical and experimental observations. Archives of Physical Medicine and Rehabilitation, *63*:97–102, 1982a.

Tardieu, C, Tabary, JC, Tabary, C, & Tardieu, G. Adaptation of connective tissue length to immobilization in the lengthened and shortened positions in the cat soleus muscle. Journal de Physiologie, *78*:214–220, 1982b.

Tardieu, C, Tardieu, G, Colbeau-Justin, P, & Huet de la Tour, E. Trophic muscle regulation in children with congenital cerebral lesions. Journal of the Neurological Sciences, *42*:357–364, 1979.

Tardieu, G, Tardieu, C, Colbeau-Justin, P, & Lespargot, A. Muscle hypoextensibility in children with cerebral palsy: II. Therapeutic implications. Archives of Physical Medicine and Rehabilitation, *63*:103–107, 1982.

Thompson, WJ. Changes in the innervation of mammalian skeletal muscle fibers during postnatal development. Trends in Neurosciences, *9*:25–28, 1986.

Thompson, WJ, Condon, K, & Astrow, SH. The origin and selective innervation of early muscle fiber types in the rat. Journal of Neurobiology, *21*(1):212–222, 1990.

Thompson, WJ, & Jansen, JKS. The extent of sprouting of remaining motor units in partly denervated immature and adult rat soleus muscle. Neuroscience, *2*:523–535, 1977.

Thomson, JD. Mechanical characteristics of skeletal muscle undergoing atrophy of degeneration. American Journal of Physical Medicine, *34*:606–611, 1955.

Trueta, T. The growth and development of bone and joints: Orthopedic aspects. In Davis, JA, & Dobbing, J (Eds.), Scientific Foundations of Paediatrics. Philadelphia: WB Saunders, 1974.

Walker, JM. Musculoskeletal development: A review. Physical Therapy, *71*:878–889, 1991.

Ward, SS, & Stickland, NC. Why are slow and fast muscles differentially affected during prenatal under-nutrition? Muscle and Nerve, *14*(3):259–267, 1991.

Waugh, KG, Minkel, JL, Parker, R, & Coon, VA. Measurement of selected hip, knee, and ankle joint motions in newborns. Physical Therapy, *63*:1616–1621, 1983.

Williams, PE, & Goldspink, G. Longitudinal growth of striated muscle fibers. Journal of Cell Science, *9*:751–767, 1971.

Williams, PE, & Goldspink, G. The effect of immobilization on the longitudinal growth of striated muscle fibers. Journal of Anatomy (London), *116*:45–55, 1973.

Williams, PE, & Goldspink, G. Changes in sarcomere length and physiological properties in immobilized muscle. Journal of Anatomy (London), *127*:459–468, 1978.

Williams, PE, & Goldspink, G. Connective tissue changes in immobilized muscle. Journal of Anatomy (London), *138*:342–350, 1984.

Williamson, GG (Ed.). Children with Spina Bifida. Baltimore: Brookes, 1987, p. 97.

Yagi, N, & Matsubara, I. Cross-bridge movements during a slow length change of active muscle. Biophysical Journal, *45*:611–614, 1984.

Chapter 5

Physical Fitness During Childhood and Adolescence

JEAN L. STOUT, PT, MS

Physical fitness is a construct that is difficult to define because it cannot be measured directly. Physical fitness is generally viewed as having two facets—health-related fitness and the more traditional motor fitness. Motor fitness generally includes physical abilities that relate to athletic performance, whereas health-related fitness includes abilities related to daily function and health maintenance. Experts believe that disease prevention in adulthood is correlated with health-related fitness (Pate & Shephard, 1989). For example, adults who are physically active have a lower risk of severe coronary artery disease (CAD) (Morris et al., 1953). Many of the risk factors that lead to CAD in adults have also been identified as risk factors in children (Despres et al., 1990; Montoye, 1985), but it is not known whether physical activity in childhood is associated with reduced health risks in adulthood. Furthermore, physical activity and physical fitness are not synonymous terms. We do not know how much physical activity is necessary for health and fitness in children.

For clinicians who design exercise programs and treat children with disabilities, it is important to have an understanding of childhood physical fitness. With this knowledge we can assess patients' level of fitness in relation to overall health and establish appropriate goals of fitness and training for our patients' specific disabilities. This chapter provides the reader with an understanding of (1) physical fitness and the cardiopulmonary response to exercise in children of different ages who do not have disabling conditions, (2) the components of physical fitness (cardiorespiratory endurance, muscular strength and endurance, flexibility, and body composition; Table 5–1), (3) the standards of fitness components consistent with good health, and (4) the effects of training and conditioning on overall physical fitness. Assessment of the components of fitness in various special populations will also be addressed. The chapter includes a review of the current physical fitness tests.

HEALTH, PHYSICAL ACTIVITY, AND PHYSICAL FITNESS

Health-related fitness is defined as a state characterized by 1) an ability to perform daily activities with vigor and 2) traits and capacities that are associated with low risk of premature development of hypokinetic disease (i.e., disease due to physical inactivity) (Pate, 1983).

TABLE 5–1. **HEALTH-RELATED FITNESS COMPONENTS AND THE RATIONALE FOR IMPORTANCE TO HEALTH PROMOTION AND DISEASE PREVENTION**

Component	Rationale
Cardiorespiratory endurance	Improved physical working capacity
	Reduced fatigue
	Reduced risk of coronary heart disease
	Optimal growth and development
Muscular strength and endurance	Improved functional capacity for lifting and carrying
	Reduced risk of lower back pain
	Optimal posture
	Optimal growth and development
Flexibility	Enhanced functional capacity for bending and twisting
	Reduced risk of lower back pain
	Optimal growth and development
Body composition	Reduced risk of hypertension
	Reduced risk of coronary heart disease
	Reduced risk of diabetes
	Optimal growth and development

Adapted from Pate, RR, & Shephard, RJ. Characteristics of physical fitness in youth. In Gisolfi, CV, & Lamb, DR (Eds.), Perspectives in Exercise Science and Sports Medicine, Vol. 2: Youth, Exercise, and Sport. Indianapolis, IN: Benchmark Press, 1989, pp. 1–45.

As mentioned previously, physical activity and physical fitness are not synonymous terms. Physical activity refers to the amount of exercise in which an individual engages. Studies suggest that a positive correlation exists between activity and fitness, but at least 80% of the variability in fitness measures cannot be explained (Pate et al., 1990; Ross & Gilbert, 1985; Ross & Pate, 1987). Physical activity may improve physical fitness and health at the same time, but the improvement in health may be caused by biologic changes different from those responsible for improvement in physical fitness (Haskell et al., 1985). Corbin (1987) suggested that some of the benefits from physical activity that are important to health have no relationship to what is defined as physical fitness per se. One example is the importance of regular exercise to a reduced risk of osteoporosis; osteoporosis is related to health but not to the components of physical fitness.

The premise is that physical activity is the path to both physical fitness and good health. Many believe that promotion of lifelong habits of physical activity in childhood will have direct and indirect effects on health and prevention of disease (Blair et al., 1989; Haskell et al., 1985; Simons-Morton et al., 1987; Strong, 1990). The major federal planning document for health promotion and disease prevention for children, Healthy Children 2000 (United States Department of Health and Human Services, 1990), includes specific objectives to increase the physical activity and fitness levels of youth. Eight objectives are outlined, with a target date of their attainment by the year 2000 (Table 5–2). In 1985, the Centers for Disease Control put forth a specific activity plan for youth through old age to attain specific health fitness goals and achieve optimal health benefits. Developing lifelong physical activity patterns was one of the specific goals for children (Haskell et al., 1985).

The major health problem for adults in North America is CAD. The main identified risk factors in adults are high levels of cholesterol, high blood pressure, obesity, inactivity, smoking, and high

TABLE 5–2. **OBJECTIVES FOR IMPROVED PHYSICAL ACTIVITY AND FITNESS**

Risk Reduction Objectives
1. Increase to at least 30% the proportion of people aged 6 and older who engage regularly, preferably daily, in light to moderate physical activity for at least 30 minutes daily.
2. Increase to at least 20% the proportion of people aged 18 and older and to at least 75% the proportion of children and adolescents aged 6 through 17 who engage in vigorous physical activity that promotes the development and maintenance of cardiorespiratory fitness 3 or more days per week for 20 or more minutes per occasion.
3. Reduce to no more than 15% the proportion of people aged 6 and older who engage in no leisure time physical activity.
4. Increase to at least 40% the proportion of people aged 6 and older who regularly perform physical activities that enhance and maintain muscular strength, muscular endurance, and flexibility.
5. Increase to at least 50% the proportion of overweight people aged 12 and older who have adopted sound dietary practices combined with regular physical activity to attain an appropriate body weight.

Service and Protection Objectives
6. Increase to at least 50% the proportion of children and adolescents in 1st through 12th grade who participate in daily school physical education.
7. Increase to at least 50% the proportion of physical education class time that students spend being physically active, preferably engaged in lifetime physical activities.

Health Status Objective
8. Reduce overweight to a prevalence of no more than 20% among people aged 20 and older and no more than 15% among adolescents aged 12 through 19.

From United States Department of Health and Human Services. Healthy Children 2000: National Health Promotion and Disease Prevention Objectives Related to Mothers, Infants, Children, Adolescents, and Youth. Washington, DC: Public Health Service, 1990.

levels of fat intake. Many of these risk factors have also been identified in children (Despres et al., 1990; Montoye, 1985). The International Atherosclerosis Project reported that fatty streaks are present in the aortas of almost all children by the age of 3 years (McGill, 1968). The presence of fatty streaks in coronary arteries in childhood is correlated with the incidence of lesions in middle age (Montoye, 1985). Evidence suggests that some risk factors identified as early as age 12 years can be followed into adulthood (Kemper et al., 1989). Despite this evidence, screening by primary care physicians for risk factors in children is highly variable (Kimm et al., 1990). The evolution of cardiac risk factors during growth and the impact of physical activity on those factors will now be presented.

Cardiac Risk Factors

PLASMA CHOLESTEROL

The body has two types of cholesterol—low-density lipoprotein (LDL) cholesterol and high-density lipoprotein (HDL) cholesterol. High serum levels of LDL cholesterol are associated with a high incidence of CAD, whereas high levels of HDL cholesterol are associated with a low incidence of disease. At birth, total cholesterol and LDL cholesterol levels are low, but they increase sharply during the first year of life (Depres et al., 1990). Levels then remain relatively stable into adulthood. Boys, however, experience a reduction of HDL cholesterol during puberty. The ability to track cholesterol levels in children to identify future risk of adult disease improves after puberty (Kemper et al., 1989), but few primary care physicians monitor cholesterol levels in their pediatric patients (Kimm et al., 1990).

Little research is available on the effects of physical activity on lipoprotein levels in children. Fit and active children tend to have higher HDL cholesterol levels than do less active or inactive children (Despres et al., 1990).

GLUCOSE AND INSULIN METABOLISM

Plasma insulin has been found to be positively correlated with blood pressure, LDL cholesterol levels, and obesity and negatively correlated with HDL cholesterol levels in children of 5 to 17 years of age. Insulin level, therefore, could be a useful indicator of cardiovascular risk. Fasting plasma insulin levels generally increase with age throughout childhood (Despres et al., 1990). Glucose tolerance and physical activity appear to be unrelated in healthy children, but increased physical activity is

an important tool for management of hyperinsulinemia in children. Physical activity can also contribute to weight control in the child with obesity as well as reduce the risks of hyperinsulinemia associated with obesity.

BLOOD PRESSURE

Measurement of blood pressure in children tracks poorly into adulthood. Tracking refers to the consistency of a risk factor over time; therefore, an individual with high blood pressure as a child may or may not have high blood pressure as an adult. Both systolic and diastolic blood pressures increase throughout childhood; systolic pressure increases 2 mm Hg/yr and diastolic increases 1 mm Hg/yr. Because blood pressure measurements exhibit wide variation among children as well as day-to-day variation in a particular child, the effects of exercise or activity on blood pressure are difficult to determine. Physically active children have lower resting and exercise blood pressures, and physical activity helps to control blood pressure (Fraser et al., 1983; Hagberg et al., 1984; Hoffman et al., 1987; Treiber et al., 1989).

OBESITY AND REGIONAL BODY FAT DISTRIBUTION

Obesity is a major marker for the clustering of other risk factors during growth (Despres et al., 1990; Gutin et al., 1990; Smoak et al., 1987). It is often associated with elevated blood pressure and levels of lipids and plasma glucose and insulin. During growth, adiposity gradually increases in both sexes until the age of 8 or 9 years, when it begins to increase at a faster rate in girls. As a cardiac risk factor in adults, regional abdominal fat distribution is more important than obesity per se (Depres et al., 1990; Gutin et al., 1990). Whether a high percentage of abdominal fat in childhood is associated with increased risk for cardiac disease as an adult is unknown. Regular physical activity is important in the management of obesity.

Overall, little is known about the effects of physical activity on cardiovascular risk factors in children. The obese child, however, seems to be at most risk of carrying risk factors into adulthood because of clustering effects. How much exercise is required for health maintenance is not known. Healthy Children 2000 (United States Department of Health and Human Services, 1990), however, puts forth some objectives. If physical activity is the path to physical fitness and disease prevention, what is the prospect for the child who is less active because of disability? The next sections begin to answer that question.

Definition of Physical Fitness

As defined previously, health-related fitness is a state characterized by 1) an ability to perform daily activities with vigor and 2) traits and capacities that are associated with low risk of premature development of hypokinetic disease (i.e., physical inactivity) (Pate, 1983). Physical fitness is multidimensional. A combination of traits and capacities contributes to physical fitness, and the interaction among them creates true fitness. Each facet is a unique, independent characteristic or ability that is not highly correlated with other components. As the concept of health-related fitness has gained acceptance, four basic components have been identified: cardiorespiratory endurance, muscular strength and endurance, flexibility, and body composition. The rationale for the importance of these parameters in day-to-day functional capacity, health promotion, and disease prevention, and therefore physical fitness, is presented in Table 5–1. The relative independence of the components from one another has been verified by low correlations between components. Of the 60 possible correlation coefficients among test items for these components, only 6 were greater than .35 (Ross & Gilbert, 1985; Ross & Pate, 1987).

The remainder of this chapter will be directed toward reviewing the components of health-related fitness along with a review of current physical fitness tests. First, however, cardiopulmonary response to exercise in the growing child is reviewed.

Cardiopulmonary Response to Exercise

As in adults, the response of a child to exercise (a single event or repeated exercise) includes physiologic changes in the cardiovascular and pulmonary systems as well as metabolic effects. In children, however, differences in physiologic changes are seen as growth and development occur. Physiologic capacities are dependent on growth of the myocardium, skeleton, and skeletal muscle. Maturation and improved efficiency of the cardiovascular, pulmonary, metabolic, and musculoskeletal systems are also important. The physical work capacity of children increases approximately 8-fold in absolute terms between the ages of 6 and 12 years, partially as a result of growth and maturation (Adams, 1973). The absolute exercise capacity of children may be less than that of adults, but relative exercise capacity is similar.

Any exercise, be it in a child or an adult, increases the energy expenditure of the body. The energy for muscle contraction and exercise depends upon splitting of adenosine triphosphate (ATP) at the cellular level. ATP is available in small quantities in resting muscle, but once contraction starts, additional sources are required if contraction is to be maintained. Three sources of ATP are available: 1) creatine phosphate (CP), 2) glycolysis, and 3) the tricarboxylic acid, or Krebs's cycle. it is beyond the scope of this chapter to describe these mechanisms in detail. The reader is referred to a standard textbook of exercise physiology (Astrand & Rodahl, 1986).

CP and glycolysis as sources of ATP are referred to as anaerobic pathways because they do not require the presence of oxygen. CP is found in the sarcoplasm of the muscle cell. During breakdown it releases a high-energy phosphate bond that can be combined with adenosine diphosphate (ADP) to create ATP.

$$CP \rightarrow C + P_i + \text{energy} \qquad [1]$$

$$ADP + P_i + \text{energy} \rightarrow ATP \qquad [2]$$

CP breakdown together with ATP production provides enough energy for 10 to 15 seconds of exercise. Glycolysis, the other anaerobic pathway, breaks down glucose to produce pyruvic acid or lactic acid and ATP. This reaction takes place in the sarcoplasm of the cell. Together, glycolysis and CP breakdown are methods of anaerobic energy production that can sustain energy for muscle contraction for 40 to 50 seconds.

Energy production by the tricarboxylic acid cycle is called an aerobic pathway because it requires oxygen. A supply of oxygen is required for sustained exercise and depends on the aerobic pathway. Most, if not all, activities use both aerobic and anaerobic pathways for supply of ATP, but often tasks are more highly dependent upon one type of pathway than the other.

Because aerobic pathways must be used to sustain exercise, an index of maximal aerobic power is used to reflect the highest metabolic rate made available by aerobic energy. The most common index is maximal oxygen uptake (Vo_2max), or the highest volume of oxygen that can be consumed per unit time. Oxygen supply to muscle is described by the Fick equation: oxygen uptake (Vo_2) is equal to cardiac output (CO) times the difference in oxygen content between arterial (Ca_{O_2}) and mixed venous ($C\bar{v}_{O_2}$) blood, or

$$Vo_2 = CO \times (Ca_{O_2} - C\bar{v}_{O_2})$$

Because CO is the product of heart rate and stroke volume, the following relationship is also true:

Vo_2 = heart rate × stroke volume ×

arteriovenous O_2 difference

For Vo_2 to increase, one or more of these factors must increase. During exercise, CO is elevated by increases in both heart rate and stroke volume. Elevated blood flow to the muscles increases the difference in oxygen content between arterial and venous blood.

Vo_2max increases throughout childhood from approximately 1 l/min at age 5 years to 3 to 4 l/min at puberty (Braden & Strong, 1990). These changes occur as a result of maturation of the cardiovascular, pulmonary, metabolic, and musculoskeletal systems. As a child grows, the cardiopulmonary and musculoskeletal systems are integrated so that oxygen flow during exercise optimally meets the energy demands of the muscle cells, regardless of body size (Cooper et al., 1984).

CARDIAC OUTPUT

CO in children, as in adults, rises at the beginning of exercise or upon transition from a lower to a higher level of exercise. CO increases by an increase in both stroke volume and heart rate. CO in children is similar to that in adults despite the fact that stroke volume in a 5-year-old is about 25% of the stroke volume in an adult (Godfrey, 1981). Stroke volume increases as total heart volume increases. At all levels of exercise, stroke volume in boys is somewhat higher than it is in girls (Bar-Or, 1983c). CO levels in children are similar to those in adults because of an increased heart rate throughout childhood. Maximal heart rates in children vary between 195 and 215 beats per minute and decrease by 0.7 to 0.8 beats per minute per year after maturity (Braden & Strong, 1990).

ARTERIOVENOUS DIFFERENCE AND HEMOGLOBIN CONCENTRATION

At rest, the difference between arterial and mixed venous blood oxygen content is the same in children as in adults (Sproul & Simpson, 1964). Research suggests, however, that children have a higher blood flow to muscles after exercise than do young adults, resulting in a higher arteriovenous oxygen difference (Koch, 1974). Greater muscle blood flow facilitates increased oxygen transport to exercising muscles and, thus, a decrease in the oxygen content of the mixed venous blood.

Hemoglobin concentration is lower in children than in the average adult and thus affects the oxygen transport capacity of the blood in children (Krahenbuhl et al., 1985). Studies suggest that total hemoglobin concentration in 11- and 12-year-olds is in the range of 78% of that in adults (Krahenbuhl et al., 1985).

ARTERIAL BLOOD PRESSURE

Lower exercise blood pressure is seen in children than in adults, a finding consistent with a lower CO and stroke volume. Blood pressure may also be reduced because of lower peripheral vascular resistance secondary to shorter blood vessels (Bar-Or, 1983c).

VENTILATION

Ventilation is the rate of exchange of air between the lungs and ambient air, measured in liters per minute. In absolute terms, ventilation increases with age. Ventilation normalized by body weight is the same for children and adults at maximal activity (Bar-Or, 1983c). At submaximal exercise levels, ventilation is higher in children and decreases with age, suggesting that children have a lower ventilatory reserve than do adults. Studies suggest that children have less efficient ventilation than do adults (i.e., more air is needed to supply 1 liter of oxygen in a child than in an adult) (Bar-Or, 1983c).

VITAL CAPACITY

Vital capacity in a 5-year-old child is about 20% of that in an adult and increases with age. It is highly correlated with body size, particularly height (Godfrey, 1981), and generally has not been found to be a limiting factor of exercise performance.

RESPIRATORY RATE

Children have a higher respiratory rate than do adults during both maximal and submaximal exercise. A high rate of respiration compensates for decreased lung volume; respiratory rate decreases as lung volume increases (Bar-Or, 1983c).

BLOOD LACTATE

Blood and muscle lactate levels are lower in children than in adults (Astrand, 1952; Eriksson et al., 1971, 1973). It has been suggested but not confirmed that lactate production is related to testosterone production and, therefore, to sexual maturity in boys. Low lactate production in children could limit glycolytic capacity and thus contribute to reduced anaerobic capacity.

A summary of comparisons between children and adults for various cardiopulmonary variables is found in Table 5–3. Growth and maturation play a vital part in determining the values of these variables. Despite size differences between adults and children (which might lead one to believe that oxy-

TABLE 5-3. **CARDIOPULMONARY FUNCTION VARIABLES AND RESPONSE TO EXERCISE IN CHILDREN**

Function	Child vs. Adult Response	Sex Differences
Heart rate (Max, Submax)	Higher	M = F (Max); F > M (Submax)
Stroke volume (Max, submax)	Lower	M > F
Cardiac output (Max, Submax)	Lower, similar	M > F
Arteriovenous difference (Submax)	Similar	
Blood flow to active muscle	Higher	
Blood pressure	Lower	M = F
Hemoglobin concentration	Lower	
Ventilation/kg body wt (Max)	Similar	
Ventilation/kg body wt (Submax)	Higher	
Respiratory rate (Max, Submax)	Higher	
Tidal volume & vital capacity (Max)	Lower	
Tidal volume and vital capacity (Submax)	Similar/lower	
Blood lactate levels (Max, Submax)	Lower	M > F after puberty

Max = maximal exercise; Submax = submaximal exercise.
Adapted from Bar-Or, O. Pediatric Sports Medicine for the Practitioner. New York: Springer-Verlag, 1983, pp. 19, 31, 46.

gen transport in children is less efficient because they are smaller), optimal oxygen transport is maintained by highly integrated functions between the cardiopulmonary and musculoskeletal systems.

Review of Tests of Physical Fitness

Numerous physical fitness tests have been developed and are in use in physical education curricula across the country. Five tests are worthy of review because of their nationwide use and the likelihood that they will constitute the standards for future testing of youth and children. One of these tests, the National Children and Youth Fitness Study Tests I and II (Ross & Gilbert, 1985; Ross & Pate, 1987), was used as the basis for current levels of fitness across the country by the U.S. Department of Health and Human Services (1990) in drafting objectives for Healthy Children 2000. Each test reviewed in this chapter emphasizes health-related fitness components. Most tests provide some information regarding inter-rater reliability, but none specifically includes information on the validity of individual test items. Most information on the validity of individual test items has been provided by separate investigators or published separately subsequent to the development of the test batteries (Cureton & Warren, 1990; Going, 1988; Jackson, AS, & Coleman, 1976; Jackson, AW, & Baker, 1986; Safrit, 1990). A comparison of all five tests and their components is presented in Table 5-4.

CURRENT TESTS

AAHPERD Physical Best Program. This test was developed by the American Alliance for Health, Physical Education, Recreation, and Dance (AAHPERD) (1988). Four components are tested by the five items composing the battery. The test is criterion referenced, but no evidence to support the validity and reliability of the standards is presented in the manual. Information on the validity of the body composition component can be found in a study by Going (1988). The program is designed to be both a physical fitness assessment and an educational program to promote health and prevent disease.

Chrysler Fund–Amateur Athletic Union Physical Fitness Program. The Physical Fitness Program by Chrysler Fund–Amateur Athletic Union (1987) consists of four required items and one optional item. Although the test battery is norm referenced, it is referenced by test administrators. The sample, therefore, is not systematically representative of the nation. A critique of the test suggests that not all data are externally valid. Significant differences in mean values in test items were noted when compared with those of other tests and when compared with results among different test administrators (Safrit, 1990; Sodoma, 1986). The test items show some variation from other tests (see Table 5-4), and the absence of a standard testing protocol among test administrators raises questions about the reliability and thus the validity of the test.

FITNESSGRAM Program. This test is a battery that uses criterion-referenced standards. The program was developed by the Institute for Aerobics Research (1987). Limited information is available on the reliability and validity of the specific standards in the test manual. Research on the validity and reliability of the cardiorespiratory endurance standards has been published separately (Cureton & Warren, 1990). Development of the standards

TABLE 5 — REVIEW OF CURRENT PHYSICAL FITNESS TESTS

Test	Component of Fitness	Test Items	Standard	Reliability/Validity
AAHPERD Physical Best Program (AAHPERD, 1988)	Cardiorespiratory endurance Body composition Lower back flexibility Muscular strength/endurance	1-mile walk-run Sum of skinfolds (triceps/calf) Sit and reach Modified sit-up, pull-up	Criterion	No specifics reported Some available in supporting research (Going, 1988)
Chrysler-AAU Physical Fitness Program (1987)	Cardiorespiratory endurance Lower back flexibility Muscular strength/endurance Upper body muscle strength/endurance	Endurance run V-sit and reach Bent knee sit-up Pull-up/flexed arm hang	Normative (for ages 6–16 (not nationwide)	Not all data externally valid
FITNESSGRAM Institute for Aerobics Research, 1987)	Cardiorespiratory endurance Lower back flexibility Upper body strength Abdominal strength Body composition Agility (K-3)	1-mile run Sit and reach Pull-up/flexed arm hang Sit-ups Skinfold measurement Shuttle run	Criterion	Not in manual Partial work reported 1990 (Cureton & Warren, 1990)
National Child and Youth Fitness Study (Ross & Gilbert, 1985) (Ross & Pate, 1987)	Cardiorespiratory endurance Lower back flexibility Upper body strength/endurance Abdominal strength/endurance Body composition	1-mile walk-run Half-mile walk-run Sit and reach Modified pull-up Bent knee sit-up Sum of skinfolds (triceps/subscapular/calf)	U.S. norms (for ages 6–18)	(Ross, Katz, & Gilbert, 1985) (Ross, et al., 1987)
Presidential Physical Fitness Program (President's Council, 1987)	Cardiorespiratory endurance Lower back flexibility Upper body strength/endurance Abdominal strength/endurance Ability/power	1-mile walk-run Sit and reach Pull-up Bent knee sit-up/curl-up Shuttle run	U.S. norms for ages 6–18 y.	General terms of validity reported; no specifics

was based on determining 1) the lowest level of the laboratory standard for cardiorespiratory endurance, that is, Vo_2max, consistent with minimal risk of disease and adequate functional capacity; 2) the timing standards of the field standard of cardiorespiratory endurance , the mile walk-run, consistent with the minimal Vo_2max; and 3) a comparison of the standards with available national normative data to evaluate both consistency and accuracy.

National Children, Youth, and Fitness Study (NCYFS) I and II. These tests were national studies undertaken to assess current levels of physical fitness of children and youth in the United States. Initiated by the U.S. Office of Disease Prevention and Health Promotion (Pate et al., 1987; Ross et al., 1985), the results have been used to set appropriate targets for improved health and fitness. The NCYFS I produced normative data by sex and age and sex and grade for children and youth aged 10 to 18 years, and NCYFS II provided the same information for children aged 6 to 9 years. Training procedures were developed for test administrators and inter-rater reliability estimates were found to be .99 for body composition measurements. Concurrent validity for some test items had already been established (Jackson, AS, & Coleman, 1976).

Presidential Physical Fitness Program. This is a norm-referenced test created by the President's Council on Physical Fitness and Sports (1987). Validity is not addressed, but some reliability information is provided.

COMPARISON OF TESTS

All the tests measure similar components of health-related fitness. Each includes items for testing cardiorespiratory endurance, muscular strength and endurance, and flexibility. Only three of the five tests measure body composition. The tests differ in the reference standard used. Tests are either norm referenced, in that performance is compared with that of a national U.S. sample of children taking the same test, or criterion referenced, in that performance is compared with a preset standard consistent with fitness. The criterion for each item is independent of the performance of other children on the same test. Two of the tests reviewed are criterion referenced, but they use different criterion measures.

Appropriate reliability and validity data are not available for any of the tests reviewed, and thus the tests do not meet standards for measurement required of scientific clinical tools (American Psychological Association, 1985). Users must be cautious in the interpretation of scores and their meaning. Strict and rigid interpretation of the test results

would be incorrect and should be avoided until further evidence of reliability and validity is available. Procedures for evaluating reliability and validity of criterion-referenced tests are available (Safrit, 1989).

▌ COMPONENTS OF PHYSICAL FITNESS

The components of health-related fitness, as mentioned earlier, are cardiorespiratory endurance, muscular strength and endurance, flexibility, and body composition. The following information will be reviewed for each component

1. The criterion measure of the component
2. Laboratory measurement
3. Developmental aspects of the component and standards by age
4. Field measurement of the component and its validity in relation to the criterion measure
5. Standards by age as determined by FITNESS-GRAM, a computer-scored fitness test with a health-related focus
6. Physical activities with high correlation to the particular fitness component
7. Response to training
8. Assessment of the component in children with disabilities

Cardiorespiratory Endurance

CRITERION MEASURE

The most widely used criterion measure for cardiorespiratory endurance is directly measured Vo_2max, sometimes referred to as maximal aerobic power. This component measures the capabilities of the cardiovascular and pulmonary systems and is significant because oxygen supply to the tissues depends on the efficiency and capacity of these systems. Vo_2max is the highest rate of oxygen consumed by the body in a given time period during exercise of a significant portion of body muscle mass (Krahenbuhl et al., 1985). Cardiorespiratory endurance is so important to overall fitness that many people view physical fitness as being synonymous with cardiorespiratory endurance (Simons-Morton et al., 1987).

LABORATORY MEASUREMENT

Laboratory measurement techniques include measurement of Vo_2 during progressive exercise to the point of exhaustion with the use of an ergometer. This method is referred to as direct determination of Vo$_2$max. Indirect determination methods predict Vo$_2$max from submaximal exercise.

Direct Determination

An ergometer is a device that measures the amount of work performed under controlled conditions. The two devices commonly available are a cycle ergometer and a treadmill. The cycle ergometer has the advantage of being relatively inexpensive and portable, but compared with the treadmill, it exercises a smaller total muscle mass. With the cycle ergometer, local fatigue develops (primarily in knee extensors), resulting in premature termination of the testing (Bar-Or, 1983a; Braden & Strong, 1990; Krahenbuhl et al., 1985). Depending on the source, values of Vo$_2$max are reported to be 5 to 30% lower on a cycle ergometer than on a treadmill (Bar-Or, 1983a; Braden & Strong, 1990; Krahenbuhl et al., 1985). For children, the coordination and rhythm, or cadence, required on a cycle ergometer are sometimes difficult to achieve. Both the treadmill and the cycle ergometers present problems when used to test populations with disabilities, in particular those with impairments of balance or coordination.

A variety of protocols for direct determination can be used with children. The most common protocol is one in which resistance, inclination, speed, or height is increased every 1 to 3 minutes without interruption until the child can no longer maintain the activity. In interrupted protocols, which are sometimes used, there is an interruption between each successive increment of exercise. Examples of some common direct determination protocols are given in Table 5-5. The main criterion for indicating that Vo$_2$max has been achieved during a progressive protocol is that an increase in power load is not accompanied by an increased Vo$_2$ (usually 2 ml/kg/min or higher) (Krahenbuhl et al., 1985). Astrand (1952), however, reported that 5% of all children tested failed to reach a plateau in Vo$_2$, even though evidence from secondary criteria suggested that exhaustion had been reached.

Despite the difficulty of determining attainment of Vo$_2$max, studies suggest that the reliability of direct determination testing with children is high. Coefficients of variation of 3, 5, and 8% for Vo$_2$max determined by treadmill walk-jogging, running, and walking, respectively, have been reported (Paterson & Cunningham, 1978). A mean variation of 5.3% was reported for children exercising to exhaustion on a cycle ergometer on 12 different occasions (Cumming et al., 1967).

Indirect Determination

As the name implies, indirect determination of Vo$_2$max is its calculation indirectly from submaxi-

TABLE 5-5. DIRECT DETERMINATION ALL-OUT PROTOCOLS

Bruce Treadmill Protocol

STAGE	SPEED (MPH)	GRADE (%)	DURATION (MIN)
1	1.7	10	3
2	2.5	12	3
3	3.4	14	3
4	4.2	16	3
5	5.0	18	3
6	5.5	20	3
7	6.0	22	3

McMaster Progressive Continuous Cycling Test

BODY HEIGHT (CM)	INITIAL LOAD (WATTS)	INCREMENTS (WATTS)	DURATION (MIN)
<119.9	12.5	12.5	2
120–139.9	12.5	25.0	2
140–159.9	25.0	25.0	2
>160	25.0	25.0 (F) 50.0 (M)	2

Adapted from Bar-Or, O. Appendix II: Procedures for exercise testing in children. In Bar-Or, O, Pediatric Sports Medicine for the Practitioner. New York: Springer-Verlag, 1983, pp. 315–341.

Watts = joules/second.

mal exercise. The child is not taken to his or her self-imposed maximum. Heart rate during one or more stages is the variable most commonly used to derive the index of Vo$_2$max. Step tests for children are usually submaximal tests, using recovery heart rate to predict Vo$_2$max. Evidence suggests that height-specific step tests can be reliable predictors of Vo$_2$max (Francis & Feinstein, 1991). Important limitations exist, however, in predicting Vo$_2$max from submaximal exercise data, and these should always be kept in mind (Wyndham, 1976). Examples of test protocols are presented in Table 5-6.

The W$_{170}$ is an index used to predict mechanical power in a submaximal test. Two or more measurements of heart rate are obtained at different power or workloads, and heart rate is then extrapolated to 170 beats per minute. The corresponding power is W$_{170}$. This index, originally described by Wahlund (1948), is based on the assumption that heart rate is linearly related to power at 170 beats per minute or less. To minimize error, more than two heart rate measurements are taken, one of which is as close as possible to 170 beats per minute.

DEVELOPMENTAL ASPECTS OF CARDIORESPIRATORY ENDURANCE

Absolute maximal aerobic power, or Vo$_2$max, increases with age throughout childhood and is

TABLE 5–6. **INDIRECT DETERMINATION PROTOCOLS**

Adams Submaximal Progressive Continuous Cycling Test*

BODY WEIGHT (KG)	STAGE 1 (WATTS)	STAGE 2 (WATTS)	STAGE 3 (WATTS)
<30	16.5	33.0	50.0
30–39.9	16.5	50.0	83.0
40–59.9	16.5	50.0	100.0
>60	16.5	83.0	133.0

Stage duration = 6 min.
Performance by W_{170}.

Modified Three-Minute Step Test†

STAGE	DURATION (MIN)	ASCENT RATE (ASCENTS/MIN)
1	3	22
2	3	26
3	3	30

Step height dependent upon height.
Performance by recovery heart rate.

*Adapted from Bar-Or, O. Appendix II: Procedures for exercise testing in children. In Bar-Or, O. Pediatric Sports Medicine for the Practitioner. New York: Springer-Verlag, 1983, pp. 315–341; and

†Adapted and reprinted by permission from Francis, K, & Culpepper, M. Height adjusted, rate specific, single stage, step test for predicting maximal oxygen consumption. Southern Medical Journal, 82:602–606, 1989.

slightly higher in boys than in girls (Krahenbuhl et al., 1985; Rutenfranz et al., 1990; Shvartz & Reibold, 1990). Initial differences during early childhood are approximately 10%, increasing to 25% by age 14 years, and exceeding 50% by age 16 (Krahenbuhl et al., 1985). The development of a greater muscle mass in boys and increasing differences in the amount of time spent in vigorous physical exercise are the most commonly given explanations. Overall, the physical working capacity of children increases approximately 8-fold between the ages of 6 and 12 years. Few data are available on VO_2max for children younger than age 6 (Adams, 1973).

Relative to body weight, only a 1% change in VO_2max is noted between the ages of 6 and 16 years for boys (52.8 ml/kg/min at age 6; 53.5 ml/kg/min at age 16), whereas girls display a 12% reduction between the same ages (52.0 ml/kg/min at age 6; 40.5 ml/kg/min at age 16) (Krahenbuhl et al., 1985; Shvartz & Reibold, 1990). VO_2max is highly correlated with lean body mass. The decline in VO_2max in girls begins around age 10, when changes in body composition occur as girls develop a relatively increased amount of subcutaneous fat. When VO_2max is measured with reference to lean body mass, the differences in values between the sexes disappears (Braden & Strong, 1990).

Increases in body dimensions, however, do not account for all changes in VO_2max that occur with growth. When comparing same-sex adolescents of different ages with the same body weight or body height, the positive relationship with age remains (Sprynarova & Reisenauer, 1978). Functional changes in cardiovascular, pulmonary, and musculoskeletal systems resulting in improved efficiency with maturity may play a role. Cooper and colleagues (1984), however, suggested that the functional components of body systems are integrated so that aerobic capacity is optimized throughout the growth process.

MEASUREMENT IN THE FIELD

The most common measure of cardiorespiratory fitness in the field is a long-distance run of various structures or lengths. All the physical fitness batteries reviewed previously have a distance run test, commonly a 1-mile run. Test-retest reliability of VO_2max during field testing has been shown to be between .60 and .95 (Cunningham et al., 1977; Safrit, 1990). Jackson, AS, and Coleman (1976) studied the construct validity of various distance run tests and the concurrent validity of the 9- and 12-minute run tests in elementary schoolchildren. Results suggested that both the 9- and 12-minute distance runs were valid measures of the construct and displayed concurrent validity with $VO_2 max$. Safrit (1990) suggested that a 9-minute run is a distance of at least 1 mile. Both the 1200- and 1600-meter runs were significantly related to VO_2max, but only the 1600-meter run had correlation coefficients above .60, which is generally accepted as the lower limit for a useful fitness test (Krahenbuhl et al., 1978; Mathews, 1973). Validation values in the range of 0.40 to 0.80 between corresponding performance and weight-relative VO_2max have been reported (Safrit, 1990).

STANDARDS BY AGE

Standards of performance are determined by ranking a child's performance in relation to the performance of a group of children tested on the same test (norm-referenced) or against an established criterion found to be consistent with good health (criterion-referenced). One of the advantages of criterion-referenced standards is that they are independent of the proportion of the population that meets the standards. A ranking by a norm-referenced standard does not necessarily represent a desirable level of fitness or performance. The limitation of criterion-referenced standards, however, is that they are somewhat arbitrary and that the criteria used in the current physical fitness tests differ from one another (Cureton & Warren, 1990). Establishing the validity of criterion-referenced standards for performance is in progress.

Both the AAHPERD Physical Best Program (American Alliance for Health, Physical Education, Recreation, and Dance, 1988) and the FITNESS-GRAM Program (Institute for Aerobics Research, 1987) have developed criterion-referenced standards for all items in their fitness tests, including the 1-mile walk-run. Cureton and Warren (1990) described the procedures for development of criterion standards for the FITNESSGRAM Program. Comparisons between those adopted by the FITNESSGRAM Program and those of the Physical Best Program indicate that FITNESSGRAM walk-run standards result in a lower percentage of incorrect classifications of children in comparison with the laboratory criterion of Vo_2max than do those of the Physical Best Program. Incorrect classification results when performance is found to be above one of either the field or the laboratory standard but below the other standard. A high validity of a test is one that has a low percentage of incorrect classifications. Validity coefficients for the FITNESSGRAM Program range from .73 to 1.00 when compared with the criterion standard of Vo_2max. The actual percentage of Vo_2max that is used during the walk-run test, however, is unknown, which makes evaluation of any or all values difficult. A comparison of walk-run standards by age is provided in Table 5-7.

PHYSICAL ACTIVITIES

Activities that are highly correlated with development of cardiorespiratory endurance are boxing, running, rowing, swimming, cross-country skiing, and bicycling. The common component among these activities is a prolonged, sustained demand on the cardiorespiratory system that requires general stamina.

RESPONSE TO TRAINING

Debate exists over whether maximal aerobic power of prepubescents is a component that can be affected by training. Research results are equivocal. Those studies that report improvement in aerobic power with training suggest that the principles of training of prepubescents, that is, frequency, intensity, and duration, are similar to those for adults (Simons-Morton et al., 1987). The functional results of conditioning on the cardiorespiratory system include decreased heart rate, increased stroke volume, improved respiratory muscular endurance, and decreased respiration rate (Bar-Or, 1983c; Braden & Strong, 1990). A more specific focus on conditioning and training will be found later in this chapter.

TABLE 5-7. **ONE-MILE WALK-RUN STANDARDS**

Age (y)	Criterion* Standard		FITNESSGRAM† Field Standard		AAHPERD† Field Standard		NYCFS I, II‡ Percentiles	
	M	F	M	F	M	F	M	F
5	42.0	40.0	16:00	17:00	13:00	14:00	—	—
6	42.0	40.0	15:00	16:00	12:00	13:00	—	—
7	42.0	40.0	14:00	15:00	11:00	12:00	—	—
8	42.0	40.0	13:00	14:30	10:00	11:30	15	15
9	42.0	40.0	12:00	13:00	10:00	11:00	20	20
10	42.0	39.0	11:00	12:00	9:30	11:00	25	35
11	42.0	38.0	11:00	12:00	9:00	11:00	20	40
12	42.0	37.0	10:00	11:30	9:00	11:00	30	30
13	42.0	36.0	9.30	10:30	8:00	10:30	20	35
14	42.0	35.0	8:30	10:30	7:45	10:30	35	50
15	42.0	35.0	8:30	10:30	7:30	10:30	25	55
16	42.0	35.0	8:30	10:30	7:30	10:30	20	50
17	42.0	35.0	8:30	10:30	7:30	10:30	30	50

*Criterion standard as set by FITNESSGRAM in ml/kg/min of oxygen uptake.
†Minutes required to complete a 1 mile walk-run.
‡Percentile rank of children performing this standard in NCYFS I, II.
Adapted from Cureton, KJ, & Warren, GL. Criterion referenced standards for youth health related fitness tests: A tutorial. Research Quarterly for Exercise and Sport, 61:7–19, 1990; Ross, JG, Dotson, CO, Gilbert, CG, & Katz, SI. The national youth and fitness study I: New Standards for fitness measurement. Journal of Physical Education, Recreation and Dance, 56:62–66, 1985; Ross, JG, Delpy, LA, Christenson, GM, Gold, RS, & Damberg, CL. The national youth and fitness study II: Study procedures and quality control. Journal of Physical Education, Recreation and Dance, 58:57–62, 1987.

ASSESSMENT OF CARDIORESPIRATORY ENDURANCE IN CHILDREN WITH DISABILITIES

Children with disabilities often exhibit decreased or limited exercise capacity relative to their nondisabled peers. This can result from either their limited participation in exercise, which leads to deconditioning, or the specific pathologic factors of their disability that limit exercise-related functions. Regardless of the cause, children with disabilities often enter a cycle of decreased activity that precipitates a loss of fitness and further decreases in activity levels.

Pathophysiologic factors that may limit cardiorespiratory endurance can sometimes be separated by the specific component of the Fick equation that they affect. This provides a convenient way to categorize conditions or diseases by the fitness components they affect most (Bar-Or, 1983c, 1986; Fig. 5–1). Studies suggest that maximal aerobic uptake is limited not only by central mechanisms of the cardiopulmonary system but also by peripheral mechanisms controlling blood flow, excitation processes in the muscle fiber, local fatigue, and enzyme availability (Green & Patla, 1992; Saltin & Strange, 1992; Sutton, 1992). When considering the limitations or reductions in VO_2max in children with disabilities, both central and peripheral limitations must be considered.

Cerebral Palsy

Directly measured maximal aerobic capacity of children and adolescents with cerebral palsy (CP) is 10 to 30% less than that of controls (Bar-Or et al., 1976; Lundberg, 1978; Lundberg et al., 1967). It would seem that peripheral mechanisms related to the neuromuscular disorder itself are more likely to contribute to decreased capacity than are central cardiopulmonary mechanisms, although this has not been studied. When indirectly assessed from submaximal heart rate, aerobic capacity of adolescents was found to be reduced by 50% (Lundberg et al., 1967). Low mechanical efficiency creates disproportionately high submaximal heart rates in individuals with CP, making submaximal heart rate a poor predictor of maximal aerobic power (Bar-Or, 1983b). Submaximal exercise tests, in general, underestimate aerobic capacity in poorly trained individuals (Astrand & Rodahl, 1986; Wyndham, 1976). Numerous studies suggest that heart rate is a good predictor or an appropriate substitute clinical measure of VO_2 because of its linear relationship to heart rate (Rose et al., 1989, 1990). It is not a measure of maximal aerobic capacity, however, and therefore it is not an alternative measure of cardiorespiratory fitness.

An increase in blood flow to exercising muscles after conditioning is a response observed in children with CP but not seen in able-bodied children (Lundberg & Pernow, 1970). Spastic muscles of individuals with adult-onset brain damage exhibit subnormal blood flow during exercise (Landin et al., 1977). (Whether the rate of blood flow changes after conditioning in individuals with adult-onset brain injury is not known.) One hypothesis to explain the increase in blood flow in conditioned individuals with CP is that it results from a decrease

$$\dot{V}O_{2max} = SV_{max} \times HR_{max} \times (CaO_2 - C\bar{v}O_2)_{max}$$

Aortic Stenosis
Cardiomyopathy
Detraining
Hypohydration · severe
Pulmonary Stenosis
Tetralogy of Fallot
Vent. Septal Defect

Anemia
Asthma · severe
Cystic Fibrosis
Hemoglobinopathies
Obesity · extreme
Right-to-Left Shunt
Scoliosis · severe

β blockers
Cong. Compl. Heart Block

Detraining
Malnutrition · severe
Muscle Atrophy
Muscle Dystrophy
Spina Bifida
2·3 DPG Deficiency

FIGURE 5–1. Maximal aerobic power (VO_2max) and pathology. The Fick equation and specific pathologic conditions that affect its variables and reduce VO_2max are shown. (From Bar-Or, O. Exercise as a diagnostic tool in pediatrics. In Bar-Or, O. Pediatric Sports Medicine for the Practitioner. New York: Springer-Verlag, 1983, p. 72.)

in spasticity. More rapid deterioration of maximal aerobic uptake is seen after discontinuation of training in children with CP than in able-bodied children (Bar-Or, 1983b).

Juvenile Rheumatoid Arthritis

Measurement of maximal aerobic capacity by cycle ergometry in children with juvenile rheumatoid arthritis has been measured to be 15 to 30% lower than in their peers matched by age, sex, and body surface area (Giannini & Protas, 1991, 1992). No correlation was found between severity of articular disease and aerobic capacity, however. Children with juvenile rheumatoid arthritis have a shorter duration of exercise before exhaustion, which occurs at a lower than normal work rate with a lower peak heart rate. Deficient oxygen extraction from exercising muscles or low blood flow to exercising muscles has been postulated to occur in this population as a result of decreased activity levels (Bar-Or, 1983b, 1986).

Scoliosis

Chest deformity, decreased lung size, and decreased physical activity are believed to contribute to the lower maximal aerobic capacity of children with advanced scoliosis. No functional or exercise-related deficits are found in children with minor or moderate scoliosis (Bar-Or, 1983b). For those with advanced scoliosis, limitations of 50 to 70% in Vo_2max have been reported. Vo_2 and minute ventilation are decreased, and pulmonary artery pressure increased at maximal exercise relative to able-bodied standards. Some improvements are seen with conditioning.

Mental Retardation

Most studies indicate that individuals with mental retardation display lower Vo_2max scores than do their nondisabled peers (Lavay et al., 1990); however, significant variability has been reported among individuals with the same level of disability. Technical problems associated with testing individuals with mental retardation are encountered that create difficulties in establishing reliable and valid information. Treadmill testing appears to be the most reliable form of testing.

Muscular Strength and Endurance

The second component of physical fitness is muscular strength and endurance. Strength is required for movement and has a direct impact on effective performance. Strength is also important for optimal posture and reduced risk of lower back pain. Muscular strength, muscular endurance, and muscular power are not synonymous terms. Muscular strength refers to maximal contractile force. Muscular endurance is the ability of muscles to perform work and assumes some component of muscular strength. Muscular power refers to the ability to release maximal muscular force within a specified time. As velocity increases or time decreases (for maximal muscular force to be obtained), power increases. Because muscular endurance and muscular power have their basis in muscular strength, strength will be the primary point of this discussion.

LABORATORY MEASUREMENT

The laboratory standard for muscular strength is strength measured by dynamometry. Tests include isometric dynamometry, isokinetic dynamometry, and single-repetition maximal isotonic dynamometry. Most measurements are made on specific, selected muscles, and then results are extrapolated to give "whole body" strength. Unfortunately, a limitation for setting standards of strength is that force measurements are dependent on the type of dynamometer used (Blimkie, 1989). The most commonly selected measures are hand grip, elbow flexion and extension, knee flexion and extension, and plantar flexion strength. The reliability of maximal voluntary isokinetic strength measures has been addressed in the pediatric population. Coefficients of variation from 5 to 11% have been reported (Blimkie, 1989). Children demonstrate the capacity to perform consistent maximal voluntary contraction under controlled conditions by age 6 to 7 years.

Developmental Aspects and Standards by Age

Grip Strength. Grip strength is the most commonly reported upper extremity strength measure in children. Absolute strength scores, however, are highly sensitive to the type of dynamometer used and to its positioning, making the results of studies difficult to compare. In general, single-hand grip strength increases from an average of approximately 5 kg for children at age 3 years to 45 kg for boys at age 17 and 30 kg for girls at age 17. Bilateral grip strength has been measured at a mean of 25 kg for children at age 7 years, increasing to an average of 95 kg for boys and 50 kg for girls by age 17 years (Blimkie, 1989). The rate of increase in strength for boys rises dramatically at puberty.

Elbow Flexion and Extension Torque. Elbow flexion strength is greater than isometric elbow extension strength throughout childhood and adolescence, and the difference between them increases with increasing age (Fowler & Gardner, 1967). The extension/flexion strength ratio for boys is approximately 0.76 at the age of 7.5 years and decreases to

0.57 during late adolescence. No data are available for girls.

Shoulder Flexion and Extension. A single study has addressed isokinetic strength values for shoulder flexion and extension in children (Brodie et al., 1986). Twenty-four untrained, prepubescent boys with an average age of 11.7 years were tested on a Cybex II (Ronkonkoma, NY) at 6 different velocities. Mean values for peak torque for shoulder extension were relatively constant at speeds of between 60 and 150°/s (13.2–13.7 N·m); mean values for shoulder flexion increased as speed increased (12.5–24.3 N·m.)

Knee Flexion and Extension. Isokinetic knee flexion strength and knee extension strength also increase throughout childhood. Results from Alexander and Molnar (1973) and Molnar and Alexander (1973) indicated that knee extension strength exceeds knee flexion strength for both sexes at all ages. Average knee flexion strength varies from 30 to 50% of average knee extension strength for girls and 28 to 65% for boys. Boys have slightly greater strength than do girls before puberty but consistently greater strength from the age of 10 years onward.

Trunk Flexion and Extension. Few data are available for laboratory dynamometry standards for trunk strength in children. Clinical data have been collected for the ability of children to sustain isometric trunk flexion (actually a test of muscular endurance) between the ages of 3 and 7 years (Lefkof, 1986). An isotonic test of the number of hook-lying sit-ups performed was also included in the study. Both the endurance for isometric trunk flexion and the ability to perform sit-ups improved with age. The greatest improvement occurred between the ages of 5 and 6 years, when average performance at least doubled. These results are important because the typical field test for muscular strength and endurance is performance of sit-ups.

Composite Strength. Composite strength provides a measure of overall or general strength and consists of a total strength score from several muscle groups. Usually, grip strength, thrust strength, (shoulder girdle), and shoulder pull measures are included in composite strength scores (Carron & Bailey, 1974; Faust, 1977). Unfortunately, no measures of composite strength that include lower extremity or trunk strength could be found by this author. The pattern of increase in composite strength during childhood is similar to that of grip strength.

Evoked Responses

A second method for muscular function assessment in the laboratory is by evoked responses from electrical stimulation. Muscle contractile characteristics are studied with this methodology, including force production. Few data are available for children (Blimkie, 1989).

DEVELOPMENTAL ASPECTS OF MUSCULAR STRENGTH AND ENDURANCE

Gajdosik and Gajdosik described the development of the musculoskeletal system in Chapter 4 of this volume. Development of strength depends on the development of force production and is influenced by numerous factors, for example, the muscle's cross-sectional area (Malina, 1986). Muscular strength in absolute terms increases linearly with chronologic age from early childhood in both sexes to approximately age 13 to 14 years. Increases in strength are closely related to increases in muscle mass during growth. Boys have greater strength than do girls at all ages (seen as early as age 3 years) and have larger absolute and relative amounts of muscle (kilogram of muscle per kilogram of body weight) (Blimkie, 1989; Malina, 1986). The sex difference in relative strength (per kilogram of body mass) before puberty is at least in part caused by a higher proportion of body fat in girls from mid-childhood onward, a difference similar to the trend in cardiorespiratory endurance (Faust, 1977; Malina, 1986). Rarick and Thompson (1956) suggested that boys are 11 to 13% stronger than girls during childhood. This value reaches 20% by adulthood for strength per cross-sectional area of muscle (Maughan et al., 1983). Correlates and determinants of strength are thought to include age, body size, muscle size, muscle fiber type and size, muscle contractile properties, and biomechanical influences.

During adolescence, there is a marked acceleration in development of strength, particularly in boys. Boys between the ages of 10 and 16 years who were followed longitudinally showed a 23% increase in strength per year. Peak growth in muscle mass occurred during and after peak weight gain, but maximal strength development occurred after peak velocity of growth in height and weight, suggesting that muscle tissue increases first in mass and then in strength (Carron & Bailey, 1974; Malina, 1986). Girls generally show peak strength development before peak weight gain (Faust, 1977). Overall muscle mass increases more than 5 times in males from childhood to adulthood; the increase in females is 3.5 times.

Differentiation in strength between the sexes at puberty is, at least in part, caused by differences in hormonal concentrations, particularly testosterone. Hormones other than the male sex steroids also make an important contribution (Florini, 1987). Unfortunately, no pediatric studies to date have correlated age-associated changes in endocrinologic function with muscle size and muscular strength.

MEASUREMENT IN THE FIELD

Field measurements of muscular strength usually entail movement of part or all of the body mass against gravity. The two common tests for muscular strength are the flexed arm hang and the sit-up. All the fitness tests previously reviewed include a sit-up test and a pull-up or flexed arm hang test. The correlation between abdominal strength and endurance and shoulder girdle strength as measures of absolute strength for physical fitness is not well established. Although strength is considered an important part of physical fitness, the standards to meet minimal fitness requirements in this area are the least clear. This may result from lack of quantitative research in this area.

Sit-Ups. The exact relationship between sit-up performance and abdominal strength and endurance is unclear. How abdominal strength is related to a given number of sit-ups is unknown. Test-retest reliability estimates for sit-ups measured for 11- to 14-year-olds range from .64 to .94 for both boys and girls (Safrit & Wood, 1987).

Standards of performance as determined by the FITNESSGRAM battery are listed in Table 5–8.

The percentage of children who achieved criterion ranged from 80% at age 7 years to 62% at age 16 to 17 years (Blair et al., 1989). These results are slightly different from those attained on the NCYFS I and II (Ross & Gilbert, 1985; Ross & Pate, 1987).

Chin-Ups and Flexed Arm Hang. The validity of chin-ups and the flexed arm hang as measures of upper body strength is questionable. Berger & Medlin (1969) suggested that the number of chin-ups as a measure of absolute strength is not valid because body weight is inversely related to the number of chin-ups performed. Considine (1973) demonstrated that pull-ups do not provide an indicator of shoulder girdle strength. The NCYFS II developed a modified pull-up test for 6- to 9-year-olds to overcome the problems associated with body weight (Pate et al., 1987).

Standards by Age

The standards of performance for the FITNESS-GRAM Program are listed in Table 5–8. No data are available on the validity or reliability of these standards.

Branta and colleagues (1984) assessed the performance of children on the flexed arm hang as part of a longitudinal study of age changes in motor skills during childhood and adolescence. The minimum standards for fitness on the flexed arm hang set by the FITNESSGRAM Program are less than

TABLE 5–8. SIT-UP STANDARDS

Age (y)	FITNESSGRAM* Sit-ups F	M	FITNESSGRAM Pull-ups F	M	FITNESSGRAM Flexed Arm Hang F	M	NCYFS I, II† Sit-ups F	M
5	20	20	1	1	5	5	—	—
6	20	20	1	1	5	5	60	60
7	20	20	1	1	5	5	35–40	35–40
8	25	25	1	1	8	10	45–50	45–50
9	25	25	1	1	8	10	45–50	35–40
10	30	30	1	1	8	10	30–40	30–40
11	30	30	1	1	8	10	25–30	25–30
12	30	35	1	1	8	10	30	40
13	30	35	1	2	12	10	40	30
14	35	40	1	3	12	15	50	50
15	35	40	1	5	12	25	50	40
16	35	40	1	5	12	25	50	40

*Number of sit-ups performed in 1 min.
†Percentile rank of children performing FITNESSGRAM standards from NCYFS I, II.

Data from Blair, SN, Falls, HB, & Pate, RR. A new physical fitness test. In Boileau, RA (Ed.). Advances in pediatric sport sciences, Vol. 1. Biological issues. Champaign, IL: Human Kinetics Press, 1984, pp 101–130; Ross, JG, Pate, RR, Corbin, CB, Delpy, LA, & Gold, RS, & Leonard, WR. The national youth and fitness study II. Study procedures and quality control. Journal of Physical Education, Recreation and Dance, 58:57–62, 1987; and Ross, JG, Dotson, CO, Gilbert, GG, & Katz, SJ. The national youth and fitness study II. New standards for fitness measurement. Journal of Physical Education, Recreation and Dance, 56:62–66, 1985.

the measured performance for children at each age in this study. A general increase in the mean performance was noted throughout childhood in both sexes. The greatest gains occurred between the ages of 5 and 6 years and 12 and 13 years for girls and between 5 and 6, 7 and 8, and 13 and 14 years for boys. Both groups showed substantial improvements in performance at puberty. Sex differences were apparent by age 8 years. Relative gains across the age span were substantially higher for boys than for girls.

PHYSICAL ACTIVITIES

Activities that have a high correlation with muscular strength are gymnastics, jumping, sprinting, weight lifting, and wrestling. Local muscular endurance is affected by cycling, figure skating, and middle-distance running.

RESPONSE TO TRAINING

Training-induced increases in strength can be influenced by numerous factors, including enhancement of motivation, improvement in coordination, increase in number of contractile proteins per cross-sectional area of muscle, and hypertrophy of muscle (Mersch & Stoboy, 1989). Gains in strength and muscle mass can be achieved by children with training at or after puberty. Prepubescent children also show improvements in force output with training but appear to have difficulty in increasing muscle mass (Bar-Or, 1983c; Sale, 1989). Strength improvements in prepubescent children have thus been attributed to neurologic adaptations to training and improved motor unit activation rather than to increased cross-sectional area of muscle (Blimkie et al., 1989; Komi, 1986; Weltman et al., 1986). Mersch and Stoboy (1989) demonstrated hypertrophy of muscle mass in preadolescent boys, so whether prepubescent children can achieve significant gains in strength and muscle mass by resistance training remains controversial.

ASSESSMENT OF MUSCULAR STRENGTH AND ENDURANCE IN CHILDREN WITH DISABILITIES

Muscular strength and endurance are crucial fitness components for walking, lifting, and performing most daily functions. Deficits of muscular strength in children with disabilities are a primary focus for the clinician in an attempt to improve (or sustain) maximum function.

Muscular Dystrophy

Strength measurements by dynamometry in children with muscular dystrophy (MD) exhibit progressive deterioration as compared with healthy children (Fowler & Gardner, 1967). A failure of muscular strength to increase with growth is seen. The result is that the absolute strength in a child with MD at the age of 16 years is similar to that of a healthy 5-year-old.

Muscular endurance, the ability to sustain static or rhythmic contraction for long periods, is also affected in children with MD. Ninety-two percent of the children tested by Hosking and colleagues (1976) scored below the 5th percentile for strength in holding the head 45° off the ground. Measurement on the Wingate anaerobic cycling test indicates that both peak muscular power and mean muscular power output are significantly less than normal (Bar-Or, 1986). The test-retest reliability of this test for various neuromuscular and muscular disease conditions has been established (Tirosh et al., 1990).

Cerebral Palsy

Strength deficits in children with CP are common. Whether voluntary strength can be accurately measured in the presence of spasticity is controversial. As methods for distinguishing spasticity from strength improve (possibilities include use of isokinetic equipment), new information may become available. Inadequate joint moment and power production as measured by computerized gait analysis are seen in children with CP (Gage, 1991; Olney et al., 1988). These measures provide indirect evidence in a functional context of decreased strength, because strength is a prerequisite for moment and power production. Power production by the ankle plantar flexor muscles in terminal stance phase provides a key source of power for forward motion during the normal walking cycle. Power production in terminal stance phase is often reduced in children with CP. Occasionally, inappropriately timed power production results in excessive, but nonproductive, energy expenditure during gait (Gage, 1991; Fig. 5–2).

Muscular endurance is also decreased in CP. Performance on the Wingate anaerobic test in a group of children with CP resulted in averages that were 2 to 4 standard deviations below the mean (Bar-Or, 1986).

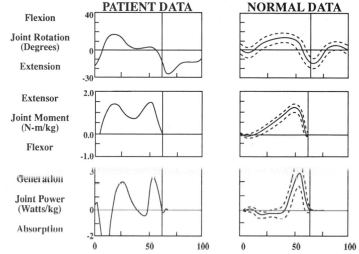

FIGURE 5–2. Sagittal plane joint rotation (kinematic), joint moment and power (kinetics) of a child with cerebral palsy versus a normal child. The child's joint moment is biphasic, and the power graph indicates two distinct bursts of power generation instead of one. The first burst is abnormal and functions to drive the center of gravity upward, not forward, which is nonproductive energy expenditure. (From Gage, JR. Gait Analysis in Cerebral Palsy. London: MacKeith Press, 1991, p. 145.)

Flexibility

The importance of flexibility as a component of health-related fitness is related to prevention of orthopaedic impairments later in life, especially lower back pain (United States Department of Health and Human Services, 1990). Flexibility of the lower back, legs, and shoulders contributes to reduction of injury (Haskell et al., 1985). Limitations in spinal mobility can interfere with activities of daily living, such as dressing, turning, and driving. Restrictions in back mobility can also contribute to abnormalities in walking.

CRITERION MEASURE

Joint range of motion is the criterion used for standards of flexibility. Although the range of motion measures for adults are well established and can be found in various textbooks (Norkin & White, 1985), range of motion information for the pediatric population correlated with changes in stature is limited. Upper extremity range of motion data for children are not well documented. The typical measurement tool is the universal goniometer. Gajdosik and Gajdosik have reviewed the reliability of goniometry in Chapter 4 of this volume.

LABORATORY MEASUREMENT/
DEVELOPMENTAL ASPECTS OF FLEXIBILITY

Extremity Range of Motion

Lower extremity passive range of motion measurements have been described in the newborn,

infant, and toddler (Drews et al., 1984; Phelps et al., 1985; Waugh et al., 1983). Newborn infants exhibit hypoextensibility of both hip and knee flexor muscles and increased popliteal angles consistent with the flexed posture in utero. Range increases in the first months of life. Ranges of hip abduction and rotations also differ from adult values.

Little to no information has been reported for range of motion during childhood. Unpublished data from the author's laboratory on lower extremity range of motion measurements in 140 children between the ages of 2 and 18 years suggest variation in some joints throughout childhood and relative stability in others (Stout, JL, Phelps, JA, Koop, SE, unpublished data, 1991; Table 5–9). (Test-retest reliability 0.95; Inter-rater reliability 0.90). Results suggested age and sex differences, with females exhibiting a trend toward more flexibility at all ages. Greater flexibility of the hamstring muscles in females is especially apparent during the teenage years in straight leg raising and popliteal angle measurements.

Posture and Spinal Mobility

Spinal mobility has been assessed in both young children and adolescents (Haley et al., 1986; Moran et al., 1979). The technique of measurement of back mobility uses tape measure distance changes in bony landmark relationships before and after a standardized spinal movement. The concurrent validity of this measurement technique has been established (Moll & Wright, 1971; Moran et al., 1979). Anterior spinal flexion appears to remain relatively stable throughout childhood and adoles-

TABLE 5–9. **SELECTED RANGE OF MOTION MEASUREMENTS DURING CHILDHOOD**

Range of Motion Measure	2–5 Years		6–12 Years		13–19 Years	
	M	F	M	F	M	F
Straight leg raise	70	75	65	75	60	70
Popliteal angle (unilateral)*	15	10	30	25	40	25
Abduction†	60	60	50	55	45	50
Internal Rotation‡	45	50	50	55	45	45
Femoral anteversion§	10	15	7	7	0	0

*Supine position
†Measured with hip extension.
‡Prone position.
§Prone position by lateral placement of the greater trochanter.
All measurements in degrees.

cence, but lateral flexion increases linearly with age through adolescence and into early adulthood. Girls were significantly more flexible than boys in both anterior flexion and lateral flexion in the 5- to 9-year-old age group (Haley et al., 1986).

The relationship of posture to physical fitness is not often addressed in today's emphasis on health-related fitness. Previous research discussing the relationship of posture to fitness included the importance of posture to trunk strength and the potential for imbalance, back pain, headaches, foot pain, and orthopaedic deformities (Clarke, 1979; Kendall & Kendall, 1952). Each aspect of posture may be important to mobility and cosmesis in children but becomes of greater importance in adulthood when impairment can lead to further deformity and loss of function.

The New York State Physical Fitness Test. This test includes a posture assessment method consisting of three profiles of 13 posture areas. The test is used for children in grades 4 through 12. The 13 areas include head, shoulder, spine, hips, feet, and arches in the coronal plane and neck, chest, shoulders, upper back, trunk, abdomen, and lower back in the sagittal plane. The 50th percentile requires good posture scores on more than half the posture items (Clarke & Clarke, 1987).

The Posture Scale for Children. This test is a static postural alignment scale being developed at the University of Illinois at Chicago for use with children between the ages of 4 months and 8 years (Levine, SB, personal communication, 1992). The scale, like the posture portion of the New York State Physical Fitness Test, includes a series of profiles for each of five positions, including supine, prone-on-elbows, bench sitting, floor sitting, and standing. Each position has one normal profile and four increasingly abnormal profiles for each body part to be rated. Preliminary data from testing with the prone-on-elbows scale indicate that the scale differentiates between the posture of normal children and children with CP (Levine, 1991).

The Adams Forward Bending Test. This test is a commonly used screening test for scoliosis. The back is viewed as the individual bends the trunk forward to 90°. The classic sign of scoliosis is the presence of a posterior rib hump during this motion (Bleck, 1991). Although children with scoliosis often develop lack of spinal mobility if the scoliosis becomes severe, the Adams Forward Bending Test is not a test of trunk flexibility per se. Posture is often assessed in children with scoliosis for the presence of lordosis to assess hip flexibility; the presence of pelvic obliquity to assess flexibility of the adductors, abductors, and tensor fasciae latae; and the presence of a posterior pelvic tilt to assess hamstring flexibility. For more information on scoliosis, see Chapter 10.

MEASUREMENT IN THE FIELD

The field test for measurement of flexibility in tests of physical fitness is the sit and reach test, a measure of hamstring muscle and lower back flexibility. All physical fitness batteries used in the United States include a sit and reach test. The test-retest reliability of the sit and reach test has been found to be high; coefficients between .94 and .99 have been reported (Flint & Gudgell, 1966; Jackson, AW, & Baker, 1986; Macrae & Wright, 1969). AW Jackson & Baker (1986) assessed the criterion-related validity of the sit and reach test both for hamstring flexibility and for lower, upper, and total back flexibility. A moderate correlation was found with hamstring flexibility (.64) and a low correlation with lower back flexibility (.28). Upper back flexibility and total back flexibility were not correlated with the sit and reach scores.

Branta and colleagues (1984) found sex differences in the performance on the sit and reach test in children between 5 and 14 years of age, with girls showing better flexibility than boys at all ages. Girls showed little variability in flexibility from the ages of 5 to 11 years. Boys experienced a net loss of flexibility between the ages of 5 and 15. This is consistent with the gonoimetric measures of hamstring flexibility noted in this author's laboratory (Stout, JL, Phelps, JA, & Koop, SE, unpublished data, 1991).

STANDARDS BY AGE

The criterion standard of performance on the FITNESSGRAM Program for the sit and reach test is 10 inches from the ages of 5 to 16 years. No variability with age or sex is allowed by the criterion. The FITNESSGRAM Program criterion is well below the average score obtained on the NCYFS I and II (Ross et al., 1985, 1987).

PHYSICAL ACTIVITIES

Activities that require a high degree of flexibility include figure skating, gymnastics, jumping (track and field), and judo. Stretching is an important part of any exercise program for general warm-up before vigorous activity and to reduce the potential for injury. Possible physiologic mechanisms for the benefits of stretching include increased blood flow to muscles, increased mechanical efficiency of muscle and tendon, and reduction of viscosity within the muscle (Bar-Or, 1983c). Decreased resistance to extension of connective tissue leads to increased efficiency and power output by muscles. Much of this research has studied the adult population, but the same principles are believed to apply to children (Bar-Or, 1983c; Kuland & Tottossy, 1985; Yamashita et al., 1992).

ASSESSMENT OF FLEXIBILITY IN CHILDREN WITH DISABILITIES

For clinicians involved in the rehabilitation (or "habilitation") of children with musculoskeletal disorders, maintenance of flexibility or joint range of motion is often a primary concern. Almost any musculoskeletal or neuromuscular disorder for which physical therapy is recommended includes treatment for loss of flexibility. Conditions such as CP, juvenile rheumatoid arthritis, MD, or long bone fracture are common examples.

In Chapter 4, Gajdosik and Gajdosik addressed both the measurement and the effects of intervention on improving joint range of motion in children. The inter-rater reliability of joint range of motion measurements in children with spasticity has been found to be within the range of .60 to .85 (Ashton et al., 1978; Harris et al., 1985). Similar results have been found in adults (Boone et al., 1978; Ekstrand et al., 1982). Because maintenance of flexibility is an important component of most physical therapy programs for children with disabilities, methods for more reliable assessment of joint range of motion are needed.

Body Composition

The term body composition is understood to mean total body content of water, protein, fat, and minerals (Dell, 1989). In reference to health-related fitness, body composition is used as a measure of body fatness or obesity. Attainment of appropriate body weight for overweight individuals is an explicit objective of Healthy Children 2000 (United States Department of Health and Human Services, 1990). Because of the clustering effects of obesity with other risk factors for CAD, the relevance of obesity to a child's present and future health cannot be overemphasized. It has been suggested that regional distribution of abdominal fat is an important predictor of mortality, stroke, heart disease, and diabetes (Bray & Bouchard, 1988). Obesity rates for juveniles range between 10 and 25% in North America and appear to be increasing (Bar-Or, 1987; Ross & Gilbert, 1985; Ross & Pate, 1987).

LABORATORY MEASUREMENT

The purposes of body composition measurement, whether in the laboratory or in the field, is to obtain a measure of fat-free or lean body mass. Chemical analysis is the only direct method to measure body composition (Klish, 1989). Because this is expensive and impractical, even laboratory standards of measurement are from indirect assessment. Most standards rely on formulas and models of composition that assume fat and lean body mass are constant. Because infants and children exhibit variable, not constant, body composition throughout childhood (Boileau et al., 1988; Haschke, 1989; Lohman, 1986; Spady, 1989), numerous problems in determining body composition in children are encountered. Use of adult standards leads to overestimation or underestimation of body fatness, depending upon the technique (Boileau et al., 1988). All methods presented have some limitations for use with children, but all have been used. There is no one "gold standard" for children.

Densitometry

More commonly referred to as underwater or hydrostatic weighing, densitometry determines the density of an individual by dividing actual body weight by the decrease in weight when the person is completely submerged in water. The densities of fat and lean body mass are assumed to be constant and can be calculated for an individual when the density of the whole body is known. Although it is considered the gold standard for measurement of body composition in adults, it has limited applicability to young children.

Total Body Water

The measurement of total body water is used as a means of estimating the nonfat portion of the body because neutral fat does not bind water. Stable isotopes of hydrogen or oxygen are administered orally and then measured to determine the amount of dilution in a body fluid.

Bioelectric Impedance Analysis

This method is based on the principle that impedance to electrical flow varies in proportion to the amount of lean tissue present. A weak electric current is passed through the body and its impedance is measured.

DEVELOPMENTAL ASPECTS OF BODY COMPOSITION

From birth through adolescence, body composition is constantly changing. Part of this change is caused by chemical maturation as a result of increasing mineral mass and hydration of adipose tissue (Spady, 1989). Chemical maturation occurs after adolescence, when the constants relating one component of body composition to another stabilize, until the last decades of life (Boileau et al., 1984, 1988; Lohman, 1986; Slaughter et al., 1984).

The four major components of body composition are water, protein, fat, and mineral. Reference models describe the body composition of these components in the child at various ages (Fomon, 1967; Fomon et al., 1982; Haschke, 1989; Haschke et al., 1981; Ziegler et al., 1976). A composite of these reference models and changes with growth in males appears in Figure 5–3.

Fat is the most variable component of body composition during infancy and childhood. Increases begin in utero when fat content changes from 2.5% at 1 kg of body weight to 12% at term gestation (Spady, 1989). The proportion of body fat rises from 12% to an average of 25% from birth to 6 months of age. Fat content decreases during early childhood as muscle mass increases. Sex differences are noted early in childhood; girls exhibit a greater percentage of fat content than do boys. At 6 to 8 years of age, the average fat content for boys is 13 to 15% and for girls, 16 to 18% (Lohman, 1987). During adolescence, fat content increases in girls so that between the ages of 14 and 16 years the mean percentage of fat content is 21 to 23%.

Water content of the body is approximately 89%

FIGURE 5–3. The normal body composition of male children as it changes with age. Data derived from data found in the descriptions of the reference fetus, infant, male child at 9 years, children from birth to 10 years, and the adolescent male. CHO = carbohydrate; tbw = total body water. (From Spady, DW. Normal body composition of infants and children. 98th Ross Laboratories Conference on Pediatric Research, *98*:67–73, 1989. Used with permission of Ross Products Division, Abbott Laboratories, Columbus, OH 43216. © 1989 Ross Products Division, Abbott Laboratories.)

of body weight at 24 weeks of gestation and drops to 75% at 40 weeks (Spady, 1989). By 4 months of age, water content stabilizes at approximately 60 to 65% and remains at that level until puberty. Protein content as a proportion of body weight increases from approximately 13% at birth to 15 to 17% at age 10 years. Mineral content of the body rises from 3% at birth to 5% at age 18 years.

Differences between the sexes exist in each major component of body composition throughout childhood and are magnified at adolescence. The major changes during adolescence in both sexes are a decrease in the percentage of water and an increase in the percentage of osseous minerals (Haschke, 1989; Lohman et al., 1984).

MEASUREMENT IN THE FIELD

Assessment of body composition in the field is by measurement of skinfold thickness. The validity of this measure is suspect, just as the validity of laboratory methods is in question. The major problem is that skinfold measurement is based on the assumption that body surface measures and body density relationships are stable throughout childhood (Lohman, 1982). Two other threats to the validity of this measurement are that use of skinfold thickness implies that the subcutaneous fat layer reflects the total amount of fat in the body, and that selected measurement sites reflect average thickness. These assumptions may not be true (Klish, 1989); however, Lohman and colleagues

(1984) and Slaughter and colleagues (1984) did not find large deviations in skinfold distribution.

Despite this controversy, measurement of body composition is an important part of almost all health-related fitness tests. Concurrent validity has been demonstrated consistently with moderately high correlations of .70 to .85 between measurements of skinfolds and densitometry or potassium spectrometry (Going, 1988).

The typical sites for measurement of skinfold thickness are the triceps brachii, subscapular area, and calf. Usually these areas are measured in some combination. Lohman (1987) has designed a series of charts for easy evaluation of skinfold thickness and percent body fatness based on either triceps and subscapular or triceps and calf skinfold measures. The method of estimation of percent body fatness from skinfold measurements involves estimating density from skinfold measurements and then converting density to percent body fatness. The reader is referred to other sources for more detailed information (Lohman, 1982, 1986; Slaughter et al., 1984). A 3 to 5% error is reported for adults when estimating body fatness from skinfold measurements (Lohman, 1982).

STANDARDS BY AGE

The criterion values for ranges of body fatness conducive to optimal health in children are 10 to 25% for boys and 15 to 25% for girls (Lohman, 1987). Values higher than 25% in boys and 30% in girls are considered to place the child at risk for associated morbidity. This standard is consistent with the cutoffs at body composition of 32% for females and 25% for males set by the FITNESS-GRAM Program (Blair et al., 1989). Results from the NCYFS I and II studies suggest that children within the 40th to 50th percentiles on the test items fall within the optimal ranges described earlier (Ross et al., 1985, 1987).

RESPONSE TO TRAINING

Conditioning and training programs may or may not affect body composition. If changes are to occur, the type of exercise must entail high-energy expenditure of high or intense effort. Appropriate activities include swimming, running, or weight training. Evidence of program effects on body composition is inconclusive in adults. Little information is available on children, but what is available indicates that percentage of body fatness can be reduced during training for specific sports but rises again when programs are discontinued (Parizkova, 1977; VonDobelin et al., 1972). General

physical activity is associated with reduced body fatness as compared with physically inactive peers (Parizkova, 1974). Evidence is inconclusive as to whether obese children are less physically active than nonobese children.

ASSESSMENT OF BODY COMPOSITION IN CHILDREN WITH DISABILITIES

Premature Infants

Clinicians treat many children with disabilities who were born prematurely. Premature birth has been shown to affect body composition (Spady et al., 1987). Compared with a "reference" fetus of similar weight, the premature infant has a higher total fat content and lower total body water content. These differences in composition are likely the result of living outside the womb and being faced with the necessity of increasing body fat for temperature regulation. The implications of this altered body composition during growth have not been studied, nor has body composition been studied in premature infants who experience neonatal complications. They may or may not have effects on composition throughout childhood and into adulthood.

Cerebral Palsy

Two studies have been conducted on body composition of individuals with CP (Bandini et al., 1991; Berg & Isaksson, 1970). Both studied adolescents but used different methods. Each reported that adolescents with CP are shorter and typically weigh less than their age-matched peers. The fat-free mass in adolescents with CP was found to be significantly lower than that in the adolescent population without disabilities (Bandini et al., 1991) and may be consistent with reduced muscle mass. Berg and Isaksson reported reduced body fatness in relation to norms but provided no percentages based on body weight. Bandini and colleagues reported an increased percentage of body fat in the subjects with CP when compared with adolescents without disability. Resting metabolic rate was found to be lower than the norm in both studies. The samples were relatively small and included children with a variety of types of CP and of functional levels. Both type of CP and functional level are likely to be important variables affecting body composition, but the conflicting results of the two studies cannot be resolved without further research.

Myelodysplasia

The study by Bandini and colleagues (1991) also included individuals with myelodysplasia. This group, on average, showed decreased stature, reduced fat-free mass, and increased percentage of body fat as compared with able-bodied peers. The percentage of body fat was above the 95th percentile for all subjects with myelodysplasia. A significant correlation was not found between skinfold thickness and body composition, which suggests that fat distribution may be altered because of the type of paralysis. A previous study had also suggested that skinfold measurements and fat distribution may be altered in myelodysplasia (Hayes-Allen & Tring, 1973). Both studies indicate that children with myelodysplasia are at risk for obesity.

CONDITIONING AND TRAINING

Whether the components of physical fitness can be affected by training programs is an important question, especially to clinicians who are designing programs for children with disabilities. Bar-Or (in 1983c) differentiated between the terms conditioning and training, which are often used interchangeably. Physical conditioning is defined as the process by which exercise, repeated over a specified duration, induces morphologic and functional changes in body systems and tissues. The tissues and systems can include skeletal muscles, the myocardium, adipose tissue, bones, tendons, ligaments, the central nervous system, and the endocrine system. Bar-Or (1983c) considered conditioning to consist of general exercise for overall physical fitness. Training, by contrast, is specific exercise designed to promote changes in performance of a particular type of activity. In the context of this chapter, training will be discussed in relation to specific fitness components, but overall conditioning will be discussed in reference to children with disabilities.

Fitness Components and Training in Children

Many of the physiologic changes that result from training and conditioning in adults also take place during the process of growth and maturation in childhood. These naturally occurring changes make it difficult to study the specific effects of conditioning and training. The primary components of physical fitness of interest to trainers are cardiorespiratory endurance and physical strength.

CARDIORESPIRATORY ENDURANCE

Some controversy exists over whether maximal aerobic power or Vo_2max can be increased by car-

diorespiratory training in children (Bar-Or, 1983c; Krahenbuhl et al., 1985). Besides the improvements seen to occur naturally during growth and maturation, other problems in assessing the effects of training include seasonal differences in activity, difficulty in ensuring that a true Vo_2max has been reached during the testing process, and the already high level of physical activity in young children.

Krahenbuhl and colleagues (1985), in a review of training programs, concluded that maximal aerobic power can be significantly increased after regular intensive training in children of 8 to 14 years of age. Endurance exercise appeared more effective than intermittent exercise. General physical education programs alone were not effective in improving Vo_2max. Effective activities included running, cycle ergometry, and swimming. Increases of 8 to 10% were measured in effective programs. Some studies reported little or no change in Vo_2max despite improved long-distance running performance after training programs lasting 1 to 9 weeks (Bar-Or, 1983c; Cumming et al., 1967).

Less controversy exists over whether training is effective in improving cardiorespiratory endurance in adolescence. The effects of training in adolescents appear to be similar to those in adults. The functional and morphologic changes of the cardiovascular and pulmonary systems that take place as a result of training are listed in Table 5–10. Training effects usually include increases in myocardial mass, stroke volume, ventilation, and respiratory muscular endurance.

TABLE 5–10. **CARDIORESPIRATORY FUNCTION VARIABLES AND RESPONSE TO TRAINING IN CHILDREN**

Function/Variable	Change with Training
Heart volume	Increase
Blood volume	Increase
Total hemoglobin	Slight increase
Stroke volume (max, submax)	Increase
Cardiac output (max, submax)	Increase, no change, or decrease
Arteriovenous difference (submax)	No change
Blood flow to active muscle	No change
Ventilation/kg body wt (max)	Increase
Ventilation/kg body wt (submax)	Decrease
Respiratory rate (submax)	Decrease
Tidal volume (max)	Increase
Respiratory muscle endurance	Increase

Max = maximal exercise; submax = submaximal exercise.
Adapted from Bar-Or, O. Physiologic responses to exercise in healthy children. In Bar-Or, O. Pediatric Sports Medicine for the Practitioner. New York: Springer-Verlag, 1983, p. 49.

MUSCULAR STRENGTH AND ENDURANCE

Muscular strength is a component of fitness that can be affected by training, especially in children at or after puberty. Resistance strength training refers to training for improved muscular strength by repeatedly overcoming heavy resistance. The practice of resistance strength training is problematic in preadolescent children because controversy exists regarding 1) whether children can make gains in strength and muscle mass, 2) whether gains improve athletic performance, and particularly 3) whether children are more susceptible to injury when participating in such training. Despite the controversy, resistance strength training has been shown to increase voluntary force production at all ages and may reduce the risk of injury during athletic participation (Sale, 1989).

In a review of strength training studies, Sale (1989) concluded that children can increase voluntary strength as a result of training, and, furthermore, children show a greater increase in strength than do adults when training-induced strength improvements are expressed as a percentage of change. During maximal voluntary contraction, children can develop the same force per unit of muscle cross-sectional area as adults despite differences in absolute strength and muscle size.

As previously described, the strength increases associated with growth are closely related to increases in muscle mass, including an increase in the number of both sarcomeres and fibrils per muscle fiber (Malina, 1986). The enhancement of muscular strength caused by growth is estimated to be approximately 1.5 kg/y from the age of 6 to 14 years (Mersch & Stoboy, 1989). In conjunction with "muscular" adaptations, neural adaptations associated with improved coordination and motor learning may also play a role. For example, the increases in voluntary strength noted with training in prepubescent children have been found to be independent of increased muscle mass or hypertrophy such as that seen in postpubescent children or adults (Blimkie et al., 1989; Sale, 1989; Weltman et al., 1986). Improved motor unit activation and neural adaptations (including more appropriate co-contraction of synergist muscles and inhibition of antagonist muscles as well as improvements in motor unit recruitment order and firing frequency within the prime movers) are believed to play a role in producing training effects in both adults and children (Kuhl, 1986; Moritani & DeVries, 1979). It has been suggested that, during the early stages of training, neural adaptation predominates in producing altered performance. Muscular adaptation contributes in the later stages of training (Sale, 1989; Fig. 5–4).

FIGURE 5–4. Relative roles of neural and muscular adaptation in strength training. Neural adaptation plays the biggest role in the early phase of training, which can last up to several weeks. Muscular adaptation predominates later and is limited by the extent that muscles can hypertrophy. (From Sale, DG. Strength training in children. In Gisolfi, CV, & Lamb, DR (Eds.), Perspectives in Exercise Science and Sports Medicine, Vol. 2: Youth, Exercise, and Sport. Indianapolis, IN: Benchmark Press, 1989, p. 180.)

Principles of Training

The principles of an effective training program include specificity as well as guidelines for intensity, frequency, and duration of exercise. Rules for children are essentially the same as those for adults.

SPECIFICITY

The changes that take place in the body as a result of training are specific to the type of exercise performed and to the tissue involved. Myocardial tissue, for example, is affected by long-distance running but not by resistance strength training. The type of contraction (concentric, eccentric, or isometric), the number of repetitions performed, the velocity of muscle contraction, and the particular muscles exercised all influence the results of a strength training program. Different sports develop different components of fitness.

INTENSITY

Activity at a certain intensity is required to achieve conditioning or training effects. Intensity should be determined as a percentage of the individual's maximum because the same amount of activity can represent two entirely different levels of intensity for two different individuals. For example, a child with CP who walks at the same velocity as an able-bodied child may consume twice as much oxygen, so walking as a form of exercise for the child with CP is more intense. Although Vo_2

depends on the square of velocity, an average 6- to 12-year-old walking at an average velocity consumes about 25% of Vo_2max; for a child with CP, Vo_2 can be as high as 75 to 90% of Vo_2max (Stout, JL, unpublished observation, 1992).

Intensity threshold refers to the intensity of exercise below which few or no training or conditioning effects are observed (Bar-Or, 1983c). The intensity threshold of maximal aerobic power in adults required to produce a training effect is 60 to 70% of Vo_2max. The threshold for strength is approximately 60 to 65% of maximal voluntary contraction. The principle of overload in strength training is in part related to the intensity threshold of exercise. Overload refers to a task that requires considerable voluntary effort to complete. No specific data are available for intensity thresholds for children, but they are thought to be at least equal to those of adults. Whether intensity thresholds for children with various disabilities are the same as those for able-bodied children is also unknown.

FREQUENCY

The optimal frequency of training depends on the type of program, and frequency is interrelated with intensity and duration. Two or three times per week is a general rule of thumb (Bar-Or, 1983c).

DURATION

Any program, whether a therapeutic program or a fitness program, requires a minimum implementation time before benefits are seen. Most effective conditioning programs last at least 6 to 8 weeks. The optimal duration of an exercise session is dependent on the type of program. In general, the session should consist of a warm-up phase of 10 minutes, an exercise phase above the exercise threshold for 15 to 30 minutes, and 5- to 7-minute cool-down period. The warm-up phase has been shown to be important for increasing performance of both aerobic and anaerobic tasks in children (Bar-Or, 1983c). The warm-up period should include 1) activities to raise core body temperature, 2) stretching exercises, and 3) activities specific to the exercise task. The American Academy of Pediatrics (1983) recommends that strength-training regimens for children include activities to provide strength training for all parts of the body to ensure balanced development.

The duration of the exercise phase in strength training is sometimes associated with the goal of achieving maximal overload. This is usually done in one of two ways—either by repeating brief maximal contractions or by repeating submaximal contractions to the point of fatigue.

PROGRESSION

A conditioning or training program must be progressive in its demands for continued improvement. The intensity threshold, the duration of exercise sessions, the number of repetitions performed during a session, or the frequency of exercise sessions may need to be increased. All contribute individually and collectively to the progression of the exercise program.

Conditioning in Children with Disabilities

CEREBRAL PALSY

As children with CP approach and move through adolescence, an important aspect of function is the ability to maintain ambulation. Vo_2 during ambulation in preadolescent children with CP (ages 6–12 y) is more than twice that of able-bodied children walking at the same velocity (Koop et al., 1989). If body weight and adiposity increase in adolescence without an increase in muscular strength, maximal aerobic capacity decreases, and the task of walking becomes more and more difficult. Growth in mass is a cubic function (volume) and growth in strength is a function of the square (cross-sectional muscle area). As previously mentioned, muscles increase in mass first, then in strength (Malina, 1986). During the adolescent growth spurt, mass increases at a faster rate than does strength. For able-bodied children, this process occurs without noticeable deficit or loss of function, but for children with CP, loss of function sometimes occurs because the rate of increase in strength is inadequate to support the rate of increase in muscle mass. A major goal of physical therapy for adolescents with CP is maintenance of the ability to ambulate throughout the growth spurt. If a child has maximal strength and aerobic capacity upon entering the growth spurt, function is also likely to be at maximal capacity. Conditioning in a child with CP could play a vital role in the process of maximizing the potential not only of the adolescent but of the preadolescent as well.

The ultimate goal of conditioning programs for children with CP is to retard or reverse the deterioration of capacity expected during adolescence. In a longitudinal study of adolescents with CP, Lundberg (1973) found that heart rate at a given power load increased an average of 10 beats per minute per year, implying decreasing efficiency. Studies have demonstrated that conditioning effects in the population of children and adolescents with CP are similar to those of children without disability (Bar-

Or et al., 1976; Berg, 1970b; Lundberg & Pernow 1970; Lundberg et al., 1967). Increased strength, range of motion, and functional endurance have also been reported as a result of a strengthening program (Horvat, 1987). One study that addressed the issue of changes in body composition as a result of conditioning showed no change in the percentage of body fat after a 4-month program (Berg, 1970a). A conditioning response unique to individuals with CP is an increase in blood flow to exercising muscles (Lundberg & Pernow, 1970). This may reflect a physiologic mechanism in which conditioning and strengthening decrease the effects of spasticity.

Evidence suggests that neither regular physical education classes nor habitual activities is sufficient to induce conditioning changes in children with CP (Berg, 1970b; Dresen, 1985). The program must increase intensity beyond habitual exercise levels. The duration of the overall program should be longer than 6 weeks; results of 6-week training programs are equivocal (Ekblom & Lundberg, 1968). Target heart rate was typically maintained for 15 to 30 minutes in most studies. Activities in accordance with the child's ability were used; examples are cycle ergometry, swimming, running, and jogging.

CYSTIC FIBROSIS

Cystic fibrosis is a hereditary disease affecting the exocrine glands. The lungs, gastrointestinal tract, and sweat glands produce excessive secretion. Airway obstruction, infection, and respiratory failure result from excess viscous mucus in the respiratory tract. Results of studies emphasizing aerobic conditioning for 3 to 5 months suggest that Vo_2max, endurance of respiratory muscles, and pulmonary function all show improvement (Jankowski, 1986; Orenstein et al., 1981; Zach et al., 1982). Jogging, cycling, swimming, weight lifting, and calisthenics of various durations and combinations were used.

In addition to the positive effects of conditioning on physical fitness, clinical benefits in the management of the disease are also reported (Bar-Or, 1985). Increased coughing and mucous clearance may reduce the need for chest therapy to manage secretions (Zach et al., 1982).

The effects of exercise on children with cystic fibrosis and other clinical populations must be closely monitored to reduce or avoid potential detrimental effects. Particular concerns in the population with cystic fibrosis are dehydration (especially in high heat) and oxygen desaturation (Bar-Or, 1985).

MUSCULAR DYSTROPHY

The effects of conditioning patients with MD have been evaluated in numerous studies, which produced equivocal results (Abrahamson & Rogoff, 1952; DeLateur & Giaconi, 1979; Fowler et al., 1965; Vignos & Watkins, 1966). Evaluation of the results must take into account that many of the studies were inadequately controlled for threats to internal validity. Results suggest that modest gains in strength can be made or the rate of deterioration retarded. In one study, DeLateur and Giaconi found no significant change in strength of the quadriceps femoris muscle after 6 weeks of a 6-month conditioning program of submaximal exercise. A modest, but not significant, increase in strength was found after 6 months. Each subject served as his or her own control. No deleterious effects of a strengthening program were found. Despite the lack of statistically significant effects, the increase in strength may be enough to deter future deterioration.

▌ CONCLUSION

This chapter was designed to provide information on physical fitness and conditioning in the able-bodied child for promoting health and preventing disease. The components of fitness, how they are tested, and how they contribute to health were reviewed. An understanding of physical fitness, physical activity, and conditioning is valuable for appreciating the impact of disabling conditions on these variables. Health-related physical fitness is important for reducing future health risks in every child, regardless of the presence or absence of disability. Preadolescent fitness may be especially important to the child with a disability because of the effects the particular disability may have on the child as he or she enters puberty and adulthood. The design of exercise programs (their intensity, frequency, and duration) should encompass the minimal requirements for physical fitness as well as incorporate therapeutic goals. Exercise programs should be designed so that the energy requirements for accomplishing day-to-day activities through the growth period are met. Meeting this goal is likely to require additional exercise beyond current therapy or physical education. One of our goals as pediatric therapists should be to ensure, to whatever extent possible, that our clients enter adulthood with a fitness level suitable to a healthy adulthood. Research is needed to document the extent to which this goal can be met for specific populations and levels of disability.

Much research remains to be done in the able-bodied population as well. Reliability and validity studies need to continue on criterion-based measures now being used to determine minimal fitness levels. Research needs to establish reliable, valid, and universal criteria, both in the laboratory and in the field. Continued identification of the relationship between childhood physical activity and fitness and health in adulthood is vital to our overall understanding of health-related fitness.

Research to benefit populations with disabilities or children with special needs has barely begun. With the inadequate base of research in children without disability, developing standards of fitness for specific disabled populations begins at a disadvantage. A question that remains to be answered is whether the fitness performance criteria for children without disabilities are valid for children with disabilities or special needs. Experience with development of testing and measurement tools for other purposes would suggest they are not. Are children with disabilities such as CP more fit because they expend in walking an amount of energy equivalent to that of an able-bodied person walking up and down stairs all day long? Are the thresholds and target zones for fitness improvement the same for children with a variety of disabilities as for able-bodied children? How are conditioning and training programs best designed for children with disabilities? Do conditioning programs initiated before the onset of puberty help to maintain fitness during and after puberty? What are the physiologic and behavioral factors that limit a child's capacity to improve fitness variables or to exercise? How much exercise is detrimental? How do presurgical strengthening programs affect the recovery of strength after surgery? Questions such as these are at only the beginning of our quest for understanding. The journey has just begun.

References

Abrahamson, AS, & Rogoff, J. Physical treatment in muscular dystrophy (Abstract). In Proceedings of the 2nd Medical Conference. Muscular Dystrophy Association, 1952, pp. 123–124.

Adams, FH. Factors affecting the working capacity of children and adolescents. In Rarick, GL (Ed.), Physical Activity: Human Growth and Development. New York: Academic Press, 1973, pp. 89–90.

Alexander, J, & Molnar, GE. Muscular strength in children: Preliminary report on objective standards. Archives of Physical Medicine and Rehabilitation, 54:424–427, 1973.

American Academy of Pediatrics. Weight training and weightlifting: Information for the pediatrician. Physician and Sports Medicine, 11(3):157–161, 1983.

American Alliance for Health, Physical Education, Recreation, and Dance. The AAHPERD Physical Best Program. Reston, VA, 1988.

American Psychological Association. Standards for Educational and Psychological Testing. Washington, DC, American Psychological Association, 1985.

Ashton BB, Pickles, B, & Roll, JW. Reliability of goniometric measurements of hip motion in spastic cerebral palsy. Developmental Medicine and Child Neurology, 20:87–94, 1978.

Astrand PO. Experimental Studies of Physical Working Capacity in Relation to Sex and Age. Copenhagen: Ejnar Munksgaard, 1952.

Astrand, PO, & Rodahl, K (Eds.). Textbook of Work Physiology: Physiological Bases of Exercise. New York: McGraw-Hill, 1986.

Bandini, LG, Schoeller, DA, Fukagawa, NK, Wykes, LJ, & Dietz, WH. Body composition and energy expenditure in adolescents with cerebral palsy or myelodysplasia. Pediatric Research, 29:70–77, 1991.

Bar-Or, O. A commentary to children and fitness: A public health perspective. Research Quarterly for Exercise and Sport, 58:304–307, 1987.

Bar-Or, O. Appendix II: Procedures for exercise testing in children. In Bar-Or, O. Pediatric Sports Medicine for the Practitioner. New York: Springer-Verlag, 1983a, pp. 315–341.

Bar-Or, O. Neuromuscular diseases. In Bar-Or, O. Pediatric Sports Medicine for the Practitioner. New York: Springer-Verlag, 1983b, pp. 227–249.

Bar-Or, O. Physiologic responses to exercise in healthy children. In Bar-Or, O. Pediatric Sports Medicine for the Practitioner. New York: Springer-Verlag, 1983c, pp. 1–65.

Bar-Or, O. Physical conditioning in children with cardiorespiratory disease. Exercise and Sport Sciences Reviews, 13:305–334, 1985.

Bar-Or, O. Pathophysiological factors which limit the exercise capacity of the sick child. Medicine and Science in Sports and Exercise, 18:276–282, 1986.

Bar-Or, O, Inbar, O, & Spira, R. Physiological effects of a sports rehabilitation program on cerebral palsied and poliomyelitic adolescents. Medicine and Science in Sports, 8:157–161, 1976.

Berg, K. Effect of physical activation and improved nutrition on the body composition of school children with cerebral palsy. Acta Paediatrica Supplement, 204:53–69, 1970a.

Berg, K. Effect of physical training of school children with cerebral palsy. Acta Paediatrica Supplement, 204:27–33, 1970b.

Berg, K, & Isaksson, B. Body composition and nutrition of school children with cerebral palsy. Acta Paediatrica Supplement, 204:41–52, 1970.

Berger, RA, & Medlin, RL. Evaluation of Berger's 1-RM chin test for junior high school mates. Research Quarterly, 40:460–463, 1969.

Blair, SN, Clark, DG, Cureton, KJ, & Powell, KE. Exercise and fitness in childhood: Implications for a lifetime of health. In Gisolfi, CV, & Lamb, DR (Eds.), Perspectives in Exercise Science and Sports Medicine, Vol. 2: Youth, Exercise, and Sport. Indianapolis, IN: Benchmark Press, 1989, pp. 401–430.

Bleck, E. Adolescent idiopathic scoliosis. Developmental Medicine and Child Neurology, 33:167–173, 1991.

Blimkie, CJR. Age and sex associated variation in strength during childhood: Anthropometric, morphologic, neurologic, biomechanical, endocrinologic, genetic, and physical activity correlates. In Gisolfi, CV, & Lamb, DR (Eds.), Perspectives in Exercise Science and Sports Medicine, Vol. 2: Youth, Exercise, and Sport. Indianapolis, IN: Benchmark Press, 1989, pp. 99–163.

Blimkie, CJR, Ramsay, J, Sale, D, MacDougall, D, Smith, K, & Garner, K. Effects of 10 weeks of resistance training on strength development in prepubertal boys. In Osteid, S, & Carlsen, K-H (Eds.), Children and Exercise XIII. Champaign, IL: Human Kinetics, 1989, pp. 183–197.

Boileau, RA, Lohman, TG, & Slaughter, MH. Exercise and

body composition in children and youth. Scandinavian Journal of Sport Sciences, 7:7–17, 1985.

Boileau, RA, Lohman, TG, Slaughter, MH, Ball, TE, Going, SB, & Hendrix, MK. Hydration of the fat-free body in children during maturation. Human Biology, 56:651–666, 1984.

Boileau, RA, Lohman, TG, Slaughter, MH, Horswill, CA, & Stillman, RJ. Problems associated with determining body composition in maturing youngsters. In Brown, EW, & Branta, CF (Eds.), Competitive Sports for Children and Youth: An Overview of Research and Issues. Champaign, IL: Human Kinetics, 1988, pp. 3–16.

Boone, DC, Azen, SP, Lin, CM, Spense, C, Baron, C, & Lee, L. Reliability of goniometric measurements. Physical Therapy, 58:1355–1360, 1978.

Braden, DS, & Strong, WB. Cardiovascular responses to exercise in childhood. American Journal of Diseases of Children. 144:1255–1260, 1990.

Branta, C, Haubenstricker, J, & Seefeldt, V. Age changes in motor skills during childhood and adolescence. Exercise and Sport Sciences Reviews, 12:467–520, 1984.

Bray, GA, & Bouchard, C. Role of fat distribution during growth and its relationship to health. American Journal of Clinical Nutrition, 47: 551–552, 1988.

Brodie, DA, Burnie, J, Eston, RG, & Royce, JA. Isokinetic strength and flexibility characteristics in preadolescent boys. In Rutenfranz, J, Mocellin, R, & Klimt, F (Eds.), Children and Exercise XII. Champaign, IL: Human Kinetics, 1986, pp. 309–319.

Carron, AV, & Bailey, DA. Strength development in boys from 10–16 years. Monographs of the Society for Research in Child Development, 39:1–37, 1974.

Chrysler Fund–Amateur Athletic Union. Physical Fitness Program. Bloomington, IN: Chrysler Fund–Amateur Athletic Union, 1987.

Clarke, HH. Posture. Physical Fitness Research Digest, 9:1–23, 1979.

Clarke, HH, & Clarke, DH. Application of Measurement in Physical Education. Englewood Cliffs, NJ: Prentice-Hall, 1987, pp. 93–99.

Considine, WJ. An Analysis of Selected Upper Body Tasks As Measures of Strength (Abstract). American Association of Health, Physical Education and Recreation, 1973.

Cooper, DM, Weiler-Ravell, D, Whipp, BJ, & Wasserman, K. Growth-related changes in oxygen uptake and heart rate during progressive exercise in children. Pediatric Research, 18:845–851, 1984.

Corbin CB. Youth fitness, exercise and health: There is much to be done. Research Quarterly for Exercise and Sport, 58:308–314, 1987.

Cumming, GR, Goodwin, A, Baggley, G, & Antel, J. Repeated measurements of aerobic capacity during a week of intensive training at a youth track camp. Canadian Journal of Physiology and Pharmacology, 45:805–811, 1967.

Cunningham, DA, MacFarlane-VanWaterschoot, B, Paterson, DH, Lefcoe, M, & Sangal, SP. Reliability and reproducibility of maximal oxygen uptake in children. Medicine and Science in Sports, 9:104–108, 1977.

Cureton, KJ, & Warren, GL. Criterion-referenced standards for youth health-related fitness tests: A tutorial. Research Quarterly for Exercise and Sport, 61:7–19, 1990.

DeLateur, BJ, & Giaconi, RM. Effect on maximal strength of submaximal exercise in Duchenne muscular dystrophy. American Journal of Physical Medicine, 58:26–36, 1979.

Dell, RB. Comparison of densitometric methods applicable to infants and small children for studying body composition. Ross Laboratories Conference on Pediatric Research, 98:22–38, 1989.

Despres, JP, Bouchard, C, & Malina, RM. Physical activity and coronary heart disease risk factors during childhood and ado-

lescence. Exercise and Sport Sciences Reviews, 18:243–263, 1990.

Dresen, MHW. Physical and psychological effects of training on handicapped children. In Binkhorst, RA, Kemper, HCG, & Saris, WHM (Eds.), Children and Exercise XI, Champaign, IL: Human Kinetics, 1985, pp. 203–209.

Drews, J, Vraciu, JK, & Pellino, G. Range of motion of the joints of the lower extremities of newborns. Physical and Occupational Therapy in Pediatrics, 4:49–62, 1984.

Ekblom, B, & Lundberg, A. Effect of training on adolescents with severe motor handicaps. Acta Paediatrica Scandinavica, 57:17–23, 1968.

Ekstrand, J, Wiktorsson, M, Oberg, B, & Gillquist, J. Lower extremity goniometric measurements: A study to determine their reliability. Archives of Physical Medicine and Rehabilitation, 63:171–175, 1982.

Erickkson, BO, Gollnick, PD, & Saltin, B. Muscle metabolism and enzyme activities after training in boys 11–13 years old. Acta Physiologica Scandinavica, 87:485–487, 1973.

Eriksson, BO, Karlsson, J, & Saltin, B. Muscle metabolites during exercise in pubertal boys. Acta Paediatrica Scandinavica Supplement, 217:154–157, 1971.

Faust, MS. Somatic development of adolescent girls. Society for Research in Child Development, 42:1–90, 1977.

Flint, MM, & Gudgell, J. Electromyographic study of abdominal muscular activity during exercise. Research Quarterly, 36:29–37, 1966.

Florini, JR. Hormonal control of muscle growth. Muscle and Nerve, 10:577–598, 1987.

Fomon, SJ. Body composition of the male reference infant during the first year of life. Pediatrics, 40:863–867, 1967.

Fomon, SJ, Haschke, F, Ziegler, EE, & Nelson, SE. Body composition of reference children from birth to age 10 years. American Journal of Clinical Nutrition, 35:1169–1173, 1982.

Fowler, WM, & Gardner, GW. Quantitative strength measurements in muscular dystrophy. Archives of Physical Medicine and Rehabilitation, 48:629–644, 1967.

Fowler, WM, Pearson, CM, Egstrom, GH, & Gardner, GW. Ineffective treatment of muscular dystrophy with an anabolic steroid and other measures. New England Journal of Medicine, 272:875–882, 1965.

Francis, K, & Feinstein, R. A simple height-specific and rate-specific step test for children. Southern Medical Journal, 84:169–174, 1991.

Fraser, GE, Phillips, RL, & Harris, R. Physical fitness and blood pressure in school children. Circulation, 67:405–412, 1983.

Gage, JR. Gait Analysis in Cerebral Palsy. London: MacKeith Press, 1991.

Giannini, MJ, & Protas, EJ. Aerobic capacity in juvenile rheumatoid arthritis patients and healthy children. Arthritis Care and Research, 4:131–135, 1991.

Giannini, MJ, & Protas, EJ. Exercise response in children with and without juvenile rheumatoid arthritis: A comparison study. Physical Therapy, 72:365–372, 1992.

Godfrey, S. Growth and development of the cardiopulmonary response to exercise. In Davis, JA, & Dobbing, J (Eds.), Scientific Foundations in Paediatrics. London: William Heinemann Medical Books, 1981, pp. 450–460.

Going, S. Physical best: Body composition in the assessment of youth fitness. Journal of Physical Education, Recreation and Dance, 59(9):32–36, 1988.

Green, HJ, & Patla, AE. Maximal aerobic power: Neuromuscular and metabolic considerations. Medicine and Science in Sports and Exercise, 24:38–46, 1992.

Gutin, B, Basch, C, Shea, S, Contento, I, DeLozier, M, Rips, M, Irigoyen, M, & Zybert, P. Blood pressure, fitness, and fatness in 5 and 6 year old children. Journal of the American Medical Association, 264(9):1123–1127, 1990.

Hagberg, JM, Ehsani, AA, Goldring, B, Hernandez, A, Sinacore, DR, & Holoszy, JO. Effect of weight training on blood pressure and hemodynamics in hypertensive adolescents. Journal of Pediatrics, 104:147–151, 1984.

Haley, SM, Tada, WL, & Carmichael, EM. Spinal mobility in young children: A normative study. Physical Therapy, 66:1697–1703, 1986.

Harris, SR, Smith, LH, & Krukowski, L. Goniometric reliability for a child with spastic quadriplegia. Journal of Pediatric Orthopedics, 5:348–351, 1985.

Haschke, F. Body composition during adolescence. Ross Laboratories Conference on Pediatric Research, 98:76–82, 1989.

Haschke, F, Fomon, SJ, & Ziegler, EE. Body composition of a nine year old reference boy. Pediatric Research, 15:847–850, 1981.

Haskell, WL, Montoye, HJ, & Orenstein, D. Physical activity and exercise to achieve health-related fitness components. Public Health Reports, 100:202–212, 1985.

Hayes-Allen, MC, & Tring, FC. Obesity: Another hazard for spina bifida children. British Journal of Preventive and Social Medicine, 27:192–196, 1973.

Hoffman, A, Walter, HJ, Connelly, PA, & Vaughan, RD. Blood pressure and physical fitness in children. Hypertension, 9:188–191, 1987.

Horvat, M. Effects of a progressive resistance training program on an individual with spastic cerebral palsy. American Corrective Therapy Journal, 41:7–10, 1987.

Hosking, GP, Bhat, US, Dubowitz, V, & Edwards, HT. Measurement of muscle strength and performance in children with normal and diseased muscle. Archives of Disease in Childhood, 51:957–963, 1976.

Institute for Aerobics Research. FITNESSGRAM Users Manual. Dallas, TX: Institute for Aerobics Research, 1987.

Jackson, AS, & Coleman, AE. Validation of distance run tests for elementary school children. Research Quarterly, 47:86–94, 1976.

Jackson, AW, & Baker, AA. The relationship of the sit and reach test to criterion measures of hamstring and back flexibility in young females. Research Quarterly for Exercise and Sport, 57:183–186, 1986.

Jankowski, JW. Exercise testing and exercise prescription for individuals with cystic fibrosis. In Skinner, JS (Ed.), Testing and Exercise Prescription for Special Cases. Philadelphia: Lea & Febiger, 1986.

Kemper, HCG, Storm–van Essen, L, & Verschuur, R. Tracking of risk indicators for coronary heart disease from teenager to adult: The Amsterdam growth and health study. In Osteid, S, & Carlsen, K-H (Eds.), Children and Exercise XIII. Champaign, IL: Human Kinetics, 1989, pp. 235–245.

Kendall, HO, & Kendall, FP. Posture and Pain. Baltimore: Williams and Wilkins Company, 1952, p. 104.

Kimm, SYS, Payne, GH, Lakotas, E, Darby, C, & Sparrow, A. Management of cardiovascular disease risk factors in children. American Journal of Diseases of Children, 144:967–972, 1990.

Klish, WJ. The "gold standard." Ross Laboratories Conference on Pediatric Research, 98:4–7, 1989.

Koch, G. Muscle blood flow after ischemic work during bicycle ergometer work in boys aged 12. Acta Pediatrica Belgica Supplement, 28:29–39, 1974.

Komi, PV. Training muscle strength and power: Interaction of neuromotoric, hypertrophic, and mechanical factors. International Journal of Sports Medicine, 7(suppl):10–15, 1986.

Koop, SE, Stout, JL, Drinken, WH, & Starr, RC. Energy cost of walking in children with cerebral palsy (Abstract). Physical Therapy, 69:386, 1989.

Krahenbuhl, GS, Pangrazi, RP, Peterson, GW, Burkett, LN, & Schneider, MJ. Field testing of cardiorespiratory fitness in primary school children. Medicine and Science in Sports, 10:208–213, 1978.

Krahenbuhl, GS, Skinner, JS, & Kohrt, WM. Developmental aspects of maximal aerobic power in children. Exercise and Sport Sciences Reviews, 13:503–538, 1985.

Kuland, DN, & Tottossy, M. Warm-up strength and power. Clinics in Sports Medicine, 4:137–158, 1985.

Landin, S, Hagenfeldt, L, Saltin, B, & Wahren, J. Muscle metabolism during exercise in hemiparetic patients. Clinical Science and Molecular Medicine, 53:257–269, 1977.

Lavay, B, Reid, G, & Cressler-Chaviz, M. Measuring the cardiovascular endurance of persons with mental retardation: A critical review. Exercise and Sport Sciences Reviews, 18:263–290, 1990.

Lefkof, MB. Trunk flexion in healthy children aged 3 to 7 years. Physical Therapy, 66:39–44, 1986.

Levine, SB. Development of a posture scale for children: Preliminary analysis of concurrent validity of the posture scale for children (Abstract). Pediatric Physical Therapy, 3:212, 1991.

Lohman, TG. Measurement of body composition in children. Journal of Physical Education, Recreation and Dance, 53(7):67–70, 1982.

Lohman, TG. Applicability of body composition techniques and constants for children and youth. Exercise and Sport Sciences Reviews, 14:325–357, 1986.

Lohman, TG. The use of skinfold to estimate body fatness on children and youth. Journal of Physical Education, Recreation and Dance, 58(9):98–102, 1987.

Lohman, TG, Slaughter, MH, Boileau, RA, Bunt, J, & Lussier, L. Bone mineral measurements and their relation to body density in children, youth, and adults. Human Biology, 56:667–679, 1984.

Lundberg, A. Changes in the working pulse during the school year in adolescents with cerebral palsy. Scandinavian Journal of Rehabilitation Medicine, 5:12–17, 1973.

Lundberg, A. Maximal aerobic capacity in young people with spastic cerebral palsy. Developmental Medicine and Child Neurology, 20:205–210, 1978.

Lundberg, A, Ovenfors, CO, & Saltin, B. The effect of physical training on school children with cerebral palsy. Acta Paediatrica Scandinavica, 56:182–188, 1967.

Lundberg, A, & Pernow, B. The effect of physical training on oxygen utilization and lactate formation in the exercising muscle of adolescents with motor handicaps. Scandinavian Journal of Clinical and Laboratory Investigation, 26:89–96, 1970.

Macrae, I, & Wright, V. Measurement of back movement. Annals of the Rheumatic Diseases, 52:584–589, 1969.

Malina, RM. Growth of muscle and muscle mass. In Falkner, F, & Tanner, JM (Eds.), Human Growth: A Comprehensive Treatise, Vol. 2: Postnatal Growth. New York: Plenum Press, 1986, pp. 77–99.

Mathews, DK. Measurement in Physical Education (4th ed.). Philadelphia: WB Saunders, 1973, pp. 28–29.

Maughan, RJ, Watson, JS, & Weir, J. Strength and cross-sectional area of human skeletal muscle. Journal of Physiology, 338:37–49, 1983.

McGill, HC. The geographic pathology of atherosclerosis. Laboratory Investigation, 18:463–502, 1968.

Mersch, F, & Stoboy, H. Strength training and muscle hypertrophy in children. In Osteid, S, & Carlsen, K-H (Eds.), Children and Exercise XIII. Champaign, IL: Human Kinetics, 1989, pp. 165–182.

Moll, JMH, & Wright, V. Normal range of spinal mobility: An objective clinical study. Annals of the Rheumatic Diseases, 30:381–386, 1971.

Molnar, GE, & Alexander, J. Objective, quantitative muscle

testing in children: A pilot study. Archives of Physical Medicine and Rehabilitation, 54:224–228, 1973.

Montoye, HJ. Risk factors for cardiovascular disease in relation to physical activity in youth. In Binkhorst, RA, Kemper, HCG, & Saris, WHM (Eds.), Children and Exercise XI. Champaign, IL: Human Kinetics, 1985, pp. 3–25.

Moran, HM, Hall, MA, Barr, A, & Ansell, B. Spinal mobility of the adolescent. Rheumatology Rehabilitation, 18:181–185, 1979.

Moritani, T, & DeVries, HA. Neural factors versus hypertrophy in the time course of muscle strength gain. American Journal of Physical Medicine, 58:115–130, 1979.

Morris, JN, Heady, JA, Raffle, PAB, Roberts, CG, & Parks, JW. Coronary heart disease and physical activity of work. Lancet, 2:1053–1057, 1953.

Norkin, CC, & White, DJ. Measurement of Joint Motion: A Guide to Goniometry. Philadelphia: FA Davis, 1985.

Olney, SJ, Boyce, WF, & Wright, M. Lower extremity work patterns in gait of diplegic CP children (Abstract). Physical Therapy, 68.847, 1988.

Orenstein, DM, Franklin, BA, Doershuk, HK, Hellerstein, KJ, Germann, KJ, Horowitz, JG, & Stern, RC. Exercise conditioning and cardiopulmonary physical fitness in cystic fibrosis. The effects of a three-month supervised running program. Chest, 80:392–398, 1981.

Parizkova, J. Interrelationships between body size, body composition and function. Advances in Experimental Medicine and Biology, 49:119–123, 1974.

Parizkova, J. Body Fat and Physical Fitness: Body Composition and Lipid Metabolism in Different Regimes of Physical Activity. The Hague: Martinus Nijhoff, 1977, pp. 152–156.

Pate, RR. A new definition of youth fitness. Physician and Sports Medicine, 11:77–83, 1983.

Pate, RR, Dowda, MD, & Ross, JG. Associations between physical activity and physical fitness in American children. American Journal of Diseases of Children, 144:1123–1129, 1990.

Pate RR, Ross, JG, Baumgartner, TA, & Sparks, RE. The national children and youth fitness study II: The modified pull-up test. Journal of Physical Education, Recreation and Dance, 58:71–73, 1987.

Pate, RR, & Shephard, RJ. Characteristics of physical fitness in youth. In Gisolfi, CV, & Lamb, DR (Eds.), Perspectives in Exercise Science and Sports Medicine, Vol. 2: Youth, Exercise, and Sport. Indianapolis, IN: Benchmark Press, 1989, pp. 1–45.

Paterson, DH, & Cunningham, DA. Maximal oxygen uptake in children: Comparison of treadmill protocols at various speeds. Canadian Journal of Applied Sport Sciences, 3:188, 1978.

Phelps, E, Smith, LJ, & Hallum, A. Normal ranges of hip motion of infants between 9 and 24 months of age. Developmental Medicine and Child Neurology, 27:785–792, 1985.

President's Council on Physical Fitness and Sports. The Presidential Physical Fitness Program. Washington, DC, President's Council on Physical Fitness and Sports, 1987.

Rarick, GL, & Thompson, JAJ. Roentgenographic measures of leg size and ankle extensor strength of 7 year old children. Research Quarterly, 27:321–332, 1956.

Rose, J, Gamble, JG, Burgos, A, Medeiros, J, & Haskell, WL. Energy expenditure index of walking for normal children and children with cerebral palsy. Developmental Medicine and Child Neurology, 32:333–340, 1990.

Rose, J, Gamble, JG, Medeiros, J, Burgos, A, & Haskell, WL. Energy cost of walking in normal children and in those with cerebral palsy: Comparison of heart rate and oxygen uptake. Paediatric Orthopaedics, 9.276–279, 1989.

Ross, JG, Delpy, LA, Christenson, GM, Gold, RS, & Damberg, CL. The national youth and fitness study II: Study procedures

and quality control. Journal of Physical Education, Recreation and Dance, 58:57–62, 1987.

Ross, JG, Dotson, CO, Gilbert, GG, & Katz, SJ. The national youth and fitness study I: New standards for fitness measurement. Journal of Physical Education, Recreation and Dance, 56:62–66, 1985.

Ross, JG, & Gilbert, GG. The national children and youth fitness study: A summary of findings. Journal of Physical Education, Recreation and Dance, 56:45–50, 1985.

Ross, JG, Katz, SJ, & Gilbert, GG: The national youth and fitness study I: Quality control. Journal of Physical Education, Recreation and Dance, 56:57–61, 1985.

Ross, JG, & Pate, RR. The national children and youth fitness study II: A summary of findings. Journal of Physical Education, Recreation and Dance, 58:51–56, 1987.

Ross, JG, Pate, RR, Delpy, LA, Gold, RS, & Svilar, M. The national children and youth fitness study II: New health related fitness norms. Journal of Physical Education, Recreation and Dance, 58:66–70, 1987.

Rutenfrunz, J, Macek, M, Lange-Anderson, A, Bell, RD, Vavra, J, Radvansky, J, Klimmer, F, & Kylian, H. The relationship between changing body height and growth related changes in maximal aerobic power. European Journal of Applied Physiology, 60:282–287, 1990.

Safrit, MJ. Criterion-referenced measurement: Validity. In Safrit, MJ, & Wood, TM (Eds.), Measurement Concepts in Physical Education and Exercise Science. Champaign, IL: Human Kinetics, 1989, pp. 119–135.

Safrit, MJ. The validity and reliability of fitness tests for children: A review. Pediatric Exercise Science, 2:9–28, 1990.

Safrit, MJ, & Wood, TM: The test battery reliability of the health-related physical fitness test. Research Quarterly for Exercise and Sport, 58:160–167, 1987.

Sale, DG. Strength training in children. In Gisolfi, CV, & Lamb, DR (Eds.), Perspectives in Exercise Science and Sports medicine, Vol. 2: Youth, Exercise, and Sport. Indianapolis IN: Benchmark Press, 1989, pp. 165–222.

Saltin, B, & Strange, S. Maximal oxygen uptake: Old and new arguments for a cardiovascular limitation. Medicine and Science in Sports and Exercise, 24:30–37, 1992.

Shvartz, E, & Reibold, RC. Aerobic fitness norms for males and females aged 6 to 75 years: A review. Aviation Space and Environmental Medicine, 61:3–11, 1990.

Simons-Morton, BG, O'Hara, NM, Simons-Morton, DG, & Parcel, GS. Children and fitness: A public health perspective. Research Quarterly for Exercise and Sport, 58:295–302, 1987.

Slaughter, MH, Lohman, TG, Boileau, RA, Stillman, RJ, VanLoan, M, Horswill, CA, & Wilmore, JH. Influence of maturation on relationship of skinfolds to body density: A cross-sectional study. Human Biology, 56:681–689, 1984.

Smoak, CG, Burke, GL, Webber, LS, Harsha, DW, Srinivasan, SR, & Berenson, GS. Relation of obesity to clustering of cardiovascular risk factors in children and young adults. The Bogalusa heart study. American Journal of Epidemiology, 125:364–372, 1987.

Sodoma, CJ. Amateur Athlete Union physical fitness program validity for selected age group test results. Bloomington: Indiana University, 1986. Thesis.

Spady, DW. Normal body composition of infants and children. Ross Laboratories Conference on Pediatric Research, 98:67–73, 1989.

Spady, DW, Payne, PR, Picou, D, & Waterlow, JC. A description of the changing composition of the growing premature infant. Journal of Pediatric Gastroenterology and Nutrition, 6:730–739, 1987.

Sproul, A, & Simpson, E. Stroke volume and related hemodynamic data in normal children. Pediatrics, 33:912–916, 1964.

Sprynarova, S, & Reisenauer, R. Body dimensions and physiological indicators of physical fitness during adolescence. In Shephard, RJ, Lavallee, H (Eds.), Physical Fitness Assessment. Springfield, IL: Charles C Thomas, 1978, pp. 32–37.

Strong, WB. Physical activity and children. Circulation, *81*:1697–1701, 1990.

Sutton, JR. Vo₂max–New concepts on an old theme. Medicine and Science in Sports and Exercise, *24*:26–29, 1992.

Tirosh, E, Bar-Or, O, & Rosenbaum, P. New muscle power test in neuromuscular disease. American Journal of Diseases of Children, *144*:1083–1087, 1990.

Treiber, FA, Strong, WB, Arensman, FW, & Gruber, M. Relationships between habitual physical activity and cardiovascular responses to exercise in young children. In Osteid, S, & Carlsen, K-H (Eds.), Children and Exercise XIII. Champaign, IL: Human Kinetics, 1989, pp. 285–294.

United States Department of Health and Human Services. Healthy Children 2000: National Health Promotion and Disease Prevention Objectives Related to Mothers, Infants, Children, Adolescents, and Youth. Washington, DC: Public Health Service, 1990.

Vignos, PJ, & Watkins, MP. The effect of exercise in muscular dystrophy. Journal of the American Medical Association, *197*:843–848, 1966.

VonDobelin, W, & Eriksson, BO. Physical training maximal oxygen uptake and dimensions of the oxygen transporting and metabolizing organs in boys 11–13 years of age. Acta Paediatrica Scandinavica, *61*:653–657, 1972.

Wahlund, H. Determination of the physical working capacity. Acta Medica Scandinavica Supplement, *215*:5–108, 1948.

Waugh, KG, Minkel, JL, Parker, R, & Coon, VA. Measurement of hip, knee, and ankle joints in newborns. Physical Therapy, *63*:1616–1621, 1983.

Weltman, A, Janny, C, Rians, CB, Strand, K, Berg, B, Tippitt, S, Wise, J, Cahill, BR, & Katch, FI. The effects of hydraulic resistance strength training in pre-pubertal males. Medicine and Science in Sports and Exercise., *18*:629–638, 1986.

Wyndham, C. Submaximal test for estimating maximal oxygen intake. Canadian Medical Association Journal, *96*:736–742, 1976.

Yamashita, T, Seiichi, I, & Isao, O. Effect of muscle stretching on the activity of neuromuscular transmission. Medicine and Science in Sports and Exercise, *24*:80–84, 1992.

Zach, MS, Oberwalder, J, & Hausler, F. Cystic fibrosis: Physical exercise vs chest physiotherapy. Archives of Disease in Childhood, *57*:587–589, 1982.

Ziegler, EE, O'Donnell, AM, Nelson, SE, & Fomon, SJ. Body composition of the reference fetus. Growth, *40*:329–334, 1976.

Chapter 6

Motor Learning: Theories and Strategies for the Practitioner

HÉLÈNE M. LARIN, PT, PhD

Learning or relearning motor tasks is a significant element of the rehabilitation process for a child with a neurologic or orthopaedic impairment. Physical therapists continue to search for a better understanding and application to rehabilitation of the phenomenon of *motor learning*. The recent development of models for analyzing tasks and structuring instruction to promote motor learning may provide a helpful perspective for the pediatric physical therapist. Such models offer a means to systematically organize knowledge of movement, skill acquisition, and development.

In the past 100 years, researchers from various fields have investigated aspects of motor learning. They conducted studies primarily with persons without disabilities, with adults more than with children, and in laboratories more than in naturalistic environments; and they addressed isolated performance or learning behaviors. Despite working in these somewhat restricted milieux, researchers developed theories and models representing the body of knowledge of their time and also proposed a series of related instructional strategies. Physical therapists must integrate the latest findings from research on motor learning into their working knowledge.

A psychologically based approach to motor learning has increasingly been adopted and applied in physical education, adapted physical education, and rehabilitation. Such an approach may be reflected in the explicit as well as implicit knowledge of practitioners. In a recent study, for example, Larin (1992) investigated how physical therapists, in practice and procedures, explicitly or implicitly based their interventions and rationales on concepts of motor learning. Review of videotapes of these pediatric physical therapists during individual treatment sessions of preschool children with cerebral palsy (moderate spastic diplegia) revealed that they implemented most of the recognized strategies for motor learning and teaching. Throughout the sessions, therapists kept the children active, emphasized mobility over stability activities, and took periodic breaks. To a high degree, they maintained a stimulating environment related to the task at hand. The frequency of use for each instructional strategy, assessed with the Motor Teaching Strategy Coding Measure (MTSCM-1), however, varied among therapists; the level of experience with neurologically impaired individuals was a factor in some cases. In a content analysis of recordings during two subsequent interviews, therapists demonstrated varying degrees of awareness or, sometimes, implicit knowledge of particular motor learning strategies. For example, the use of active mode, stimulating environmental conditions, waiting periods, assisted types of movements, and positive feedback received greater acknowledgment than the use of movement goals, specific task descriptions, or quantitative types of feedback to the child.

The relationship between clinicians' practice and implicit professional knowledge presented a mixed pattern that appeared to vary according to the characteristics of the (self-selected) tasks performed and the therapists' cognition of the motor learning strategies (Larin, 1992). Overall, they were aware of scientific knowledge of diverse origins, including some in motor learning, but particularly ecologic, motivational, and developmental theories. Thus a greater awareness and understanding of the contemporary body of knowledge on motor learning may help practitioners to maximize therapeutic opportunities. It may help therapists to 1) engage in self-analysis of their practice and identification of new or less exploited strategies; 2) adapt the information to their individual needs; 3) plan and perform assessment and treatment sessions from a new perspective; and 4) engage in research documenting the applicability of principles of motor learning to intervention with children with disabilities.

To these ends, literature on concepts and strategies of motor learning and teaching is reviewed in the three main sections of this chapter; throughout, research findings on the learning process of children are highlighted. In the first section, a brief historical summary of the development of motor control and motor learning theories is presented. In the second, motor learning models from three authors who attempted to bridge the gap between theory and practice are briefly introduced. These models form the basis for a third section in which a series of instructional strategies are reviewed along with presentation of examples from pediatric clinical practice.

MOTOR CONTROL AND MOTOR LEARNING THEORIES: A HISTORICAL PERSPECTIVE

How does a person learn to control a new movement? How does one account for the complexity and variety of motor behavior in the process? These are some of the major questions theorists in motor control and motor learning have attempted to answer. The evolution of these concepts has gradually come to influence the body of knowledge, as well as the practice, of physical therapy.

Theoretical Groundwork

According to early views on the subject, motor learning was a process of "habit" formation (James, 1890); recently more sophisticated approaches have dealt with motor control and motor learning in terms of information processing theories and ecologic theories. The development of information processing theories can be related to the study of both slow and fast movements. The closed-loop theories of movement control (Adams, 1971; Mott & Sherrington, 1895; Thorndike, 1927) emphasized the need for sensory input, sensory feedback, and rewards during repetition of movements that are slow and self-paced, the goal being to augment the intrinsic feedback and develop a perceptual memory trace of movements. These instructional strategies were considered necessary as event reinforcers.

In contrast, theorists who studied quickly executed movements discovered the existence of a structured, linear, hierarchical organization within the central nervous system (CNS) (Sheridan, 1984) and minimized the importance of the role of feedback. "Open-loop" or "motor program" theories attributed skill acquisition to a central, executive motor program responsible for producing and executing selected, sequential subroutines in a top-down fashion for short, fixed, repeatable, automatic sequences of movements (e.g., Marteniuk, 1976). Consequently, step-by-step instructional strategies were promoted following systematic, developmental stages, with elicited movements prevailing over spontaneous movements and a preference for reflex activity over self-initiated activity. In yet a third point of view, McCulloch (1945), among others, proposed a "heterarchical" view of information processing: different levels of control interact, cooperate, and transfer control according to the need at hand rather than being subservient to an executive (Sheridan, 1984).

Schema Theories and Later Developments

Another concept, "schema," was to become significant in our understanding of information processing. In 1899, Woodworth and followers had enunciated the concept of schema as a set of rules serving as instructions for producing unique sequences of motor commands applicable to a variety of similar actions, referred to as a movement class. In 1975, Schmidt revived and expanded this concept in a schema theory. Schmidt emphasized the role of memory in motor learning and proposed the notion of two states of memory: recall and recognition schemas "stored" or programmed in the CNS as sets of rules. In the case of rapid, ballistic movements, motor experiences and memories would activate the recall schema (rule for movement production) and recognition schema (rule for establishing the relation between knowledge of the initial conditions, the environmental outcomes, and the expected sensory consequences for the purpose of response evaluation), resulting in the formation of motor learning structures.

From the original schema theory of Schmidt, certain predictions relating to motor learning have emerged: 1) practice variability promotes the building of a schema, especially for children; 2) after varied practice, novel responses in open-skills situations can be produced about as accurately as they can be after repeated practice (more so in children); and 3) the capability for error detection should exist mostly after fast movement and not after slow movement; in the latter case the recognition schema is said to be used to govern the ongoing production of the movement, leaving no more error detection capability after a slow movement (Schmidt, 1988).

To account for the great adaptability of the CNS, theorists attempted to marry the previous positions to develop what may be referred to as sensorimotor theories (e.g., Abbs et al., 1984; Marteniuk et al., 1988; Schmidt, 1991). They maintained the concepts of *heterarchy*, *schema*, a form of *motor program* and added an *ecologic element* (from evolving behavioral theories mentioned later). Concepts such as *feedforward* and *feedback* processes within the CNS were also included.

Feedforward processes involve preparation of the system for anticipated consequences of movements that, in part, provide a postural set. Feedback regarding what is happening (or has happened) makes possible changes or mid-course correction of movement to bring about convergence to a goal. If the movement occurs too quickly for feedback to be used effectively for correction during the course of a movement, feedback information can be used as instructional information in the planning of a more refined set of commands the next time.

A sensorimotor integration, referred to as "multimovement coordination" is also argued (Abbs et al., 1984; Marteniuk et al., 1988). It is proposed that sensory events are coded in efferent terms, specific to each learned task, and have the function of modifying the central storage of information.

Among other issues, contemporary theorists have attempted to resolve the problem of storage of large amounts of information in the CNS and the problem of coping with the immense and complex variability of parameters in movement production, referred to as degrees of freedom. To solve this problem, Asatryan and Feldman (1965) advanced the mass-spring model, which hypothesizes that equilibrium points between the torques of agonist and antagonist muscles are programmed for efficiency. In 1967, Bernstein revived the original Ferrier concept of *synergy*, a phenomenon in which groups of muscles and joints are coupled with a common pool of afferent and efferent information to produce coordinated patterns of movement. See Chapter 2 for further discussion of these concepts.

The development of instructional strategies paralleled the expansion of these integrative theories of motor control and motor learning. Emphasis on the role of memory outlined the significance of the cognitive element in motor learning. The constructs of schema and motor program reinforced the need for repetition to enhance motor learning. Finally, the concepts of coordinating multiple degrees of freedom and synergy brought a greater focus on action specificity in practice.

Ecologic Approaches

Parallel to these developments and in reaction to the "habit" theory and information processing motor theories, Gibson (1966) and others (e.g., Michaels & Carello, 1981; Turvey & Carello, 1986) proposed action systems or environment-related theories of motor control. For example, the direct perception theory (Gibson, 1966; Michaels & Carello, 1981), a pure ecologic approach, considers the learning environment as specific to the child who actively and continuously explores and "picks up" the information "afforded" by the environment. Information is not presumed to be "processed" through memory or cognitive representation. Instead, according to the measure of attraction to the child, the biologic systems are said to "resonate" the information the environment "broadcasts." According to this theory, perception and action form a closed unity; functional and relevant contexts for movement are, therefore, essential to promote motor learning.

Another aspect of this approach proposes that muscle groups and joints act as units, termed *muscular collectives* or *coordinative structures*; consequently, movements are said to be closely connected to the dynamic, mechanical properties of coordinative structures (e.g., length–tension and force–velocity relations), as opposed to a central representation. The formulation of these concepts has pointed toward more specific intervention strategies, such as 1) choosing or adapting individual, attractive sensorimotor environments, 2) respecting the child's interest in the selection of functional activities, and 3) promoting opportunities for muscle strengthening in particular needed ranges of movement, varied speeds, or coordinated movement patterns.

Recent Synthetic Theories

In the past decade, further "action systems" have been proposed (Reed, 1982), but the latest theory developed, elaborated, and promoted is the dynamic pattern theory of Kelso and colleagues (Scholz, 1990; Thelen et al., 1987), also referred to as the dynamical systems approach (Kamm et al., 1990). According to this theory, motor behavior is said to emerge from the dynamic cooperation of all subsystems within the context of a specific task: CNS, biomechanical, psychological, and social-environmental components. Each component is perceived as necessary but insufficient to explain movement changes. Patterns of movement are portrayed not as rigidly fixed or programmed in the CNS but as flexible, adaptable, and dynamic, yet having "preferred" paths. Functional movement synergies are self-assembled according to the interaction between the environment and the individual's intention. Dynamical theory emphasizes function more than instruction as the driving force for motor behavior (motor learning) and stresses the study of movement pattern transitions ("phasing" phenomena) rather than regular, repetitive occurrences.

The identification of critical variables leading to motor changes or motor learning becomes the focus of dynamical theory. The provision of specific instructional strategies (verbal and nonverbal) to the learner is dependent on a detailed assessment, which includes 1) observable collective variables called "order parameters," such as temporal and spatial phasing between limbs and interjoint relationships; and 2) the dynamics of variables called "control parameters," such as speed, loudness of voice, or surface (Heriza, 1991; Scholz, 1990). Further work on these and other variables will continue to expand our knowledge of motor learning and guide, to some extent, our therapeutic interventions by providing instructional models.

FROM MOTOR LEARNING TO MOTOR TEACHING MODELS

Learning or relearning motor skills and improving the performance of motor skills are two main effects of practice of particular interest to physical therapists. Learning occurs through an interaction of external and internal factors that influence the ability to process information (Toglia, 1991), and motor learning is a set of processes associated with practice that lead to relatively permanent changes in performance capability (Schmidt, 1991). That is, temporarily improved *performance* observed immediately following practice does not automatically equate to motor *learning* or necessarily imply that learning has occurred. Motor learning may be measured by the degree of long-term retention of performance capability, although the amount of transfer to different settings (near transfer) or to some different activity (far transfer) is the more accepted measure of motor learning as well as of effective training. In therapeutic intervention, therefore, a conscious choice must be made between promoting motor learning and promoting performance; this choice determines the selection of instructional strategies. Systems for guidance in the selection and organization of relevant strategies in a comprehensive, coherent, and practical way have resulted from the development of models of motor teaching.

Models of motor teaching based on models of motor learning are few and relatively recent. They aim at improving the impact of motor teaching on persons with and without disabilities. The models have followed earlier work in the cognitive, educational domain. Orme's General Model of Teacher Behavior in Instruction (1978), including his series of practical teaching strategies, is one such source. Within this teaching model, the "teaching act" is described in six phases that are held to be necessary to elicit learning: 1) motivation, 2) presentation, 3) response guidance, 4) practice, 5) feedback, and 6) transfer. To be effective, these phases must be combined with arresting stimuli, including surprise, novelty, conflict, complexity, intensity, uncertainty, duration, and repetition. A close relationship exists between these cognitive concepts and those of the psychomotor-teaching models proposed by Gentile (1972, 1987), Marteniuk (1976, 1979), and Schmidt (1991).

The Gentile (1987) model for acquisition of motor skills is based on the proposition that skill learning takes place in two stages: initial and late. In the initial stage of learning of motor skills, the learner discovers a reasonably effective approach to desired movement patterns. In the later stage, the learner concentrates on achieving *skilled* performance (i.e., goal attainment and economy of effort). The latter processes are said to be task dependent, changing according to the environmental context and the function of the action. It follows that instructional interventions should be based on the structure of the task and on the environmental context in which it is to be performed while assisting the learner to move from the initial stage of motor learning to the stage of skill acquisition.

The information processes involved in Gentile's initial stage are also reflected in the Marteniuk model of motor teaching based on his description of information processes of motor skill acquisition in the Human Perceptual-Motor Performance Model (Marteniuk, 1976) (summarized in Fig. 6–1). Marteniuk recognizes attention (alertness) and anticipation (expectation) as being of utmost importance for CNS preparation to receive and process perceptual information. Preparation includes potential factors affecting arousal for the therapeutic instruction such as stimulus intensity, variety, complexity, uncertainty, and meaningfulness; induced muscle tension; and physical exertion. Thus perception, decision, and action form the three basic components of the model.

The perceptual mechanisms include information detection, comparison and recognition of kinesthetic information, selective attention (through meaningfulness) and short-term memory (assisted by knowledge of performance [KP]), knowledge of result (KR), noninterference, motor sequencing, coding and "chunking," and rehearsal, all concepts that are discussed later in this chapter. The second component, the decision mechanism, is influenced by certain information characteristics and measured by the reaction time (RT), which is the interval of time between the presentation of an unanticipated stimulus and the initiation of a motor response. RT decreases with increased anticipation and with decreased temporal and spatial (event) uncertainty, amount of information, number of possible alternative movements, movement precision demand (e.g., target size), and directional accuracy demand (Schmidt, 1991; Sideway, 1991). Other influential factors in decreasing RT are increased level of cognitive processes in mediating environmental stimuli and action (Weeks & Proctor, 1990), increased consistent practice, increased compatibility of information, and successively presented signals. Finally, the effector mechanism is said to contain a large number of motor commands; it organizes these commands to produce movement by activating muscles in correct sequential and temporal order.

Finally, the Schmidt Conceptual Model of Human Performance (Fig. 6–2) forms the basis for Schmidt's comprehensive instructional guidebook, which summarizes the current body of knowledge relating to motor learning (for able-bodied individuals) (Schmidt, 1991). Three main areas are proposed for consideration in composing instructional strategies: 1) preparation and design of practice, 2) organization and scheduling of practice, and 3) feedback for skill learning. It is suggested that relevant instructional strategies be adapted to the learner's stage of learning, in this case, as defined by Fitts and Posner (1967): verbal-cognitive, motor, and autonomous stages. A concise survey follows of the suggested, theoretically based, strategies that have been studied with different populations by various investigators. The applicability of these strategies to the pediatric population has been tested in some cases, but in other cases is assumed and remains to be verified. Overall, there is a high degree of consensus about the appropriate use of strategies of motor teaching among the promoters of these strategies; minor conflicts exist in certain instances.

MOTOR LEARNING AND TEACHING STRATEGIES IN PEDIATRICS

During a therapeutic session, each activity trial of the child becomes a unit of potential motor learning for which the therapist must decide on appropriate strategies. The selection of instructional

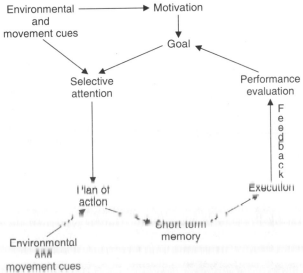

FIGURE 6–1. Motor-teaching model: information processes in motor learning.

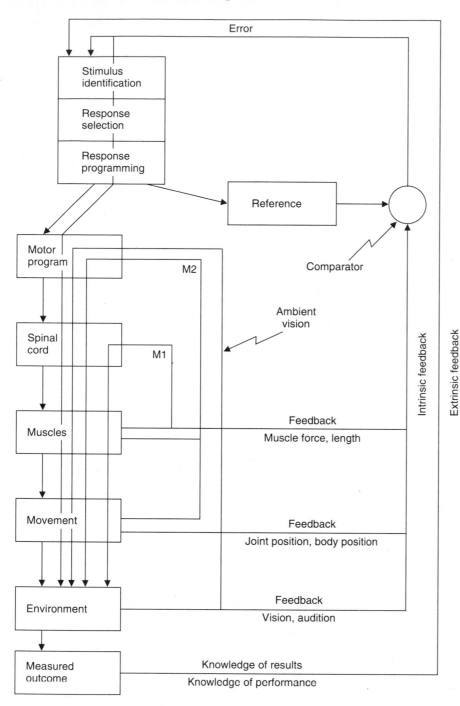

FIGURE 6-2. Conceptual model of human performance: a basis for the organization of practice. (Redrawn from Schmidt, RA. Motor Learning and Performance. Champaign, IL: Human Kinetics Publishers, 1991, p. 265. Copyright 1991 by Richard A. Schmidt. Reprinted by permission.)

strategies should reflect the *stage of learning* of the child (earlier or verbal-cognitive, later or motor, autonomous) for the motor task practiced. In addition, the potentially dichotomous goals of practice should be clear to the therapist: to optimize the child's *motor learning* (long-term retention and transfer to other tasks or settings) *or* the child's *motor performance* (greater ability within a task) during the treatment session. The specific goal of practice must be clear because instructional strategies effective in promoting retention of particular tasks, near transfer to a similar task, or far transfer to different activities will not necessarily lead to better performance during practice (Schmidt,

1991). In addition, the therapist needs to consider three potential sensitive periods for instructional intervention: before, during, and after the execution of *each* activity trial, whether the activity is static or dynamic.

Context

Before and during a treatment session, the overall *context* must be set and remain adequate and conducive to the child's learning. To a high degree, therapists have been found to maintain a stimulating environment and to motivate the child through verbal and visual stimuli during a treatment session (Carter, 1989; Larin, 1992).

First, the physical aspects of the environment must be considered. "Children learn more rapidly in stimulating and varied physical environments which meet basic human needs"; these include health/safety function, psychological comfort, and aesthetic satisfaction, according to the "habitability" framework (Taylor & Gousie, 1988, p. 23). Because the physical aspects of the environment may be potential stressors on the child, more or less noise, light, color, and space cannot be ignored and may exert a direct effect on the child's level of motivation during a treatment session. Understanding of the child's attentional abilities and level of sensory processing and organization, as well as the influence of the environmental changes on movement production, is also crucial in enabling the therapist to modify and adapt the environment appropriately and individually for each child (Cook Merrill et al., 1990).

Both children and adults have been found to respond positively to a multicontext treatment approach. In this approach, the individual is required to apply the newly learned skill to multiple situations (Toglia, 1991). Consequently, one goal is to bring the child to a "context-independent state," decreasing the likelihood of association between a particular piece of information and a particular context. In some clinical settings, an appropriate response has been the renovation of the traditional, contained treatment room with its standard equipment into various playground or household simulation contexts. Therapy may not begin and end at the threshold of a treatment room or even a treatment mat. The interaction milieu of home, school, and community remains the child's most functional context where varied practice and learning for transfer are most liable to occur. Direct therapeutic intervention and program management ought to reflect this reality. For example, sitting in the waiting room, sitting for fine motor tasks or

self-help, and sitting to pedal a tricycle become linked and provide real contexts for varied practice leading to motor learning of postural body control under a variety of conditions. Similarly, the same principle may be applied to climbing a bed, a chair, a step, or someone's lap. Another outcome in using the "multicontext treatment approach" is to enhance movement that is of interest to the child. Engaging in social interaction with puppets, other children, or adults may modify a child's level of participation in an activity (positively or negatively, depending on interest level).

Second, the socioculturoeducational aspect of the context that pertains to the quality of the instructor–learner interaction also affects the child's learning with respect to the amount and type of information transmitted (Simpson & Galbo, 1986). Effective *learning contexts* are those that promote initiations by the learner, reciprocity and shared control over the interaction between the less skilled (child) and the more skilled (therapist) party, and provision of responsive or content feedback rather than simply corrective feedback to the learner. In such contexts, children, whether mildly or moderately disabled, may gain more control over their own learning and reduce their level of dependence on adult control (Glynn, 1985).

The therapist seeks an integration and a balance between the dichotomous roles of playmate and instructor in his or her therapeutic intervention with the child. The playmate's role needs to feel genuine and pleasing to the child, and the instructor's role denotes supportive, confident, and effective guidance toward improved capabilities with a shared control of decision-making. Therapeutic power is real and must be used with prudence. For example, the therapist may offer predetermined choices of activities to the child or take turns with the child in the decision-making in an obvious, concrete, fair manner; above all the therapist should address the child within the "higher order thinking skills" of the child (Ritson, 1987) and incorporate risk-taking behaviors (Cintas, 1992). In a treatment session, this may translate into the therapist's setting a challenging game, verbalizing the action or movement goal, and providing some timely, explicit feedback to the child, in spite of the child's minimal or delayed verbal and nonverbal communication skills and while being acutely attentive to the child's level of active participation.

Motivation

In the pretask execution period, the child should gain *motivation* and clear, purposeful *prior knowl-*

edge of the activity through auditory, visual, or proprioceptive signals (Higgins, 1991). The instructional strategies that relate to motivation include, for instance, action goal setting, preferably by or in conjunction with the child; selective attention (e.g., instructions, demonstration-modeling, and interference); and rehearsal (e.g., mental practice).

Motivated learning is intentional learning for improvement. The learner needs to have 1) the perception of a skill as meaningful, useful, desirable, and having personal implications; 2) the experience of satisfaction from executing a movement; and 3) encouragement toward higher, achievable goals after task execution. The therapist may indirectly but positively influence the child's personal goals, self-perceptions, and cognitive-affective experiences through verbal and nonverbal communication. For example, counting out loud (with a meaningful tone of voice) the seconds spent in stride-standing, moving back and forth to place a basketball in the basket, marking points, and raising the basket or stepping back a step are ways to further challenge the child. Such strategies, however, may not be successful in motivating all children in spite of similar cognitive levels. Motivated learning is an individual process. To optimize this process, further insight is necessary into the learner's individual motivational variables relevant to physical skills, movement behavior in different contexts, and personal strategies, thoughts, and emotional responses during the learning process (Pohl et al., 1992).

CREATIVE BEHAVIOR

Besides altering context, encouraging creative behaviors is a powerful means of enhancing the child's motivation. These primarily include fluency (e.g., movement variability); flexibility (e.g., movement independence); originality (e.g., in movement sequences); and elaboration. To gain fluency, the child needs to solve the same movement problem or goal through a number of different organizational approaches (i.e., motor equivalence). For example, the practice of going up the stairs for a child who has not yet mastered this skill may involve supervised creeping on hands and knees, hands and feet, sideways cruising up while holding onto the rail, and forward walking up with assistance (a device or manually). Promoting flexibility in therapy could entail allowing and acknowledging a child's independent thinking and creative movement response. Providing some basic movement information to the child such as "Let's find a way to twist your shoulders" may support this behavior as well as allow originality in the child's movement se-

quences and may result in the production of a completely novel response. Asking appropriate questions that require the child to think at his or her cognitive level and to perform the results of that thought process may lead to the fourth factor of movement creativity—elaboration. Such motor instructional strategies that go beyond the command style and promote process-oriented rather than product-oriented approaches constitute in themselves sources of motivation and enhance the desired, perceived internal control of the child (Ritson, 1987).

GOAL-SETTING

Setting goals is still another major, motivational, instructional strategy available for use during a therapy session. First the therapist must consider the child's social influences, such as gender, age, cultural background, and personal socialization experiences. For example, knowing that children up to the age of approximately 11 tend to hold "mastery goals" may guide the therapist in providing self-referenced achievement tasks rather than social comparison. In addition, the therapist's assessment of the child's cognitive ability to understand the task or goal will have a direct impact on potential learning of motor skills. Realizing that immediate social environmental conditions can override some preexisting goals of the child, the therapist may choose to provide a goal. Two types of goals may be provided: The goal may be related to the action (e.g., "Let's go slide") or to the movement itself, in this case, climbing the steps leading to the slide (e.g., "Let's see you bring one foot up very high and quickly"). As observed in Larin's (1992) study, therapists offered a verbal goal in 44 to 88% (average, 75%) of the activity trials during treatment sessions; the action goal accounted for 43% and the movement goal made up 47% of the verbal goals.

It is recommended that either type of goal be specific, consistent, attainable, and short in duration and that the standards be high enough to foster improved performance but not so high as to provoke discouragement by repeated failure (Edwards, 1988). Error awareness is a necessary element of the learning process. However, to ensure a successful learning experience, the therapist should guide the learner to make a decision on (evaluate) the environmental goal or related movement in a systematic, comparative fashion. Gentile (1972) suggests such an approach:

- If a goal and movement are successful, use repetition.
- If a goal is unsuccessful in spite of apparent

good movement, help the learner in identifying relevant environmental conditions.

- If a goal is successful but the movement produced a surprise success, describe the movement to the learner.
- If both the goal and the movement are unsuccessful, encourage the learner and analyze further the task at hand.

Overall, the therapist should continue to explore movement options with the learner until repeated success in both movement and goal attainment are achieved.

Another useful tactic of the therapist is to ask the learner to set the goal. Movements "preselected" by the child result in greater goal clarity, increased energy production, and success, as well as superior reproduction of movements as compared with "constrained" movements selected by the instructor (Lewthwaite, 1990; Runnings & Diewert, 1982; Sage, 1984; Schempp, 1983; Schmidt, 1988). Preselection by the child has been found to be especially effective for children with low ability (Goldberger & Gerney, 1990). Once again, the experience of personal "locus of control" during an instructional session is of great importance for motor learning (Coster & Jaffe, 1991).

Instructions

The therapist's instructions before practice are critical for motivational purposes but also as feedforward input to convey information about the task requirements. This information should include a description of the task based on the learner's competencies as well as on relevant environmental elements. It may be verbally presented and/or modeled (Schmidt, 1991). The therapist's verbal instructions have the potential to bring the child's attention to different levels of information about a movement task. This information is closely associated with feedback information and with the environment. Examples include the following (Newell et al., 1990):

1. Intrinsic, sensorimotor information may address precise muscle-response organization, such as "Feel the muscles of your toes and legs pushing hard as you reach up."

2. Movement patterns or performance direction such as segmental body organization may be provided (e.g., "Bring your arm up, elbow straight, and open your hands to reach up")

3. The end result in the form of the action goal (e.g., "Let's decorate the top of the mirror") may activate the desired pattern of movement of reaching up.

4. Environmental information related to the action may guide the child's visual and auditory attentiveness (e.g., "The mirror is taller than you and is on wheels; the decorations are sticky and a bit heavy").

Appropriate instruction can enhance the child's selective attention and foster his or her ability to separate task-relevant information from task-irrelevant information, an integral part of the motor learning process. With regard to the developmental, restrictive scanning strategies of younger children (Vurpillot, 1968), Stratton (1978) believes that lack of training and experience rather than processing capacity is the cause of children's deficits in information processing and attention capability. Children deserve to be given a chance to acquire strategies for improved selective attention. Along with instruction, distractions may be provided: interferences, such as people talking or walking or the therapist referring to other activities, may be presented to the child; these simulate a real world environment. Introducing this strategy early in the learning situation appears to produce the best results in improved ability to deal with irrelevant information (Stratton, 1978). Neurologically impaired children, however, may display sensorivisual loss and cognitive deficits in the selective attentional system (Hood & Atkinson, 1990). Such a tactic, of course, must be used carefully with these children, for whom the addition of extraneous information may be overwhelming and counterproductive.

Verbal instructions about the motor activity (prior knowledge) should be offered, first, about the entire movement, describing the same speed and accuracy required in the desired skill (Gentile, 1987). According to the child's level of selective attention and capability of processing information, the therapist has the option to break down the verbal instructions, with an initial emphasis on only one or two essential elements of the skill; brevity and meaningfulness are important in this case. Minimal guidance from research is available because only limited data have been gathered on individual needs and the complexity and distribution of instructions appropriate for different age groups. A combination of distance and location information, however, has been found to allow greater accuracy of movement reproduction, whether the movement practiced in active or passive (Runnings & Diewert, 1982). Allowing further trial-and-error (no prompting) attempts before providing feedback or further instructions has also been reported to be superior to use of a guiding stimulus (prompting) exclusively. Children with learning disorders (cognitive and motor) may benefit from the same opportunity.

However, children with cerebral palsy have been reported to respond with greater movement excursions (forearm pronation or supination) to concrete instructions (e.g., "Bang the drums."), rather than abstract instructions (e.g., "Turn the handle back and forth as far as possible.") when compared with nondisabled children, who showed no difference between tasks (van der Weel et al., 1991). Verbal prompting is a useful strategy but should not be provided in proportion to the learning difficulty (Koegel & Rincover, 1976). Nonverbal prompting should also be considered.

Demonstration or Modeling

Demonstration or modeling may complement or replace verbal instructions. Children tend to be more visually dependent than adults, who rely more on a combination of proprioceptive and visual input (Shumway-Cook & Woollacott, 1985). Observational motor learning is thus an effective strategy for developing the perceptual skills necessary for children to selectively attend to environmental cues (Arend, 1980). Modeling is task-specific and may be enhanced by verbal labeling, rehearsal, temporal spacing of demonstrations, and verbal pretraining (i.e., the child verbally cueing himself or herself about movement demands) (Gould & Roberts, 1982). With low-skilled subjects, however, peer modeling (i.e., watching an unskilled person learning a motor skill) has been found to be more effective than instructor modeling (Landers & Landers, 1973; Lee et al. 1991). Therapists were observed to use demonstrations minimally in the treatment of preschool children with a diagnosis of cerebral palsy, although they claimed greater use with children 6 years of age and older (Larin, 1992). Coordinating therapy sessions among therapists with similar clients to encourage reciprocal peer modeling should be recognized as a potentially valuable tool of motor teaching.

Purposeful Tasks

"Given appropriate tasks and sufficiently guided practice, gross motor skill learning in young children can be effectively enhanced through planned instruction" (Haubenstricker & Seefeldt, 1986, p. 65). Purposeful tasks are more appropriate than reflexive or passive behaviors (Bernstein, 1967). Purposeful tasks are active, voluntarily regulated (from initiation to termination), goal directed (Croce & DePaepe, 1989), and meaningful to the learner (van der Weel et al., 1991). Heart rates and perceived exertion ratings are significantly lower during purposeful tasks than during nonpurposeful activities (Bakshi et al., 1991). In addition, the individual's freely chosen work rate (preferred rhythm) has been found to be the most efficient for performance across a variety of tasks (Fetters, 1991; Sparrow, 1983), particularly for 5-year-old children (Williams, 1985). Purposeful tasks of individuals with neuromotor disorders, however, do not necessarily lead to the same level of movement efficiency achieved by nondisabled individuals. Gait studies in children with cerebral palsy, for example, have revealed reduced muscle activity, uneven kinetic energy patterns, and mechanical energy cost above normal values (Olney, 1989).

The "will to act" on the part of the learner builds up over a long time before a movement begins (120 msec); in fact it is longer than reaction time to a stimulus (30 to 80 msec) (Kelso, 1991). Hence, the pretask period is important for information processing, decision-making, and response programming. The ability to rapidly process information increases progressively up to 18 years of age, reducing response latency (Clark, 1982); this phenomenon has been found to be more prevalent in males than females (Thomas et al., 1981). In addition, the speed of the reaction time is related to a series of factors as previously mentioned. Both children's and adults' most accurate anticipations, when confronted with velocity problems, are made when they experience them in the context of their daily activities (Wade, 1980), a natural phenomenon referred to as stimulus–response compatibility (Schmidt, 1991). Certain biomechanical parameters have also been identified as decisive in achieving optimum anticipatory postural adjustments and motor outcome (e.g., configuration of the base of support before moving) (Brenière et al., 1987). Moreover, feedback anticipation seems to emerge from feedback experiences (Haas et al., 1989). Individuals with verbal-motor performance deficits, however, take longer to organize and initiate movements (Elliot et al., 1991). Children with cerebral palsy show deficits in the sensorimotor organization and muscular coordination of their anticipatory activities (Nashner et al., 1983); they tend to compensate with early onset of force production and overall high force outputs (Eliasson et al., 1991, 1992).

Based on this research, the therapist would do well to promote practice of relevant, functional, purposeful tasks; to use spatial and temporal anticipation strategies to increase the readiness of the child to respond (i.e., informing the child of what will occur [and when]); and to use routine rather than random activities to influence reaction time and facilitate anticipation skills (Schmidt, 1991). Permitting information processing to occur requires a "waiting" period on the part of the therapist. Therapists have been observed waiting for the child's action or reaction in an average of 66% of activity trials in a treatment session (range, 48–93%). Most therapists (85% of the sample) were aware of their use of this strategy, but various rationales were offered (Larin, 1992).

Task Sequencing and Related Issues

Information processing demands vary with the type of task, making task classification taxonomies useful as an adjunct to planning a developmentally appropriate motor learning program. Purposeful tasks have been classified as continuous, serial, or discrete; open or closed; and complex or simple (Schmidt, 1988, 1991) (Table 6–1).

The sequencing of tasks plays an important role in motor learning and teaching. Different paradigms exist for sequencing tasks and instructions effectively. Gentile's (1987) taxonomy of tasks is one guide for the evaluation and selection of functionally appropriate activities, and for planning therapeutic interventions (Table 6–2).

Other systems also exist to assist practitioners in the sequencing of motor skill learning. Bressan and Woollacott (1982) proposed a paradigm in which skill construction, stabilization, and differentiation represent phases in the progressive control of the muscle synergies' program for motor skill acquisition. Wickstrom (1977) and Roberton and Halverson (1977) broke down skills into components of movement (intratask) and determinants of movement sequences relevant to other tasks (intertask), the former leading to the latter. More recently, in 1991 and 1992, Davis and Burton proposed an ecologic task analysis system based on the dynamic relationship between task environmental and performer factors. They suggested four instructional guidelines: 1) identify the task in terms of function (rather than perfection), 2) allow the learner choices and freedom to use movements, 3) identify and manipulate the relevant and critical task dimensions and performer's variables, and 4) provide direct instruction on the movement pattern using performer-scaled or intrinsic units of measure (e.g., ratio, rather than comparative, normative units).

Overall task sequencing has been considered according to various dimensions: general or specific, more or less complex, blocked or random, and part or whole. Schema theory supports the approach of developing a general base of motor activities before developing specific skilled activities (Kerr, 1978) for both open and closed skills. Referring to developmentally delayed children, Croce and DePaepe (1989) have suggested teaching sequentially less

complex patterns before more complex skills. Winstein (1991b), however, has cautioned against reducing the difficulty of a task to the point where the inherent nature of the task is altered. Such a practice could be detrimental to transfer of motor learning to the intended task. For example, emphasizing weight shift in standing as a subtask of locomotion did not achieve improved gait in adults with hemiparesis (Winstein et al., 1989). In pediatrics, one might extrapolate that children may not learn to kick in standing from practicing kicking in a sitting position or even performing pendular movements of the lower extremity in one-leg standing.

In general, therapists have been reported to adhere, more or less consciously, to the concepts of general or specific and more or less complex task sequencing, based on maturational and developmental theories (Larin, H, unpublished data, 1992). For example, a therapist may promote gross mobility before specific gait activities (e.g., initial heel contact), practice walking while holding onto a ball before free walking, or practice forward directional progression before changes of direction.

BLOCKED VS. RANDOM

Task sequencing may also be "blocked," that is, practiced in drill-type repetition where all trials of a given task are completed before another task is undertaken (intratask processing), or in "random" sequence (i.e., mixed repetition of various tasks [intertask processing]). In the early, verbal-cognitive stage of motor learning, blocked practice is slightly more effective than random practice. Random sequencing, however, has proven more beneficial than blocked sequencing for motor learning, measured on *retention* tests of motor skills. Random sequencing requires a greater number of trials, however, and typically degrades performance during the practice session; hence the acquisition–retention paradox known as the "contextual interference effect" (Battig, 1979; Gabriele et al., 1987, 1989; Shea & Morgan, 1979; Wright, 1991).

Furthermore, repetitions lead to the acquisition of a motor skill if they occur under conditions that most closely resemble those normally encountered during the performance of that skill. Through repetition children have shown considerable improvement, as compared with older individuals, in learning a demanding movement (Nicolson, 1982). Children with motor delay as well as children presenting a diagnosis of cerebral palsy have yielded similar findings from intensive, individual physical therapy sessions (Bower & McLellan, 1992, Mayo, 1991). One may conclude that, during a treatment session, it is important for the therapist to regard repetition as a means to 1) explore move-

TABLE 6–1. **TASK CLASSIFICATION: TYPES, CHARACTERISTICS, AND IMPLICATIONS**

Type	Continuous	Discrete	Serial	Open	Closed	Complex	Simple
Characteristics	Series of ongoing modifications No recognizable beginning or end Longer movement time Fatiguing Example: swim, run	Minimal feedback information effect Recognizable beginning and end Shorter movement time Minimal fatigue Example: kick, write signature	Combination of continuous and discrete	Constant unpredictable, and uncertain environment Needs to adapt behavior to changing environment Cannot effectively plan the response (on the spot decisions) Example: walk and step over obstacle	Stable predictable environment Allow advance organization of movement Can plan in advance Can learn with practice Example: Put hat on	Requires more coordination or more body parts Requires longer time to initiate	Requires less coordination and body parts Requires less time to initiate
Practical, instructional implications	Focus = sensory information and how to modify More time for rest between trials Error detection *during* movement	Focus = preplanning and production No attempt to modify during movement Less time for rest Increased number of trials Develop error detection through own response-produced feedback after movement		Focus = nature of environment (try to learn irregularities) Variable practice Flexibility	Focus = generation of preprogrammed actions Stability and consistency	Focus: keep arousal level fairly low More attention to describe and demonstrate Provide more feedback Budget more time	Focus: bring up arousal level More direct practice repetitions Provide less feedback

TABLE 6–2. GENTILE TAXONOMY OF TASKS

Environmental Context	Body Stability		Body Transport	
	NO MANIPULATION	**MANIPULATION**	**NO MANIPULATION**	**MANIPULATION**
Stationary No intertrial variability	Closed Body stability	Closed Body stability plus manipulation	Closed Body transport	Closed Body transport plus manipulation
Stationary Intertrial variability	Variable Motionless Body stability	Variable Motionless Body stability plus manipulation	Variable Motionless Body transport	Variable Motionless Body transport plus manipulation
Motion No intertrial variability	Consistent Motion Body stability	Consistent Motion Body stability plus manipulation	Consistent Motion Body transport	Consistent Motion Body transport plus manipulation
Motion Intertrial variability	Open Body stability	Open Body stability plus manipulation	Open Body transport	Open Body transport plus manipulation

Adapted from Gentile, AM. Skill acquisition: Action, movement, and neuromotor processes. In Carr, JA, & Shepherd, RB (Eds.), Movement Science: Foundations for Physical Therapy in Rehabilitation. Rockville, MD: Aspen Publishers, 1987, p. 115. With permission of Aspen Publishers, Inc., © 1987.

ment options until there are one or more occurrences of total success (Gentile, 1987) and 2) practice several skills, rotating among them. The therapist should explain the paradoxical phenomenon to the child or caretaker (i.e., the tradeoff between poorer, immediate performance versus long-term learning and retention performance as it is likely to affect motivation and motor learning). In general, however, therapists who stress the importance of repetition and claim to use this strategy have been observed to practice, on average, only four repetitions per activity, whether in a blocked or random sequencing (Larin, 1992). The principle of variety appears independent and of higher order than the principle of repetition; this may be related to a misunderstanding of the criteria associated with effective random sequencing, in which a large number of trials is necessary.

PART VS. WHOLE

The sequence of the components of a task may also be presented in "parts" or as a "whole," depending on the nature of the skill. For rapid, discrete skills of short duration (less than 1 second), practice of the whole task from the outset leads to the best results. If the learner has the prerequisite skills to master the new skill in its entirety, or if the degree of cognitive processing is minimal, the "whole" method is reported to be far superior to one based on "parts" (Croce & DePaepe, 1989). On the other hand, for slower, serial skills of long duration (more than 10 seconds) and for very complex tasks, the most time-efficient approach is to first practice the most troublesome parts of the task. "Progressive part practice" follows to gradually integrate the parts as acquired into the whole task so as to minimize transfer problems between the two. According to the "specificity of learning hypothesis," intertask transfer between two tasks does not happen or is very small if the two tasks are different in only very minor ways. It is therefore essential to use correct techniques during practice to master a motor skill (Ashy et al., 1988). To do so, it seems imperative for the therapist to differentiate skill characteristics and adopt the use of a taxonomy to guide practice.

Mental Practice

Practice is usually thought of as being physical (i.e., execution of a task with one's body); however, both physical and mental practice are useful strategies of motor teaching. Furthermore, a combination of mental and physical practice seems to be the most productive. Mental practice, also called "cognitive rehearsal" or "imagery practice," is imagining one's correct performance of a motor task without any associated overt movement. This strategy has been mainly designated as an end result of practice, but it may be used in the pre- or posttask execution period, or between physical trials to enhance performance over motor learning. Using 3 to 5 minutes of mental practice, beginners and highly skilled performers have been reported to benefit from this type of practice, particularly in correcting errors in execution, increasing concentration, and strategy rehearsal. Random imagery practice has been found to facilitate retention better than blocked imagery (Gabriele et al., 1989). This strategy may also increase speed (Rawlings et al., 1972, in Maring, 1990), balance (Fansler et al., 1985), and accuracy and efficiency (Maring, 1990). Mental practice can also be left to the learner to use outside of coaching sessions. Despite the usefulness of mental practice, however, the emphasis should be on physical practice during a session.

Therapists generally do not use much mental practice in treatment sessions. Having a child anticipate a movement through mental practice is not considered a concrete enough activity for children younger than 5 years of age. When employed, however, therapists have reported using it occasionally with older children in practicing specific gross motor tasks, such as wheelchair transfers (Larin, 1992). Given that planning a movement is, in itself, beneficial to motor learning, therapists may find that mental practice (adapted to the child's cognitive level) may be particularly effective in early practice, as findings with young adults have indicated (Schmidt, 1988). For example, the therapist might say "Let's think how it feels when you . . ., first you . . ., then you . . .," or "Try to imagine you watch yourself on television," or "Pretend you are doing it like in a dream, close your eyes. . . ." For brief periods of time, in a random fashion, children should be given the chance to experience and learn from mental practice.

Physical Practice: Determinants of Effectiveness

Physical practice remains essential to motor learning. Previously discussed aspects of such practice include the selected criterion (goal), task classification and dimensions, sequencing of tasks, and repetition. In addition, scheduling of practice and fatigue effects, degree of variability, physical guidance, and concurrent feedback also play important roles.

SCHEDULING

With regard to scheduling of practice trials, in general, "distributed" practice (i.e., when the amount of rest between trials equals or exceeds the amount of time in a trial) has been found to improve performance; and "massed" practice (i.e., when the amount of practice time in a trial is greater than the amount of rest between trials) enhances learning, in spite of fatigue (Gentile, 1987). More specifically, massed practice is advocated for discrete tasks, in which the skill level of the learner is higher and in which peak performance on a well-learned skill is needed. For continuous tasks, however, only slight negative effects of massed practice on learning are reported. In this case, distributed practice is most beneficial, as the tasks require greater energy demands. The same is true for complex tasks and in the presence of a lower level of motivation from the learner (Sage, 1984).

Realistically, motor activities are usually performed under gradually increasing amounts of fatigue; and Schmidt (1991) suggested that, to be effective, practice needs to be somewhat difficult and effortful. In addition, for children with cerebral palsy, increased fatigue caused by repetition of activities has been found to be associated with progress toward certain motor goals (Bower & McLellan, 1992). One concludes that some degree of fatigue is a necessary element in motor learning and should be explained to the child and caretaker. Therapists need to ensure that treatment sessions contain sufficient rest to remain energizing and challenging for the child and, importantly, to avoid accidents. In therapy sessions as in sport training, practice periods tend to be fixed in length; no single, optimal practice/rest ratio has been determined to be most effective in maximizing learning in all types of tasks. Each task must, therefore, be analyzed, and the analysis used to guide decisions about practice scheduling.

VARIABILITY

Another determinant of motor learning is the amount of variability—rehearsal of many variations of the same movement class. Actions within a movement class are said to share a particular relative timing and similar sequences of movements (Schmidt, 1991); for example, clapping hands and making music banging objects together or altering a parameter or a part of an action such as throwing (e.g., higher, faster, longer). There are two main purposes for using variability: first, to enhance generalizability and adaptability when one task-practice contributes to the performance of another in the same class of movement; and second, to establish competence throughout a dimension (i.e., altering either distance, speed, direction, or timing) while maintaining the same fundamental pattern.

The variability strategy has been more effective for children and female subjects than for male adults (Sage, 1984; Schmidt, 1988). Overall, low-variable practice (overlearning through practice of the same task) translates into greater performance on the practiced task; high-variable practice yields high performance on task transfer within a similar movement class and better retention learning (Carson & Wiegand, 1979; Shea & Kohl, 1990). Furthermore, high-variable practice leads to more generalizability, adaptability, and competence throughout a dimension (i.e., distance, speed, direction, or timing) while maintaining the same fundamental pattern. A caveat is that "similar" may mean different things at different ages (van Rossum, 1980); the breadth of a class of "similar" movements under a given motor program remains equivocal (Schmidt, 1977). For example, slowing down a movement too much might destroy its essential dynamics (Fetters, 1991; VanSant, 1990).

Optimum variability of practice for open or closed motor skills also differs. For open tasks, practice should be diversified, providing the learner with variations encountered in the habitual environment. Recently, however, Eidson and Stadulis (1991) reported no significant effect from the type of practice for an open skill in children with a moderate mental handicap; variable practice, however, reduced error in a closed skill. In general, practice for closed tasks should be consistent, enabling the learner to refine the movement pattern (i.e., decrease the variability of the movement trajectory [Darling & Cooke, 1987]), particularly after the acquisition phase during the later stages of motor learning (Gentile, 1987). In early learning, for example, therapists may slow down the activity somewhat while practicing small blocks of several trials of an activity (open or closed). Soon after, one needs to shift to random practice of two or more movement classes with variable practice on each (Sage, 1984). Besides undertaking variable tasks, the learner needs to apply the newly learned skill to multiple situations or environments; both children and adults respond positively to a multicontext treatment approach (Toglia, 1991).

Guidance

Guidance from the instructor or from mechanical equipment (e.g., metronome) is an effective method to restrict movement errors during the performance of a task. Physical or verbal guidance techniques assist the learner, in varying degrees, through the proper movements of the task. Physical and/or verbal guidance, often referred to as "facilitation" in the therapeutic milieu, has traditionally been a major strategy used by therapists in neurorehabilitation. Carter's (1989) findings, however, indicated that therapists spend more time in handling behaviors (facilitation, stimulation, inhibition, passive movements, and other maneuvers) than in using verbal behaviors (instructions, praise, criticism). Therapists have also been observed to provide physical guidance during 78% of the activity trials in a treatment session while spending 11% on passive, task-related activities and 11% on allowing independent movements (Larin, 1992).

Guidance has a considerable positive effect on performance during the trials of the practiced task (i.e., in the acquisition phase) but not on learning. It modifies the feel of the task, and the learner relies too strongly on it, developing a dependency (Salmoni and colleagues' "guidance hypothesis," 1984). Continuous guidance alters the task, greatly reducing its specificity and transfer potential. Trial-and-error or "discovery" procedures, however, result in learning (i.e., more effective retention and transfer performance). Providing a relative frequency of guidance (i.e., for a certain percentage of trials during practice), however, contributes more to learning than use of continuous input, as will relative frequency rather than continuous feedback (Lee et al., 1990). Moreover, with able-bodied individuals, guidance has been found most effective: 1) in early practice of unfamiliar tasks, 2) for slower rather than rapid and ballistic tasks, and 3) in the prevention of injury and reduction of fear (Schmidt, 1991).

The therapist should generally aim at reducing the use of guidance while increasing independent practice; this goal was noted to be predominant in therapists' current professional knowledge base (Larin, H, unpublished data, 1992). When needed, the therapist should provide a "relative frequency" of guidance rather than continuous input and possibly alternate between trial and error, independent movements, and guided movements. Reduced guidance in therapy may progress from firm physical handling with verbal input to a lesser, modified physical contact and verbal input, to minimal verbal input with supervision.

Feedback

Some form of feedback is essential for motor learning. Feedback may occur before, during (concurrent), or after (terminal) and be immediate or delayed, with respect to the task execution. Terminal feedback has been studied the most (Salmoni et al., 1984) and is the most frequently used in therapy (Larin, 1992).

TWO TYPES OF FEEDBACK

Two types of feedback are recognized: intrinsic and extrinsic. Intrinsic feedback is related to the child's inherent, rich, and varied sensory channels involved in practicing a task, provided the CNS is intact. Intrinsic feedback may be augmented by information concerning the movement or the degree of goal attainment (Holding, 1965). Extrinsic feedback, also called "augmented" or "enhanced" feedback, speeds up the learning rate, while no feedback and irrelevant feedback conditions do not result in learning. Any feedback has the potential to generate rapid and permanent motor learning if it adds essential information to intrinsic feedback, but it is not needed in all learning tasks.

Feedback may be provided verbally or nonverbally. The latter refers to artificial, sensory feedback, such as proprioceptive, auditory, visual, tactile, and electromyographic inputs, through the use of manual "handling" devices or media. Extrinsic feedback may be of several types: qualitative (e.g., "good," "right," "no") or quantitative feedback related to distance or magnitude of error (e.g., "three more steps"). It may trigger motivation and provide reinforcement. Therapists, however, tend to provide primarily positive, qualitative verbal feedback (in Larin's study, 47% of activity trials compared with 6% of negative reinforcement and 9% of quantitative feedback). Furthermore, according to Carter's (1989) findings, therapists' "praise" may reinforce abnormal as much as normal movements and their "criticism" may act as punishment for abnormal movements.

One purpose of extrinsic feedback is to give the child information (success or error) on the environmental outcome and on his or her movement patterns. Outcome information is termed *knowledge of result* (KR) and refers to direction and magnitude (Schmidt, 1991) or superficial movement features such as topology, timing (duration and speed), direction, amplitude or distance, or forcefulness (Gentile, 1987). Information on kinetics and kinematics is termed *knowledge of performance* (KP). Kinematic feedback is information on positions, time, velocities, patterns of coordination, or movement patterning; kinetic measures are descriptors of the forces that produce the kinematic variables (Schmidt, 1988). For Gentile (1987), kinematic feedback is mainly information on fundamental movement patterns such as timing or sequencing information.

There are inconsistencies between authors in their definitions of KR and KP, but they generally agree that KR does not always ensure learning enhancement and that KP is the most powerful form of feedback for motor learning and the most useful in motor teaching (Gentile, 1987; Sage, 1984; Schmidt, 1991). Overall, a combination of KP and KR is superior to one or the other form of feedback alone for both open and closed skills. KP is particularly suggested for closed skills, and KR plus KP, including information on anticipatory functions, for open skills (Gentile, 1987).

Adolescents with a diagnosis of cerebral palsy have shown improvement in the accuracy of their performance of a simple arm movement when provided with feedback on their actual time of movement, as have nondisabled individuals (Harbourne, 1991). At any time, feedback should focus on only one or two movement features and should be easily understood by the learner (e.g., "I like your quick reaching up above your head to catch the butterfly," or "It is good to push hard with your feet on the floor and keep a tall, straight back") and accompanied by nonverbal cueing.

PRECISION OF FEEDBACK

More precise, more frequent, and more immediate feedback during practice facilitates performance, but each has been found to be detrimental to learning and to produce dependency in the same way as physical guidance (see Salmoni and colleagues' "guidance hypothesis," 1984). Increased precision of feedback content may lead to increased learning, but the precision level of the verbal feedback must be adapted to the learner's level (i.e., less precision earlier, somewhat more precision later). An optimal level of precision has been hypothesized. If feedback is more or less precise than the optimum, subsequent performance is less accurate.

The optimal level of precision has been shown to increase with age. Young children naturally tend to ignore relevant information and respond immediately without using feedback (Barclay & Newell, 1980). Children, however, *can* use feedback to improve their learning, when required. Between the ages of 3.5 and 5 years, they have been reported to make fewer errors when provided with more precise feedback (Shapiro, 1977). Increasingly precise feedback, however, tends to result in more error for younger children (grade 2) but in more accuracy for older children (grade 4).

The choice of wording and the format of presentation are critical. Verbal feedback should be presented in key words and short phrases whether it is about the environmental goal (e.g., "It is great you put your hat on") or about the movement itself (e.g., "Your feet are nice and straight and no kissing knees," "It is very good holding your arms out with elbows straight like an airplane; let's count to twenty moving your wings up and down," "This was too fast and your chin was poking out").

TIMING OF FEEDBACK

Frequent feedback distracts and interferes with the information-processing activities leading to learning (retention). Concurrent feedback and terminal, continuous feedback (after each trial), while more effective for performance during practice and for guiding directly to the environmental goal, maximize dependency. The use of "relative" frequency is advocated over continuous feedback (Lee et al., 1990); for example, providing 50% relative feedback resulted in significantly better learning as measured by retention than 100% frequency feedback and concurrent feedback in Vander Linden and associates' (1993) study.

In a one-to-one learning situation (such as a therapy session), reducing the relative frequency of feedback (i.e., increasing the number of no-feedback trials [blank trials]) not only increases learning but also helps the learner to develop an error-detection mechanism and to become more active in problem solving. In addition, asking the child to guess the performance *before* feedback is given helps him or her to focus attention on the task and its sensory qualities (Gentile, 1987). The optimum frequency appears to vary in direct proportion to the complexity of the task.

Various methods exist to use a relative frequency of feedback in practice. Intermittent (occasional) feedback may be provided in several different, systematic ways. In *summary* feedback, feedback is withheld for a predetermined number of trials (e.g., 15 to 16 trials during a simple task or in the early part of practice or 5 trials during a complex task or as proficiency increases) (Gable et al., 1991). In the practice of a complex perceptuomotor skill, however, adults have been found to learn equally well when summary feedback ranged between 1 and 20 trials (Christensen et al., 1992). In *average* feedback, an average score is provided after a set of trials (e.g., "The last five times, you sat down slowly and gently all throughout with no flop").

In using feedback, the goals are improved learning and performance without feedback, with the child being capable of detecting his or her own errors. One approach consists of a *fading* procedure in which feedback usage is arbitrarily decreased, on an individual basis, from higher to lower relative frequency during the practice session, leading finally to a complete withdrawal. Still another approach is *bandwidth* corrective feedback, which is particularly useful in the earlier stage of learning. Informative feedback is provided only when the learner performs outside a preset band of accuracy (motivational feedback may be used within the bandwidth). For example, a therapist may decide to provide quantitative feedback (KR/KP) only when the child rotates the head less than 45° to look to the right and left sides. This procedure allows for a certain margin of error, and the absence of informative feedback helps reinforce the learner to exe-

cute repetitions. For movement tasks, bandwidth feedback has been reported to enhance accuracy and stability better than a pure, relative frequency condition (Winstein, 1991a).

Finally, the temporal aspect of extrinsic feedback after a trial is another factor influencing learning. Three distinct periods of time may be considered: *feedback delay*, *postfeedback delay*, and *intertrial interval* (Fig. 6–3). Extrinsic feedback provided immediately after a trial (a frequent schedule in physical therapy) is actually detrimental to learning, whereas feedback delayed by several seconds to several minutes has no significant negative effect on learning. Learning happens as long as competing events do not occur and interfere during the delay interval. Feedback delay allows the child to engage in the appropriate information processing and retention learning.

The postfeedback delay interval (time between the provision of feedback and the next trial) does not appear as a powerful factor in learning as long as the interval is longer than approximately 5 seconds, allowing for planning the next movement. Extremely short (less than 5 seconds) or long (days or weeks) postfeedback delay intervals were reported to have a detrimental effect on performance accuracy, more so in children than in adults. A 12-second processing time, however, was found to reduce performance variability, thereby increasing performance stability in children and adults (Gallagher & Thomas, 1980; Schmidt, 1991). Other motor activities (interferences) performed during this interval also have a negative effect on the next performance but, in contrast to a feedback-delay interval, do not affect learning negatively and may even produce retention learning (Lee & Magill, 1985).

The effects of the intertrial interval, that is, the time between two trials (the sum of the feedback delay and postfeedback delay intervals) have been the subject of controversy. If too short, inputs conducive to learning may not be processed; if too long, forgetting may occur. Practically, as long as the interval is not too short, this does not appear to affect motor learning adversely (Schmidt, 1988). Therapists, therefore, might optimally delay their intermittent feedback several seconds to several minutes and wait about 12 seconds before engaging the child in the next trial of activity.

Session Length and Frequency

Some considerations are now presented regarding the *length* (duration) and *frequency* of the whole therapeutic (practice) session from a motor learn-

FIGURE 6–3. Knowledge of result (KR): periods of time. (Redrawn from Schmidt, RA. Motor Control and Learning: A Behavioral Emphasis. Champaign, IL: Human Kinetics Publishers, 1988, p. 428. Copyright 1988 by Richard A. Schmidt. Reprinted by permission.)

ing perspective. Length and frequency may vary for three main reasons: 1) the level of demands of the task and related fatigue of the child (i.e., physical, attention, processing, and performance in general); 2) the skill level of the child (i.e., beginner, intermediate, advanced); and 3) the nature of the skill. For beginners, sessions that are demanding should generally be short at first, gradually increasing with the skill level, but frequent and spaced over a long period of time. The intensity of therapy should be purposefully determined. Treatment goals should be functionally oriented and consequently require numerous hours of practice based on sound motor control and pedagogic principles (Croce & DePaepe, 1989; Singer, 1990).

Findings from a study on the delivery mode of physical therapists in Ontario treatment centers indicated that individual therapy sessions for preschool children with moderate spastic diplegia last an average of 48 minutes, including 20% (about 10 minutes) of rest; they have an average frequency of 1.4 sessions per week (Larin, 1992). Determining treatment intensity tends to be the privilege of institutional policy-makers and individual therapists. In spite of tools such as the Pediatric Screening manual (Taylor et al., 1983) to assist in this task, therapists stated rationales for treatment frequency and duration that appeared to be primarily based on economic, logistic, and experiential factors (Larin, 1992). Variations in the intensity of therapeutic intervention have been related to therapist availability and severity of infant motor delay; that is, infants with more delayed development tend to receive a greater amount of individual therapy time (Haley, 1988).

Recent meta-analyses have suggested that a high level of intensity and duration may have a positive effect on the efficacy of early intervention, particularly for populations with disabilities (Casto, 1985; Innocenti, 1991). More specifically, in neuropediatrics, Mayo (1991) and Bower and McLellan (1992) provided evidence that increasing the intensity, duration, and frequency of individual therapy sessions

produced substantial change in children's motor development and accelerated acquisition of motor skills. In Mayo's study, infants younger than 18 months of age with delayed or abnormal motor behavior who received weekly, individual, neurodevelopmental therapy for 1 hour over a period of 6 months showed greater changes in their motor development than those who received monthly, individual, 1-hour periods of intervention. In Bower and McLellan's study, children 2 to 12 years old with a diagnosis of cerebral palsy of various types and learning difficulties were involved in individual, 1-hour therapy sessions each school day for 3 weeks; these children demonstrated accelerated acquisition of motor skills during the intervention period compared with before and after. Individual intensive treatment sessions cannot be excluded from a child's management program. Benefits and constraints must be carefully weighed in making decisions regarding the frequency and intensity of interventions to promote motor learning. Periods of time when movement patterns are in transition during the child's development may potentially emerge as sensitive periods for intervention.

Frequency of intervention may not, however, be limited to direct, individual, 1-hour treatment sessions. The daily activities of the child offer numerous occasions for intervention and should be viewed as an indispensable part of the child's total management. In these instances, the child's motor learning and motor performance may be enhanced or impaired. It is of utmost importance that the instructions provided to the parents or caretakers for addressing the child's functional motor activities reflect motor learning principles and employ relevant motor teaching strategies.

▌ CLINICAL EXAMPLE

In an attempt to unify the various theoretical and instructional concepts presented in this chapter, clinical scenarios intended to foster motor learning and motor performance are now presented. Therapists are encouraged to develop other scenarios based on their clinical experience, reinforcing certain aspects of their professional knowledge and practice and modifying and improving others.

A pediatric physical therapist is engaged in an individual, 1-hour, direct treatment session with a 5-year-old preschool child of average cognitive function who presents a movement dysfunction (diagnosis: moderate spastic diplegia). Without underestimating other potential mechanical or physiologic needs pertinent to the management of this child, the following functional goal is selected for its potentially broad application in daily activities: following 6 months of intensive therapy and management, the child will be able to walk with a posterior walker the length of the linear corridor from the classroom to the gym (approximately 50 feet) together with other classmates (nondisabled children) in a more efficient manner as measured by a 25% increase in step length and speed (distance/minutes) and a 25% decrease in cadence (steps/minutes).

The therapist's associated, movement-oriented therapeutic goal, in this case, is to obtain greater selective control (dissociation) of the lower extremities during gait as related to 1) range of movement (i.e., hip and knee flexion and extension); 2) muscle activity (i.e., stability and mobility; stance and swing); and 3) compensatory movement patterns (i.e., upper trunk, upper extremity excess-assistance).

The child is functioning at the early stage or verbal-cognitive to motor stages of motor learning in which he or she needs to discover a reasonable, effective approach to the desired movement pattern of walking. Walking is a dynamic, continuous, complex, open-type, functional activity. The objectives are, in one scenario, to gain a short- and long-term skilled "performance" and, in a second scenario, to "learn" the multiple facets of gait. First, the similarities of therapeutic, instructional strategies used in the two scenarios are presented, followed by their respective particularities.

Similarities

In both scenarios, the therapist pays attention to the physical aspect of intervention, planning and preparing the different functional areas to ensure security, fun, and appropriateness for the child's motivational level, attentional abilities, and sensory processing status. To this end, the playroom (treatment room) is organized into three ecologically valid stations entailing use of upright movement: cafeteria, library, and dance floor; the corridor

leading to the washroom and classroom is also selected as a therapeutic environment.

In a friendly, respectful, and "partnership" manner, the therapist presents in an exciting and genuine way (verbal and nonverbal) the various predetermined, novel play areas. First, the therapist asks the child what he or she would like to do in each area, with more rather than fewer details (promoting preselected goals). On the child's response, the therapist encourages the child through verbal guidance, for about 3 to 5 minutes, to imagine himself or herself doing the chosen activity. Then, as necessary, the therapist describes some of the possible movement activities in each (using modeling and verbal labeling) (e.g., "You may pick some food around the display, moving sideways," "You may reach up or down for your preferred books, going up and down the stool," or "You may dance with slow or fast music, rocking"). The therapist adds her choice to the list, incorporating certain risk-taking behaviors (e.g., "I would really like ballet dancing, on one foot, like that!"), and then negotiates, takes turns in the decision-making, and gradually fades out the directives to the child.

The therapist's instructions to the child throughout the session incorporate elements of arresting stimuli (e.g., surprise or uncertainty) and are often presented in "chunks." These instructions relate to the child's preselected environmental goals (e.g., "Let's go get your Sesame Street book from the top shelf") but also, if not more, to increasing the child's awareness of certain aspects of the movement pattern. The therapist questions the child (e.g., "How do you reach it so high?" [climbing up on bench with one foot], "What do you do not to fall? [keep feet apart and stay up straight], or "How does it feel to go so fast?").

Alternating with questions, the therapist also provides relevant information directly about the skill of walking to increase the child's selective attention to critical features. At times this information is about aspects of the environment affecting gait (e.g., "The floor is hard, let's walk on the carpet, it feels soft," or "Watch for the door, which may open quickly; walk more to the side"). At other times, it is about the whole movement (e.g., "Let's walk nice and straight") and, as necessary, about one or two aspects of the movement practiced (e.g., "Keep your feet straight pointing toward Big Bird [touching them] and three fingers further [showing on one's hand]," or "Arms down and knees up straight").

Apart from providing a combination of these two forms of information (environment and movement), the therapist fosters the child's self-correction in different ways. The therapist asks the child:

"Tell me what you need to remember and be attentive to before you begin walking" (verbal pretraining). The therapist models some of the correct or incorrect movements and labels certain important features (e.g., "Look, my toes are all stretched out"). At times, without physical prompting, the therapist asks the child to correct his or her posture or movement (e.g., "Tell me what you need to change"). At other times, the therapist points out to the child how his or her friend performs certain aspects of gait when meeting the friend in the corridor or when in the same playroom area.

In addition, functional selective attention is enhanced by introducing distractions early on and randomly in the treatment session, according, of course, to the child's response (level of confusion and attentiveness) and also to the objective of the practice session (i.e., performance or learning). These might be people walking by, talking, playing, or singing (opened window or door or shared playroom) or using a combination of activities, such as entertaining a conversation or singing while walking. First distractions are gradually introduced (i.e., the child can anticipate them), but as soon as possible they are randomly presented (i.e., unanticipated) to promote greater adaptability and function.

Different activities are practiced in a random fashion, and each one is repeated several times, maintaining a reasonably high level of complexity. Such a sequence might comprise: the child sits at the edge of a small rocking chair, one foot slightly in front of the other, stands up and climbs up and down a stool several times to reach different books, coming down through half kneel, and reaching down to give them to Miss Piggy sitting nearby; then the child stands up the same way, picks up a baton and walks forward, sideways, and then backward to the dance floor where ballet starts! Since the child may not be performing optimally during the session, the paradox of performance and learning is explained and encouragement given to the child.

Most activities are generated voluntarily with particular attention to the initiation of the movements for the purpose of attaining shorter reaction times and decreased use of compensatory synergies. In addition to setting relative daily living contexts, the therapist instructs the child (with and without the use of modeling) on how to prepare for movement, with an emphasis on adequate base of support and postural, biomechanical alignment (e.g., "One foot behind, one in front, and lean forward to stand up," or "Hip up and straight to bring other foot up on stool and climb," "Pretty tall back to walk backward"). Acknowledging the latency period of the child's reactions, the therapist waits for the child's voluntary initiation of movement. Then, the therapist gradually reduces the anticipatory input to the child (fading process) and requests more accuracy and speed in performing the activities, increasing the child's adaptability through use of a greater level of uncertainty (random activities).

Walking and related activities are complex skills to practice. In spite of this, when possible, each activity sequence is practiced in its entirety from the beginning (e.g., kneel to half kneel to stride standing, climbing up and down, walking in different directions). However, if an activity is too complex for the child and totally unsuccessful (goal and movement), the most troublesome parts of the activity are practiced individually, alternating regularly with practice of the whole activity (with physical guidance) for gradual integration and function (progressive part practice). For example, working toward climbing up could involve practicing sustaining weight transfer on one leg for short periods of time, maintaining an erect trunk while bringing the other leg up and down at different heights, transferring weight onto the other leg while placing a foot on the stool and swinging back and forth, and trunk leaning forward over a leg using momentum to climb up. In addition, mental practice is occasionally used between physical trials.

Differences

The practice of walking and related activities for the alternative purposes of performance or learning requires different practice scheduling, degrees of variability, application of physical guidance, and provision of feedback to the child. The differences particular to the two motor teaching scenarios follow.

In the scenario aiming at short- and long-term performance, the therapist chooses a distributed scheduling of practice in which the amount of rest between trials equals or exceeds the amount of time in a trial; hence, fatigue building to the point of impairing performance during the treatment session is avoided. Overlearning an activity becomes the goal; therefore, the therapist does not vary greatly among activities, and, in this case, the time spent walking forward predominates in the treatment session.

In the early stage of motor performance, the therapist uses a high degree of verbal and physical guidance to correct most of the child's movement errors and to obtain an immediate performance. Precise, extrinsic feedback is offered frequently and immediately to the child during (concurrent) and after (continuous terminal) activity trials. The therapist praises the child's success, referring to the goal or movement, and indicates mistakes in a corrective and encouraging manner. In addition, the therapist supplies KR and KP focused on one or two movement features (including anticipatory function) easily understood by the child (e.g., "Great, you kept your hip straight and moved your foot gently up," reinforced by facial expression, and look and touch of the hip, or "Oh! What a little step that was; let's stand nicely up tall on this [touch] leg to help take a bigger step to dance with the Sesame Street music!"). Another tactic used might be asking the child to "guess" the level of his or her performance before providing feedback. The feedback is not offered immediately after the performance but rather is delayed several seconds to several minutes and the next trial initiated another 5 to 12 seconds after the feedback. At all times interferences (distractions) are minimized to strengthen the performance. In the later stage of refined motor performance, however, practice is associated primarily with intrinsic feedback and minimal therapist input.

In the scenario aiming at learning, the therapist first chooses a massed scheduling of practice in which the amount of practice time in a trial is greater than the amount of rest between trials, in spite of fatigue building up and the likelihood that performance will deteriorate during the treatment session. However, distributed scheduling is also advantageous in the practice of complex, continuous activities such as walking. The therapist then begins using a distributed practice schedule and gradually increases the intensity of practice with repetitions; the practice remains somewhat difficult and effortful and generates fatigue.

High-variable practice leads to learning for retention and transfer, particularly in the case of open skills such as walking. The therapist diversifies the activities in two ways: 1) the practice of different but similar actions (intertask with the same movement class) (e.g., marching, standing up from half kneeling, climbing up a stool or even stairs [if one concedes that they all require various types of dissociation]); and 2) the practice of the same task altering one characteristic such as distance, speed, direction, or timing of the movement pattern (intratask), for example, walking a moderate and long distance, at moderate and fast speeds (not too slow), forward, sideways, and backward and on varied surfaces. In the early learning of an activity, the therapist may reduce somewhat the speed and sequence of practice into small blocks of several trials, breaking down the activity; soon after, the therapist shifts to random, variable practice, using the same speed and accuracy of the entire, desired, age-appropriate gait and practicing in different situations and environments.

In practice for learning, the therapist uses the least possible amount of verbal and physical guidance (relative frequency) in a fading manner. A combination of trial-and-error, guided, and independent movements is incorporated in the child's practice session. When guidance is used, the degree and the timing are adjusted to the child's need at the different periods of a task practice (i.e., pre-set anticipatory postural adjustments, movement initiation, sustained control, or termination). In the early stage of practice, however, when movements are somewhat slower and activities unfamiliar (e.g., half-kneeling or walking backward) and the child is more fearful and at risk of injury, the therapist employs a greater amount of guidance while attempting to gradually reduce it as much as possible. This is achieved by offering less manual support or more distal assistance or by using a medium between the therapist and the child (e.g., baton, ball, book, walker).

Extrinsic feedback provided for learning purposes is of the same types as for performance (i.e., qualitative and quantitative [KR + KP]); the level of precision and frequency, however, differs. Earlier in practice, the precision of the feedback is minimal, offered in key words or short sentences, and then increased as the child progresses. The therapist presents feedback in a relative frequency during the treatment session; and the higher the task complexity for the child, the more feedback is provided. The therapist chooses among four ways to determine this relative frequency: 1) fading (i.e., gradually reducing to no feedback); 2) average (e.g., after every fifth trial, giving feedback about that trial); 3) summary (e.g., after a predetermined number of five trials, giving feedback about all the previous trials); or 4) bandwidth technique (i.e., only after trials in which performance is outside a predetermined acceptable range, allowing for a margin of error). The timing of the feedback for learning remains the same as for performance purposes (i.e., several seconds to several minutes after a trial with a delay of 5 to 12 seconds before the next trial). Finally, to heighten learning, the therapist introduces other motor activities or distractors (interferences) at a higher rate than in the performance scenario.

CONCLUDING REMARKS

Future Research

Clinical and laboratory research is required to further document the factors of critical importance in motor learning of children. Normative data are greatly needed on information processing, particularly during the early stage of skill acquisition in young children. Comparative and single-subject data banks on the motor learning processes of children with motor impairment would assist the practitioner and researcher in their respective and collaborative activities. Instructional strategies for motor learning and performance need to be tested on large populations of children at varied ages and presenting different motor, cognitive, and social levels of functioning.

Clinical research is also required to further understand therapists' practice and knowledge (explicit and implicit) of the motor learning framework. The study of groups of therapists treating various populations of children with neurologic and orthopaedic impairment would reveal a more comprehensive picture of motor teaching patterns used in pediatric physical therapy. More specifically, investigation may address how therapists formulate goals (action or movement) for treatment sessions as a whole, as well as for each task practiced, with regard to emphasis on performance versus motor learning, function, or neuromuscular needs. Further insight into the therapists' taxonomy of tasks is necessary to ascertain the appropriateness and sequencing of strategies and optimal types of scheduling practice. Through research with control and experimental groups, the optimal proportions of strategies for different populations could be determined.

Implications

The motor learning framework has direct implications for the physical therapist as clinical educator interacting with the child, the child's parents or caretakers, colleagues, and students. In the learning–teaching relationship, guidelines from models are useful to provide sound principles for adapting tested strategies to the learner. A motor learning approach is pertinent to each of these interactions.

Motor learning theories have been transposed into motor teaching models, and numerous instructional strategies have been suggested. Therapists already use many of the strategies with varying degrees of conscious selection and competency. Their professional working knowledge, however, does not usually incorporate all of the important elements of the theoretical motor learning framework. The professional challenge is to continuously relate new theories to knowledge derived from practice. This chapter on motor learning may provide pediatric physical therapists with useful information for such a process. It may also offer a means to guide therapists' systematic reflection on their practice and to foster renewed energy in therapy.

References

Abbs, JH, Gracco, VL, & Cole, KJ. Control of multimovement coordination: Sensorimotor mechanisms in speech motor programming. Journal of Motor Behavior, 16:195–231, 1984.

Adams, JA. A closed-loop theory of motor learning. Journal of Motor Behavior, 3:111–149, 1971.

Arend, S. Developing perceptual skills prior to motor performance. Motor Skills: Theory into Practice, 4:11–17, 1980.

Asatryan, DG, & Feldman, AG. Biophysics of complex systems and mathematical models. Biophysics, 10:925–935, 1965.

Ashy, MH, Lee, AM, & Landin, DK. Relationship of practice using correct technique to achievement in a motor skill. Journal of Teaching in Physical Education, 7:115–120, 1988.

Bakshi, R, Bhambhani, Y, & Madill, H. The effects of task preference during purposeful and nonpurposeful activities. American Journal of Occupational Therapy, 45:912–916, 1991.

Barclay, C, & Newell, K. Children's processing of information in motor skill acquisition. Journal of Experimental Child Psychology, 30:98–108, 1980.

Battig, WF. The flexibility of human memory. In Cermack, LS, & Craik, FI (Eds.): Levels of Processing in Human Memory. Hillsdale, NJ: Erlbaum, 1979, pp. 23–44.

Bernstein, N. The Co-ordination and Regulation of Movements. Oxford: Pergamon Press, 1967.

Bower, E, & McLellan, DL. Effect of increased exposure to physiotherapy on skill acquisition of children with cerebral palsy. Developmental Medicine and Child Neurology, 34:25–39, 1992.

Brenière, Y, Cuong Do, M, & Bouisset, S. Are dynamic phenomena prior to stepping essential to walking? Journal of Motor Behavior, 19:62–76, 1987.

Bressan, ES, & Woollacott, MH. A prescriptive paradigm for sequencing instruction in physical education. Human Movement Science, 1:155–175, 1982.

Burton, AW, & Davis, W. Optimizing the involvement and performance of children with physical impairments in movement activities. Pediatric Exercise Science, 4:236–248, 1992.

Carson, LM, & Wiegand, RL. Motor schema formation and retention in young children: A test of Schmidt's schema theory. Journal of Motor Behavior, 11:247–251, 1979.

Carter, RE. A behavioral analysis of interactions between physical therapists and children with cerebral palsy during treatment. Unpublished doctoral dissertation, Northern Illinois University, 1989.

Casto, G. The relationships between program intensity and efficacy in early intervention. Unpublished manuscript, Utah State University, Early Intervention Research Institute, Logan, Utah, 1985.

Christensen, S, Fitch, N, & Winstein, C. Acquisition and retention of a partial weight bearing skill: Effect of practice with summary knowledge of results (Abstract). Physical Therapy, 72(Suppl. 6):S51–S52, 1992.

Cintas, HM. The relationship of motor skill level and risk-taking during exploration in toddlers. Pediatric Physical Therapy, 4:165–170, 1992.

Clark, JE. Developmental differences in response processing. Journal of Motor Behavior, 14:247–254, 1982.

Cook Merrill, S, Slavik, B, Holloway, E, Richter, E, & David, S. Environment: Implications for Occupational Therapy Practice. Rockville, MD: American Occupational Therapy Association, 1990.

Coster, WJ, & Jaffe, LE. Current concepts of children's perceptions of control. American Journal of Occupational Therapy, 45:19–25, 1991.

Croce, R, & DePaepe, J. A critique of therapeutic intervention programming with reference to an alternative approach based on motor learning theory. Physical and Occupational Therapy in Pediatrics, 9(3):5–33, 1989.

Darling, WG, & Cooke, JD. Changes in the variability of movement trajectories with practice. Journal of Motor Behavior, 19:291–309, 1987.

Davis, WE, & Burton, AW. Ecological task analysis: Translating movement behavior theory into practice. Adapted Physical Activity Quarterly, 8:154–177, 1991.

Edwards, R. The effects of performance standards on behavior patterns and motor skill achievement in children. Journal of Teaching in Physical Education, 7:90–102, 1988.

Eidson, TA, & Stadulis, RE. Effects of variability of practice on the transfer and performance of open and closed motor skills. Adapted Physical Activity Quarterly, 8:342–356, 1991.

Eliasson, A, Gordon, AM, & Forssberg, H. Basic co-ordination of manipulative forces of children with cerebral palsy. Developmental Medicine and Child Neurology, 33:661–670, 1991.

Eliasson, A, Gordon, AM, & Forssberg, H. Impaired anticipatory control of isometric forces during grasping by children with cerebral palsy. Developmental Medicine and Child Neurology, 34:216–225, 1992.

Elliot, D, Gray, S, & Weeks, DJ. Verbal cuing and motor skill acquisition for adults with Down syndrome. Adapted Physical Activity Quarterly, 8:210–220, 1991.

Fansler, CL, Poff, CL, & Shepard, KF. Effects of mental practice on balance in elderly women. Physical Therapy, 65:1332–1338, 1985.

Fetters, L: Cerebral palsy: Contemporary treatment concepts. In Lister, MJ (Ed.): Contemporary Management of Motor Control Problems: Proceedings of the II Step Conference. Alexandria, VA: Foundation for Physical Therapy, 1991, pp. 219–224.

Fitts, PM, & Posner, MI. Human Performance. Belmont, CA: Brooks/Cole, 1967.

Gable, CD, Shea, CH, & Wright, DL. Summary knowledge of results. Research Quarterly for Exercise and Sport, 62:285–292, 1991.

Gabriele, TE, Hall, CR, & Buckolz, EE. Practice schedule effects on the acquisition and retention of a motor skill. Human Movement Science, 6:1–16, 1987.

Gabriele, TE, Hall, CR, & Lee, TD. Cognition in motor learning: Imagery effects on contextual interference. Human Movement Science, 8:227–245, 1989.

Gallagher, JD, & Thomas, JR. Effects of varying post-KR intervals upon children's motor performance. Journal of Motor Behavior, 12:41–56, 1980.

Gentile, AM. A working model of skill acquisition with application to teaching. Quest, 44:3–23, 1972.

Gentile, AM. Skill acquisition: Action, movement, and neuromotor processes. In Carr, JA, & Shepherd, RB (Eds.): Movement Science: Foundations for Physical Therapy in Rehabilitation. Rockville, MD: Aspen Publications, 1987, pp. 93–154.

Gibson, JJ. The Senses Considered as Perceptual Systems. Boston, Houghton-Mifflin, 1966.

Glynn, T. Contexts for learning: Implications for mildly and moderately handicapped children. Australian and New Zealand Journal of Developmental Disabilities, 10:257–263, 1985.

Goldberger, M, & Gerney, P. Effects of learner use of practice time on skill acquisition of fifth grade children. Journal of Teaching in Physical Education, 10:84–95, 1990.

Gould, DR, & Roberts, GC. Modeling and motor skill acquisition. Quest, 33:214–230, 1982.

Haas, G, Diener, HC, Rapp, H, & Dichgans, J. Development of feedback and feedforward control of upright stance. Developmental Medicine and Child Neurology, 31:481–488, 1989.

Haley, SM. Patterns of physical and occupational therapy implementation in early motor intervention. Topics in Early Childhood Special Education, 7:46–63, 1988.

Harbourne, RT. Error detection skills in cerebral palsy (Abstract). Physical Therapy, 71(Suppl. 6):S9, 1991.

Haubenstricker, J. & Seefeldt, V. Acquisition of motor skills during childhood. In Seefeldt, V. (Ed.): Physical Activity and Well Being. Reston, VA: American Alliance for Health, Physical Education, Recreation and Dance, 1986, pp. 41–104.

Heriza, CB. Implications of a dynamical systems approach to understanding infant kicking behavior. Physical Therapy, 71:222–235, 1991.

Higgins, S. Motor skill acquisition. Physical Therapy, 71:123–139, 1991.

Holding, DH. Principles of Training. Oxford, England: Pergamon Press, 1965.

Hood, B, & Atkinson, J. Sensory visual loss and cognitive deficits in the selective attentional system of normal infants and neurologically impaired children. Developmental Medicine and Child Neurology, 32:1067–1077, 1990.

Innocenti, MS. More or less: A review of intensity as a program variable in early intervention. Paper presented at the meeting of the Society for Research in Child Development, Seattle, April 1991.

James, W. The Principles of Psychology (Vol. 1). New York: Holt, 1890.

Kamm, K, Thelen, E, & Jensen, JL. A dynamical systems approach to motor development. Physical Therapy, 70:763–775, 1990.

Kelso, JAS. Anticipatory dynamical systems, intrinsic patterns dynamics and skill learning. Human Movement Science, 10:93–111, 1991.

Kerr, R. Schema theory applied to skill acquisition. Motor Skills: Theory into Practice, 3:15–20, 1978.

Koegel, RL, & Rincover, A. Some detrimental effects of using extra stimuli to guide learning in normal and autistic children. Journal of Abnormal Child Psychology, 4:59–71, 1976.

Landers, DM, & Landers, DM. Teacher versus peer model: Effects of model presence and performance level on motor behavior. Journal of Motor Behavior, 5:129–140, 1973.

Larin, H. Knowledge in practice: Motor learning theories in pediatric physiotherapy. Unpublished doctoral dissertation, University of Toronto, 1992.

Lee, TD, & Magill, RA. Can forgetting facilitate acquisition? In Goodman, D, Wilberg, RB, & Franks, IM (Eds.): Differing Perspectives in Motor Learning, Memory, and Control. North Holland: Elsevier Science, 1985, pp. 3–22.

Lee, TD, Swanson, LR, & Hall, AL. What is repeated in a repetition? Effects of practice conditions on motor skill acquisition. Physical Therapy, 71:150–156, 1991.

Lee, TD, White, MA, & Carnaham, H. On the role of knowledge of results in motor learning: Exploring the guidance hypothesis. Journal of Motor Behavior, 22:191–208, 1990.

Lewthwaite, R. Motivational considerations in physical activity involvement. Physical Therapy, 70:808–819, 1990.

Maring, JR. Effects of mental practice on rate of skill acquisition. Physical Therapy, 70:165–172, 1990.

Marteniuk, RG. Information Processing in Motor Skills. New York: Holt, Rinehart, & Winston, 1976.

Marteniuk, RG. Motor skill performance and learning: Considerations for rehabilitation. Physiotherapy Canada, 31:187–202, 1979.

Marteniuk, RG, Mackenzie, CL, & Leavitt, JL. Representational and physical accounts of motor and learning: Can they account for the data? In Colley, AM, & Beech, JR (Eds.): Cognition and Action in Skilled Behaviour. North-Holland: Elsevier Science, 1988, pp. 173–190.

Mayo, NE. The effect of physical therapy for children with motor delay and cerebral palsy. American Journal of Physical Medicine and Rehabilitation, 70:258–267, 1991.

McCulloch, WS. A heterarchy of values determined by the topology of nervous nets. Bulletin of Mathematical Biophysics, 7:89–95, 1945.

Michaels, CF, & Carello, C. Direct Perception. Englewood Cliffs, NJ: Prentice-Hall, 1981.

Mott, FW, & Sherrington, CS. Experiments on the influence of sensory nerves upon movement and nutrition of limbs: Preliminary communication. Proceedings of the Royal Society of London, 57:481–488, 1895.

Nashner, LM, Shumway-Cook, A, & Marin, O. Stance posture control in select groups of children with cerebral palsy: Deficits in sensory organization and muscular coordination. Experimental Brain Research, 49:393–409, 1983.

Newell, KM, Carlton, MJ, & Antoniou, A. The interaction of criterion and feedback information in learning a drawing task. Journal of Motor Behavior, 22:536–552, 1990.

Nicolson, RI. Cognitive factors in simple reactions: A developmental study. Journal of Motor Behavior, 14:69–80, 1982.

Olney, S. New developments in the biomechanics of gait in children with cerebral palsy. In Topics in Pediatrics: Lesson 1. Alexandria, VA: American Physical Therapy Association, 1989.

Orme, M. Teaching Strategies Kit. Toronto, Ontario: Ontario Institute for Studies in Education, 1978.

Pohl, PS, Winstein, C, & Lewthwaite, R. Processes underlying motor learning: A methodological perspective (Abstract). Physical Therapy, 72(suppl. 6):S10, 1992.

Reed, ES. An outline of a theory of action systems. Journal of Motor Behavior, 14:98–134, 1982.

Ritson, RJ. Psychomotor skill teaching: Beyond the command style. Journal of Physical Education, Recreation, and Dance, 58:36–37, 1987.

Roberton, MA, & Halverson, LE. The developing child—His changing movement. In London, B (Ed.): Physical Education for Children: A Focus on the Teaching Process. Philadelphia, PA: Lea & Fabiger, 1977.

Runnings, DW, & Diewert, GL. Movement cue reproduction under preselection. Journal of Motor Behavior, 14:213–227, 1982.

Sage, GH. Motor Learning and Control: A Neuropsychological Approach. Dubuque, IA: Wm. C. Brown, 1984.

Salmoni, AW, Schmidt, RA, & Walter, CB. Knowledge of results and motor learning: A review and critical reappraisal. Psychological Bulletin, 95:355–386, 1984.

Schempp, PG. Enhancing creative thinking: A study of children making decisions in human movement programs. Human Movement Science, 2:91–104, 1983.

Schmidt, RA. A schema theory of discrete motor skill learning. Psychological Review, 82:225–260, 1975.

Schmidt, RA. Schema theory: Implications for movement education. Motor Skills: Theory into Practice, 2:36–48, 1977.

Schmidt, RA. Motor Control and Learning: A Behavioral Emphasis. Champaign, IL: Human Kinetics Publishers, 1988.

Schmidt, RA. Motor Learning and Performance. Champaign, IL: Human Kinetics Publishers, 1991.

Scholz, JP. Dynamic pattern theory: Some implications for therapeutics. Physical Therapy, 70:827–843, 1990.

Shapiro, DC. Knowledge of results and motor learning in preschool children. Research Quarterly for Exercise and Sport, 48:154–158, 1977.

Shea, CH, & Kohl, RM. Specificity and variability of practice. Research Quarterly for Exercise and Sport, 61:169–177, 1990.

Shea, CH, & Morgan, RL. Contextual interference effects on the acquisition, retention, and transfer of motor skill. Journal of Experimental Psychology: Human Learning and Memory, 5:179–187, 1979.

Sheridan, MR. Planning and controlling simple movements. In

Smyth, MM, & Wing, AM (Eds.). The Psychology of Human Movement. London: Academic Press, 1984, pp. 47–82.

Shumway-Cook, A, & Woollacott, MH. The growth of stability: Postural control from a developmental perspective. Journal of Motor Behavior, 17:131–147, 1985.

Sideway, B. Motor programming as a function of constraints on movement initiation. Journal of Motor Behavior, 23:120–130, 1991.

Simpson, RL, & Galbo, JJ. Interaction and learning: Theorizing on the art of teaching. Interchange, 17:37–51, 1986.

Singer, RN. Motor learning research: Meaningful ways for physical educators or waste of time? Quest, 42:114–125, 1990.

Sparrow, WA. The efficiency of skilled performance. Journal of Motor Behavior, 15:237–261, 1983.

Stratton, RK. Information processing deficits in children's motor performance: Implications for instruction. Motor Skills: Theory into Practice, 3:49–55, 1978.

Taylor, A, & Gousie, G. The ecology of learning environments for children. CEFP Journal, July–August 1988, pp. 23–28.

Taylor, D, Christopher, M, Freshman, S. Pediatric Screening: A Tool for Occupational and Physical Therapists. Seattle: University of Washington, 1983.

Thelen, E, Kelso, JAS, & Fogel, A. Self-organizing systems and infant motor development. Developmental Review, 7:39–65, 1987.

Thomas, JR, Gallagher, JD, & Purvis, GJ. Reaction time and anticipation time: Effects of development. Research Quarterly for Exercise and Sport, 52:359–367, 1981.

Thorndike, WL. The law of effect. American Journal of Psychology, 39:212–222, 1927.

Toglia, JP. Generalization of treatment: A multicontext approach to cognitive perceptual impairment in adults with brain injury. American Journal of Occupational Therapy, 45:505–516, 1991.

Turvey, MT, & Carello, C. The ecological approach to perceiving-acting: A pictorial essay. Acta Psychologica, 63:133–155, 1986.

van der Weel, FR, van der Meer, ALH, & Lee, DN. Effect of task on movement control in cerebral palsy: Implications for assessment and therapy. Developmental Medicine and Child Neurology, 33:419–426, 1991.

van Rossum, JHA. The level of organization of the motor schema. Journal of Motor Behavior, 12:145–148, 1980.

Vander Linden, DW, Cauraugh, JH, & Green, TA. The effect of frequency of kinetic feedback on learning an isometric motor force production task in nondisabled subjects. Physical Therapy, 73:79–87, 1993.

VanSant, AF. Life-span development in functional tasks. Physical Therapy, 70:788–798, 1990.

Vurpillot, E. The development of scanning strategies and their relation to visual differentiation. Journal of Experimental Child Psychology, 6:632–650, 1968.

Wade, MG. Coincidence anticipation of young normal and handicapped children. Journal of Motor Behavior, 12:103–112, 1980.

Weeks, DJ, & Proctor, RW. Salient-features coding in the translation between orthogonal stimulus and response dimensions. Journal of Experimental Psychology: General, 119:355–366, 1990.

Wickstrom, RL. Fundamental Motor Patterns. Philadelphia: Lea & Febiger, 1977.

Williams, K. Age difference on a coincident anticipation task: Influence of stereotypic or "preferred" movement speed. Journal of Motor Behavior, 17:389–410, 1985.

Winstein, CJ. Knowledge of results and motor learning: Implications for physical therapy. Physical Therapy, 71:140–149, 1991a.

Winstein, CJ. Designing practice for motor learning: Clinical implications. In Lister, MJ (Ed.), Contemporary Management of Motor Control Problems. Proceedings of the II Step Conference. Alexandria, VA: Foundation for Physical Therapy, 1991b, pp. 65–76.

Winstein, CJ, Gardner, ER, McNeal, DR, Barto, PT, & Nicholson, DE. Standing balance training: Effect on balance and locomotion in hemiparetic adults. Archives of Physical Medicine and Rehabilitation, 70:755–762, 1989.

Woodworth, RS. The accuracy of voluntary movement. Psychological Review, 3(suppl. 2), 1899.

Wright, DL. The role of intertask and intratask processing in acquisition and retention of motor skills. Journal of Motor Behavior, 23:139–145, 1991.

Chapter 7

Clinical Decision-Making in Pediatric Physical Therapy

ROBERT J. PALISANO, PT, ScD
SUZANN K. CAMPBELL, PT, PhD, FAPTA
and SUSAN R. HARRIS, PT, PhD, FAPTA

Every day, pediatric physical therapists must make decisions that affect the lives of children and their families. On what basis do we make these important decisions? Physical therapy has long used the empirical base of collective experience in clinical practice that is passed down from clinicians and educators to successive generations of new practitioners. Although this knowledge has served clinicians and their clients well throughout the brief history of our discipline, today's health care climate requires more. Increasingly, physicians and other health professionals, third-party payers, and the public expect that physical therapists will use scientific evidence and more valid and reliable decision methods as the basis for their practice.

In general, pediatric physical therapists make four major types of decisions: 1) who needs treatment and why; 2) how a client in need of treatment should be served, for example, which treatments should be applied or home exercises prescribed, which appliances or other assistive devices are needed, and who else should be consulted or involved in the management of the case; 3) how outcomes of intervention should be documented; and 4) how the overall clinical program should be evaluated for success in treatment and cost-effective-

ness (Magistro, 1989). The purpose of this chapter is to describe the problems inherent in making decisions in each of these categories and to review the methods that pediatric physical therapists have available to them for making these four types of decisions.

Discussion of these topics can best be made in an overall conceptual framework of the disabling process. Thus, before embarking on our task of analyzing decision-making, we describe such models.

MODELING THE DISABLING PROCESS

Two similar but complementary approaches exist for classifying functional performance in the presence of potentially disabling conditions. They are general conceptual models but can be elaborated for description of specific disorders. One is the World Health Organization's International Classification of Impairments, Disabilities, and Handicaps (Grimby et al., 1988; World Health Organization, 1980); the other is the four-dimensional classification of pathology, impairment,

Impairment

Functional Limitation

Pathophysiology

Disability

The Person with a Disability and the Rehabilitation Process

Societal Limitation

FIGURE 7-1. Domains of science relevant to medical rehabilitation and the disabling process. (From National Institutes of Health. Research Plan for the National Center for Medical Rehabilitation Research. Bethesda, MD: National Institutes of Health, 1993, p. 34.)

functional limitations, and disability developed by Nagi and elaborated by others (Guccione, 1991; Nagi, 1969, 1991, n.d.; Schenkman & Butler, 1989). These two models have been integrated by the National Center for Medical Rehabilitation Research (NCMRR) (National Institutes of Health, 1993) to form a five-dimensional model (Fig. 7-1). The five dimensions of the disabling process are pathophysiology, impairments, functional limitations, disabilities, and societal limitations. The focus of the classification is the person with a disabling condition, and the five dimensions interact in complex ways rather than form a simple hierarchy.

The five dimensions are defined here and then elaborated on in examples related to decision-making in the sections that follow. The key concepts in the conceptual model are illustrated by means of two examples: one, a condition that can be diagnosed at birth, and the other, one in which diagnostic uncertainty may remain for many months. The examples used are the child with myelodysplasia and the child with spastic diplegia, emphasizing the motor dysfunction characteristic of these conditions (Molnar, 1992). The framework for classifying the disabling process, however, can be broadened to include all types of disability or multiple aspects of disability within any given condition.

The conceptual framework for understanding the disabling process begins with *pathophysiology*, the underlying medical or injury processes at the cellular and tissue levels that are primarily studied and managed by basic scientists or medical specialists, such as the neonatologist or the neurosurgeon. In the child with myelodysplasia, a failure of neural tube closure results in an open spine with neural tissues extruded into a myelomeningocele. In the child who will develop spastic diplegia, a white matter infarct in the periventricular areas caused by hypoxia is an example of a pathophysiologic condition leading to this particular type of cerebral palsy. Damage to the corticospinal tracts and other nervous system pathways traveling through the periventricular areas is a likely result of hypoxic effects on these areas. Primary prevention strategies at this level are currently aimed at understanding nutritional deficiencies that might cause neural tube defects and at discovering means of preventing hypoxic-ischemic events that lead to cerebral palsy.

The complexity of modeling the disabling process can be appreciated if we remind ourselves that many children born prematurely who demonstrate pathologic findings on ultrasound examination of the periventricular area do not develop cerebral palsy. The challenge for clinical practitioners is to understand the signs and symptoms that verify a diagnosis of developmental impairment or to identify a child who is recovering from such a potentially disabling event. Similarly, for myelodysplasia, level of the lesion does not correlate perfectly with functional capabilities because of individual variations in nerve root innervation of muscles.

The second dimension of the model is *impairment*. Present at this level are the organ and system disorders that potentially will impair functioning at the organism or person level. Impairments are not necessarily recognized in the lesioned area (the brain and spinal cord in our examples) but result from it. In myelodysplasia, sensorimotor impairments include lack of sensation, total or partial denervation of muscles, and muscle atrophy, resulting in paralysis of the lower extremities. In spastic diplegia, sensorimotor impairments include decreased force and power output by the neuromuscular system, poor selective control of movements, and poor anticipatory regulation of postural set for movement, all well-known abnormalities resulting from periventricular damage to the corticospinal tracts or damage to the supplementary cortical motor areas involved in motor planning and coordination (Campbell, 1992). Impaired balance, efficiency, endurance, and coordination of movement are seen in both conditions. These impairments are known effects of cerebral palsy that all physical therapists can recognize once they are fully present; however, definitive diagnosis may not be apparent until some months after birth.

An important concept for therapists to understand is that of secondary prevention (Pope & Tarlov, 1991). Early in the course of a disabling condition, the pathophysiologic process results in identifiable impairments that may or may not be permanent or even affect function. The purpose of secondary prevention efforts is to limit impairment and thereby preserve as much function as possible. Parents of children with myelodysplasia must be taught proper handling and skin care to prevent fractures and skin breakdown. Scoliosis and decreased pulmonary function may be late-appearing secondary impairments that can seriously affect overall functional performance and quality of life. In the province of physical therapy, secondary prevention clearly involves the role of early intervention. For children with spastic diplegia, it also involves education for parents that enables them to avoid allowing their child to fall into movement habits that may later impair function by leading to muscle hypoextensibility (e.g., W-sitting) and that provides them with advice about when to seek medical attention for developing problems, such as worsening contractures.

The combination of impairments in one or more systems may lead to *functional limitations*, the third dimension of the conceptual framework. Functional limitations involve whole body function, for example, slow and inefficient gait and tendency to lose one's sitting balance while using the arms for dressing. Functional limitations result from impairments and are typically assessed in a clinical setting but may or may not be remediable. By contrast, not all impairments result in limitations of function. For example, a slight contracture of the hamstring does not cause obvious functional limitation; at some level, however, tight hamstrings begin to impair gait and other activities. The problems of children with various types of disabilities begin to become more similar at this level of the disabling process, although unique characteristics of both children and conditions dictate individualized treatment planning and intervention. For example, children with myelodysplasia must have individualized attention to deal with bowel and bladder functions. Functional limitations of gait in myelodysplasia and spastic diplegia may be relatively similar (poor endurance and balance, for example), yet because different impairments cause the functional limitations, children with these two conditions require different types of assistive devices and intervention strategies.

When functional limitations persist for long periods and are not remediable or cannot be compensated for by use of assistive devices or orthoses, *disabilities* result. At this level, children fail to fulfill normal life roles, such as participation in school,

play, or family activities, and quality of life may be seriously affected for both children and their families. For children with myelodysplasia, social consequences of bowel and bladder dysfunction can be serious if not adequately handled, even resulting in anorexia in a misguided attempt to decrease incontinence. For children with spastic diplegia, disabilities might include lack of independence in dressing or mobility, learning problems because of perceptual impairments, or inability to participate in sports with able-bodied peers. It is important to note that the degree of disability does not necessarily follow directly from functional limitations and shows high individual variability. Depression and low self-esteem, for example, if not recognized and treated, can impair social interaction and lead to decreased participation in activities that are functionally possible for the individual.

The most severe dimension of dysfunction in the disabling process is called *handicap* in the World Health Organization's model (World Health Organization, 1980) or *societal limitations* in the NCMRR model (National Institutes of Health, 1993). Handicaps result when societal barriers prevent an individual from functioning at the highest level of which he or she is capable. Societal limitations might include architectural barriers to mobility, inability to attend a day care center because of rules that exclude children who are incontinent, or the need for special equipment that is prohibitively expensive or not covered by insurance. Problems such as these often fall outside the usual purview of rehabilitation specialists and must be addressed through problem identification and action at the community and societal level.

The dimensions of the disabling process encompassed by the practice of pediatric physical therapy are most likely to be those of impairment, functional limitation, and disability. These dimensions will be considered further when problems and processes for making diagnostic, prescriptive, outcome assessment, and program evaluation decisions are discussed.

PHYSICAL THERAPY DIAGNOSIS

Historically, answers to the question, Who needs treatment by a physical therapist and what for? were simple to obtain. Physicians identified the problem—the medical diagnosis—and referred children to physical therapists, sometimes with a specific prescription, at other times for "evaluation and treatment" at the therapist's discretion. For many of the disorders treated by pediatric physical therapists, physicians remain the primary diagnosticians, especially at the level of identification of pathophysiologic processes. Few standardized practice guidelines exist, however, to guide physicians in deciding who would benefit or when to refer children with developmental disabilities, and physicians' practices vary widely. For example, research on physicians' decisions regarding referral for physical therapy of children with suspected cerebral motor dysfunction indicates that the decision to refer is related to the physician's diagnostic certainty, perceived severity of the child's involvement, and belief in the value of physical therapy (Campbell & Gardner, 1992). The diagnostic certainty expressed by physicians in the study who reviewed a series of standardized videotaped cases varied widely. Furthermore, the probability of referral varied with physician specialty. Orthopaedists were less likely and physiatrists more likely to refer a child younger than 2 years of age for physical therapy than were pediatricians or neurologists.

Under the current health care model and evolving state licensure laws, however, physical therapists increasingly serve as the point of entry into physical therapy services, either as independent practitioners, as part of a comprehensive diagnostic and intervention team, as related service providers in educational settings, or as practitioners in other venues. To be deemed worthy of such a powerful role, physical therapists need valid and reliable decision-making procedures that result in the provision of truly necessary services in the most cost-effective manner.

The diagnostic decisions that physical therapists make are typically in the realm of impairments and functional limitations. For example, therapists are best qualified to make decisions regarding whether a client has impairments of strength or passive range of motion, the presence of and degree to which a client has functional limitations of mobility, and the presence of developmental gross motor delay and the types of impairments contributing to that delay. The diagnostic tests that are available, however, frequently lack adequate sensitivity and specificity for identifying and defining the impairments and functional limitations we hope to diagnose.

The Problem of Predictability

Most often, the decision regarding who needs treatment revolves around the diagnosis of developmental delay or the presence of signs of aberrant development, such as those seen in the motor control dysfunction associated with cerebral palsy. The most useful means for assessing delayed or aberrant development are likely to be standardized developmental scales that have been normed on large populations. The predictive validity of those tests that currently exist, however, has been problematic.

What do we know about prediction of outcomes from early assessment? The bulk of the literature on assessment in infancy suggests that little regarding outcome in later years can be successfully predicted for individual children and certainly little from typical developmental assessment scales (Harbst, 1990; Kopp, 1987; Piper et al., 1991; Rosenblith, 1992). For example, poor motor performance scores early in life have some capacity for identifying children at risk for developmental problems but in a nonspecific way. Poor motor scores may later be associated with cerebral palsy, mental retardation, or even blindness and behavioral problems (Campbell & Wilhelm, 1985; Ferrari et al., 1990; Nelson & Ellenberg, 1982). The process of recovery from early medical complications and the role of the environment a family provides for optimal recovery and facilitation of development also contribute to the difficulty in predicting developmental outcomes. Test scores at any single point in time may be inadequate for making a decision regarding whether a child's development is permanently impaired until the time for maximally effecting important long-term outcomes has already passed. A conceptual framework that encompasses the complexity involved in early brain lesions or abnormal development is needed. Aylward and Kenny (1979) and Gordon and Jens (1988) have suggested models for early identification of developmental disabilities (Campbell, 1993). Models are also available from the work of other disciplines that, if fully implemented in clinical practice, might make decision-making more systematic and more precise and accurate (Watts, 1985, 1989). These models can help us to decide whom to treat and for what, can aid communication with other health professionals, and can explicitly allow for input from the child's family.

CLINICAL DECISION THEORY

One conceptual framework for developing new diagnostic procedures and measurement instruments is clinical decision theory (Dowie & Elstein, 1988). This theory assumes that clinical judgment encompasses such a complex set of tasks that mathematic algorithms and decision models incorporating the results of research on important clinical problems are likely to be more successful than is clinical judgment for making diagnostic and treatment decisions.

In decision theory, probabilities of various outcomes are assessed based on variables such as previous historical events or assessments, potential negative results of various decisions, and patient or family judgments regarding the value of various potential positive and negative outcomes. In the diagnostic area, for example, risk for cerebral palsy or motor developmental delay could be estimated based on a combination of findings such as ultrasound results at birth, general movement assessment, and tests of postural control and motor milestone achievement at successive ages. Bayesian statistical models allow the degree of risk calculated at earlier points in time to be incorporated as factors in an equation using current test results, thus establishing a cumulative risk probability that takes into account prior history as well as current functioning (Slovik & Lichtenstein, 1971). Studies of decision equations based on variables such as these have almost universally found that diagnostic decisions made with such algorithms are much more reliable than those based on clinicians' judgments (Dawes et al., 1989).

Decision models such as those just described do not currently exist for pediatric physical therapy, but it is entirely possible to develop them. What is needed is data from large research studies on the variables believed to be important that can then be developed into probability-of-outcome equations. The data needed may actually be available in the literature and in large clinical centers for several conditions, such as spastic diplegia. For this condition, many long-term follow-up studies using sophisticated imaging techniques and developmental assessment have already been published. Longitudinal assessment records available in many large centers should help to identify developmental test scores at particular ages that are likely to suggest ominous outcomes or significant milestones that can be used as markers of developmental progress in prediction equations. Even the imperfection of prediction that is likely to exist, given the data currently available, is likely to be better than current methods involving even more imperfect clinical judgment. Furthermore, deciding to try such a method will lead to the gradual development of a clinical database that will improve the methods used to make decisions.

Why have decision models proved to be better than experienced clinicians' judgments? As Goldberg (1991) suggested, rehabilitation specialists tend to base decisions on personal clinical experience, intuition, and hunches. Studies of clinical judgment suggest the many ways in which bias is introduced into the assessment and decision-making process when operating in such a mode (Sackett et al., 1985). Practitioners are liable to make errors of both omission and commission in assessment, and judgments made from data collected tend to be overly affected by recent experiences with other clients. Furthermore, the sensory perception of clinicians varies from time to time, owing to fatigue and other factors, including assumptions made from client history and from biased expectations. Studies have also revealed that practitioners immediately formulate hypotheses regarding what is wrong (or right) and then collect data to rule out or in the various hypotheses entertained (Dowie & Elstein, 1988). Obviously, if the true situation is not one of the entertained hypotheses, judgment is likely to go awry. Experienced clinicians tend to have a broader base of knowledge from which to generate appropriate hypotheses than do novices; nevertheless, their clinical decisions can still be impaired by any of the various factors just mentioned. Use of standardized assessments, a systematic data-gathering protocol, and decision algorithms can guard against such unreliability in clinical judgment.

CLASSIFICATION OF IMPAIRMENT AND ITS CONSEQUENCES

Use of taxonomic classification systems for describing disability is another means to improve clinical decision-making. All clinicians know that no two clients with the same disorder are exactly alike. Establishing taxonomies for the description of constellations of impairments presenting in particular conditions can lead to improved diagnosis and can generate studies of differential treatment effects for subcategories of disability and studies of whether different types of treatments are most appropriate for different subcategories. But do we have ways to identify the underlying impairments at the systems level, and are there clinically practical means for measuring them?

Work on developing diagnostic systems for classifying patients with low back pain is already well under way in physical therapy (Binkley et al., 1993). Experts in orthopaedic physical therapy participated in a consensus-building exercise to determine levels of agreement on diagnostic classes of low back pain and associated clinical findings. Further research is under way to identify proportions of patients in each diagnostic class from an existing clinical database and to study the reliability with which physical therapists use the classification system and relate diagnostic class to patients' complaints.

Recent research on neonates and young infants also suggests that we may, indeed, have the means for identifying the primary impairments in cerebral palsy at an early age. All clinicians know that children with cerebral palsy are characterized by stereotypic movement patterns and lack of selective control. Prechtl and his colleagues have developed an assessment of general movement that characterizes the movement pattern in cerebral palsy as being one of "cramped synchrony," with a paucity of selective joint movements, especially in the rotational components (Ferrari et al., 1990). Their work has also demonstrated that clinical assessment of children with known signs of brain pathophysiologic impairment can identify the effects of such lesions on movement, that these effects can be qualitatively and quantitatively described longitudinally and used to predict recovery or nonrecovery from early nonoptimal medical conditions and events. The test is totally noninvasive because it involves observation of spontaneous movement from 1-hour videotapes. Although more documentation of the reliability and validity of this approach is needed, it appears to be promising. If successful, this method is likely to alleviate the problem of late referral because of diagnostic uncertainty (Campbell & Gardner, 1992).

Crenna and colleagues (1992) have demonstrated that cerebral palsy can also be described on the basis of a constellation of impairments, leading to a taxonomic classification system that differs greatly from traditional ways of classifying cerebral palsy by area of involvement and presence of spasticity or movement dysfunction. In this system, categories of the taxonomy have been related to functional performance capabilities. Although still under development, such taxonomies show promise for use in diagnosis and for studying the effects of different types of treatments on variations in the underlying impairment.

The classification of impairments, functional limitations, and disabilities within the framework of the disabling process can be used to develop a comprehensive clinical assessment protocol, either for determining whether a disabling condition exists or for developing treatment goals appropriate for various levels of dysfunction. Tests at the level of impairment are likely to be the most discipline-specific, whereas assessments of problems along the dimension of disability heavily involve the client and family and are most often interdisciplinary.

▌TREATMENT PRESCRIPTION

Having identified the need for intervention for the presence of impairments or functional limitations, the therapist's next important decision is related to how to treat the patient. What approach should be implemented, how often and for how long, and which goals should be established?

Depending on the family's needs and goals and the child's age, overall developmental level, and specific problems and competencies identified by the physical therapist and other members of the assessment team, treatment goals might focus on various aspects of the disabling process. For example, treatment emphasis might be aimed at reducing impairment (emphasizing strength, endurance, tone, postural control, or other factors), at overcoming functional limitations through practice of the tasks or use of compensatory strategies, or at reducing or preventing disability through provision of assistive devices. Use of the conceptual model of the disabling process helps to clarify which treatment goals are most appropriate for any developmental stage and disability and to identify the methods to be applied.

Such decisions are frequently sources of professional conflict because members of each discipline view the disabling process from their unique perspectives and may develop entirely different goals and potential solutions for the same constellation of impairments, functional limitations, and disabilities. Even when clinicians agree on overall goals, priorities may differ (Butler, 1991). The resolution of such conflicts through the use of effective team consensus-building processes, however, can lead to elegant program plans that truly meet clients' needs. Both preventive and ameliorative approaches may be necessary; however, both stages of life and stages of the disease or condition affect the decision regarding which goals are the most important to attain in the limited time that is likely to be available.

For example, if primary impairments can be limited by early therapy, some functional limitations that would otherwise result as a part of the natural history of a condition may be avoided. Thus, prevention at this level of the disabling process involves attempts to limit impairment resulting from the lesion and to promote developmentally appropriate functional capabilities. For example, most therapists believe that early intervention for children with spastic diplegia produces a more efficient gait later. Little research exists to document such effects, however. One of the few studies that suggests such a result is a comparison of early (before 9 months) versus late Vojta therapy that reported that children whose treatment began before 9 months of age walked earlier, on average, and with better postural alignment than did those treated later (Kanda et al., 1984). Theoretically, early treatment should also result in prevention or reduction of secondary impairments, such as contractures and deformities, that are not generally present as primary impairments in children. Rather, they develop later as a result of habitual movement using abnormal compensatory patterns or overactive muscles with paretic antagonists or as a result of overall poverty of movement and disuse. Until we develop tests that clearly separate elements of underlying impairment from functional limitations that may be primary or may result from use of compensatory strategies to enhance function, we will be unable to document the value of early or preventive intervention for cerebral palsy and other conditions present in early childhood. With appropriate measurement tools available, studies of the efficacy and effectiveness of early intervention at the impairment level will be possible. Until such time as this information is available, however, therapists will continue to come into conflict with physicians and other professionals (including other therapists!) who believe that intervention does not need to begin early or can be carried out by parents, does not need to include hands-on treatment by therapists, and should be aimed at provision of compensatory strategies to increase function rather than at treatment of underlying impairment.

When functional limitations persist for long periods and are not remediable or cannot be compensated for, children may fail to succeed in normal life roles, such as participation in school, play, or family activities. Therapy planning should start with interdisciplinary assessment at the disability level when a condition that impairs developmental progress and functional capabilities is already well established. This involves asking which roles and skills are needed and appropriate for a specific child at his or her particular stage of life and must involve the family as full participants in the assessment process. When disabilities are present or can be prevented, each discipline considers what contributions it has to make and plans further exploratory assessment or intervention accordingly, again in concert with the family and other team members. In the case of our example of the child with spastic diplegia, a therapist may decide that independent locomotion is a future goal but that the child needs an assistive device at the moment to allow him or her to keep up with ambulatory peers. Other members of the rehabilitation team will have their own unique contributions to make to the solution of the problems of lack of mobility and other functional limitations.

The setting in which treatment is to be provided also shapes the goals and treatment methods to be used. For example, care of children in educational settings is by law aimed at preventing disabilities in learning and educational attainment. Related services are provided in the nation's public schools solely for this purpose, so the goals of therapy must be targeted at disability-level problems and competencies. Therapists, teachers, families, and other professionals must all be clear regarding these priorities and realize that decision-making for school therapy may not meet all of the needs for intervention that children with disabilities have. Impairments may not be treated at all in such settings, and only functional limitations that can be directly related to the prevention or alleviation of educational disabilities will be managed under the public law mandate.

Decision theory can again be helpful in making choices for intervention strategies. Specific models are available in the clinical literature for involving patients and their families in making decisions regarding which treatments should be applied (Watts, 1985, 1989; Weed & Zimny, 1989). These models incorporate both research-based knowledge regarding the possible costs and benefits of implementation of different approaches to the problem under consideration and also the values clients place on differing outcomes and the risks they are willing to incur, given the probabilities of both positive and negative outcomes. Such models have been discussed in the physical therapy literature for years, but little use has been made of such strategies for improving the decision-making process and involving clients more in deciding the course of their own treatment.

Although explicit conceptual models for describing various disabling conditions along with fully elaborated assessment and decision protocols are not currently available in pediatric physical therapy, treatment of patients must, of course, continue. Using an available model as a framework for clinical decision-making, however, can still be fruitful. The model, for example, can guide the problem-solving process, aid identification of which impairments are primary and which may be most responsible for limiting the client's function, indicate whether to refer to or consult with other professionals, and aid in deciding when to help a client develop compensatory strategies for dealing with a permanent functional limitation rather than attempt to treat the underlying impairment.

The Hypothesis-Oriented Algorithm for Clinicians

To the extent that decision-making in physical therapy is complex and that in many cases there is no single solution to a problem, decision models can be particularly helpful. The experienced therapist may find decision models of value in organizing and externalizing thought processes. Models are also of value in bridging the theory-practice gap in the clinical education of physical therapy students and recent graduates. The Hypothesis-Oriented Algorithm for Clinicians (HOAC) (Rothstein & Echternach, 1986) was selected for presentation in this chapter because it is specific to physical therapy and compatible with the NCMRR model of the disabling process. In presenting the HOAC, application will be made to children receiving physical therapy.

The HOAC was developed by Rothstein and Echternach (1986) to provide physical therapists with a systematic method for clinical decision-making and patient care that is independent of methods of assessment and treatment philosophy. An algorithm uses a branching approach to decision-making, involving several steps that are intended to narrow the focus of the problem and direct the practitioner to the appropriate plan of action. Echternach and Rothstein (1989) stated that their interest in decision-making was stimulated by observations that assessments performed by physical therapists did not always appear to have a direct bearing on the treatment plan and that the use of treatment protocols in physical therapy seemed to replace the thought process associated with *individualizing* treatment to the patient's unique set of problems. The HOAC is not supported by a database, computer generated, or intended to provide specific guidelines for assessment and treatment decisions. Rather, the HOAC provides a format to guide the physical therapist through the decision-making process.

The HOAC consists of two parts. The first part addresses assessment and treatment planning and consists of eight steps: initial data collection, problem statement, goals, examination, generation of a hypothesis, plan reevaluation methodology, plan treatment strategy and tactics, and implementation of treatment (Fig. 7–2). The second part is a branching program that consists of a series of questions that serve to direct the physical therapist in further problem solving when goals have not been achieved (Fig. 7–3). Successful application of the HOAC lies in the ability of the physical therapist to define goals and to evaluate whether the goals have been achieved.

The first step in part one is the initial data collection. Sources of information include a review of medical records and the patient interview. Information should be collected in the context of the patient's reasons for seeking assistance from a physical therapist. In pediatrics, the interview includes the family and addresses parent questions and concerns. Pertinent information that is obtained both from medical and educational records and from the interview includes knowledge of a diagnosis; health precautions; development, including the child's age of achievement of motor milestones and present motor abilities; previous medical interventions, including orthopaedic surgery; whether the child has special equipment such as a walker, wheelchair, or orthosis; and the professionals and agencies currently providing service to the family. The therapist is also interested in the composition of the family unit, the family's understanding of the child's development, and a description of the child's daily routines, behavior, and play style. The initial data collection provides the therapist with insights about the child's motor development and the potential impact of functional limitations and disability upon other areas of development and family function.

In step 2, the physical therapist generates a problem statement to guide the selection of goals. The problem statement should reflect the patient's reasons for seeking help. This practice is based on the authors' belief that the initial focus should be on the needs identified by the patient and on research indicating that physicians and physical therapists begin to generate problem lists *before* performing the formal assessment (Elstein et al., 1972; Payton, 1985). The rationale for step 2 corresponds with the practice of collaboration between professionals and the family that is mandated by part H of the Education of the Handicapped Act Amendments of 1986 (Public Law 99-457) and the Individuals with Disabilities Education Amendments of 1991 (Public Law 102-119).

The problem statement is the basis for step 3, the selection of goals that are measurable and functional and include a time frame for achievement. Although physical therapists typically determine goals after the assessment has been completed, Rothstein and Echternach (1986) cited three advantages to selection of goals before examination of the patient: 1) The therapist is more likely to state problems and goals that represent what is important to the patient. 2) The therapist and the patient are more likely to delineate what the patient expects from treatment and what functional outcomes are important to the patient. 3) Through understanding the patient's expectations in the patient's terms, the therapist can treat and advise the patient more appropriately. The process of goal selection supports professional-family collaboration and empowerment of families to act as advocates for their child through active participation in decision-making.

HYPOTHESIS-ORIENTED ALGORITHM FOR CLINICIANS

PART ONE

1. Collect initial data (eg, interview, history, chart review, subjective information)

2. Generate a problem statement

Establish goals (measurable and functional with a temporal element)

3. Examination (collection of data)

Referral to other practitioner (if no hypotheses can be generated)

4. Generate working hypotheses about why goals are or cannot be met at the present time (establish testing criteria for each hypothesis)

Ask whether goals are viable
• if no, modify
• if yes, proceed

5. Plan reevaluation methodology (schedule dates for reevaluations)

Consultation, if needed

6. Plan treatment strategy based on hypotheses (overall treatment approach)

7. Plan tactics to implement strategy (specifics of treatment plan)

8. Implement tactics (treatment)

FIGURE 7–2. Hypothesis-Oriented Algorithm for Clinicians. Part One: Guidelines for evaluation and treatment planning. (From Rothstein, JM, and Echternach, JL. Hypothesis-oriented algorithm for clinicians: A method for evaluation and treatment planning. Physical Therapy, *66*:1389, 1986. Reprinted from *Physical Therapy* with the permission of the American Physical Therapy Association.)

After goals have been established, the examination (step 4) is performed. Methods of examination are not specified in the HOAC but can include administration of standardized motor developmental and functional assessments, quantitative motion analysis, and measurement of energy cost. Clinical observations can include the quality of a child's self-initiated movements, how effectively a child uses movement during play and when performing functional tasks, and how a child's motor ability influences interaction with parents, siblings, and friends. The HOAC stresses the importance of assessment of skeletal alignment, range of motion, muscle performance, and sensation to identify impairments that contribute to functional limitation or disability. After the examination is completed, goals should be reevaluated and modified as necessary.

In step 5, the therapist formulates a hypothesis (clinical impression) about the cause of the patient's problem in motor function. The hypothesis is based on integration of all available data including the assessment results. Multiple hypotheses may be generated for a problem. Although physical therapists have traditionally emphasized musculo-skeletal, neuromotor, and cardiopulmonary im-

HYPOTHESIS-ORIENTED ALGORITHM FOR CLINICIANS
PART TWO

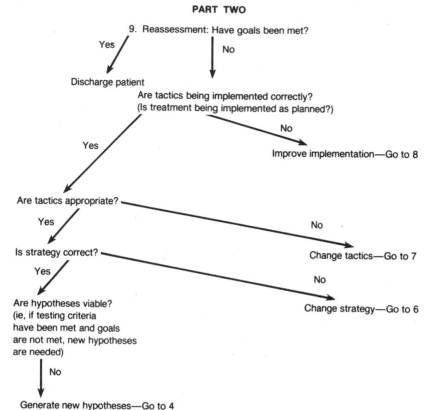

FIGURE 7–3. Hypothesis-Oriented Algorithm for Clinicians. Part Two: Branching program. (From Rothstein, JM, and Echternach, JL. Hypothesis-oriented algorithm for clinicians: A method for evaluation and treatment planning. Physical Therapy, *66*:1389, 1986. Reprinted from *Physical Therapy* with the permission of the American Physical Therapy Association.)

pairments as causes of problems in motor function, systems theories (Heriza, 1991; Horak, 1991) suggest that therapists should also consider behavioral, cognitive, perceptual, social, and environmental causes as well. The major premise of the HOAC is that treatment should not be provided unless the therapist is able to generate a hypothesis about the cause of the patient's problem in motor function. The therapist who is unable to formulate a testable hypothesis should consult with either another therapist or some other health care professional.

In step 6, the therapist determines criteria for evaluation of treatment goals and the date for reexamination. In steps 7 and 8, treatment is planned and implemented, respectively. Based on each functional goal and hypothesis regarding the cause of the patient's problem, a treatment strategy is planned and tactics are selected. In the HOAC, a strategy is defined as the overall treatment approach and tactics are the specific means of implementing the strategy (procedure or techniques). Treatment, or the implementation of tactics, is prescribed for a finite time period, the end of which corresponds to reexamination date.

After treatment has been implemented, the ther-

apist refers to the branching program (see Fig. 7–3). The branching program requires the therapist to respond to a series of questions regarding treatment. Questions are posed in the reverse order of the steps in part one. If the response to a question is yes, the algorithm directs the therapist to the next question in the hierarchy. If the response to a question is no, the therapist is referred back to the appropriate step in part one. The therapist then analyzes whether the step was completed successfully and, if not, what action to take before proceeding to the next question.

The first question of the branching program asks whether, upon reassessment, the goals have been met. If the goals have been achieved, either the patient is discharged or the process is repeated and new problems and goals are identified. If the goals have not been achieved, the therapist begins to problem solve using the branching program. The therapist first considers whether the treatment is being implemented as planned. In pediatrics this question has several facets that depend on the management plan and method of service delivery. Questions regarding implementation include whether the child has regularly attended therapy sessions and whether therapy has been incorporated into home, school, and community activities. The therapist must also consider how the child's behavior and motivation have affected the treatment plan. Finally, the therapist needs to verify whether treatment procedures have been performed correctly. If treatment is not being performed as planned, the therapist is referred back to step 8 to improve implementation.

Next, the branching program asks the therapist whether the treatment procedures are appropriate. In pediatrics, this might involve deciding for a particular child whether prolonged static stretch of the hamstring muscles is an appropriate procedure for increasing passive range of motion, whether resistive exercise is an appropriate procedure for strengthening leg muscles, whether reaching for objects positioned beyond arm's length is an appropriate procedure to improve sitting balance, or whether a postural control walker is an appropriate assistive device for gait training. If the therapist concludes that a treatment procedure is not appropriate, then the action is to go back to step 7 and change the treatment procedure.

The next question asks whether the treatment strategy is correct. Rothstein and Echtnernach (1986) indicated that the strategy (overall approach) and tactics (treatment procedures) are closely linked and may be considered identical by some therapists. Approaches used in pediatric physical therapy such as neurodevelopmental treatment (NDT) (Bobath & Bobath, 1984), proprioceptive neuromuscular facilitation (Voss et al., 1985), and sensory integration (Fisher et al., 1992) are examples of strategies as defined in the HOAC. A contemporary strategy might also be based on theories of motor development, motor control, and motor learning. If the therapist deems that the strategy is incorrect, then the action is to go back to step 6 and change the strategy.

The last question of the branching program prompts the therapist to consider whether the hypothesis is viable. If treatment is being implemented as planned and the strategy and procedures are appropriate but the goal has not been achieved, then the therapist is instructed to go back to step 4 and generate a new hypothesis. For example, a therapist might have identified muscle hypertonia as the primary cause of a child's inability to walk using a reciprocal leg pattern. Therapy was initiated and emphasized reduction of hypertonia. Upon reassessment, the child's ability to walk with a reciprocal pattern had not improved despite the therapist's having judged that therapy was implemented correctly and that the treatment strategy and procedures were appropriate. In reconsidering the cause of the problem, the therapist hypothesizes that poor ability to shift weight and unload the leg for swing phase is the primary cause of the child's inability to walk using a reciprocal leg pattern. The treatment strategy and procedures are modified accordingly.

The HOAC has several features that are advantageous for use by pediatric physical therapists. The child and parents are involved in the decision-making process. In addition, problems and goals must be functional and meaningful to the child and family. Formulation of a hypothesis about the cause of a child's problems requires the physical therapist to make inferences regarding the impact of impairment on functional limitations and disability. Furthermore, the hypothesis is integral to the development of an individualized treatment plan that emphasizes functional problems and goals rather than treatment approaches and procedures. Upon reassessment, if goals have not been achieved, the branching program guides the therapist through a problem-solving process to determine how to modify the management plan.

Although the HOAC is a systematic approach to decision-making, the complex and diverse nature of physical therapy assessment and treatment is not fully captured. This is not surprising considering the uncertainty that confronts the experienced physical therapist in attempting to select goals that the child is capable of achieving, formulate a hypothesis about the cause of the problem that has a high probability of being accepted, develop a successful intervention plan, and select an appropriate treatment strategy and procedures. Weed and Zimny (1989) have expressed their concern that algorithms simplify decision-making and require the practitioner to make choices before giving adequate consideration to possible alternative choices. They proposed that a more effective model is one that allows the therapist to ask all relevant questions, hold all possible options open until the end, and recognizes the uncertainty that frequently accompanies clinical decisions. This perspective is particularly germane to the formulation of a hypothesis about the cause of a functional problem. Physical therapists frequently treat children who have several primary and secondary impairments that can cause limitations in function and disability. When using the HOAC, therefore, therapists are encouraged to consider all possible hypotheses, to prioritize multiple hypotheses, and to consider how each hypothesis relates to the others.

Clinical Reasoning

Although decision models can be helpful for physical therapy management, they do not eliminate the need for physical therapists to have a strong knowledge base, problem solve, and make sound clinical judgments. Indeed, research on problem solving has repeatedly confirmed that skill in problem solving is problem specific, indicating that one can solve problems better with a comprehensive base of knowledge about the problem. Clinical reasoning refers to the many ways a practitioner thinks about and interprets an idea or phenomenon and incorporates knowledge, experience, problem solving, judgment, and decision-making (Fleming, 1991). Watts (1985) described decision-making as both an art and a science. She suggested that many decisions are made with a degree of uncertainty and reflect intuitive thought processes. Magistro (1989) proposed that clinical decisions in physical therapy are derived from both theoretic knowledge and practice experiences that intelligently influence our courses of action. He discussed the role of intuition and suggested that practice decisions are not always apparent as rational thought processes. Magistro's perspective is consistent with Brenner's (1984) conceptualization of professional development. Brenner described the transition from novice to expert as involving a shift from the use of explicit, verbally based theoretic knowledge to the use of highly implicit and embodied practical knowledge.

Mattingly (1991) has proposed an interpretive or meaning-centered model of clinical reasoning in occupational therapy that emphasizes implicit and embodied knowledge. She conceptualized clinical reasoning as the process of deciding on the appropriate action for an individual patient at a particular time. Theoretic knowledge is viewed as a starting point but not as a strict plan for action. As part of the process of individualizing treatment, the therapist makes judgments and improvises in moving from general practice guidelines to the requirements of a specific situation. Mattingly suggested that the knowledge that guides judgment and improvisation is often embodied in the therapist's hands or eyes in a manner that is difficult to translate into words. Part of the therapist's expertise, therefore, is reflected in implicit thought processes that are translated into habitual ways of observing and interacting with patients. The perspective that clinical reasoning involves more than the ability to apply theory and learned technical skill may explain the frustration of physical therapy students when they first attempt to apply classroom material to the clinical setting.

Mattingly (1991) proposed that through experience therapists develop the implicit knowledge that is integral to clinical reasoning. The therapist learns to attend to relevant cues and modify therapeutic interventions in response to these cues. Furthermore, therapists are often not completely aware of how they use implicit knowledge to identify problems, develop treatment plans, and engage the patient in the therapeutic process. On the basis of the results of a study in which occupational therapists described their assessment practices (Rogers & Masagatani, 1982), Mattingly suggested that pediatric therapists incorporate a minimum of five domains of knowledge into their thought processes: 1) understanding of the child's motivation, commitments, and tolerances; 2) assessment of the environment in which the task is taking place; 3) knowledge of the child's physical and cognitive deficits and capacities; 4) perception of the therapeutic relationship; and 5) immediate and long-term goals. Effective clinical reasoning enables the occupational therapists to improvise treatment and address the unique meaning of disability as it relates to a particular patient.

The results of two studies provide insight into clinical reasoning in pediatric physical therapy. Carter (1989) examined the behavioral interactions between physical therapists and children with cerebral palsy during an NDT session. The behaviors of an experimental group of seven physical therapists who attended an 8-week NDT certification course were compared with those of a control group of six physical therapists who were not certified in NDT. Therapists in the experimental and control groups were videotaped before and after the NDT certification course. The interactions of the experimental and control groups were also compared with those of seven physical therapists who were NDT course instructors. The rates and durations of the therapists' verbal and physical handling behaviors and the children's movement behaviors were operationally defined and coded from videotape using a portable laptop microcomputer with a program specifically designed for the study.

There were no statistically significant differences between the behavioral interactions of therapists in the experimental and control groups after the NDT course. Physical therapists in both groups employed facilitation procedures with little reinforcement of the children's responses, and inhibition procedures were followed by abnormal movement a significant number of times. The behaviors of the experimental and control groups were in contrast to those of the NDT instructors. NDT instructors produced more normal movement responses from the children, and facilitation procedures were followed by normal movement a significant number of times. Furthermore, the NDT instructors anticipated abnormal movements before they were observed and responded with inhibition procedures.

Carter (1989) concluded that the manner in which the NDT instructors used facilitation and inhibition procedures was in accordance with behavioral learning principles.

Although Carter (1989) did not formally assess clinical reasoning, his results support Brenner's distinction between novice and expert practitioners. Comments from the physical therapists in the experimental group suggested that after the NDT course, they were more concerned with their hand placement and the particulars of movement than with the response they obtained from the children. This implies that during treatment, the physical therapists in the experimental group focused their thought processes on explicit knowledge, which is characteristic of the novice practitioner. By contrast, the treatment behaviors of the NDT instructors suggested that they thought less about the psychomotor aspects of treatment and attended to relevant cues about the children's responses. The NDT instructors' ability to anticipate abnormal movement suggested that they used implicit knowledge to select treatment procedures, a characteristic of the expert practitioner. If NDT instructors use implicit knowledge to make treatment decisions and are not fully cognizant of their thought processes, then perhaps they are unable to impart their treatment skills fully to other therapists. Alternatively, therapists may first have to become proficient in their psychomotor skills before they can effectively acquire and apply implicit knowledge, a process that might not have occurred in the experimental group after completion of the NDT course.

In the second study, Larin (1992) investigated physical therapists' explicit and implicit knowledge of motor learning and the relationship between this knowledge and their practice. The subjects were 21 Canadian pediatric physical therapists who had between 8 months and 27 years of experience. The physical therapists were videotaped during individual treatment sessions with preschool-aged children who had a diagnosis of spastic diplegia. After the treatment session, the therapists viewed the videotape and a stimulated-recall interview was held. The therapists were asked to identify and describe treatment activities, indicate goals, and report what they were thinking about during treatment. During a second interview, the therapists were asked to comment on their ideas, beliefs, theories, and the sources of knowledge they had used in their treatment sessions. The Motor Teaching Strategies Coding Instrument, an observational recording instrument developed by Larin (1992) for the study, was used to code from the videotapes the type, frequency, and timing of selected strategies of motor learning that the therapists used during the treatment sessions.

The physical therapists were found to have implemented most of the motor-learning strategies that researchers and theorists in the field have identified as important in the teaching of motor skills but to have done so in varying degrees. More-experienced therapists promoted more independent movements, whereas less-experienced therapists treated the children in a richer environment, employed more nonverbal cues, and more frequently assisted a child's self-initiated movement. A clear relationship between implicit professional knowledge and practice was not found. Qualitative analysis suggested that motor-learning strategies were frequently not organized in a consistent, effective framework of knowledge. This implies that many of the strategies were implemented incidentally and, therefore, did not represent meaningful integration of motor-learning strategies into pediatric physical therapy. In addition, the therapists provided an overwhelming impression that they did not routinely stop and think about what they were doing in their treatment sessions. The therapists indicated that their main sources of knowledge were clinical experience, continuing education, interaction with colleagues, and readings. Professional education was the source of knowledge that was least often mentioned.

On the basis of her findings, Larin (1992) offered several recommendations pertinent to the theory-practice issue in physical therapy education. Therapists are encouraged to reflect upon their treatment practices and rationales for clinical decisions. Larin advocated providing therapists with resources to enhance professional development, including continuing education programs and a greater opportunity for on-the-job information exchange with peers and mentors. In addition, she proposed that frequent information exchange between researchers and practitioners may foster a role for the practitioner as "research translator." Larin also recommended development of movement science curricula in physical therapy education programs that strive to recognize similarities and reflect upon differences among theory, research, and clinical approaches and strategies. A goal is for academic faculty and clinical educators to incorporate motor-learning and motor-teaching theory into student instruction and to model strategies for clinical application of this information with specific reference to pediatrics.

A great deal remains to be learned about clinical reasoning in pediatric physical therapy. The results of the studies by Carter (1989) and Larin (1992) provide preliminary support for the concept that clinical reasoning involves the application not only of theory and psychomotor skill but also of intuitive or implicit thought processes. The results of Larin's study, however, suggest that a therapist's implicit knowledge may not be organized into an effective framework consistent with theory and that therapists have difficulty in explaining their thought processes during treatment. Entry-level physical therapy education programs have traditionally focused on teaching multiple overlapping therapeutic exercise approaches and techniques. As a consequence, the early professional development of many physical therapists has centered on comparing and contrasting approaches in attempts to develop a preferred treatment style. Perhaps the focus on understanding and mastering treatment approaches and techniques has hindered the development of theory and models for clinical reasoning and decision-making that emphasize the problems and needs of the children and families who are the recipients of physical therapy. Pediatric physical therapists are encouraged to understand their thought processes better not only to enhance their own professional development but also to serve their clients and educate physical therapy students more effectively. A better understanding of clinical reasoning is essential for the development of comprehensive decision models for treatment planning, implementation, and evaluation that reflect the broad scope of pediatric physical therapy.

ASSESSING INTERVENTION OUTCOMES

Physical therapists typically assess outcomes by comparing client performance with preset short- and long-term goals developed on the basis of patient testing and observation. How can we guarantee, however, that the outcomes we identify are really the result of our intervention and not the effect of other interventions, of natural development, or of recovery? And how can we be sure that our interventions do not result in unintended negative consequences?

One clinical decision tool that has been used increasingly by pediatric physical therapists to assess the effectiveness of their interventions is the single-subject research design. The single-subject design is an experimental paradigm that is particularly useful for practicing clinicians who wish to study intensively the effects of treatment on individual clients within their caseload (Gonnella, 1989; Harris, 1993).

Nearly all pediatric physical therapists must develop individualized, measurable objectives for the children with whom they work as part of "best-practice" procedure, and the single-subject design represents a logical extension of this procedure. In developing individual behavioral objectives, therapists are required to specify client outcomes that are expected to change as a result of introducing treatment. These behavioral objectives are analogous to outcome measures that are a form of dependent variable, a term that is universal to all types of experimental research designs.

A second major component of experimental research is selection of the independent variable or, in the case of physical therapy, the specific treatment technique that is being applied in an effort to effect positive change in the outcome variable. Obviously, careful treatment planning for the pediatric client involves not only the selection of the outcome or target behavior, as represented in the individualized therapy objective, but also selection of a specific treatment technique that is designed to enhance change or facilitate improvement in the outcome behavior. To return to the HOAC example, the selection of measurable, functional objectives (target or outcome behaviors) is analogous to step 3 of assessment and treatment planning, whereas the selection of the appropriate intervention strategies evolves from steps 5 through 8 (developing a hypothesis about the cause of the problem, determining criteria for evaluating the treatment, and planning and implementing the treatment).

In comparing the single-subject research design to physical therapy as it is typically provided in a clinical setting, Gonnella (1989) has stated that the first few steps are similar: the problem behavior is identified, baseline data are collected on the problem behavior, a treatment plan is developed and implemented, and changes in the problem behavior are assessed. However, several important differences exist between the single-subject design and the therapeutic model.

Whereas typically only one baseline assessment is taken in the therapeutic model, single-subject design mandates that a minimum of three data points must be collected on the outcome behavior before treatment is introduced (Barlow et al., 1984). A second criterion of single-subject research is that a very specific design should be implemented that involves sequential application and withdrawal of the intervention. Finally, performance must be measured repeatedly (and frequently) throughout each phase of the design. For a visual comparison of these two models as described and depicted by Gonnella (1989), Figure 7–4.

Other important criteria of single-subject research designs are that the data collection procedures are both replicable and reliable (Ottenbacher,

THERAPEUTIC MODEL	SINGLE-SUBJECT EXPERIMENTAL PARADIGM
1. Evaluate patient's status	Evaluate patient's status
One baseline measure (BL)	*Three or more BLs
Specify problem(s)	Same
Measure problem(s)	Same
Specify goal(s)	Same
Specify therapeutic intervention (TI)	Same
	*Specify design to assess efficacy
2. Apply TI	*Apply TI within design strategy
Adjust TI to patient's response	Same
3. Evaluate patient's response	Evaluate patient's response
	*Repeated measures

*Indicates absence of difference in approach from the current model.

FIGURE 7-4. Comparison of therapeutic process with single-subject paradigm. (From Gonnella, C. Single-subject experimental paradigm as a clinical decision tool. Physical Therapy, 69:603, 1989. Reprinted from *Physical Therapy* with the permission of the American Physical Therapy Association.)

1986). Percent agreement is typically used to assess consistency of scoring the behavioral objectives or outcome measures between two or more independent raters.

In his excellent text on single-subject designs for occupational and physical therapists, Ottenbacher (1986) has outlined six important steps for setting up such designs: 1) determining the setting in which the behavior or performance will be observed and recorded; 2) deciding on the method to collect data; 3) determining the length of time that the behavior will be observed and measured; 4) observing and recording client behavior; 5) recording and plotting the data collected; and 6) continuing measurement and recording procedures until requirements of the design have been satisfied. Pediatric physical therapists who wish to set up single-subject designs in their own clinical settings are advised to consult the Ottenbacher text as well as other references in the physical therapy literature that describe this important clinical decision tool (Gonnella, 1989; Harris, 1993).

Since the early 1980s, pediatric physical and occupational therapists have used single-subject designs to examine the effects of "tone-reducing" (inhibitive) casts and orthoses in improving gait and standing balance in children with cerebral palsy (Harris & Riffle, 1986; Hinderer et al., 1988); to evaluate the influence of some specific well-defined NDT techniques on increasing heel contact (Laskas et al., 1985) and decreasing knee flexion during gait (Embrey et al., 1990) in children with cerebral palsy; to assess the effects of two different treatment approaches (behavior modification and a neurophysiologic approach) in reducing tongue protrusion in young children with Down syndrome (Purdy et al., 1987); and to examine the effects of different modes of mobility on school performance

of children with myelodysplasia (Franks et al., 1991). These are but a sampling of the published reports that have used single-subject designs to examine treatment effectiveness.

In keeping with the pediatric examples outlined at the beginning of this chapter, two published single-subject studies will be described—one involving 2 children with spastic diplegia and the other involving 3 children with myelodysplasia. Reference will be made to the NCMRR model of the five dimensions of the disabling process in discussing the goals and outcomes of each of these studies.

In a single-subject study published in 1988, Hinderer and colleagues set out to evaluate the relative effects of tone-reducing casts and standard plaster casts on gait characteristics and functional locomotor activities in 2 young children with cerebral palsy. The first child (Case 1) was a 3.5-year-old boy with mild spastic diplegia and mild mental retardation; spasticity was greater on the right. Some of the impairments noted in this child included gait deviations such as moderate in-toeing on the right, decreased stride length on the left, toe-dragging, forefoot weight-bearing, limited trunk rotation, and high-guard posture of the upper extremities. Functional limitations included the inability to walk up and down stairs without support as well as the inability to squat or rise to standing without support.

The second child (Case 2) was a girl, aged 5 years 9 months, with asymmetric spastic diplegia (greater involvement on the left), moderate ataxia, and normal intelligence quotient (IQ). Impairments included poor static and dynamic balance and unsteady gait with frequent falling. Specific gait deviations consisted of mild in-toeing on the left and difficulty with left toe clearance, limited trunk rotation, and a wide base of support. Functional limitations that resulted from these impairments included the inability to walk backward and balance on one leg and the need for upper extremity support to climb stairs and to move from squatting to standing.

An A-B-A-C crossover single-subject design was used in this study to evaluate the effects of the two different types of casts (the independent variables or specific intervention techniques). Tone-reducing casts were defined as those that "maintain the ankle at zero degrees and stabilize the toes and foot in neutral alignment by incorporating a footplate which supports the toes and the metatarsal, peroneal and longitudinal arches of the foot" (Hinderer et al., 1988, p. 371). Standard plaster casts held the ankle in neutral alignment but did not include a footplate.

The study began with both children in a baseline (A1) phase (no casts). In the second phase of the study, Case 1 wore tone-reducing casts (B) and Case 2 wore standard casts (C). Then the baseline condition (A2) was reinstituted for both subjects, after which the crossover of treatments occurred so that the design for Case 1 was A1-B-A2-C and the design for Case 2 was A1-C-A2-B.

Outcome measures (target behaviors) included footprint data used to analyze various gait parameters, specific developmentally appropriate fine motor tasks, and videotaped ratings by an interdisciplinary panel of experts of gait and functional motor activities. Data were collected two or three times per week for 19 weeks. The number of data points per phase ranged from 5 to 12. Inter-rater percent agreement for the gait measures was 96.1% and for the fine motor measures was 97.4%. Subjective impressions were also obtained from parents of the 2 children and their treating therapists.

One of the benefits of sequential application and withdrawal of interventions, as occurs in single-subject designs, is the ability to control for natural history, developmental maturation, and practice effects. Analysis of the fine motor data for the children in this study revealed that their performance continued to improve even during the baseline (no-cast) phases—thus suggesting that practice of these tasks was contributing more to their improvement than were the specific interventions. In a typical therapeutic model as described by Gonnella (1989) (see Fig. 7–4), such control is not possible and the treating therapist might assume that the improvements are due to the intervention itself whereas they may, in fact, be due to practicing the task or to other intervening variables such as developmental maturation.

Another benefit of this particular crossover design is the opportunity to compare two different interventions. Greater increases in stride length were noted for both children during the tone-reducing cast phases as compared with the standard cast condition. Blinded videotape analysis by the panel of experts revealed mild gait improvements for Case 2 during the tone-reducing cast phase as well as functional improvements in standing balance, ability to walk backward, and ability to squat and return to upright. Owing to poor compliance by Case 1, a standardized sequence of gait and functional motor activities was not obtained.

Although this study provided some limited support for the relative benefits of tone-reducing casts as compared with standard casts, the authors concluded their paper by making a plea for practitioners to document their own outcomes of tone-reducing casts and orthoses: "Single-subject research designs offer a clinically appropriate means for reliably studying their effectiveness, and are particularly indicated when studying a heterogeneous population, such as individuals with cerebral palsy, whose clinical presentation varies from day to day" (Hinderer et al., 1988, p.375).

Another single-subject study compared the relative effects of assistive device ambulation (walker or crutches) and wheelchair mobility on three school performance measures for children with myelodysplasia (Franks et al., 1991). Subjects were students aged 9, 10, and 15 years with L-4 or L-5 level myelomeningocele, all of whom had a physiologic cost index (an indicator of energy efficiency) of greater than 1.00 beat per meter when ambulating with assistive devices. The independent variables or specific interventions in this study were the assistive ambulation devices and the wheelchair. Outcomes assessed were reading fluency, visuomotor accuracy, and manual dexterity. A convincing rationale for this study was the frequent encouragement of ambulation for children with lumbar-level lesions in spite of the high energy costs (Waters & Lunsford, 1985).

In the case of these children with lumbar-level lesions, the pathophysiologic condition (myelodysplasia) led to impairments, including lower extremity paralysis, which had then resulted in functional limitations in gait and upright mobility. Basically, this study sought to examine whether secondary functional limitations that can result from ambulation, such as high energy cost, had a negative effect on school performance. If assisted ambulation does, in fact, result in greater energy costs, which in turn lead to poorer school performance, could such a decline in school performance actually lead to school failure, which might then be considered a long-term disability?

To examine these questions, an alternating condition single-subject design was used in which phase 1 was wheelchair propulsion, phase 2 was ambulation with crutches or walker, and phase 3 was again wheelchair propulsion. Each phase was 1 week in length (5 school days), with data collected daily on the three outcome measures: correct words per minute of a 100- to 200-word reading passage (reading fluency); visuomotor accuracy as assessed by the Motor Accuracy Test, Revised (Ayres, 1972); and manual dexterity as assessed on the Purdue Pegboard Assembly subtest (Tiffin, 1968).

Although reading fluency was unaffected by the method of mobility and manual dexterity varied across the 3 subjects and the two treatment conditions, visuomotor accuracy scores were significantly lower for all 3 subjects during the assistive ambulation phase.

In an accompanying commentary on this article, Haley concluded that "implications of this study may cause us to step back from our often aggressive posture toward functional ambulation at all costs. If assisted ambulation is not energy efficient, time efficient, or safe or leads to an interruption in social, emotional, or cognitive growth, then alternate means of mobility must be considered. Is not the aim of the physical therapist to promote overall development rather than to promote ambulation at a significant cost? Is not efficient, independent mobility the real functional goal for children and their families?" (Haley, 1991, p. 578).

It is exactly these types of questions that we face daily in our clinical decision-making as pediatric physical therapists. Using single-subject studies to examine effects of specific interventions systematically and replicating these studies across other subjects in other clinical settings will assist in allowing us to answer such questions. It is the responsibility of all practicing therapists, be they clinicians, researchers, or educators, to provide ethically responsible and efficacious treatment for their clients. Systematic examination of treatment outcomes, through such strategies as the single-subject design, can assist us in attaining this goal.

▌ PROGRAM EVALUATION

Although individual physical therapists frequently believe that they have done their professional jobs thoroughly when they have appropriately assessed outcomes in individual clients, professional practice requires additional evaluation of the overall impact and costs of physical therapy programs. Goldberg (1991), for example, suggested that therapeutic and surgical outcomes for children with cerebral palsy include technical outcomes of

typical interventions, functional outcomes, parent and child satisfaction with both outcome and service delivery, and cost-effectiveness relative to other intervention approaches. Here, the tools include formal program evaluations and quality assurance programs involving evaluation of record keeping; monitoring of therapist adherence to program policies; assessment of interactions with clients, other providers, and third-party payers; and evaluation of client satisfaction and long-term outcomes.

Monitoring Services with a Database

Developments in the area of monitoring services and tracking outcomes include computerized approaches to creating a database on clients served that may also provide systematic, structured individual patient reports to guarantee uniform reporting of significant information across both therapists and types of patients (Jenkins, 1989; Lehmann et al., 1984; Shurtleff, 1991; Slagle & Gould, 1992). A database is a generalized set of computer programs that allows 1) entry of a variety of data by different authorized users; 2) organization of the data for storage; and 3) retrieval, updating, reorganization, and printing of output in the form of summary reports (Lehmann et al., 1984). Yearly statistics can be rapidly collated, care trends can be monitored across time, and data can be used for prospective or retrospective research (Slagle & Gould, 1992). Use of a database approach can guard against errors of both omission and commission by structuring therapists' reports and by automatically providing checks of entered data against a range of appropriate responses. When a database is developed along the lines of the conceptual framework of the disabling process, studies can be undertaken of how impairments or their alleviation affect functional limitations and whether disability in the client's natural environment is reduced by the therapy provided. Such a system allows comparison of the performances of both clients and therapists across a range of functions and allows easy access to comparison of the processes and outcomes of contemporary patient care with that in historical populations. Development of national databases on specific client populations can form the basis for improving practice through comparison of institutional or regional differences in management strategies, identifying infrequent negative outcomes, and studying low-incidence conditions.

Slagle and Gould (1992) emphasized that only 27% of tertiary care neonatal units responding to a national survey of database use monitored the accuracy of their data, an essential element of a high-quality plan. Users liked their system best if it generated patient records, such as discharge summaries. In addition to these critical issues, Jenkins (1989) suggested that database developers should consider what aspects of care are likely to change over time in order to develop a system that is flexible in meeting long-term needs. Developers should consider how to collect enough data to be maximally useful for meeting such diverse needs as preparing annual reports and answering important research questions, while eliminating large amounts of data that are easy to collect but unlikely to be used (Slagle & Gould, 1992). In addition, a specific plan for maintaining overall quality of the database should be developed (Slagle & Gould, 1992).

Formal Program Evaluation

A more comprehensive approach to assessing program effectiveness is formal program evaluation (Shadish et al., 1991). Although frequently using well-known social science methodology, formal evaluation practice since the 1960s has developed into a discipline in its own right. The explicit purpose of program evaluation is to assess the effects of programs in meeting their stated goals for the purpose of improving subsequent decision-making about the program and, in a broader sense, for improving future program planning. Evaluation theory, although initially idealistic, has been expanded and revised based on the experience of program evaluators operating in the real world. These experiences have led to the recognition that 1) the achievement of stated goals may not be the only useful product of a social program; 2) there are many stakeholders involved in the typical program, some of whom are more concerned that the interests of their particular group are addressed than that program goals have been achieved; and 3) politics always acts on programs in ways that may be difficult to identify but may mean that program evaluation results are not likely to change programs effectively in major ways. Because of these real world complications, new evaluation theories have arisen, some complementary and some in more direct opposition to others.

"Theory connotes a body of knowledge that organizes, categorizes, describes, predicts, explains, and otherwise aids in understanding and controlling a topic" (Shadish et al., 1991, p. 30). Ideal evaluation theory describes and justifies why certain evaluation practices lead to particular types of results; clarifies the activities, processes, and goals of evaluation; explicates relationships among evaluative activities and the processes and goals they facilitate; and empirically tests propositions to identify and address those that conflict with research or other knowledge about evaluation (Shadish et al., 1991). The purpose of program evaluation theory is to specify the practices that are feasible for evaluators to use to garner evidence for the value of programs and to reduce identified problems of relevance to the program. Formulation of an appropriate methodology for evaluating a program depends on proper identification of the uses to which the evaluation results will be put. The prospective program evaluation planner needs to know who wants to know what and to what end.

The uses of evaluation results are usually considered to be of two major types: summative (outcomes or products) and formative (evaluation for the purpose of improving the program and understanding the processes by which the program operates). The former makes the supposition that an outcome of the evaluation itself might be abolition of the program; the latter generally assumes that the program will continue to exist and that better ways of improving the product or the provision of services are sought. Because studies of the uses to which evaluation results are put have generally shown that effects trickle down into new-generation programs, producing slow, incremental change rather than resulting in revolutions in thinking and implementation, recent theorists have emphasized that evaluation results may be most usefully thought of as being "enlightening," that is, having future use for program planners in thinking about issues, defining problems, and developing new perspectives and ideas. Those who formulate policy and implement programs seldom actively search for evidence, or if they do, tend to use whatever fits with their current understanding of the problem under study. Information such as this has led to important studies of the uses of program evaluation and theoretic formulations regarding how information can be most usefully disseminated. In any case, whatever the purpose, program evaluation must be conducted based on the identified need for the program and how well it satisfies the needs identified as well as meets the needs that might not have been previously identified but happen to be satisfied by the program. The best program evaluation designs also search for potential negative effects, such as those identified by the study of Franks and colleagues (1991) on mobility in children with myelodysplasia.

Arguments have arisen among program evaluation theorists regarding the value of quantitative versus qualitative evaluation methods. The randomized, controlled clinical trial remains, at least in medical areas, the most highly valued summative assessment of intervention outcomes, and it is especially valuable in studies of intervention with children because of the control needed to rule out the effects of maturation and other threats to internal validity (Norton & Strube, 1989; Shadish et al., 1991). Combined with causal modeling of the theoretically and empirically derived processes and factors influencing outcomes, clinical trials are most powerful in studies with large numbers of subjects or in studies seeking to identify low-incidence but potentially highly dangerous unintended negative effects. Qualitative methods, however, offer flexibility, a dynamic quality, and a unique ability to reflect the world from the perspective of multiple program stakeholders and participants. They are especially well suited for gathering answers to formative questions about the quality of program implementation and its meaning to participants. They may also be highly useful for studying the processes by which programs achieve useful outcomes in meeting needs of clients and society. Of most importance, however, are the use of methods appropriate to the level of development of the program (early development stage program, innovative demonstration project, established ongoing program), the problematic issues of concern to program stakeholders of various types, decisions under the control of the program to be made at a time when evaluation results will be available, and the level of uncertainty regarding critical program features. Methods tailored to these factors are most likely to result in effective use of program evaluation results.

Methods of program evaluation that emphasize the process of service delivery are well suited for examining the overall effectiveness of therapy programs. Wang and Ellett (1982) used the term "program validation" to describe a form of evaluative research useful in the development and refinement of innovation educational programs. The major purposes of program validation are to 1) obtain empirical evidence of the effectiveness of an innovative program, 2) identify aspects of the program that require improvement in order to achieve the intended outcomes, and 3) evaluate the feasibility of implementing the innovative program. Wolery and Bailey (1984) have proposed that a comprehensive program evaluation of early intervention programs addresses the following questions:

1. Does the method of service delivery represent the best educational practice?
2. Is the intervention being implemented accurately and consistently?

3. Is an attempt being made to verify the effectiveness of intervention objectively?
4. Does the program carefully monitor client progress and demonstrate a sensitivity to points at which changes in service need to be made?
5. Does a system exist for determining the adequacy of client progress and service delivery?
6. Is the program accomplishing its goals and objectives?
7. Does the service delivery system meet the needs and values of the community and clients it serves?

The questions proposed by Wolery and Bailey offer a framework for program evaluation of physical therapy services provided in a variety of settings, including the school system, acute care and rehabilitation hospitals for children, and private practices.

Three studies will serve to illustrate the scope of program evaluation and how questions are developed specific to particular programs. Haley and colleagues (1988) evaluated how physical therapy and occupational therapy services were implemented in six publicly funded early intervention programs in the greater Boston area. The authors examined the influences of infant, family, and program variables on the therapy services provided over a 6-month period. Dependent variables included intensity of individual therapy, intensity of group therapy, ratio of direct therapy to group therapy, ratio of home therapy to center therapy, and ratio of therapy time to total program time. Therapist availability predicted best whether an infant received individual therapy. Infants with more delayed motor development tended to receive more individual therapy and more total therapy. Infants received a higher proportion of therapy when 1) motor quotient was low and parent education was high, 2) infants were younger and therapist availability was high, and 3) infants were younger and parent education was high. Diagnostic risk factor and age did not predict type or intensity of therapy. Although the study was exploratory in nature and should not be generalized to other early intervention programs, the results contribute to the understanding of how infant characteristics and therapist availability influence the degree and types of intervention.

Holmes and colleagues (1987) evaluated the developmental progress of 64 of 203 infants who attended a publicly funded early intervention program in the Kansas City, MO, area during a 5-year period. The program included an intradisciplinary developmental assessment; development of an individualized educational and therapy program in conjunction with the parents; weekly or twice-weekly center-based physical therapy, speech therapy, and educational activities; monthly parent discussion groups; and home program activities planned by the staff and parents. The Early Intervention Developmental Profile (Rodgers et al., 1977), a multiple developmental domain curriculum-based assessment, was used to assess each infant. Infants were classified into five diagnostic groups to compare rates of development among infants receiving early intervention. Infants in the myelodysplasia, cerebral palsy, developmental delay, and multiple handicap diagnostic groups maintained their developmental rates during intervention, whereas the development quotient of infants in the Down syndrome group declined. Younger infants and infants with higher overall developmental quotients and higher developmental quotients in the cognitive domain on admission to the early intervention program demonstrated higher rates of developmental change. The authors concluded that although cause and effect relationships were not determined, the results suggested intervention efficacy for four of the groups. They recommended investigating the curricula for the infants with Down syndrome.

In the third study, Palisano (1989) evaluated two methods of therapy service delivery provided to students with learning disabilities who attended public school during the 1986–1987 school year. To serve adequately approximately 500 students receiving occupational and physical therapy, the therapy staff of the Delaware County, PA, Intermediate Unit had instituted group and consultation methods of providing services to students with learning disabilities who met eligibility criteria. The therapists and teachers of students who participated in the study had worked together during the previous school year using the two methods of service delivery. Students in classrooms that received a combination of large group and small group therapy were compared with students in classrooms that received large group therapy and consultation. Methods of evaluation included student progress in motor, visuomotor, and visuoperceptual skills; the therapy needs of each group; teacher satisfaction; and use of available therapy resources. Both methods appeared to represent sound therapy practice. Interaction between the therapist and the teacher in establishing goals and planning group sessions was identified as integral to the success of both methods of service delivery. Recommendations for the following year included placing greater emphasis on achievement of functional goals, establishing group behavioral objectives, and examination of similarities and differences between the services provided by occupational and physical therapy.

SUMMARY

Decision-making is integral to determining who needs physical therapy and why, how cases should be managed, how outcomes should be documented, and what methods should be used for evaluating the effectiveness of clinical services. Clinical decision models for diagnosis, prediction of developmental or treatment outcome, and treatment prescriptions that are based on data from large research studies and statistical models have not been developed for pediatric physical therapy. Although models supported by a database are not currently available, conceptual models and objective methods of documentation and program evaluation can improve the decision-making process. The NCMRR model provides a conceptual framework for relating decision-making to the disabling process. The NCMRR model is applied in subsequent chapters on treatment of children with specific musculoskeletal, neurologic, and cardiopulmonary impairments. The HOAC provides specific guidelines for assessment and treatment decisions that are compatible with the NCMRR model. Although conceptual models are advantageous for organizing and externalizing thought processes, they do not eliminate the need for therapists to have a strong knowledge base, problem solve, and make sound clinical judgments. The limited research suggests that clinical reasoning involves the application not only of theory and psychomotor skill but also of intuitive or implicit thought processes.

Although physical therapists typically evaluate outcomes on the basis of whether children achieve short- and long-term goals or demonstrate improvement on standardized assessments of motor development and function, these methods do not indicate whether the outcomes were the result of intervention, because children are also expected to change as a result of maturational processes. Single-subject research designs are a clinical decision tool that enables pediatric physical therapists to evaluate the efficacy of their interventions for individual clients and to discover information of use in future research. In addition to evaluations of individual client outcomes, professional practice requires evaluation of the overall effectiveness and costs of physical therapy programs. Monitoring of program inputs, implementation, and outputs is enhanced by computerized programs that allow the creation of databases on patient populations and provide a systematic, structured individual client report. Formal methods of program evaluation provide information for assessing whether programs meet important consumer and societal needs, are properly implemented for maximal impact, and actually serve targeted populations. Use of formal experiments and data collection provides the opportunity to study cause and effect relationships among program inputs, interventions, and outcomes. Given the changing and complex nature of health care, pediatric physical therapists are challenged to enhance their use of more scientific evidence and more valid and reliable decision methods as the basis for their practice.

Acknowledgments

The work reported in this chapter was partially supported by a grant to SK Campbell from the Agency for Health Care Policy and Research. Appreciation is expressed to Darl Vander Linden for his suggestions regarding classification of impairments, functional limitations, and disabilities in children with myelodysplasia. Robert J. Palisano was Associate Professor, Program in Pediatric Physical Therapy, Hahnemann University, Philadelphia, at the time this chapter was written.

References

Aylward, GP, & Kenny, TJ. Developmental follow-up: Inherent problems and a conceptual model. Journal of Pediatric Psychology, 4:331–343, 1979.

Ayres, AJ. Southern California Sensory Integration Tests. Los Angeles: Western Psychological Services, 1972.

Barlow, DH, Hayes, SC, & Nelson, RO. The Scientist Practitioner: Research and Accountability in Clinical and Educational Settings. Emsford, NY: Pergamon Press, 1984.

Binkley, J, Finch, E, Hall, J, Black, T, & Gowland, C. Diagnostic classification of patients with low back pain: Report on a survey of physical therapy experts. Physical Therapy, 73:138–155, 1993.

Bobath, B, & Bobath, K. The neurodevelopmental treatment. In Scrutton, D (Ed.), Management of the Motor Disorders of Children with Cerebral Palsy. Philadelphia: JB Lippincott, 1984, pp. 6–18.

Brenner, P. From Novice to Expert: Excellence and Power in Clinical Nursing Practice. Reading, MA: Addison-Wesley, 1984.

Butler, C. Augmentative mobility: Why do it? Physical Medicine and Rehabilitation Clinics of North America, 2:801–815, 1991.

Campbell, SK. Measurement of motor performance in cerebral palsy. In Forrsberg, H, & Hirschfeld, H (Eds.), Movement Disorders in Children. Basel, Switzerland: Karger, 1992, pp. 264–271.

Campbell, SK. Future directions for physical therapy assessment in early infancy. In Wilhelm, IJ (Ed.), Physical Therapy Assessment in Early Infancy. New York: Churchill Livingstone, 1993, pp. 293–308.

Campbell, SK, & Gardner, HG. Physician opinions on referral of children with cerebral palsy to physical therapy. Final Report of Grant R01 HS06429. Bethesda, MD: Agency for Health Care Policy and Research, 1992.

Campbell, SK, & Wilhelm, IJ. Development from birth to three years of fifteen children at high risk for central nervous system dysfunction. Physical Therapy, 65:463–469, 1985.

Carter, RE. A behavioral analysis of interactions between physical therapists and children with cerebral palsy during treatment. Unpublished doctoral dissertation. Dekalb, IL: Northern Illinois University, 1989.

Crenna, P, Inverno, M, Frigo, C, Palmieri, R, & Fedrizzi, E. Pathophysiological profile of gait in children with cerebral palsy. In Forrsberg, H, & Hirschfeld, H (Eds.), Movement Disorders in Children. Basel: Karger, 1992, pp. 186–198.

Dawes, RM, Faust, D, & Meehl, PE. Clinical versus actuarial judgment. Science, 243:1668–1674, 1989.

Dowie, J, & Elstein, A (Eds.). Professional Judgment: A Reader in Clinical Decision Making. New York: Cambridge University Press, 1988.

Echternach, JL, & Rothstein, JM. Hypothesis-oriented algorithms. Physical Therapy, 69:559–564, 1989.

Elstein, AS, Kagan, N, Shulman, LS, Jason, H, & Loupe, MJ. Methods and theory in the study of medical inquiry. Journal of Medical Education, 47:85–92, 1972.

Embrey, DG, Yates, L, & Mott, DH. Effects of neuro-developmental treatment and orthoses on knee flexion during gait: A single subject design. Physical Therapy, 70:626–637, 1990.

Ferrari, F, Cioni, G, & Prechtl, HFR. Qualitative changes of general movements in preterm infants with brain lesions. Early Human Development, 23:193–231, 1990.

Fisher, A, Murray, AE, & Bundy, A. Sensory Integration. Theory and Practice. Philadelphia: FA Davis, 1992.

Fleming, MH. Clinical reasoning in medicine compared to clinical reasoning in occupational therapy. American Journal of Occupational Therapy, 45:988–996, 1991.

Franks, CA, Palisano, RJ, & Darbee, JC. The effect of walking with an assistive device and using a wheelchair on school performance in students with myelomeningocele. Physical Therapy, 71:570–577, 1991.

Goldberg, MJ. Commentary: Measuring outcomes in cerebral palsy. Journal of Pediatric Orthopedics, 11:682–685, 1991.

Gonnella, C. Single-subject experimental paradigm as a clinical decision tool. Physical Therapy, 69:601–609, 1989.

Gordon, BN, & Jens, KG. A conceptual model for tracking high-risk infants and making early service decisions. Journal of Developmental and Behavioral Pediatrics, 9(5):279–286, 1988.

Grimby, G, Finnstam, J, & Jette, AM. On the application of the WHO handicap classification in rehabilitation. Scandinavian Journal of Rehabilitation Medicine, 20:93–98, 1988.

Guccione, AA. Physical therapy diagnosis and the relationship between impairments and function. Physical Therapy, 71:499–503, 1991.

Haley, SM. Commentary on "The effect of walking with an assistive device and using a wheelchair on school performance in students with myelomeningocele." Physical Therapy, 71:577–578, 1991.

Haley, SM, Stephens, TE, & Larsen, AM. Patterns of physical and occupational therapy implementation in early motor intervention. Topics in Early Childhood Special Education, 7(4):46–63, 1988.

Harbst, KB. Indicators of cerebral palsy 1985-1988. Physical and Occupational Therapy in Pediatrics, 10(3):85–107, 1990.

Harris, SR. Research techniques for the clinician. In Connolly, BH, Montgomery, PC (Eds.), Therapeutic Exercise in Developmental Disabilities (2nd ed.). Hixson, TN: Chattanooga Group, 1993, pp. 211–220.

Harris, SR, & Riffle, K. Effects of inhibitive ankle-foot orthoses on standing balance in a child with cerebral palsy. Physical Therapy, 66:663–667, 1986.

Horak, C. Motor development: Traditional and contemporary theories. In Lister, MJ (Ed.), Contemporary Management of Motor Control Problems, Proceedings of the II STEP Conference. Alexandria, VA: Foundation for Physical Therapy, 1991, pp. 44–126.

Hinderer, KA, Harris, SR, Purdy, AH, Chew, DE, Staheli, LT, McLaughlin, JF, & Jaffe, KM. Effects of 'tone-reducing' vs. standard plaster-casts on gait improvement of children with cerebral palsy. Developmental Medicine and Child Neurology, 30:370–377, 1988.

Holmes, GE, Britain, LA, Simpson, RL, & Hassanein, RS. Developmental progress of five groups of disabled children attending an early intervention program. Physical and Occupational Therapy in Pediatrics, 7(1):3–18, 1987.

Horak, FB. Assumptions underlying motor control for neurologic rehabilitation. In Lister, MJ (Ed.), Contemporary Management of Motor Control Problems: Proceedings of the II STEP Conference. Alexandria, VA: Foundation for Physical Therapy, 1991, pp. 11–27.

Jenkins, D. A practical introduction to databases: Part 2. Biomedical Instrumentation and Technology, 23:109–112, 1989.

Kanda, T, Yuge, M, & Yamori, Y. Early physiotherapy in the treatment of spastic diplegia. Developmental Medicine and Child Neurology, 26:438–444, 1984.

Kopp, CB. Developmental risk: Historical reflections. In Osofsky, JD (Ed.), Handbook of Infant Development. New York: John Wiley & Sons, 1987, pp. 881–912.

Larin, HM. Knowledge in practice: Motor learning theories in pediatric physiotherapy. Unpublished doctoral dissertation. University of Toronto, 1992.

Laskas, SA, Mullen, SL, Nelson, DL, & Willson-Broyles, M. Enhancement of two motor functions of the lower extremity in a child with spastic quadriplegia. Physical Therapy, 65:11–16, 1985.

Lehmann, JF, Warren, CG, Smith, W, & Larson, J. Computerized data management as an aid to clinical decision making in rehabilitation medicine. Archives of Physical Medicine and Rehabilitation, 65:260–262, 1984.

Magistro, CM. Clinical decision making in physical therapy. Physical Therapy, 69:525–534, 1989.

Mattingly, C. What is clinical reasoning? American Journal of Occupational Therapy, 45:979–986, 1991.

Molnar, GE (Ed.). Pediatric Rehabilitation (2nd ed.). Baltimore: Williams & Wilkins, 1992.

Nagi, SZ. Disability and Rehabilitation. Columbus, OH: Ohio State University Press, 1969.

Nagi, SZ. Disability concepts revisited: Implications for prevention. In Pope, AN, & Tarlov, AR (Eds.), Disability in America: Toward a National Agenda for Prevention. Washington, DC: National Academy Press, 1991, pp. 309–327.

Nagi, SZ. Some conceptual issues in disability and rehabilitation. In Sussman, MB (Ed.), Sociology and Rehabilitation. New York: American Sociological Association, n.d., pp. 100–113.

National Institutes of Health. Research Plan for the National Center for Medical Rehabilitation Research. NIH Publication No. 93–3509. Bethesda, MD: National Institutes of Health, 1993.

Nelson, KB, & Ellenberg, JH. Children who "outgrew" cerebral palsy. Pediatrics, 69:529–536, 1982.

Norton, BJ, & Strube, MJ. Making decisions based on group designs and meta-analysis. Physical Therapy, 69:594–600, 1989.

Ottenbacher, KJ. Evaluating Clinical Change: Strategies for Occupational and Physical Therapists. Baltimore: Williams & Wilkins, 1986.

Palisano, RJ. Comparison of two methods of service delivery for students with learning disabilities. Physical and Occupational Therapy in Pediatrics, 9(3):79–100, 1989.

Payton, O. Clinical reasoning process in physical therapy. Physical Therapy, 65:924–928, 1985.

Piper, MC, Darrah, J, Pinnell, L, Watt, MJ, & Byrne, P. The consistency of sequential examinations in the early detection of neurological dysfunction. Physical & Occupational Therapy in Pediatrics, 11(3):27–44, 1991.

Pope, AN, & Tarlov, AR (Eds.). Disability in America: Toward a National Agenda for Prevention. Washington, DC: National Academy Press, 1991.

Public Law 99-457, Education of the Handicapped Act Amendments of 1986.

Public Law 102-119, Individuals with Disabilities Education Amendments of 1991.

Purdy, AH, Deitz, JC, & Harris, SR. Efficacy of two treatment approaches to reduce tongue protrusion of children with Down syndrome. Developmental Medicine and Child Neurology, 29:469–476, 1987.

Rodgers, SJ, Donovon, CM, D'Eugenio, DB, Brown, SL, Lynch, EW, Moersch, MS, & Schafer, DS. Early intervention developmental profile. In Schafer, DS, Moersch, MS (Eds.), Developmental Programming for Infants and Young Children, Vol. 2. Ann Arbor, MI: University of Michigan Press, 1977.

Rogers, J, & Masagatani, G. Clinical reasoning of occupational therapists during the initial assessment of physically disabled patients. Occupational Therapy Journal of Research, 2:195–219, 1982.

Rosenblith, JF. A singular career: Nancy Bayley. Developmental Psychology, 28:747–758, 1992.

Rothstein, JM, & Echternach, JL. Hypothesis-oriented algorithm for clinicians: A method for evaluation and treatment planning. Physical Therapy, 66:1388–1394, 1986.

Sackett, DL, Haynes, RB, & Tugwell, P. Clinical Epidemiology: A Basic Science for Clinical Medicine. Boston: Little, Brown, 1985.

Schenkman, M, & Butler, RB. A model for multisystem evaluation, interpretation, and treatment of individuals with neurologic dysfunction. Physical Therapy, 69:538–547, 1989.

Shadish, WR Jr., Cook, TD, & Leviton, LC. Foundations of Program Evaluation: Theories of Practice. Newbury Park, CA: Sage Publications, 1991.

Shurtleff, DB. Computer data bases for pediatric disability: Clinical and research applications. Physical Medicine and Rehabilitation Clinics of North America, 2:665–687, 1991.

Slagle, TA, & Gould, JB. Database use in neonatal intensive care units: Success or failure. Pediatrics, 90:959–965, 1992.

Slovick, P, & Lichtenstein, S. Comparison of Bayesian and regression approaches to the study of information processing in judgment. Organizational Behavior and Human Performance, 6:649–744, 1971.

Tiffin, J. Purdue Pegboard Examiner Manual. Chicago: Scientific Research Associates, 1968.

Voss, DE, Ionta, MK, & Myers BJ. Proprioceptive Neuromuscular Facilitation (3rd ed.). Philadelphia: Harper & Row, 1985.

Wang, MC, & Ellet, CD. Program validation: The state of the art. Topics in Early Childhood Special Education, 1(4):35–49, 1982.

Waters, RL, & Lunsford, BR. Energy cost of paraplegic locomotion. Journal of Bone and Joint Surgery (American), 67:1245–1250, 1985.

Watts, N. Decision analysis: A tool for improving physical therapy practice and education. In Wolf, SL (Ed.), Clinical Decision Making in Physical Therapy. Philadelphia: FA Davis, 1985, pp. 7–23.

Watts, N. Clinical decision analysis. Physical Therapy, 69:569–576, 1989.

Weed, LL, & Zimny, NJ. The problem-oriented system, problem-knowledge coupling, and clinical decision making. Physical Therapy, 69:565–568, 1989.

Wolery, M, & Bailey, DD. Alternatives to impact evaluation: Suggestions for program evaluation in early intervention. Journal of the Division for Early Childhood, 4:27–37, 1984.

World Health Organization. International Classification of Impairments, Disabilities, and Handicaps. Geneva: World Health Organization, 1980.

Section Two

Management of Musculoskeletal Impairment

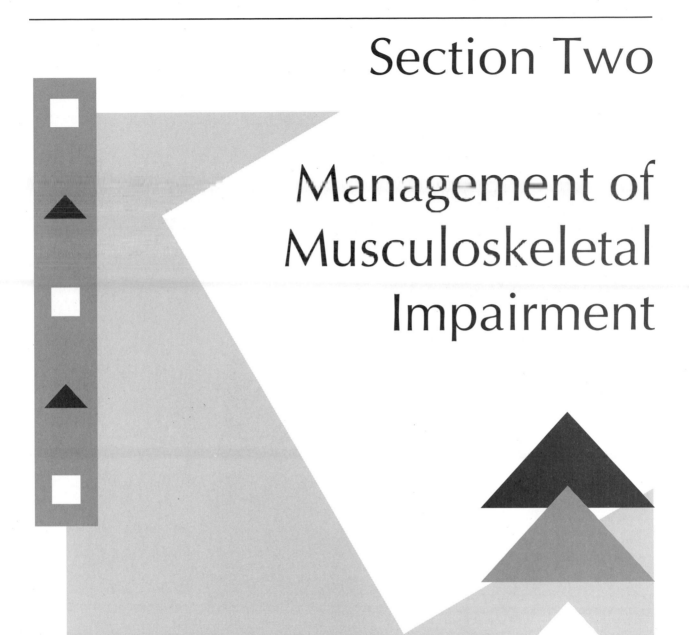

DARL W. VANDER LINDEN, PT, PhD
Section Editor

Chapter 8

Juvenile Rheumatoid Arthritis

SHIRLEY A. SCULL, PT, MS

Chronic childhood arthritis can result from many different disorders, of which juvenile rheumatoid arthritis (JRA) is one of the most common. Other rheumatic diseases that cause joint pathology include systemic lupus erythematosus, Lyme disease, juvenile ankylosing spondylitis, scleroderma, and dermatomyositis. Children with hemophilia may also suffer recurrent hemarthroses resulting in arthritis (see Chapter 9).

A team of professionals is required to manage the musculoskeletal complications of these disorders. The pediatric rheumatologist, orthopaedist, physical therapist, and occupational therapist all contribute to the decision-making process regarding musculoskeletal problems. Parent education about the disease as well as case management is often provided by a nurse or social worker. Consultation may be obtained from psychologists, ophthalmologists, and cardiologists, depending on the child's needs (Rhodes, 1991).

ROLE OF THE THERAPIST

The physical therapist and occupational therapist often share responsibility for musculoskeletal evaluation and treatment of the child with JRA. They instruct the child and parent in a home-care program that includes splinting, exercises, positioning, joint conservation, activities of daily living (ADL), and advice regarding recreational activities. Direct treatment may be carried out intensively in an inpatient rehabilitation facility with the goals of improving functional skills and of maximizing flexibility and strength. More often, children with JRA are treated regularly as outpatients or receive physical therapy services at school.

On the basis of a comprehensive musculoskeletal assessment, the therapist develops a problem list for each patient. Impairments such as loss of motion, weakness, postural deviations, and pain are analyzed for their impact on present function as well as their potential for creating future problems. Relationships between impairments and functional limitations are identified. Examples include muscle weakness secondary to disuse with an antalgic gait or knee flexion contracture secondary to leg length discrepancy. Part of the role of the physical therapist is early recognition of potential problems and development of a treatment plan that involves prevention of secondary impairments.

The patient's goals and the family supports must be understood. The child's developmental age is used as a yardstick to assist in determining appro priate functional goals and treatment methods. Guidance by the therapist may be necessary if the child's or the family's goals are unrealistic. Goals are prioritized so that the therapy program and home instructions are focused on those impairments and functional limitations that contribute most to current disabilities in daily life. Measurable goals that the patient understands and can monitor provide incentive toward further effort.

INCIDENCE AND DIAGNOSTIC CLASSIFICATIONS

JRA is one of the more frequently occurring chronic illnesses of childhood. A study in 1983 at the Mayo Clinic estimated the annual incidence to be 13.9 per 100,000. The prevalence was found to be 113.4 cases per 100,000 (Towner et al., 1983). There are 160,000 to 190,000 children with JRA in the United States (Cassidy & Petty, 1990).

The diagnostic criteria for JRA have been defined by the American Rheumatism Association (Brewer et al., 1977). The age at onset is arbitrarily set at younger than 16 years to distinguish JRA from adult-onset disease. Arthritis is evidenced by joint swelling or effusion and the presence of two or more of the following signs: heat, limitation of range of motion (ROM), and tenderness or pain on motion. Symptoms must persist for a minimum of 6 weeks but preferably for 3 months. Because no definitive laboratory tests are available to identify JRA, the diagnosis is made by exclusion of other diseases, such as joint infections, trauma, malig-

nancies, or systemic illnesses, depending on the presenting symptoms.

Clinical signs during onset, defined as the first 6 months of the disease, are used to classify three distinct subtypes of JRA (Table 8–1) (Cassidy & Petty, 1990). Pauciarticular JRA is the most common subtype, affecting one to four joints, often a knee, ankle, or wrist. Patients with pauciarticular JRA have a 20% chance of developing inflammation of the iris and ciliary body known as anterior uveitis or iridocyclitis (Petty, 1987). Eye involvement is often asymptomatic, and therefore slit lamp biomicroscopy by an ophthalmologist is required at the time of diagnosis and periodically thereafter. Complications of iridocyclitis include synechiae, band keratopathy, and cataract. Functional blindness has been reported in 15 to 40% of eyes with uveitis, although routine screening and earlier diagnosis are improving these statistics (Petty, 1987). Topical corticosteroids are prescribed to control inflammation and prevent blindness.

Polyarticular disease onset (involving 5 or more joints) occurs in 40% of children with JRA. The number of joints involved can be 20 or more in some children. Joints commonly affected include the knees, ankles, elbows, wrists, cervical spine, and temporomandibular joint; a symmetric distribution is typical.

Systemic disease is the least common subtype, occurring in 10% of cases. As the name implies, systemic JRA is characterized by severe constitutional symptoms, including intermittent fevers to 40°C (104°F), rash (erythematous macules on the trunk and proximal extremities), hepatosplenomeg-

TABLE 8–1. **CLASSIFICATION OF THE TYPES OF ONSET OF JUVENILE RHEUMATOID ARTHRITIS**

Criterion	Polyarthritis	Oligoarthritis (Pauciarticular Disease)	Systemic Disease
Frequency of cases	40%	50%	10%
Number of joints involved	≥5	≤4	Variable
Age at onset	Throughout childhood; peak at 1–3 years	Early childhood; peak at 1–2 years	Throughout childhood; no peak
Sex ratio (F:M)	3:1	5:1	1:1
Systemic involvement	Moderate involvement	Not present	Prominent
Occurrence of chronic uveitis	5%	20%	Rare
Frequency of seropositivity			
Rheumatoid factors	10% (increases with age)	Rare	Rare
Antinuclear antibodies	40–50%	75–85%*	10%
Prognosis	Guarded to moderately good	Excellent except eyesight	Moderate to poor

*In girls with uveitis.
From Cassidy, JT, & Petty, RE. Textbook of Rheumatology (2nd ed.). New York, Churchill Livingstone, 1990.

aly, lymphadenopathy, pleuritis, and pericarditis. Onset of joint involvement may lag behind these systemic symptoms by months or, occasionally, 1 or 2 years.

ETIOLOGY AND PATHOPHYSIOLOGY

Multiple etiologies may be responsible for the various subtypes of diseases classified together as JRA, or a single cause may evolve into different clinical patterns as it interacts with the host (Cassidy & Petty, 1990). The etiology of JRA is unknown, although it is considered an autoimmune disorder and is probably multifactorial in origin. There are very few reports of cases of JRA in more than one member of the family. Studies of human leukocyte antigen types, however, show a probable correlation between genetic predisposition to the disease and specific subtypes.

Often an environmental trigger such as infection or trauma precedes the onset of JRA, although the precise relationship between these events is not clear (Cassidy & Petty, 1990). Despite intensive efforts, no specific infectious agent has been identified in the blood or synovial tissue. Whatever the inciting event, joint inflammation is initiated and perpetuated by immunologic mechanisms.

The predominant cells in the joint fluid are neutrophils. These cells release a number of chemicals after ingesting immune complexes and cell debris. The chemicals cause pain, swelling, warmth, and effusion into the joint.

In the synovial membrane, the predominant cells are lymphocytes, mostly T cells. These cells are probably activated by the persistence of putative antigen. This, in turn, leads to production of antibodies by B cells and stimulation of macrophages. Cytokines produced by macrophages cause proliferation of fibroblasts, production of prostaglandins, and bone resorption. The inflammatory response causes the subsynovial tissues to become edematous and hyperemic. The synovium begins to proliferate, resulting in massive overgrowth called pannus. The pannus can actually invade the adjacent cartilage and bone, resulting in erosions.

Late joint changes include adhesions and osteophytes. Surrounding tissues such as tendons and ligaments undergo fibrosis, resulting in contracture. The underlying bone is scarred and damaged (Fig 8-1), and the joint shape may become irregular. Subluxation can occur at the wrists and small joints

FIGURE 8-1. Synovial hypertrophy and destruction of cartilage and bone.

of the hands and feet, or less commonly, there may be posterior subluxation of the tibia on the femur.

MEDICAL MANAGEMENT

A variety of medications are used to control joint inflammation (Table 8-2) (Cassidy & Petty, 1990). The first-line medication is a nonsteroidal anti-inflammatory drug such as a salicylate, naproxen, or tolmetin. A slow-acting antirheumatic drug (SAARD) such as a gold salt, an antimalarial agent, or sulfasalazine may be added to the drug program. Corticosteroids are potent and effective anti-inflammatory agents, but long-term use is avoided because of side effects such as growth retardation and Cushing's syndrome. Methotrexate has been shown to have a dramatic effect in controlling this disease, although long-term follow-up is needed to rule out the possibility of adverse side effects (Giannini et al., 1992). Newer experimental approaches include cytotoxic agents and immune-modulation therapy (Athreya & Cassidy, 1991). Frequent laboratory testing is required to monitor for toxic side effects of any drug program.

PROGNOSIS

The number of children with JRA who enter into remission varies with the subtype. Wallace and Levinson (1991) reviewed long-term outcome stud-

TABLE 8-2. **DRUG THERAPY FOR JUVENILE RHEUMATOID ARTHRITIS**

Medication	Dose	Indication	Toxicity
Aspirin	75–90 mg/kg/d	Control of pain, stiffness, and inflammation	Salicylism (lethargy, hyperpnea, tinnitus), gastrointestinal irritation, bleeding, hepatitis
Nonsteroidal anti-inflammatory agents	Varies with drug	Control of pain, stiffness, and inflammation	Gastrointestinal irritation, hepatitis, decreased renal function
Hydroxychloroquine	7 mg/kg/d	Selective use for arthritis	Dermatitis, keratopathy, retinopathy
Gold salt	0.75 mg/kg/mo	Polyarthritis unresponsive to nonsteroidal anti-inflammatory agents	Dermatitis, nephritis, stomatitis, bone marrow suppression
D-Penicillamine	10 mg/kg/d	Polyarthritis unresponsive to other regimens	Dermatitis, nephritis, lupus-like syndrome
Sulfasalazine	40–60 mg/kg/d	Polyarthritis unresponsive to other regimens	Bone marrow suppression, dermatitis, gastrointestinal irritation
Corticosteroid drugs			
Systemic	Prednisone, 1 mg/kg/d (as low a dose as possible)	Life-threatening systemic disease, chronic uveitis	Growth retardation, infection, Cushing's syndrome
Ophthalmic	4 drops/d	Chronic uveitis	Cataracts, glaucoma
Intra-articular	30-mg prednisolone–TBA	Selective use for arthritis	Infection
Immunosuppressive agent	Varies with drug	Life-threatening systemic disease	Infection, bone marrow suppression, sterility, oncogenesis

From Cassidy, JT, & Petty, RE. Textbook of Rheumatology (2nd ed.). New York, Churchill Livingstone, 1990.

ies and discussed implications for early and aggressive medical management of inflammation before onset of joint destruction. Ten years after onset, 22 to 71% of children with pauciarticular JRA had active disease, 40 to 50% of children with polyarticular JRA had active disease, and 25 to 58% of children with systemic JRA had active disease. Studies focusing on functional outcome are limited by the use of the older Steinbrocker classification system (Steinbrocker et al., 1949), which groups all children with mild to severe functional limitations into class III (Table 8–3). An average of 31% of

patients showed severe functional deficits (class III or IV) when followed for more than 5 years. Children with polyarticular disease who are rheumatoid factor positive have the worst prognosis for unremitting arthritis with joint erosions (Schaller, 1983). Children with pauciarticular JRA do well functionally, except for possible complications related to vision. Even children whose disease remits may have long-term musculoskeletal complications of contractures, postural deviations, and localized growth disturbances.

TABLE 8-3. **STEINBROCKER CLASSIFICATION FOR RHEUMATOID ARTHRITIS**

I = Complete functional capacity with ability to carry on all usual duties without handicaps
II = Functional capacity adequate to conduct normal activities despite handicap or discomfort or limited mobility of one or more joints
III = Functional capacity adequate to perform only few or none of the duties of usual occupation or of self-care
IV = Largely or wholly incapacitated with patient bedridden or confined to wheelchair, permitting little or no self-care

From Steinbrocker, O, Traeger, CH, & Batterman, RC. Therapeutic criteria in rheumatoid arthritis. Journal of the American Medical Association, *140*:659–662, 1949. Copyright 1949, American Medical Association.

▌DISABILITIES

The type and degree of disability vary depending on the age of the child, the severity of the disease, and the family's coping strategies.

A nondisabled toddler or preschooler begins to achieve separation from the parent and some independence with ADL such as feeding, dressing, and toileting. A child with JRA who is in pain and refuses to cooperate, or one who gains attention because of his or her need for help, may cause difficulty with parent-child interactions. Parents may be frustrated, be tired, or feel guilty. Some parents adopt a style of being overprotective, discouraging their child's engagement in appropriate tasks such as playground activities with peers. Opportunities to master certain gross motor skills such as bike riding may be missed because of fear of injury.

The school-aged child may have poor school attendance because of morning stiffness and time-consuming morning care. Some children are unable to walk on arising and must take a bath or do exercises to loosen up. Difficulty with mobility, such as needing to use an elevator instead of stairs, or inability to dress or toilet independently may lead to the child's rejection by other students. Postural deviations and other cosmetic differences have an impact on the child's self-esteem. Participation in physical education classes to the student's tolerance should be encouraged, but activities need to be monitored to protect the joints (Scull & Athreya, in press). Some children require a special, individualized education plan at school to address transportation, time requirements for examinations, adaptive physical education, or other related services. Physical therapists and occupational therapists in schools may provide direct services or consultation. Appropriate goals relate to attaining an optimal education by providing assistance with handwriting, mobility skills, physical education, or ADL (Whitehouse et al., 1989).

The adolescent's social roles in dating, driving, and entering the work force are affected by functional impairments. Career selection must take into account the physical limitations of the individual. College plans may be complicated by the need for wheelchair accessibility and assistance from attendants. The ability to become fully independent from the family will be tested at this time.

The mature patient who becomes sexually active may require counseling to be comfortable during sexual activities. Pregnancy requires special consideration because of the effects on the arthritis. Medications may need to be altered because of the effects on the fetus. Delivery by cesarean section may be recommended.

▮ MUSCULOSKELETAL IMPAIRMENTS

Joint Pathology

Joint pathology produces restricted ROM and, typically, flexion contractures, which should be assessed using a goniometer. Measurements of active ROM provide functional data but may be limited by joint pathology, weakness, or pain. Passive ROM provides a more accurate baseline for joint pathology and should be reliable for most joints to within ±5°. Additional assessment of the joints should include ligamentous laxity and postural def-

icits, such as valgus or varus. Measurements of circumference can document swelling but are confusing in the presence of bony overgrowth. Synovial thickness, heat, or redness is also noted.

Inactivity stiffness can interfere with the ability to walk for up to 2 hours each morning. A warm tub bath is recommended on arising, with exercises performed in the water to decrease morning stiffness. The use of a small whirlpool may decrease pain since sensory receptors are fired that compete with pain signals (Michlovitz, 1986). In my experience, however, the primary benefits are the warmth and buoyancy of the water rather than its aeration. Other methods used to manage morning stiffness include resting night splints for the knees and a sleeping bag or blanket sleeper pajamas that provide neutral warmth (Scull, 1989).

Early radiographic changes include soft tissue swelling about the joints, widening of the joint space, osteoporosis near the joint, and periosteal new bone formation, especially in the phalanges, metacarpals, and metatarsals (Cassidy & Petty, 1990). After 2 or more years of active disease, radiographic changes may include marginal erosions and joint space narrowing secondary to loss of articular cartilage. Bony ankylosis may be seen, especially of the carpal or tarsal joints or cervical spine. Loose bodies that mechanically block joint motion may also be present.

Abnormalities of the hip occur in about 35% of cases. In young children, coxa valga may occur. Forces across the femoral epiphysis may cause widening of the femoral neck, resulting in restricted motion. Avascular necrosis can occur, sometimes as a complication of corticosteroid use, resulting in disabling hip pain and decreased function. Hip motion should be closely monitored because children with active hip disease often develop difficulty with ambulation.

Loss of normal flexibility can also be caused by muscle imbalance around a joint. This typically occurs in the hip flexors, adductors, hamstrings, and gastrocnemius of the lower extremities and in the wrist and finger flexors of the upper extremities. Tendon sheaths, which are lined with synovium, can develop tenosynovitis, typically manifested in the flexors and extensors extrinsic to the hand, resulting in loss of gliding motion.

Contractures

Contractures occur in a majority of cases of JRA. Minor contracture in joints of the lower extremities (less than 10°) may not have functional significance. However, if allowed to progress toward 15°

to 20°, contractures can cause dysfunctional mobility or problems with ADL. Long-standing contractures may lead to growth abnormalities of the joint, the limb, or the spine, since secondary postural compensations are adopted because of abnormal alignment. Useful physical therapy techniques include exercise and splinting designed to lengthen the antagonist and strengthen the agonist (Scull, 1989). Later in the chapter, the use of continuous passive motion (CPM) for early deformities and of surgery for those that are fixed is discussed.

EXERCISE

Active ROM exercises are extremely important in the management of JRA. The patient should move all the joints through their full available ROM at least once a day. Combinations of movement patterns are taught for efficiency. Passive stretching exercises are avoided for acutely inflamed joints as well as for those that show signs of instability or mechanical derangement. Gentle, passive ROM exercise is indicated for contractures if joint inflammation is under medical control and if the restriction is believed to be at least partially muscular, with a stretchy end-feel.

Flexion contractures of the hips and knees may be managed by gravity-assisted stretching in the prone position for 20 minutes per day, with feet suspended over the edge of the support (Fig. 8–2) (Scull et al., 1986). The weight of the lower leg drops the knee into extension. A sandbag may be placed over the buttocks for stabilization. If the patient lacks full neck rotation, a towel roll applied at the forehead may provide comfort.

Hand placement when passively stretching a knee flexion contracture must avoid use of a long lever arm because of the potential for posterior subluxation of the tibia on the femur. In addition, the patient may not tolerate hand placement over the patella.

If shoulder motion is available above 90°, exercise while in the supine position will allow gravity to assist the shoulder stretch. A baton held in both hands allows the patient to perform active assisted shoulder flexion. Proprioceptive neuromuscular facilitation patterns may also be taught.

At the neck, ROM should be assessed in both supine and sitting positions, with manual stabilization of the shoulders. A kyphotic sitting posture often interferes with optimal neck ROM. Apophyseal joint involvement may result in torticollis, with unilateral restriction of rotation, lateral flexion, and extension and can proceed to fusion (Fried et al., 1983). Moist heat applied before the exercise program may be helpful in obtaining improved ROM. Clinicians must be mindful of the potential for atlantoaxial subluxation, which is a contraindication for exercise and should be identified by radiographs. In this instance, a cervical collar is recommended for car travel to avert deceleration injury in case of an impact.

SPLINTING

Slow prolonged stretch such as that provided by a dynamic splint is often more effective for reducing flexion contractures than exercise (Hepburn, 1987), although this has not yet been documented by clinical research for children with JRA. I have used dynamic splints (Fig. 8–3) successfully on elbow and knee flexion contractures for children aged 2 years and older. The tension is set to patient tolerance and can be advanced as the contracture improves. Results should be measurable (greater than 10°) within 2 weeks. Some patients are able to tolerate splints during the hours of sleep, which gives maximum benefit. Others wear them two or three times a day for 1-hour periods. Traction may also be used to provide a prolonged stretch to flexion contractures but requires confinement to bed.

Serial casting or drop-out casts are used occasionally for knee flexion contractures that do not respond to exercise, positioning, or dynamic splinting. However, the patient is at risk for losing flexion when the joint is placed in a cast in extension. Therefore, the cast should be bivalved for daily exercise or changed every 3 days with an exercise session scheduled before reapplying the cast. This treatment option is typically selected as a last resort before surgery and would increase compliance for the patient who refused a home exercise program of exercise or splinting. Careful measurement of the ROM at the time of cast change provides evidence regarding the need to continue the treatment.

FIGURE 8–2. The prone position is used to stretch hip and knee flexion contractures.

FIGURE 8–3. Dynamic splinting is effective in stretching knee flexion contractures.

Weakness

Secondary changes are seen in the muscles, especially atrophy due to disuse. Assessment should include manual muscle testing of key functional groups and may be done by isometric testing if resistance through the range increases discomfort (Scull, 1989). Strength ratings of less than 4 on a scale of 1 to 5 in lower extremity antigravity muscles may be expected to result in gait deviations and functional limitations, such as inability to climb stairs. If the child is younger than 5 years of age, manual muscle testing may be difficult, and the ability to perform certain developmental skills is a more useful way to test strength.

Strengthening exercises may be done isometrically if active exercise causes pain. Concentric and eccentric contractions are taught, if tolerated. Resisted exercises are restricted to weights less than a few pounds; Theraband (Hygenic Corporation, Akron, OH) is a useful product in pediatric treat-

ment programs and can be progressed by choosing the next color of resistance. Play activities such as bicycle or tricycle riding are also useful for strengthening the lower extremities. Exercise in water can improve both strength and flexibility while reducing pain.

Growth Disturbances and Postural Abnormalities

JRA may affect posture and growth since the epiphyseal plates are open in children (White, 1990). Generalized growth retardation may be the result of the basic disease process or may be related to the side effects of use of corticosteroids. Small stature may be compounded by premature closure of the epiphyses. Proper attention to nutrition has to be incorporated into a management program (Henderson et al., 1992). Research protocols using growth hormone are in the process of being tested.

Local growth disturbances may result in leg length discrepancy. An increase in blood supply to the epiphysis because of inflammation results in overgrowth of the limb, especially with unilateral knee involvement. Posture should be assessed periodically and leg lengths measured for symmetry. A shoe lift can be added to correct leg length if it improves posture or gait.

Scoliosis, kyphosis, torticollis, and cervical lordosis may be the result of spinal involvement or habitual posture secondary to pain. Leg length discrepancy may also cause an oblique pelvis and secondary scoliosis.

Undergrowth of the mandible, called micrognathia, is seen in about 20% of cases of JRA, usually in children with polyarticular disease (White, 1990). Radiographic changes show shortening of the body and vertical rami of the mandible with widening of the mandibular notch. Orthodontic work may be required to correct for resultant malocclusion (Mayro et al., 1991).

Pain

Pain is assessed in children in a variety of ways, depending on the child's age (McGrath, 1990; Varni et al., 1987). One option is use of a visual analogue scale, which is a 10-cm line anchored at one end with the words "No pain" and at the other end with "Pain as bad as it could be." The child draws a line through the estimated amount of pain. Good correlation has been demonstrated between the child, parent, and physician's estimates of the

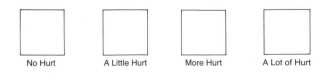

| No Hurt | A Little Hurt | More Hurt | A Lot of Hurt |

Pick the colors that mean *No Hurt, A Little Hurt, More Hurt,* and *A Lot of Hurt* to you and color in the boxes. Now, using those colors, color in the body to show how you feel. Where you have no hurt, use the *No Hurt* color to color in your body. If you have hurt or pain, use the color that tells how much hurt you have.

FRONT   BACK

FIGURE 8–4. Pain may be assessed by allowing a child to color a body map. Intensity of pain is matched with four separate colors.

present pain (Varni et al., 1987). A body outline can be given to the child to draw the location of pain (Fig. 8–4). Four developmentally appropriate labels of pain intensity are discussed, and the child selects a crayon color to represent each one. A list of pain descriptors has also been developed for pediatrics as part of the Pediatric Pain Questionnaire developed by Varni and associates (1987).

Because children with JRA are already taking one or more medications, the physician has few choices for ongoing management of chronic pain. Behavioral management techniques involving muscle relaxation, meditative breathing, and guided imagery can be taught to the child. Parents may also be instructed in appropriate behavior modification techniques that involve encouraging adaptive behaviors and discouraging maladaptive pain behaviors.

FUNCTIONAL LIMITATIONS

The combination of pain, restricted ROM, muscle weakness, and skeletal deformities may result in significant functional limitations for the patient. The patient with mild involvement may show some gait deviations but be fully functional in the home and school environment. The patient with more severe involvement may require a wheelchair for community mobility and be dependent for many ADL. The American College of Rheumatology has proposed four categories of disabilities based on functional deficits (Hochberg et al., 1992):

Class I   Completely able to perform usual ADL (self-care, vocational, and avocational)

Class II   Able to perform usual self-care and vocational activities but limited in avocational activities

Class III   Able to perform usual self-care activities but limited in vocational and avocational activities

Class IV   Limited in ability to perform usual self-care, vocational, and avocational activities

These global functional categories have been studied in adults but not in children.

Two tools called the Juvenile Arthritis Functional Assessment Scale (JAFAS) (Lovell et al., 1989) and the Childhood Health Assessment Questionnaire (CHAQ) (Singh et al., in press) are specifically designed to assess the functional limitations for children with arthritis. The JAFAS is a list of 10 activities with accompanying criterion times (Fig. 8–5). A child is graded a 0 when he or she meets or exceeds a criterion, 1 if he or she completes the activity slowly, and 2 if he or she is unable to perform. The test takes less than 10 minutes to complete and requires a minimum of simple equipment. A version is also designed to be scored by parental report and is called the Juvenile Arthritis Functional Assessment Report (JAFAR) (Howe et al., 1991).

The CHAQ (Fig. 8–6) covers dressing and grooming, arising, eating, walking, hygiene, reaching, gripping, and community mobility. The parent or child completes a checklist with four scoring choices:

1. Unable to do
2. Does with much difficulty
3. Does with some difficulty
4. Does without any difficulty

A list of aids or devices may be checked off to document which assistive devices are used.

For each activity, please record how long the child took to perform the activity. If the activity was completed in less than or equal to the criterion time, then score the item as 0; if completed but requiring longer than the criterion time, score the item as 1; if unable to perform the activity, score the item as 2.

Activity	Criterion Time (seconds)	Observed Time (seconds)	Item Score 0	1	2
1. Button shirt/blouse	22.4	_____	_____	_____	_____
2. Pull shirt or sweater over head	14.6	_____	_____	_____	_____
3. Pull on both socks	27.2	_____	_____	_____	_____
4. Cut food with knife and fork	12.8	_____	_____	_____	_____
5. Get into bed	3.4	_____	_____	_____	_____
6. Get out of bed	2.9	_____	_____	_____	_____
7. Pick something up off of floor from standing position	2.4	_____	_____	_____	_____
8. From standing position sit on floor, then stand up	4.0	_____	_____	_____	_____
9. Walk 50 feet without assistance	15.1	_____	_____	_____	_____
10. Walk up flight of 5 steps	3.7	_____	_____	_____	_____
		TOTAL SCORE	_____		

FIGURE 8–5. The Juvenile Arthritis Functional Assessment Scale (JAFAS) is a list of 10 functional activities that must be completed within the criterion time. (Reprinted with permission from Lovell, DJ, Howe, S, Shear, E, Hartner, S, McGirr, G, Schultz, M, & Levinson, J. Development of a disability measurement tool for juvenile rheumatoid arthritis: The Juvenile Arthritis Functional Assessment Scale. Arthritis and Rheumatism, *32*:1390–1395, 1989.)

Gait Abnormalities

Gait deviations are often the primary functional problem addressed by the physical therapist. Lechner and colleagues (1987) studied 30 children with JRA using the gait laboratory and described common deviations, such as decreased velocity, cadence, and stride length, as compared with controls. They also documented increased anterior pelvic tilt throughout the gait cycle, with decreased hip extension and decreased plantar flexion at toe-off (Fig. 8–7). Gait deviations may be caused by one or a combination of impairments such as contractures, weakness, or pain. The clinician can develop hypotheses for treatment by analyzing the cause of the dysfunctional gait. Assessment must also incorporate climbing activities such as ascending and descending stairs, ramps, and curbs.

Common foot deformities include loss of subtalar motion, such as a valgus hindfoot, combined with pronation (Fig. 8–8). Forefoot involvement is common and may be responsible for gait deviations such as lack of push-off, shortened stride length, and stiff-legged gait. The great toe may lose extension at the metatarsophalangeal joint or may deviate into a valgus position. The toes often develop a hammer toe posture.

Selecting comfortable yet supportive footwear is important for gait. Sneakers are generally the preferred footwear because they have a good arch support and cushioning throughout the sole. Special shoe modifications may need to be added, such as a metatarsal bar to provide a rocker-like surface to the sole of the forefoot, allowing a mechanical means to toe-off without requiring hyperextension of the toes (Fig. 8–9). Ankle-foot orthoses may be useful if the patient has pain in the ankles on weight bearing. Newer orthotic packages allow the therapist to experiment with a variety of custom-molded modifications to the shoes at a minimal cost.

A small percentage of children require an assistive device for ambulation. This may be indicated if lower extremity pain, contracture, or weakness prevents efficient weight bearing. Typically, such a child has polyarticular disease with significant upper extremity involvement necessitating the use of platform crutches (Lofstrand or axillary) or a wheeled walker with platform attachments to avoid weight bearing on the small joints of the wrist and hand.

Community Mobility

Children who are unable to achieve community mobility may require a wheelchair for outings. In this instance, lightweight wheelchairs are medically justifiable for joint conservation. In my clinic population, fewer than 5% of children require wheelchairs for community access or as their sole means of mobility. In the preschool years, occasional use of a stroller may be necessary, a child's wagon and tricycle are other alternatives. By the time of entrance to high school, a power wheelchair may be needed for distances. Patients with adequate lower extremity alignment and upper extremity strength

In this section, we are interested in learning how your child's illness affects his/her ability to function in daily life. Please feel free to add any comments on the back of this page. In the following questions, please check the one response that best describes your child's usual activities (averaged over an entire day) *OVER THE PAST WEEK*. If your child has difficulty in doing a certain activity or is unable to do it because he/she is too young but NOT because he/she is RESTRICTED BY ARTHRITIS, please mark it as "Not Applicable." ONLY NOTE THOSE DIFFICULTIES OR LIMITATIONS THAT ARE DUE TO ARTHRITIS.

	Without ANY Difficulty	With SOME Difficulty	With MUCH Difficulty	UNABLE To Do	Not Applicable
DRESSING & GROOMING					
Is your child able to:					
• Dress, including tying shoelaces and doing buttons?					
• Shampoo his/her hair?					
• Remove socks?					
• Cut fingernails/toenails?					
ARISING					
Is your child able to:					
• Stand up from a low chair or floor?					
• Get in and out of bed or stand up in crib?					
EATING					
Is your child able to:					
• Cut his/her own meat?					
• Lift a cup or glass to mouth?					
• Open a new cereal box?					
WALKING					
Is your child able to:					
• Walk outdoors on flat ground?					
• Climb up five steps?					

*Please check any AIDS or DEVICES that your child usually uses for any of the above activities.

_____Cane   _____Devices used for dressing (button hook, zipper pull, long-handled shoe horn, etc.)
_____Walker   _____Built-up pencil or special utensils
_____Crutches   _____Special or built-up chair
_____Wheelchair   _____Other (Specify:_____)

*Please check any categories for which your child usually needs help from another person BECAUSE OF ARTHRITIS:

_____Dressing and Grooming   _____Eating
_____Arising   _____Walking

	Without ANY Difficulty	With SOME Difficulty	With MUCH Difficulty	UNABLE To Do	Not Applicable
HYGIENE					
Is your child able to:					
• Wash and dry entire body?					
• Take a tub bath (get in and out of tub)?					
• Get on and off the toilet or potty chair?					
• Brush teeth?					
• Comb/brush hair?					
REACH					
Is your child able to:					
• Reach and get down a heavy object such as a large game or books from just above his/her head?					
• Bend down to pick up clothing or a piece of paper from the floor?					
• Pull on a sweater over his/her head?					
• Turn neck to look back over shoulder?					
GRIP					
Is your child able to:					
• Write or scribble with pen or pencil?					

FIGURE 8-6. The Childhood Health Assessment Questionnaire (CHAQ) is a checklist completed by the parent or child assessing functional activities. (Reprinted with permission from Singh, G, Athreya, B, Fries, JF, & Goldsmith, DP. Measurement of functional status in JRA. Arthritis and Rheumatism. In press.)

	Without ANY Difficulty	With SOME Difficulty	With MUCH Difficulty	UNABLE To Do	Not Applicable
GRIP (*Continued*)					
• Open car doors?	_____	_____	_____	_____	_____
• Open jars that have been previously opened?	_____	_____	_____	_____	_____
• Turn faucets on and off?	_____	_____	_____	_____	_____
• Push open a door when he/she has to turn a door knob?	_____	_____	_____	_____	_____
ACTIVITIES					
Is your child able to:					
• Run errands and shop?	_____	_____	_____	_____	_____
• Get in and out of car or toy car or school bus?	_____	_____	_____	_____	_____
• Ride bike or tricycle?	_____	_____	_____	_____	_____
• Do household chores (e.g., wash dishes, take out trash, vacuuming, yardwork, make bed, clean room)?	_____	_____	_____	_____	_____
• Run and play?	_____	_____	_____	_____	_____

*Please check any AIDS or DEVICES that your child usually uses for any of the above activities:

_____ Raised toilet seat   _____ Bathtub bar
_____ Bathtub seat   _____ Long-handled appliances in reach
_____ Jar opener (for jars opened previously)   _____ Long-handled appliances in bathroom

*Please check any categories for which your child usually needs help from another person BECAUSE OF ARTHRITIS?

_____ Hygiene   _____ Gripping and Opening Things
_____ Reach   _____ Errands and Chores

We are also interested in learning whether your child has been affected by pain because of his or her illness.

*How much pain do you think your child has had because of his or her illness IN THE PAST WEEK?

Place a mark on the line below to indicate the severity of the pain.

No pain   Very severe pain

|——|
0   100

HEALTH STATUS

1. Considering all the ways that arthritis affects your child, rate how your child is doing on the following scale by placing a mark on the line.

|——|
0   100
Very well   Very poor

2. Is your child stiff in the morning?   _____ Yes   _____ No
   If YES, about how long does the stiffness usually last (in the past week)?
   Hours/Minutes_____

FIGURE 8–6. *Continued*

---

may transfer with a stand-pivot-sit method, perhaps using an assistive device such as platform crutches.

Children with severe hand involvement may be unable to propel a manual wheelchair but may propel it by walking their feet on the floor or use a power wheelchair. Seat height from the floor has a critical effect on function, including propulsion and transfer. Posture in the chair should optimally be erect in order to prevent hip asymmetry or spinal deformity. Accessories such as brake extensions provide leverage for weak upper extremities.

Swing-away or desk arms ensure close access to school desks.

The school or home should be evaluated for architectural barriers, and modifications recommended to facilitate mobility and transfer. A wheelchair-dependent child should have his or her living space on one floor, if possible. Electric-powered wheelchairs require ramps and a van for transportation, as well as a back-up manual chair. Outings using a manually propelled chair need to be planned in advance to allow for reasonable distances and frequent rests.

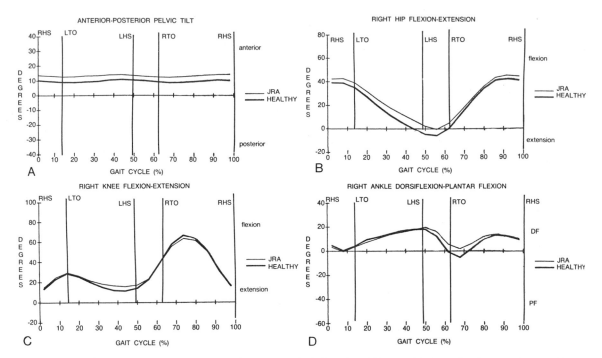

FIGURE 8-7. Gait lab studies have demonstrated common deviations in children with juvenile rheumatoid arthritis (JRA), including: *(A)*, Angle of anteroposterior pelvic tilt in the sagittal plane as a function of percentage of the gait cycle for both JRA group and healthy group subjects. *(B)*, Angle of right hip flexion-extension as a function of percentage of the gait cycle for both JRA group and healthy group subjects. *(C)*, Angle of right knee flexion-extension as a function of percentage of the gait cycle for both JRA group and healthy group subjects. *(D)*, Angle of right ankle dorsiflexion (DF) and plantar flexion (PF) as a function of percentage of the gait cycle for both JRA group and healthy group subjects. (From Lechner, DE, McCarthy, CF, & Holden, MK. Gait deviations in patients with juvenile rheumatoid arthritis. Physical Therapy, *67*:1335–1341, 1987. Reprinted from Physical Therapy with the permission of the American Physical Therapy Association.)

FIGURE 8-8. A common foot deformity is hindfoot valgus with pronation.

FIGURE 8-9. A metatarsal bar has been added to the sneaker to provide a rocker-like surface on the sole of the foot, allowing a mechanical means of toe-off.

Self-Care Activities

Children's skills should be evaluated within the context of both the home and the school environments. Simple solutions such as a backpack for carrying books or asking the school to issue two sets of textbooks are well-accepted options. Other recommendations such as use of dressing aids may not be so readily accepted when they differ from the norm.

Training in ADL can be time consuming, and counseling may be required to obtain the cooperation of the parent. Special devices for dressing may include a dressing stick to assist with reaching the feet to don pants or underwear, a zipper pull, a button hook, a sock aid, a long-handled shoehorn, or elastic shoelaces (Scull et al., 1986). Grooming the hair may require use of assistive devices as well.

Enlarging the handles of utensils and brushes makes gripping these objects easier. A variety of writing aids have enlarged diameters that improve writing endurance. In addition, the student may use a computer or a dictating device for many written tasks.

An area needing special attention is the bathroom. The tub may need to be equipped with a special seat and a grab bar to ensure safety. A long hose attached to the shower allows the child to bathe from a seated position. A long-handled sponge on a stick allows the child to reach more areas with ease. The toilet seat may need to be raised to a specific height to facilitate transfer. Sinks should be fitted with lever-type handles rather than knobs.

Principles of joint conservation are taught, including instruction on how to use the large joints of the body so as to avoid stress on the small joints of the wrists and hands. Books are carried in a backpack close to the center of gravity rather than in a briefcase. Some tasks can best be accomplished by increasing the lever arm, such as using a jar opener rather than twisting off a lid. Teaching patients to listen to their bodies and pace themselves is incorporated, as developmentally appropriate.

Avocational Activities

Because JRA interferes with normal mobility, the child does not have the usual opportunity to maintain cardiopulmonary endurance. Giannini and Protas (1992) studied 30 patients with JRA who were matched with controls for age, sex, and body surface area. An exercise tolerance test using cycle ergometry demonstrated deconditioning of the JRA group. Peak oxygen consumption, highest workload, exercise duration, and peak heart rate were all significantly lower in children with JRA as compared with their controls. Surprisingly, the decreased aerobic capacity was unrelated to the severity of the articular disease as measured by the global articular disease severity score. This score is derived by summing all involved joints for swelling, pain on passive ROM, tenderness to palpation, and passive limitation of motion but is probably not specific enough to show correlation with endurance. Giannini and Protas concluded that aerobic conditioning programs should be started soon after diagnosis to prevent hypoactivity leading to deconditioning.

Klepper and colleagues (1992) corroborated the results of this study on 20 children with JRA, aged 6 to 11 years, using the Health-Related Physical Fitness Test (Table 8–4). A planned program of recreation such as swimming, cycling, or dance should achieve cardiopulmonary training effects if scheduled for 15 to 20 minutes three times per week. Further study is needed, however, to document that intervention with a consistent conditioning program improves endurance.

Guided selection of recreational activities can also assist in reinforcing exercise goals, such as improving lower extremity ROM or strength. Young children enjoy upper extremity games such as "Simon Says." A special exercise videotape has been prepared by the Texas Scottish Rite Hospital (Carman, 1991) in which various ROM dances are performed to stories and music. Other home exercise programs are designed in a coloring book format, such as *Exercise with Kela* (Pediatric Arthritis Center of Hawaii, 1985), or as part of a parent information book, such as *We Can* (Arthritis Foundation, 1985).

School-aged children are encouraged to participate in physical education classes to their tolerance. Certain activities are contraindicated, such as tumbling (especially headstands or somersaults), weight bearing on the upper extremities, contact sports, and high-impact activities such as jogging. Consultation between the physical therapist and the physical education teacher usually helps to clarify the optimal exercise prescription for each child (Scull & Athreya, in press).

▌ SURGICAL PROCEDURES AND ▌ POSTSURGICAL REHABILITATION

Patients with mild involvement are managed by medication, splints, and therapy. Surgery may be considered, however, if conservative treatment fails to prevent joint contractures or if joint erosion is severe.

TABLE 8–4. **FITNESS SCORES FOR CHILDREN WITH JUVENILE RHEUMATOID ARTHRITIS (JRA) AND CONTROLS**

	Number	Means	SD	Range	Percentile
(1) Run (yards)					
JRA	20	1093	243	691–1824	15.5
Controls	20	1456	198	1068–1824	49.6
		t(19) = − 5.20*			
(2) Sit-ups (no.)					
JRA	20	24.8	7.0	13–38	31.8
Controls	20	39.6	10.4	23–60	75.4
		t(19) = − 5.61*			
(3) Reach (cm)					
JRA	20	19.5	7.8	7–35	24
Controls	20	25.3	6.6	9–36	45.8
(4) Skinfolds†					
JRA	20	19.0	7.4	8–36	50.4
Controls	20	18.0	8.0	12–45	54.6

*$p \leq .0005$.
†Sum of triceps and subscapular skin thickness in millimeters.
From Klepper, SE, Darbee, J, Effgen, SK, & Singsen, BH. Physical fitness levels in children with polyarticular juvenile rheumatoid arthritis. Arthritis Care and Research, 5:93–100, 1992.

Soft tissue releases of the hip flexors, hamstrings, hip adductors, or heel cords are indicated for contractures that are resistant to conservative measures. Decompression of the joint and improved ROM also improve joint nutrition, and sometimes fibrocartilage is laid down (Swann, 1990). Occasionally, a simple manipulation under anesthesia is sufficient to regain motion, especially in a child who has been unwilling to cooperate with therapy.

Synovectomy may be performed arthroscopically, but the long-term effects may be disappointing (Jacobsen et al., 1985). It may be considered for a single joint, particularly the knee, which has active disease, effusion, and overgrowth of synovium in spite of adequate medical therapy. However, the degree of postoperative pain and muscle spasm often gives a poor outcome in children. Jacobsen's review (1985) of 41 procedures showed relief of swelling but no long-term changes in pain, ROM, or function.

Osteotomies are sometimes required to correct valgus or flexion contractures at the knee. Epiphysiodesis, or stapling of the growth plate, is occasionally used to correct limb length discrepancy or valgus deformity. Arthroplasty, or less frequently distal arthrodesis, may be required for the severely damaged joint that interferes with function and causes pain. Adolescents may be candidates for replacements of hips, knees, shoulders, elbows, or ankles. Wrist fusion or other types of hand surgery may improve ADL. Ankle fusion may be required to obtain a pain-free joint in neutral alignment.

Indications for arthroplasty include marked functional impairment, especially inability to ambulate, and disabling pain (Hyman & Gregg, 1991; Scott, 1990). Loss of motion, subluxation, and deformity are secondary reasons. Other selection criteria include ability to bear weight on the upper extremities with an assistive device and alignment of other lower extremity joints for weight bearing, both ipsilateral and contralateral. If multiple joints must be replaced, the hips are usually done before the knees. Rehabilitation is easier if the procedures are staged so that one joint is replaced at a time. The goals of rehabilitation are to achieve pain-free ROM and functional ambulation, usually with an assistive device.

Total hip prostheses are custom-designed in smaller sizes and ideally are porous allowing biologic fixation because cement may not last sufficiently long. Although skeletal maturity is desirable, children as young as 12 years of age have received total hip replacements (Hyman & Gregg, 1991).

The postoperative program includes passive ROM exercise with precautions to avoid hip flexion past 90°, adduction, and internal rotation. A foam abduction pillow is worn for 6 weeks, alternating with use of a continuous passive motion (CPM) machine. Isometrics are started early for strengthening of hip extensors and abductors and knee extensors. Gait training with an assistive device begins with weight bearing as tolerated during the first week. Stationary cycling may be attempted after several weeks if the seat height is set high and supervision is used to maintain hip precautions. Aquatic therapy consisting of exercises while sitting in shallow water and ambulation in chest-deep water are begun as soon as wound healing is complete and the staples are removed. Special pools

FIGURE 8–10. Aquatic therapy ideally includes shallow water exercises for flexibility and strengthening *(A)*, as well as ambulation in deep water *(B)*.

with a movable floor allow gradual progression of the water depth to increase weight bearing (Fig. 8–10) (AFW of North America, Olean, NY).

Total knee arthroplasty is usually done with a cemented procedure and may be combined with release of posterior structures, such as the hamstrings, the capsule, and the proximal gastrocnemius, if knee flexion contractures exist. The patella is routinely resurfaced with a plastic button cemented to the undersurface, and the lateral retinaculum is released to prevent further valgus deformity. The tibial tubercle must undergo osteotomy and fixation to gain exposure to the knee. Therefore, early strengthening programs using isometrics and straight leg raising exercises are tolerated better than short arc quadriceps exercises.

Patients are bearing full weight with a knee immobilizer on the second postoperative day. When the bulky dressing is removed by day 4, CPM is begun if sufficient wound healing is present. The ROM goal is 0 to 100° of knee motion. Ambulation aids are discontinued when the knee flexes to 90° and the quadriceps strength grades 4/5. Stationary cycling may be done if a range limiter is applied to the pedal to shorten the shank and allow the therapist to control the amount of knee flexion required during cycling (Fig. 8–11).

Complications of arthroplasty include loosening of components and infection. Wear of components is less problematic in this group because patients with JRA are typically small and have decreased activity levels. In a group of patients with a total of 72 hip replacements, 30% required revision after 10

years of follow-up (Swann, 1989). Nevertheless, keeping the patient ambulatory during the young-adult years was believed to be beneficial. The increased use of biologic fixation should improve these long-term results.

CONTINUOUS PASSIVE MOTION

CPM has been studied in animals as an alternative to rest and immobilization in the care of articular defects, fractures, septic arthritis, and tendon lacerations (Salter, 1989). Basic science studies have involved the creation of cartilaginous defects in rabbit joints and comparison of their gross and histologic differences following treatment with either immobilization in a cast, intermittent active motion (cage activity), or CPM. The results show that CPM 1) is well tolerated by rabbits and seems to be pain free; 2) has a significant healing effect on cartilage, tendon, and ligamentous tissues; 3) prevents adhesions and joint stiffness; 4) does not interfere with healing incisions; and 5) is superior to rest for tissue healing. One week of immediate postoperative CPM at a slow speed was found to be as effective as 3 weeks of CPM.

Salter (1989) recommends early use of CPM following synovectomy, soft tissue releases, or arthroplasty. Units are available for the lower extremities, and CPM may be integrated with electrical stimulation of the quadriceps, for example, to facilitate full knee extension and prevent atrophy. Upper ex-

FIGURE 8–11. This ergometer *(A)* is equipped with a range limiter on the pedal *(B,C)*, which shortens the shank and allows the patient with limited knee flexion to cycle.

tremity units or universal joint units are also available to treat the shoulder and elbow.

CPM may also be an effective treatment adjunct in management of contractures or morning stiffness. Because no bilateral pediatric units are presently manufactured, however, its use for patients with morning stiffness is limited. Furthermore, confinement to bed or loss of sleep limits its acceptance. Further clinical trials are needed to fully understand the benefit of CPM in the care of children with JRA.

Most recently, animal research is exploring the biologic resurfacing of joints in rabbits with periosteal grafts, including both autogenous grafts and allografts (Zarnett et al., 1987). Studies have demonstrated that articular cartilage can regenerate with CPM, with or without the additional periosteal grafts. Further study is needed before this approach is applied to humans, but the potential exists for future treatment of the young, active JRA patient who may wear out a prosthetic joint at an early age.

CASE HISTORY: AMANDA

Amanda is a 6-year-old girl with polyarticular JRA. She has involvement of multiple joints, including the neck, temporomandibular joint, elbows, wrists, hands, knees, ankles, and toes. She is taking 14 mg/d of naproxen to control inflammation. She has 15° hip and knee flexion contractures bilaterally and is unable to extend the great toes. Cervical spine motion is limited in rotation and extension by 50%. Muscle strength grades 4/5 in the antigravity muscles of both lower extremities. Grip strength measured by a hand-held dynamometer is 9 lbs on the right and 8 lbs on the left. Leg lengths are equal, and there are no postural deviations except a slightly forward head.

Amanda ambulates independently, but her gait shows bilateral gluteus medius lurch, decreased hip extension at toe-off, decreased stride length, and poor push-off. She shifts her weight to the lateral borders of her feet. She is not able to keep up with the family on outings to the local mall.

Her ADL were assessed by the occupational therapist using the CHAQ. Amanda can complete all dressing in a reasonable amount of time except for donning her shoes and socks. Her mother shops carefully for clothing that is loose fitting with elastic rather than fasteners. Amanda has significant stiffness following any period of inactivity. In the morning, she must be carried to the tub because she cannot walk for up to an hour. In class, she becomes stiff after sitting for circle time. She is unable to carry her tray in the cafeteria and often asks to be excused from recess.

Problem No. 1: Dysfunctional gait

Impairment 1-A. Metatarsophalangeal joint pain especially during toe-off.
Goal. Improve gait, specifically increase stride length, increase push-off, decrease Trendelenburg sign.
Plan:

1. Recommend sneakers for footwear.
2. Use cushioned insoles to decrease metatarsophalangeal pain.
3. Add metatarsal bar to shoe to allow rolling over forefoot.

Impairment 1-B. Weakness of lower extremity muscles.
Goal. Increase strength of antigravity muscles to 5/5.
Plan:

1. Perform Theraband exercises for increased strength of gluteus medius, maximus, and quadriceps muscles.
2. Issue adaptive tricycle for use in school, especially during recess.
3. Encourage use of swings on school playground.

Impairment 1-C. Inactivity stiffness, especially on arising.
Goal. Decrease inactivity stiffness so that child will be able to ambulate on arising and move freely in classroom.
Plan:

1. Wear posterior knee splints, of low temperature thermoplastics, at night, allowing the knees to rest in extension.
2. Take morning tub bath and perform active ROM exercises to decrease morning stiffness.
3. Encourage ambulating in the classroom every hour to avoid stiffness from inactivity.

Impairment 1-D. 15° hip and knee flexion contractures of both lower extremities.
Goal. Maintain/improve lower extremity ROM: hip and knee extension to 5°, great toe extension to 50°.

Plan:

1. Recommend prone positioning for 20 minutes a day to decrease hip and knee flexion contractures.
2. Use passive ROM performed by mother after bath to increase metatarsophalangeal extension.

Problem No. 2: Dependent for ADL

Limitation 2-A. Dressing skills are not age appropriate.
Goal. Develop ability to don/doff shoes and socks independently with a sock aid and elastic shoelaces.
Plan:

1. Train for use of sock aid and shoe donning.
2. Provide dressing frame or doll as a toy to learn how to tie and lace shoes.
3. Continue to select clothes for ease of donning and doffing.

Impairment 2-A. Decreased grip strength.
Goal. Increase grip strength to 11 lb on the right and 9 lb on the left.
Plan. Perform exercises with playdough involving pinching and grasping.

Impairment 2-B. Daily activities can stress joints or cause postural deviations.
Goal. Prevent stress to involved joints and postural abnormalities.
Plan:

1. Avoid tailor-sitting during circle time. Encourage use of small stool.
2. Have occupational therapist make resting cock-up splint for wrists to be used during writing tasks.
3. Adapt pencils with soft build-up to increase diameter.
4. Recommend large-diameter crayons.

Problem No. 3: Psychosocial Adjustment to Disease
Societal Limitation 3-A. Potential for child to be excluded from children in peer group secondary to their lack of understanding of JRA.
Goal. Integrate child into school setting for as normal a social experience as possible.
Plan:

1. Counsel teacher and school nurse about JRA.
2. Arrange for child to educate peers regarding JRA in appropriate method, such as show-and-tell session.
3. Provide written pamphlets from the Arthritis Foundation.

Reassessment of ROM, strength, and gait is done every other month at a rheumatology clinic where the child is seen by the rehabilitation team. If the knee flexion contractures do not improve with the home program, then consideration will be given to prescribing a dynamic splint to be worn during the hours of sleep.

Amanda is still young and is not yet showing disabilities in carrying out her life roles at home and in school. The therapist should work intensively on this child's impairments of ROM and strength to prevent further functional limitations in gait or ADL. Continued assessment of Amanda's school attendance and her psychosocial interactions with peers and family will be needed to ensure that she does not develop any disabilities. The plan for education of school professionals and peers is aimed at prevention of social isolation to promote Amanda's full inclusion in school activities.

Acknowledgments

With special thanks to Balu H. Athreya, MD, and Greg Keenan, MD, for their editorial assistance, to Margi Ide for photography, and to Janice Lockhart for manuscript revisions.

References

Arthritis Foundation. We Can: A Guide for Parents of Children with Arthritis. Atlanta: Arthritis Foundation, 1985.

Athreya, BH, & Cassidy, JT. Current status of the medical treatment of children with JRA. Rheumatic Disease Clinics of North America, 17: 871–889, 1991.

Brewer, EJ, Bass, J, Baum, J, Cassidy, JT, Fink, C, Jacobs, J, Hanson, V, Levinson, JE, Schaller, J, & Stillman, JS. Current proposed revision of JRA criteria. Arthritis and Rheumatism 20:195–199, 1977.

Carman, D. Where Are the Indians? An Exercise Video for Children. Dallas: Scottish Rite Hospital for Children, 1991.

Cassidy, JT, and Petty, RE. Textbook of Rheumatology (2nd ed.). New York: Churchill-Livingstone, 1990.

Fried, JA, Athreya, BH, Gregg, JR, Das, M, & Doughty, R. The cervical spine in juvenile rheumatoid arthritis. Clinical Orthopedics and Related Research, 179:102–106, 1983.

Giannini, EH, Brewer, EJ, Kuzmina, N, Shaikov, V, Maximov, A, Vorontsov, I, Fink, CW, Newman, AJ, Cassidy, JT, & Zemel, LS. Methotrexate in resistant juvenile rheumatoid arthritis: Results of the USA-USSR double-blind, placebo-controlled trial. New England Journal of Medicine, 326:1043–1049, 1992.

Giannini, MJ, & Protas, EJ. Comparison of peak isometric knee extensor torque in children with and without juvenile rheumatoid arthritis. Arthritis Care and Research, 6:82–87, 1993.

Giannini, MJ, & Protas, EJ. Exercise response in children with and without juvenile rheumatoid arthritis: A case comparison study. Physical Therapy, 72:365–372, 1992.

Henderson, CJ, Lovell, DJ, & Gregg, DJ. A nutritional screening test for use in children and adolescents with juvenile rheumatoid arthritis. Journal of Rheumatology, 19:1276–1281, 1992.

Hepburn, GR. Case studies: Contractures and stiff joint management with Dynasplint. Journal of Orthopedic and Sports Physical Therapy, 8:498–504, 1987.

Hochberg, MC, Chang, RW, Dwosh, F, Lindsey, S, Pincus, T, & Wolfe, F. The American College of Rheumatology 1991 revised criteria for the classification of global functional status in rheumatoid arthritis. Arthritis and Rheumatism, 35:498–502, 1992.

Howe, S, Levinson, J, Shear, E, Hartner, S, McGirr, G, Schulte, M, & Lovell, D. Development of a disability measurement tool for juvenile rheumatoid arthritis. The Juvenile Arthritis Functional Assessment Report for Children and Their Parents. Arthritis and Rheumatism, 34:873–880, 1991.

Hyman, BS, & Gregg, JR. Arthroplasty of the hip and knee in juvenile rheumatoid arthritis. Rheumatic Disease Clinics of North America, 17:971–983, 1991.

Jacobsen, ST, Levinson, JE, & Crawford, AH. Late results of synovectomy in juvenile rheumatoid arthritis. Journal of Bone and Joint Surgery (American), 67:8–15, 1985.

Klepper, SE, Darbee, J, Effgen, SK, & Singsen, BH. Physical fitness levels in children with polyarticular juvenile rheumatoid arthritis. Arthritis Care and Research, 5:93–100, 1992.

Lechner, DE, McCarthy, CF, & Holden, MK. Gait deviations in patients with juvenile rheumatoid arthritis. Physical Therapy, 67:1335–1341, 1987.

Lovell, DJ, Howe, S, Shear, E, Hartner, S, McGirr, G, Schulte, M, & Levinson, J. Development of a disability measurement tool for juvenile rheumatoid arthritis: The Juvenile Arthritis Functional Assessment Scale. Arthritis and Rheumatism, 32:1390–1395, 1989.

Mayro, RF, DeLozier, JB III, & Whitaker, LA. Facial reconstruction consideration in rheumatic diseases. Pediatric Rheumatology, 17:943–969, 1991.

McGrath, PA. Pain in Children: Nature, Assessment, Treatment. New York: Guilford Press, 1990.

Michlovitz, SL. Thermal Agents in Rehabilitation. Philadelphia: FA Davis, 1986, p. 123.

Pediatric Arthritis Center of Hawaii. Exercise with Kela. Kapiolani Women's and Children's Medical Center, Honolulu, HI, 1985.

Petty, RE. Current knowledge of the etiology and pathogenesis of chronic uveitis accompanying juvenile rheumatoid arthritis. Rheumatic Disease Clinics of North America, 13:19–31, 1987.

Rhodes, VJ. Physical therapy management of patients with juvenile rheumatoid arthritis. Physical Therapy, 71:910–919, 1991.

Salter, RB. The biologic concept of continuous passive motion of synovial joints: The first 18 years of basic research and its clinical application. Clinical Orthopedics, 242:12–25, 1989.

Schaller, JG. Chronic arthritis in children. Clinical Orthopedics, 182:79–89, 1983.

Scott, RD. Total hip and knee arthroplasty in juvenile rheumatoid arthritis. Clinical Orthopedics and Related Research, 259:83–91, 1990.

Scull, S. Juvenile rheumatoid arthritis. In Tecklin, JS (Ed.), Pediatric Physical Therapy. Philadelphia: JB Lippincott, 1994.

Scull, SA, & Athreya, BH. Exercise and sports in childhood arthritis. In Goldberg, B (Ed.), Sports and Exercise for Chronically Ill Children. Champaign, IL: Human Kinetics. In press.

Scull, SA, Dow, MB, & Athreya, BH. Physical and occupational therapy for children with rheumatic diseases. Pediatric Clinics of North America, 33:1053–1077, 1986.

Singh, G, Athreya, B, Fries, JF, & Goldsmith, DP. Measurement of functional status in JRA. Arthritis and Rheumatism. In press.

Steinbrocker, O, Traeger, CH, & Batterman, RC. Therapeutic criteria in rheumatoid arthritis. Journal of the American Medical Association, 140:659–662, 1949.

Swann, MC. The surgery of juvenile chronic arthritis. Clinical Orthopedics and Related Research, 259:70–75, 1990.

Towner, SR, Michet, CJ, O'Fallon, WM, & Nelson, AM. The epidemiology of juvenile arthritis in Rochester, Minn. Arthritis and Rheumatism, 26:1208, 1983.

Varni, JW, Thompson, KL, & Hanson, V. The Varni/Thompson Pediatric Pain Questionnaire: I. Chronic musculoskeletal pain in juvenile rheumatoid arthritis. Pain, 28:27–38, 1987.

Wallace, CA, & Levinson, JE. Juvenile rheumatoid arthritis: Outcome and treatment for the 1990s. Rheumatic Disease Clinics of North America, *17*:891–905, 1991.

White, PH. Growth abnormalities in children with juvenile rheumatoid arthritis. Clinical Orthopedics and Related Research, *259*:46–50, 1990.

Whitehouse, R, Shope, JT, Sullivan, DB, & Kulik, CL. Children with juvenile rheumatoid arthritis at school. Clinical Pediatrics, *28*:509–514, 1989.

Zarnett, R, Delaney, JR, O'Driscoll, SW, & Salter, RB. Cellular origin and evolution of neochondrogenesis in major full-thickness defects of a joint surface treated by free autogenous periosteal grafts and subjected to continuous passive motion in rabbits. Clinical Orthopedics, *222*:267, 1987.

Chapter 9

Hemophilia

SANDRA M. McGEE, PT

INCIDENCE AND ETIOLOGY

Hemophilia is the term used to collectively identify several X-linked disorders of blood coagulation. The most common of these are factor VIII deficiency, or hemophilia A, composing 80 to 90% of the population with hemophilia, and factor IX deficiency, or hemophilia B. Hemophilia is present in approximately 1 in 10,000 males, and 60 to 65% of the patients will have a positive family history (Karayalcin, 1985).

The severity of the disorder is determined by the amount of factor activity in the blood (Table 9–1). Over 60% of males with hemophilia A and 50% with hemophilia B have the severe form of the disorder. These patients are subject to recurrent hemorrhages that may occur spontaneously or as a result of minor trauma. Infants and toddlers may develop subcutaneous ecchymosis over bony prominences or large hematomas after intramuscular injections for vaccination against childhood diseases. By 3 to 4 years of age, bleeding into muscles and joints begins to present problems because of increased activity level, and it continues to be a major problem throughout childhood and adolescence.

In the moderate form of hemophilia A or B the patient may have spontaneous hemorrhages, but more frequently bleeding occurs as a result of trauma. The child with the mild form, however, will bleed only after severe trauma, and, consequently, hemophilia may not even be diagnosed in infancy or childhood (Buchanan, 1980).

Hemorrhages may occur anywhere in the body but most often are in the joint cavities. Muscles are the second most common site of bleeding, particularly in the iliopsoas, gastrocnemius, and forearm flexor muscle compartment. Hemorrhages within muscles can be dangerous owing to the risk of nerve compression from the hematoma. Patients with hemophilia may also be susceptible to hematuria, mucous membrane hemorrhages, and central nervous system hemorrhages. Fortunately, central nervous system hemorrhages are uncommon, developing in approximately 3% of the hemophilic population, but they are the major cause of death from these bleeding disorders (Buchanan, 1980).

HEMOPHILIC ARTHROPATHY

Pathophysiology

Hemarthrosis is the most clinically significant problem in hemophilia. It affects the hinge joints (knees, elbows, and ankles) most frequently because these joints have less muscular padding and a decreased ability to withstand lateral and rotary forces. When bleeding occurs into a joint, the joint becomes swollen, warm, and painful and range of motion (ROM) is restricted (Corrigan, 1990). A

TABLE 9–1. RELATION OF FACTOR LEVELS TO SEVERITY OF CLINICAL MANIFESTATIONS OF HEMOPHILIA A AND B

Type	Factor Levels (VIII/IX) (Percent of Normal)	Type of Hemorrhage
Severe	<1	Spontaneous; hemarthroses and deep tissue hemorrhages
Moderate	1–5	Gross bleeding following mild to moderate trauma; some hemarthrosis; seldom spontaneous hemorrhage
Mild	5–25	Severe hemorrhage following moderate to severe trauma or surgery
High-risk carrier females	30–50	Gynecologic and obstetric hemorrhages

single or infrequent bleeding episode will usually resolve without complication as the blood is resorbed. Recurrent hemarthroses, however, can lead to chronic synovitis and degenerative arthropathy. Although the mechanisms of recurrent bleeding leading to degenerative arthropathy are not well understood, Joist and Ameri (1990) have outlined a reasonable hypothesis (Fig. 9–1). Recurrent hemarthroses cause synovial hypertrophy with formation of villi, as well as pannus formation on the joint cartilage. The hypertrophic, hyperemic synovium is more susceptible to mechanical trauma, leading to further bleeding. In addition, capsular stretching and muscle atrophy from immobilization and disuse increase joint instability, creating a vicious cycle that is difficult to break. The chronic synovitis and chemical reactions related to the breakdown of the blood in the joint eventually lead to cartilage damage, bone erosion, and bone remodeling.

In 1977, Arnold and Hilgartner classified hemophilic arthropathy into five stages based on roentgenographic findings (Fig. 9–2). In stage 1, no bony abnormalities are seen but soft tissue swelling is present. Stage 2 is characterized by osteoporosis and overgrowth of the epiphyses, but the joint integrity is maintained. In stage 3, subchondral cysts are visible, squaring of the patella is evident when the knee is involved, and the intercondylar notch of the knee and the trochlear notch of the elbow are widened. The articular cartilage, however, is still intact. By stage 4, the joint space has narrowed and there is damage to the cartilage. In stage 5, there is fibrous joint contracture, loss of joint space, extensive enlargement of the epiphyses, and total destruction of the articular cartilage.

All children with moderate or severe hemophilia will suffer from hemarthroses. The aim of treatment is to slow down or halt the progression of joint destruction.

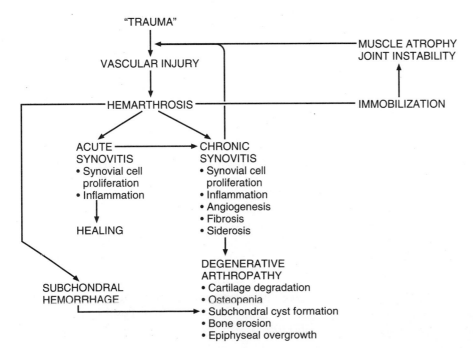

FIGURE 9–1. Joist and Ameri's concept of the pathogenesis of hemophilic arthropathy. (Redrawn from Joist, JH, & Ameri, A. Pathogenesis of hemophilic arthropathy. In Gilbert, MS, & Greene, WB [Eds.], Musculoskeletal Problems in Hemophilia. New York: National Hemophilia Foundation, 1990, pp. 20–25.)

FIGURE 9-2. Hemophilic arthropathy. In stage 1, soft tissue swelling occurs without bony changes. Stage 2 consists of early osteoporosis and epiphyseal overgrowth. *A* to *C* illustrate stages 3 to 5. *A*, Stage 3: Joint disorganization, with patellar squaring and subchondral cysts but intact articular cartilage. *B*, Stage 4: Narrowing of joint space and damage to cartilage. *C*, Stage 5: Loss of joint space, fibrous joint contracture, and total destruction of cartilage. (From Arnold, WD, & Hilgartner, MW. Hemophilic arthropathy. Journal of Bone and Joint Surgery [American], 59:288-305, 1977.)

Medical Management

Bleeding episodes are managed medically by intravenous factor replacement, extracted from normal plasma. Factor replacement should occur as soon as the patient feels stiffness or discomfort in a joint. These "prodromal" sensations can precede objective signs of bleeding by 4 to 6 hours. In an effort to control the bleeding as quickly as possible, many families are taught to perform infusions at home. Factor replacement may also be given before vigorous exercise, such as participation in intramural sports or intensive physical therapy. Some patients with frequent bleeding episodes may be placed on long-term prophylactic factor replacement (Corrigan, 1990).

In addition to factor replacement, hemarthroses are treated with rest, through immobilization and avoidance of weight bearing, until bleeding has resolved. Aspiration of the blood from the joints as a treatment modality has been reported in the literature after 1 to 2 decades of disuse (Corrigan, 1990; Gregosiewicz et al., 1989).

Orthopaedic surgery may be indicated in patients with chronic synovitis or severe joint destruction. Synovectomy, both open and by arthroscopy, is frequently performed on knees and elbows in an effort to reduce bleeding episodes by removing fragile, hypertrophic synovium (Atkins et al., 1987). "Medical synovectomies" by intra-articular injection of radionucleotides are also being performed to ablate the synovium (Erken, 1991). Arthrodeses, osteotomies, and arthroplasties have been used when severe joint destruction causes intractable pain and disability.

Prognosis

Despite more aggressive and earlier home treatment of hemarthroses, severe joint arthropathy remains a major disabling consequence of hemophilia. Although the incidence of joint hemorrhages declines in late adolescence and early adulthood, joint destruction has already occurred in a large percentage of those patients with severe hemophilia (Joist & Ameri, 1990).

Between 10% and 15% of patients with hemophilia A develop antibodies (inhibitors) that are directed against the activity of factor VIII. Hemostasis is more difficult to achieve in patients with inhibitors. These patients are treated with high doses of factor VIII when major bleeding episodes occur, but they are not candidates for prophylactic infusions or elective surgery (Karayalcin, 1985).

Since the late 1970s, secondary complications of hemophilia have become a more significant health problem than the primary impairment. The child with severe hemophilia can use from 50,000 to 100,000 units of factor concentrate annually. (One unit is the amount of clotting activity in 1 mL of fresh pooled plasma.) The complications from receiving that amount of pooled human plasma are numerous (Corrigan, 1990). Eighty to 90% of all patients with severe hemophilia A and 55% of those with severe hemophilia B who received factor re-

placement between 1979 and 1984 test positive for human immunodeficiency virus (HIV) (Hilgartner, 1991). In addition, 80% of patients with severe hemophilia have hepatitis B surface antibodies and more than 50% have persistently elevated liver function test results that indicate chronic liver disease from hepatitis. Both the advent of a hepatitis B vaccine and the screening and heating of blood products have diminished the incidence of hepatitis B and HIV infection as consequences of factor replacement therapy. No documented cases of HIV seroconversion in patients with hemophilia have been reported since 1985 (Corrigan, 1990). To further reduce the risks from factor replacement, factor VIII concentrate has been made in culture by recombinant DNA techniques and has been in prelicensure clinical trials since 1987; approval for licensure was granted by the Food and Drug Administration for the first of these recombinant factors in December 1992 (Butler, R, personal communication, 1993).

▌ DISABILITIES

For the child with hemophilia, the degree and type of disability are similar to those of the child with juvenile rheumatoid arthritis and are dependent on the age of the child, on the severity of the disease, and often on the emotional support provided by the family.

The child with moderate or severe hemophilia is usually diagnosed shortly after birth or within the first few months of life. Parents are counseled to watch for signs of hemorrhages and to treat all head injuries as potentially life threatening. As the child begins to pull to stand, a lightweight protective helmet is usually prescribed; and parents may be advised to use knee and elbow pads to protect the joints of children who are learning how to walk. Understandably, parents may become overprotective and discourage peer group activities and playground play, such as swinging and sliding, that helps to develop balance and coordination.

The child with severe hemophilia will begin to have more frequent joint and muscle hemorrhages by 3 years of age, as his activity level increases and he becomes physically able to run and jump, which may increase the incidence of direct trauma. Pain and frequent visits to the emergency department for factor replacement therapy may become the norm for many of these children and their families. Varied responses to their pain may cause differing disabilities. Some children may use their pain to maintain dependency on their parents by refusing to participate in normal activities of daily living

(ADL). Other children may deny their pain because they know it means they will receive an intravenous injection and be immobilized. The young child may not understand that prompt treatment will relieve the pain and limit the need for more infusions (Holdredge & Cotta, 1989).

The school-aged child with frequent hemorrhages may have poor school attendance because of time spent in emergency departments and the need to immobilize the joint. With the advent of home replacement therapy, time lost from school has become less of a problem, although special arrangements may need to be made for transporting the child on crutches. Children will need to be excused from physical education classes when acute hemarthroses occur and may need adaptive physical education programs if chronic arthropathy is present. Participation in organized sports is an important aspect of the school-aged child's and adolescent's social life that may not be available for the child with hemophilia. Certain sports are absolutely contraindicated, and participation in other sports must be carefully evaluated by the entire medical team and family.

By late adolescence, many young men with severe hemophilia will have at least one arthropathic joint that causes chronic pain and stiffness, which may be disabling. The Musculoskeletal Committee of the World Federation of Hemophilia developed a scale for evaluating chronic pain using a 0 to 3 rating:

0. No pain; no functional deficit; no analgesic use needed (except for acute hemorrhage)

1. Mild pain; does not interfere with occupation or with ADL; may require occasional relief by a nonnarcotic analgesic

2. Moderate pain; causes partial or occasional interference with occupation or ADL; may require occasional narcotics for relief

3. Severe pain; interferes with performing occupation or carrying out ADL; requires frequent use of nonnarcotic or narcotic medication for relief (Holdredge & Cotta, 1989)

Many adolescents and young adults not only face the above-mentioned problems of the school-aged child but also face peer and even community ostracism because of their HIV-positive status. At a time when peer acceptance and increasing independence are so important, they may face rejection and an increasing dependence on others as the HIV-related disease progresses.

Little published data exist on the degree of disability resulting from the musculoskeletal complications of hemophilia. Weinman (1977) reported on a study conducted by Ahlberg in 1966 on 250 boys and men with hemophilia. On a scale of 0 to 3, with 0 representing no disability and 3 representing severe arthropathy and wheelchair-dependent mobility, 50% scored 0 and less than 10% scored 3. As factor replacement products have become more available, the clinical impression is that the degree of disability has diminished. In my clinic, in which children with hemophilia are followed until their late teens, less than 5% of patients require assistive devices or orthoses for ambulation on a continuous basis and no patients are wheelchair-dependent.

Primary Musculoskeletal Impairments

In 1987, Atkins and colleagues reported that the prevalence of joint contracture in patients with the severe form of hemophilia is between 50% and 95%. These contractures are the result of recurrent hemarthroses and intramuscular bleeding episodes and most frequently involve knee and elbow flexion and ankle plantar flexion. Although recurrent intramuscular hemorrhages are rare, a single large hematoma can cause permanent joint contracture because the large volume of blood will cause localized necrosis; and as the blood is reabsorbed the dead muscle fibers are replaced by fibrous tissue in a shortened position. This occurs in about 10% of all muscle hemorrhages and is most common in the plantar flexor and forearm muscles.

Contractures secondary to recurrent hemarthroses are related to a number of factors. Acute bleeding episodes are painful, and the patient is placed in a splint in the position of comfort, which at the knee and elbow is typically in flexion. Multiple hemorrhages, with frequent immobilization, can result in muscle shortening around a joint. As hemarthroses recur, with synovial hypertrophy and eventual articular cartilage destruction, bony changes, such as genu valgus, posterior subluxation of the tibia, and osteophytes, may occur. These changes may restrict ROM in a more permanent manner.

Muscle weakness is usually found around affected joints. In a study by Pietri and associates (1992), 10 patients (from 8 to 23 years of age) with unilateral knee involvement were strength tested on a Cybex 340 (Cybex, Division of Lumex, Ronkonkoma, NY) for knee strength (as measured by peak torque), total work, and average power output. The average number of knee hemarthroses per patient was seven, and minimal or no radiographic changes were seen in any patient. Peak torque at 60°, total work, and average power were all significantly lower in the involved knee. The decreased muscle function was attributed to immobilization resulting in muscle atrophy, as well as reflex inhibition of the alpha motoneuron of the quadriceps muscle and facilitation of the hamstrings from slowly adapting capsular receptors sensitive to pressure and distention.

Another study by Strickler and Green (1984) looked at isokinetic torque levels in the quadriceps and hamstrings muscles of males with hemophilia, aged 7 through adult. All their subjects demonstrated knee flexor and extensor strength deficits when compared with age-matched healthy subjects. Additionally, they found that as the degree of arthropathy and flexion deformities increased, muscle strength decreased, with a relatively greater decrease in extensor torque, resulting in a higher than normal flexor-extensor ratio. Normally, knee flexors are approximately 60% as strong as extensors. In the patients with hemophilia, flexor strength averaged 70% of extensors in those with no arthropathy and was greater than extensor strength in adolescents and adults with stage 4 arthropathy.

Peripheral nerve lesions are a potential consequence of large intramuscular hemorrhages, owing to compression on the nerve from the rapidly expanding hemorrhage. The highest incidence of lesions is to the femoral nerve after iliacus muscle hemorrhages. Fortunately, in the majority of cases, nerve function returns to normal within a few weeks or months, but the limb affected must be protected until full function returns (Houghton & Duthie, 1979).

Postural deviations may also be seen in the child with hemophilia. Leg-length discrepancies can occur with epiphyseal overgrowth from hyperemia. Mechanical, or apparent, discrepancy can occur from a pelvic obliquity caused by psoas shortening after one or more hemorrhages. Whether real or apparent, this discrepancy may result in a postural scoliosis (Fernandez-Palazzi et al., 1990).

Hemarthroses, intramuscular hemorrhages, and hemophilic arthropathy are all sources of pain. The pain of an acute hemorrhage is usually relieved shortly after hemostasis is achieved by factor replacement. The chronic pain associated with a severely damaged joint is much more difficult to alleviate. Analgesics that contain aspirin or antihistamines must be avoided because they inhibit platelet function necessary for clotting. Narcotics may be necessary for severe, chronic pain but must be prescribed cautiously. Drug abuse among adolescents and adult males with hemophilia is a recognized problem, with one study finding that 21% of older patients with severe hemophilia abused drugs, including alcohol and prescribed pain killers, as well as illegal drugs (Jonas, 1989). Transcutaneous electrical nerve stimulation, biofeedback, relax-

ation, and guided imagery may be used for pain relief. Orthopaedic surgery may be necessary to reduce unremitting pain by fusing a painful joint or replacing it (Corrigan, 1990).

Functional Limitations

The functional limitations for the child with hemophilia are dependent on the number of joints involved and the severity of the joint arthropathy. Gait deviations are seen most often and result from frequent immobilizations with subsequent weakness, joint changes, muscle shortening, and pain. Even mild gait deviations can create additional stress on joints and contribute to perpetuating the cycle of vulnerability to stress, recurrent hemarthrosis, synovitis, and further joint destruction. Weight bearing on a flexed knee not only increases the stress on the tibiofemoral and patellofemoral surfaces but also increases the quadriceps force required to maintain available extension against gravity. Despite the greater force required, Strickler and Greene (1984) found that subjects with arthropathy and knee flexion contractures demonstrated significantly reduced knee extension torque values.

Wheelchairs are usually not needed for children with hemophilia, except when acute hemorrhages in more than one joint prohibit the use of assistive devices for ambulation. As the child progresses to adulthood, more orthoses or ambulation aids may be used; but even in the adult population, less than 10% of persons with severe hemophilia will need wheelchairs for mobility (Ahlberg, 1965).

ADL such as dressing, grooming, and hygiene may be problematic for the child with frequent elbow hemorrhages and decreased elbow extension and forearm pronation and supination. Carrying schoolbooks may stress the elbow joints and lead to bleeding. Although there are no functional assessment scales specific to the hemophilia population, evaluation using the Functional Independence Measure (FIM) or Wee-FIM (for children younger than age 7) will provide a numerical score and an objective way to measure functional progress (State University of New York, 1991).

Cardiopulmonary endurance is frequently impaired in children with hemophilia. Koch and colleagues (1984) evaluated response to exercise in 11 boys with factor VIII deficiency, ranging in age from 8 to 15.5 years, according to a uniform bicycle protocol and compared their performances with data available for healthy children. All the boys had previously been encouraged to participate in the physical education program at school, as well as after-school activities. Although none of the patients had acute bleeding problems, pain, significant weakness, or orthopaedic deformities, several had previously sustained lower extremity hemorrhages. Their performance on bicycle ergometry demonstrated that peak heart rate, minutes of exercise, physical working capacity (maximum workload per weight in kilograms), and mean power were all significantly lower than for a population of healthy children whose physical activities did not exceed age-appropriate recreation. The clinical implication stated by the authors was that physical education alone does not provide aerobic conditioning, so it is imperative to supplement physical education with an individualized exercise program for fitness.

The physical therapist may be involved in counseling the child and family about appropriate recreational activities to maintain cardiopulmonary and muscular fitness. Before beginning participation in any sport, a child should be evaluated for joint motion, muscle strength, flexibility, and ligament stability, with particular attention paid to those joints that are likely to be stressed by the chosen sport. Any deficiencies should be eliminated before participation in the sport begins. In addition, a sport-specific conditioning program should be implemented and appropriate protective wear discussed. (See Chapter 16 on sports injuries for additional relevant information.)

Participation in certain sports is contraindicated owing to the danger of traumatic hemorrhages. The National Hemophilia Foundation, in association with the American Red Cross, published a booklet in 1985 entitled "Hemophilia and Sports." In this booklet, sports activities are divided into three categories: 1) recommended sports with minimal risks, such as swimming and cycling; 2) sports in which the physical, social, and psychological benefits usually outweigh the risks; and 3) sports in which the risks outweigh the benefits. Contact sports, such as boxing, football, hockey, racquetball, and skateboarding, are in the highest risk category and not recommended for patients with hemophilia. Participation in most other sports can be considered, but the decision to participate should be made jointly by the child, his parents, and the members of a comprehensive hemophilia clinic team.

THE ROLE OF PHYSICAL THERAPY

Physical therapy for the child with hemophilia is aimed at maintaining strength and a good ROM in all joints, and at preventing or diminishing disability. The majority of this therapy will occur in a clinic or outpatient setting with adjunctive home

exercise programs. Unless the child has neurologic involvement from a central nervous system hemorrhage, his limitations rarely affect his educational abilities, so school physical therapy is not indicated.

Kasper and Dietrich (1985) recommend that a daily exercise program be followed from early childhood and encouraged with as much enthusiasm as other medical care. Clinical observations would suggest that strong muscles help support joints and decrease the frequency of hemorrhages, and several studies have demonstrated that participation in strengthening programs resulted in reduced bleeding episodes (Koch et al., 1984; Greene & Strickler, 1983; Timmermans, 1990). The specific type of strengthening program appears to be less important than daily participation. In Koch and colleagues' case studies, two preteen boys attended physical therapy 1 to 2 times per week for 12 to 18 months, beginning with active assistive exercises and progressing to active resistive exercises and daily participation in aerobic activities, such as jogging, swimming, or cycling. Greene and Strickler's 32 patients (aged 7 to 51 years) participated in 6 months of modified isokinetic strengthening for 15 minutes a day. Thirty patients seen by Timmermans (1990) were involved in physical therapy treatments of stretching and strengthening, joint stability training, joint mobilization, postural and gait correction, and functional training for ADL and sports. In all these studies, strength improved in all patients, and bleeding frequency decreased in all but two of Timmermans' patients.

Assessment

Assessment of the child with hemophilia should include gathering subjective information about the location and frequency of bleeding episodes and the patient's normal activities. This information is essential in identifying the causative factors of hemorrhage and in designing a program to reduce the frequency and severity of hemorrhages. Objective data should include goniometric evaluation of active and passive ROM and joint deformities, such as genu valgus. Valgus and varus stress tests and assessment of calcaneal and subtalar mobility should be performed to determine ligamentous integrity.

Muscle strength is assessed functionally in the child who is too young to participate in manual muscle testing; otherwise, manual muscle testing is performed. Isokinetic testing may be performed in the older child if more sensitive strength measures are desired, such as for postoperative rehabilitation or to assess readiness to participate in organized sports.

Leg lengths, both from the anterior-superior iliac spine to the medial malleolus and from the umbilicus to the medial malleolus, should be measured to rule out leg-length discrepancy, either actual or apparent secondary to pelvic obliquity. Girth measurements at joints may reveal swelling, although they are more useful when done serially on one joint than in comparison to the contralateral limb, since repeated hemarthroses can cause bony overgrowth. Muscle girth measurements may be indicative of muscle atrophy.

In my clinic, gait is evaluated visually for gross abnormalities, including posture, stride length, stance time, and heel-toe progression. If a treadmill is available, increases in speed and elevation often reveal more subtle differences.

Balance and coordination can be screened quickly by observing stair climbing, single-limb stance, hopping, and skipping (if appropriate for age). Parental reports are usually accurate in identifying coordination problems, at which time more formal testing (e.g., with the Bruininks-Oseretsky Test of Motor Proficiency [Bruininks, 1978]) can be completed.

Gross motor development is assessed annually in our clinic for the first few years of life using the Peabody Developmental Motor Scales (Folio & Fewell, 1983) if developmental problems are suspected. Otherwise, a simple screening tool such as the Denver II (Frankenburg et al., 1990) will give information about development in gross motor, fine motor, cognitive, and ADL skills.

Pain assessment must include the nature and severity of pain. The pain of an acute bleeding episode must be distinguished from the chronic pain of arthropathy. In the very young child who cannot verbalize his pain, the parents are instructed to watch for decreased use of a limb or changes in activity patterns or personality as signs of an acute bleeding episode. The chronic pain of arthropathy will not be evident until joint destruction has progressed to stage 4 or 5, which usually does not occur before the end of the first decade or into the second decade of life. For these preadolescent and older boys, visual analogue or numerical (0–10) scales can be used to measure pain (see Chapter 8).

Treatment

When hemostasis has been achieved after an acute hemorrhage, the child and family should be instructed in active exercises for ROM and strengthening. Koch and colleagues (1982) describe a physical therapy program for the knee with the following rules:

1. Passive ROM is contraindicated.
2. The isometric technique of alternating muscle contraction and relaxation is beneficial.
3. When the quadriceps muscle strength is in the fair range, the patient is encouraged to achieve full active knee extension in supine and sitting.
4. Active resistive exercises may be initiated when available knee flexion is at least 90° and there is less than a 15° flexion contracture.

During this subacute phase, factor replacement therapy is usually given before participation in physical therapy to minimize the risk of rebleeding and may be continued at regular intervals until the hemorrhage resolves. The exercise program must be individualized to progress from isometric to active-assistive, active, and, finally, resistive mode as the pain and swelling diminish and ROM and strength increase. Modalities such as ice, transcutaneous electrical nerve stimulation, and splints may be used to decrease joint pain, and hydrotherapy will allow for ROM, strengthening, and gait training activities to be performed with minimal stress to the joints.

CONTRACTURE MANAGEMENT

If the patient has recurrent hemarthroses without achieving full ROM and strength between bleeding episodes, a contracture will develop. Exercise alone may not be able to overcome the muscle shortening and intracapsular adhesions that may have formed. The Dutch physical therapist Hanke Timmermans has described a program using manual traction and mobilization techniques to relax the joint capsule, increase ROM, and decrease painful movements (1989). Her method, as described below, is one way of approaching contracture management, although it has not been shown to be more effective than other methods.

Manual traction is applied in the position of comfort, taking care that there are no angular movements. With traction maintained, gentle manipulations may be performed to facilitate the restricted motion (e.g., anterior shifting of the tibia facilitates knee extension). Such techniques should only be used when the patient has received factor replacement and the therapist is experienced in both mobilization and management of hemophilia. They should never be used in the presence of severe instability or synovitis.

If full ROM cannot be achieved through exercise, several nonsurgical options are available. Although purely passive manual stretching is rarely indicated, slow stretching of joint contractures over relatively long periods has been shown to be effective (Weiss-man, 1977). Dynamic splints can provide a low intensity, prolonged stretch and can be used in the patient's normal environment without difficulty. To reduce the risk of inducing a bleeding episode, tension on the dynamic splint is started at 0 or 0.5 and increased very slowly. If joint hemorrhage should occur, the dynamic splint is discontinued until the hemorrhage has resolved and then reapplied at a reduced tension. In one study, seven patients with chronic knee flexion contractures of greater than 15° were fitted with dynamic splints (Lang, 1990). The patients wore the dynamic splints at night for several months (range: 4–10), and all demonstrated ROM increases of at least 5°. Although three of these patients experienced knee hemarthroses during the study, each was able to resume use of the splint without restrictions. Despite modest increases in ROM, 5 of the 7 patients reported decreased stiffness and subjective improvement in ambulation.

Dynamic sling traction has also been used to provide prolonged stretch but requires hospitalization and confinement to bed for an average of 2 weeks (Duthie, 1990). The Quengel cast-brace may be used when posterior subluxation of the tibia accompanies a knee flexion contracture. This cast brace has offset subluxation hinges that correct the subluxation while a toggle stick corrects the flexion contracture.

Serial casting and drop-out casts are another option for contracture management. My experience has been limited to use in patients who have severe gastrocnemius muscle hemorrhages with resultant decreased ROM. In one patient, a 70° knee flexion contracture present 1 month after hemorrhage was reduced to his prehemorrhage range of −15° of extension in 6 days by use of a drop-out cast and active knee extension exercises.

ORTHOTICS

Splints and orthoses are commonly used in the management of joint and muscle hemorrhages, but their use must be carefully monitored to prevent overuse. The general rule is to use the least restrictive means necessary to protect the joints and to discontinue this use when the joint is strong enough to be without the extra protection, which is usually when strength and joint stability are in the good range. Therapists may be involved in the fabrication of splints to provide rest to a joint after a bleeding episode or surgery; to prevent or decrease the number of hemorrhages in a chronic joint, prevent or correct joint deformity, or improve function; or to provide support for weak or unstable joints (Holdredge, 1989). The splints are used as an adjunct to therapy and should not be used without a comprehensive program of strengthening exercises and joint stability, gait, and functional training.

STRENGTHENING

Strengthening can be achieved through isometric, isotonic, or isokinetic exercise. The choice of type of exercise depends on the patient's ability to move the joint without pain, particularly after an acute hemarthrosis, or if there is need for immobilization. Isometrics are prescribed immediately after an acute hemarthrosis and continued until the joint is no longer tensely swollen and hot and can be moved without pain. Concentric exercises are then begun and progressed through active-assistive, active, and resistive modes. If the equipment is available, isokinetic exercises can be initiated when muscle strength is in the good range. If the equipment is unavailable, Greene and Strickler (1983) have described a "modified isokinetic" knee strengthening program that consists of using simultaneous contraction of the flexors of one leg against the extensors of the other leg. The patient is instructed to push with as much force as tolerated while allowing the legs to fully extend over a 5- to 10-second period and then to switch position of the legs. The benefit of isokinetic exercise is that resistance is accommodated to maintain maximum muscle tension throughout the full arc of motion, regardless of the relative strength of the muscle at any point along the arc.

Exercises prescribed should not jeopardize an unstable joint by overly stressing it, and thereby increasing the risk of bleeding. For that reason, slow-speed isokinetics (below 180° per second) should be used cautiously or avoided. Progressive resistive exercise (isotonic or isokinetic) in the open chain provide both concentric and eccentric strengthening and are preferred initially to closed-chain eccentric exercise that could produce exercise-induced joint tissue damage from compressive forces. All exercise programs should be advanced slowly to allow for monitoring of effects on the joints (Pietri et al., 1992). Any signs of bleeding, such as increased swelling or pain or decreased ROM, will necessitate reducing the intensity of the exercise program and possibly exercising only under cover of factor replacement until supporting muscles are stronger.

GAIT TRAINING

Gait training focuses on correct positioning of the lower extremities and use of all joints and muscle groups. The patient should be taught a springy way of moving by pushing with the ankle and forefoot to allow the shock absorption of walking to be transferred to the muscles rather than the joints. Temporary use of crutches will transfer some of the weight bearing to the arms, which will decrease the load and pain on an affected lower extremity joint and allow for a more normal gait pattern to be simulated. Orthoses, such as the University of California Biomechanical Laboratory foot orthosis, are helpful when ankle laxity leads to hindfoot valgus, with weight bearing causing abnormal stresses all the way up the lower extremity (Timmermans, 1990).

POSTSURGICAL REHABILITATION

Physical therapists in the pediatric setting will usually be involved only in rehabilitation after synovectomy in the child with hemophilia. Osteotomies and arthrodeses are performed for severe chronic arthropathy with marked deformity, instability, and pain, but there are no references in the literature to these procedures being performed on children. Similarly, arthroplasties of the hip and knee are being performed on adults with severe arthropathy but have not been reported in the pediatric literature.

CASE HISTORY: JIMMY

Jimmy is a 12-year-old boy with severe factor VIII deficiency. Two years ago, with a stage 3 arthropathy and 6-month history of chronic synovitis, he had arthroscopic synovectomy of the right knee with excellent results: ROM of 0 to 130°; quadriceps and hamstring muscle strength both 4+/5 (good+); and only two right knee hemorrhages, 6 months and 10 months earlier. He has been able to resume his favorite sport of tennis in the past year. He has noticed an increase in the incidence of left knee hemarthroses, and in the past month has had five knee bleeding episodes. He has been put on every-other-day factor replacement and referred to physical therapy for intensive rehabilitation.

Current evaluation reveals a boggy, swollen but cool left knee. ROM is −30° of extension to 70° of flexion in the left knee. Within available range, quadriceps strength is 2/5 and hamstring strength is 3/5. Jimmy is ambulating with bilateral axillary crutches, with toe-touch weight bearing on the left. He scores a 6 of 7 (independent with assistive device) on all the mobility and transfer items on the FIM except tub transfers, which are scored a 4 (require moderate assistance). He denies resting pain but does have pain with motion.

Problem 1: 30° left knee flexion contracture

Goal. Improve ROM of both knees to 0 to 140°.
Plan.

1. Fabricate resting knee splint for hours of sleep to maintain maximum available extension at night. Revise splint as extension returns.
2. Use dynamic splinting during the day for prolonged stretch.
3. Perform active ROM exercises.

Problem 2: Decreased strength in both knees

Goal. Increase strength of quadriceps and hamstrings muscles of both legs to normal.
Plan.

1. For left knee, begin with isometric exercises and contract and relax techniques for ROM and strengthening. Begin active-assistive and active exercises when pain abates. When ROM is 15 to 90°, begin resistive exercises and advance slowly using low weights and high repetitions.
2. For right knee, isokinetic strengthening at 180°, 240°, and 300° per second and joint stability activities, such as progressive resistive straight-leg raises and single-limb minisquats.
3. For both lower extremities, strengthening and joint stability activities for hips and ankles (e.g., straight-leg raises in prone and sidelying positions, heel raises, Biomechanical Ankle Platform System [BAPS] board [Camp, Jackson, MI]).

Problem 3: Ambulation dysfunction: toe-touch weight bearing on left using bilateral axillary crutches

Goal. Independent community ambulation without assistive devices.
Plan.

1. Maintain left weight bearing as tolerated in crutch ambulation until knee range is no less than 10 to 100° and quadriceps muscle strength is at least 3+/5.
2. Practice gait training on the treadmill at slow speeds to encourage heel-toe gait pattern and equal stride and step lengths.
3. Progress to independent household ambulation and then community ambulation as ROM and strength improve.

Problem 4: Inability to participate in physical education classes and other athletic functions with friends

Goal. Maintain cardiovascular fitness and resume tennis.
Plan.

1. Aquatic therapy and swimming, 3 times per week for 20 to 30 minutes.

2. Contact school physical education teacher and discuss alternatives to regular physical education program.

3. Consider taping or knee cage for both knees to reduce rotary forces while playing tennis, when able.

Jimmy will be seen three times a week in physical therapy until his ROM and strength return to normal and he is ambulating without an assistive device. He will also be given a home exercise program to supplement his physical therapy sessions. The decision to discontinue factor replacement therapy before physical therapy sessions will be made jointly by the physical therapist and hematologist. Because Jimmy's left knee flexion contracture is an acute problem, his range is expected to return quickly and he should be off crutches in 2 to 3 weeks. His strength will return more slowly, but if he is compliant with his home program he can be cut back to once-a-week physical therapy for monitoring progress and adjusting the home program. Current radiographs will be reviewed with the orthopaedist to determine if playing tennis is an appropriate expectation; if so, Jimmy should be able to resume playing tennis within 3 months.

References

Ahlberg, A. Hemophilia in Sweden: VII. Incidence, treatment, and prophylaxis of arthropathy and other musculoskeletal manifestations of hemophilia A & B. Acta Orthopaedica Scandinavica, 77:3–132, 1965.

Arnold, WD, & Hilgartner, MW. Hemophilic arthropathy. Journal of Bone and Joint Surgery (American), 59:288–305, 1977.

Atkins, RM, Henderson, NJ, & Duthie, RB. Joint contractures in the hemophilias. Clinical Orthopedics and Related Research, 219:97–105, 1987.

Bruininks, RH. Bruininks-Oseretsky Test of Motor Proficiency, Examiners Manual. Circle Pines, MN: American Guidance Service, 1978.

Buchanan, GR. Hemophilia. Pediatric Clinics of North America, 27(2):309–326, 1980.

Corrigan, JJ. Coagulation disorders. In Miller, DR, & Bachner, RL (Eds.), Blood Disorders of Infancy and Childhood. St. Louis: CV Mosby, 1990, pp. 849–859.

Duthie, RB. Dynamic sling traction. In Gilbert, MS, & Greene, WB (Eds.), Musculoskeletal Problems in Hemophilia. New York: National Hemophilia Foundation, 1990, pp. 67–68.

Erken, EHW. Radiocolloids in the management of hemophilic arthropathy in children and adolescents. Clinical Orthopedics and Related Research, 264:129–134, 1991.

Fernandez-Palazzi, F, Rupcich, M, Rivas, S, & Bosch, N. Biomechanical alterations that impair evolution and prognosis of haemophilic arthropathy. In Gilbert, MS, & Greene, WB (Eds.), Musculoskeletal Problems in Hemophilia. New York: National Hemophilia Foundation, 1990, pp. 34–44.

Folio, MR, & Fewell, RR. Peabody Developmental Motor Scales and Activity Cards. Allen, TX: DLM Teaching Resources, 1983.

Frankenburg, WK, Dodds, JB, Archer, P, Bresnick, B, Maschka, P, Edelman, N, & Shapiro, H. Denver II Screening Manual. Denver: Denver Developmental Materials, 1990.

Greene, WB, & Strickler, EM. A modified isokinetic strengthening program for patients with severe hemophilia. Developmental Medicine and Child Neurology, 25:189–196, 1983.

Gregosiewicz, A, Wosko, I, & Kandzierski, G. Intraarticular bleeding in children with hemophilia: The prevention of arthropathy. Journal of Pediatric Orthopedics, 9:182–185, 1989.

Hilgartner, MW. AIDS in the transfusion recipient. Pediatric Clinics of North America, 38:121–129, 1991.

Holdredge, S. Thermoplastic splints. In Funk, S (Ed.), Rehabilitation in Hemophilia: Proceedings of a Conference. New York: National Hemophilia Foundation, 1989, pp. 38–44.

Holdredge, S, & Cotta, S. Physical therapy and rehabilitation in the care of the adult and child with hemophilia. In Hilgartner, MW, & Pochedly, C (Eds.), Hemophilia in the Child and Adult. New York: Raven Press, 1989, pp. 235–262.

Houghton, GR, & Duthie, RB. Orthopedic problems in hemophilia. Clinical Orthopedics and Related Research, 138:197–216, 1979.

Joist, JH, & Ameri, A. Pathogenesis of hemophilic arthropathy. In Gilbert, MS, & Greene, WB (Eds.), Musculoskeletal Problems in Hemophilia. New York: National Hemophilia Foundation, 1990, p. 20–25.

Jonas, DL. Drug abuse in hemophilia. In Hilgartner, MW, & Pochedly, C (Eds.), Hemophilia in the Child and Adult. New York: Raven Press, 1989, pp. 229–234.

Karayalcin, G. Current concepts in the management of hemophilia. Pediatric Annals, 14:640–655, 1985.

Kasper, CK, & Dietrich, SL. Comprehensive management of hemophilia. Clinics in Haematology, 14:491–492, 1985.

Koch, B, Cohen, S, Luban, NC, & Eng, G. Hemophiliac knee: Rehabilitation techniques. Archives of Physical Medicine and Rehabilitation, 63:379–382, 1982.

Koch, B, Galioto, FM, Jr, Kelleher, J, & Goldstein, D. Physical fitness in children with hemophilia. Archives of Physical Medicine and Rehabilitation, 65:324–326, 1984.

Lang, L. Dynasplint for knee flexion contractures in hemophilia. In Gilbert, MS, & Greene, WB (Eds.), Musculoskeletal Problems in Hemophilia. New York: National Hemophilia Foundation, 1990, pp. 83–86.

National Hemophilia Foundation. Hemophilia and Sports. New York: National Hemophilia Foundation, 1985.

Pietri, MM, Frontera, WR, Pratts, IS, & Suarez, EL. Skeletal muscle function in patients with hemophilia A and unilateral hemarthroses of the knee. Archives of Physical Medicine and Rehabilitation, 73:22–26, 1992.

State University of New York at Buffalo, Center for Functional Assessment Research, Department of Rehabilitation Medicine. Guide for the Use of the Uniform Data Set for Medical Rehabilitation Including the Functional Independence Measure for Children (WeeFIM), 1991.

Strickler, EM, & Greene, WB. Isokinetic torque levels in hemophiliac knee musculature. Archives of Physical Medicine and Rehabilitation, 65:766–770, 1984.

Timmermans, H. Severe arthropathy of the hemophilic joint: a comprehensive rehabilitation program. In Funk, S (Ed.), Rehabilitation in Hemophilia: Proceedings of a Conference. New York: National Hemophilia Foundation, 1989, pp. 11–15.

Timmermans, H. The role of the physiotherapist. In Gilbert, MS, & Greene, WB (Eds.), Musculoskeletal Problems in Hemophilia. New York: National Hemophilia Foundation, 1990, pp. 115–121.

Williamson, J. Rehabilitation medicine and the hemophilia patient. Mt. Sinai Journal of Medicine, 44:359–370, 1977.

Chapter 10

Spinal Conditions

CHERYL PATRICK, PT

The spine is the framework for our posture and our movement. It supports our cranium, extremities, and spinal cord; allows for trunk flexibility; acts as a shock absorber; and provides structural support for normal chest and respiratory development. Orthopaedic concerns arise when spinal alignment is altered by congenital or progressive changes, producing scoliosis, kyphosis, or lordosis.

Each one or a combination of these conditions, if left untreated, directly affects a child's pulmonary function, psychosocial well-being, potential for back pain, and mortality rate. We, as physical therapists, play a vital role in the detection and treatment of spinal conditions because 2 to 3% of the population of school-aged children (7–16 years) are at risk for adolescent idiopathic scoliosis, the most common form of scoliosis. The prevalence of other spinal conditions varies with the condition and underlying disease process (Bleck, 1991; Weinstein, 1989).

In this chapter the prevalence and natural history, identification, examination, and treatment of these spinal conditions are addressed. Specific case histories are presented to discuss impairments, functional limitations, and disabilities of children with spinal conditions. Emphasis is on physical therapy intervention with nonsurgical and surgical management of these spinal conditions.

Because pathologic spinal conditions are discussed in this chapter, it is necessary for the reader

Proliferation of the somites occurs, developing to have some knowledge of normal spinal development (Fig. 10–1). Therefore, development in the embryologic, fetal, and childhood stages is briefly discussed.

Fetal development is divided into three stages. The first 3 weeks after fertilization are termed the *pre-embryonic period.* The *embryonic period* is next, lasting from week 3 to week 8 of gestation, and it is during this stage that the organs of the body develop. The *fetal period* lasts from week 8 until term, and during this stage maturation and growth of all structures and organs occur (Moe et al., 1987).

Early development of the skeletal, muscular, and neural systems is related to the notochord. Cell proliferation occurs at approximately 3 weeks, forming a trilaminar structure with layers of ectoderm, mesoderm, and endoderm. Proliferation of the mesodermal tissue continues, forming 29 pairs of somites in the fourth week and the remainder, 42 to 44 total, in the fifth week. Differentiation of the somites then occurs, producing 4 occipital, 8 cervical, 12 thoracic, 5 lumbar, 5 sacral, and 8 to 10 coccygeal somites. The occipital somites form a portion of the base of the skull and the articulation between the cranium and cervical vertebrae while the last 5 to 7 coccygeal somites disappear. Cervical, thoracic, lumbar, and sacral somites form the structures of the spine (Winter, 1983).

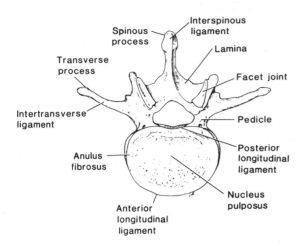

FIGURE 10–1. The L-2 vertebra viewed from above. (From Moe, JH, Winter, RB, Bradford, DS, Ogilvie, JW, & Lonstein, JE. Scoliosis and Other Spinal Deformities, [2nd ed.]. Philadelphia: WB Saunders, 1987, p. 8.)

three distinct areas. Dorsally the cells become dermatome, giving rise to the skin. Medially to the dermatome, cells migrate deep to give rise to skeletal muscle. The ventral and medial cells migrate toward the notochord and neural tube to form the sclerotome (Moe et al., 1987; Winter, 1983).

The sclerotomal cells proliferate and differentiate, giving rise to rudimentary vertebral structures, including rib buds. Chondrification begins at the cervicothoracic level, extending cranially and caudally. Centers of chondrification allow for formation of the solid cartilage model of a vertebra with no line of demarcation between body, neural arch, or rib rudiments (Moe et al., 1987).

Ossification occurs at primary and secondary centers. Ossification begins during the late fetal period and continues after birth. Primary centers of ossification extend to the spinous, transverse, and articular processes. Secondary ossification centers develop at the upper and lower portions of the vertebral body, at the tip of the spinous processes, and at each transverse process. These centers expand in late adolescence. Secondary ossification centers also develop in the ribs—one at the head of the rib and two in the tubercle. Ossification of the axis, atlas, and sacrum differs slightly from that of the other vertebrae. The atlas has two primary centers and one secondary center of ossification, while the axis has five primary and two secondary centers of ossification. Ossification of the axis begins near the end of gestation with fusion of the two odontoid centers and is completed in the sec-

ond decade of life with fusion of the odontoid and centrum. Fusion of the sacrum begins in adolescence and is completed in the third decade of life (Moe et al., 1987).

Spinal growth occurs throughout adolescence. A knowledge of spinal growth is essential in nonsurgical and surgical treatment of spinal deformities. Spinal growth does not proceed in a uniform linear pattern (Tanner et al., 1966; Tanner & Whitehouse, 1976). Two periods of rapid spinal growth occur, the first from birth to age 3 years and the second at the adolescent growth spurt. Between 3 years and the onset of puberty, growth is linear.

The spinal pubertal growth spurts occur at different chronologic and Tanner ages for females and males. In females, the growth spurt coincides with Tanner 2 or a chronologic age of 8 to 14 years, with the maximum growth occurring at a mean of 12 years of age. The spurt lasts 2.5 to 3 years (Calvo, 1957). The growth spurt occurs later in males, at Tanner 3 or chronologic age 11 to 16 years, with the maximum growth at age 14 years. These values are average values based on white Anglo-Saxon populations (Duval-Beaupere, 1972).

A fused area of the spine does not grow longitudinally, as documented by Moe and colleagues (1964). The information, therefore, on spinal growth potential is taken into account by the surgeon for each individual case.

SCOLIOSIS

Detection and Clinical Evaluation

Detection of scoliosis is primarily by identification of trunk, shoulder, or pelvic asymmetries. Children who present with asymmetries should be referred for a baseline evaluation to an orthopaedic surgeon with an interest and knowledge of scoliosis. Ideally, the surgeon should specialize in pediatrics or pediatric spines, be affiliated with a reputable medical center, and be part of a team that includes an orthotist, a nurse, and a physical therapist.

An evaluation begins with a complete patient history to obtain information regarding curve detection, familial conditions, general health, and physical maturity. Clinical examination includes evaluation of the deformity, general alignment, shoulder and pelvic symmetry, spinal alignment by forward bend test, trunk compensation using a plumb line, and leg length measurement. The examiner also evaluates signs and symptoms of any underlying disease and neurologic status. Rotation of the spine is quantified using a scoliometer with the forward bend test (Moe et al., 1987). This instrument works like a level placed astride the spinous processes to measure rotation of a rib hump or prominent lumbar paraspinal musculature.

Radiographs (initially two views: anterior-posterior and lateral) are used to determine location, type, and magnitude of the curve as well as skeletal age. Skeletal maturity is determined using the Risser sign, which quantifies the amount of ossification of the iliac crest, using grades 0 to 5. Grades 1 to 4 are excursions from 25 to 100%, starting at the anterior-superior iliac spine. Grade 5 categorizes fusion of the iliac crest with the ileum (Zaouss & James, 1958). Grade 0 represents absence of ossification. Grades 0, 1, and 2 correlate with skeletal immaturity, grade 3 with progressing skeletal maturity, grade 4 with cessation of spinal growth, and grade 5 with cessation of increase in height.

The spinal curvature is measured using the Cobb method. To complete the measurement, one must first identify the end vertebrae. The end vertebrae are described as the most cephalad vertebra of a curve whose upper surface maximally tilts toward the curve's concavity and the most caudal vertebra with maximal tilt toward the concavity. Lines are drawn as extensions of the end vertebra from either end-plate or pedicle. The degree of curvature is measured as the angle formed by the intersection of lines perpendicular to these end vertebral lines (Dickson et al., 1984; Goldstein & Waugh, 1973). Minimal degree of curvature for diagnosis is 10° (Fig. 10–2). Computed tomography, conventional tomography, magnetic resonance imaging, myelography, and bone scanning provide additional information if necessary to aid in diagnosis and detection of spinal conditions.

Terminology

Spinal deformities are classified according to magnitude, location, direction, and etiology. Curvatures may be idiopathic, neuromuscular, or congenital and may further be classified by the area of the spine in which the apex of the curve is located: (1) cervical curve, between C-1 and C-6; (2) cervicothoracic curve, between C-7 and T-1; (3) thoracic curve, between T-2 and T-11; (4) thoracolumbar curve, between T-12 and L-1; (5) lumbar curve, between L-2 and L-4; and (6) lumbosacral curve, between L-5 and S-1. Direction of the curve is designated right or left by the side of the convexity of the deformity (Rothman & Simeone, 1982).

Essentially there are two major types of curvatures: structural and nonstructural. A nonstructural curve fully corrects clinically and radiographically on lateral bend toward the apex of the curve and lacks vertebral rotation. A nonstructural curve is

FIGURE 10–2. A, Cobb's method of measuring the angle of the curve in scoliosis. Please refer to text for explanation. (From Tachdjian, MO. Pediatric Orthopedics [2nd ed.]. Philadelphia: WB Saunders, 1972, p. 2385.) B, The Cobb method of measuring the curve angle of scoliosis as seen on a radiograph.

usually nonprogressive and is most often caused by a shortened lower extremity on the side of the apex of the curve. It is essential, however, to watch these curves during growth because occasionally they may develop into structural deformities.

A structural curve cannot be voluntarily, passively, or forcibly fully corrected. Rotation of the vertebrae is present toward the convexity of the curve. A fixed thoracic prominence or rib hump in a child with a thoracic deformity or a lumbar paraspinal prominence in a child with a lumbar curve is evidence of rotation when seen on clinical examination (Rothman & Simeone, 1982).

Idiopathic Scoliosis

Idiopathic scoliosis denotes a lateral curvature of the spine of unknown cause and is the most common form of scoliosis in children.

ETIOLOGY, INCIDENCE, AND PATHOPHYSIOLOGY

Infantile idiopathic scoliosis develops in children younger than age 3, usually presenting shortly after birth. The majority of the curves are left thoracic and occur more frequently in male infants. Eighty to ninety percent of these curves spontaneously resolve. Most of the remainder of cases progress throughout childhood, resulting in severe deformity. Because infantile idiopathic scoliosis is common in England and Northern Europe, but rare in the United States, research suggests environmental factors in the development of the deformity (Rothman & Simeone, 1982).

Juvenile idiopathic scoliosis develops between age 3 years and before the onset of puberty. The most common curve is right thoracic, presenting in males and females with equal frequency and most often recognized around age 6 years. Juvenile idiopathic curves have a high rate of progression and result in severe deformity if untreated. A study by Wynne-Davies (1974) found the incidence of children younger than the age of 8 years who have scoliosis to be 1.3%.

Adolescent idiopathic scoliosis categorizes curves presenting at or around the onset of puberty. The prevalence of idiopathic scoliosis is 2 to 3% of children aged 7 to 16, with the majority of curves presenting at the onset of puberty, therefore classified as being adolescent idiopathic scoliosis (Bleck, 1991). Three to nine percent of these children have curves greater than 10° and require treatment (Dickson, et al., 1984; Weinstein, 1989). The overall female/male ratio for prevalence of adolescent

idiopathic scoliosis is 3.6:1. The female/male ratio is roughly equal (1.4:1) in curves of approximately 10°. With curve magnitude of 20° or greater, the female/male ratio increases to 6.4:1 (Weinstein, 1989). A greater percentage of curves will progress in the female patient, 19.3% compared with 1.2% of males. A large number of adolescent idiopathic scoliosis curvatures are structural at the time of detection, although flexibility and the progression of these curves vary. Structural curves have a greater tendency to progress throughout adolescence at an average rate of 1° per month if untreated, while the nonstructural curves may remain flexible enough to avoid becoming problematic (Rothman & Simeone, 1982).

An extensive amount of research has been devoted to discovering the cause of idiopathic scoliosis, but the mechanics and specific etiology are not clearly understood. A number of theories have been proposed that attempt to explain the mechanics of vertebral column failure and decompensation of the spine as seen in idiopathic scoliosis. These include insufficiency of the costovertebral ligaments, asymmetric weakness of the paraspinal musculature, unequal distribution of type I and type II muscle fibers, and collagen abnormalities. Clinical studies have focused on deviations in vibratory responses, proprioceptive deficits, and neurologic or vestibular dysfunction. No conclusive evidence has been found to indicate any of these factors as a cause of idiopathic scoliosis. In fact, it is now proposed that some of the clinical changes such as vibratory and proprioceptive deficits are actually secondary to, rather than a cause of, the existing spinal deformity (Dickson et al., 1984; McInnes et al., 1991).

Although the specific etiology of idiopathic scoliosis is not known, data from studies by Wynne-Davies (1966, 1968) and Cowell and colleagues (1972) reflect the existence of a familial tendency. Familial prevalence of idiopathic scoliosis may reflect a growth pattern shared by families. The growth pattern and effects of biplanal spinal asymmetry during growth are discussed in a study by Dickson and associates (1984), which specifically examines the growth factors in the coronal and sagittal planes and their effect on progressive idiopathic scoliosis.

Structural changes vary with the degree of scoliosis and affect the anatomy and physiology of the spine, with the greatest change at the apex of the curve (Tachdjian, 1990). Compression and distraction forces act on the growing spine to produce wedge-shaped vertebrae (larger on the convex side and smaller on the concave side). Associated changes are seen in the intraspinal canal and poste-

FIGURE 10–3. Anatomic specimen of the spine demonstrating structural changes of right thoracic scoliosis. Note vertebral wedging on the concave side and rotation of the vertebral bodies to the convexity of the curve. (From James, JIP. Scoliosis. Baltimore: Williams & Wilkins, 1967, p. 13. © 1967, the Williams & Wilkins Co., Baltimore.)

rior arch, which may cause angulation and stretch on the spinal cord but very rarely cause functional disturbances. Cord compression and functional changes occur most often secondary to an unusually tight dura mater, as seen in spines with marked dorsal kyphosis. Changes occurring on the concave side of the curvature include compression and degenerative changes of intravertebral discs and shortening of muscles and ligaments (Fig. 10–3). Changes in the thoracic spine directly affect the rib cage. The translatory shift of the spine causes an asymmetrically divided thorax, producing decreased pulmonary capacity on the convex side and increased pulmonary capacity on the concave side. Severe curves in the thoracic spine associated with increased angulation of the ribs posteriorly further reduce aeration of the lung on the convex side, potentially causing abnormal stresses on the heart and disturbed cardiac function (Dickson et al., 1984; Tachdjian, 1990). Structural changes cause cosmetic deformity that, in turn, affects appearance and may affect psychosocial well-being.

NATURAL HISTORY

A progressive curve is defined by a sustained increase of 5° or more on two consecutive examinations occurring at 4- to 6-month intervals. An untreated progressive curve has the potential to increase in magnitude in adult life. The following are the main factors that influence the probability of progression in the skeletally immature patient (Weinstein, 1989):

1. The younger the patient at diagnosis, the greater the risk of progression.
2. Double curve patterns have a greater risk for progression than single curve patterns.
3. The lower the Risser sign, the greater the risk of progression.
4. Curves with greater magnitude are at a greater risk to progress.
5. Risk of progression in females is approximately 10 times that of males with curves of comparable magnitude.
6. Greater risk of progression is present when curves develop before menarche.

Congenital Scoliosis

ETIOLOGY, INCIDENCE, AND PATHOPHYSIOLOGY

Congenital scoliosis curves are caused by anomalous vertebral development. Congenital anomalies of the vertebrae can be attributed to failure of ver tebral segmentation or failure of vertebral formation. Both pathologic processes are frequently seen in the same spine and may occur either at the same or at different levels. Location on the vertebrae (anterior, posterior, lateral, or a combination) determines the congenital deformity. Purely lateral deformity produces congenital scoliosis, while anterolateral and posterolateral deformities produce congenital kyphoscoliosis and lordoscoliosis, respectively (Winter, 1983, 1988).

A defect of segmentation is seen when adjacent vertebrae do not completely separate from one another, thereby producing an unsegmented bar, with no growth plate or disc between the adjacent vertebrae. A lateral, one-sided defect of segmentation produces severe progressive congenital scoliosis, Circumferential failure of segmentation produces en bloc vertebrae, an anomaly that results in loss of segmental motion and loss of longitudinal vertebral growth but no rotational or angular spinal deformity (Winter, 1983).

Defects of formation may be partial or complete. An anterior failure of formation of all or part of the vertebral body produces a kyphosis. A partial unilateral defect of formation of a vertebra produces a wedge-shaped hemivertebra (Fig. 10–4) with one pedicle and only one side with growth potential. A nonsegmented hemivertebra is completely fused to the adjacent proximal and distal vertebrae. A semisegmented hemivertebra is fused to only one adjacent vertebra and separated from the other by a normal end-plate and disc. A segmented hemivertebra is separated from both the proximal and distal vertebrae by a normal end-plate and disc. Hemivertebrae may be unbalanced, with the defect present on one side of the spine, or balanced, with different hemivertebrae present with defects on opposite sides of the spine compensating any curves (Winter, 1983, 1988).

The etiology of congenital scoliosis involves fetal environmental factors that affect development at 45 to 60 days after fertilization (Winter, 1988). A study by Wynne-Davies (1975) represents a comprehensive review of 337 patients with congenital spinal anomalies and their families. She found that an isolated anomaly, like a hemivertebra, is a sporadic lesion with no increased risk of spinal deformities for subsequent births or for children of parents who have the deformity. Multiple spinal anomalies, with or without the presence of spina bifida, are believed to be related etiologically to spina bifida and therefore carry a 5–10% risk to subsequent siblings for any one of the anomalies. A review by Winter (1983) of 1250 patients with congenital spinal anomalies, however, found few familial relationships (only 13 of 1250). Conclusions

FIGURE 10–4. Radiograph of congenital scoliosis due to hemivertebrae of thoracic vertebrae. Compensatory scoliosis in the lumbar spine. (The arrow on the left indicates the hemivertebrae.)

were drawn that hemivertebrae carry an approximate 1% chance of occurring in a first-degree relative of a patient with a hemivertebra. A relationship between multiple congenital anomalies and spina bifida was not noted.

Other spinal anomalies or other organ system anomalies may be associated with congenital spinal malformations. One of these anomalies is diastematomyelia, a congenital malformation of the neural axis in which there is sagittal division of the spinal cord. Diastematomyelia is often associated with an osseous, fibrous, or fibrocartilaginous spur attached to one or more vertebral bodies and the dura mater. Clinical signs of a spinal dysraphism include a hair patch, unequal foot size, various foot deformities (e.g., cavus feet), and asymmetric lower extremity circumference and strength. Other associated defects include urinary tract anomalies, hearing deficits, facial asymmetries, and Sprengel's deformity, which is a partially undescended scapula that may cause apparent webbing or shortening of the neck as well as limited shoulder range of motion (ROM) (Winter, 1983).

The risk of progression can be analyzed by examining the growth potential of the congenital anomaly. Many congenital curves become stable and do not progress. The highest risk of progression is when there is asymmetric growth in which the convexity outgrows the concavity. This usually occurs when the anatomy of the convex side is relatively normal and the concave side is deficient. A shortened trunk may be the main deformity if both convex and concave growth deficiencies occur over multiple levels (Winter, 1988).

Treatment of Idiopathic and Congenital Scoliosis

Treatment decisions are based on skeletal maturity of the child, growth potential of the child, and curve magnitude. Options include nonsurgical methods, such as exercise, orthotic treatment, and electrical stimulation, and surgical treatment.

NONSURGICAL METHODS

Idiopathic curves of less than 25°, curves of nonsurgical magnitude of any type in a skeletally mature patient, and nonprogressive congenital curves are evaluated by clinical examination every 4 to 6 months. Radiographs are obtained for congenital curves at each visit; however, unchanged results of a scoliometer examination may reduce the frequency of radiographs to every other visit depending on individual physician and institution practice.

A home exercise program designed to maintain or improve trunk and pelvic strength and flexibility is often prescribed for children with idiopathic or congenital scoliosis. Exercises include postural exercises (trunk extensor control, abdominal strengthening, gluteal strengthening), lateral flexion exercises, trunk shifts, stretching of pectorals and lower extremities, and respiratory exercises to increase chest capacity and maximize volume. In my clinical experience, compliance is often poor unless the child experienced back pain before diagnosis of scoliosis. Exercise as the sole treatment for prevention of progression of scoliotic curves has not been shown to be effective (Lonstein & Renshaw, 1987).

Electrical Stimulation

The use of electrical stimulation versus orthotic management is often physician and rehabilitation center specific. Electrical stimulation is used on the convex side of the curve, in theory to produce sufficient stimulation to alter the direction of the deformity, decrease the pressure on the concave side of the curve, and allow for more normal vertebral growth. The stimulator is worn at night, and treatment continues until growth ceases, skin complications prevent further use, or curve progression continues. Indications for use are a skeletally immature child with an idiopathic curve of 10 to 40°. (Eckerson & Axelgaard, 1984; Farady, 1983). Contraindications include inability of the patient to operate the unit, curves greater than 40°, heart disease, or thoracic hypokyphosis (Tachdjian, 1990).

Controversy surrounds the use of electrical stimulation as a viable treatment method for idiopathic scoliosis. Early studies indicated that curve stabilization occurred in 70 to 75% of patients (Brown et al., 1984) with good compliance and that potential for retention of curve correction was good (Eckerson & Axelgaard, 1984). More recent studies have found that electrical stimulation did not arrest progression or change the natural history of the curves, when compared with control groups (Bertrand et al., 1992; Bylund et al., 1987). Electrical stimulation was found to be ineffective for double curves, and noncompliance rates were comparable to those of orthotic wear (Bertrand et al., 1992). Recent research, therefore, concluded that electrical stimulation had no effect on prevention of idiopathic curve progression, especially for patients with high-risk factors.

Orthotic Management

Goals of orthotic management include halting curve progression, gaining some permanent correction, and allowing for continued spinal growth (Renshaw, 1985).

The principles of orthotic management are based on the biomechanical hypothesis that spinal stability is directly proportional to the end support of the spine and inversely proportional to spinal flexibility and the approximate square of its length. Therefore, the amount of load that may be placed on the spine before collapse can be increased by firm support at the upper and lower ends. An orthosis provides this support at the lower end of the spine anteriorly and laterally on the abdomen, posteriorly and laterally on the buttocks and by contour over the iliac crests, effectively decreasing the lumbar lordosis. The upper end is supported by neck, shoulder, and spinal musculature, by central nervous system reflexes, and possibly by a throat mold. These end supports result in a functional shortening of the spinal column, decreased spinal flexibility, and increased resistance to buckling. Indirect forces are applied laterally by pads, flanges, or slings, thus providing lateral and rotational correction (Kehl & Morrissey, 1988; Renshaw, 1985).

The indication for orthotic use is dependent on curve type, magnitude, and location. Indications for orthotic management for children with idiopathic scoliosis are skeletal immaturity, a documented progressive curve of 20 to 29° or a curve at presentation of 30 to 40°, curve flexibility, and patient compliance (Green, 1986; Renshaw, 1985). A progressive curve is one that has increased at least 5° since detection. Rigid congenital curves do not respond well to orthotics, but an orthosis may be used to control compensatory, flexible curves resulting from a congenital anomaly in another part of the spine (Renshaw, 1985; Winter, 1988).

A Milwaukee brace or cervical-thoracic-lumbar-sacral orthosis (CTLSO) best treats a curve with an apex of T8 or above. A CTLSO consists of a pelvic girdle, throat mold, and a metal suprastructure. Axillary slings, shoulder flange, and pads provide lateral or horizontal corrective forces giving three-point axially directed pressure. The Milwaukee brace was the only spinal orthosis available until the 1970s when the Boston bracing system was developed (Kehl & Morrissy, 1988; Renshaw, 1985).

The Boston system was designed to decrease costs, improve the acceptability of orthotic wear, and simplify construction (Farady, 1983). A series of 24 prefabricated polypropylene pelvic molds lined with polyethylene foam constitute the Boston system (Fig. 10-5). An orthotist molds the brace to

FIGURE 10-6. The Wilmington brace—a custom-molded, total contact TLSO.

the patient, adding lumbar pads and relief areas. The rigid shell provides a firm support while the foam lining allows for comfort. A Boston brace is an example of a thoracolumbosacral orthosis (TLSO) and best treats a curve with an apex lower than T-9 (Farady, 1983). A Boston brace may be modified by the addition of an extension on the concave side to achieve improved correction for curves with an apex at T-7 to T-9 (Kehl & Morrissy, 1988).

Other TLSO types include the Wilmington, Lyon, and Charleston models. A Wilmington TLSO (Fig. 10-6) is a total contact, custom-molded orthosis that achieves maximal spinal correction by the tight contact and fit, not by pads and relief areas (Kehl & Morrissy, 1988). A Lyon orthosis is used to treat idiopathic scoliosis presenting with thoracic hypokyphosis. A Charleston orthosis is used for idiopathic curves and worn only at night, since it is fabricated in the position of maximum side bend correction. Preliminary results are promising, especially for single curves, with 87% (166 of 191) of curves either improving or not progressing more than 5° from the initial measurement. Results, however, cannot be considered conclusive until all patients in the study have reached skeletal maturity (Price et al., 1990).

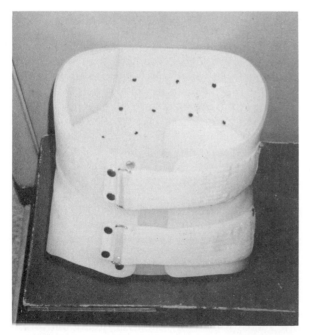

FIGURE 10-5. The Boston brace, underarm TLSO. Note pads for relief and pressure areas.

The active theory of orthotics is that curve progression is prevented by muscle contractions responding to the brace wear. A study by Wynarsky and Schultz (1989), however, showed no statistical difference between myoelectrical activity during braced and unbraced states of female patients being treated with the Boston brace for idiopathic scoliosis. The passive theory is that curve progression is prevented through the external forces of the brace on the spine.

Exercises to be performed while wearing the brace, such as pelvic tilts, thoracic flexion, and lateral shifts, are often taught to patients to improve the active forces. Studies have shown no statistical difference in curve stability between those patients who comply with orthotic wear and exercises and those who comply only with orthotic wear (Carman et al., 1985). A physical therapist's main role is to encourage physical activity of the patient (e.g., during physical education class, aerobics, dance) while wearing the orthosis to maintain balance, coordination, and strength and to develop good habits of achieving and maintaining cardiorespiratory fitness. Specific trunk exercises, such as those for unbraced scoliosis, may be taught to the patient to perform while out of the brace and are designed to maintain trunk strength and flexibility.

Orthotic treatment continues until the curve is no longer controlled (usually 40-45° or higher), curve progression persists, or skeletal maturity occurs, at which time weaning may begin. Twenty to twenty-six percent of orthotically treated curves will progress enough to require spinal fusion (Piazza & Basset, 1990). High-risk factors include younger age at curve detection, higher magnitude, and low Risser sign just as for untreated idiopathic scoliosis, although orthotic wear can positively influence the natural history of idiopathic scoliosis (Basset et al., 1986; Kehl & Morrissy, 1988).

The weaning process takes about 12 months from the time of skeletal maturity and consists of gradually decreasing the amount of time wearing the brace. An orthotic treatment is considered successful if the curve magnitude at the end of treatment is within 5° of the magnitude at the start of treatment. Three studies by Carr and associates (1980), Basset and colleagues (1986), and Emans and co-workers (1986) have shown that a gradual loss of curve correction occurs over 2 to 5 years following successful orthotic management.

SURGICAL METHODS

The major indication for spinal fusion is a documented progressive idiopathic curve that reaches 45° or greater. Curves greater than 40° are increasingly difficult to manage orthotically and also present with significant risk of progression after skeletal maturity (Kostuik, 1990). The goals of spinal fusion are to halt the progression of the deformity to avoid the sequelae of pain and pulmonary dysfunction, achieve maximal correction in all three planes with minimal surgical risk, obtain a balanced trunk, and obtain a solid spinal arthrodesis (Drummond, 1991). The main objective of any scoliosis surgery is to obtain a solid arthrodesis because the fusion mass is ultimately what prevents further progression of the deformity (Drummond, 1991; Kostuik, 1990).

A posterior surgical approach is most often used for spinal fusion. Bone graft is packed into disc spaces and facet joints of the vertebrae after surgical exposure and preparation. The differences in posterior spinal fusions lie with the instrumentation used to obtain correction and protect the fusion. The Harrington rod system is the standard for comparison with newer instrumentation, although this system is rarely used today. The system consists of a distraction rod to the concave side and compression rod to the convex. The rods are attached to posterior spinal elements by hooks. This technique always requires postoperative immobilization of the trunk, does not allow for sagittal plane correction, and produces a flattened lumbar lordosis secondary to the distraction forces.

The Luque instrumentation consists of two L-shaped rods attached with sublaminar wiring. This system allows for load sharing as multiple segments are wired and is therefore best suited to patients with poor bone quality, anomalies of the posterior spinal elements, or poor muscle or skin quality (Drummond, 1991; Kostuik, 1990). The Luque system (Fig. 10–7) can prevent loss of lumbar lordosis and provide stabilization to the pelvis. The disadvantage is a risk of neurologic damage (Tachjdian, 1990). The Cotrel-Dubousset system (Fig. 10–8) uses two rods and compression or distraction hooks attached to either laminae or pedicles. The rods can be contoured to obtain sagittal plane correction, that is, restoring lumbar lordosis and thoracic kyphosis (Drummond, 1991; Kostuik, 1990).

An anterior surgical approach includes opening of the thoracic cavity, resection of a rib, and excision through the diaphragm to expose the necessary vertebrae. To obtain correction and protect the spinal fusion, either Zielke or Dwyer screws are used on the vertebral bodies. Zielke screws are newer, provide control at each segment with a rod and screw, and allow for prevention of postinstrumentation kyphosis (Tachdjian, 1990). An anterior approach may be used to fuse a thoracolumbar or lumbar idiopathic scoliosis.

FIGURE 10-7. Radiograph of the Luque rod instrumentation system for corrective spinal surgery. Note the segmental wiring.

A two-staged procedure is used for higher magnitude curves of severe kyphoscoliotic curves. An anterior approach is used for the release of anterior spinal ligaments, a discectomy, or a fusion with or without instrumentation. The procedure is completed by a posterior spinal fusion with instrumentation (Kostuik, 1990). Two procedures are necessary to gain range of the vertebral column for maximal correction of the curve and to provide fusion stability to prevent instrumentation failure or pseudarthrosis.

Anterior or posterior surgical approaches are used for fusion or congenital curves depending on the area of the spine where the anomaly occurs. Surgical methods for congenital scoliosis may include excision of the anomalous vertebrae or spinal fusion or both. The fusion most often is performed in situ or without instrumentation on the convex side of the curve to prevent further curve progression because the goal of surgery is curve stabilization, not correction (Winter, 1983; 1988).

If a very young, skeletally immature patient presents with a significant curve that is not responsive to orthotic management, a procedure known as "rod without fusion" may be performed. A single, subcutaneous rod without compressive or distractive forces is placed along the scoliotic curve to control the direction of spinal growth. A fusion is not performed because this causes a cessation of growth at the fused segments of spine. An orthosis is prescribed for the patient for full-time wear to protect the instrumentation and control any decompensation of the trunk (Rothman & Simeone, 1982).

POSTOPERATIVE MANAGEMENT

The postoperative use of an orthosis is dependent on the type of curve that was fused, the type of instrumentation used, and the postoperative alignment of the trunk. Nearly all congenital scoliosis curves require postoperative orthotic or plaster cast treatment to protect the in situ fusion, to promote

FIGURE 10-8. Cotrel-Dubousset instrumentation system implanted on a plastic spine.

healing or the fusion, and to help correct any compensatory curves. Idiopathic scoliotic curves managed with a two-staged procedure, Luque rods, or an anterior spinal fusion with instrumentation require orthotic use until the fusion mass is well formed as determined by radiographs. Currently, a child with idiopathic scoliosis who is treated with posterior spinal fusion and Cotrel-Dubousset instrumentation does not require postoperative bracing if the trunk is compensated and the correction is satisfactory.

The average length of a hospital stay for a posterior spinal fusion (or a one-stage procedure) is 7 to 10 days, with physical therapy initiated on the second postoperative day. A physical therapist's role following any spinal fusion procedure includes patient instruction in body mechanics for bed mobility, transfers, dressing, and ambulation. Trunk rotation is contraindicated; therefore the therapist must instruct the patient in log-rolling and in coming from a supine position to sitting without rotation. Shoes and socks are donned or doffed with the legs in tailor position, with negligible forward flexion. The therapist may also instruct the patient in donning or doffing of the orthosis while in bed, while from a sidelying to a supine position, or while standing with assistance (if not contraindicated by physician's orders). For the acute stage, donning or doffing of the orthosis in bed is preferable. The patient is instructed in general ROM and strengthening exercises (without resistance) for the extremities such as isometric quadriceps sets, straight leg raises, supine abduction, and isometric gluteal sets. Because the patient's functional activities for the first 2 postoperative weeks are limited to showering and walking, the therapist's role is to encourage ambulation. Not only does this enable the patient to experience fewer side effects from bed rest, but it is also beneficial to the development of a strong, healthy fusion mass or arthrodesis.

On discharge from the hospital, the patient's postoperative activity remains restricted. In 1 month, the patient usually returns to school and can lift objects up to 5 pounds. At 3 months following surgery, bicycling, driving, swimming and light jogging are allowed. The patient is able to lift objects weighing up to 10 pounds and also participate in noncontact sports (with physician approval) by 6 months postoperatively. By 1 year the patient may be involved in routine physical education classes, may lift more than 10 pounds, and may be active in other activities, such as skating, skiing, bowling, and amusement park rides. These guidelines are appropriate for the majority of patients with fusion of congenital and idiopathic curves regardless of which instrumentation is used.

Adults and Scoliosis

Two long-term longitudinal studies have been completed on scoliosis into adulthood. The first (Nachemson, 1968) reviewed 130 patients with untreated scoliosis of all types. Ninety percent (117 patients) were followed for 35 years. The results showed an overall mortality rate of twice normal, with the group that had thoracic curves having a rate of four times the norm. There was an increase in death or disability at age 40, with 80% of the causes being cardiorespiratory conditions. The results also included the presence of back pain in 39 of 97 surviving patients.

In the second study Nilsonne & Lundgren (1968) investigated 117 patients with idiopathic scoliosis with a maximal follow-up time of 50 years. The results showed a mortality rate 2.2 times higher than that of a control group. Pulmonary or cardiac failure was the cause of death in 60% of the scoliotic group, while 50% of the surviving scoliotic group were unable to work secondary to disabling symptoms. This study also reported that 70% of the female patients did not marry, perhaps because of cosmetic concerns.

The natural history of idiopathic scoliosis continues into adult life, because curves can progress after skeletal maturity. Risk of progression is dependent on curve magnitude and location (Lonstein, 1988). Curves of greater than 45° at the time of skeletal maturity have a higher risk of progressing and producing complications. Although thoracic and lumbar curves can both progress, progression in the thoracic region causes significant complications because of the effects on the heart and lungs. Complications of untreated scoliosis include severe cosmetic deformity and major disability, which may include pain, respiratory insufficiency, or right-sided heart failure (Rothman & Simeone, 1982). Considerations for adult treatment include back pain, compromised pulmonary function, psychosocial effects, and increased risk for mortality. The treatment plan is consistent with that for adolescent idiopathic scoliosis (Weinstein, 1989).

Neuromuscular Scoliosis

The terms *neuromuscular* and *myopathic scoliosis* describe curves that are due to neurologic or muscular disorders (Raimondi et al., 1989). The curve presentation and risk of progression of neuromuscular scoliosis differ from idiopathic or congenital curves in some cases. Curves may be secondary to pelvic obliquity (Lonstein & Renshaw, 1987),

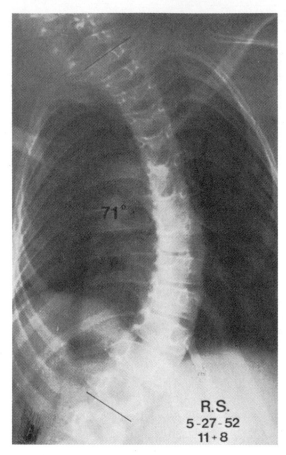

FIGURE 10–9. Severe neuromuscular scoliosis. (From Moe, JH, Winter, RB, Bradford, DS, Ogilvie, JW, & Lonstein, JE. Scoliosis and Other Spinal Deformities, [2nd ed.]. Philadelphia: WB Saunders, 1987, p. 277.)

unilateral or asymmetric spasticity of trunk musculature, athetosis, or asymmetric movement patterns (Tachdjian, 1990). Often a long "C-type" curve characterizes a neuromuscular curvature, but as compensatory curves become structural the pattern may change to an "S-type" curve (Fig. 10–9). A neuromuscular curve typically develops at a young age and tends to be progressive (Fisk & Bunch, 1979). The prevalence of spinal deformities varies with the type of neuromuscular disease.

The highest prevalence of spinal deformities (90–100%) occurs with a dystrophy diagnosis, such as spinal muscular atrophy or muscular dystrophy, and in spinal cord injuries that result in quadriplegia in infants or young children. There is a 60% prevalence of spinal deformity in patients with myelomeningocele and a 25% prevalence in patients with cerebral palsy (Lonstein & Renshaw, 1987).

ETIOLOGY AND RISK OF PROGRESSION

The direct cause of neuromuscular scoliosis is unknown. One hypothesis is that spinal stability, which is directly proportional to the condition of the end support of the spine and inversely proportional to spinal flexibility and to the approximate square of spinal column length, is reduced in children with neuromuscular disease. Loss of muscle strength and loss of proprioception may also be factors in the development of scoliosis when occurring in the relatively flexible and elongating spinal column of a child with a neuromuscular disease (Lonstein & Renshaw, 1987).

TREATMENT

Nonsurgical treatment of neuromuscular spinal curvatures includes clinical observation, radiograph examination, and orthotic management. Clinical observation allows thorough assessment of the child's present and potential function, level of comprehension, and ability to cooperate (Fisk & Bunch, 1979). Although no research studies have shown that custom seating is effective in reducing or preventing progression of curves, it is an important part of clinical treatment in which the physical therapist plays a vital role. A good postural support system allows the child to interact with the environment. These children often have multiple disabilities, which are best addressed by the team approach of a physical therapist, occupational therapist, physician, equipment vendor, and orthotist. In Chapter 23, considerations are presented regarding seating options appropriate for this population.

The child with a neuromuscular curvature managed by orthotics has special needs that must be considered when ordering or fabricating seating systems. The orthosis eliminates the normal flexibility of the spine, which potentially reduces the child's ability to adjust the footrests, operate the brakes, and propel the chair. A child with a neuromuscular curve may demonstrate pelvic obliquity requiring specialized custom-molded seating to provide adequate support and pressure relief. Because these children may require lower extremity orthotics, adequate clearance in the seating device is necessary to accommodate orthoses.

Orthotic management might include the custom-molded, total contact TLSO, underarm TLSO, or Milwaukee brace (Lonstein & Renshaw, 1987). The orthosis is worn during all upright (i.e., sitting or standing) activities and is usually not worn at night.

The use of an orthosis must provide curve stabilization without limiting the child's functional abilities. For example, attempting to control the lordosis in an ambulating child with muscular dystrophy would eliminate compensatory functional posture and result in earlier use of a wheelchair. An orthosis may be used before any measurable deformity to support the trunk. For example, a young child with spinal muscular atrophy may be fitted with a TLSO that has the anterior rib portion relieved and covered with elastic material to provide support for use during therapy, during feeding, and while standing in a standing frame. The use of a TLSO can improve head and upper extremity control. An orthosis should also be used to maintain alignment and provide trunk support for children with quadriplegic paralysis secondary to birth injuries or acquired spinal cord injuries. In these children the use of an orthosis allows for upright orientation and may provide the support necessary for the child to operate a head switch or sip-and-puff mechanism to control an electric wheelchair.

If a neuromuscular scoliosis continues to progress, hygiene, nursing care, functional abilities, pulmonary function, and life expectancy may be affected. Once again, a team approach is preferred for optimal management of children with neuromuscular disease.

SURGICAL OPTIONS

Surgical methods for neuromuscular scoliosis are similar to those for idiopathic scoliosis. The curve may require both anterior and posterior fusion with instrumentation, posterior fusion with instrumentation, or fusion to the pelvis to correct obliquity and maintain symmetry. The goal of surgery is to achieve a stable and compensated spine.

An orthosis is always used postoperatively for support and immobilization of the fusion. Occasionally the patient may be placed in a body cast (Risser cast) in the operating room to protect against potential sheer stresses before the fabrication of a custom orthosis (Fisk & Bunch, 1979). The orthosis must be on the patient before initiation of out-of-bed mobility, unless otherwise specified by the physician.

The role of the physical therapist is similar to that for postoperative treatment of other curve types. The treatment may need to be modified to adjust to a patient's motor and cognitive abilities.

KYPHOSIS

A kyphosis is an abnormal posterior convexity of a segment of the spine. A spinal kyphosis may occur as a result of trauma, congenital conditions, or Scheuermann's disease or secondary to previous

treatment of spinal tumors with laminectomy or to lumbosacral anomalies. Spinal kyphosis may also be found in children with osteochondrodystrophies, rickets, osteogenic imperfecta, idiopathic juvenile osteoporosis, neurofibromatosis, myelomeningocele, and spondyloepiphyseal dysplasia. Spinal kyphosis should be differentiated from postural roundback (Rothman & Simeone, 1982; Winter et al., 1973). The discussion in this section focuses on congenital kyphosis, Scheuermann's disease, and kyphosis in children with myelomeningocele.

Congenital Kyphosis

Congenital kyphosis results when the anterior part of the vertebra is aplastic or hypoplastic and posterior elements form normally. An anterior unsegmented failure of formation, or unsegmented bar, leads to progressive kyphosis. Congenital kyphoscoliosis or lordoscoliosis is the result when a combination of defective segmentation occurs at more than one location (Winter, 1983, 1988).

The natural history of congenital kyphosis includes progression, cosmetic deformity, back pain, and neurologic deficit. Congenital kyphosis is the most common cause of spinal cord compression caused by a spinal deformity (Winter et al., 1973). It is a potentially more debilitating deformity than congenital scoliosis without kyphosis. An anterior unsegmented bar at the thoracolumbar junction produces mild to moderate deformities but no reported paraplegia. Paraplegia is frequently noted with a progressive congenital kyphosis located in the upper thoracic spine when the posterior elements grow unaccompanied by anterior growth. The treatment of congenital kyphosis is surgery to prevent further progression (Winter, 1983).

Scheuermann's Disease

Scheuermann's disease is an often neglected deformity that develops during childhood and adolescence and is usually ascribed to poor posture. Diagnosis is made by these radiographic criteria: 1) irregular vertebral end-plates, 2) narrowing of the intervertebral disc space, 3) anterior wedging 5° or greater of one or more vertebrae, and 4) kyphosis greater than 40° that is uncorrected on active hyperextension. Scheuermann's disease can be found in the thoracic spine, producing an increased kyphosis, in the thoracolumbar and lumbar spine, producing a neutral appearance in the sagittal plane, and, more rarely, in the cervical spine (Rothman & Simeone, 1982).

Little has been published on the pathophysiology of Scheuermann's disease. Cadaver dissections show that the anterior longitudinal ligament is thickened and taut as in other kyphoses and that the vertebral bodies are wedged and the disc spaces narrowed. The spongiosa and bone are irregular and can show disruption where Schmorl's nodules have fractured the bony tubercle. Growth plates are disorderly as a result of this disruption (Rothman & Simeone, 1982; Tachdjian, 1990).

Clinical findings include tight pectorals and hamstrings. An increased thoracic kyphosis with a compensatory increased lumbar lordosis and forward head posture are seen. Associated scoliosis is present in 30–40% of children with Scheuermann's disease. The disease has also been reported to be transmitted as an autosomal dominant trait with an incidence of 0.4–8.3%. Males and females are affected equally. Radiographic findings are often not seen until age 11 (Tachdjian, 1990). The chief complaint of patients is pain at the apex of the kyphosis.

TREATMENT

Treatment of Scheuermann's disease includes exercise, orthotic management, and surgical management. The prescribed exercises are specific for active trunk extensor strengthening, passive trunk stretching into extension, and general postural exercise (abdominals and gluteals). The child must be instructed to extend at the kyphotic section of the spine (usually thoracic) while maintaining a neutral or slightly flexed cervical and lumbar spine. Exercises addressing abdominal strengthening, especially of lower abdominals, are important to help maintain an upright posture and decrease lumbar

lordosis. A patient may present with hip flexion contractures from increased lumbar lordosis and increased anterior pelvic tilt, and limited hamstring length by straight leg raising due to kyphotic and crouched posture in sitting and standing. Stretching exercises are incorporated to improve overall alignment (Fig. 10–10). Exercise as the sole treatment has not been established as effective, although it has been shown to be beneficial in conjunction with other methods of treatment (Moe et al., 1987; Tachdjian, 1990).

Orthotic treatment is used when the kyphosis is greater than 50° to 60°. The use of a modified Milwaukee-type brace has a high reported success rate in the skeletally immature patient. The procedure is considered to be successful when the kyphosis decreases and vertebral bodies appear less wedge shaped on radiographs (Moe et al., 1987).

Surgical management is often a two-stage procedure, with anterior discectomy and intravertebral grafting coupled with a posterior compression arthrodesis. Posterior fusion alone in a child with a fixed kyphosis greater than 60° may be associated with significant complications and loss of correction of kyphosis with instrumentation failure (Rothman & Simeone, 1982).

Postoperative treatment includes plaster casting and/or orthotic wear. The orthotic of choice is usually a Milwaukee-type brace that may be modified to a TLSO after a 2- to 5-month postoperative period.

POSTURAL ROUNDBACK

Postural roundback may often be confused with Scheuermann's disease; however, the kyphosis of postural roundback is not fixed and vertebrae show

FIGURE 10–10. Active trunk extensor and abdominal strengthening for kyphosis.

no end-plate irregularity. Exercise alone, as described for treatment of Scheuermann's disease, is the treatment of choice for this condition. If the kyphosis progresses to more than 60°, it may be treated with a Milwaukee brace to prevent permanent structural changes (Moe et al., 1987).

Kyphosis and Myelomeningocele

Spinal deformities are common in children with myelomeningocele. A congenital lumbar kyphosis, involving the portion of spine from the thoracolumbar junction to the sacrum, is unique to children with myelomeningocele.

Congenital kyphosis is easily recognized at birth because it is rigid and resistant to passive correction. Anatomically the pedicles are widely separated and protrude posterolaterally, accentuating the kyphotic appearance. The pedicles and laminae are splayed, pushing the deep back muscles to an anterior position. These deep back muscles may then serve as pathologic flexors of the lumbar spine. Often, owing to the level of deficit, the psoas muscle is the only innervated muscle. The force of the psoas, coupled with activity in the quadratus lumborum and anterior abdominals, may cause progressive deformity (Rothman & Simeone, 1982).

The congenital kyphosis may produce closure problems, caused by size and rigidity of the lesion, at primary meningocele closure. Orthopaedic surgery, a kyphectomy or spinal osteotomy, may be done at the time of closure to help facilitate the procedure (Sharrad, 1968). Recurrent skin breakdown problems are common; therefore, special attention must be taken for the use of adaptive equipment.

The kyphosis usually remains relatively stable until the child sits, using the hands for support. The child's sitting posture is marked by a forward trunk and sacral or lumbar, instead of ischial, spine weight-bearing, and there may be a compensatory thoracic lordosis. These children often develop respiratory complications when the anterior rib cage lies on the pelvic brim, causing the abdominal contents to be forced against the diaphragm, restricting excursion and respiratory function (Rothman & Simeone, 1982) (Figs. 10–11 and 10–12).

TREATMENT

Treatment of congenital kyphosis in children with myelomeningocele is limited. Bracing and stretching exercises are of no use because of the rigidity of the deformity and potential for skin breakdown. Exercises are useful in maintaining

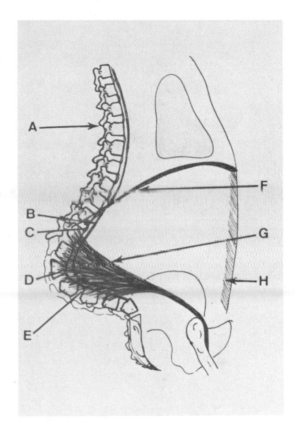

FIGURE 10–11. Drawing illustrating the deforming forces found in congenital lumbar kyphosis. *A*, Compensatory dorsal lordosis. *B*, Contracted anterior longitudinal ligament. *C*, Contracted anulus fibrosus. *D*, Wedge-shaped vertebral bodies. *E*, Intervertebral discs narrowed anteriorly with the nucleus pulposus shifted posteriorly. *F*, Diaphragm attached to the apex of the deformity. *G*, Psoas muscle is hypertrophied and bowstrings across the curve. *H*, Anterior abdominal musculature. (From Rothman, RH, & Simeone, FA. The Spine, [2nd ed.]. Philadelphia: WB Saunders, 1982, p. 252.)

good range of motion at the hips and shoulders. The surgical procedure, a kyphectomy, is controversial and may only produce limited correction. The procedure and results require further research.

Postoperative treatment may include plaster casting or orthotic treatment to protect the fusion. Physical therapy is often involved to maximize endurance and mobility, as outlined in the section on surgery for idiopathic scoliosis.

LORDOSIS

An anterior convexity (or a posterior concavity) of a segment of spine is described as a lordosis. Congenital lordosis is the result of bilateral posterior failure of segmentation (Winter, 1983). Lor-

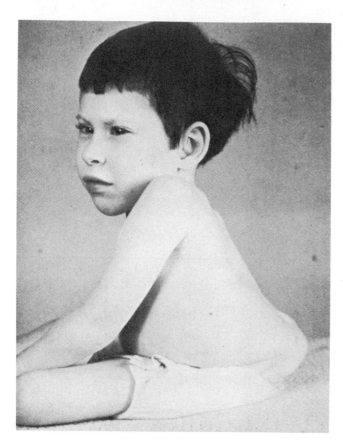

FIGURE 10–12. Nine-year-old with a congenital lumbar kyphosis. Typical sitting posture serves to accentuate the kyphosis. The child is sitting directly on the sacrum and the lower portion of the lumbar spine. (From Rothman, RH, & Simeone, FA. The Spine, [2nd ed.]. Philadelphia: WB Saunders, 1982, p. 252.)

dosis, both fixed and flexible, may be found in children with a variety of diagnoses. Lordosis in children with myelomeningocele usually occurs in the lumbar spine secondary to use of a tripod gait pattern. A lordosis may develop in the thoracic vertebrae to compensate for an increased lumbar kyphosis (Rothman & Simeone, 1982).

Children without motor deficits may present with an increased lumbar lordosis. Assessment includes testing of lower extremity ROM, spinal flexibility, trunk and lower extremity strength, posture, and gait. Treatment includes abdominal strengthening (curls, crunches, and pelvic lifts), pelvic tilts in a supine position and standing, trunk extensor strengthening, and appropriate lower extremity stretching.

Spondylolisthesis

Spondylolisthesis is a term for the forward translatory displacement of one vertebra on another, usually occurring at the fifth lumbar vertebra. Five types of spondylolysis and spondylolisthesis are classified by Wiltse and associates (1976). They include the following:

1. *Dysplastic*, developing secondary to congenital malformations of the sacrum and posterior vertebral arch of L-5. These malformations may include hypoplasia of the superior surface of the body of S-1, hypoplasia-aplasia of the facets, elongation of the pars interarticularis, and spina bifida. The malformations decrease the efficiency of the posterior stabilizing system (Wiltse et al., 1976). The degree of slippage is usually severe and may produce neurologic deficits as the laminae of L-5 are pulled against the dural sac (Tachdjian, 1990).

2. *Isthmic* describes slippage occurring secondary to an elongation of the pars interarticularis, a break of the pars interarticularis, or a combination of both with the facets intact. A stress or fatigue fracture of the pars interarticularis is the basic pathologic occurrence. These pathogenic factors can cause elongation of the pars secondary to repeated microfractures that heal with the pars in an attenuated-elongated position. An isthmic spondylolisthesis may also be caused by an acute fracture of the pars (Tachdjian, 1990).

3. A *degenerative* type occurs in adults older than the age of 50 years and is caused by the structural destruction of the capsule and ligaments of the posterior joints producing hypermobility of the segment.

4. A *traumatic* type, more correctly defined as a fracture, is caused by a sudden fracture of the posterior arch of a vertebral segment. The fracture may occur at the pedicle, laminae, or facet, leaving the pars interarticularis intact.

5. *Pathologic* spondylolisthesis occurs most often secondary to an infectious disease that destroys the posterior arch of the vertebra (Wiltse et al., 1976).

Dysplastic and isthmic spondylolisthesis types are the most common in the pediatric population. Spondylolisthesis is further described by degree of severity as described by percentage of slippage, grades I to IV. Grade I is the mildest slippage at less than 25%. Grade II is 25–50% slippage. Grade III is 50–75%, and grade IV is greater than 75% slippage (Tachdjian, 1990; Wiltse et al., 1976).

CLINICAL SYMPTOMS

A spondylolisthesis is often discovered on a radiograph taken for some other purpose. The clinical picture includes poor posture and increased lumbar lordosis in mild slippage. Higher-grade slippage may produce a flattened lumbar spine, a crease anteriorly at the umbilicus, and a prominent sacrum (Fig. 10–13). Symptoms may include low back pain relieved by rest, sciatic-type pain, local

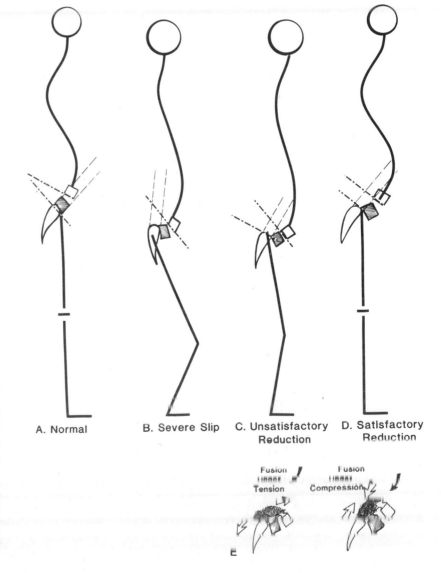

FIGURE 10–13. *A*, Normal sagittal plane spinal alignment. *B*, Loss of alignment can be visualized following a severe L-5 spondylolisthesis. The sacrum becomes vertical, and the resultant lumbosacral kyphosis "pushes" the lumbar spine forward. *C*, An unsatisfactory reduction occurs when L-5 has little mobility and L-4 lies anterior to the "anatomic zone" and is kyphotic in relationship to the sacrum. The fusion in this case will be under tension and less likely to hold. *D*, A satisfactory reduction occurs when L-4 can be placed in the "anatomic zone" and oriented lordotic in relation to the sacrum. *E*, The more L-4 can be positioned over the sacrum, the greater posterior compressive forces will be directed across the fusion. In this position, sagittal plane alignment and hence deformity will be corrected. (From Moe, JH, Winter, RB, Bradford, DS, Ogilvie, JW & Lonstein, JE. Scoliosis and Other Spinal Deformities, [2nd ed.]. Philadelphia: WB Saunders, 1987, p. 418.)

A. Normal   B. Severe Slip   C. Unsatisfactory Reduction   D. Satisfactory Reduction

Fusion under Tension   Fusion under Compression

E

tenderness, hamstring spasm or tightness, and, in severe cases, torso shortening (Tachdjian, 1990).

RISK OF PROGRESSION

The risk factors, clinically and radiographically, are similar to those for idiopathic scoliosis. Clinically, adolescents who are symptomatic are at a higher risk for increased slippage during their growth spurt. Females are at a greater risk than males, as are patients with increased ligament laxity, as in Down's syndrome or Marfan's syndrome. Radiographically, dysplastic types or patients with a 50% slippage, with a slip angle over 40° to 50°, or with bony instabilities or decreased anatomic stability of L-5 and S-1 are at greater risk for increased slippage (Moe et al., 1987; Tachdjian, 1990).

NONSURGICAL TREATMENT

Observation is the treatment of choice, with asymptomatic spondylolisthesis presenting with less than 50% slippage. These children are routinely followed two times per year with clinical and radiographic examinations. Normal activities are allowed if the degree of slippage is less than 25%. Activities such as weight-lifting and contact sports are restricted in patients with a slippage greater than 25%. Patients also learn lumbar stabilization exercises in which they are taught to maintain pain-free, neutral alignment of the pelvis and lumbar spine while they vary their positions. Exercises include bridging, wall-squats, abdominal strengthening, prone gluteal strengthening, and supine exercises. A therapeutic exercise ball may be incorporated into the exercise session to allow patients to achieve and maintain neutral lumbar spine stabilization on a mobile surface.

A lumbosacral orthosis is used to manage the symptomatic patient with a slippage percentage of less than 25%. This treatment form is initially also used to conservatively treat patients with a slippage of 25–50%. If symptoms persist, surgery is indicated.

SURGICAL TREATMENT

The indications for surgery are persistent back pain despite conservative measures including physical therapy, greater than 50% slippage and associated gait deviations unresponsive to physical therapy, marked instability of the defect with slip progression, neurologic deficit, and persistent sciatic symptoms unresponsive to conservative measures (Tachdjian, 1990). The goals of surgery are to prevent further slippage, immobilize the unstable

segment, prevent further neurologic deficit and relieve any nerve root irritation, and correct clinical symptoms of poor posture, gait, and decreased hamstring length (Tachdjian, 1990).

The surgical procedure most often performed is a posterolateral alar transverse process fusion. The fusion usually extends to L-4 and is performed with an iliac bone graft. The patients are immobilized in a TLSO brace with a thigh extension for 6 weeks to 3 months and then in a TLSO until the fusion is solid (VanRens & Van Horn, 1982; Verbeist, 1979). Physical therapy is indicated for bed mobility, gait training, and activities of daily living and may be initiated to regain normal hamstring flexibility.

In severe cases associated with significant neurologic deficit, a decompression and posterior fusion procedure is indicated. A decompression consists of removal of the bony anatomy that is causing nerve root irritation. The segments are then fused posteriorly to prevent further slippage (VanRens & Van Horn, 1982; Verbeist, 1979). Anterior fusions have been performed with good results (Freebody, 1962); a posterior fusion is usually preferred, however, because it is less hazardous.

A reduction of the spondylolisthesis is indicated in cases in which the sacrum is in a vertical position causing a severe lumbosacral kyphosis that displaces the lumbar spine anteriorly (see Fig. 10–13). The result is a marked compensatory lumbar lordosis. A reduction of the slippage is followed by posterior fusion, anterior fusion, or a combination of surgical approaches.

CASE HISTORY: ANN

Ann, a 15-year-old girl with a diagnosis of idiopathic scoliosis (curves measuring 45° right thoracic and 42° left lumbar) was referred to physical therapy for assessment and treatment. She was also being treated with full-time orthotic wear (Lyon-type TLSO) and has a curve that will require posterior spinal fusion in the future.

Assessment included testing of: 1) lower extremity ROM; 2) lower extremity manual muscle; 3) trunk strength; 4) trunk flexibility; 5) trunk symmetry, including levels of bony prominences (i.e., iliac crest, inferior border of scapulae); 6) activity level; 7) posture; and 8) gait. The assessment revealed decreased trunk flexibility in all planes (forward flexion by one half, lateral flexion by one third, and extension by one fourth) and limited hamstring length, (145° popliteal angle bilaterally). Cosmetically, she was well compensated in her trunk with curves of essentially equal magnitude.

Ann's disabilities or inabilities to fulfill life roles included: 1) limited participation in extracurricular activities; 2) limitations in choice of clothes secondary to orthotic wear, which caused her to become self-conscious and limit her social activities: and 3) potential for progression that may limit physical endurance. Ann was interested in playing basketball and volleyball as well as babysitting so the disability issue addressed was limited participation in extracurricular activities.

Ann was instructed in proper body mechanics to adjust to limited trunk mobility and in trunk strengthening and flexibility exercises to be performed daily when not wearing the orthosis. The exercises (knees to chest, pelvic tilts, four-point trunk extensor strengthening, curl-ups, oblique curl-ups, lateral flexion, and trunk shift) were specifically designed to address trunk flexion, trunk rotation, abdominal strength, and trunk extensor–hip extensor strength while avoiding hyper extension of the spine. Her physical therapy also addressed her cardiorespiratory status. She was started on a daily walk/run program with a goal of 45 minutes three to five times per week. She also rode a stationary bicycle for 20 to 30 minutes during each treatment session.

Impairments included primary anatomic changes of the vertebrae and surrounding structures; decreased spinal, trunk, and lower extremity ROM secondary to full-time orthotic wear; decreased trunk strength secondary to inactivity; and decreased endurance secondary to limited activity due to orthotic wear. Primary changes of the vertebrae could not be made, but through instruction in the home exercise program the issues of trunk strength, flexibility, and cardiorespiratory endurance were addressed.

In most instances, Ann was allowed to participate in noncontact, organized sports activities. The physical therapist encouraged wearing the orthosis when possible during these activities. The physical therapist also played an important role in helping Ann to understand the importance of maintaining flexibility and strength in preparation for a faster recovery following her anticipated posterior spinal fusion.

A checklist system was used to follow Ann's compliance with home exercises and orthotic wear. After initial sessions for evaluation and teaching of a home program, Ann was followed clinically at regular intervals (6 to 8 weeks) to re-evaluate strength, flexibility, and ROM as additional indicators of compliance.

Ann was very compliant with her flexibility and strengthening exercises. Her hamstring length improved to normal as measured by straight leg raise, her forward flexion was limited by one third, and she played on her school's basketball team. She was discharged from therapy after 3 months because she was continuing with a home program. She will undergo a posterior spinal fusion with Cotrel-Dubousset instrumentation in the future.

CASE HISTORY: KATIE

Katie, a 14-year-old girl with a diagnosis of athetoid cerebral palsy and a scoliosis measuring 54° (right thoracolumbar) out of brace and 42° in brace (custom-molded TLSO), was seen in a scoliosis clinic. Katie received physical therapy twice weekly at her home. Her highest level of function was limited household ambulation. She is a potential surgical candidate.

A physical therapy assessment included testing of 1) posture in prone, supine, sitting, and standing; 2) lower extremity ROM; 3) lower extremity manual muscle strength, including cortical control and in-pattern grades; 4) balance in sitting and standing; 5) tone; and 6) primitive reflexes. Findings included bilateral hip flexion contracture of 15°, poor voluntary control of distal lower extremity musculature, ability to move from sitting to standing with minimal to moderate assistance by one person, athetoid/fluctuating tone, and present, but not obligatory, right asymmetric tonic neck reflex.

Katie's disabilities and functional limitations included 1) inability to perform independent self-care owing to decreased balance; 2) inability to efficiently propel her manual wheelchair owing to orthotic wear; and 3) inability to independently obtain and maintain proper postural alignment of the trunk because of the influence of primitive reflexes, trunk weakness, abnormal tone, and decreased proprioception. Physical therapy was used to address 1) assisted training in activities of daily living, 2) independent mobility with wheelchair modifications or change to an electric device, 3) balance, 4) endurance for facilitated ambulation, and 5) postural alignment and midline orientation in all positions.

Impairments included 1) primary anatomic changes in the vertebrae, supporting structures, and musculature of the trunk; 2) decreased midline orientation abilities due to spinal deformity and cerebral palsy; 3) decreased spinal mobility due to orthotic wear; and 4) decreased ability to use compensations of the trunk during household ambulation due to orthotic restrictions.

Physical therapy was used to address impairment through services two to three times per week, emphasizing trunk strengthening (abdominals, gluteals, extensors), active-assistive ROM of bilateral lower extremities, and facilitated weight bearing and ambulation to improve endurance and function. Over 4 months, she progressed to require only minimal assistance for household ambulation.

The physical therapist plays a role in determining function, the effect of an orthosis on function, and the potential effect of surgical fusion on the child's function. To accomplish these objectives it is necessary to maintain verbal or written contact regarding the child's progress or regression with the child's orthopaedic physician. In this particular case, surgery was postponed because the child was making improvements in independent household ambulation. Katie is expected to require surgery in the future, but her improved endurance and independence will give her an advantage for the procedure itself as well as for recovery time.

CASE HISTORY: ABBEY

Abbey, a 12-year-old girl with a diagnosis of grade III spondylolisthesis, was seen in scoliosis clinic. Her clinical examination revealed 1) tight hamstrings with decreased ROM to 40° as measured by straight leg raising, 2) antalgic, crouch-type gait, 3) anterior abdominal crease at the level of the umbilicus, and 4) posterior pelvic tilt with prominent "heart-shaped" sacrum due to spasticity of the hamstrings because of nerve root irritation. Surgery was recommended for reduction of the spondylolisthesis coupled with a fusion. Postoperatively this child wore a TLSO for immobilization. Physical therapy included hamstring stretching, body mechanics instruction, and gait re-education.

Her pathophysiologic features included 1) primary anatomic changes of the vertebrae and surrounding structures, 2) neurologic changes of the lower extremities secondary to nerve rootlet pressure caused by the primary slippage of the vertebrae, and 3) potential for permanent neurologic changes of lower extremities and bowel and bladder if no intervention occurred. The associated impairments and functional limitations expected if there was no surgical intervention include 1) low back pain; 2) potential for decreased lower extremity function due to neurologic changes; 3) altered gait; and 4) altered alignment of spine and pelvis causing difficulties with clothing, sitting for long periods of time, and endurance. After surgical intervention functional limitations included decreased trunk strength and limited participation in extracurricular activities.

Physical therapy addressed the postsurgical issues through rehabilitation exercises once the fusion was stable. The child participated in pool activities, lumbar stabilization activities utilizing the Swiss ball, and cardiovascular endurance activities after permission from her orthopaedic surgeon. Proper surgical management and rehabilitation can allow the child to return to pain-free function.

CONCLUSION

Scoliosis, kyphosis, and lordosis are common pediatric orthopaedic conditions of the spine. We, as pediatric physical therapists, often concentrate our therapy for many types of patients on the trunk for midline activities, symmetry, and stability for movement, and, therefore, we can play a vital role in early detection of spinal deformities. We encourage children to become active to allow for improved cardiorespiratory function, muscle strength, and endurance. We can provide a referral source for families, instruction in home exercises, input for selecting appropriate adaptive equipment and seating, and rehabilitative treatment following injury or surgery. We address issues concerning the spine on a daily basis and play an important role in achieving and maintaining good health through maximizing proper alignment and function.

References

Basset, GS, Burness, WP, & MacEwen GD. Treatment of scoliosis with a Wilmington brace: Results in patients with 20–29 degree curves. Journal of Bone and Joint Surgery (American), 68:602–605, 1986.

Bleck, E. Annotation—Adolescent idiopathic scoliosis. Developmental Medicine and Child Neurology, 33:167–176, 1991.

Bertrand, SL, Drvaric, DM, Lange, N, Lucas, PR, Deutsch, SD, Herdon, JH, & Roberts, JM. Electrical stimulation for idiopathic scoliosis. Clinical Orthopedics and Related Research, 276:176–181, 1992.

Brown, JC, Alexgaard, J, & Howson, DC. Multicenter trial of a non-invasive stimulation method for idiopathic scoliosis: A summary of early treatment results. Spine, 9:382–387, 1984.

Bylund P, Aaro, S, Gottfries, B, & Jansson, E. Is lateral electric surface stimulation an effective treatment for scoliosis? Journal of Pediatric Orthopedics, 7:298–300, 1987.

Calvo, JJ. Observations on the growth of the female adolescent spine and its relationship to scoliosis. Clinical Orthopedics, 10:40, 1957.

Carman, D, Roach JW, Speck, G, Wenger, DR, & Herring JA. Role of exercises in the Milwaukee brace treatment of scoliosis. Journal of Pediatric Orthopedics, 11:65–68, 1985.

Carr, WA, Moe, JH, & Winter, RB. Treatment of idiopathic scoliosis in the Milwaukee brace, long term results. Journal of Bone and Joint Surgery (American), 62:8–15, 1980.

Cowell, HR, Hall, JN, & MacEwen, GD. Genetic aspects of idiopathic scoliosis. Clinical Orthopedics, 86:121–132, 1972.

Dickson, RA, Lawton, JD, Archer, JA & Butt, WP. The pathogenesis of idiopathic scoliosis. Journal of Bone and Joint Surgery (British), 66:8–15, 1984.

Drummond, DS. A perspective on recent trends for scoliosis correction. Clinical Orthopedics and Related Research, 264:90–102, 1991.

Duval-Beaupere, G. The growth of scoliosis patients: Hypothesis and preliminary study. Acta Orthopaedica Belgica, 38:365–376, 1972.

Eckerson, LF, & Axelgaard, J. Lateral electrical surface stimulation as an alternative to bracing in the treatment of idiopathic scoliosis: Treatment protocol and patient acceptance. Physical Therapy, 64:483–490, 1984.

Emans, JB, Kaelin, A, Bancel, P, Hall, JE, & Miller, ME. The Boston bracing system for idiopathic scoliosis: Follow-up results in 295 patients. Spine, 11:792–801, 1986.

Farady, JA. Current principles in the non-operative management of structural adolescent idiopathic scoliosis. Physical Therapy, 63:512–523, 1983.

Fisk, JR, & Bunch, WH. Scoliosis in neuromuscular disease. Orthopedic Clinics of North America, 10(4), 1979.

Freebody, D. Lumbosacral fusion by the transperitoneal approach. Journal of Bone and Joint Surgery (British), *44*:217, 1962.

Goldstein, LA, & Waugh, TR. Classification and terminology of scoliosis. Clinical Orthopedics, *93*:10, 1973.

Green, N. Part-time bracing of adolescent idiopathic scoliosis. Journal of Bone and Joint Surgery (American), *68*:738–742, 1986.

Kehl, DK, & Morrissy, RT. Brace treatment in adolescent idiopathic scoliosis: An update on concepts and technique. Clinical Orthopedics and Related Research, *229*:34–43, 1988.

Kostuik, JP. Current concepts review operative treatment of idiopathic scoliosis. Journal of Bone and Joint Surgery (American), *72*:1108–1113, 1990.

Lonstein, JE, & Renshaw TS. Neuromuscular Spine Deformities. Instructional Course Lectures, Vol. 36. St. Louis, MO: CV Mosby, 1987, pp. 285–304.

Lonstein, JE, & Winter RB. Adolescent idiopathic scoliosis. Orthopedic Clinics of North America, *19*:239–246, 1988.

McInnes, E, et al. Vibratory response in adolescents who have idiopathic scoliosis. Journal of Bone and Joint Surgery (American), *73*:1208–1212, 1991.

Moe, JH, Sundberg, AB, & Gustlio, R. A clinical study of spine fusion in the growing child. Journal of Bone and Joint Surgery (British), *46*:784–785, 1964.

Moe, JH, Winter, RB, Bradford, DS, Ogilvie, JW, & Lonstein, JE. Scoliosis and Other Spine Deformities. (2nd ed.) Philadelphia: WB Saunders, 1987, pp. 162–228, 237–261, 347–368, 403–434.

Nachemson, A. A long term follow-up study of non-treated scoliosis. Acta Orthopaedica Scandinavica, *39*:466–476, 1968.

Nilsonne, V, & Lundgren, KD. Long-term prognosis in idiopathic scoliosis. Acta Orthopaedica Scandinavica, *39*:456–465, 1968.

Piazza, MR, & Basset, GS. Curve progression after treatment with the Wilmington brace for idiopathic scoliosis. Journal of Pediatric Orthopedics, *10*:39–43, 1990.

Price CT, Scott, DS, Reed, FE, Jr, & Riddick, MF. Nighttime bracing for adolescent idiopathic scoliosis with the Charleston bending brace: Preliminary report. Spine, *15*:1294–1299, 1990.

Raimondi, AJ, Choux, M, & Dirocco, C. The Pediatric Spine: II. Developmental Anomalies. New York: Springer-Verlag, 1989, pp. 189–220.

Renshaw, TS. Orthotic treatment of idiopathic scoliosis and kyphosis. Instructional Course Lectures, Vol. 34. St. Louis, Mo; CV Mosby, 1985, pp. 110–118.

Rothman, RH, & Simeone, FA. The Spine. (2nd ed.). Philadelphia: WB Saunders, 1982, pp. 239–255, 263–282, 316–439.

Scoliosis Research Society, Terminology Committee. A glossary of scoliosis terms. Spine, *1*:57, 1976.

Sharrad, WJW. Spinal osteotomy for congenital kyphosis in myelomeningocele. Journal of Bone and Joint Surgery (British), *50*:466–471, 1968.

Tachdjian, MO. Pediatric Orthopedics. (2nd ed.) Philadelphia: WB Saunders, 1990, pp. 1747, 2201–2320, 2380–2387.

Tanner, JM, & Whitehouse, RH. Clinical longitudinal standards for height, weight, height velocity and stages of puberty. Archives of Disease in Childhood, *51*:170–179, 1976.

Tanner, JM, Whitehouse, RH, & Takaisni, M. Standards from birth to maturity for height, weight, height velocity and weight velocity: British children, 1965. Archives of Disease in Childhood, *47*:454–471, 613–635, 1966.

VanRens, JG, & VanHorn, JR. Long-term results in lumbosacral interbody fusion for spondylolisthesis. Acta Orthopaedica Scandinavica, *53*:383, 1982.

Verbeist, H. The treatment of lumbar spondyloptosis or impending lumbar spondyloptosis accompanied by neurologic deficit and/or neurogenic intermittent claudication. Spine, *4*:68, 1979.

Weinstein, SL. Adolescent idiopathic scoliosis: Prevalence and natural history. Instructional Course Lectures, Vol. 38, chap. 6. St. Louis, MO: CV Mosby, 1989.

Wiltse, LL, Newman, PH, & MacNab, I. Classification of spondylolysis and spondylolisthesis. Clinical Orthopedics, *117*:23, 1976.

Winter, RB. Congenital Deformities of the Spine. New York: Thieme-Stratton, 1983, pp. 6–10, 43–49.

Winter, RB. Congenital scoliosis. Orthopedic Clinics of North America, *19*(2), 1988.

Winter, RB, Moe, JH, & Wang, JF. Congenital kyphosis: Its natural history and treatment as observed in a study of one hundred and thirty patients. Journal of Bone and Joint Surgery (American), *55*:223–256, 1973.

Wynarsky, GT, & Schultz, AB. Trunk muscle activities in braced scoliosis patients. Spine, *14*:1283–1286, 1989.

Wynne-Davies, R. Congenital vertebral anomalies: Etiology and relationship to spina bifida cystica. Journal of Medical Genetics, *12*:280–288, 1975.

Wynne-Davies, R. The aetiology of infantile idiopathic scoliosis. Journal of Bone and Joint Surgery (British), *56*:565, 1974.

Wynne-Davies, R. Genetic and environmental aspects. Journal of Bone and Joint Surgery (British), *50*:24–30, 1968.

Wynne-Davies, R. Familial (idiopathic) scoliosis. Journal of Bone and Joint Surgery (British), *48*:583, 1966.

Zaouss, AL, & James, JIP. The iliac apophysis and the evolution of curves in scoliosis. Journal of Bone and Joint Surgery (British), *40*:442–453, 1958.

Chapter 11

Arthrogryposis Multiplex Congenita

MAUREEN DONOHOE, PT
DEBRA ANN BLEAKNEY, PT

Arthrogryposis multiplex congenita (AMC) is a nonprogressive neuromuscular syndrome that is present at birth. AMC is characterized by severe joint contractures, muscle weakness, and fibrosis and is present in 1 of every 3000 to 4000 live births in the United States (Goodman & Gorlin, 1983). The etiology of AMC is unknown, but many different factors have been implicated. The insult, however, is believed to occur during the first trimester of pregnancy (Wynne-Davies et al., 1981). The various forms of arthrogryposis include a neuromuscular syndrome (7%); congenital anomalies (6%); chromosomal abnormalities (2%); contracture syndromes (35%); amyoplasia (43%), which is considered the "classic arthrogryposis"; and distal arthrogryposis (7%). Distal arthrogryposis, which affects primarily the hands and foot and is quite responsive to treatment, has a genetic basis and is inherited as an autosomal dominant trait (Hall et al., 1982).

Although the child's condition does not deteriorate as a result of the primary diagnosis, the long-term sequelae of AMC can be very disabling. Func-

tional limitations occur in mobility and activities of daily living (ADL), rendering the child dependent. Proper therapeutic and medical intervention, however, can ameliorate this otherwise devastating disability by helping children to capitalize on opportunities to achieve independence.

In this chapter, we address the pathophysiology of AMC, its management from a medical and surgical perspective, therapeutic assessment, and specific physical therapy and team interventions from infancy to adulthood. The chapter concludes with presentation of two case histories.

ETIOLOGY

Many theories exist regarding the cause of AMC, but most researchers agree that the primary insult occurs during the first trimester of pregnancy. Insults occurring early in the first trimester have the potential for creating more involvement of the child than those that occur late in the first trimester. The basic pathophysiologic mechanism for the multiple joint contractures appears to be the lack of fetal movement (Tachdjian, 1990).

AMC is associated with neurogenic and myopathic disorders in which motor weakness immobilizes the fetal joints leading to contracture. It is not known whether all those with the neuropathic form of AMC have degeneration of the anterior horn cell, but of those studied post-mortem, this is a consistent finding. A neurogenic disorder of the anterior horn cell is believed to cause muscle weakness with subsequent periarticular soft tissue fibrosis (Drummond et al., 1978; Goodman & Gorlin, 1983; Hall, 1989; Wynne-Davies et al., 1981). Because of the failure of the muscle to function, the joints in the developing fetus lack movement, which probably explains the stiffness and deformities of the newborn's joints. The fetus may have an imbalance in strength of oppositional muscle groups, creating the tendency toward a certain posture. For example, the fetus with good strength in the hamstrings and triceps brachii but weakness in the quadriceps and biceps brachii will have a flexed knee and extended elbow posture in utero. Decreased amniotic fluid throughout the pregnancy, but especially during the last trimester when the fetus is largest, may further inhibit freedom of movement in utero.

Although the etiology of AMC remains unknown, several factors have been implicated. Hyperthermia of the fetus is caused by a maternal fever greater than 37.8°C (100°F). Some mothers of children with AMC report having an illness with a fever for 1 to 2 days during the first trimester. Prenatal viral infection, vascular compromise between mother and fetus, or a septum in the uterus have all been suspected as causes of AMC (Wynne-Davies et al., 1981).

PROGRESS IN PRIMARY PREVENTION

Arthrogryposis appears to be a disorder of fairly recent origin since very few middle-aged or elderly patients are reported (Wynne-Davies et al., 1981). Little progress has been made in the prevention of this rare disorder, given its nonspecific etiology. However, significant improvements have been made in the management of a child with AMC.

DIAGNOSIS

No definitive laboratory studies exist that can diagnose AMC prenatally. The majority of AMC cases are not genetically based and, therefore, prenatal amniocentesis or chorionic villous sampling may be inconsequential. If a parent or physician suspects that something is amiss, a detailed ultrasound evaluation can be helpful in identifying anomalies and decreased fetal movements. Ultrasound studies in subsequent pregnancies would help to relieve parental anxiety.

During the first 6 months of life an immunoglobin study may identify evidence of a viral infection. After that time, an ophthalmologist can examine the eye for pigment clumps on the retina, called chorioretinitis. This has no effect on vision but will establish if the insult was a prenatal viral process.

Muscle biopsy in AMC varies with the muscle under study. Histologic analysis reveals that relatively strong muscles will appear virtually normal while very weak muscles reveal fibrofatty changes but may have normal muscle spindles. Embryologically, the muscles are formed normally but are replaced by fibrous and fatty tissue during fetal development (Hall, 1981, 1985). Neuropathic and myopathic changes can be seen in different muscles in the same patient with electromyographic testing (Sarwark et al., 1990). Muscle biopsies along with blood tests and clinical findings rule out progressive and fatal disorders while providing evidence to support the diagnosis of AMC.

CLINICAL MANIFESTATIONS

Clinical manifestations of AMC demonstrate great variability but generally include severe joint contractures and lack of muscle development or amyoplasia. The typical severely affected body parts in the AMC population include, in decreasing order of prevalence, the foot (67%), the hip (50%), the wrist (43%), the knee (41%), the elbow (30%), and the shoulder (4%) (Scott & Nicholson, 1992). One may see these percentages vary in the literature based on how the cases have been ascertained (i.e., care centers will see different mixes based on their specialty).

There are two commonly seen variations of AMC. In one type, the child presents with flexed and dislocated hips, extended knees, clubfeet (equinovarus), internally rotated shoulders, flexed elbows, and flexed and ulnarly deviated wrists (Fig. 11–1). In another type, the child presents with abducted and externally rotated hips, flexed knees, clubfeet, internally rotated shoulders, extended elbows, and flexed and ulnarly deviated wrists (Fig. 11–2). Parents often describe the legs in the first type as jackknifed and in the second type as froglike. Because of the stiffness of the joints, extremity movements are described as wooden or marionette-like. The position of the upper extremities in the second type is described as the "waiter tip position" owing to the internally rotated shoulder, ex-

example, clubfoot surgery, performed to allow plantigrade feet, is often deferred until the child is both able to pull to stand and is interested in standing. The child can then easily self-stretch when standing and walking. One common clubfoot surgery is the posteromediolateral release. The entire hindfoot is opened during surgery so as to shorten the lateral column, lengthen the medial column, and lengthen the tendo Achillis. Occasionally, this procedure includes using wires to realign the talus and the calcaneus. In severe cases of equinovarus and where this procedure fails, a talectomy is performed.

Children with AMC often have subluxed or dislocated hips. Dislocation is as frequently bilateral as unilateral. Generally, if both hips are dislocated, they are not surgically reduced. One dislocated hip is usually relocated to prevent secondary pelvic obliquity and scoliosis, unless the hip is extremely stiff (Sarwark et al., 1990; Staheli et al., 1987). The most common approach to relocating the hips is through an anterolateral approach (MacEwen & Gale, 1983;

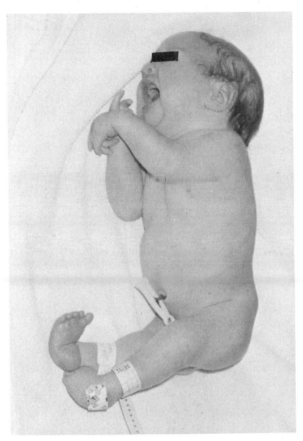

FIGURE 11–1. Infant with AMC with flexed and dislocated hips, extended knees, clubfeet (equinovarus), internally rotated shoulders, flexed elbows, and flexed and ulnarly deviated wrists.

tended elbow, pronated forearm, and flexed wrist. Common to both types are clubfeet, flexed and ulnarly deviated wrists, and internally rotated shoulders. Other associated characteristics may include scoliosis, dimpling of skin over joints, hemangiomas, absent or decreased finger creases, congenital heart disease, facial abnormalities, respiratory problems, and abdominal hernias. Intelligence and speech are usually normal.

▌ MANAGEMENT

The main components of medical treatment include well-timed orthopedic, therapeutic, and surgical management (Hall, 1989; Palmer et al., 1985; St. Clair & Zimbler, 1985). Interventions include vigorous therapy such as stretching, strengthening, and positioning for improved range of motion (ROM) and motor control to enhance functional skill development.

Specific operations should be timed so that the child optimally benefits from the procedure. For

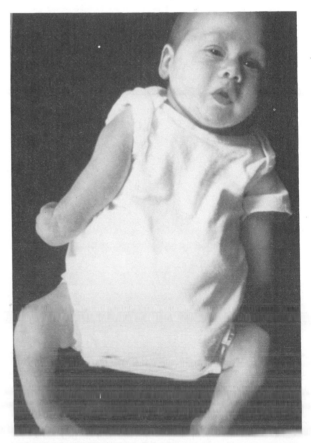

FIGURE 11–2. Infant with AMC with abducted and externally rotated hips, flexed knees, clubfeet, internally rotated shoulders, extended elbows, and flexed and ulnarly deviated wrists.

Sarwark et al., 1990; Staheli et al., 1987; St. Clair & Zimbler, 1985). It is more important to have mobile, painless, yet dislocated hips than to have very stiff but located ones. Prolonged immobilization following open or closed techniques can lead to the serious sequela of fused or stiff hips.

Moderate to severe contractures of the knee joint can be addressed surgically but, in the conservative approach, one waits until the child is ambulating comfortably before surgical correction. Knee flexion contractures are most commonly associated with capsular changes within the joint. Medial and lateral hamstring lengthenings or sectioning (if the muscle is fibrosed) along with a posterior capsulotomy of the knee joint may be performed (Tachdjian, 1990). These contractures inconsistently respond to hamstring lengthenings and posterior capsulotomy because there is a subsequent loss of muscle strength and risk of scar tissue leading to further joint stiffness and recurrence of the contracture. A distal femoral osteotomy is more frequently successful in realigning the joint and changes the arc of motion without risk of increased scar tissue and loss of strength (Jayakumar, 1992) (Fig. 11–3).

Knee extension contractures are frequently addressed by quadriceps lengthening if there is at least 25° of ROM in the knee. Intra-articular procedures such as a capsulotomy may be necessary if the knee is stiff. Some evidence suggests that knee extension contractures tend to have better results than knee flexion contractures when addressed surgically (Sodergard & Ryoppy, 1990). An important consideration before surgical intervention is determination of whether the limitation in ROM is creating functional problems with sitting or walking and if, indeed, the surgical intervention is likely to improve the child's function. For example, if the legs extend straight out when sitting, this position will interfere with sitting at school desks, in the car, and so on and may inhibit community involvement. The child participates in this decision-making process.

Restrictions in shoulder movement are rarely addressed through surgical interventions such as capsular or soft tissue releases because the musculature is usually inappropriate for transfer. If adequate muscle strength and control are present, surgery may be indicated to place wrists and elbows in positions of optimal function. One scenario involves a child with symmetrical weakness or severe contractures of the upper extremities. In this case, a dominant arm can be identified for feeding (postured in flexion) and the other one for hygiene care (postured in extension) (Williams, 1973). If both arms are postured in extension, surgery would be necessary to position one arm in a functional flexion position. Such surgical considerations would include a pectoralis or triceps brachii transfer to give a child active elbow flexion with a posterior capsulotomy to allow for elbow flexion (Tachdjian, 1990). The muscle under consideration for transfer would need to be strong before transfer with adequate passive elbow flexion present. A consistent passive ROM and stretching program from birth is essential to maintain elbow motion for this type of surgery to be successful.

Wrists can be fused in positions for function if conservative splinting and stretching management have been unsuccessful. Wrists are fused in the dissimilar positions. Before a surgical wrist fusion, casting of the wrist for 1 week in the position of the potential fusion is suggested. During this time, the child's functional ADL skills are assessed while wearing the cast to ascertain the appropriateness of this potential surgery.

Scoliosis is frequently managed conservatively with bracing. In about one-fifth of the children or adolescents with AMC, a long-C thoracolumbar scoliosis develops (Tachdjian, 1990). If the curve continues to progress, surgical fusion is considered. Most commonly, a posterior spinal fusion is performed. On large stiff curves, an anterior release of structures limiting spinal mobility may be necessary before the posterior spinal fusion to obtain satisfactory results. The type of fixation used is based on the orthopaedist's preference (see Chapter 10).

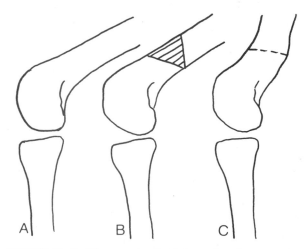

FIGURE 11–3. Diagram of a distal femoral wedge osteotomy performed to realign the contracted knee joint. *A*, Knee flexion contracture deformity before surgery. *B*, Distal femoral wedge osteotomy for reduction of the knee flexion deformity. *C*, Realignment after surgery.

IMPAIRMENT

Diagnosis and Problem Identification

The primary impairments in the child with AMC are joint limitations of movement and decreased muscle strength and bulk. Joint contractures are evident at birth, although a formal diagnosis of AMC may not be given at that time. In AMC, limitation of movement typically is seen in two or more joints in different body areas (Hall, 1989). No data are available to determine whether flexor or extensor musculature is most likely to be affected. From our experience, we have observed that approximately 65% of the children with AMC seen in our clinic have extended elbows; 35% have flexed elbows; 55% have extended knees; and 45% have flexed knees (Jayakumar, 1992). Contractures can develop from an imbalance in muscle pull of agonist and antagonist but also when symmetric weakness is present on all sides of the joint, thus hindering movement. Theoretically, this may be indicative of the point in fetal development that the insult occurs. For example, since flexors develop before extensors in the upper extremity, a child may develop elbow flexion contractures but does not develop the usual strength in either the biceps or triceps brachii subsequent to the time of insult.

Decreased muscle bulk is evidence of muscle weakness secondary to decreased motor units in a muscle. Histologic analysis of muscles reveals nonspecific changes in the muscle such as fibrofatty scar tissue. Weakened muscles often have a fat layer around the muscle with dimpling of the skin. A muscle with a contracture but of normal strength through its available ROM may not have normal muscle bulk secondary to its inability to be active throughout the entire ROM.

Problem Identification by the Team

The team evaluation establishes a baseline from which to set realistic and functional goals. In addition to physical therapists, the primary intervention team consists of patients and their families and such medical professionals as orthopaedists and geneticists, occupational therapists, and orthotists. Occasionally, speech pathologists, dentists or oral surgeons and ophthalmologists are consulted as well. One of the goals of the primary team is to educate the family about AMC. Families are taught that arthrogryposis is a nonprogressive disorder but that without positioning, stretching, and strength-

ening, or possible surgery, the child's impairments could lead to further functional limitations and disability in daily life.

During the initial assessment by the team, photographs and videos are taken of the child depicting the child's position of comfort as well as detailing specific contractures such as clubfeet. This is an objective way to document changes that occur during growth and throughout splinting procedures and should be repeated every 4 months for the first 2 years.

In physical therapy, baseline goniometry is performed, documenting passive ROM as well as the resting position of each joint. ROM can be measured with a standard goniometer cut down to pediatric size. Active ROM is measured at the hips, knees, shoulders, elbows, and wrists. If possible, the same therapist consistently measures ROM for the child. Intratester and intertester reliability is determined for all therapists who evaluate children with AMC and should be checked annually. Functional ROM is also assessed to assist with visualizing the whole composite of motions and evaluating functional abilities. For example, functional active ranges include assessment of the hand to the mouth, ear, forehead, top of head, and back of neck.

A formal manual muscle test is performed when appropriate. Ascertaining muscle grades for infants and very young children is performed by using palpation, observation of the ability of extremities to move against gravity, and evaluation of gross motor function. The strength of the extensor muscles of the lower extremities is especially important to determine the appropriate level of bracing. Less than fair (grade 3/5) muscle strength in hip extensors will require bracing above the hip. Less than fair (grade 3/5) strength in knee extensors requires bracing above the knee. Corrected clubfeet require molded braces during growth to minimize problems of recurrent clubfeet. Children with poor upper extremity function and weak lower extremities may not be functional community ambulators as a result of decreased motor control and protective responses. Power mobility may be the most functional means of community locomotion.

Gross motor skills and functional levels of mobility and ADL are assessed. There are no current developmental tests that have been designed for children with AMC, but these children usually score lower than average in formal gross motor tests secondary to inadequate strength and ROM in their extremities. Certain gross motor skills may never be attained owing to physical limitations. For example, some developmental milestones such as creeping may not be attained even though the child is able to stand and start to walk. Cognitively, AMC children tend to score average to above average in formal developmental tests (Sarwark et al., 1990; Williams, 1978).

The therapist assesses the child for current and potential modes of functional mobility. This may include ambulation with assistive devices or the use of manual or power wheelchair or mobility devices. The therapist evaluates movement patterns and muscle substitutions used to accomplish each motor task or ADL skill.

A team treatment plan is established, incorporating the family early on as part of the team. The ultimate goal is to maximize the child's independence in ADL and mobility.

THERAPY IN INFANCY

One type of physical limitation and deformity seen in an infant with AMC includes clubfeet, hip flexion contractures, knee extension contractures, shoulder tightness (especially internal rotation), and elbow and wrist flexion contractures. At birth these children were commonly breech presentations. In another type, common posturing includes abducted and externally rotated hips, flexed knees, internally rotated shoulders, extended and pronated elbows, and flexed wrists. There may be asymmetric posturing of the extremities, which is especially problematic at the hip when dislocation of only one hip is present. The resulting asymmetry makes surgical correction the treatment of choice to relocate the hip and secondarily prevent pelvic obliquity and scoliosis.

Assessment

Formal assessment of an infant with AMC begins as soon as possible after birth. The assessment consists of goniometry of passive ROM with re-evaluation of ROM done on a monthly basis during this period. The therapist also documents the presence and strength of muscles based on observation of the child's movements and palpation of muscle contractions. Muscles of the trunk and upper and lower extremities are evaluated. Formal developmental assessment tools are occasionally used but reflect poorly on a child with AMC because strength and ROM limitations preclude the achievement of many motor milestones. These are the functional limitations and disabilities stemming from the initial impairments. Motor milestones in these children are often delayed or skipped. For

example, because of development of good trunk control and balance and the ability to "hitch" on their buttocks, these children often bypass the creeping stage. Functional mobility and the mechanism used in attaining this mobility are more important to evaluate than is assignment of a developmental level or score. The therapist assesses rolling, prone tolerance, sitting control, scooting, creeping, crawling, transitional movements, and standing tolerance and upright mobility. Occupational therapy plays a key role in assessing feeding, ADL skills, and manipulation of objects. Physical therapists also assess the fit of any supportive or assistive devices that may have been issued.

Although it is not imperative to use formal scales in assessing these skills, some useful tests include the Alberta Infant Motor Scale, an observational tool for assessing motor milestones; the Pediatric Evaluation of Disability Inventory geared for tracking progress in children with disabilities and assessing functional limitations; the Bayley Scales of Infant Development; and the Peabody Developmental Motor Scales, where gross motor change over time is assessed (see Chapters 1 and 2 on motor development and motor control).

Physical therapy goals for very young children include maximizing strength, improving ROM, and enhancing general sensorimotor development. Education of the family emphasizes instruction in proper positioning, stretching techniques, and the avoidance of potentially harmful activities.

Intervention Strategies

Treatment strategies focus on reducing the physical impairments through stretching, thermoplastic serial splinting, positioning, and strengthening activities. Treatment also addresses the functional limitations and disability through facilitation of developmental activities and teaching compensatory strategies especially in ADL and alternative modes of mobility.

DEVELOPMENT, STRENGTH, AND MOBILITY

Infants with the first type of AMC described earlier begin life with limited positioning options as a result of hip flexion contractures. Consequently, stretching hip flexors and prone positioning are encouraged within the first 3 months of life. Developmentally, these infants learn to roll or scoot on their bottoms as their primary means of floor mobility, since it is nearly impossible to comfortably assume the quadruped position without reinforcing a flexed posture of the upper extremities. Although delayed in their ability to obtain sitting independently, they are often able to do so by 15 months through trunk flexion and rotation. These children typically are able to stand when placed for over a year before pulling to stand is initiated by the child. Usually, the child attempts walking after clubfoot surgery is completed and the child has definitive bracing. In the past, clubfoot surgery was performed early but most often required revisions by the time the child was developmentally ready to walk. In our facility, we suggest postponement of surgery until after the first year of life so that the child has an opportunity to develop strength and a readiness to walk. Furthermore, the child is able to stand after clubfoot surgery and cast removal, which assists in stretching the feet into a plantigrade position and eliminates the need to perform multiple surgical revisions. Clubfoot surgery should be performed before 2 years of age when bony changes may occur that would necessitate more extensive osteotomy procedures rather than soft tissue releases. Also, most children begin some form of independent ambulation by the middle of their second year.

Infants with the second type of AMC posturing (hips externally rotated and flexed, knees flexed, elbows extended) have more positioning options. However, these children become frustrated with prone positioning secondary to their decreased ability to comfortably prop themselves up because of extended elbows. A towel roll or wedge under the infant's chest assists with increasing tolerance for this position. Positioning the hips in neutral rotation and neutral abduction is encouraged. Towel rolls can be placed along the lateral aspect of the thighs when the infant is sitting, and a wide Velcro band can be strapped around the thigh when the child is lying supine to keep the legs in more neutral alignment (Fig. 11–4). Developmentally, these children tend to be a little slower in attaining rolling but faster in attaining sitting and scooting than the children with the first type of posturing. Although assuming the quadruped position and creeping are often feasible for this type of child, sitting and scooting are more energy efficient. Depending on muscle strength and the amount of bracing needed for standing, these children may never perform transitional movements from sitting to standing independently. They begin ambulating, as do their able-bodied counterparts, by the middle of their second year. Therapy focuses on establishing some key functional motor skills, such as rolling, sitting, hitching on the buttocks, standing, and strengthening those muscles that assist in maintaining posture. The goal is reducing disability related to mobility.

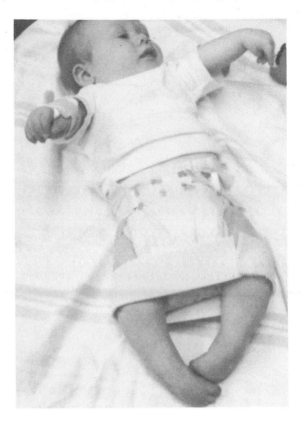

FIGURE 11–4. This child with AMC is wearing a wide Velcro band strapped around the thigh to keep the legs in more neutral alignment.

Strengthening during the first 2 to 3 years is most frequently addressed through developmental facilitation and play. Dynamic strengthening of the trunk can be achieved by having the child reach for, swipe at, or roll toys in the positions of sitting and static standing or while straddling the therapist's leg so that the child must rotate the trunk. These maneuvers incorporate stretching and strengthening into the therapeutic play activity. One way to determine whether functional training is having a strengthening effect is to ascertain the child's improved ability to perform the task.

Self-care skills, feeding, and manipulation of objects are dependent on hand function and elbow flexibility. Those children with limited upper extremity strength may have significant functional limitations because of decreased ability to manipulate objects. Fortunately, these children tend to be resourceful in using other body parts, such as their feet or mouth, to manipulate objects when hands have inadequate strength and ROM. If the child has adequate ROM but inadequate strength, the child learns to support the arm on a leg or a table to assist in bringing the hand to the mouth. If the child is unable to get the hand to the mouth, adaptive equipment may make it possible to do some self-feeding. For example, if shoulder power is absent, overhead arm slings are fashioned out of polyvinyl chloride piping and added to the high chair to permit finger feeding. If the upper extremities are postured in elbow extension, a typical and effective method of grasping an object is a hand cross-over maneuver, which affords some control and strength in holding or lifting an object. Toys can be adapted so that the child can operate them by use of a mercury switch attached to the head, whereby the erectly held head activates the toy. These compensatory treatment strategies help to decrease the child's disability in accomplishing ADL.

Standing is an important component of therapy during the first and second years. Families are encouraged to begin standing the child around 6 months of age, as is normally done with nondisabled children. During standing, lower extremities are held in as optimally corrected a position as possible before surgery through the use of splints. The sneakers can be wedged to accommodate the plantar flexion deformity and allow the child to bear weight throughout the plantar surface of the foot. Standing is initiated in a standing frame and progresses to independent static standing in the frame (Fig. 11–5). By 1 year of age, a child should be able to tolerate a total of 2 hours a day in the standing frame. This standing helps the child begin self-stretching of the feet and encourages the child to begin independent standing and walking. Dynamic standing is encouraged through games such as kicking a soccer or beach ball. Floor-to-stand activities usually do not begin to emerge until the child is ambulating securely, while sit-to-stand activities from a low chair usually begin to emerge when ambulation begins. Limitations in lower extremity strength and ROM can be addressed through splinting and bracing while the child is standing. Knee extension splints may be worn to compensate for muscle weakness and mediolateral instability of the knees.

STRETCHING AND SPLINTING

Because stretching programs for joint contractures are imperative, parents and caregivers are taught a stretching regimen from the time of the initial evaluation. This treatment strategy addresses the primary impairment. A stretching program is divided into three to five sets a day with three to five repetitions during each set. Each repetition is held for 20 to 30 seconds. With the realization that this is a huge time commitment, families are taught to incorporate stretching into times that the child would normally have one-on-one time with the

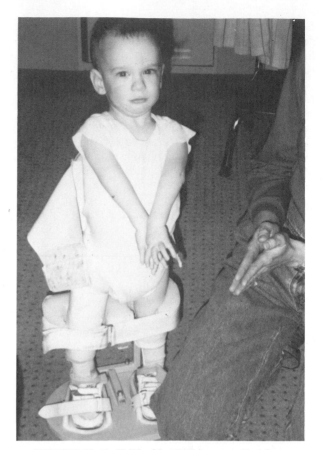

FIGURE 11–5. Child with AMC in a standing frame.

caregiver. A frequently used example includes lower extremity stretches during diaper changes and upper extremity stretches during feeding. Dressing and bath times are also opportunities for stretching, especially once the child is self-feeding and out of diapers. Stretching needs to be a daily lifelong commitment for a person with arthrogryposis, but consistent stretching is most critical during the growing years and especially within the first 2 years of life.

To maintain the prolonged effect of the stretch, the extremity is maintained in a comfortable position of stretch with thermoplastic splints. Attempting to maintain the maximum stretch, rather than a comfortable position, over prolonged periods will cause skin breakdown and intolerance to splints. Splints are adjusted for growth and improvements in ROM, usually every 4 to 6 weeks during infancy. When fabricating ankle-foot orthoses (AFOs) for clubfeet, the calcaneus must be aligned in a neutral position because this will impact on the entire foot's position. If the calcaneus is allowed to move medially with respect to the talus, the forefoot will fall into an undesirable varus position. When the hindfoot and forefoot are in a neutral position between varus and valgus, splinting can address insufficient dorsiflexion of the hindfoot rather than forefoot. This will avoid the potential problem of a rocker-bottom foot. To be maximally effective, AFOs are worn 22 hours per day.

Knee contractures are addressed early using splinting and stretching. For the first 3 to 4 months, anterior thermoplastic knee flexion splints for extension contractures or posterior knee extension splints for knee flexion contractures are worn up to 20 hours per day. When the infant is older, we advise that children not wear a knee flexion splint at greater than 50° of flexion for sleeping because this may encourage hip flexion contractures. Knee extension splints are worn for standing activities and sleeping, after 4 months, to encourage improved lower extremity positioning during independent floor mobility. Knee extension splints worn while sleeping also help to stretch the hip flexors.

Newborns are provided with cock-up wrist splints, but splints for hands are generally provided only after 3 months of age. This allows the child to integrate the normal physiologic flexion before placing a stimulus across the palm. Two sets of hand splints are fabricated. For day use, the child wears dorsal cock-up splints with a palmar arch in a position of neutral deviation and a slight stretch into extension as tolerated. This allows the child to have fingers available to manipulate toys. For night wear, the splint is a dorsal cock-up splint with a pan to allow finger stretching when the child is sleeping.

When considering elbow splinting, note that function and independence in ADL are improved when one elbow is able to flex adequately to reach the mouth and one elbow is in adequate extension to reach the perineum. Other factors to consider include available muscle strength and ROM, response to stretching, and potential future surgical procedures. Elbow extension splints are best worn while sleeping, but elbow flexion splints and elbow flexion-assist splints tend to be most functional when worn during the day. This allows the child to experiment with the hand in a more functional position for most play activities.

In our experience, young children respond most readily to conservative treatment using serial splinting, frequent stretching, and proper positioning. In Figure 11–6A, the infant's posture is shown without leg splints. In Figure 11–6B, the infant's

FIGURE 11–6. A, A child with AMC without leg splints. B, The same child's lower extremity is held out of the deforming positions through use of molded thermoplastic knee splints and AFOs.

lower leg is held out of the deforming postures through molded thermoplastic knee and AFO splints. The key to this success is family training. Family training begins during the initial evaluation. The caretakers not only are given general information about arthrogryposis but they also receive information regarding their child's specific needs. Appropriate stretching exercises for involved joints are given with sketches or photographs to supplement the training. Subsequent visits work on splint fabrication and modification and positioning. Developmental play ideas are incorporated into the exercises to help the child progress developmentally. Therapists also work with the family to adapt age-appropriate toys to stimulate the child physically and mentally.

THERAPY IN THE PRESCHOOL PERIOD

During the preschool period, the child's functional abilities and disabilities vary based on the degree of involvement. Poor upper extremity function from the contractures and lack of muscle power limit the child's independence in feeding, dressing, and playing at a time when nondisabled peers are relishing their independence. This may be particularly distressing for the parents, who are struck with the magnitude of the child's limitations when the child is no longer an infant in whom dependency is expected.

The impairments and functional limitations during this stage are similar to those found in the younger child. Restriction in joint ROM continues to be a problem secondary to rapid growth changes. Ambulation is often limited by decreased use of upper extremities and poor protective responses.

Assessment

Passive and active ROM continue to be closely monitored by the therapist and caregivers. Monitoring proper fit of the splints is imperative in providing adequate stretch and positioning to impede the development of further deformities.

Functional muscle strength is an important component in the preschooler because it determines to a great degree the extent of bracing necessary and level of independence in self-care skills. Formal manual muscle testing, as defined by Kendall and colleagues (1993) or Daniels and Worthingham (1986), becomes more appropriate during this period because the child can comprehend verbal instructions. When testing strength, it is important to grade the resistance throughout the arc of motion because the child with AMC will frequently be strong in the midrange but unable to move the extremity to the shortened end range. This finding is significant because the end range is where the child needs to work the muscle to maintain stretch of the antagonist muscles.

Gait assessment should include distance, use of assistive devices, speed, symmetry of step length, gait deviations, and muscle activity. Some children will ambulate as their primary means of locomotion, while others will rely on a stroller for community mobility. Mobility with wheelchairs is not usually addressed until school age when slow speed of ambulation, endurance, and safety concerns may preclude the child from interacting with peers.

Goals

Ability rather than disability must be stressed with a strong emphasis on assisting the child through problem-solving rather than through physical assistance. The ultimate goals for this age are aimed at reducing the disability and enhancing independent ambulation and mobility with minimum bracing and use of assistive devices. Physical and environmental structural barriers may limit achievement of some fine and gross motor skills, but social skill attainment is paramount. Another goal is for the team to work together to improve the child's function in basic ADL challenges.

Intervention Strategies

The team will work together during the preschool period to solve basic ADL challenges, such as independent feeding and toileting. For example, the use of a lightweight reacher may assist with dressing skills. Preschoolers usually can self-feed with adaptive equipment. These children are often toilet trained but lack the ability to perform the task independently.

STRETCHING

The need for stretching at this age continues to be addressed despite the preschooler's decreased tolerance to three to five times a day. Two times a day for the stretching program is more realistic and, in our experience, maintains ROM adequately in most cases. Families report that the best time for this is during dressing and bathing, which incorporates the program into an automatic part of the daily routine. Children can be taught how to assist with stretching through positioning. The child is also encouraged to verbally participate in the program, for example, by counting the number of repetitions. AFOs and positional splints continue to be worn to maintain the achieved positions.

Independent mobility in a safe and efficient manner is important for the preschooler to achieve to enhance social skills as well as allow functional mobility. Independent ambulation with supportive bracing and with as minimal assistive devices as possible is stressed. Children with adequate strength and ROM who do not require bracing to walk generally need an AFO to prevent recurring clubfeet deformities. An articulating AFO, which provides forefoot control but allows for ankle dorsiflexion and stretch of the hindfoot during gait, is sometimes appropriate. Older preschoolers with AMC are generally in the level of bracing that will be continued throughout school age.

BRACING

Most braces now used are made of lightweight polypropylene and are more durable, less cumbersome, and more adjustable than the metal braces used previously. Children with knee extension contractures tend to require less bracing than those with knee flexion contractures. If there is any question about the child's ability to maintain upright without hip support, the child's first set of long leg braces, a hip-knee-ankle-foot orthosis, will include a pelvic band. This type of orthosis is used for several reasons. The family may perceive that the child is regressing if a pelvic band is found to be needed and then added after unsuccessful ambulation without the pelvic band. The pelvic band encourages neutral rotation and abduction of the lower extremities. The pelvic band can also facilitate full available hip extension, and the hips can be locked in that position for prolonged standing. Once the child is ambulating with both hips unlocked, without jackknifing at the hips during stance, the pelvic band can be removed.

Maintaining hip strength, especially when the pelvic band is removed, continues to be important. One activity is to have the child begin static and dynamic standing on the tilt board. The child also begins taking steps forward, backward, and sideways. Strengthening, as with progressive resisted exercises, may be appropriate at this time. Our clinical experience suggests that muscles may increase in strength by 1/2 muscle grade with exercise.

Ideally, the least amount of bracing is optimal, but if decreasing the bracing requires the child to use an assistive device that was previously unneces-

sary, the increased bracing may be more appropriate. A child with strong extensors such as the gluteus maximus and quadriceps is more functional than a child who requires bracing as a functional substitute for the extensors. The child with a good deal of bracing has difficulty donning and doffing braces and is usually dependent for locking and unlocking hip and knee joints for standing and sitting.

Those children learning to walk may be limited in their independence if they do not have adequate strength and ROM to manipulate the assistive device, like a walker, that is required to ambulate. Walkers are often heavy and cumbersome for the child who may have inadequate protective responses in standing and upper extremity limitations. Thermoplastic material can be molded to the walker for forearm support when hand function is limited, affording the child added support and control (Fig. 11–7). Many children prefer to walk with

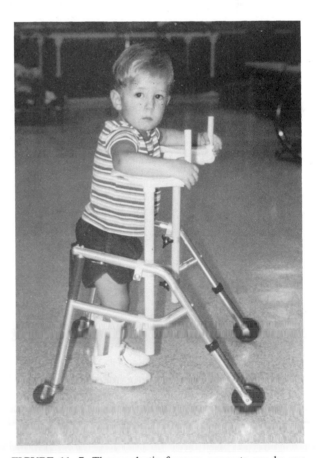

FIGURE 11–7. Thermoplastic forearm supports can be customized to the walker.

someone rather than use a walker while they are gaining confidence in ambulatory skills.

Children with weak quadriceps and knee flexion contractures tend to ambulate with locked knee and ankle-foot orthoses. These braces can be fabricated with dial knee locks so that the knee position can be adjusted to coincide with the changing state of the knee flexion contracture. This will afford the ongoing opportunity to stretch out the contracture. Shoes may need external wedges to compensate for hip and knee flexion contractures that interfere with static standing. The child should be able to comfortably balance with the feet plantigrade without upper extremity support. For walking, assistive devices can be customized with thermoplastic material to allow for less awkward hand grips. Very lightweight crutches can be custom-made of polyvinyl chloride pipe and thermoplastic material to give the child maximal independence (Fig. 11–8). Families may require assistance in identifying and removing environmental barriers that block the child's independence.

FIGURE 11–8. Child with AMC wearing polypropylene braces and using lightweight custom-made crutches constructed with PVC pipe.

Children in this age group are encouraged to participate in activities with children the same age in day care, swimming classes, and other peer group activities. They are encouraged to develop relationships with children who do not have disabilities as well as those who do. These relationships may influence the children to think and act not out of a response to disabilities but toward creative solutions. During the preschool period, many states mandate therapy services for children with special needs. These preschool services as well as additional therapy services are imperative for maximizing these children's skills for the demands they will encounter during school.

THERAPY DURING THE SCHOOL AGE AND ADOLESCENT PERIOD

The focus of physical therapy moves from the outpatient clinic into the classroom at this stage. The majority of children are mainstreamed, although they may have adaptive physical education, physical therapy, occupational therapy, and speech services to enhance the educational process.

Disabilities include limitations in mobility, now with the added constraints of needing to quickly traverse greater distances, which complicates the independent mobility issue. Efficient and independent dressing, feeding, and toileting abilities take on a more compelling nature. Joint contractures continue to be problematic, and appropriate intervention often is postponed because of time and social considerations.

Assessment

The school therapist acts as a team member addressing goals of the child and family in regard to enhancing the child's educational experience. The evaluation determines what type of training and adaptive equipment are needed to achieve educational objectives. Functional ADL skills are assessed to ascertain how efficiency and independence can be improved.

Goals

During this period, the child with AMC needs to be responsible for self-care and for an exercise program to be performed to the best of the child's ability. The family must also become more responsible for expecting and allowing the child to be more independent. Addressing these goals reduces the overall disability. The goal of independence in mobility and keeping up with friends is important in the development of peer relationships. ROM continues to be a focus in management of impairment because a child with AMC will lose motion if he or she does not continue to stretch throughout the growing years.

Intervention Strategies

Dressing, toileting, and feeding may require adaptive equipment and/or setup for the child to be independent. Children with AMC require some collective pieces of adaptive equipment for achieving independence, but most are quite adaptable and innovative in using compensatory strategies versus relying on assistive devices to achieve their goals. Frequently, classroom chairs and tables must be at custom-made heights to accommodate rising from a chair without manipulating brace knee locks. The desk top may need to be adjusted so that the child, by using a mouthstick or a wrist aid to hold crayons, can maneuver items on the desk or write (Fig. 11–9). Implementation of ideas such as these

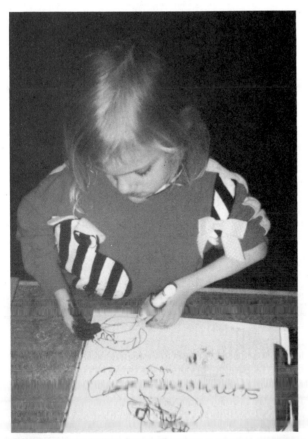

FIGURE 11 9. Child with AMC using a wrist aid to hold a crayon.

limits disability by providing the child with successful compensatory strategies.

Continued compliance with the customized splinting and stretching program is expected. Children at this age may lose a few degrees of motion during growth, but further regression may result in loss of function and of independence. Surgical intervention may then be necessary to improve joint position. A self-stretching program, utilizing assistive straps, braces, and positioning, can be incorporated into the child's routine to promote independence in attaining goals. The adolescent must be permitted to plan his or her schedule or compliance can be expected to be poor. Adaptive physical education in school can be an adjunct to physical therapy for promoting strength, endurance, and mobility.

Speed and safety in independent mobility are important in the development of peer relationships. Families may be counseled during this time to look toward electrically powered mobility devices as an adjunct to previous mobility devices. Cumbersome bracing, inefficient gait, and poor upper extremity function can limit a child's ability to participate in playground or social activities. Alternative modes of mobility may allow the child to participate safely. Use of alternative modes need not preclude ambulation but rather provides supplemental mobility for safety and energy conservation. From our experience, most children can achieve functional household ambulation but require a wheelchair for efficient community mobility.

TRANSITION TO ADULTHOOD

We could find no published studies that address the transition to adulthood for children with AMC. Much of what we present in this section is derived from interviews with individuals with AMC. Disabilities in adulthood relate to continued problems achieving independence in ADL, ambulation, and mobility. Those who required assistance with ADL during their school-age years continued to require assistance throughout their lifetime but were able to achieve a degree of independence with feeding, dressing, and grooming using selected assistive ADL devices.

Problems

Some specific problems that occur in adults are arthritic changes in weight-bearing joints and overuse syndromes in muscles that are used for compensation or unique postures. Carpal tunnel problems and neuropathies may develop as a result of prolonged joint constrictions and deformities. Mobility problems emerging later in life may stem from secondary degenerative changes and muscle overuse syndrome (Hall, 1989). Manually or electrically powered wheelchairs, therefore, may be more commonly used than during the school-age years. From our experience, adults with AMC used a wheelchair as their primary mode of mobility.

Advanced education is of utmost importance so that the adult with AMC becomes trained in a specialized skill or field. The type of work chosen will depend on the degree of functional limitations, education, and marketable skills. Desk work and computer work tend to be high employment options.

Many of the barriers that the adult with AMC will meet are physical barriers. Through the enactment of the Americans with Disabilities Act, attempts are being made to reduce the presence of these physical barriers. Through advancements in technology, patients with arthrogryposis have opportunities available to them to enhance their freedom of mobility and their career options. Assistive technology can be of value in helping the patient safely and efficiently achieve work and leisure goals. Rehabilitation adult facilities, although probably unfamiliar with AMC owing to the small numbers of adults, can provide services regarding assistive technology and orthotics.

Technology for independent driving can provide customized equipment to accommodate to the special needs of these drivers. Computerization and voice-activated equipment may provide new freedoms for this population.

Intervention Strategies

Once skeletal growth has stopped, stretching is not as imperative, but maintaining flexibility and proper positioning is encouraged to impede the further development of deformities. Those with AMC who used orthoses during the school-age years continue to do so throughout adulthood. Those who used only ankle-foot orthoses for clubfoot control tend not to need these orthoses once growth is complete. One intervention required is joint conservation, which addresses the secondary impairments due to degenerative changes.

Information about the long-term sequelae of AMC in relation to degenerative changes, mobility levels, and use of adaptive ADL devices is critical to providing the most effective therapy to persons with AMC. However, there is a lack of research regarding the extent of independence of these children, adolescents, and adults in the area of ADL,

use of manual or power chairs, and ambulation ability. This lack of data may be because the children are followed early on within a medical model addressing their primary orthopaedic concerns but when they transfer to the educational setting and to less medical intervention they are lost to follow up. To meet the objective of providing the most appropriate therapy to these children, a nationwide database on functional independent outcomes, mobility, and associated long-term problems needs to be established.

CONCLUSION

Arthrogryposis poses a variety of challenges for the health care team throughout the client's lifetime. Although AMC is nonprogressive, its sequelae can be quite disabling. There is variability in clinical manifestations, but severe joint contractures and lack of muscle development are hallmarks of the disease. Each stage of development requires special attention for maximizing the child's function. An early goal of the team is to educate the family about AMC and to create the understanding that, without intervention, the child's impairments could lead to further functional limitations and disability. Early medical and therapeutic management includes vigorous stretching, splinting, positioning, and strengthening, which allow the child to develop optimal positions for functional ADL and enhance motor skill development. Timing of surgical procedures is critical to minimize intervention while maximizing benefits.

During infancy, motor milestones are often delayed or skipped and determining functional mobility is more important than ascribing a developmental level. The intervention strategies focus on reducing physical impairments through serial splinting and strengthening and on facilitating developmental activities. Ambulation is a preliminary primary goal, but once the child reaches school age, the focus shifts toward more independent, functional, and safe mobility. During the school-age years, once the child can begin to participate in an exercise program, the child needs to be responsible for stretching exercises because stretching is an integral part of the program throughout the growing years. The team emphasizes assisting the child with problem solving and working toward independent mobility. Adaptive equipment is often necessary to allow the child with AMC to be independent in mobility and self-care. A comprehensive and integrated team approach is critical in developing strategies to meet these challenges.

CASE HISTORY: WILL

Will was first seen by a physical therapist at 12 days of age. He was referred to physical therapy by our orthopaedic department. During the initial evaluation, photographs were taken to document positions of his extremities. Will exhibited postures with extended elbows, flexed and pronated wrists, and hips in flexion, abduction, and external rotation. An x-ray examination determined that the right hip was dislocated. The ROM was as follows:

	Right	Left
Shoulder flexion	0–150°	0–130°
Shoulder abduction	0 90°	0–140°
Elbow flexion	0–15°	0–20°
Wrist flexion	5–130°	5–95°
Hip flexion	70–105°	65–120°
Hip abduction	30–55°	20–50°
Hip internal rotation	0–20°	0–15°
Hip external rotation	0–60°	0–90°
Knee flexion	55–135°	65–130°
Ankle plantar flexion	40° (fixed)	35° (fixed)
Forefoot adduction	25–40°	35–65°

The family was instructed in passive ROM of the lower extremities during diaper changes and of the upper extremities during feeding. The following week, therapists fabricated customized low-temperature thermoplastic splints. These included AFOs, knee extension splints, and wrist splints. The infant was treated by physical therapists and occupational therapists every 3 to 4 weeks to adjust the splints and monitor the home program.

At 3 months of age, the therapists initiated the use of elbow flexion splints worn 23 hours per day. The family was taught to position the legs in a less abducted posture by wrapping a wide Velcro band around the thighs. At 3 months, the ROM of the lower extremities was as follows:

	Right	Left
Hip flexion	25–120°	25–120°
Hip abduction	0–75°	0–60°
Hip internal rotation	0–40°	0–50°
Hip external rotation	0–90°	0–70°
Knee flexion	30–95°	25–125°
Ankle plantar flexion	25–45°	25 50°
Forefoot abduction	0–5°	0–10°
Forefoot adduction	0–45°	0–40°

There was a marked decrease in hip flexion contractures bilaterally, improvement to neutral hip adduction, marked reduction in knee flexion contractures, improved forefoot abduction, and reduced ankle plantar flexion contractures.

Muscle testing determined by palpation and observation of active movement revealed active hip flexion, extension, and abduction. The hamstrings were active against gravity. The contractions of the quadriceps and plantar flexors were palpable. No biceps brachii contraction was palpable. There was, however, active shoulder flexion against gravity as well as at least fair strength of the pectoralis and triceps brachii.

At 6 months of age, Will began use of a standing frame using knee extension splints, AFOs and wedged sneakers. At 7 months of age, Will began sitting independently once placed in that position. At 10 months, he was rolling for locomotion and was able to "commando" crawl occasionally. He was able to sit in a straddle position on the floor and tolerate dynamic challenges to his balance. He could move from supine to sitting while the lower extremities were stabilized.

Will was enrolled in a center-based early intervention program at 12 months of age. In this program, he received physical therapy three times a week with the goals of independent mobility, improving ROM through stretching and positioning, and work on preambulation activities. Will was treated on a monthly outpatient basis through our clinic for program updates, and the family continued the stretching program two to three times per day. During this time, the potential use of adaptive equipment such as slings for play and feeding was explored. Splints were adjusted to accommodate the improving ROM.

At 14 months of age, Will independently maneuvered from prone to sitting by widely abducting his hips and using his arms to raise and lower his trunk. By 16 months of age, he could stand independently in leg splints and wedged sneakers, but his hips were very abducted and he required upper extremity support. A wide elastic strap was used in a figure-eight pattern around his thighs to reduce the abducted posture. Once this excessively abducted posturing was prevented, he was able to achieve a step but needed facilitation for weight shifting.

By 20 months of age, Will was excited about standing and wanted to stand all the time. When he was supported under the axillae, he would walk. At 22 months of age, Will underwent bilateral posterior mediolateral releases for his clubfeet, which were subsequently placed in casts for 8 weeks. During that time, he used a cart for mobility. After cast removal, custom-made hip-knee-ankle-foot orthoses were fabricated and preambulation training began. He started standing with a posterior walker with the braces unlocked at the hips and rapidly progressed to taking 2 steps with the walker. During this period, Will received physical therapy three times per week, with concentration on independent standing and walking and adaptive aquatics two times per week. By 27 months of age, he was able to stand independently with both hips unlocked and could take 2 steps without upper extremity support.

At 30 months, Will's current ROM is as follows:

	Right	Left
Shoulder flexion	0–140°	0–160°
Shoulder abduction	0–130°	0–140°
Elbow flexion	0–50°	0–80°
Wrist flexion	0–90°	0–90°
Wrist extension	0–20°	0–30°
Hip flexion	0–140°	0–140°
Hip abduction	0–45°	0–45°
Hip internal rotation	0–25°	0–20°
Hip external rotation	0–55°	0–70°
Knee flexion	10–120°	20–120°
Ankle plantar flexion	0–30°	0–30°
Forefoot abduction	0–15°	0–25°
Forefoot adduction	0–20°	0–20°

At 30 months, Will is able to walk 600 feet with a walker and unlocked hip joints. He is also able to walk 6 feet without any assistive device. Gait training without the pelvic band on his braces has begun but requires verbal cues to avoid abducting the lower extremities during gait.

CASE HISTORY: ERICA

Erica is a 17-year-old female with AMC. She was one of a pair of twins who was placed in foster care at an early age and eventually was adopted at the age of 5.

At the age of 15, Erica was seen in our clinic and found to be nonambulatory with severe equinovarus feet and bilateral knee flexion contractures. An orthopaedist was consulted to determine the extent of surgery necessary to attain ambulation if, indeed, it were feasible at all.

Before any surgical or therapeutic intervention, Erica had independent bed mobility, independent scooting transfer ability from the wheelchair with the armrest removed, and independence in moving from supine to sitting. She was unable to assume or maintain high kneeling or standing. She was dependent on a caregiver for all self-care skills except feeding, for which she used a ball bearing feeder. She required moderate to maximal assistance with toilet transfers. Her initial ROM revealed primary limitations at the knee: 30° to 70° on the right and 40° to 70° on the left. Strength was in the 3+/5 range bilaterally throughout the hip musculature, 4/5 in the hamstrings, and 1/5 in the quadriceps and plantar flexors.

An intensive stretching and strengthening program was initiated before surgical intervention. Erica was treated in physical therapy two times per week for stretching of the lower extremities, strengthening of hip and knee muscles, and high kneeling activities. Knee extension splints were fabricated by the therapist to passively stretch her contractures at night. An active exercise program including functional activities such as high kneeling progressing to knee walking was accomplished. After 3 months of this program, she underwent bilateral triple arthrodesis. She was in a cast for 8 weeks and then placed into bilateral knee-ankle-foot orthoses with dial locks to allow for gradual adjustments of the knee angle for progressive stretching. Her sneakers were wedged to give her a plantigrade surface for weight-bearing.

Ten weeks after surgery, Erica ambulated in locked orthoses and wedged sneakers for 15 feet with contact guard supervision. She progressed to ambulating 100 feet with close supervision over a few months.

Currently, Erica continues to have no active use of her upper extremities, with the exception of shoulder depressors. She has bilateral elbow flexion contractures, and her wrists are held stiffly in 20° of flexion. She continues to have knee flexion contractures of 30° bilaterally and 10° plantar flexion contractures. Lower extremity strength consists of 4/5 hip extensors, 4/5 hip flexors, 3/5 hip adductors, 5/5 hip abductors, 4/5 hamstrings through the available ROM, 1+/5 quadriceps, and 1/5 plantar flexors. Hip musculature improved strength generally by 1/2 muscle grade. She has no active dorsiflexion bilaterally.

Erica's current ambulation status is independent on level surfaces indoors using her orthoses. She requires moderate assistance to ascend and descend stairs. She is working on dynamic standing balance on the tilt board and outdoor ambulation on uneven surfaces. She continues to need assistance to lock and unlock her braces. She performs toilet transfers with stand-by assistance and transfers independently from the wheelchair to bed and back using trunk movements while stabilizing with her feet. Erica uses her power wheelchair with joystick control as her primary means of mobility outside the home but now is able to walk within the home environment. Some of her expectations were met when she achieved this long-desired goal. Walking has not made her the equal of her peers, and society still identifies her with her wheelchair. Erica has a helper dog that is trained to assist her at school and in the community.

In the area of communication, because Erica has no hand function, she uses a mouth stick for most of her writing and drawing. She uses a voice-activated computer at school. Despite physical limitations, Erica's ambitions are to become a medical illustrator and she is making plans for hiring a companion to assist her with self-care when she attends college.

References

Daniels, L, & Worthingham, C. In Venable, B (Ed.), Muscle Testing: Techniques of Manual Examination (5th ed.). Philadelphia: WB Saunders, 1986.

Drummond, DS, Siller, TN, & Cruess, RL. Management of arthrogryposis multiplex congenita. In AAOS Instructional Lectures, Montreal, Canada, 1978.

Goodman, RM, & Gorlin, RJ. Arthrogryposis. In Goodman, RM, & Gorlin, RJ (Eds.), The Malformed Infant and Child. New York: Oxford University Press, 1983, pp. 42–43.

Hall, JG. An approach to congenital contractures (arthrogryposis). Pediatric Annals, 10:249–257, 1981.

Hall, JG. Genetic aspects of arthrogryposis. Clinical Orthopedics, 194:44, 1985.

Hall, JG. Arthrogryposis. American Family Physician, 39(1):113–119, 1989.

Hall, JG, Reed, SD, & Green, G. The distal arthrogryposis: Delineation of new entities—review and nosologic discussion. American Journal of Medical Genetics, 1:185–239, 1982.

Jayakumar, S. Personal communication. Alfred I. duPont Institute, Department of Orthopedics, Wilmington, DE: 1992.

Kendall, FP, McCreary, EK, & Provance, PG. Muscle and Function (4th ed.). Baltimore: Williams & Wilkins, 1993.

MacEwen, GD, & Gale, DI. Hip disorders in arthrogryposis multiplex congenita. In Katz, J, & Siffert, R (Eds.), Management of Hip Disorders in Children. Philadelphia: JB Lippincott, 1983, pp. 209–228.

Palmer, PM, MacEwen, GD, Bowen, JR, & Matthews, PA. Passive motion therapy for infants with arthrogryposis. Clinical Orthopedics and Related Research, 194:54–59, 1985.

Sarwark, JF, MacEwen, GD, & Scott, CI. Amyoplasia (a common form of arthrogryposis). Journal of Bone and Joint Surgery (American), 72:465–469, 1990.

Scott, CI, & Nicholson, L. Personal communication. Alfred I. duPont Institute, Genetics Department, Wilmington, DE, 1992.

Sodergard, J, & Ryoppy, S. The knee in arthrogryposis multiplex congenita. Journal of Pediatric Orthopedics, 10:177–182, 1990.

Staheli, LT, Chew, DE, Elliot, JS, & Mosca, VS. Management of hip dislocations in children with AMC. Journal of Pediatric Orthopedics, 7:681–685, 1987.

St. Clair, HS, & Zimbler, S. A plan of management and treatment results in the arthrogrypotic hip. Clinical Orthopedics and Related Research, 194:74–80, 1985.

Tachdjian, MO. Arthrogryposis multiplex congenita (multiple congenital contractures). In Tachdjian, M (Ed.), Pediatric Orthopedics. Philadelphia: WB Saunders: 1990, pp. 2086–2114.

Williams, PF. The elbow in arthrogryposis. Journal of Bone and Joint Surgery (British), 55:834, 1973.

Williams, P. The management of arthrogryposis. Orthopedic Clinics of North America, 9:67–88, 1978.

Wynne-Davies, R, Williams, PF, & O'Conner, JCB. The 1960's epidemic of arthrogryposis multiplex congenita. Journal of Bone and Joint Surgery (British), 63:76–82, 1981.

Bibliography

Brown, LM, Robson, MJ, & Sharrard, WJW. The pathophysiology of arthrogryposis multiplex congenita neurologica. Journal of Bone and Joint Surgery (British), 62:291–296, 1980.

Davidson, J, & Beighton, P. Whence the arthrogrypotic? Journal of Bone and Joint Surgery (British), 58:492–495, 1976.

Fisher, RL, Johnstone, WT, Fisher, WH, & Goldkamp, OG. Arthrogryposis multiplex congenita: A clinical investigation. Journal of Pediatrics, 76:255, 1970.

Hageman, G, Ippel, EP, Beemer, FA, DaPater, JM, Lindhout, D, & Willemse, J. The diagnostic management of newborns with congenital contractures and nosologic study of 75 cases. American Journal of Medical Genetics, 30:883–904, 1988.

Hall, JG, Reed, SD, & Driscoll, EP. Amyoplasia: A common sporadic condition with congenital contractures. American Journal of Medical Genetics, 15:579–590, 1983.

Hall, JG, Reed, SD, Scott, CI, Rogers, JG, Jones, KL, & Camarano, A. Three distinct types of X linked AMC seen in 6 families. Clinical Genetics, 21:81–97, 1982.

Kamil, NI. A dynamic elbow flexion splint for an infant with arthrogryposis. American Journal of Occupational Therapy, 44:460–461, 1990.

Lai, MM, Tettenborn, MA, Hall, JG, Smith, LJ, & Berry, AC. A new form of autosomal dominant arthrogryposis multiplex congenita. Journal of Medical Genetics, 28:701–703, 1991.

Lloyd-Roberts, GC, & Lettin, AWF. Arthrogryposis multiplex congenita. Journal of Bone and Joint Surgery (British), 52:494, 1970.

Mead, NG, Lithgaw, WC, & Sweeney, HJ. Arthrogryposis multiplex congenita. Journal of Bone and Joint Surgery (American), 40:1285, 1958.

Robinson, RO. AMC: Feeding, language and other health problems. Neuropediatrics, 21:177–178, 1990.

Sack, GH. A dominantly inherited form of AMC with unusual dermatoglyphics. Clinical Genetics, 14:317–323, 1978.

Schiulli, C, Corradi-Scalise, D, & Donatelli-Schulthiss, ML. Powered mobility vehicles as aides in independent locomotion for very young children. Physical Therapy, 68:997–999, 1988.

Chapter 12

Osteogenesis Imperfecta

DEBRA ANN BLEAKNEY, PT,
MAUREEN DONOHOE, PT

Osteogenesis imperfecta (OI) is an inherited disorder of connective tissue. Other terms in the literature used to describe OI include fragilitas ossium and brittle bones. OI has an incidence of 1 in 20,000 live births. Its prevalence in the population is 16 per million (Wynne-Davies & Gormley, 1981). This disorder comprises a number of distinct syndromes and has great variability in its manifestations. The salient impairments of OI are lax joints, weak muscles, and diffuse osteoporosis, which results in multiple recurrent fractures. These recurring fractures, sustained from even minimal trauma, coupled with weak muscles and lax joints, result in major deformity. Additional impairments in OI with variable presentation include blue sclerae, dentinogenesis imperfecta, deafness, hernias, easy bruising, and excessive sweating. Without early and adequate intervention, these problems in children with OI may lead to irreversible deformities and disability.

Too often children and adolescents with OI are overprotected as a result of the recurring fractures, leading to social isolation. This contributes to difficulty in interacting in peer play, adjusting to regular school, and achieving an independence level necessary to accomplish vocational plans. Because most children with OI have average or above-average intelligence, they may greatly benefit from a stimulating educational environment. These chil-

dren usually become productive members of society. The management of their disabilities should therefore be directed toward obtaining optimal independence, social integration, and educational achievement. The overall prognosis of OI and its long-term sequelae depend on the severity of the disease, which ranges from severe to very mild. Likewise, the range of disability is from extremely severe, with death occurring at birth or shortly thereafter, to relatively mild with no deformities.

CLASSIFICATION

OI presents as a group of impairments that vary in severity and that are marked by fragility of bone. It is not a single genetic disorder but is heterogeneous.

Because of the wide spectrum of this disease, there are many proposed classifications (Falvo et al., 1974; Sillence, 1981). In 1906, Looser classified OI into two types: OI congenita and OI tarda. Seedorf (1949) further subclassified OI tarda into two types: tarda gravis and tarda levis. Historically OI was classified based on clinical and descriptive characteristics (i.e., fracture healing and spinal deformities). The OI congenita and tarda classification system has clinical usefulness but does not reflect the scope of OI from a genetic or pathogenetic standpoint; however, the clinician will often see this classification system referenced in the literature and in patients' medical records.

Osteogenesis imperfecta congenita (OIC), the most severe and disabling form, is characterized by numerous fractures at birth, dwarfism, bowing or deformities of the long bones, blue sclerae (80% of cases), and dentinogenesis imperfecta (80% of cases). Infants with OIC have a poor prognosis, with a high mortality rate resulting from either intracranial hemorrhage at birth or recurring respiratory tract infections during infancy (Tachdjian, 1990).

Osteogenesis imperfecta tarda (OIT), considered the milder form of OI in which fractures occur after birth, has been subclassified based on either the degree of bowing of the extremities or the number of fractures. Bowing is a good measure of the severity of OI because it correlates with the number of fractures and the severity of subsequent deformity (Tachdjian, 1990). The degree of bowing also indicates the potential need for surgical intervention. The clinical characteristics of OIT type I include dentinogenesis imperfecta, short stature, and bowing of lower extremities, but the upper extremities are not bowed. Most children with OIT type I can ambulate but may need bracing. Surgery is often indicated for correction of the long bone deformity.

OIT type II is the least disabling form of OI in which fractures can occur in the first year of life or later. In contrast to OIT type I, there is no bowing of the long bones and no deformities of the upper limbs are present. Most of these children approach average height. Prognosis for ambulation is excellent.

The classification system of OIC and OIT, although descriptive, has been deemed oversimplified by clinicians, geneticists, and biochemists. As a result of a comprehensive survey done by Sillence and Danks (1978), four distinct genetic types of OI have been delineated. This classification system includes clinical presentation, radiologic criteria, and mode of inheritance. The Sillence classification uses a numerical system rather than the more cumbersome descriptive classifications and correlates with morphologic and biochemical studies of OI (Sillence, 1981). A more recent theory suggests that the mode of inheritance in all forms of OI is dominant (Scott, CI, & Nicholson, L, personal communication, 1993).

OI type I shows an autosomal dominant inheritance (Sillence, 1981; Sillence & Danks, 1978; Sillence et al., 1979). It is characterized by markedly blue sclerae throughout life, generalized osteoporosis with bone fragility, joint hyperlaxity, and pre-senile conductive hearing loss. These patients are generally short but are not as short as those with other forms of OI. At birth, weight and length are normal; short stature occurs postnatally. Dentinogenesis imperfecta is variably present. If dentinogenesis is not present, then this type of OI is further subclassified as OI type IA; if dentinogenesis imperfecta is present, the subclassification is OI type IB. Fractures may be present at birth (10%) or may appear at any time during infancy and childhood (Sillence, 1981). The frequency and development of skeletal deformity are also variable. The birth and population incidence of OI type I is 1 in 30,000.

Based on the Sillence classification, OI type II is either a common autosomal dominant form or a rare autosomal recessive form. OI type II is lethal in the perinatal period. These infants may be stillborn. There is extreme bone fragility with minimal mineralization. Marked delay of ossification of the skull and facial bones is noted, and the long bones are crumbled (Tachdjian, 1990). The infants are small for their age and have characteristic short, curved, and deformed limbs. The incidence as reported by Sillence is 1 in 62,487 live births.

According to the Sillence classification, OI type III can be autosomal dominant or recessive but is heterozygous. This form is severe, and there is progressive deformity of the long bones, skull, and spine, resulting in very short stature. Usually, there is severe bone fragility, moderate bone deformity at birth, multiple fractures, and severe growth retardation. OI type III appears similar to the lethal perinatal OI type except that the lack of skull ossification is not as marked and birth weight and length are within normal range. Sclerae have a variable hue, tending to be bluish at birth but becoming less so with age. Dentinogenesis occurs in 45% of patients with OI type III. Hearing loss is common. As a result of the complications of severe kyphoscoliosis and resulting respiratory compromise, death occurs in childhood. OI type III is rare, and the exact incidence is not documented (Tachdjian, 1990).

OI type IV is rare and is inherited by autosomal dominant transmission. It is characterized by mild to moderate deformity and postnatal short stature. There is bone fragility and deformities of the long bones of variable severity. Sclerae tend to be normal and dentinogenesis is common. Hearing loss is variable. The prognosis for ambulation is excellent (Byers, 1988). The exact incidence of OI type IV is unknown (Tachdjian, 1990).

Sillence (1981) has compared his proposed nomenclature with the congenita or tarda classification. He relates type I to the congenita and tarda form of OI, type II to the congenita form (always), and types III and IV to both congenita and tarda forms. Silence acknowledges that difficulty exists in this comparison because any syndromes accompanied by the onset of fractures at birth may be classified as congenita, whereas children with types I, III, or IV could have their first fracture at any time.

PATHOPHYSIOLOGY

In all forms of OI, a defect in collagen synthesis results from an abnormality in processing procollagen to type I collagen, apparently causing the bones to be brittle. This defect affects the formation of both enchondral and intramembranous bone. The collagen fibers fail to mature beyond the reticular fiber stage. Studies show that osteoblasts have normal or increased activity but fail to produce and organize the collagen (Ramser & Frost, 1966). Histologically, there is variability among the different types of OI. In the more severe congenita form, the proportion of primitive osseous tissue with a woven matrix is markedly greater than in the tarda form (Bullough et al., 1981; Falvo & Bullough, 1973). A relative abundance of osteocytes is present, but intracellular matrix is deficient. In Sillence classification OI type I, morphologic findings include an increased amount of glycogen in osteoblasts, mild hypercellularity of bone (Albright et al., 1975), and no abnormality in collagen fiber diameter (Doty & Matthews, 1971). In OI type II, morphologic findings include poorly ossified cortical bone (Follis, 1952), abnormally thin corneal and skin collagen fibers (Bluemcke et al., 1972), hypercellularity of secondary bone trabeculae and cortical bone (Sillence & Danks, 1978), and deficient osteoid with deposition of argyrophilic material or primary trabeculae (Follis, 1952). In types III and IV, morphologic findings include an increased amount of woven bone, increased cellularity, increased number of resorption surfaces, and wide osteoid seams (Falvo & Bullough, 1973).

Those persons who have inherited OI tend to have a similar, if not the same, collagen defect as their parent. First-generation OI tends to be caused by a novel mutation of the gene. This specific gene mutation can then be passed to offspring. Genetic counseling when OI is found gives parents an accurate estimate of the risk of recurrence and an understanding of clinical variabilities in their family. The degree of severity in families is also variable. A mildly affected patient could give birth to a severely affected child. Describing to the parents the lifestyle of a child with OI may have more meaning than quoting risk figures (Solomons & Millar, 1973).

MANAGEMENT

Medical Management

No consistently effective medications are available to strengthen skeletal structures and prevent fractures. Improvements in medical care for the treatment of respiratory tract infections and in orthopaedic management contribute to the improved outlook for a child with OI. Life expectancy appears to be increasing, but limited gains have been made in improving functional abilities (Albright, 1981).

Pharmacologic Management

Pharmacologic management for recurring fractures has included numerous medications and dietary supplements, all of dubious efficacy. Magnesium oxide, calcitonin, and fluoride have been administered in an attempt to decrease the frequency of fractures, but with inconsistent results. Sex hormones have been tried as a result of the clinical observation that fracture incidence diminishes after puberty. All of these regimens have been deemed ineffective as primary treatments in the prevention of fractures. Despite the fact that no dietary alterations have been shown to be effective, eating a well-balanced diet is highly recommended (Albright, 1981).

Surgery

Once a fracture occurs, the bone is more susceptible to refracture. The already weakened structure predisposes the child to limb deformities from bowing of the long bones. Immobilization to assist in setting the bone in proper alignment can cause disuse osteoporosis, which, in turn, puts those fragile bones at greater risk of fracturing. Hence, a vicious cycle is created: osteoporosis leads to fractures, and immobilization secondary to fracture creates disuse osteoporosis, which leads to further fractures. The goal then, is to limit immobilization of the extremities as much as possible to prevent exacerbation of osteopenia and risk of more fractures.

Fractures in patients with OI generally heal within the normal healing time, although the resultant callus may be large but of poor quality. These fractures need to be immobilized for pain relief and to promote healing in the correct alignment. Pseudarthrosis may occur when the fracture is not immobilized. Immobilization may be in the form of splinting with thermoplastic materials, orthoses, hip spica posterior shells, or casting. When there is malunion of fractures, angulation and bowing of the long bones occur, frequently accompanied by joint contractures. There may be disruption of the physis, resulting in asymmetric growth and deformity. When angulation occurs, mechanical forces tend to increase the deformity, thus aggravating the overall problem (Albright, 1981). The cartilaginous ends of the long bones are disproportionately large and have irregular articular surfaces. Fortunately, in nearly all patients with OI, the fracture rate diminishes near or after puberty.

The most successful means of fracture stabilization in weight-bearing long bones in OI is internal fixation with intermedullary rods. Although this method of stabilization is not without complications, the intramedullary rod can be helpful in preventing long bones from bowing after fractures and provides internal support to prevent further fractures. Indications for stabilization with rods include multiple recurring fractures and increasing long bone deformity that is interfering with orthotic fit and impairing function. The age of the patient and the size of the bone determine the type and timing of surgery. Intermedullary rod fixation of the femur is best done after 4 or 5 years of age when the thigh is not so short as to complicate surgery by compounding the technical difficulty. Surgical insertion of the rod in thin bones is also technically difficult.

The type of rod used depends on the type and severity of fracture. When a solid rod is used, bone growth may occur beyond the ends of the rods, necessitating reoperation later for placement of a longer rod. Because children with severe OI are at greater than normal anesthetic risk from potential respiratory compromise, the number of operative procedures is best kept to a minimum. Special instrumentation has been designed that "elongates" with the child's growth, eliminating the need for multiple reoperations as the bone grows (Fig. 12-1). These extensible intramedullary fixation devices were introduced by Bailey and Dubow (1965). They are used more frequently in the femur and humerus and less often in the tibia and forearm. Problems exist with the control of rotation and migration when using extensible rods; thus postoperative casting may be necessary. Orthoses may be needed after insertion of the rod for further external support. Early weight bearing with orthotic support is initiated as soon as possible.

FIGURE 12-1. Extensible intramedullary fixation rods that elongate as the bone grows in a child with OI.

Spinal deformities, including scoliosis and kyphosis, occur in 50% of the patients with OI, as a result of osteoporosis and vertebral compression fractures. Kyphoscoliosis can be disabling and may be present in 20 to 40% of patients (Tachdjian, 1990). The kyphoscoliosis further compounds the patient's short stature. The most common curve is that of thoracic scoliosis. Scoliotic and kyphotic curves in patients with OI are not usually amenable to conservative bracing. The bones in children with OI usually cannot withstand the forces of the brace, and the result is rib deformities rather than the intended effect on the spine (Albright, 1981). In adolescents and adults with severe OI, the incidence of scoliosis is 80 to 90%. Surgical stabilization is often advocated for the management of these deformities, but there is little documentation of long-term outcome (Hanscom et al., 1992).

IMPAIRMENT

Diagnosis and Problem Identification

In the most severe forms of OI, the infant is born with multiple fractures sustained in utero or during the birth process. The prognosis of OI depends on its type. In the most severe forms these multiple fractures that have occurred in utero and during birth are associated with a high mortality rate. Prognostic indicators concerning survival and ambulation are the time of the initial fracture and the radiologic appearance of long bones and ribs at the time of the initial fracture. Spranger and associates (1982) devised a scoring system for providing an accurate prognosis for newborns with OI. This system coded the degree of skeletal changes based on clinical and radiographic findings in 47 cases. These investigators found that newborns who had marked bowing of their lower extremities but less severe changes in the skull, ribs, vertebrae, and arms and who had normal sclerae survived and had fewer fractures as they grew older. In the moderate and mild types, although the prognosis varies, there is a gradual tendency toward improvement when the incidence of fractures decreases after puberty.

If a family is known to be at risk of having a child with OI and the collagen defect has been identified in the parent, human chorionic villus biopsy can be done prenatally at 10 weeks' gestation to determine if the child has the same defect. A prenatal ultrasound examination at 15 weeks' gestation can be helpful in identifying fractures as well as possible mineralization problems (Byers, 1988).

The infant is usually of normal size at birth, but postnatal growth is impaired. Although no conclusive causative factors for this impaired growth are known, possible factors are the deformities themselves or abnormalities in the epiphyseal growth plates. The radiologic appearance of long bones associated with the most severe cases indicates bones with a thin radiolucent appearance. The malformed ribs affect respiratory function, which may lead to respiratory tract infections and reduced functional potential of the child.

Children with moderate OI are often identified after there have been several fractures from seemingly slight trauma. An example is a fractured humerus caused by the child holding onto a car seat while the caretaker is trying to get the child out of the car. Those children who begin having fractures of unknown origin at a young age can have collagen and biochemical studies done, usually from a skin biopsy. The tests can also be helpful in ruling out other disorders, such as idiopathic juvenile osteoporosis, leukemia, and congenital hypophosphatasia (which is lethal). No specific diagnostic abnormality indicating OI appears in laboratory tests; the diagnosis is made primarily from clinical and radiographic findings. In the infant, OI and achondroplasia are often confused because, in both conditions, children have large heads and short limbs.

Radiographic reports, however, distinguish between the two.

Collagen and biochemical studies can assist in differentiating a battered infant from an infant with OI. Radiographic studies are helpful because fractures at the epiphysis are rare in OI but common in child abuse, in which there is also evidence of soft tissue trauma. Bruising is common to both the infant with OI and the battered infant, but the bruising will disappear when the battered infant is in a safe environment. Three of the most helpful radiographic views in diagnosing OI are those of the skull (Wormian bones), the lateral view of the spine (biconcave vertebrae or platyspondyly), and the pelvis (the beginnings of protrusio acetabuli) (Wynne-Davies & Gormley, 1981).

In the moderate to severe forms of OI, early childhood fractures lead to multiple recurring fractures because of the already weakened structure. The child develops limb deformities from bowing, which leads to impairment of mobility and of other functional skills. In the least severe forms of OI, because the first pathologic fractures occur later in childhood, there is less likelihood of recurring fractures with associated long bone deformities and therefore the best overall prognosis.

Team members other than physical therapists who have an important role in the management of OI are orthopaedists, orthotists, occupational therapists, audiologists, dentists, and genetics professionals. Little progress has occurred in the primary prevention of this disorder, nor has there been much improvement in the medical management. With technologic enhancements and advances in neonatal care, more of these infants are surviving and presenting a management challenge to health care professionals.

Infancy

Typical disabilities seen in an infant with OI depend on the severity. In severe cases, the most serious impairments are those of rib and skull fractures, which could compromise pulmonary status and neural status, respectively. Because of possible cardiopulmonary compromise, time may be spent in the neonatal intensive care unit, which could lead to decreased parental interaction and bonding. If OI is moderate to severe, parents have increased anxiety about holding the infant for fear of fracturing the infant's bones. This may result in minimal contact and may decrease the mutually nurturing interaction vital to both parent and child. Children with severe OI who have reduced mobility from skeletal deformities may be unable to achieve age-appropriate activities of daily living (ADL) or play in the normal peer environment.

Infants with OI are at a very delicate stage of life. They are completely dependent on their caregivers and have special needs regarding handling, positioning, and playing. During this stage, minimizing fractures, the development of further muscle weakness, and joint laxity are paramount. This is accomplished primarily through a physical therapy home program and parental education for proper positioning and handling.

At birth the infant may be of normal size, but postnatal growth is almost always stunted. The infant tends to have a relatively large head with a soft and membranous skull. The limbs are usually deformed and short in the more severe forms of OI. Other features include a broad forehead and faciocranial disproportions, which give the face a triangular shape. Radiographically, fractures present at birth may be in varying stages of healing. The bones of infants with severe OI are short and wide with thin cortices, and the diaphyses are as wide as the metaphyses. Crepitation can be palpated at fracture sites.

ASSESSMENT

The physical therapist should be aware of the infant's medical history of past and present fractures and know the types of immobilizations employed before beginning the assessment. The caregiver's handling and positioning techniques during dressing, diapering, and bathing are evaluated. Assessing active, but not passive, range of motion (ROM) is essential. A standard goniometer can be used for measuring active ROM but may need to be cut down to a size suitable for the infant. Active ROM is measured at the hips, knees, ankles, shoulders, and elbows by lining up the goniometer at the axis of motion and, while observing the infant's movements, moving the goniometer through the observable range. Because passive ROM testing is contraindicated in these children, active ROM provides, at best, a close estimate and may vary during successive assessments. Functional ROM may prove more useful because it will assist in visualizing the whole composite of motions needed in functional abilities. For example, functional active ranges would include the extent to which the child can bring the hand to the mouth or reach to the top of the head. If possible, the same therapist measures ROM during re-evaluations. Intrarater and inter-rater reliability is determined for therapists and is checked annually.

Assessing muscle strength is done through observation of the infant's movements and palpation of contracting muscles rather than by use of formal muscle tests. A gross motor developmental evaluation should also be performed because these children often have delayed development of gross motor skills secondary to fractures and muscular weakness. Delayed gross motor skills are functional limitations involving impaired achievement of motor milestones. Some formal tests used include the Peabody Developmental Motor Scales (Folio & Fewell, 1983), which are normed and standardized; the Pediatric Evaluation of Disability Inventory (Haley et al., 1989), which is designed for tracking progress and assessing functional limitations; and the Bayley Scales of Infant Development (1993). Finally, it is important to assess the appropriateness of equipment used for seating, transporting, and encouraging independent mobility of the infant.

THERAPEUTIC INTERVENTION

Physical therapy includes early parent education in proper handling and positioning techniques. Bathing, dressing, and carrying the infant are critical times when the infant is at risk for fractures (Binder et al., 1984). When handling the infant it is important that force not be put across the long bones; instead the head and trunk should be supported with the arms and legs gently draped across the supporting arm. Some parents feel most comfortable supporting the infant on a standard-size bed pillow for carrying at home. It is important, however, to change the carrying position of the infant periodically because he or she develops strength by accommodating to postural changes. Dressing and undressing can be facilitated by using loose clothing and front or side Velcro closures. Overdressing should be avoided to reduce excessive sweating. Proper diapering includes a technique of rolling the infant off the diaper and supporting the buttocks with one hand with the infant's legs supported on the caregiver's forearm while the other hand positions the diaper. The infant should never be lifted by the ankles. Bathing is done in a padded, preferably plastic, basin. Infant carriers that are designed to safely support the head, trunk, and extremities are frequently used for household transporting. A customized carrier, a one-piece molded thoracolumbosacral orthosis (TLSO) fabricated from polyethylene, is used at our facility (Fig. 12–2). This carrier can incorporate the legs so they will not dangle and sustain injury. The carrier is helpful in positioning and transporting the infant while minimizing stresses to the fragile bones.

Proper positioning of the infant is a critical component of the home program and management of the infant with OI. One supported position is side-

FIGURE 12–2. Molded thoraco-lumbosacral orthosis carrier for a child with OI.

lying with towel rolls along the spine and extremities so that they are aligned and protected while the child is allowed active movement (Fig. 12–3). A prone position over a towel roll or with a wedge under the chest (if prone position is tolerated) is an alternative. When supine, the infant needs support for the arms, and the hips should be in neutral rotation with the knees over a roll (Fig. 12–4). Positions should be changed frequently and should not restrict active spontaneous movement because this affords muscle strengthening and bone mineralization (Binder et al., 1984). Positioning is useful not only for the purpose of protection from fractur-

FIGURE 12–4. Infant positioned supine with hips in neutral rotation, with knees flexed, and supported through the trunk.

FIGURE 12–3. Infant positioned lying on side using rolls. Emphasis is on maintaining trunk alignment while allowing for active and spontaneous but safe movement.

ing but also for minimizing joint malalignment and deformities. Varying the position promotes the development of age-appropriate development skills.

Promotion of sensorimotor developmental skills is an ongoing component in the management of the infant and child. Identification of appropriate and safe toys for a child, as well as comfortable play positions that promote development, is often ad-

FIGURE 12–5. Infant positioned prone on a roll encourages weight bearing, extremity and trunk alignment, and strengthening of extensor musculature during developmental play.

dressed jointly by the occupational therapist and physical therapist. For example, prone-on-a-roll positioning can allow for weight-bearing use of the arms with co-contraction of shoulder musculature as well as promote active neck and back extensor muscle control (Fig. 12–5). Increasing muscle strength and support around the joint in activities such as this is especially important because the joint ligaments are lax. The prone-on-a-roll positioning also maintains good alignment of the extremities.

Developmental activities such as rolling and supported sitting should be encouraged as tolerated. In encouraging rolling, the infant's arm is placed alongside his or her head, and then he or she attempts to roll over. Supported sitting is accomplished with seat inserts or corner chairs. Upright unsupported sitting can begin on the parent's lap with a pillow. When the child exhibits appropriate head control, short-sit and straddle activities can be done over the caregiver's leg or a roll. These activities promote the development of protective and equilibrium responses and the beginning of protected weight bearing of the lower extremities. Many children with OI spend much time scooting on their buttocks before crawling is accomplished.

Awareness of proper handling while encouraging these developmental skills is of key importance. For instance, a pull-to-sit maneuver is contraindicated when using a distraction pull on the hands. Rather, this maneuver should be modified and facilitated by supporting the child around the shoulders while the child attempts to sit up. In working on trunk control over a ball, the therapist's hands are positioned on the pelvis and trunk rather than supporting or facilitating movement from the legs. Parents should be cautioned against using baby walkers and jumping seats because they do not foster proper positioning and weight bearing. Baby walkers tend to give parents a false sense that the infant is protected. The child may have difficulty controlling these devices, resulting in unnecessary fractures. A

car seat can be adapted with foam behind the cover to ensure that the infant fits snugly in the seat with limited ability to fall sideways. The legs should be supported and not left to dangle. Padding can be rearranged in the seat to accommodate the various devices the child may be in for immobilization of fracture sites.

Active, spontaneous activity and exercise are encouraged in side-lying and supine positions, and in supported sitting, with the child reaching for, swiping at, rolling, and lifting lightweight toys of different textures. Pool exercises may begin as early as 6 months of age with the goals of promoting active exercise and weight bearing (Binder et al., 1984). Extremity movement may occur unobstructed as the child is supported in a neck or trunk flotation device accompanied by a parent or the therapist. Long-sleeved clothing may be used to distribute the absorbed water weight evenly over the length of the limb, thus introducing a resistive component to the exercise.

At this stage, goals include use of safe handling and positioning techniques by the caregivers and providing opportunities for development of age-appropriate skills. The intensity of treatment varies with the individual needs of the infant and family, but providing a home program and regular home visits by a physical therapist at least weekly is essential in ensuring that the environment is suitable for sensorimotor and cognitive development. The therapist can act as a resource and support for the caregivers as together they develop strategies to meet the challenges of safe caregiver handling, mobility, and developmental facilitation.

When fractures do occur, they may require splinting using a variety of materials such as perforated orthoplast or fiberglass. An Ace wrap has been used to support and protect a limb in mild cases and in the young infant. Fractures may heal within 2 weeks for the newborn and generally within the same time frame as other fractures in infancy (usually 6 weeks).

Preschool Period

The primary impairments of bone fragility, joint laxity, and reduced muscle strength continue to be present but are now accompanied by secondary impairments of disuse atrophy and osteoporosis from fracture immobilization (Fig. 12–6). Typical disabilities include the inability of the child to be as mobile as his or her peers, which will hamper play and socialization. This may affect the child's adjustment to regular school and hinder academic progress.

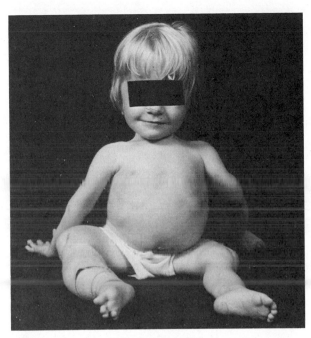

FIGURE 12–6. Child with OI showing joint laxity and bony deformities: femoral anterolateral bowing and tibial anterior bowing.

At this stage, muscles are usually weak as a result of immobilization and disuse. Developmental skills may continue to lag in the presence of frequent fractures and subsequent immobilizations, but cognitive skills should be appropriate for the child's age. When sustaining a fracture, these children complain of little pain and usually have minimal soft tissue trauma. There may be microfractures from repeated trauma at the epiphyseal plates, resulting in arrested growth and potential leg-length discrepancy. In childhood, "popcorn calcifications" appear in the metaphyseal and epiphyseal areas of long bones (Goldman et al., 1980). It is postulated that these are fragmentations of the cartilaginous growth plate.

If the child begins to walk without adequate support, there is further bending of the long bones as a result of abnormal stress on the weakened structure. Bowing occurs in the anterolateral direction in the femur and anteriorly in the tibia. In those children who do not walk, lack of the normal weight-bearing stress leads to a honeycomb pattern in the long bones.

Emphasis at this stage is on protected weight bearing and self-mobility for enhanced independence. Although proper positioning, handling, and transferring are still important, the emphasis shifts to the child's active participation in his or her care and safe independence. During this period, the

child with OI should have adequate upright control and, at the very least, should be held in standing, since early weight bearing appears to have some beneficial effect on progress of the condition. When comparing radiographs of children with OI from the time of birth and later, the changing levels of bone density suggested that progressive osteoporosis had been superimposed on the basic bone defect (Bleck, 1981). Upper extremity bones were frequently more dense than those of the lower limbs and were less likely to fracture. This finding may be related to the use and stress put on upper extremity bones during ADL. A study by King and Bobechko in 1971 concluded that limb immobilization caused osteoporosis; thus, in the prevention of secondary impairment by osteoporosis in OI, stress on the bone through weight bearing is advocated. The management principle used to implement appropriate weight bearing is to stress the lower limb bones while supporting the weakened structures through compression of the musculature around the bone. Contour-molded orthoses can be used to provide this compression and support.

Assessment tools used at this stage include an evaluation of modes of mobility and of equipment and environmental modification needs for supported sitting and mobility. Equipment requires constant updating because of the changing positional needs related to mobilization–immobilization status. Splinting needs and adaptive ADL equipment are assessed for fit and usefulness. Developmental assessment tools used may include the Peabody Developmental Motor Scales and the Pediatric Evaluation of Disability Inventory to assess gross motor function and functional limitations in children with disabilities, respectively.

THERAPEUTIC INTERVENTION

Active exercise continues to be emphasized to increase muscle strength of the weakened muscles. Usually the hip extensor and abductor muscles are weak. Active exercise can be achieved primarily through developmental play. One developmental activity to increase weight bearing and maintain or increase strength in the quadriceps and hip extensor musculature involves having the child straddle a roll and come to stand with the therapist supporting the child's pelvis (Fig. 12–7). The therapist begins with the child sitting on a high roll that requires a small excursion of movement to come from sitting to standing and then gradually changes to using a lower roll. An active-resistive program graded for the patient's tolerance should be cautiously established. Use of light weights may be incrementally increased, but they should be at-

FIGURE 12–7. Straddle roll activity of supported sit-to-stand for lower extremity strengthening and weight bearing.

tached close to large joints so as to avoid a long lever arm that increases the potential for fracture.

An aquatic exercise program is an excellent therapeutic program for the child with OI. It can be started at an early age and continue for a lifetime. There are many benefits to aquatic therapy, including the opportunity to socialize with peers in a safe environment, a safe method of strengthening muscles through resistance and assistance of the water, and the opportunity to improve cardiovascular fitness and to bear weight in a protected environment. The therapist can finely grade the progression of exercises in the pool by first using the buoyancy effect of the water to assist weak movements and then support and, finally, resist the movements. Exercises can be modified with floats by changing the length of the lever arm of the moving body part, through use of turbulence, and through altering the speed and direction of the movement. Pool exercises can also promote deep breathing to facilitate chest expansion and overall respiratory function, a goal that is especially important because chest deformities that may compromise breathing capacity are common. Certain precautions should be taken when considering pool therapy for the child with OI. The heat of the water creates a rise in body temperature and increases metabolism, which is frequently already elevated in these children. It is

suggested, therefore, that the time, water temperature, and exercise activity level be closely monitored for each child. Pool sessions are generally limited to 20 to 30 minutes.

Pool exercise therapy may interrupt the cycle of further disuse and secondary complications from immobilization. Aquatics therapy is not only an ideal therapeutic modality for the child with OI but can also be a therapeutic, lifelong avocational activity that can ameliorate the effects of the disabling process.

One key goal to be emphasized for the preschool child is safe, independent mobility, which is certainly a challenge if the child has frequent fractures. The aim is to prevent a functional limitation of reduced mobility resulting from the initial impairment. Researchers such as Perrin and Gerrity (1984) theorize that disabilities in intellectual development may occur when children have limited mobility. Opportunities for multiple safe modes of mobility should be explored to expand the child's repertoire of environmental experiences.

The degree of ambulation attainable varies for preschool children with OI. Those children with limited ambulatory skills may need formal gait training as well as instruction of family members. Interest in standing often occurs in the child's second year of life. Factors affecting this ability include the degree of bowing in the extremities and the muscle strength of the limbs. Ambulation is often introduced in the pool, for protected weight bearing. Because the buoyancy of water provides support for the body, weight bearing on weakened extremities and unstable joints can be gradually introduced without fear of causing trauma. Weight relief depends on the proportion of the body below the water level. For maximum weight relief for ambulation, the child begins standing in the deeper end of the pool where the water level is at the child's neck. Over time, the child gradually progresses to bearing more weight in shallow water. If the child with OI is recovering from a fracture, it is recommended that thermoplastic splints be used to further protect the extremity while in the pool. General guidelines for walking re-education in water according to Duffield (1983) suggest that a patient start in parallel bars or a walking frame with the therapist initially supporting the pelvis from the front. The patient practices weight shifts from side to side, forward, and backward and progresses to walking forward. The therapist cues the patient to lean slightly forward to counteract the upthrust of buoyancy, which tends to cause the child to overbalance backward. In this manner, protected walking for a child with OI can start much earlier than on a solid surface. Unsupported standing on solid ground is not recommended because it leads to rapid bowing of the long bones. When severe bowing of the extremities occurs, the child usually undergoes orthopaedic surgery in the form of osteotomies. Age-appropriate lower extremity weight bearing is encouraged, although the child with moderate to severe OI needs external devices such as splints or braces to protect fragile long bones. Supported standing frames or orthoses such as hip-knee-ankle-foot orthoses (HKAFOs) are used.

In moderate to severe OI, braces and splints are usually required to begin standing activities on solid surfaces. Use of orthotics provides protected weight bearing needed to reduce the impact of stress on the osteoporotic bony deformities. Braces or splints are first used in conjunction with a standing frame. Prone standers with orthoses are used to grade the amount of weight born on the lower extremities with progression from an inclined position to upright. The child may be fitted with a containment-type brace fabricated of lightweight thermoplastic material. These plastic orthoses can be fabricated to conform to the contours of the limb to provide support for the weakened structures around the bone. Often the first braces used during the toddler stage are made without knee joints and may have a pelvic band for maximal support. The pelvic band and locked hips minimize femoral rotation (Gerber et al., 1990). Knee joints can be added to the orthosis when the limb grows and strength increases (Fig. 12–8). Some braces use a lightweight plastic clamshell design and are contoured for ischial weight bearing. The child usually progresses from maximally supportive bracing to less cumbersome bracing as bony alignment and strength factors permit.

Air splints have been used either to prevent fractures or as a fracture management tool, either as a substitute for bracing or as a transition to bracing. Types of splinting include pneumatic trouser splints, which are used extensively in Europe. These air-filled trouser splints were introduced by Morel and Houghton (1982) for the support of the fragile long bones in OI. Morel has recommended that following the healing of the osteotomy for correction of long bone deformity these pneumatic splints be used for support. Letts and colleagues (1988) described pant orthoses called "vacuum pants" that were used in children with OI to enable weight bearing in a functional position during transition to knee-ankle-foot orthoses (KAFOs). Pneumatic trouser splints are not used in the United States, in part because of commercial unavailability and lack of familiarity with the splint. Therapy air splints such as the URIAS Pediatric C.P. Therapy Splints (J. A. Preston Corp., Jackson, MI) are read-

FIGURE 12–8. Child with OI in plastic contoured hip-knee-ankle-foot orthoses and pelvic band.

ily available, need not be custom-made, and afford some flexibility when inflated to allow ambulation. Scott (1990) used these splints for instituting graded weight bearing and gait training in a child with OI. Drawbacks of the air splints and pneumatic trousers are that they may be bulky and hot so the child may not always tolerate them well.

The child graduates from using a standing frame with orthoses to ambulating in long-leg braces with the knees locked in full extension. He or she then progresses from parallel bars to various walkers or crutches as limb strength and ability improve. A walker that supports the majority of body weight through the trunk and pelvis is often used to assist in weight bearing during initial overland ambulation. This walker supports weight by means of a trunk support cuff and a padded pommel that is positioned between the child's legs. Rollators and four-point walkers followed by canes or crutches (depending on the type and severity of OI) may be used (Fig. 12–9). Forearm attachments to walkers or crutches afford a degree of weight bearing distributed throughout the forearm to reduce stress on the arm and wrist as well as to relieve some weight bearing on the lower extremities. Some children ambulate without braces when their fracture rate decreases in later years.

Customized mobility caster carts may be fabricated to encourage independent mobility when the child is immobilized (Fig. 12–10), enabling the child to explore his or her environment, gain some independence, and maintain strength in the upper extremities. When there is good head and trunk control and the child can cognitively and safely handle a mobility device, power mobility may be an adjunct to preventing disability by allowing the child to keep up and interact with peers. These alternative mobility modes do not preclude ambulation but are useful additional mobility options. Regardless of the mode of mobility used, it is imperative to provide the child with a degree of functional independence in the home and preschool environments.

FIGURE 12–10. Drawing of a mobility cart that a child with OI can propel using the upper extremities.

School Age and Adolescence

Typical disabilities seen at this stage include inability to keep up with peers as a result of reduced mobility and limited independence in ADL. Social skill development may also be hampered if the school-aged child has been overprotected because of overwhelming fear and anxiety by caregivers regarding fracturing. This may have an impact on the school-aged child's scholastic endeavors and future vocational achievements. Studies show that children with OI tend to be intelligent and cheerful (Rezte, 1972). Parents and educators need to encourage a positive attitude and excellence in school performance to prepare the child for a productive future.

At this age, the spine may show varying degrees of deformity. Usually there is scoliosis, kyphosis, or both, resulting from compression fractures of the vertebrae, osteoporosis, and ligamentous laxity. The child with moderate to severe OI shows marked bowing of the long bones from the multiple fractures and growth arrest at the epiphyseal plates. In the femur the neck-shaft angle is decreased with a coxa vara deformity and acetabular protrusion.

FIGURE 12–9. Child with OI with long-leg braces and rollator posture walker.

The tibia is anteriorly angulated, which in combination with the angulation of the femur results in an apparent knee flexion contracture. The patellofemoral joint frequently dislocates, predisposing the patient to falls and fractures. Pes valgus frequently occurs at the ankle. In the upper extremities, the humerus is angulated laterally or anterolaterally and the forearms are limited in rotation. The elbows often exhibit cubitus varus deformities, and elbow flexion contractures may be present.

Fractures tend to decrease markedly in frequency after puberty. Possible causes may be hormonal changes, increased awareness of how to prevent fractures, improvement in coordination, and increasing bone strength. Paradoxically, the adolescent who senses his or her increased stability and emerging independence may maximize involvement in activities, which increases the risk of more severe types of fractures. In an effort not to discourage these activities and independence, ongoing use of safe methods of mobility, caution, and responsible behavior should be stressed in patient instruction throughout childhood.

THERAPEUTIC INTERVENTION

Physical therapy management at this stage involves other team members, including professionals in orthopaedics, orthotics, occupational therapy, and rehabilitation engineering, to maximize the child's independence in ADL, mobility, endurance, problem solving, and adjustment to the school environment.

Children and adolescents should be encouraged to do their share of the chores at home within their functional capacity. This allows the child to feel valued and lessens sibling rivalry (Thompson, 1990).

In this period, physical therapy may be helpful in returning the child to premorbid mobility status after a series of immobilizations from prepubertal fractures. The child may also require changes in bracing to accommodate growth and body changes, such as increased or decreased mass. Lower extremity bracing continues to be of the lightweight plastic HKAFO or KAFO clamshell design, usually with joints.

Management of scoliosis and kyphosis is usually addressed by a spinal fusion, but the long-term results in maintaining alignment are questionable (Benson & Newman, 1981). Orthotic devices such as the Milwaukee brace and orthoplast jackets have been deemed ineffective in controlling scoliosis and kyphosis.

Along with occupational therapy, physical therapy can help to maximize the child's independence by identifying safe, energy-efficient positions in which the child can work. Adaptive equipment is imperative for those with severe involvement. Occupational therapists, physical therapists, and rehabilitation engineers work together to adapt wheelchairs and seating and mobility devices to accommodate skeletal deformity, scoliosis, and kyphosis. A variety of lightweight and easily maneuverable manual wheelchairs can be adapted with seating inserts for trunk control and proper positioning. Plastic upholstery is usually unsatisfactory for the child with OI because of the propensity for excessive perspiration. Proper wheelchair positioning is critical for prevention of further disabling deformities and for protection of the exposed extremities from trauma.

Physical therapy continues throughout this stage to work on ambulation, endurance, and strength. Household ambulation is usually achieved with assistive devices if adequate upper extremity strength is present. Walkers with progression to canes or crutches are used. Toward adolescence, ambulation without braces is more conceivable than before because the fracture rate decreases. Many children with OI who have primarily used the wheelchair for mobility are now able to ambulate about the house without any special change in their program. It is important to emphasize the maintenance of adequate skeletal alignment and maximal muscular strength throughout childhood to prepare for this improved function as an adolescent and adult. Community ambulation without braces, however, is not practical, given the patient's short stature, the energy expenditure required, and the reduced muscle power. Most school-aged and older children with OI use wheelchairs for community ambulation (Bleck, 1981). Independence in mobility is paramount because it has been shown to correlate with the degree of adaptation to the community environment. In Bachman's study (1972) of the variables in children with disabilities that affected adaptation outside the school environment, it was reported that independence in travel away from home was the most significant factor.

Strengthening and endurance programs can be most successful when the child participates in developing a program that suits his or her interests and schedule. Programs can consist of progressive resistive exercises using incremental weights or adaptive sport activities. Enjoyable avocational activities that incorporate functional strengthening and mobility also need to be stressed at this age. Although contact sports such as football, soccer, and baseball must be avoided, customized athletic and fitness programs are vital for youngsters with OI. These adaptive physical education activities can assist in improving physical health, finding a competitive outlet, helping to discover one's potential, and providing an opportunity to make friends (Patti, 1990). Activities may include swim team competition and wheelchair court sports such as tennis, badminton, and ping pong. The physical therapist's role is to set appropriate parameters for participation, to provide precautions, and to upgrade the level of activity progressively. Volunteer jobs and social opportunities, such as the Boy and Girl Scouts, encourage emotional growth and develop leadership skills. Volunteer jobs for the adolescent can be helpful when applying for future employment (Fehribach, 1990).

In an 8-year cumulative management program, Gerber and colleagues (1990) found that a comprehensive rehabilitation program, long-leg bracing, and surgical procedures on the femur resulted in a high level of functional activity for children with OI along with an acceptable level of risk for fractures. The three-part program consisted of early intervention emphasizing positioning and handling, muscle strengthening and aerobic conditioning, and protected ambulation. Included in the program were strengthening exercises for the pelvic girdle and lower extremity musculature, pool exercises, molded seating, long-leg bracing, and gait training. Of the 12 children studied, 10 became functional ambulators, whereas 2 were household ambulators. Five children walked or took steps without braces, and 6 ambulated without gait aids. No child primarily used a wheelchair. All children of school age were enrolled in regular neighborhood schools. The physical activity of these children was high in that they participated in peer activities and some sports. Fractures were not eliminated through bracing, but the fracture rate was deemed acceptable.

Transition to Adulthood

In the transition to adulthood, patients with OI are dealing with the secondary effects of disease because the fracture rate has declined or ceased by the late teen years. The onset of deafness in some children with OI will occur in adult life. Scoliotic curves are usually severe and continue to progress. The incidence of scoliosis approaches 80 to 90% in teenagers and adults (Albright, 1981). Patients with OI are especially susceptible to postmenopausal osteoporosis or the osteoporosis of immobilization (Sillence, 1981). No scientific data have been published on long-term sequelae for adults with OI. Adults with OI do, however, report problems with arthritic changes and back pain.

Emphasis of intervention during the transition to adulthood is on appropriate career placement, given the patient's intellectual capacity and consideration of the physical constraints. Because most patients with OI become productive members of society, optimal academic, social, and physical development will facilitate their opportunities to succeed in a competitive job market (Bleck, 1981). It is difficult to compete for jobs with physically healthy persons when life is complicated by repeated fractures, hospitalizations, and absences from work or school. Despite these problems, adults with OI tend to be ambitious and have low hostility levels. Half of adults with OI choose to marry and have children (Kiley et al., 1976). In a 1981 study by Bleck, 10 of 12 patients with OIC who had undergone early weight-bearing, orthotic, and mobility management programs attended regular educational facilities. Twelve patients with OIT who were managed by this program all attained complete independence in ADL, mobility, and ambulation (Bleck, 1981).

By the time these children reach adulthood, most use either manual or power wheelchairs for community mobility. Ambulation consists of household walking with an assistive device. Many of the children who previously relied on wheelchairs for household ambulation no longer needed them because they improved in functional mobility as adults.

CASE HISTORY: RACHEL

Rachel is a 13-year-old girl with the diagnosis of osteogenesis imperfecta tarda I. She was born after a 38-week gestation with apparently normal fetal movements, and no abnormalities were perceived at birth. By the end of her second year, the diagnosis of OI was made based on clinical and radiographic findings. Before this her parents were questioned to rule out child abuse. Rachel's mother reports feeling high anxiety over the inherent accusations and her helplessness in explaining the fractures. Once the diagnosis was made, her anxiety was reduced so that education and training could be more effective.

Pathophysiologically, Rachel demonstrated general osteopenia and severe demineralization of the bilateral lower extremities with evidence of prior fractures of the shafts of long bones. This underlying pathophysiologic condition set the stage for her primary impairments — reduced mobility and strength as a result of the series of fractures.

Her early fractures, involving the clavicle and scapula, resulted from a fall she sustained at 18 months. At age 4, she fractured her right ulna, radius, and left tibia and fibula when she fell approximately 1½ feet. At age 8, she sustained a fracture of the left tibia and growth plate. At age 9, she fractured her right tibia. Her fractures at age 10 involved the left distal femur and right distal tibia, both sustained while transferring from her wheelchair to a toilet. The patient again sustained a hairline fracture of her right distal tibia when her foot caught in a towel while showering.

The combination of these impairments, resulting in the cycle of immobilization and further disuse, rendered her condition disabling. Rachel was referred to our facility at age 10.

Femur fractures sustained at age 10 were managed with hip spica casts to allow continued weight bearing while the fractures were healing. Nevertheless, this series of fractures left Rachel virtually nonambulatory and with decreased ADL skills. In addition, she was afraid of attempting to walk again. At this point, Rachel's initial impairments had resulted in functional loss.

Rachel's disabilities included nonambulatory status, reduced endurance for community mobility using a wheelchair, and reduced independence at home in all of her self-care needs, such as toileting and bathing.

Specific impairments, functional limitations, and disabilities that physical therapy was intended to change included reduced ambulatory ability, reduced endurance and skill in wheelchair mobility, reduced strength in both the lower and upper extremities, and reduced ADL skills, particularly toileting and bathing. It was deemed necessary to provide Rachel with intensive rehabilitation with the goals of regaining lost ambulatory ability and functional ADL skills. In addition, weight management became a goal because she had gained weight secondary to her decreased activity level. Another complication to address was that of low back pain.

Physical therapy was used to prevent further secondary impairment with the goal of preserving and regaining as much function as possible. Specifically, for Rachel this was intended to retard the impairment and loss of function that had ensued from immobilization following the fractures.

The physical therapy program initially consisted of preambulation weight bearing and exercises (active, active-assisted, and active-resistive when possible). This was initiated in the pool, where protected weight bearing and graded resistive exercise could safely be monitored. Through the aquatics program, general conditioning, strengthening, and endurance could also be enhanced, thus addressing the weight and back pain concerns.

In conjunction with the aquatic program, Rachel gradually progressed to standing with a left HKAFO with drop-lock hinge for protected weight bearing and

musculature support. During this time, graded manual and skateboard exercises (done in an antigravity horizontal plane) were accomplished primarily for lower extremity musculature strengthening and flexibility. Independence in a strengthening and flexibility (other than passive ROM) program was emphasized. Upper extremity exercises and activities were emphasized as well to improve strength needed for use in ambulation training with crutches and for wheelchair propulsion and transfer skills.

Ambulation training progressed from use of maximal support in which the HKAFO was locked at the knee and a walker was used as the assistive device with contact guard. The goal was to progressively reduce the support of assistive devices and wean Rachel from use of the brace while she progressed in ambulatory endurance. During her 4-week admission, Rachel achieved household ambulation with the HKAFO on the left leg (knee unlocked) using Lofstrand crutches. She continued to use her wheelchair, which was once her major mode of mobility but was now primarily for community mobility. Wheelchair adjustments were addressed, such as installing proper footrests to prevent a hyperextension injury, to prevent possible fracture to the ankles from otherwise dangling extremities, and to accommodate a leg-length discrepancy. ADL were addressed in collaboration with the occupational therapist, and improvements were made in safer but independent transfer ability to the tub and toilet. An elevated toilet seat and nighttime commode helped to achieve independence in toileting.

Also investigated was the use of hormonal therapy to either stimulate or arrest linear growth. A pediatric endocrinologist was consulted to consider the use of estrogen therapy to enhance her pubertal process and therefore reduce the likelihood of fractures. The conclusion from the endocrinologist was that he did not recommend use of estrogen therapy for Rachel because she had not yet completed 90% of her linear growth and estrogen therapy may decrease ultimate adult height.

In conclusion, Rachel benefited from the intensive and structured rehabilitation program in which she was an active participant both in the setting of her goals and in carrying them out now and in the future. Ultimately, she attained household ambulation status with braces and crutches, improved wheelchair propulsion skill and endurance for community mobility, and independence in ADL with the use of selected adaptive devices.

Although Rachel has endured setbacks, she has achieved greater independence in function and participated in community-based activities culminating in receipt of outstanding recognition and a medal in the state's annual wheelchair games. Academically and socially, Rachel interacts well with her peers and is attaining educational goals that will allow her to progress vocationally.

References

Albright, JA. Management overview of osteogenesis imperfecta. Clinical Orthopedics, *159*:80–87, 1981.

Albright, JP, Albright, JA, & Crelin, ES. Osteogenesis imperfecta tarda: The morphology of rib biopsies. Clinical Orthopedics, *108*:204–213, 1975.

Bachman, WH. Variables affecting post school economic adaptation of orthopedically handicapped and other health-impaired students. Rehabilitation Literature, *3*:98, 1972.

Bailey, RW, & Dubow, HI. Experimental and clinical studies of longitudinal bone growth utilizing a new method of internal fixation crossing the epiphyseal plate. Journal of Bone and Joint Surgery (American), *47*:1669, 1965.

Bayley, N. Bayley Scales of Infant Development (2nd ed.). San Antonio: Psychological Corporation, 1993.

Benson, DR, & Newman, DC. The spine and surgical treatment in osteogenesis imperfecta. Clinical Orthopedics, *159*:147–153, 1981.

Binder, H, Hawkes, L, Graybill, G, Gerber, NL, & Weintrob, JC. Osteogenesis imperfecta: Rehabilitation approach with infants and young children. Archives of Physical Medicine and Rehabilitation, *65*(9):537–541, 1984.

Bleck, EE. Nonoperative treatment of osteogenesis imperfecta: Orthotic and mobility management. Clinical Orthopedics, *159*:111–122, 1981.

Bluemcke, S, Niedorf, HR, Thiel, HJ, & Langness, U. Histochemical and fine structural studies on the cornea in osteogenesis imperfecta. Virchows Archiv. B. Cell Pathology, *11*:124–132, 1972.

Bullough, PG, Davidson, DD, & Lorenzo, JC. The morbid anatomy of the skeleton in osteogenesis imperfecta. Clinical Orthopedics, *159*:42–57, 1981.

Byers, PH. Osteogenesis Imperfecta: An Update: Growth, Genetics and Hormones, Vol. 4, Part 2. New York: McGraw-Hill, 1988.

Doty, SB, & Matthews, RS. Electronmicroscopic and histochemical investigation of osteogenesis imperfecta tarda. Clinical Orthopedics, *80*:191–201, 1971.

Duffield, MH. Physiological and therapeutic effects of exercise in warm water. In Skinner, AT, & Thomson, AM (Eds.), Duffield's Exercise in Water. (3rd ed.). London: Baillière Tindall, 1983.

Falvo, KA, & Bullough, PG. Osteogenesis imperfecta: A histometric analysis. Journal of Bone and Joint Surgery (American), *55*:275–286, 1973.

Falvo, KA, Root, L, & Bullough, PG. Osteogenesis imperfecta: A clinical evaluation and management. Journal of Bone and Joint Surgery (American), *56*:783–793, 1974.

Fehribach, G. Independent living. Presented before the Osteogenesis Imperfecta Foundation National Convention, Pittsburgh, 1990.

Folio, M, & Fewell, R. Peabody Developmental Motor Scales and Activity Cards. Allen, TX: DLM Teaching Resources, 1983.

Follis, RH, Jr. Osteogenesis imperfecta congenita: A connective tissue diathesis. Journal of Pediatrics, *41*:713–721, 1952.

Gerber, LH, Binder, H, Weintrob, J, Grenge, DK, Shapiro, J, Fromherz, W, Berry, R, Conway, A, Nason, S, & Marini, J. Rehabilitation of children and infants with osteogenesis imperfecta: A program for ambulation. Clinical Orthopaedics and Related Research, *251*:254–262, 1990.

Goldman, AB, Davidson, D, Pavlov, H, & Bullough, PG. "Popcorn" calcifications: A prognostic sign in osteogenesis imperfecta. Radiology, *136*:351–358, 1980.

Haley, SM, Faas, RM, Coster, WJ, Webster, H, & Gans, BM. Pediatric Evaluation of Disability Inventory. Boston: New England Medical Center, 1989.

Hanscom, DA, Winter, RB, Lutter, L, Lonstein, JE, Bloom, B, & Bradford, DS. Osteogenesis imperfecta. Journal of Bone and Joint Surgery (American), *74*:598–616, 1992.

Kiley, L, Sterne, R, & Witkop, CJ. Psychosocial factors in low-incidence genetic disease: The case of osteogenesis imperfecta. Social Work in Health Care, *1*:409–420, 1976.

King, JD, & Bobechko, WP. Osteogenesis imperfecta: An orthopedic description and surgical review. Journal of Bone and Joint Surgery (British), *53*:72–86, 1971.

Letts, M, Monson, R, & Weber, K. The prevention of recurrent fractures of the lower extremities in severe osteogenesis imperfecta using vacuum pants: A preliminary report in four patients. Journal of Pediatric Orthopedics, *8*(4):454–457, 1988.

Looser, E. Zur Kenntnis der Osteogenesis imperfecta congenita und tarda (sogenannte idiopathische Osteopsathyrosis). Mitteilungen Grenzgebieten Medizin und Chirurgie, *15*:161, 1906.

Morel, G, & Houghton, GR. Pneumatic trouser splints in the treatment of severe osteogenesis imperfecta. Acta Orthopaedica Scandinavica, *53*:547–552, 1982.

Patti, G. Sports and OI. Presented before the Osteogenesis Imperfecta Foundation National Conference, Pittsburgh, 1990.

Perrin, EC, & Gerrity, PS. Development of children with a chronic illness. Pediatric Clinics of North America, *31*:19–31, 1984.

Ramser, JR, & Frost, HM. The study of a rib biopsy from a patient with osteogenesis imperfecta: A method using in vivo tetracycline labeling. Acta Orthopaedica Scandinavica, *37*:229–240, 1966.

Rezte, L. Osteogenesis imperfecta: Psychological function. American Journal of Psychiatry, *128*(12):1446–1540, 1972.

Scott, EF. The use of air splints for mobility training in osteogenesis imperfecta. Clinical Suggestions, *2*(1):52–53, 1990.

Seedorf, KS. Osteogenesis imperfecta: A study of clinical features and heredity based on 55 Danish families comprising 180 affected members. Opera ex Domo Biologiae Hereditariae Humanae Universitatis Hafniensis, Arhus: Universitetsforlaget, *20*:1–229, 1949.

Sillence, DO. Osteogenesis imperfecta: Expanding panorama of variants. Clinical Orthopaedics and Related Research, *159*:11–25, 1981.

Sillence, DO, & Danks, DM. The differentiation of genetically distinct varieties of osteogenesis imperfecta in the newborn period. Clinical Research, *26*:178A, 1978.

Sillence, DO, Senn, A, & Danks, DM. Genetic heterogeneity in osteogenesis imperfecta. Journal of Medical Genetics, *16*:101–116, 1979.

Solomons, CC, & Millar, EA. Osteogenesis imperfecta: New perspectives. Clinical Orthopaedics and Related Research, *96*:299–303, 1973.

Spranger, J, Cremin, B, & Beighton, P. Osteogenesis imperfecta congenita. Pediatric Radiology, *12*:21–27, 1982.

Tachdjian, MO (Ed.). Pediatric Orthopedics (2nd ed.), Vol. 2. Philadelphia: WB Saunders, 1990.

Thompson, CE. Raising a handicapped child. Presented before the Osteogenesis Imperfecta Foundation National Conference, Pittsburgh, 1990.

Wynne-Davies, R, & Gormley, J. Clinical and genetic patterns in osteogenesis imperfecta. Clinical Orthopaedics and Related Research, *159*:26–35, 1981.

Chapter 13

Muscular Dystrophy and Spinal Muscular Atrophy

WAYNE A. STUBERG, PT, PCS, PhD

Neuromuscular diseases include disorders of the motor neuron (anterior horn cells and peripheral nerve), neuromuscular junction, and muscle. Muscular dystrophy (MD) and spinal muscular atrophy (SMA) are two prevalent, progressive neuromuscular diseases that require physical therapy. Both diseases are characterized by progressive weakness, atrophy, contracture, deformity, and progressive disability. No cure is available for either disease. "Incurable," however, is not synonymous with "untreatable," and the physical therapist can be influential in prevention of complications, preservation of function, and issues concerning quality of life.

ROLE OF THE PHYSICAL THERAPIST

As a member of the management team in either the educational or medical setting, the physical therapist assists in the identification and amelioration of impairments, functional limitations, disabilities or handicaps for persons with MD or SMA. The team often includes a physician (neurologist, orthopaedist, or physiatrist), physical therapist, oc-cupational therapist, speech therapist, educator, social worker, genetic counselor, psychologist, and orthotist. Because therapists typically maintain a higher frequency of contact with families, referral to and ongoing communication with other team members becomes an important issue in maintaining continuity of care.

The team approach should be family-centered with a focus on collaborative goal setting among individuals with the disorder, family members, and professionals to ensure optimal care. By providing care using a family-centered philosophy, the pivotal role of the family is recognized and respected in the lives of persons with special health care needs (Brewer et al., 1989; Kolobe, 1992).

In addition to providing ongoing input on physical management, the role of the physical therapist becomes particularly important at times of increased stress on the family caused by progression of the disease and resultant increased disability. For example, increased input is needed before the loss of major functional skills such as walking, before the need for architectural modifications to accommodate adaptive equipment for mobility, during transition from the educational environment, or during the terminal stages of the disease.

Providing information to family members, persons with MD or SMA, and other members of the team regarding physical limitations and expected disabilities is also an important role for the physical therapist. Resource materials for families (Ringel, 1987), teachers (Bleck & Nagel, 1982), or other members of the team can often eliminate misconceptions or false expectations. Many resource materials are available through the National Muscular Dystrophy Association (MDA) office (3300 East Sunrise Drive, Tucson, AZ 85718) or through state chapter MDA offices.

PHYSICAL THERAPY ASSESSMENT AND EVALUATION

Physical therapy assessment and evaluation for MD and SMA should be systematic and objective. Although the progression of MD and SMA is relatively well known, the clinician needs to be careful in observing for changes that require interventional modifications. As stated by Thomas McCrae (1870–1935), "More is missed by not looking than by not knowing" (Siegel, 1986). Ongoing dialogue with families is invaluable in identifying family-centered goals and the need for program modification.

The physical therapy assessment should include the following major areas:

1. Background information with identification of the individual's or families' major concerns
2. Developmental level in the infant or young child
3. Mobility, including ambulation and transfers in the older child
4. Muscle strength
5. Range of motion (ROM) and postural alignment
6. Respiratory function
7. Equipment, if used
8. Independence in activities of daily living (ADL), such as grooming, dressing, feeding, and hygiene.

Systematic documentation of disease progression is essential in timing of interventions during transitions from one functional status to another or during times of increased family need. An example of a transition period in MD would include the termination of independent walking.

The objective of this chapter is to present an overview of the childhood forms of MD and SMA and the role of the physical therapist as a member of the management team. The clinical presentation of the diseases is reviewed and assessment procedures are presented to assist the clinician in identifying impairments, functional limitations, and disabilities associated with MD and SMA. Guidelines for physical therapy management are also outlined based on my clinical experience and review of related literature.

MUSCULAR DYSTROPHY

The cause of all forms of MD that have been classified to date is genetic inheritance. The pathophysiology underlying the disease is progressive loss of muscle contractility due to the destruction of myofibrils. The specific cellular mechanism behind the destruction in Duchenne's muscular dystrophy (DMD) and Becker's MD has been partially identified and is discussed later in the chapter. The rate of progression of myofibril destruction is variable among the various forms of MD, giving evidence for the possibility of more than one cellular mechanism in the destructive process.

The diagnosis of MD is confirmed by clinical examination and laboratory procedures, including electromyography, muscle biopsy, DNA analysis, and selected enzyme levels assayed from blood samples (Siegel, 1986). The criteria for classification of the various forms of MD include the mode of inheritance, age at onset, rate of progression, localization of involvement, muscle morphologic changes, and associated involvement of other organ systems. The MDA recognizes nine primary classifications of MD (MDA, 1991). Table 13–1 lists the six types that exhibit initial clinical signs in infancy, childhood, or adolescence. Emery-Dreifus MD (humeroperoneal) is very rare and is only discussed briefly. Limb-girdle MD may exhibit signs in the teenage years but more typically in early adulthood, and, therefore, along with the adult-onset forms of MD, is not discussed. The reader should refer to texts on neuromuscular diseases by Brooke (1986), Siegel (1986), and Harper (1989) for further information on clinical presentation and general management of MD.

The primary impairment in MD is insidious weakness secondary to progressive loss of myofibrils. In the case of the congenital forms of MD the weakness is pronounced at birth and easily recognizable. In DMD, the weakness becomes evident by the age of 3 to 5 years. In congenital and congenital myotonic MD, contractures present at birth also cause primary impairment. The incidence of mental retardation is highest in congenital myotonic MD but is less frequently reported in DMD or the other childhood forms.

Secondary impairments in all forms of MD in-

TABLE 13–1. **CLASSIFICATION OF MUSCULAR DYSTROPHY**

Type	Onset	Inheritance	Course
Duchenne's	1-4 years	X-linked	Rapidly progressive; loss of walking by 9 to 10 years; death in late teens
Becker's	5-10 years	X-linked	Slowly progressive; maintain walking past early teens; life span into third decade
Congenital	Birth	Recessive	Typically slow but variable; shortened life span
Congenital myotonic	Birth	Dominant	Typically slow with significant intellectual impairment
Childhood-onset facioscapulohumeral	First decade	Dominant/recessive	Slowly progressive loss of walking in later life; variable life expectancy
Emery-Dreifus	Childhood to early teens	X-linked	Slowly progressive with cardiac abnormality and normal life span

clude the development of contractures and postural malalignment. Postural malalignment is seen in antigravity positions of sitting and standing and often includes development of scoliosis. Other secondary impairments include decreased respiratory capacity, easy fatigability, and, occasionally, obesity. Although significant intellectual impairment is not usual, IQ is commonly below average and reported in the range of 70 to 80 in DMD (Cohen, et al., 1968; Leibowitz & Dubowitz, 1981; Prosser et al., 1969).

With the progression of muscle weakness, increasing caregiver assistance is required for persons with MD to carry out ADL. Progressive disability is a hallmark of MD and requires multidisciplinary team management to minimize handicaps through the use of adaptive equipment and environmental adaptations.

Physical management in the treatment of MD is a key intervention since no drug has been found to be curative (Brooke, 1986; DeSilva et al., 1987). Physical therapy has been used to prolong the child's independence, slow the progression of complications, and improve the quality of life.

Duchenne's Muscular Dystrophy

Duchenne's muscular dystrophy is the most common X-linked disorder known, with an incidence of about 1 in 3500 live male births. The prevalence of DMD in the general population is generally reported at about three cases per 100,000 (Moser 1984; Mostacciuolo et al., 1987). Longevity is variable from the late teens to early 20s up to the third decade, dependent on the rate of disease pro-

gression, presence of complications, and aggressiveness of respiratory care, including the use of assisted ventilation (Curran & Colbert, 1989; Inkley et al., 1974; Vignos et al., 1963; Ziter & Allsop, 1976).

In 1985, Kunkel and associates identified the gene on the X chromosome that, when defective, causes DMD and Becker's MD. Hoffman and associates (1987a) then reported the identification of the missing protein of the locus for human DMD and Becker's MD. The protein was named dystrophin. This finding was followed within a short period of time by the cloning of the complete gene that produces dystrophin to be used in either prenatal or postnatal diagnosis (Koenig et al., 1987). However, the amount of dystrophin in an individual's muscle assay has not been found to directly correlate with the severity of DMD or Becker's MD. Therefore, a biochemical test to predict the rate of progression is not available, and careful clinical examination with objective documentation continues to be the "best practice" in program planning and prediction of evolving disability.

Further work on the cause of muscle cell destruction in DMD and Becker's MD has demonstrated that the lack of dystrophin exhibits its primary effect at the surface membrane of the skeletal muscle cell (Arahata et al., 1988; Bonilla et al., 1988; Hoffman et al., 1988). Research has demonstrated that dystrophin is localized to the sarcolemmal membrane of the muscle cell and that its absence allows increased permeability of the cell (Arahata et al., 1988). Because several lytic enzymes within the muscle cell are activated by calcium, it is now hypothesized that necrosis may be due to an uncontrolled rise of calcium concentration in the cell, thereby activating proteolytic enzymes leading to cell destruction (Cullen & Fulthorpe, 1975; Mokri & Engel, 1975).

The focus of research in the treatment of DMD involves gene replacement therapy and myoblast transfer therapy. Both therapies are in the experimental stage, with only myoblast transfer currently being evaluated in humans.

Gene therapy involves the introduction of the dystrophin gene to a recipient with MD. Lee and colleagues (1991) have produced an entire dystrophin gene and have shown that the gene was taken up by the muscle cell membrane in an animal model. No studies on humans have been published.

In myoblast transfer therapy the embryologic precursor cells of skeletal muscle (i.e., myoblasts) are obtained from a histocompatible donor. The cells are then injected into the muscle of the individual with DMD with the hope that the normal myoblasts will grow, mutate with the surrounding cells that are lacking dystrophin, and result in development of dystrophin. The results of the research in animals have shown that donor myoblast cells fuse with the dystrophic cells to form a hybrid multinucleated cell that produces dystrophin (Partridge et al., 1978). Clinical experiments using myoblast therapy are underway in the United States and Canada under the funding of the MDA.

Medical management of DMD has also included clinical trials of prednisone therapy; the drug is being evaluated with double-blind studies sponsored by the MDA. DeSilva and colleagues (1987) have demonstrated initial evidence of significantly prolonged survival (up to 2 years) in a prednisone-treated versus control group study.

Although it is commonly agreed that the prevention of contractures and deformity and the preservation of independent mobility are primary goals of a physical management program (Gucker, 1964; Vignos, 1983), the prolongation of ambulation through surgery or orthotics has been controversial

in DMD (Gardner-Medwin, 1977; Gardner-Medwin, 1980a). Some authors promote the use of surgery and lightweight bracing (Bach & McKeon, 1991; Heckmatt et al., 1985; Miller & Dunn, 1982; Siegel, 1975; Ziter & Allsop, 1979); others, however, express skepticism about prolonging the inevitable in a progressive disease when the financial and emotional costs to the family may be very high (Gardner-Medwin, 1979).

Surgical management has focused on the control of lower extremity contractures, use of orthoses in conjunction with surgery to prolong ambulation, and spinal stabilization for control of scoliosis. Achilles tendon lengthenings and fasciotomies of the tensor fascia lata and iliotibial bands are two procedures commonly reported to be used in conjunction with orthotics and physical therapy to prolong ambulation (Bach & McKeon, 1991). Posterior tibialis transfer into the third cuneiform to reverse equinovarus deformity has also been reported (Roy & Gibson, 1970). Surgical management of scoliosis typically includes the use of spinal instrumentation with Luque rods (Sussman, 1984).

IMPAIRMENTS

Examination of the 4- to 5-year-old child demonstrates the onset of classical clinical features of DMD and the primary impairment of muscle weakness. The posterior calf is usually enlarged as a result of fatty and connective tissue infiltration, which corresponds to the term *pseudohypertrophic* MD that is used for the eponym DMD. The pseudohypertrophy can occasionally be seen to affect the deltoid, quadriceps, or forearm extensor muscle groups. Initial weakness of the neck flexor, abdominal, interscapular, and hip extensor musculature can be noted with a more generalized distribution with progression of the disease. Figure 13–1 demonstrates the trends of muscle strength decline up to age 16 years from a study by Brooke (1986). The

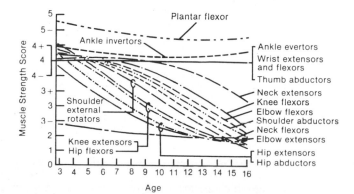

FIGURE 13–1. Muscle strength 50th percentile lines plotted against age of 150 children with DMD. (Redrawn from Brooke, MH. A Clinician's View of Neuromuscular Diseases [2nd ed.]. Baltimore: Williams & Wilkins, 1986.)

data were obtained in a multiclinic study of 150 children with DMD over a follow-up period of 3 to 4 years. The data represent approximately 15 data points per boy as recorded during follow-up visits.

Muscle strength can be documented using manual muscle testing in the young child since use of specialized devices is difficult (Kendall & McCreary, 1983; Medical Research Council, 1976; Ziter et al., 1977). Use of instruments such as a hand-held dynamometer can be used to obtain objective strength recordings in the older child to assist in prediction of disability, such as the loss of independent ambulation (Stuberg & Metcalf, 1988).

No limitations in ROM are noted typically before 5 years of age in DMD. Mild tightness of the gastrocsoleus and tensor fascia lata muscles usually presents first. The normal lordotic standing posture is increased, and mild winging of the scapulae is then seen as a compensation to keep the center of mass behind the hip joint to promote standing stability (Fig. 13–2). Scoliosis typically develops just before or during adolescence.

Infancy to Preschool-Aged Period

No significant disability is typically seen in the infant or toddler with DMD. Gardner-Medwin (1980b) reported that half of the children fail to walk until 18 months of age. Delay in walking, however, rarely leads to the diagnosis of DMD. Symptoms are seldom noted before the age of 3 to 5

years, unless there is a positive family history and caregivers are looking for early signs. The mean age at diagnosis is usually reported to be around age 5 years (Miller & Dunn, 1982).

Early School-Aged Period

The initial disability in DMD typically occurs by the age of 5 years and includes clumsiness, falling, and inability to keep up with peers while playing. The young child's gait pattern is only slightly atypical, with an increased lateral trunk sway (waddling). Attempts at running, however, accentuate the waddling progression, and neither running nor jumping is attained. The Gower sign (using the arms to push on the thighs to attain standing) is usually present after one or repeated trials of assuming standing from sitting on the floor.

Stair climbing and arising to standing from the floor become progressively more difficult and signal the first significant functional limitation by the age of 6 to 8 years. Progressive changes in the gait pattern include the deviations of an increased base of support, pronounced lateral trunk sway (compensated Trendelenburg), toe-walking, and retraction of the shoulders with lack of reciprocal arm swing. Toe-walking initially may be a compensation for weakness of the abdominal and hip extensor muscles, resulting in lordosis and forward shift of the body's center of mass with later evidence of contracture of the posterior calf musculature.

Toe-walking caused by contracture of the poste-

FIGURE 13–2. Typical standing posture of a 7-year-old boy with DMD.

rior calf musculature, in-toeing with substitution of the tensor fascia lata to compensate for weakness of the iliopsoas muscles, falls resulting from progressive weakness, and complaints of fatigue while walking become increasingly frequent from age 8 to 10 years. A restrictive pattern of pulmonary impairment and progressive decline in maximal vital capacity also becomes increasingly evident (Gardner-Medwin, 1980b; Haas & Pineda, 1979).

A functional evaluation to document disability progression is essential. Various formats have been reported (Brooke, 1986; Vignos et al., 1963) that are variations of the guidelines initially published by Swinyard and associates (1957). A simple functional classification published by Vignos and colleagues (1963) is outlined in Table 13–2. A more detailed functional testing format for DMD has been published by Brooke and associates (1981), which includes pulmonary function and timed performance of activities (see Appendix I). A functional assessment tool, such as the Pediatric Evaluation of Disability Inventory (PEDI), can also be included to give more specific information on the child's performance of ADL (Haley et al., 1992). Either the PEDI or the Brooke functional testing format can also be used for diagnoses of other types of MD or of SMA.

Muscle weakness is apparent in the school-aged child by the age of 6 to 8 years and should be objectively documented using a hand-held dynamometer (Stuberg & Metcalf, 1988), electrodynamometer (Saranti et al., 1980), isokinetic dynamometer (Molnar & Alexander, 1973; Scott et al., 1982), or other device. Use of a dynamometer in conjunction with manual muscle testing has been shown to provide reliable information on the progression of weakness in key muscle groups (Fowler & Gardner, 1967; Stuberg & Metcalf, 1988). Specific guidelines on dynamometer use should be followed to ensure reliability and validity of data (Smidt, 1984).

Contracture development should be documented

using goniometry and a standardized protocol. Numerous texts are available documenting the techniques for measuring ROM (American Academy of Orthopaedic Surgeons, 1965; Clarkson & Gilwich, 1989). Intrarater reliability of the measurements has been shown to be acceptable to provide objective information for program planning when a standardized measurement protocol is used (Pandya et al., 1985).

A clinical estimate of respiratory function can be obtained through measurement of respiratory rate and chest wall excursion (using a tape measure) and by noting the child's ability to cough and clear secretions. A portable spirometer is recommended to obtain a more direct and objective reading of expiratory capacity before the need for formal pulmonary function testing.

Physical therapy management typically begins when the child is initially diagnosed at age 3 to 5 years. Goals of the program are to provide family support and education, obtain baseline data on muscle strength and ROM, and monitor for the progression of muscle weakness that will lead to disability. Initial therapeutic input should not be burdensome to the child or family because the child is usually independent in all ADL before the age of 5 years. Information should be provided to the family pertaining to the therapist's role as a member of the management team. An appropriate activity level to avoid fatigue should be discussed with the family and school staff. Information on services through the local MDA office should be provided, including identification of support groups or contact families.

The role of exercise in the management of MD is controversial (Brooke, 1986; Fowler, 1982; Vignos, 1983). It is widely accepted that both overexertion (Bennett & Knowlton, 1958; Johnson & Braddom, 1971; Vignos et al., 1963) and immobilization (Vignos et al., 1963) are detrimental. The use of graded resistive exercise has been reported to have a range of results from good (Abramson,

TABLE 13–2. **VIGNOS FUNCTIONAL RATING SCALE FOR DUCHENNE'S MUSCULAR DYSTROPHY**

1. Walks and climbs stairs without assistance
2. Walks and climbs stairs with aid of railing
3. Walks and climbs stairs slowly with aid of railing (over 25 seconds for eight standard steps)
4. Walks, but cannot climb stairs
5. Walks assisted, but cannot climb stairs or get out of chair
6. Walks only with assistance or with braces
7. In wheelchair: sits erect and can roll chair and perform bed and wheelchair ADL
8. In wheelchair: sits erect and is unable to perform bed and wheelchair ADL without assistance
9. In wheelchair: sits erect only with support and is able to do only minimal ADL
10. In bed: can do no ADL without assistance

Data from Vignos, PJ, Spencer, GE, & Archibald, KC. Management of progressive muscular dystrophy. Journal of the American Medical Association, *184*:103–112, 1963. Copyright © 1963, American Medical Association.

1952; Vignos & Watkins, 1966; Wratney, 1967) to limited (de Lateur & Giaconi, 1979) to adverse (Hoberman, 1955). Resistive exercise would theoretically be indicated with the disproportionate loss of type II (fast-twitch) muscle fibers in DMD (Edwards, 1980). However, the use of resistive exercise in the young school-aged child should not be universally prescribed. Prescribing a submaximal exercise program early has been shown to have beneficial effects, but it should be offered only to families who have a specific desire to include it in the child's program (Fowler, 1982). Consideration should be given to the fact that significant muscle weakness is not seen in the early stage of the disease and the use of an exercise program may be burdensome to the child and family.

If exercise is initiated early, the key muscle groups to be included are the abdominal, hip extensor and abductor, and knee extensor groups. Abdominal exercises should include trunk curls as opposed to sit-ups, which will primarily strengthen the hip flexors. Assistance may be required for neck flexor weakness, as the head typically cannot be flexed from a supine position. Cycling and swimming are excellent activities for overall conditioning and are often preferred over formal exercise programs (Gardner-Medwin, 1980b; Harris & Cherry, 1974; Vignos, 1983). Standing or walking for a minimum of 2 to 3 hours daily is highly recommended (Siegel, 1978; Ziter & Allsop, 1976).

Breathing exercises have been shown to slow the loss of vital capacity and forced expiratory flow rate (Houser & Johnson, 1971). Game activities such as inflating balloons or using blow-bottles to maintain pulmonary function can easily be included in a home program and will decrease the severity of symptoms during episodes of colds or other pulmonary infections.

The use of electrical stimulation in DMD has also been suggested as a means of slowing the progression of weakness and improving function. Scott and coworkers (1986) studied the effect of low-frequency electrical stimulation on the tibialis anterior muscle of 16 children with DMD. A 47% increase in maximum voluntary contraction was observed in younger children following a stimulation protocol used for 8 weeks, with little change noted in older children. The authors concluded that the results were encouraging and that further study on muscle groups used for functional activities is needed.

One of the primary considerations in the early management program of the young school-aged child is to retard the development of contractures. Contractures have not been shown to be preventable, but the progression can be slowed with posi-

tioning and an ROM program (Dubowitz & Heckmatt, 1980; Harris & Cherry, 1974; Scott et al., 1981; Ziter & Allsop, 1976).

The initial ROM program should include the gastrocsoleus and tensor fascia lata. Progressive contracture of the gastrocsoleus and tensor fascia lata corresponds to gait deviations of toe-walking and an increased base of support. Stretching for the gastrocsoleus can be done using a standing runner's stretch. The child stands at a supportive surface, places one leg back at a time with the knee straight, and leans forward. The position also assists with maintenance of hip flexor flexibility, however, specific stretching for the hip flexors should be included when any limitation is noted. Having the child lie supine with one thigh off the edge of a mat or bed and the other held to their chest (Thomas's test position) can be used to stretch the hip flexors initially. An alternative method is discussed later for use as progression of hip extensor weakness evolves. A standing stretch for the tensor is accomplished by having the child stand with one side toward the supportive surface with the feet away from the wall and with the knee kept straight while leaning sideways toward the supportive surface.

A home ROM program should be emphasized for the young child and the family instructed in the stretching exercises. There is a lack of agreement as to the frequency and duration of the stretching program. Suggested frequency of the program varies from once daily (Gardner-Medwin, 1980b; Miller & Dunn, 1982; Scott et al., 1981; Wratney, 1967) to twice daily (Vignos et al., 1963; Ziter & Allsop, 1976), and duration from one repetition (Wratney, 1967) up to ten (Vignos et al., 1963). Other authors have suggested a time frame of 10 (Ziter & Allsop, 1976) to 20 (Gardner-Medwin, 1980b) minutes to complete the stretching exercises. As a general recommendation, each movement should be repeated for 5 to 10 repetitions and with a 10-second hold in the stretched position. The stretch should be done slowly and should not be painful. Increased risk of injury with the loss of myofibrils and replacement by connective tissue is present because of decreased muscle elasticity, and caution in using excessive passive force is advised. Reassessment of the contracture progression should be used as the final guide to stretching frequency and duration.

The ROM program can often be supplemented as part of the physical education program at school. Special instruction should be provided to the physical education teacher to develop an adapted program, particularly if the teacher does not have an adapted physical education endorsement. General physical education activities will also require modification for the child's participation and should not be exhaustive. Physical fitness test activities such as pushups, situps, or timed running for long time periods should be modified or excluded to avoid fatigue or overwork weakness.

Night splints are helpful to slow the progression of ankle contractures. Scott and associates (1981) studied the efficacy of night splints and a home ROM program in a group of 59 boys diagnosed with DMD ranging in age from 4 to 12 years. The subjects were categorized into three groups based on compliance with splint wear and use of stretching. The group that followed through on the daily passive stretching program and use of the below-knee splints over the 2 years of the study demonstrated significantly less progression of the Achilles tendon contractures and less deterioration in functional skills, leading to a longer period of independent walking. Boys in the group that did not follow through on the stretching or splint program lost independent walking at a younger age.

The use of prone positioning at night to slow progression of the hip and knee flexion contractures may be possible if tolerated by the child. The recommendation to have the child sleep prone with the ankles off the edge of the bed has not been shown to effect the progression of the contractures but theoretically is sound.

Scoliosis is not common when the child is ambulatory, but the spine should be checked routinely (Wilkins & Gibson, 1976; Ziter & Allsop, 1976). Alignment of the spine should be closely monitored as weakness progresses to the stage of making walking difficult. Postural analysis using the forward bend test, which is also known as Adam's test, is recommended to monitor spinal alignment for scoliosis (Kisner & Colby, 1985). Presence of a rib hump with the forward bend test verifies a structural versus functional curve of the spine. Amendt and colleagues (1990) have demonstrated that a rib hump measuring at least 5° of inclination with a scoliometer is a reliable method and correlated to radiographic assessment. The study by Amendt and colleagues (1990) was, however, not inclusive of children with DMD but demonstrates an objective method of noninvasive screening for scoliosis. Orthopaedic referral is indicated if a rib hump is evidenced.

Falls and complaints of fatigue while walking become increasingly more frequent as the child reaches age 8 to 10 years. Guarding during stair climbing or during general walking should be considered to ensure safety as balance becomes tenuous. A manual wheelchair with appropriate fit and accessories will allow for limited mobility as walking becomes more difficult. As progression of weakness in the trunk and hip girdle begins to make walking difficult, a similar amount of weakness of the shoulder girdle musculature is also present, making propulsion of a manual wheelchair difficult except on level and smooth surfaces such as linoleum. A motorized scooter should be considered to provide the child with independence, provided that access is available in the home and school (Fig. 13–3).

Information should be made available to families concerning recreational activities provided through the local chapter of the MDA or other groups. Summer MDA camp is a wonderful experience for most children, and a support group is often developed for the child or family through participation in MDA or other group activities that provide not only physical but also emotional support.

Adolescent Period

Adolescence marks a time of significant disability progression as a result of the combined impact of muscle weakness and development of contractures. Walking is lost as a means of mobility, and increasing difficulty in general mobility with transfers is seen. Use of a manual wheelchair and/or powered mobility becomes necessary during adolescence. If powered mobility is used, then assistance with finances for purchase of equipment or home modifications for access are typically needed with coordination through a social worker or MDA patient services coordinator. Increasing difficulty with ADL, including dressing, transfers, bathing, grooming, and feeding, increases the involvement

FIGURE 13–3. Motorized three-wheeled scooter for independence in distance mobility as an adjunct to walking. (Ortho-Kinetics, Inc., Waukesha, WI.)

of the physical therapist and occupational therapist. Decisions regarding possible surgical intervention are also considered for the management of contractures or to prolong walking with the use of orthoses.

As muscle weakness becomes more pronounced in the trunk and hip musculature, and contractures of the hip flexors, tensor fascia lata, and gastrocsoleus progress, walking becomes increasingly difficult until cessation of independent walking occurs, usually by the age of 10 to 12 (Brooke, 1986; Johnson & Kennedy, 1971). If orthoses are used to maintain a standing or walking program, they should be initiated before the child reaches the stage of being nonambulatory.

Various methods to predict the termination of walking have been reported. The inability to rise from the floor or climb stairs and reports of frequent falls often signal the impending termination of independent walking. If muscle strength has been routinely recorded using a dynamometer or other instrument, Vignos and Archibald (1960) and Scott and associates (1982) have reported cessation of walking when muscle strength in the lower extremities has decreased by 50%. An alternative method as shown in Figure 13–4 has been suggested by Siegel (1977). The knee extension lag while sitting and the hip extension lag while prone are assessed to predict the cessation of independent walking. If the combined lag is greater than 90°, the

FIGURE 13–5. Prone stretching of the hip flexor, iliotibial band, and tensor fasciae lata. The hip is first positioned in abduction and then moved into maximal hip extension and then hip adduction. The knee can be extended to provide greater stretch for the iliotibial band and tensor.

termination of independent ambulation is within a few months. Ziter and Allsop (1976) have reported using the point when the child is no longer able to ambulate for more than 1 hour during the day or requires external support as a signal to initiate bracing.

Monitoring and management of contractures becomes a key element in maintaining walking when the older child spends more time in sitting. Because the hip extensor musculature is significantly weak in the early stage of the disease and weakness of the quadriceps muscles becomes pronounced by age 8 to 10 years, inability to maintain the center of gravity behind the hip joint or in front of the knee joint during stance will lead to loss of the ability to stand.

Manual stretching of the hip flexors, tensor fascia lata, and heel cords will be necessary as the older child will demonstrate difficulty in carrying out the exercises without assistance. Prone lying will help to retard the development of hip and knee flexor contractures, but stretching of the hip flexors and tensor using the method shown in Figure 13–5 is recommended. The leg is initially positioned in abduction, then brought into the maximum allowable hip extension followed by hip adduction. A hamstring stretch can also be included; however, a pattern of capsular tightness of the knee joint due to prolonged sitting is more common than excessive hamstring contracture because use of the Gower maneuver to assume standing maintains flexibility of the hamstrings during the period of independent ambulation. If a hamstring stretch is used, the leg should be slightly abducted to minimize the subluxing force placed across the hip joint that is present when the leg is in the sagittal plane during the maneuver.

FIGURE 13–4. Prognostic method used by Siegel to determine cessation of independent walking due to lack of antigravity hip and knee extensor torque. (Redrawn from Siegel, IM. Muscle and its Diseases. An Outline Primer of Basic Science and Clinical Method. Chicago: Year Book Medical Publisher, 1986.)

The use of orthoses for a standing program or continuation of supported walking is not appropriate for all individuals, and input in decision-making from the family and adolescent is essential. Opponents of braced walking point out that it is not functional nor practical since the child will eventually use a wheelchair (Gardner-Medwin, 1977). Because surgery is often required in addition to bracing for prolonged ambulation, both the parents and adolescent must agree in the management decision.

Prognostic factors for success that should be considered in making the decision to use orthoses include the residual muscle strength (approximately 50%) (Vignos, 1983); absence of severe contractures (Roy et al., 1970; Spencer & Vignos, 1962); timely application of the braces (Bach & McKeon, 1991; Spencer & Vignos, 1962); residual walking ability (Archibald & Vignos, 1959); and motivation of the child and family (Bowker & Halpin, 1978). The degree of mental retardation, if present, and obesity should also be considered. The timely use of orthoses has been shown to prolong walking (Bach & McKeon, 1991; Bowker & Halpin, 1978; Heckmatt et al., 1985; Johnson & Kennedy, 1971; Vignos & Archibald, 1960) and to increase the child's longevity (Bach & McKeon, 1991; Miller & Dunn, 1982; Vignos et al., 1963). Orthoses provide support for weak leg musculature, retard contracture formation, and provide joint stability and functional assistance for walking.

Bach and McKeon (1991) reported a significant reduction in the number of falls, maintenance of walking, and ability to use normal footwear with orthopaedic surgery and a comprehensive rehabilitation program including surgery and braced walking. A cohort of 13 boys were studied with a mean age at surgical intervention of 8.8 years (SD = 1.1 year). The prolongation of walking, although statistically significant, ranged from an increase from predicted cessation of walking by 1 year in the boys treated at a younger age versus 6 months for the boys who were older. When asked in a questionnaire whether they were satisfied with the results of the intervention, all boys in the early group and their family reported satisfaction. However, in the group treated in the later stage of walking, three of the four boys and their family were not satisfied with the intervention and would not have repeated it. The use of consumer feedback in using invasive procedures with families has not been typically included in clinical trials. The results of Bach and McKeon (1991) demonstrate the need for more consistent use of feedback in identifying key factors for consideration in the decision-making process.

If the decision to use orthoses to prolong standing or walking is made, lightweight knee-ankle-foot orthoses (KAFOs) should be prescribed (Fig. 13–6) (Bowker & Halpin, 1978; Siegel, 1975). Ankle-foot orthoses are appropriate for positioning but often interfere with compensations required for balance during walking on nonlevel surfaces. A reciprocating or rollator walker may be helpful when assistance for balance is needed. Assistive devices such as a standard walker, crutches, or canes are seldom functional because of the degree of proximal shoulder girdle and upper extremity muscle weakness. Standby assistance should be provided when KAFOs are used, owing to the risk of injury with falls. Closer guarding and increased assistance will be needed as the weakness progresses. Transfers to and from standing are dependent because the knee of the KAFO must be locked to provide stability. The KAFOs can then be used for continuation of a standing program even after walking is no longer possible.

The continued use of standing, if orthoses are prescribed, may help deter the development of osteoporosis and of flexion contractures in the legs;

FIGURE 13–6. Polypropylene knee-ankle-foot orthosis and use of a reciprocating walker to promote walking for exercise in a 14-year-old boy with DMD. The reciprocating walker allows progression without picking up the device.

however, no objective data supporting this recommendation are available for MD. In cerebral palsy, it appears that at least 1 to 2 hours, 3 to 5 times a week, is needed to have an inhibitory effect on osteoporosis and contracture formation (Stuberg et al., 1991). A tilt table, supine stander, or standing table can be used with the braces to provide support in an upright position. If KAFOs are not available, the use of knee immobilizers with a standing table can serve as an alternative for a standing program.

Surgical intervention is commonly needed in conjunction with the use of braced walking if significant contractures are present. Documented indications for surgery include ankle plantar flexion contractures of greater than 10°, iliotibial band contractures greater than 20°, or knee-hip flexion contractures greater than 20° but less than 45° (Bowker & Halpin, 1978). Subcutaneous tenotomy of the Achilles tendon and fasciotomy of the iliotibial bands are the most commonly reported surgical procedures (Bach & McKeon, 1991; Bowker & Halpin, 1978; Siegel et al. 1972; Vignos, 1983). Transfer of the posterior tibialis tendon is occasionally used for correction of the equinovarus foot posture.

An intensive postoperative management program is essential to retard the effects of immobilization (Siegel et al., 1986). Standing in the plaster casts can be done on the first or second postoperative day. Gait training is begun as tolerated, and general conditioning exercises for the hips, trunk, and upper extremities are recommended. Breathing exercises should also be stressed. A smooth transition from the casts to bracing is ensured by having the child fitted for the KAFOs before hospitalization.

Standing pivot transfers must eventually be replaced by one- or two-person lifts or use of equipment as a result of the development of knee and hip flexion contractures and pronounced weakness of the lower extremities. Transfers to and from the wheelchair, toilet, tub, car, and furniture usually become dependent by age 12 to 14. A sliding board, manual lift, or Hoyer lift can be used during transfers. Proper instruction for transfers is needed because the degree of trunk muscle weakness makes sitting balance tenuous by this stage. If the caregiver is using manual lifting for transfers, he or she should be observed for and instructed in proper body mechanics and safety. A Hoyer lift can be used for transfers to and from the wheelchair particularly when the adolescent is large or obese. A hammock-style sling should be used with the lift to provide adequate head and trunk support during transfers. A tub lift or bath bench for bathing will

be needed and a wheeled commode-shower chair considered depending on bathroom accessibility.

A power scooter as shown in Figure 13–3 should be considered as an initial power wheelchair prescription for the child who is hesitant to use a power wheelchair when walking is no longer possible. The scooter is often more easily accepted by the child and may be used for transition to a standard power wheelchair. If a power scooter is initially used, transition to a power wheelchair should be considered when the adolescent is seen propping on the arm rests for trunk control. Asymmetric sitting postures must be aggressively managed owing to the correlation of increased sitting time and poor sitting posture with the onset of scoliosis.

A manual wheelchair will be needed if nonaccessible areas for a powered wheelchair are encountered in the usual environment. Architectural barriers in the home or inability to transport a power wheelchair may also necessitate the use of a manual wheelchair. Use of a manual wheelchair is also appropriate for children with significant intellectual impairment who cannot safely use a power wheelchair.

Fit of the wheelchair must be closely monitored to provide adequate support. The reader should refer to Chapter 23 for general information on wheelchairs. Special attention should be given to alignment of the spine and the pelvis and to the need for customized accessories or modifications. Accessories to be considered for the manual or power wheelchair prescription should include a solid back and seat, lateral trunk support, lumbar support, adductor pads, seat belt, and chest strap (Fig. 13–7). The footrests should be modified to support the ankle in a neutral position. Additional items that may be appropriate include a tray; head support, if needed; or coated push rims, if the child has the strength to propel the wheelchair. A reclining back will allow a position change while sitting in the wheelchair and will help deter flexion contracture formation at the hip, or a tilt-in-space reclining option can be considered to allow for pressure relief. Midline placement of the control stick on a power wheelchair may be considered to assist in symmetric trunk alignment. If a cushion is required, it should maintain the pelvis in a level position.

Maintaining the spine in a neutral or slightly extended position is essential to retard the formation of a scoliosis. The spine should be in slight extension to increase weight bearing through the facet joints, minimize truncal rotation and lateral flexion, and slow the progression of scoliosis formation (Gibson et al., 1978; Wilkins & Gibson, 1976). Scoliosis is seen in approximately 25% of

FIGURE 13–7. Power wheelchair with cushion and trunk support. A firm back and seat insert are needed to provide midline trunk and pelvic positioning.

individuals before the cessation of walking (Miller et al., 1992). Poor sitting posture, in addition to the weakness, has been shown to accelerate scoliosis formation and progression (Gibson & Wilkins, 1975). The onset of scoliosis is typically seen by the age of 10 to 14 years (Ziter & Allsop, 1976). Spinal orthoses may also retard the progression of scoliosis, although they have not been shown to prevent development of a significant scoliotic curve (Cambridge & Drennan, 1987; Colbert & Craig, 1987). Custom-molded seating inserts, corsets, and modular seating inserts are options to provide trunk support in an attempt to slow the progression of the scoliosis. A study comparing the three methods of spinal control in a cohort of 24 boys with DMD concluded that the progression of the curvature was not significantly changed by either method, nor was one found to be superior in controlling the progression (Colbert & Craig, 1987; Seeger et al., 1984).

Early surgical intervention is gaining popularity for the control of scoliosis through the use of segmental spinal instrumentation with Luque rods (Miller et al., 1992; Sussman, 1984). Miller and associates (1992) report improved "quality of life," attainment of a balanced sitting posture, and more normal alignment following surgical intervention for scoliosis. Pulmonary complications are reported as minimal if forced vital capacity is at least 35% of normal age-predicted values.

With the cessation of walking in late childhood or early adolescence, the emphasis of an exercise program should shift from the lower extremities to active-assistive and active exercises of the upper extremities. More importantly, however, active exercise should be encouraged by having the adolescent assist as much as possible in ADL such as grooming, upper body dressing, and feeding through consultation with an occupational therapist. Key muscle groups for maintenance of strength for transfers include the shoulder depressors and triceps. The shoulder flexor and abductor and elbow flexor muscle groups are key areas for exercises to maintain routine ADL such as self-feeding and hygiene. Weakness of the upper arm musculature by 16 years of age makes ADL such as dressing, feeding, or hygiene extremely difficult.

The ROM program will require further modification as the adolescent becomes nonambulatory. Stretching of the aforementioned lower extremity ranges should be continued with stretching of the shoulder and elbow included. Limitation in shoulder flexion and abduction, elbow extension, forearm supination, and wrist extension are most common.

Additional equipment considerations for the adolescent may include the use of a stair glide for a home with stairs, although this is generally not recommended because of the number of transfers involved, inaccessibility to independent mobility when the power wheelchair is not available on the second floor, and safety concerns in the event of an emergency. A motorized scooter can be transported in a car trunk, but a van with a lift or ramp will be needed to transport a power wheelchair. Modification of the bathroom can significantly assist the family by using a wheeled commode chair for toileting and a bath chair and hand-held shower for bathing. A tub lift is a second option for bathing. A urinal should be available at home or school to decrease the frequency of transfers to the toilet. Modifications of the bed are also frequently required because the adolescent is unable to change position. An airflow mattress, egg-crate foam cushion, or hospital bed are all possibilities to be considered. A positioning program to include position changes at night is necessary for adolescents who are thin to provide comfort and ensure against skin breakdown. Customized foam wedges fabricated by the therapist may also be very helpful in positioning at night.

Transition to Adulthood

The transition to adulthood marks a time of continued progression of disability with greater reliance on assistive technology for environmental access and increased need for assistance to carry out routine ADL. Mobility using a power wheelchair is necessary because upper extremity and truncal weakness will typically not allow use of a motorized scooter. Assistance for ADL including dressing, transfers, and bathing is now required. Hygiene about the face and feeding become increasingly difficult but usually remain manageable. Many social issues also arise with the completion of educational programming and transition to a prevocational, vocational, or home environment on a more full-time basis. Another major issue that requires thoughtful consideration by the family, individual, and management team is the utilization of assisted ventilation with progressive respiratory involvement at the terminal stage of the disease.

All transfers require assistance during late adolescence and by adulthood typically require use of a Hoyer or other mechanical lift. A high-backed sling seat is indicated since head and trunk control is minimal with the progressive weakness.

Depending on the availability of funding, accessibility, and family choice, power recline on the wheelchair may have been purchased; if not, a regular schedule for pressure relief through lateral weight shifting with assistance is needed. A properly fitting and well-tolerated cushion to avoid skin breakdown becomes an area of intervention with loss of the ability to weight shift in the wheelchair. Skin breakdown is not a typical problem in DMD, but a cushion should be considered. A Jay Medical cushion (Jay Medical, Boulder, CO) is often well tolerated and provides a firm base of support to control pelvic obliquity, yet the gel inserts can be adjusted to allow for adequate pressure distribution. A customized insert will be needed if deformity becomes severe (e.g., severe scoliosis without surgical stabilization).

A ball-bearing feeder may be required to assist arm movement when progression of upper extremity weakness makes independent feeding difficult (Chyatte et al., 1965). The device can also be used to assist with general use of the arms in conjunction with activities at a table, such as during use of a computer. Coordination of planning with an occupational therapist to address feeding and dressing issues is needed to identify solutions to increased dependence in feeding, dressing, and hygiene.

To maintain independence in environmental access, consideration for using environmental control devices should be given. An environmental control unit included on the power wheelchair can be used to independently access the lights, telephone, television, motors on doors, or a computer, to name just a few applications. Computer access for vocational applications such as word processing or avocational activities such as games is available.

Breathing exercises, postural drainage, or intermittent pressure breathing treatments should be included in the management program based on results of pulmonary evaluation (Houser & Johnson, 1971). Specific tests of pulmonary function that document respiratory status include forced vital capacity (amount of air expired following a maximal inspiration) and peak expiratory flow rate (highest flow rate sustained for 10 ms during maximal expiration). In addition to the breathing exercises and assisted coughing, the family should be instructed in the technique of postural drainage.

Close monitoring of respiratory function should become routine with increasing age since respiratory failure or pulmonary infection is the major contributing factor to death in 75% of children with DMD (Gilroy et al., 1982; Inkley et al., 1974). The lives of individuals with DMD can be significantly prolonged by assisted ventilation (Alexander et al., 1979; Bach et al., 1987; Curran & Colbert, 1989); however, the current trend in a survey conducted of MDA-sponsored clinics reports that only 26% of clinic directors offered ventilatory aid for acute respiratory failure (Bach, 1992). Bach goes on to stress the need for health care professionals to explore attitudes toward mechanical ventilation because our perceived impression of client desires may often be incorrect. The use of intermittent positive-pressure breathing, negative pressure ventilators, and suctioning may be considered for the chronic hypoventilation related to weakness of respiratory musculature (Fairley, 1968; Hill et al., 1992).

A power-controlled bed to allow elevation of the head for respiratory management should be considered. Use of a bed with elevating capability also allows for greater ease in transfers, and height adjustment promotes use of proper body mechanics by family members for activities that require assistance such as dressing. Mattress selection should also be reviewed with the family because an airflow mattress may be needed when increasing dependence for bed mobility is encountered. Use of an airflow mattress may decrease the frequency of need for turning and repositioning at night. If sitting in a wheelchair is no longer tolerated in the later stages of the disease, elevation of the head of the bed becomes beneficial for reading or watching television. An easel will be required for reading.

Although it may be assumed by care providers that the quality of life and therefore satisfaction are significantly reduced for severely disabled individuals with DMD, this notion may be incorrect. In a survey of 82 ventilator-assisted individuals with DMD, Bach and colleagues (1991) concluded that the vast majority of individuals had a positive affect and were satisfied with life despite the physical dependence. Furthermore, it was found in a survey of 273 physically intact health care professionals that a significant underestimation of patient's life satisfaction scores was evidenced that may profoundly affect attitudes and management recommendations. The article by Bach and colleagues (1991) points out that we need to constantly inquire and objectively assess family and individual needs when interacting to provide therapeutic programs. Curran and Colbert (1989) have reported an average increase in longevity from 19 years 9 months to 25 years 9 months in individuals who use ventilatory assistance.

Respiratory insufficiency is a hallmark sign of the preterminal stage of DMD (Newsom-Davis, 1980). Progressive muscular weakness results in decreased ventilatory volumes caused by restriction of chest wall excursion. Coordination of care with the respiratory therapist is essential when clinical findings of respiratory muscle weakness, inability to cough, or chest wall restrictions are observed (Burke et al., 1971). Severe oxygen desaturation leading to a comatose state is evidence of the terminal stage of the disease.

Members of the team often become involved in answering questions regarding death. The physical therapist should be aware of the stages of disease progression and especially the preterminal signs to avoid making inappropriate comments concerning prognosis. Often little needs to be said, but rather a good listening ear is needed to help the family work through the crisis that is ever pending. It is often a comfort to individuals with DMD or family members that the end may come as a sleep without wakening (Edwards, 1989). The person with DMD and his family members may indicate the need for additional support, but if issues are not being resolved adequately by the support that is available, consideration for involvement by a psychologist, counselor, clergy member, MDA support group, or other trained professional is indicated. Literature is available through the MDA to comfort family members, and texts are available if the family is interested. (Kushner, 1981; Tatelbaum, 1980).

Becker's Muscular Dystrophy

Becker's MD, a more slowly progressive variant of DMD, has an incidence of about 1 in 20,000 births and a prevalence of 2 to 3 cases per 100,000 population (Bushby et al., 1991; Mostacciuolo et al., 1987). The impairments and disabilities of Becker's MD closely resemble those of DMD, however, the progression is significantly slower with a longevity into the 40s (Emery & Skinner, 1976; Gilroy & Holliday, 1982). The genetic defect for Becker's MD is located on the same gene as that for DMD only in a different area and therefore dystrophin is present in reduced amounts, which may explain the slower progression of clinical symptoms (Kingston et al., 1983).

Initial clinical symptoms are typically not identified in boys with Becker's MD before late childhood or early adolescence. Emery and Skinner (1976) found the mean age at onset of symptoms to be 11 years, inability to walk at 27 years, and death at 42 years; however, the authors point out that the range is very wide. Perhaps one of the best functional discriminators between Becker's MD and DMD is that 97% of adolescents with DMD are using a wheelchair for mobility by age 11 years, whereas 97% of adolescents with Becker's MD are still walking (Emery & Skinner, 1976). Another discriminator is the frequent complaint of muscle cramping in individuals with Becker's MD that is rarely reported in DMD (Dubowitz, 1992).

The impairments of Becker's MD are the same as in DMD, although less severe, and the initial disability includes frequent falls and clumsiness in the mid to late teens. The pattern of weakness is the same as in DMD, and pseudohypertrophy of the calves may be present. The incidence of contracture, scoliosis, and other skeletal deformities is lower in Becker's MD. Although not as severe as in DMD, hip, knee, and ankle plantar flexor muscle contractures can be evidenced when walking is no longer possible. The use of night splints to maintain ankle dorsiflexion ROM is often indicated, along with a home program of heel cord stretching. Significant disability will develop by the mid 20s, requiring the use of power mobility and consideration for use of orthoses to maintain walking. KAFOs can also be used to prolong walking; however, braced ambulation will not be functional for community access but rather as a means of exercise. The general goals and management procedures outlined in the section on DMD are the same for Becker's MD, including the progression from walking to use of power mobility.

Because the person with Becker's MD lives much longer than someone with DMD, transition planning following school and assistance with living arrangements into adulthood become major issues. Vocational or avocational choices should be made with the disease progression and disability level in mind. Vocational rehabilitation services should be initiated before completion of high school to allow adequate time for evaluation. Governmental support through Medicaid, Social Security benefits, or other sources may be needed to offset expenses to allow for independent living because adaptive equipment and an attendant will be needed. Ongoing medical services are available through the MDA. No data are available regarding the number of individuals who go to college or become employed following high school, but with the assistive technology available to promote independence, either option can be explored.

Congenital Muscular Dystrophy

Congenital myopathies as a diagnostic category consist of many diseases, including congenital MD. Congenital MD is not a single clinical entity, and up to four different forms have been reported. The four types reported by Brooke (1986) are 1) congenital MD with central nervous system (CNS) disease (Fukuyama type), 2) congenital MD without CNS damage, 3) atonic sclerotic type, and 4) stick man type. The last two types are extremely rare, and the reader should refer to the text by Brooke (1986) for additional information since only the first two types are discussed here. The mode of inheritance in congenital MD is reported as autosomal recessive (MDA, 1991). Although all forms are rare, the range of severity and disability varies significantly among types.

Currently, no definitive information is available regarding longevity in the various forms of congenital MD other than case reports. McMenamin and associates (1982) reported on a cohort of 24 patients with congenital MD, of whom 4 had died between the ages of 5 and 8 years, and 4 between the ages of 18 and 24 years. The oldest patient in the study was 23 years of age.

In congenital MD with associated CNS disease (Fukuyama type), mental retardation and seizures are common along with moderate to severe hypotonia at birth and the presence of contractures (Bernier et al., 1979; Fukuyama et al., 1981; Yoshioka et al., 1992). Magnetic resonance imaging reveals nonspecific cerebral malformations and occasionally lissencephaly as pathologic features of the CNS disease. Contractures typically involve the lower extremities (hips and knees) and elbows. Other commonly reported dysmorphic features include congenital dislocation of the hips, pectus excavatum, pes cavus, kyphoscoliosis, and an unusually long face. Weakness of the extraocular muscles, optic atrophy, and nystagmus have been reported (Brooke, 1986; Yoshioka et al., 1992). Children with this type of MD rarely attain the ability to walk.

The early management program in children with congenital MD with nervous system disease should focus on family instruction, developmental activities to address delays in gross motor skill development, and aggressive management of contractures. Attention to positioning is necessary to guard against secondary deformity resulting from gravitational effects on the trunk with presence of moderate to severe hypotonia. Early intervention by an occupational therapist to address feeding and oral motor control issues is commonly coordinated with physical therapy. Impaired respiratory function and pulmonary complications are hallmark features of congenital MD. The family should be instructed in chest physical therapy, such as postural drainage, and consultation with a respiratory therapist may be needed on an ongoing basis.

Because many children with congenital MD and associated nervous system disease do not attain walking, maximizing functional skills in sitting becomes a primary goal of the physical therapy management program as the child ages. Therapeutic exercise to improve head and trunk control should be aggressively addressed with use of adaptive equipment to slow the progression of spinal deformity and contractures and to maximize access to the environment. Since mental retardation is common, power mobility may not be an option. Additional management issues for children with significant hypotonia are discussed later in the chapter in the section on acute SMA.

CONGENITAL MUSCULAR DYSTROPHY WITHOUT CENTRAL NERVOUS SYSTEM DISEASE

In congenital MD without CNS disease, the typical clinical presentation includes hypotonia and weakness, frequently with contractures, and a delay in acquisition of motor milestones. Infants with this form of congenital MD may demonstrate a rapid progression of muscle weakness with loss of skills (Donner et al., 1975), slow progression, or static neuromotor status (Goebel et al., 1980; Lazaro et al., 1979; McMenamin et al., 1982), to slow improvement (Jones et al., 1979).

Jones and associates (1979) reported on a cohort of 27 children with congenital MD, all younger than the age of 18 years. The authors subdivided the group into severe (those who never walked and demonstrated severe weakness, n = 19) and mild (those who walked independently before age 7 years, n = 8). Sixteen of the children were reported to demonstrate a general improvement in strength with increasing age, 8 remained static, and 2 demonstrated progressive weakness. One child was only 2 months of age and progress was not reported. The follow-up period was 5 years.

Muscle weakness and contractures are the primary impairment; however, intellectual impairment may also limit attainment of functional skills. Muscles innervated by the cranial nerves may be involved, requiring a feeding program that is coordinated with occupational therapy. Contractures need to be managed aggressively with a home ROM program including manual stretching, positioning, and splinting. Because many of the children have a potential to develop walking, the ankle plantar flexion contractures may require orthopaedic intervention if the contractures cannot be managed conservatively. McMenamin and coworkers (1982) reported significant developmental delay in all cases of congenital MD. The average age for attainment of independent sitting was 11.5 months and 2.6 years for walking. Only 15 of the 26 infants attained independent walking.

Functional limitations, such as delayed acquisition of gross motor skills, should not be managed by extensive direct service therapy programs because a slower rate of skill progression is expected. Since many children begin to walk within the first 2 to 3 years, information can be provided to the family concerning probable rates of motor skill acquisition and unrealistic therapeutic expectations should be avoided. Because there is a wide range of functional deficits in children with congenital MD, care needs to be taken in predicting functional gross motor outcomes.

Childhood-Onset Facioscapulohumeral Muscular Dystrophy

Facioscapulohumeral MD is rare, with an incidence of 3 to 10 cases per million births (Stevenson et al., 1990). The disorder is inherited as autosomal dominant or recessive with the genetic defect on chromosome 4. The disorder affects males and females equally. Childhood-onset facioscapulohumeral MD typically demonstrates the onset of clinical signs within the first 2 years but without significant impairment or disability until later in the first decade. Contractures are seldom a problem.

Infancy and Preschool-Aged Period

The impairment of muscle weakness about the face and shoulder girdle is typically the only prominent feature of the disease during the infant and preschool-aged period. Parents report that the child may sleep with the eyes partially open and on physical examination, weakness of the facial musculature is predominant. Children are frequently unable to whistle, and drinking with a straw may be difficult. When asked to purse the lips together and puff the cheeks out, the child is unable to maintain the cheeks out when even the slightest pressure is applied. The child's smile is also masked because of the weakness, thereby hindering communication as a result of inconsistency between what is spoken and the affect displayed.

Children with childhood-onset facioscapulohumeral MD typically develop independence in walking without significant delay. An excessive lordotic posture during walking is a classic clinical feature with progression of weakness. The scapulae are widely abducted and outwardly rotated, giving evidence of the degree of interscapular muscle weakness.

School-Aged Period

Progressive disability occurs during the school-aged period, with weakness becoming more generalized throughout the trunk, shoulder, and pelvic girdle musculature. Progression of childhood-onset facioscapulohumeral MD is more insidious than the adult form, and independent walking may be lost by the end of the first decade (Gardner-Medwin, 1980b; Hanson & Rowland, 1971).

The severe winging of the scapula, a hallmark feature of the adult form of the disease, becomes more prominent with age in activities such as reaching overhead. Management should focus on instruction to the child and family on activities to avoid that promote fatigue and on guarding against heavily resisted upper extremity activity. Studies of adults with facioscapulohumeral MD comparing dominant with nondominant arm strength have shown that mechanical factors play a significant role in progression of muscle weakness (Brouwer et al., 1992; Johnson & Braddom, 1971).

As weakness of the hip and knee extensors progresses, the use of KAFOs should be considered for assisted walking and transfers. When walking becomes increasingly difficult, power mobility using a scooter or power wheelchair should be considered because the degree of upper extremity weakness will not allow independence in propulsion of a manual wheelchair.

Transition to Adulthood

No specific prognostic information on the longevity of individuals with childhood-onset facioscapulohumeral MD is available, and therefore transition planning from the educational environment should be a goal of the therapy program. If severe weakness is present and significant assistance from the family is needed, individuals may not desire to plan for living outside the family home. If independent living is desired, coordination of planning with an attendant will be necessary and evaluation for accessibility issues completed. Assistance through vocational rehabilitation services should be coordinated with transition planning if vocational goals are identified.

Congenital Myotonic Muscular Dystrophy

Myotonic MD has the highest incidence of the dystrophies at 3 to 5 cases per 100,000 population (Gardner-Medwin, 1980a). Congenital myotonic MD is rare and demonstrates severe clinical features of the adult-onset diagnosis. Inheritance is reported as autosomal dominant with genetic defect of chromosome 19 affecting males and females equally (Harley et al., 1991).

Children with congenital myotonic MD are almost exclusively born to mothers with myotonic MD, and a "maternal factor" has been hypothesized by Harper (1989). Two variations within the congenital form are reported. Most children demonstrate severe hypotonia and weakness at birth; however, a few children first present with only signs of mental retardation by age 5 years and no significant motor impairment as infants. Because the children who initially present with only mental impairment follow a progression of motor impairment similar to that of adult-onset myotonic MD, the infancy onset form is discussed in this section of the chapter.

Mental retardation in congenital myotonic MD is common. A mean IQ of 66 was reported by Harper (1975a). There is no evidence of progressive deterioration of mental function. A study by Rutherford and co-workers (1989), including 14 children, provides prognostic information regarding survival and the relationship to mechanical ventilation. No infant in the study survived who required mechanical ventilation for longer than 4 weeks.

Infancy

If the child survives the early weeks of life, the prognosis is one of steady improvement in motor function over the first decade, with most children developing independent walking (Harper, 1975a; Harper, 1989). A follow-up study by O'Brien and Harper (1984) of 46 children reported only 4 children who died outside the neonatal period at the ages of 4, 18, 19, and 22. Four additional children demonstrated a more significant disability associated with a poor prognosis, and none was older than age 30 years. Information is lacking on the longevity of individuals who survive to adulthood with congenital myotonic MD.

Severe weakness and partial paralysis of the diaphragm at birth are clinical features that often suggest the diagnosis of congenital myotonic MD. Myotonia (delay in relaxation after muscular contraction), a hallmark feature of adult myotonic MD, is typically not evident at birth in the congenital form but rather develops by 3 to 5 years of age (Brooke, 1986). Myotonia in congenital myotonic MD is typically not considered to be a significant impairment or a cause of functional limitations in comparison to the degree of weakness that is present. The symptoms of myotonia, however, are increased with fatigue, cold, or stress (Siegel, 1986). Typical facial features include a short median part of the upper lip, which gives the mouth an inverted-V shape. Facial movements are limited, with muscles innervated by the cranial nerves involved in the severe weakness pattern. Severe respiratory impairment is prominent in the newborn period, requiring resuscitation and assisted ventilation in most cases. Talipes equinovarus contractures are reported in over 50% of children, and a general pattern of arthrogryposis occurs in less than 5% (Harper, 1989).

Progressive improvement in gross motor skills can be expected if the child survives the newborn period. The presence of and degree of intellectual impairment becomes a major factor in the progression of milestone acquisition. The development of hip abduction and external rotation contractures should be closely monitored if leg movement and habitual positioning favor the development of secondary impairment.

Harper (1989), in a cohort of 70 children with congenital myotonic dystrophy, reported that hypotonia is rarely prominent beyond age 3 to 4 years. Children typically develop walking, but further motor impairment follows the clinical progression of adult-onset disease without definitive data being available into adulthood to document disease progression.

Consultation with a respiratory therapist on pulmonary care will be needed until the infant is weaned from assisted ventilation. Feeding may require the use of a nasogastric tube during the newborn period or early infancy, and initiation of a feeding program should be coordinated with an occupational therapist. A swallowing study may be indicated to evaluate potential for aspiration when the feeding program is initiated. If the newborn survives early respiratory difficulties, progressive improvement in pulmonary function is usually seen without need for ongoing intervention.

Talipes equinovarus contractures should be aggressively managed in infancy with casting, taping, and exercises but may ultimately require orthopaedic intervention. Ankle-foot orthoses or night splints may be indicated based on individual needs. In addition to home instruction for ROM activities to manage contractures, the family should be provided with a general program of activities to promote gross motor skill development. Because the natural progression of the disease is improvement of motor function, consultation rather than a direct service program is indicated, unless surgical intervention for contracture management is required.

School-Aged Period

Consultation for development of adaptive physical education activities will be needed during the school-aged period. Other physical therapy–related activities will depend on the use of orthoses and progression of gross motor skill development. Specific therapeutic exercise programs for strengthening have not been reported but may be indicated in addition to ROM activities.

Transition to Adulthood

The natural progression of myotonic MD is insidious weakness of the distal upper and lower extremity musculature and progressive increase in myotonia, leading to increasing disability. Children with congenital myotonic MD will demonstrate progression in the disease as described for adults, but typically at an earlier stage, usually by the middle of the second decade. The reader should refer to references on adult myotonic MD for further information on clinical course and management (Brooke, 1986; Harper, 1989; Siegel, 1986).

Emery-Dreifus Muscular Dystrophy

Emery-Dreifus MD is inherited as an X-linked recessive disorder characterized by weakness predominately in a humeroperoneal distribution and with variable facial involvement (Pinelli et al., 1987). Limited information is available in the literature, but the disorder resembles facioscapulohu-

meral MD in certain persons. Onset of muscle weakness is typically in the first decade, and progression is very slow (Brooke, 1986).

Ankle equinus and elbow flexion contractures are common. Contracture of muscles of the neck and spine, resulting in limited flexion ROM, is reported (Brooke, 1986). Weakness of the elbow flexor and extensor musculature presents as the initial pattern of muscle involvement. Cardiac abnormalities are common, with sudden death (in persons ranging in age from 25 to 56 years) reported by Pinelli and colleagues (1987) in a large family cohort with bradyarrhythmias.

Physical therapy management is limited during the childhood period because disability is not common. Independent walking is typically maintained into adulthood without significant disability. An ROM program for contracture prevention is advised, but orthopaedic intervention is common to correct the Achilles tendon contractures (Shapiro & Specht, 1991). Holter monitoring is advised when cardiac abnormalities are identified, and pacemakers are used to control rhythm.

▌ SPINAL MUSCULAR ATROPHY

Classification of SMA into four groups is based on clinical presentation and progression (Table 13–3). Types I and II are commonly referred to as acute and chronic Werdnig-Hoffmann disease, respectively, type III as Kugelberg-Welander disease, and type IV as adult-onset SMA.

Diagnosis and Pathophysiology

SMA comprises the second most common group of fatal recessive diseases after cystic fibrosis (Pearn, 1980). The pathologic feature of SMA is abnormality of the large anterior horn cells in the spinal cord. The number of cells is reduced, and progressive degeneration of the remaining cells is correlated with loss in function.

TABLE 13–3. **CLASSIFICATION OF SPINAL MUSCLE ATROPHY**

Type	Onset	Inheritance	Course
Acute child-onset, type I, Werdnig-Hoffmann (acute)	0–3 mo	Recessive	Rapidly progressive; severe hypotonia; death within first year
Chronic childhood-onset, type II, Werdnig-Hoffmann (chronic)	3 mo–4 yr	Recessive	Rapid progress that stabilizes; moderate to severe hypotonia; shortened life span
Juvenile-onset, type III, Kugelberg-Welander	5–10 yr	Recessive	Slowly progressive; mild impairment

The diagnosis of SMA is confirmed by clinical examination and laboratory procedures, including electromyography and muscle biopsy (Brooke, 1986; Siegel, 1986). Blood tests, although not specific for SMA, are often administered to rule out other neuromuscular diseases. Electromyographic findings include fibrillation and fasciculation potentials, repetitive discharge, excessive polyphasic potentials, and increased amplitude and duration of the motor unit potentials consistent with chronic denervation and reinnervation of muscle. Nerve conduction velocities are normal. The muscle biopsy demonstrates changes that are typical of a disease involving denervation (i.e., large groups of atrophic fibers are dispersed among groups of normal or hypertrophic fibers). The absence of fibrosis around the atrophic groups on the muscle biopsy helps to delineate SMA from DMD.

The incidence of Werdnig-Hoffmann disease is 1 in 15,000 to 25,000 live births (Pearn, 1973; Pearn et al., 1973), and the incidence of Kugelberg-Welander disease is reported as 6 cases per 100,000 live births (Winsor et al., 1971). Specific information on the incidence of the other forms is variable due to inconsistency of classification criteria and based on the clinical heterogeneity of the disease.

One criterion for classification of SMA includes the level of functional ability (Dubowitz, 1989). The more typical classification criteria are multifactorial and involve age at onset of the first clinical signs, pattern of muscle involvement, age at death, and genetic evidence (Pearn, 1980).

Contrary to the first descriptions in the literature, SMA is now believed to be a heterogeneous disorder containing several different clinical presentations, modes of inheritance, and rates of progression. Progressive SMA of early childhood (type I) was first reported by Werdnig and Hoffmann in the late 1800s (Hoffmann, 1893; Werdnig, 1894). A more slowly progressive form of SMA (type III) with onset usually between the ages of 2 to 9 years was reported by Kugelberg and Welander (1956) and also by Wohlfart and colleagues (1955) in the mid 1900s. Werdnig-Hoffmann disease and Kugelberg-Welander disease have therefore become the eponyms for early onset and juvenile onset SMA, with many authors preferring to use the numeric classification system as outlined in Table 13–3.

SMA is typically inherited as autosomal recessive with the genetic defect on chromosome 5 (Gilliam et al., 1990). An autosomal dominant inheritance has been reported that tends to present with clinical signs later in the first decade and demonstrates a slower progression (Emery et al., 1976; Pearn, 1978; Zellweger et al., 1972). The sex-linked recessive form demonstrates clinical findings similar to those of Becker's MD with onset later in the first decade, a slow progression, and calf muscle hypertrophy (Bundey & Lovelace, 1975; Gamstrop, 1967; Pearn, 1978). The greatest variation in the clinical course of SMA is seen with the autosomal recessive mode of inheritance.

Pearn (1980), in a large multicenter study in England, reported SMA type II and III to be the most frequent, accounting for approximately 47% of the population, followed by SMA type I at about 27%, adult-onset type IV at 8%, and the other 18% with mixed classifications including distal involvement, neurogenic SMA, SMA of adolescence with hypertrophied calf muscles, and childhood-onset SMA with cerebellar and optic atrophy.

No cure is available for SMA, but physical therapy is commonly advocated (Brooke, 1986; Hausmanowa-Petrusewicz, 1978; Marshall, 1984; Watt & Greenhill, 1984). The prognosis is variable, but grave indicators for long-term survival include early age at onset (before 4 months of age) that is often noted as weak fetal movement, fasciculations of the tongue in infancy, and severe, generalized weakness, particularly of the trunk and proximal musculature (Gamstrop, 1967).

Acute Childhood Spinal Muscular Atrophy (Type I)

IMPAIRMENTS

The primary impairment in all forms of SMA is muscle weakness secondary to progressive loss of anterior horn cells in the spinal cord. Weakness is particularly pronounced in the acute and chronic childhood forms (types I and II) within the first 4 months. The cranial nerves are inconsistently involved in childhood-onset SMA, with rare involvement with juvenile onset. Contractures may be a primary impairment in acute-onset SMA, with reports of talipes equinovarus or other intrauterine deformities secondary to limited fetal movement. Muscle fasciculations, including fasciculations of the tongue, are most commonly reported in children with acute-onset SMA (Namba et al., 1970). Unlike the faces of children with myotonic or facioscapulohumeral MD, children with acute childhood SMA appear alert and responsive. Respiratory distress is present early, and significant effort to augment breathing by use of the abdominal musculature is typical.

Secondary impairments in acute-onset SMA include the development of scoliosis and often contractures. It is widely reported in the literature that all children with SMA develop scoliosis, usually requiring surgical intervention (Granata et al., 1989c; Lonstein, 1989). Other secondary impairments include decreased respiratory capacity and easy fatigability. Since only the passage of time will allow differentiation of children with acute versus chronic childhood SMA, treatment should begin early with a focus on feeding, ROM, positioning, respiratory care, and selected developmental activities.

Infancy

In acute childhood SMA, weak or absent fetal movement during the last months of pregnancy is commonly reported by the mother. Significant weakness is present at birth or develops within the first 4 months, which presents as inability to perform antigravity movements with the pelvic or shoulder girdle musculature and typical posturing in a gravity-dependent position (Fig. 13–8). The proximal musculature of the neck, trunk, and pelvic and shoulder girdles demonstrates the greatest weakness. Limited antigravity movement of distal upper and lower extremity musculature is present, and a positioning program in the newborn period or at the onset of symptoms is necessary. Use of wedges should be considered to avoid supine positioning in the presence of respiratory distress. If the supine position is used, rolled towels or bolsters are

needed to keep the upper extremities positioned in midline and to prevent lower extremity abduction and external rotation. Side-lying is a position that will allow midline head and hand use for play without having to work against gravity. Prone positioning on wedges should be limited or not used owing to the effort required for head righting to interact with the environment.

Respiratory care is a central focus of the habilitation program in acute childhood SMA. Children frequently require intubation for respiratory distress and tracheostomy. Coordination with nurses and respiratory therapists on a program that includes suctioning, assisted coughing, and postural drainage is necessary. The use of supported sitting should be closely monitored for spinal alignment and respiratory response. Use of an elastic binder around the abdomen in sitting may be useful for children who demonstrate a marked reduction in oxygen saturation when seated.

ROM exercises should be carried out to ensure maintenance of flexibility and comfort. Flexion contractures of the hips, knees and elbows, hip abductors, ankle plantar flexors, and positional torticollis are deformities that can be avoided with a comprehensive ROM and positioning program (Binder, 1989). The exercise program should also include limited activities for strengthening, such as

FIGURE 13–8. Typical postures seen in a young child with SMA while supine (a), prone (b), and sitting (c). Note the limited antigravity control and dependent posturing.

lightweight toys or rattles with Velcro straps around the wrists or mobiles positioned close to the hands for easy access. The use of hammocks have also been advocated to provide the child with the opportunity for movement with only slight movements of the body (Eng, 1989a, 1989b). Developmental activities such as the use of supported sitting for the development of head control should be of short duration to avoid fatigue.

Head control fails to develop or is significantly impaired in acute childhood SMA. The child is unable to lift the head from a prone position to clear the airway. Early developmental postures such as prone on elbows are not attained. The use of developmental exercise in acute childhood SMA is controversial but should be considered if the child tolerates the activities because a few children with chronic childhood SMA demonstrate clinical signs in the first year of life also.

In conjunction with an occupational therapist, a feeding program that is safe and not excessively exhausting should be implemented. Small, frequent feedings may be necessary, and breast-feeding may be difficult (Eng, 1989b). Special care with feeding is necessary to avoid aspiration and secondary respiratory problems.

Although death secondary to pneumonia or other respiratory complications is typical within a few months to a few years in acute childhood SMA, the child's death is usually not a struggle, owing to the degree of weakness and apnea (Eng, 1989b; Gamstrop, 1967). The mean age of death is reported to be 6 months, with a range from 1 to 21 months reported by Merlini and associates (1989). Counseling and support for the parents and family is a very important component in the management of these children.

Chronic Childhood Spinal Muscular Atrophy (Type II)

IMPAIRMENTS

The onset of significant weakness in chronic childhood SMA usually appears within the first year. The course of the disease may be widely variable. Pearn and colleagues (1978) reported on the clinical progression in a cohort of 141 children and stated that 95% of the children demonstrated clinical signs before age 3 years, 46% never walked (even with orthotics), 38% were able to walk unaided at some stage, and the median age at death exceeded 10 years.

Eng (1989b) has reported three separate sub groupings within type II based on the pattern of presentation and progression. In the most severely involved group, the children never developed the ability to sit alone and respiratory capacity was significantly reduced; in the intermediate group the children sat alone but never developed the ability to walk and demonstrated a regression of forced vital capacity to 45% by age 10 years; in the last group independent walking was attained but half of the children lost this ability toward the end of the first decade. Interestingly, in the group of patients who remained ambulatory in the study by Eng (1989b), forced vital capacity was maintained at 90% as compared with 65% for those who lost independent walking during the first decade, leading Eng to conclude that forced vital capacity may be a physiologic predictor of walking duration.

Contractures are infrequently an impairment in chronic SMA. The distribution of weakness is similar to acute childhood SMA with primary proximal involvement, but of much less severe degree. Weakness is usually greatest in the hip and knee extensors and trunk musculature. Involvement of the distal musculature appears later in the course of the disease and is less severe than the proximal involvement (Namba et al., 1970). Involvement of the cranial nerves is reported but not considered to be a typical feature of SMA other than in the acute childhood form. Fasciculations of the tongue are reported in approximately one half of the children (Pearn et al., 1973). A tremor may also be noted and is considered by several authors as substantiating the diagnosis (Brooke, 1986; Moosa & Dubowitz, 1973).

Infancy

As the clinical presentation and progression of chronic childhood SMA differs widely, the management program needs to address the major disability at each point in time. Approximately 15% of children will present with impairments within the first 3 months and the remaining children present by 18 months (Merlini et al., 1989). The program for the newborn with chronic SMA should be similar to that for children with acute SMA. Some children may develop the ability to stand, but few are able to use walking as a primary means of mobility.

Sitting posture is an area of primary concern in the management program with children who demonstrate significant weakness, requiring head and trunk control in antigravity positions. A molded sitting support orthosis as shown in Figure 13–9 provides optimal contouring of the torso for support in sitting or a thoracolumbosacral orthosis (TLSO or "body jacket") can also be used. Developmental activities provided on an ongoing basis are indicated to develop gross motor skills. The impor-

FIGURE 13–9. Custom-molded sitting-support orthosis to provide trunk support in sitting.

sessions should be kept short to avoid fatigue and emphasize selected developmental areas during each session because tolerance to handling in multiple positions is usually limited. Instruction with the family for carryover and the use of adaptive equipment for proper positioning are crucial in slowing the deforming effects of gravity on the spine when the child is sitting or standing.

If the child is not standing by the age of 16 to 18 months, adaptive equipment for standing should be considered. The rate of fracture in SMA has been reported to range from 12% to 15%, and weight bearing has been shown to decrease the frequency of lower extremity fractures (Ballestrazzi et al., 1989). A supine stander is recommended for children without adequate head control. Orthopaedic consultation for a corset or TLSO should be considered for use in standing to maintain trunk alignment if the adaptive equipment does not provide adequate control.

Preschool-Aged and School-Aged Period

In the toddler, orthotics for standing might be considered (lightweight KAFOs); however, the pro-gression of weakness may make walking an unrealistic goal. In a report of promotion of walking in 12 children with intermediate SMA (aged 13 months to 3 years), Granata and associates (1989a) described success in attaining assisted ambulation with 58% of the children using orthoses. Although preliminary, these investigators also reported less severity of scoliotic curves in the children who used the orthoses in comparison to a control group of children with SMA.

If a walking program is initiated, training in the parallel bars followed by use of a walker or other device to allow greater independence is desired. Close monitoring of safety with supported walking is necessary owing to the degree of weakness present and the potential for serious injury with a fall. The incidence of hip dislocation and contractures has also been reported as less when a supported walking program is used (Granata et al., 1989b).

Independence with mobility other than walking is a primary goal for the child who will not develop independence in walking or when walking is no longer possible. Since most power scooters do not provide adequate trunk control, use of a power wheelchair is commonly indicated. If an orthopaedic appliance is not used, close attention to fit is needed with use of lateral trunk supports and a trunk harness. Consideration should also be given to changing the side of the joystick every 6 months to avoid a pattern of leaning to one side. Prognosis for children with chronic childhood SMA is dependent on frequency and severity of pulmonary complications. Severe contractures as a result of prolonged sitting and progression of scoliosis are common, necessitating use of a consistent ROM program. Surgical intervention for spinal stabilization is an option if pulmonary function testing indicates a good prognosis for survival of the surgical intervention.

Transition to Adulthood

Survival into adulthood is extremely variable in chronic childhood SMA and depends on the progression of muscle weakness and secondary deformities. Because of the significant degree of muscle weakness, assistance is typically required for transfers and many ADL. An attendant or family member is needed to provide assistance for general ADL. Intelligence is rarely affected, and therefore vocational goals in areas of interest should be explored through vocational rehabilitation services.

An aggressive program of pulmonary care is required, including breathing exercises and postural drainage. The ROM program should also be continued to control progression of the contractures unless a pattern of stability is recorded.

Juvenile-Onset Spinal Muscular Atrophy (Type III)

Juvenile-onset SMA may demonstrate symptoms of weakness within the first year of life in the proximal hip and shoulder girdle musculature, but more typically the onset is later in the first decade. Rarely are bulbar signs seen with the disease. Calf pseudohypertrophy is reported in approximately 10% of the cases. Fasciculations are noted in about half of the patients, and minimyoclonus may be a primary impairment noted on examination but rarely interferes with function (Brooke, 1986; Dorscher et al., 1991).

IMPAIRMENTS

In a study by Dorscher and colleagues (1991) reviewing the status of 31 patients with Kugelberg-Welander disease, proximal lower extremity weakness was the most common impairment reported. Secondary impairments included postural compensations resulting from the muscle weakness, contractures, and occasionally scoliosis. An increased lumbar lordosis and compensated Trendelenburg gait pattern are common postural compensations for proximal muscle weakness of the lower extremities. Ankle plantar flexion contractures are occasionally reported but not with the frequency seen in DMD, which aids differentiation of the two diseases. Scoliosis was reported in about 20% of patients by Dorscher and colleagues (1991) but was reported in all patients by other researchers (Granata et al., 1989b). In adolescents with type III SMA the incidence of scoliosis and its severity are related to the degree of weakness and functional status. Individuals who maintain independent walking may demonstrate less frequent and less severe curves.

School-Aged Period

A similar clinical presentation to DMD is seen in juvenile-onset SMA. The initial disability usually becomes apparent within the first decade and includes difficulty in arising from the floor, climbing stairs, and keeping up with peers during play and a waddling gait, which becomes more pronounced with attempts at running. Unlike DMD, no significant disability of upper extremity function is usually noted and proximal upper extremity strength is well preserved. Walking can usually be maintained lifelong as the primary means of ambulation. In those cases when weakness is noted before 2 years of age, however, a wheelchair or scooter may ultimately be required for mobility over long distances.

Management for the adolescent with juvenile-onset SMA is consistent with the concepts previously presented in this chapter. ROM exercises should be prescribed where appropriate, and selected strengthening exercises may be indicated to maintain functional skills. Adaptive equipment for mobility is not usually indicated; however, a power scooter for long-distance mobility may be needed in certain cases. If ADL become a problem, collaboration with an occupational therapist to address concerns may also be needed.

Transition to Adulthood

Difficulty in ADL that requires lifting of moderately heavy objects overhead can be expected, and vocational activities that involve manual labor are not recommended. Since life span is not significantly shortened, vocational planning is needed. No significant disability requiring adaptive equipment or environmental access is usually required until later in adulthood.

CASE HISTORY: DONALD

Donald is 21 years old and from a family with 6 siblings (3 brothers and 3 sisters). Three of the 4 boys were diagnosed with DMD. No family history of neuromuscular disease was reported, and diagnosis followed medical examination of Donald's older brother at the age of 5 years for clumsiness and frequent falls. Donald was 3 years of age at the time of diagnosis with a medical report of no significant gait deviations but presence of mild shoulder girdle and trunk flexor muscle weakness, evidence of a Gower sign after the third attempt to rise to standing from the floor, and pseudohypertrophy of the posterior calf musculature.

Physical therapy assessment at age 8 years demonstrated a gait pattern typical for DMD as previously described. No significant disability was noted, and impairments were only minimal. Donald was independent on stairs using a handrail but demonstrated a two-foot-per-step progression. Functional status corresponded to grade 2 on the scale published by Vignos and associates (1963) (see Table 13–2). ROM was within normal limits, with the exception of mild limitation of ankle dorsiflexion with the knee in extension. Muscle strength was quantified with manual muscle testing and recorded as fair plus in the shoulder and hip girdle musculature, poor in the abdominals, and good minus in the intermediate and distal upper and lower extremities. A home program was provided that included daily ROM of the posterior calf musculature and instruction on general activities to avoid excessive fatigue. Services were coordinated by the local MDA clinic with a follow-up visit every 6 months.

Donald's initial disability was related to independent mobility with progressive loss of walking, which by the age of 12 involved inability to climb stairs and increased frequency of falls with attempts to walk on uneven surfaces. Furniture around the house and walls were commonly used for balance. He was independent in scooting on the floor and used crawling for additional mobility at home. Although he was not able to stand from the middle of the floor, he was able to pull up to standing at a supportive surface. Night splints were initiated to augment the ROM program for the ankle plantar flexion contractures, and a manual wheelchair was provided for assistance with long-distance mobility. Muscle strength demonstrated progressive decline with manual muscle testing measuring poor grades for the proximal hip and shoulder girdle musculature, fair plus grade for knee extension, and a Vignos scale rating of 5. Evidence of mild tightness of the iliotibial band was present, and limitation of full hip and knee extension by 5° was noted. The ROM program was expanded to include the additional areas of tightness.

By the age of 15, Donald was walking only short distances and primarily for mobility around the home. A three-wheeled motorized scooter was provided for distance mobility, and Donald was independent in all transfers from the scooter. A raised toilet seat and tub bench were provided for the bathroom. With the passage of Public Law 94-142, physical therapy services were provided in the educational setting and Donald's home program was augmented by a school program including standing using a prone stander, ROM exercises 3 times per week, and adaptive physical education activities for general mobility and upper and lower extremity strengthening.

Progressive weakness and flexion contractures at the hip and knee resulted in the loss of walking when Donald was 17. It should be noted that this is exceptionally late for the loss of walking since 10 to 11 years is more typically reported (Brooke, 1986). Because Donald's older brother had died following complications from a fracture resulting from a fall while wearing KAFOs, Donald and the family decided against continuation of a walking program using orthoses. A daily standing program at school was maintained until progression of the contractures resulted in a need to discontinue the program since orthopaedic intervention was not desired by the family. Assistance for bathing was now required, with Donald using a tub bench and hand-held shower. Donald was independent with dressing and eating when assistance was provided for setup. Transfers to and from the scooter were independent if the transfer surfaces were level, but assistance was otherwise required. Donald was independent with bed mobility including rolling but required assistance to sit up at bed side. Mobility using the scooter was independent with infrequent use of the manual wheelchair when access or transportability problems with the scooter were en-

countered. A urinal was used to limit the need for transfers at school or home.

Currently, Donald is at stage 8 on Table 13–2. Physical therapy follow-up is provided as requested or yearly through the MDA clinic. Within the past 2 years a mild scoliosis has developed and is being radiographically monitored by an orthopaedist every 6 months. The motorized scooter has been replaced by a standard power wheelchair as seen in Figure 13–10 owing to progression of upper extremity weakness and a need to provide greater trunk support in sitting. Donald requires assistance for transfers in the bathroom but uses a sliding transfer to enter and exit from his bed (Fig. 13–11). A Hoyer lift is available if needed for transfers by the family. Minimal assistance is required for dressing and bathing. A wheeled commode chair is used at home.

Donald, or as he prefers, "the Duckman," has graduated from high school and is currently working part-time as a volunteer. He assists an art teacher at a school for children with multiple disabilities (Fig. 13–12). Donald's career goal is to pursue commercial art, and assistance has been sought through vocational rehabilitation services.

CASE HISTORY: GIDEON

Gideon is a bright and inquisitive 21-month-old boy with a diagnosis of type I SMA (see Fig. 13–8). He was born at 32 weeks' gestation without significant neonatal complications and was discharged after 4 days. The only concerns during the early neonatal period were problems tolerating formula and frequent episodes of choking. Gideon is an only child.

Gideon's mother reported that he had a spontaneous

FIGURE 13–10. Donald using power mobility for ambulation.

FIGURE 13-11. Donald demonstrating sliding board transfer technique used for chair to bed transfers.

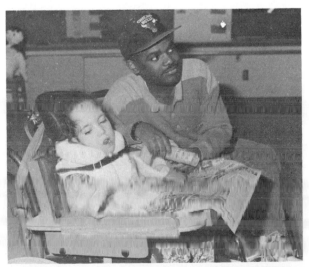

FIGURE 13-12. Donald assisting student in art class.

and interactive smile with cooing at 2 months of age, midline play with shaking and banging of toys by 5 months, but delayed head control, no rolling, and limited movement. At 5 months of age the pediatrician stated concern about Gideon's developmental delays in head control and rolling, but because of family history of later motor milestone development, further evaluation was not completed until the next well-baby checkup at 8 months of age.

At 9 months, Gideon was referred to an MDA Clinic for further assessment. He was noted to lie quietly supine with limited spontaneous movement. He would play with a toy while supine and roll to side-lying but was unable to roll to prone. Verbalizations were frequent. In the prone position, limited head righting into extension was noted and the mother reported limited use of this position because Gideon often fussed when placed prone. Head righting reactions in supported sitting were developed, and he was able to maintain prop sitting momentarily. Fasciculations of the tongue were noted. Following electromyographic testing and a muscle biopsy the diagnosis of SMA was confirmed.

Home-based physical therapy services were authorized following the diagnosis, and services were coordinated through hospital visits for medical follow-up. Equipment included a customized seating insert and mobility base for transportation. A therapy program was carried out at home with Gideon's mother as the primary caregiver. The program included instruction on positioning and handling for ADL, therapeutic exercise to facilitate head and trunk control, reaching games, and ROM. Pulmonary care instructions were given by a respiratory therapist. Routine pulmonary care included use of a percussor and nebulizer every 4 hours during the day.

Gideon has shown a regression in gross motor skill during the past 6 months with increased fatigability during activities such as sitting. He is able to prop sit when placed and rolls independently from supine to and from side-lying. Other developmental skills require assistance. A standing frame has been used for supported standing. He is very active in his chair using the tray for play, and side-lying is another positioning alternative that allows easy access to toys.

Medical intervention has been required for feeding and respiratory impairments. Choking with feeding continued to be a concern, and a fundoplication and placement of a gastric button were performed when Gideon was 11 months of age. At 20 months of age concern was expressed by Gideon's mother about his breathing at night, and after further evaluation oxygen by means of a nasal cannula has been initiated.

Even though Gideon's prognosis is not hopeful, he is a warm and intelligent child who is busy exploring his world. He takes delight in new adventures and brings great happiness to all those who care for him, especially his mother.

SUMMARY

Muscle weakness and contracture are hallmark features of the childhood forms of muscular dystrophy and spinal muscle atrophy. A background knowledge of therapeutic exercise, functional use of orthoses and adaptive equipment, and strategies to minimize disabilities secondary to these impairments allow the physical therapist to bring unique information and skills to the management team.

Many of the disorders significantly reduce longevity. Therefore, the quality of life and attention to how the family copes with the stress should be included in the team's intervention program. Providing the children and families with support and realistic expectations is an ongoing challenge. Support groups or contact with another family who has had a similar experience can often help the family work through crisis periods, particularly when extended family support is not available.

Through the combined perspectives and innovative solutions of team members, a comprehensive program can be provided that takes into consideration the multifaceted demands of each individual and family. A philosophy of using a family-centered approach to care will help to ensure that needs are met to the best of the team's ability.

Acknowledgment

My personal thanks goes to the children and their families who contributed to my knowledge of MD and SMA that made the writing of this chapter possible. Many challenges, accomplishments, disappointments, joy, and tears have paved the way. Special thanks to Donald and Gideon's family for sharing their stories and to Becky, who first inspired me to take this path of clinical work.

References

Abrahamson, AS. An approach to the rehabilitation of children with muscular dystrophy. Proceedings of the Second Medical Conference, Muscular Dystrophy Association, USA, 1952.

Alexander, MA, Johnson, EW, Petty, J, & Stauch, D. Mechanical ventilation of patients with late stage Duchenne muscular dystrophy: Management in the home. Archives of Physical Medicine and Rehabilitation, 60:289–292, 1979.

Amendt, LE, Ause-Ellias, KL, Eybers, JL, Wadsworth, CT, Nielsen, DH, & Weinstein, SL. Validity and reliability testing of the scoliometer. Physical Therapy, 70:108–117, 1990.

American Academy of Orthopaedic Surgeons. Joint Motion, Method of Measuring and Recording. Chicago: American Academy of Orthopaedic Surgeons, 1965.

Arahata, K, Ishiura, S, & Ishiguro, T. Immunostaining of skeletal and cardiac muscle surface membrane with antibody against Duchenne muscular dystrophy peptide. Nature, 333:861-863, 1988.

Bach, JR. Ventilator use by Muscular Dystrophy Association patients. Archives of Physical Medicine and Rehabilitation, 73:179-183, 1992.

Bach, JR, Campagnolo, DI, & Hoeman, S. Life satisfaction of individuals with Duchenne muscular dystrophy using long-term mechanical ventilatory support. American Journal of Physical Medicine and Rehabilitation, 70:129–135, 1991.

Bach, JR, & McKeon, J. Orthopaedic surgery and rehabilitation for the prolongation of brace-free ambulation of patients with Duchenne muscular dystrophy. American Journal of Physical Medicine and Rehabilitation, 70:323–331, 1991.

Bach, JR, O'Brien, J, Krotenberg, R, & Alba, AS. Management of end stage respiratory failure in Duchenne muscular dystrophy. Muscle and Nerve, 10:177–182, 1987.

Ballestrazzi, A, Gnudi, A, Magni, E, & Granata, C. Osteopenia in spinal muscular atrophy. In Merlini, L, Granata, C, & Dubowitz, V (Eds.), Current Concepts in Childhood Spinal Muscular Atrophy. New York: Springer-Verlag, 1989, pp. 215–219.

Bennett, RL, & Knowlton, GC. Overwork weakness in partially denervated skeletal muscles. Clinical Orthopedics, 12:22–29, 1958.

Bernier, JP, Brooke, MH, Naidich, TP, & Carroll, JE. Myoencephalopathy cerebral hypomyelination revealed by CT scan of the head in a muscle disease. Transactions of the American Neurologic Association, 104:244–246, 1979.

Binder, H. New ideas in the rehabilitation of children with spinal muscular atrophy. In Merlini, L, Granata, C, Dubowitz, V. (Eds.), Current Concepts in Childhood Spinal Muscular Atrophy. New York: Springer-Verlag, 1989.

Bleck, EE, & Nagel, DA. Physically Handicapped Children, A Medical Atlas for Teachers. New York: Grune & Stratton, 1982.

Bonilla, E, Samitt, CE, Miranda, AF, & Hays, AP. Duchenne muscular dystrophy: Deficiency of dystrophin at the muscle cell surface. Cell, 54:447–452, 1988.

Bowker, JH, & Halpin, PJ. Factors determining success in reambulation of the child with progressive muscular dystrophy. Orthopedic Clinics of North America, 9:431–436, 1978.

Brewer, EJ, McPherson, M, Magrab, PR, & Hutchins, VL. Family-centered, community-based, coordinate care for children with special health care needs. Pediatrics, 83:1055–1061, 1989.

Brooke, MH. A Clinician's View of Neuromuscular Diseases (2nd ed.). Baltimore: Williams & Wilkins, 1986.

Brooke, MH, Griggs, RC, Mendell, JR, Fenichel, GM, Shumate, JB, and Pellegrino, RJ. Clinical trial in Duchenne dystrophy: I. The design of the protocol. Muscle and Nerve, 4:186–197, 1981.

Brouwer, OF, Paderg, GW, Van Der Ploeg, RJO, Ruys, CJM, & Brand, R. The influence of handedness on the distribution of muscular weakness of the arm in facioscapulohumeral muscular dystrophy. Brain, 115:1587–1598, 1992.

Bundey, S, & Lovelace, RE. A clinical study of chronic proximal spinal muscular atrophy. Brian, 98:455–472, 1975.

Burke, SS, Grove, NM, & Houser, CR. Respiratory aspects of pseudohypertrophic muscular dystrophy. American Journal of Diseases of Children, 121:230–234, 1971.

Bushby, KM, Thambyayah, M, & Gardner-Medwin, D. Prevalence and incidence of Becker muscular dystrophy. Lancet, 337:1022–1024, 1991.

Cambridge, W, & Drennan, JC. Scoliosis associated with Duchenne muscular dystrophy. Journal of Pediatric Orthopedics, 7:436–440, 1987.

Chyatte, SB, Long, C, & Vignos, PJ. Balanced forearm orthosis in muscular dystrophy. Archives of Physical Medicine and Rehabilitation, 46:633–636, 1965.

Clarkson, HM, & Gilewich, GB. Musculoskeletal Assessment. Joint Range of Motion and Manual Muscle Strength. Baltimore: Williams & Wilkins, 1989.

Cohen, HJ, Molnar, GE, & Taft, LE. The genetic relationship of progressive muscular dystrophy (Duchenne type) and mental retardation. Developmental Medicine and Child Neurology, 10:754–765, 1968.

Colbert, AP, & Craig, C. Scoliosis management in Duchenne muscular dystrophy: Prospective study of modified Jewett hyperextension brace. Archives of Physical Medicine and Rehabilitation, 68:302–304, 1987.

Cullen, MJ, & Fulthorpe, JJ. Stages in fibre breakdown in Duchenne muscular dystrophy: An electron-microscopic study. Journal of Neurologic Science, 24:179–200, 1975.

Curran, FJ, & Colbert, AP. Ventilator management in Duchenne muscular dystrophy and postpoliomyelitis syndrome: Twelve years' experience. Archives of Physical Medicine and Rehabilitation, 70:100–186, 1989.

deLateur, BJ, & Giaconi, RM. Effect on maximal strength of submaximal exercise in Duchenne muscular dystrophy. American Journal of Physical Medicine, 58:26–36, 1979.

DeSilva, S, Drachman, DB, Mellitis, D, & Kuncl, RW. Prednisone treatment in Duchenne muscular dystrophy. Archives of Neurology, 44:818–822, 1987.

Donner M, Rapola, J, & Somer, H. Congenital muscular dystrophy: A clinico-pathological and follow-up study of 15 patients. Neuropediatrics, 6:239–258, 1975.

Dorscher, PT, Mehrsheed, S, Mulder, DW, Litchy, WJ, & Ilstrup, DM. Wohlfart-Kugelberg-Welander syndrome: Serum creatine kinase and functional outcome. Archives of Physical Medicine and Rehabilitation, 72:587–591, 1991.

Dubowitz, V. The clinical picture of spinal muscular atrophy. In Merlini, L, Granata, C, Dubowitz, V. (Eds.), Current Concepts in Childhood Spinal Muscular Atrophy. New York: Springer-Verlag, 1989, pp. 13–19.

Dubowitz, V. The muscular dystrophies. Postgraduate Medical Journal, 68:500–506, 1992.

Dubowitz, V, & Heckmatt, J. Management of muscular dystrophy. British Medical Bulletin, 36:139–143, 1980.

Edwards, RHT. Studies of muscular performance in normal and dystrophic subjects. British Medical Bulletin, 36:159–164, 1980

Emery, AEH, & Skinner, R. Clinical studies in benign (Becker-type) X-linked muscular dystrophy. Clinical Genetics, 10:189–201, 1976.

Eng, GD. Therapy and rehabilitation of the floppy infant. Rhode Island Medical Journal, 72:367–370, 1989a.

Eng, GD. Rehabilitation of the child with a severe form of spinal muscular atrophy (Type I, Infantile or Werdnig-Hoffman disease). In Merlini, L, Granata, C, & Dubowitz, V. (Eds.), Current Concepts in Childhood Spinal Muscular Atrophy. New York: Springer-Verlag, 1989b, pp. 113–115.

Fairley, HB. Principles and practice of mechanical ventilation. Applied Therapy, 10:36–40, 1968.

Fowler, WM. Rehabilitation management of muscular dystrophy and related disorders: I. The role of exercise. Archives of Physical Medicine and Rehabilitation, 63:208–210, 1982.

Fowler, WM, & Gardner, GW. Quantitative strength measurements in muscular dystrophy. Archives of Physical Medicine and Rehabilitation, 48:629–644, 1967.

Fukuyama, Y, Osaw, M, & Suzuki, H. Congenital muscular dystrophy of the Fukuyama type: Clinical, genetic and pathological considerations. Brain and Development, 3:1–29, 1981.

Gamstrop, I. Progressive spinal muscular atrophy with onset in infancy or early childhood. Acta Paediatrica Scandinavica, 56:408–423, 1967.

Gardner-Medwin, D. Objectives in management of Duchenne muscular dystrophy. Israel Journal of Medical Science, 13:229–234, 1977.

Gardner-Medwin, D. Controversies about Duchenne muscular

dystrophy: II. Bracing for ambulation. Developmental Medicine and Child Neurology, 21:659–662, 1979.

Gardner-Medwin, D. Rehabilitation in muscular dystrophy. International Rehabilitative Medicine, 2:104–110, 1980a.

Gardner-Medwin, D. Clinical features and classification of the muscular dystrophies. British Medical Bulletin, 36:109–115, 1980b.

Gibson, DA, Koreska, J, & Robertson, D. The management of spinal deformity in Duchenne's muscular dystrophy. Clinical Orthopedics, 9:437–450, 1978.

Gibson, DA, & Wilkins, KE. The management of spinal deformities in Duchenne's muscular dystrophy. Clinical Orthopedics, 108:41–51, 1975.

Gilliam, TC, Brzustowicz, LM, & Castilla, LH. Genetic homogeneity between acute and chronic forms of spinal muscle atrophy. Nature, 345:823–825, 1990.

Gilroy, J, & Holliday, P. Basic Neurology. New York: Macmillan, 1982.

Goebel, HH, Lenard, HG, Langenbeck, U, & Mehl, B. A form of congenital muscular dystrophy. Brain and Development, 2:387–400, 1980.

Granata, C, Magni, E, Sabattini, L, Colombo, C, & Merlini, L. Promotion of ambulation in intermediate spinal muscle atrophy. In Merlini, L, Granata, C, & Dubowitz, V. (Eds.), Current Concepts in Childhood Spinal Muscular Atrophy. New York: Springer-Verlag, 1989a, pp. 127–132.

Granata, C, Marini, ML, Capelli, T, & Merlini, L. Natural history of scoliosis in spinal muscular atrophy and results of orthopaedic treatment. In Merlini, L, Granata, C, & Dubowitz, V. (Eds.), Current Concepts in Childhood Spinal Muscular Atrophy. New York: Springer-Verlag, 1989b, pp. 153–164.

Granata, C, Merlini, L, Magni, E, Marini, ML, & Stagni, SB. Spinal muscular atrophy: Natural history and orthopaedic treatment of scoliosis. Spine, 14:760–762, 1989c.

Gucker, T. The orthopaedic management of progressive muscular dystrophy. Physical Therapy, 44:243–246, 1964.

Haas, A, & Pineda, H. Pulmonary Therapy and Rehabilitation: Principles and Practice. Baltimore, Williams & Wilkins, 1979, pp. 89–91.

Haley, SM, Coster, WJ, Ludlow, LH, & Haltiwanger, JT. Pediatric Evaluation of Disability Inventory (PEDI): Development, Standardization and Administration Manual. Boston: New England Medical Center Hospital, 1992.

Hanson, PA, & Rowland, LP. Moebius syndrome and facioscapulohumeral muscular dystrophy. Archives of Neurology, 24:31–39, 1971.

Harley, HG, Walsh, KV, Rundle, S, Brook, JD, Sarfarazi, M, Koch, JL, Harper, PS, & Shaw, DJ. Localization of the myotonic dystrophy locus to 19q13.2-19q13.3 and its relationship to twelve polymorphic loci on 19q. Human Genetics, 87:73–80, 1991.

Harper, PS. Congenital myotonic muscular dystrophy in Britain: I. Clinical aspects. Archives of Disease in Childhood, 50:505–513, 1975a.

Harper, PS. Congenital myotonic muscular dystrophy in Britain: II. Genetic aspects. Archives of Disease in Childhood, 50:514–521, 1975b.

Harper, PS. Myotonic Dystrophy (2nd ed.). Major Problems in Neurology, Vol. 21. Philadelphia: WB Saunders, 1989

Harris, SE, & Cherry, DB. Childhood progressive muscular dystrophy and the role of physical therapy. Physical Therapy 54:4–12, 1974.

Hausmanowa-Petrusewicz, I. Spinal Muscular Atrophy: Infantile and Juvenile Type. Springfield, VA: US Department of Commerce, National Technical Information Service, 1978.

Heckmatt, JE, Dubowitz, V, & Hyde, SA. Prolongation of walking in Duchenne muscular dystrophy with lightweight orthoses: Review of 57 cases. Developmental Medicine and Child Neurology, 27:149–154, 1985.

Hill, NS, Redline, S, Carskadon, MA, Curran, FJ, & Millman, RP. Sleep-disordered breathing in patients with Duchenne muscular dystrophy using negative pressure ventilators. Chest, 102:1656–1662, 1992.

Hoberman, M. Physical medicine and rehabilitation: Its value and limitations in progressive dystrophy. American Journal of Physical Medicine, 34:109–115, 1955.

Hoffman, EP, Brown, RH, & Kunkel, LM. Dystrophin: The protein product of the Duchenne muscular dystrophy locus. Cell, 51:919–928, 1987a.

Hoffman, EP, Fischbeck, H, & Brown, RH. Characterization of dystrophin in muscle-biopsy specimens from patients with Duchenne's or Becker's muscular dystrophy. New England Journal of Medicine, 318:1363–1368, 1988.

Hoffman, J. Ueber chronische spinale Muskelatrophie im Kindesalter, auf familiar Basis. Deutsche Zeitschrift fur Nervenheilkunde, 3:427, 1893.

Houser, CR, & Johnson, DM. Breathing exercise for children with pseudohypertrophic muscular dystrophy. Physical Therapy, 51:751–759, 1971.

Inkley, SR, Oldenburg, FC, & Vignos, DJ. Pulmonary function in Duchenne muscular dystrophy related to stage of disease. American Journal of Medicine, 56:297–306, 1974.

Johnson, EW, & Braddom, R. Over-work weakness in facioscapulohumeral muscular dystrophy. Archives of Physical Medicine and Rehabilitation, 52:333–336, 1971.

Johnson, EW, & Kennedy, JH. Comprehensive management of Duchenne muscular dystrophy. Archives of Physical Medicine and Rehabilitation, 52:110–114, 1971.

Jones, R, Khan, R, Hughes, S, & Dubowitz, V. Congenital muscular dystrophy: The importance of early diagnosis and orthopaedic management in the long-term prognosis. Journal of Bone and Joint Surgery (American), 61b:13–17, 1979.

Kendall, FP, & McCreary, E. Muscles: Testing and Function (3rd ed.) Baltimore: Williams & Wilkins, 1983.

Kingston, HM, Harper, PS, Pearson, PL, Davies, KE, Williamson, R, & Page, D: Localization of the gene for Becker muscular dystrophy. Lancet, 2:1200, 1983.

Kisner, C, & Colby, LA. Therapeutic Exercise: Foundations and Techniques. Philadelphia: FA Davis, 1985.

Koenig, M, Hoffman, EP, & Pertelson, CK. Complete cloning of the Duchenne muscular dystrophy (DMD) cDNA and preliminary genomic organization of the DMD gene in mouse and affected individuals. Cell, 50:509–517, 1987.

Kolobe, T. Working with families of children with disabilities. Pediatric Physical Therapy, 4:57–63, 1992.

Kugelberg, E, & Welander, L. Heredofamilial juvenile muscular atrophy simulating muscular dystrophy. Archives of Neurology and Psychiatry, 75:500, 1956.

Kunkel, LM, Monaco, AP, Middlesworth, W, Ochs, SD, & Latt, SA. Specific cloning of DNA fragments absent from the DNA of a male patient with an X chromosome deletion. Proceedings of the National Academy of Science, USA, 82:4778–4782, 1985.

Kushner, HS. When Bad Things Happen to Good People. London: Pan Books, 1981, pp. 54–79.

Lazaro, RP, Fenichel, GM, & Kilroy, AW. Congenital muscular dystrophy: Case reports and reappraisal. Muscle and Nerve, 2:349–1355, 1979.

Lee, CC, Pearlman, JA, Chamberlain, JS, & Caskey, CT. Expression of recombinant dystrophin and its localization to the cell membrane. Nature, 349:334–336, 1991.

Leibowitz, D, & Dubowitz, V. Intellect and behavior in Duchenne muscular dystrophy. Developmental Medicine and Child Neurology, 23:557–590, 1981.

Lonstein, JE. Management of spinal deformity in spinal muscular atrophy. In Merlini, L, Granata, C, Dubowitz, V. (Eds.),

Current Concepts in Childhood Spinal Muscular Atrophy. New York: Springer-Verlag, 1989, pp. 165–173.

Marshall, CR. Medical treatment of spinal muscular atrophy. In Gamstorp, I & Sarnat, HB (Eds.) Progressive Spinal Muscular Atrophies. International Review of Child Neurology Series. New York: Raven Press, 1984, pp. 163–171.

McMenamin, JB, Becker, LE, & Murphy, EG. Congenital muscular dystrophy: A clinical/pathological report of 24 cases. Journal of Pediatrics, 100:692–697, 1982.

Medical Research Council. Aids to the Investigation of Peripheral Nerve Injuries. London: Her Majesty's Stationery Office, 1976.

Merlini, L, Granata, C, Capelli, T, Mattutini, P, & Colombo, C. Natural history of infantile and childhood spinal muscular atrophy. In Merlini, L, Granata, C, & Dubowitz, V. (Eds.), Current Concepts in Childhood Spinal Muscular Atrophy. New York: Springer-Verlag, 1989, pp. 95–100.

Miller, F, Moseley, CF, & Koreska, J. Spinal fusion in Duchenne muscular dystrophy. Developmental Medicine and Child Neurology, 34:775–786, 1992.

Miller, G, & Dunn, N. An outline of the management and prognosis of Duchenne muscular dystrophy in Western Australia. Australian Pediatric Journal, 82:277–282, 1982.

Mokri, B, & Engel, AW. Duchenne dystrophy: Electron microscopic findings pointing to a basic or early abnormality in the plasma membrane of the muscle fiber. Neurology, 25:1111–1120, 1975.

Molnar, GE, & Alexander, J. Objective, quantitative muscle testing in children: A pilot study. Archives of Physical Medicine and Rehabilitation, 54:224–228, 1973.

Moosa, A, & Dubowitz, V. Spinal muscular atrophy in childhood: Two clues to clinical diagnosis. Archives of Disease in Childhood, 48:386–388, 1973.

Moser, H. Duchenne muscular dystrophy: Pathogenetic aspects and genetic prevention. Human Genetics, 66:17–40, 1984.

Mostacciuolo, ML, Lombardi, A, Cambissa, V, Danieli, GA, & Angelini, C. Population data on benign and severe forms for X-linked muscular dystrophy. Human Genetics, 75:217–220, 1987.

Muscular Dystrophy Association: Facts About Muscular Dystrophy, Tucson, AZ: Muscular Dystrophy Association, 1991.

Namba, T, Aberfeld, DC, & Grob, D. Chronic proximal spinal muscular atrophy. Journal of Neurologic Science, 11:401–423, 1970.

Newsom-Davis, J. The respiratory system in muscular dystrophy. British Medical Bulletin, 36:135–138, 1980.

O'Brien, T, & Harper, PS. Course, prognosis and complications of childhood-onset myotonic dystrophy. Developmental Medicine and Child Neurology, 26:62–67, 1984.

Pandya, A, Florence, JM, King, WM, Robinson, JD, Oxman, M, & Province, MA. Reliability of goniometric measurements in patients with Duchenne muscular dystrophy. Physical Therapy, 65:1339–1342, 1985.

Partridge, TA, Grounds, M, & Sloper, JC. Evidence of fusion between host and donor myoblasts in skeletal muscle grafts. Nature, 273:306–308, 1978.

Pearn, JH. The gene frequency of acute Werdnig-Hoffman's disease (SMA type 1): A total population survey in northeast England. Journal of Medical Genetics, 10:260–265, 1973.

Pearn, JH. Autosomal dominant spinal muscular atrophy: A clinical and genetic study. Journal of Neurologic Science, 38:263–275, 1978.

Pearn, JH. Classification of spinal muscular atrophies. Lancet, 1:919–922, 1980.

Pearn, JH, Carter, CO, & Wilson, J. The genetic identity of acute spinal muscular atrophy. Brain, 96:463–470, 1973.

Pinelli, G, Dominici, P, Merlini, L, DiPasquale, G, Granata, C, & Bonfiglioli, S. Cardiologic evaluation in a family with

Emery-Dreifus muscular dystrophy. Giornale Italiano di Cardiologia, 17:589–593, 1987.

Prosser, EJ, Murphy, EF, & Thompson, MW. Intelligence and the gene for muscular dystrophy. Archives of Disease in Childhood, 44:221–230, 1969.

Ringel, SP. Neuromuscular Disorders, A Guide for Patient and Family. New York: Raven Press, 1987.

Roy, L, & Gibson, DA: Pseudohypertrophic muscular dystrophy and its surgical management: Review of 30 patients. Canadian Journal of Surgery, 13:13–20, 1970.

Rutherford, MA, Heckmatt, JZ, & Dubowitz, V. Congenital myotonic dystrophy: Respiratory function at birth determines survival. Archives of Disease in Childhood, 64:191–195, 1989.

Saranti, AJ, Gleim, GW, & Melvin, M. The relationship between subjective and objective measurements of strength. Journal of Orthopedic Sports and Physical Therapy, 2:15–19, 1980.

Scott, OM, Hyde, SA, Goddard, C, & Dubowitz, V. Prevention of deformity in Duchenne muscular dystrophy: A prospective study of passive stretching and splintage. Physiotherapy, 67:177–180, 1981.

Scott, OM, Hyde, SA, & Goddard, E. Quantification of muscle function in children: A prospective study in Duchenne muscular dystrophy. Muscle and Nerve, 5:291–301, 1982.

Scott, OM, Vrbova, G, Hyde, SA, & Dubowitz, V. Responses of muscles of patients with Duchenne muscular dystrophy to chronic electrical stimulation. Journal of Neurology, Neurosurgery and Psychiatry, 49:1427–1434, 1986.

Seeger, BR, Sutherland, AD, & Clark, MS. Orthotic management of scoliosis in Duchenne muscular dystrophy. Archives of Physical Medicine and Rehabilitation, 65:83–86, 1984.

Shapiro, F, & Specht, L. Orthopaedic deformities in Emery-Dreifus muscular dystrophy. Journal of Pediatric Orthopedics, 11:336–340, 1991.

Siegel, IM. Plastic-molded knee-ankle-foot orthosis in the management of Duchenne muscular dystrophy. Archives of Physical Medicine and Rehabilitation, 56:322, 1975.

Siegel, IM. The Clinical Management of Muscle Disease: A Practical Manual of Diagnosis and Treatment. Philadelphia: JB Lippincott, 1977.

Siegel, IM. The management of muscular dystrophy: A clinical review. Muscle and Nerve, 1:453–460, 1978.

Siegel, IM. Muscle and its Diseases, An Outline Primer of Basic Science and Clinical Method. Chicago: Year Book Medical Publishers, 1986.

Siegel, IM, Miller, JE, & Ray, RD. Subcutaneous lower limb tenotomy in the treatment of pseudohypertrophic muscular dystrophy. Archives of Physical Medicine and Rehabilitation, 53:404–406, 1972.

Smidt, GL. Muscle Strength Testing: A System Based on Mechanics. Coralville, IA: Sparks Instruments and Academics, 1984.

Spencer, GE, & Vignos, PJ. Bracing for ambulation in childhood progressive muscular dystrophy. Journal of Bone and Joint Surgery (American), 44:234–242, 1962.

Stevenson, WG, Perloff, JK, Weiss, JN, & Anderson, TL. Facioscapulohumeral muscular dystrophy: Evidence for selective, genetic electrophysiologic cardiac involvement. Journal of the American College of Cardiology, 15:292–299, 1990.

Stuberg, WA, DeJong, S, & Gallagher, J. Bone density changes in nonambulatory children following immobilization of lasive standing programs. Developmental Medicine and Child Neurology, 33(suppl 64):34, 1991.

Stuberg, WA, & Metcalf, WM. Reliability of quantitative muscle testing in healthy children and in children with Duchenne muscular dystrophy using a hand-held dynamometer. Physical Therapy, 68:977–982, 1988.

Sussman, MD. Advantage of early spinal stabilization and fusion in patients with Duchenne muscular dystrophy. Journal of Pediatric Orthopedics, 4:532–537, 1984.

Swinyard, CA, Deaver, GG, & Greenspan, L. Gradients of functional ability of importance in rehabilitation of patients with progressive muscular and neuromuscular diseases. Archives of Physical Medicine, 38:574, 1957.

Tatelbaum, J. The Courage to Grieve. London: Heinemann, 1980.

Vignos, PJ. Physical models of rehabilitation in neuromuscular disease. Muscle and Nerve, 6:323–338, 1983.

Vignos, PJ, & Archibald, KC. Maintenance of ambulation in childhood muscular dystrophy. Journal of Chronic Diseases, 12:273–290, 1960.

Vignos, PJ, Spencer, GE, & Archibald, KC. Management of progressive muscular dystrophy. Journal of the American Medical Association, 184:103–112, 1963.

Vignos, PJ, & Watkins, MP. The effect of exercise in muscular dystrophy. Journal of the American Medical Association, 197:121–126, 1966.

Watt, JM, & Greenhill, B. Commentary: Rehabilitation and orthopaedic management of spinal muscle atrophy. In Gamstorp, I, & Sarnat, HB (Eds), Progressive Spinal Muscular Atrophies. International Review of Child Neurology Series. New York: Raven Press, 1984.

Werdnig, G. Eie fruhinfantile progressive spinale Amyotrophie. Archives fur Psychiatrie Nervenkrankheiten, 26:706–744, 1894.

Wilkins, KE, & Gibson, DA. Patterns of spinal deformity in Duchenne muscular dystrophy. Journal of Bone and Joint Surgery, 58:24–32, 1976.

Winsor, EJ, Murphy, EG, Thompson, MW, & Reed, TE: Genetics of childhood spinal muscular atrophy. Journal of Medical Genetics, 8:143–148, 1971.

Wohlfart, G, Fex, J, & Eliasson, S. Hereditary proximal spinal muscular atrophy: A clinical entity simulating progressive muscular dystrophy. Acta Psychiatrica Neurologica Scandinavica, 30:395–406, 1955.

Wratney, MJ. Physical therapy for muscular dystrophy. Physical Therapy Review, 38:26–32, 1967.

Yoshioka, M, Kuroki, S, Nigami, H, Kawai, I, & Nakamura, H. Clinical variation within sibships in Fukuyama-type congenital muscular dystrophy. Brain and Development, 14:334–337, 1992.

Zellweger, H, Simpson, J, McCormick, WF, & Ionaseslu, V: Spinal muscular atrophy with autosomal dominant inheritance. Neurology, 22:957–963, 1972.

Ziter, FA, & Allsop, KG. The diagnosis and management of childhood muscular dystrophy. Clinical Pediatrics, 15:540–548, 1976.

Ziter, FA, & Allsop, KG. The value of orthoses for patients with Duchenne muscular dystrophy. Physical Therapy, 59:1361–1365, 1979.

Ziter, FA, Allsop, KG, & Tyler, F. Assessment of muscle strength in Duchenne muscular dystrophy. Neurology, 27:981–984, 1977.

Appendix I

Clinical Protocol for Functional Testing in Duchenne's Muscular Dystrophy*

A. Pulmonary
1. Forced vital capacity
2. Maximum voluntary ventilation
B. Functional grade (arms and shoulders). Select one.
1. Starting with arms at the sides, the patient can abduct the arms in a full circle until they touch above the head.
2. Can raise arms above head only by flexing the elbow (i.e., shortening the circumference of the movement) or using accessory muscles.
   If 1 or 2 is entered above, how many kilograms of weight can be placed on a shelf above eye level, using one hand?
3. Cannot raise hands above head but can raise an 8-oz glass of water to mouth (using both hands if necessary).
4. Can raise hands to mouth but cannot raise an 8-oz glass of water to mouth.
5. Cannot raise hands to mouth but can use hands to hold pen or pick up pennies from the table.
6. Cannot raise hands to mouth and has no useful function of hands.
C. Pulmonary
1. Maximum expiratory pressure
D. Time to perform functions. Enter time in seconds. T = tried but failed to complete by time limit of 120 seconds.

1. Standing from lying supine.
2. Climbing four standard stairs (beginning and ending standing with arms at sides).
3. Running or walking 30 feet (as fast as is compatible with safety).
4. Standing from sitting on chair (chair height should allow feet to touch floor).
5. Propelling a wheelchair 30 feet.
6. Putting on a T-shirt (sitting in chair—see instructions).
7. Cutting a 3 × 3–inch premarked square from a piece of paper with safety scissors (lines do not need to be followed precisely).
E. Functional grade (hips and legs). Select one.
1. Walks and climbs stairs without assistance.
2. Walks and climbs stairs with aid of railing.
3. Walks and climbs stairs slowly with aid of railing (over 12 seconds for four standard stairs).
4. Walks unassisted and raises from chair but cannot climb stairs.
5. Walks unassisted but cannot rise from chair or climb stairs.
6. Walks only with assistance or walks independently with long-leg braces.
7. Walks in long-leg braces but requires assistance for balance.
8. Stands in long-leg braces but is unable to walk even with assistance.
9. Is in wheelchair.
10. Is confined to bed.

*From Brooke, MH, Griggs, RC, Mendell, JR, Fenichel, GM, Shumate, JB, & Pellegrino, RJ. Clinical trial in Duchenne dystrophy: I. The design of the protocol. Muscle and Nerve, 4:186–197, 1981.

Chapter 14

Limb Deficiencies and Amputations

MEG STANGER, PT, PCS, MS

Many different factors must be considered in the management of children with a limb deficiency or amputation. These factors differ from those involved in the management of adults with a limb deficiency or amputation because as children grow their neuromuscular systems continue to develop. Children also are emotionally immature and variably dependent on adults for care and decision-making regarding surgical and prosthetic issues (Tooms, 1985).

In this chapter the etiology of limb deficiencies and amputations in children, surgical management, physical therapy intervention relative to a child's age and developmental function, and pediatric prosthetic options are discussed. Emphasis is on the aspects of management that differ from those encountered by adults with amputations.

The child with an amputation is defined as a person with an amputation who is skeletally immature because the epiphyses of the long bones are still open (Aitken, 1963). Amputations can be classified as congenital or acquired. Annual surveys of child amputee clinics in the United States indicate that 60% of childhood amputations are congenital and 40% are acquired (Kay & Fishman, 1967; Tooms, 1992). Krebs and Fishman's (1984) study of 4105 children with limb deficiencies supports these findings. Krebs and colleagues (1991) further extrapolated from the data to estimate that the United States would be likely to experience 5525 new cases of childhood amputations per year, with 3315 of these amputations being congenital.

CONGENITAL LIMB DEFICIENCIES

Classification

Various classification systems of congenital limb deficiencies have been developed. Greek terminology has been used to describe various deficiencies but is often inaccurate and ambiguous (Day, 1991). Frantz and O'Rahilly (1961) developed a classification system based on embryologic considerations and the absent skeletal portions. Swanson and colleagues (1968) modified that system with a classification system of seven categories based on embryologic failure: 1) failure of formation of parts (arrest of development), 2) failure of differentiation (separation of parts), 3) duplication, 4) overgrowth, 5) undergrowth (hypoplasia), 6) congenital constriction band syndrome, and 7) generalized skeletal deformities. Further modifications were made by the International Society for Prosthetics and Orthotics (ISPO) in 1973 and 1989. The classification developed by the ISPO has now been accepted and published as an international standard, International Organization for Standardization (ISO) 8548-1:1989, "Method of describing limb deficiencies present at birth" (Day, 1991, 1992).

The ISO/ISPO classification of congenital limb deficiency is restricted to skeletal deficiencies described on anatomic and radiologic bases only; Greek terminology, such as hemimelia and phoco-melia, is avoided because of its lack of precision and difficulty of translation into languages that are not related to Greek (Day, 1991). Deficiencies are described as either transverse or longitudinal. In transverse deficiencies the limb has developed normally to a particular level beyond which no skeletal elements exist, although digital buds may be present. A transverse deficiency is described by naming the segment in which the limb terminates and then describing the level within the segment beyond which no skeletal elements exist (Day, 1991, 1992) (Fig. 14–1).

In longitudinal deficiencies there is as a reduction or absence of an element or elements within the long axis of a limb. Normal skeletal elements may be present distal to the affected bones. A longitudinal deficiency is described by naming the bones affected in a proximal to distal sequence and stating whether each affected bone is totally or partially absent (Day, 1991, 1992) (Fig. 14–2).

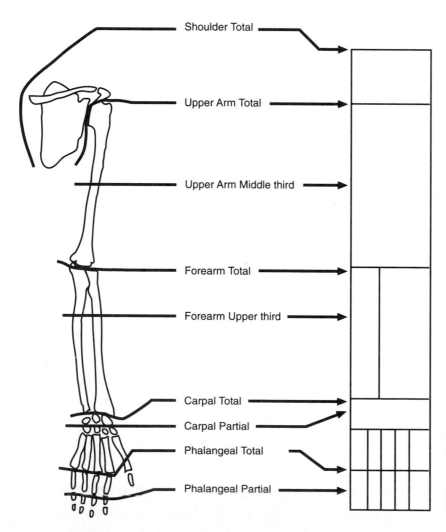

Shoulder Total
Upper Arm Total
Upper Arm Middle third
Forearm Total
Forearm Upper third
Carpal Total
Carpal Partial
Phalangeal Total
Phalangeal Partial

FIGURE 14–1. Examples of transverse deficiencies at various levels of the upper extremity. (From Day, HJ. The ISO/ISPO classification of congenital limb deficiency. In Bowker, JH, & Michael, JW [Eds.], Atlas of Limb Prosthetics: Surgical, Prosthetic, and Rehabilitation Principles [2nd ed.]. St. Louis: Mosby–Year Book, 1992, p. 747.)

Longitudinal
Tibia Total
Tarsus Partial
Ray 1 Total

FIGURE 14-2. Example of a longitudinal deficiency of the lower extremity. (From Day, HJ. The ISO/ISPO classification of congenital limb deficiency. In Bowker, JH, & Michael, JW [Eds.], Atlas of Limb Prosthetics: Surgical, Prosthetic, and Rehabilitation Principles [2nd ed.]. St. Louis: Mosby–Year Book, 1992, p. 748.)

Etiology

To fully understand the etiology of congenital limb deficiencies, a basic knowledge of embryonic skeletal development is necessary. Limb buds first appear at the end of the fourth week of embryonic development, arising from mesenchymal tissue. During the next 3 weeks the limb buds grow and differentiate into identifiable limb segments (Moore, 1982; Ogden, 1989). Development of limb buds occurs in a proximodistal sequence, with the upper limb developing ahead of the lower limb by several days. The mesenchymal tissue undergoes chondrification to become cartilaginous models of individual bones (Tooms, 1985). By the end of the seventh week a recognizable embryonic skeleton is present. Teratogenic factors must, therefore, be present at some time between the third and seventh weeks of embryonic development to produce a limb deficiency.

Brent (1985) reviewed human malformations and found that in 60 to 70% of cases the cause is unknown. Several teratogenic factors have been identified (e.g., thalidomide, contraceptives, irradiation) as possible causative factors for congenital limb deficiencies. Genetic factors have also been linked with some congenital limb deficiencies, such as Holt-Oram, Fanconi, Nager, and thrombocytopenia-absent radius syndromes (Lenz, 1980). The limb deficiency may be the result of sporadic genetic mutation (Lenz, 1980). For most children born with a limb deficiency, however, the cause is unknown.

Levels of Limb Deficiency

The clinical presentation of a child with a congenital limb deficiency depends on the type, level, and number of deficiencies. Almost any combination or variety of limb deficiency is possible, but some are more common, and these are discussed here in detail. Between 20 and 30% of children have limb deficiencies affecting more than one limb (Krebs & Fishman, 1984; Tooms, 1985) (Fig. 14-3).

Most transverse deficiencies are unilateral, with the transverse below-elbow limb deficiency being the most common (Wright & Jobe, 1991) (Fig. 14-4). Rudimentary finger vestiges called nubbins may be present. This type of deficiency occurs more frequently in females, with a left-sided predominance of almost 2:1 (Shurr & Cook, 1990).

A complex lower extremity congenital limb deficiency has been termed *proximal femoral focal deficiency* (PFFD). Aitken (1969) first described this deficiency, which includes absence or hypoplasia of the proximal femur with varying degrees of involvement of the acetabulum, femoral head, patella, tibia, and fibula. The deficiency may be unilateral or bilateral. Aitken describes four classes of severity, A through D, with class A exhibiting the least involvement (Fig. 14-5).

The clinical manifestations of a child with PFFD are relatively typical. They include a shortened thigh that is held in flexion, abduction, and external rotation; hip and knee flexion contracture; and severe leg-length discrepancy, with the foot often at the level of the opposite knee. These children also have instability of the knee joint secondary to absent or deficient cruciate ligaments and a 70 to 80% incidence of total longitudinal deficiency of the fibula. Fifteen percent of children with PFFD have bilateral involvement (Epps, 1983). The incidence of PFFD is reported to be 1 per 50,000 live births, and it is usually of unknown etiology (Herzenberg, 1991).

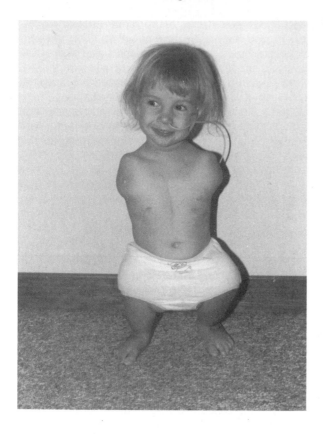

FIGURE 14-3. Child with multiple congenital limb deficiencies including bilateral transverse upper arm deficiency and bilateral proximal femoral focal deficiency.

ACQUIRED AMPUTATIONS

Acquired amputations account for approximately 40% of childhood amputations. Of these, 70 to 85% can be attributed to trauma (Challenor, 1992; Lamb & Law, 1987). The remainder of acquired amputations in children are the result of disease (most frequently tumors but also infection and vascular malformations). Ninety percent of acquired amputations involve only one limb, and the lower extremity is involved in 60% of cases (Tooms, 1985) (Figs. 14-6 and 14-7).

Traumatic Amputations

Accidents involving farm machinery and power tools are the leading causes of acquired amputations in the pediatric population, followed closely by vehicular accidents, gunshot wounds, and railroad accidents (Tooms, 1992). Incidences vary according to age and geographic location. Lawn mowers and household accidents account for most amputations in the 1- to 4-year-old population. Vehicular accidents, power tools and machinery, and gunshot wounds are common causes

FIGURE 14-4. Child with congenital transverse below-elbow limb deficiency.

TYPE		FEMORAL HEAD	ACETABULUM	FEMORAL SEGMENT	RELATIONSHIP AMONG COMPONENTS OF FEMUR AND ACETABULUM AT SKELETAL MATURITY
A		Present	Normal	Short	Bony connection between components of femur Femoral head in acetabulum Subtrochanteric varus angulation, often with pseudarthrosis
B		Present	Adequate or moderately dysplastic	Short, usually proximal bony tuft	No osseous connection between head and shaft Femoral head in acetabulum
C		Absent or represented by ossicle	Severely dysplastic	Short, usually proximally tapered	May be osseous connection between shaft and proximal ossicle No articular relation between femur and acetabulum
D		Absent	Absent Obturator foramen enlarged Pelvis squared in bilateral cases	Short, deformed	(none)

FIGURE 14-5. Aitken classification of proximal femoral focal deficiency. (From Tachdjian, MO [Ed.], Pediatric Orthopedics [2nd ed.]. Philadelphia: WB Saunders, 1990, p. 556.)

of traumatic amputations in the older child (Tooms, 1992).

Disease-Related Amputations

SARCOMA OF BONE

Primary bone tumors are rare in children, accounting for 5% of cancers in children younger than 15 years of age (Austin, 1988). Annual incidence rates for childhood bone cancers in the United States are 5.5 per million for whites and 4.3 per million for African Americans. This represents

approximately a 1 in 12,000 chance of developing a bone malignancy before 15 years of age (Robinson et al., 1991). Osteosarcoma and Ewing's sarcoma are the most common of the primary bone tumors and account for 89% of malignant bone tumors in children (Robison et al., 1991). Childhood cancer statistics are based on children younger than 15 years of age; however, both osteosarcoma and Ewing's sarcoma continue to be seen in the late teenage years and beginning of the second decade of life with incidence rates comparable to the 10 to 14-year-old population. Both are more frequent in males than females (Link et al., 1991a).

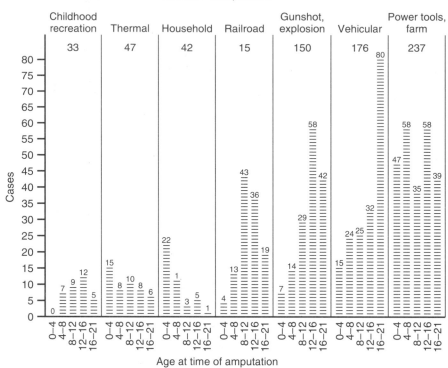

FIGURE 14-6. Etiology of acquired amputations due to trauma. (From Juvenile Amputee Course Manual. Evanston, IL: Northwestern University Medical School Prosthetic-Orthotic Program, 1983.)

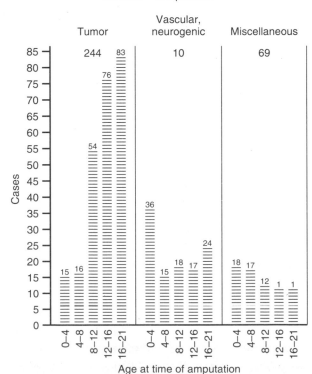

FIGURE 14-7. Etiology of acquired amputations due to disease. (From Juvenile Amputee Course Manual. Evanston, IL: Northwestern University Medical School Prosthetic-Orthotic Program, 1983.)

Osteosarcoma

Osteosarcoma is a primary malignant tumor of bone derived from bone-forming mesenchyme in which the malignant proliferating spindle cell stroma produces osteoid tissue or immature bone. The cause of osteosarcoma is unknown; however, osteosarcoma has been linked with exposure to ionizing radiation (Link et al., 1991a; Meyers, 1987a). A viral cause has also been suggested based on evidence that bone sarcomas can be induced through viruses in animals (Link & Eilber, 1988; Link et al., 1991a).

Osteosarcoma represents 50% of bone cancers in children in the United States. The annual incidence is 3.4 cases per million for whites and 2.5 for African-Americans. Annual incidences of fewer than 2 per million have been noted in Asian countries. Approximately 80% of childhood cases are diagnosed between 10 and 14 years of age (Robison et al., 1991).

The peak incidence of osteosarcoma coincides with the pubertal growth spurt, and it occurs most frequently at the metaphyseal portion of the most rapidly growing bones in adolescence. As a result, the distal femur, proximal tibia, and proximal humerus are the most common sites for osteosarcoma. This finding supports the theory that these rapidly growing cells are susceptible to oncogenic agents or mitotic errors and that osteosarcoma is the result of an aberration of the normal process of bone growth and remodeling (Link & Eilber, 1988; Link et al., 1991a; Meyers, 1987a).

Ewing's Sarcoma

Ewing's sarcoma is an undifferentiated round cell tumor. The tumor infiltrates bone marrow and, subsequently, adjacent soft tissue. Primary sites for Ewing's sarcoma are the weight-bearing bones of the lower extremity or pelvis. Ewing's sarcoma tends to occur in the diaphysis of long bones. The cause is unknown; however, radiation does not increase the risk (Link et al., 1991a).

Ewing's sarcoma is less common than osteosarcoma and represents 39% of bone tumors in children (Robison et al., 1991). The incidence in the United States is 2.4 cases per million children with an extremely low rate in African-Americans of 0.4 cases per million children. Eighty percent of patients are younger than 20 years of age; the median age is 11 years. Slightly more males than females are diagnosed with Ewing's sarcoma (Link et al., 1991a).

Diagnosis

The initial complaint for both osteosarcoma and Ewing's sarcoma is pain at the site of the tumor with or without a palpable mass. Localized swelling is present in 63% of children with Ewing's sarcoma. Systemic symptoms are rare in osteosarcoma unless widespread metastatic disease is present. On the other hand, systemic symptoms, most commonly fever and weight loss, are present in 25% of children with Ewing's sarcoma at the time of diagnosis (Link et al., 1991a). If fever is present, Ewing's sarcoma may be mistakenly suspected to be chronic osteomyelitis (Miser et al., 1988a). The most common site for tumors in children with osteosarcoma is the knee. Fifty percent of tumors arise from the distal femur and proximal tibia (Link et al., 1991a, Meyers, 1987a). Common sites for Ewing's sarcoma include the diaphyses of the weight-bearing bones of the lower extremity, the pelvis, and the humerus (Link et al., 1991a; Meyers, 1987b).

Because the initial complaint for both osteosarcoma and Ewing's sarcoma is pain at the site of the tumor, diagnosis is often delayed. Duration of symptoms before diagnosis averages 3 months for osteosarcoma and up to 6 months for Ewing's sarcoma (Link et al., 1991a). Children presenting to a physical therapist with a complaint of pain, which is often chronic, a negative history of injury, and no evidence of musculoskeletal abnormalies should be referred for further medical workup to rule out a malignant bone tumor.

The key to diagnosis of a bone tumor is a radiologic evaluation (Link et al., 1991a). Plain-view x-ray films, computed tomography, or magnetic resonance imaging will reveal evidence of a mass and bony destruction. A definitive diagnosis is made through biopsy and histologic examination (Meyers, 1987a; Meyers, 1987b). To complete the workup, a bone scan and chest computed tomography are performed to determine the extent of metastases.

Medical Management of Malignancies

Medical management of bony tumors and neoplasms includes several goals: 1) complete and permanent control of the primary tumor, 2) control and prevention of microstatic and metastatic disease, and 3) preservation of as much function as possible. Local control of the primary tumor is most often achieved through surgery and radiation therapy. Surgical options include amputation and numerous limb-sparing procedures. Which surgical procedure is selected varies depending on location and size of tumor, extramedullary extent, presence or absence of metastatic disease, and the child's age, skeletal development, and lifestyle. Control of microstatic and metastatic disease is achieved through radiation therapy and adjuvant chemotherapy (multidrug chemotherapy).

RADIATION THERAPY

Radiation therapy directs high-energy emissions at the tumor. The energy from the radiation disrupts the structure of atoms and damages essential molecules, including the chromosomes. Cell reproductive capacity is, therefore, compromised, leading to tumor cell death (Link, 1982). Damage can occur to surrounding normal tissue as well.

Osteosarcoma is generally unresponsive to radiation therapy. Osteosarcoma cells seem to repair themselves after radiation injury while Ewing's sarcoma is very responsive to radiation therapy (Link & Eilber, 1988; Link et al., 1991a; Miser et al., 1988a). Local control of Ewing's sarcoma may be achieved with moderately high doses of radiation to the entire bone and a boost of radiation to the primary tumor.

The side effects of radiation therapy are related to the primary site of the tumor, volume, dose rate, age of the patient, and use of chemotherapy. Acute side effects are seen in rapidly dividing tissues such as the skin, bone marrow, and gut. Common side effects are red and tender skin, mouth sores from irradiation to mucous membranes, and nausea and vomiting from irradiation to the abdomen. Irradiation of extremities produces few acute side effects (Link et al., 1991a). Children receiving radiation therapy may exhibit a decreased activity level secondary to nausea and vomiting, poor appetite secondary to mouth sores, and generalized malaise. Their physical therapy sessions may need to be altered on a daily basis to accommodate their changing energy levels. Children who may be wearing a prosthesis must be monitored closely for skin irritation and breakdown.

Late side effects of radiation include fibrosis of soft tissues, bony changes ranging from osteoporosis to fractures, and growth disturbances, including damage to the epiphyseal plate and bowing of the metaphysis. Greater growth disturbances are found in younger children (Goldwein, 1991). Butler and colleagues (1990) reported that 77% of patients with Ewing's sarcoma who received radiation therapy developed a leg-length discrepancy; in 58% of these patients the leg-length discrepancy was significant enough to require treatment. If possible, attempts are often made to shield the epiphyseal plate at the opposite end of the involved bone to minimize the radiation-linked growth retardation and still allow for some growth of the extremity. For some young children, an amputation may produce a more functional extremity than an extremity that is significantly shortened as the result of radiation therapy.

Secondary malignant neoplasms resulting from radiation therapy of the primary tumor are well documented. Meadows and colleagues (1985) cite data indicating that 3 to 12% of survivors of childhood cancer develop secondary neoplasms. Tucker and colleagues (1987) also report an increased risk of developing secondary bone tumors after receiving radiation therapy for childhood cancers.

CHEMOTHERAPY

The use of adjuvant chemotherapy has increased the survival rates for both osteosarcoma and Ewing's sarcoma. Children treated with surgery or radiation therapy alone have a poor prognosis, with 9 to 25% achieving 5-year survival (Link & Eilber, 1988; Miser et al., 1988b). Chemotherapy is used to control micrometastatic disease that is present but undetectable at diagnosis. It may also be used to control the size of the primary tumor. Preoperative chemotherapy may shrink the local tumor, making limb-sparing surgery a more feasible option or reducing the level of the amputation.

Five-year disease-free survival rates for children with Ewing's sarcoma treated with a combination of radiation therapy, chemotherapy, and, in some cases, surgery vary from 60 to 80% (Meyers, 1987b; Miser et al., 1988b). Survival rates are better for children whose tumors are more distal, rather than located on the axial skeleton, and for patients with no metastases at the time of diagnosis. Overall survival rates for children with osteosarcoma treated with a combination of surgery and chemotherapy have also drastically improved from 20% in the 1970s to 60 to 65% more recently (Link et al., 1991b).

Chemotherapy agents are circulated in the bloodstream and so are delivered to all tissues of the body. They enter the cells and disrupt metabolic processes, especially cell division (Link, 1982). The result is death of the invaded cells. Malignant cells are killed, but normal cells may also be damaged or killed. Typical side effects of chemotherapy include nausea and vomiting, hair loss, anemia, neutropenia, and thrombocytopenia. Most of these side effects are reversible (Link, 1982). Some chemotherapeutic agents produce more specific and dose-related side effects. Therapists treating children receiving chemotherapy should be aware of how these side effects and possible complications will affect therapy (Table 14–1).

TABLE 14–1. CHEMOTHERAPY AGENTS

Agent	Side Effects and Adverse Reactions	Therapy Concerns
Doxorubicin (Adriamycin)	Alopecia (hair loss), myelosuppression, orogastrointestinal reactions (oral reddening, ulcers, nausea, vomiting; more serious include diarrhea, dysphagia, gastrointestinal bleeding), myocardial toxicity (can lead to cardiac failure)	Extravasation can occur with intravenous administration. Reactions include stinging and burning sensation, possible cellulitis, blistering, and tissue necrosis. Life-threatening arrhythmias may occur during or within a few hours of administration. Cardiac failure is not often favorably affected by medical or physical support and must be detected early for successful treatment.
Bleomycin (Blenoxane)	Toxic to skin and lung tissues. Skin reactions include erythema, tenderness, hyperpigmentation. Pulmonary toxicities occur in 10% of patients. Pneumonitis may progress to pulmonary fibrosis and death.	Dyspnea is earliest symptom of pulmonary toxicity. Fine rales on auscultation. Pulmonary function test changes include decrease in total lung volume and decrease in vital capacity, but they are not predictive of development of pulmonary fibrosis. Pulmonary toxicity monitored through x-ray changes.
Dactinomycin (Actinomycin D), Cosmegen	Orogastrointestinal reactions, alopecia, myelosuppression, liver toxicity	Can impair wound healing. Corrosive to soft tissue. If extravasation occurs, severe damage to soft tissues will occur and can lead to contractures. Severe skin reactions occur where there has been previous irradiation.
Cyclophosphamide (Cytoxan)	Alopecia, nausea and vomiting, myelosuppression, hemorrhagic cystitis	Can impair wound healing. Must force liquids to control cystitis.
Dacarbazine (DTIC)	Myelosuppression, anorexia, nausea and vomiting, myalgias, malaise, alopecia	Extravasation after intravenous administration produces severe local pain and stinging; can result in tissue damage.
Methotrexate	Potential for serious toxicity. Toxicity is function of dose and duration of treatment. Orogastrointestinal reactions, myelosuppression, hepatic and/or renal damage occur with prolonged use. Leukoencephalopathy reported in patients with osteosarcoma. Neurologic effects include behavioral changes, abnormal reflexes, and focal sensorimotor signs. Pulmonary symptoms include dry nonproductive cough, fever, dyspnea, hypoxemia, and chest x-ray infiltrate.	After discontinuation of methotrexate, complete recovery not always noted with leukoencephalopathy. Blurred vision, headaches, aphasia, and hemiparesis are other neurologic adverse reactions seen with methotrexate. Seizures have led to coma in children. May be administered with anticonvulsants if on large doses.
Vincristine (Oncovin)	Alopecia, constipation, nausea and vomiting, hypertension and hypotension, neuromuscular side effects, cranial nerve manifestations, seizures	Monitor cardiovascular status. Neuromuscular side effects include pain distally, loss of deep tendon reflexes, footdrop, with progression to contractures, gait abnormalities, ataxia. Splinting may be helpful to avoid contractures. Extravasation during administration can lead to cellulitis. Paralysis of cranial nerves may be seen; most comonly affected muscles are extraocular and laryngeal.
Cisplatin (Platinol)	Nausea and vomiting, myelosuppression, cumulative renal toxicity, ototoxicity, peripheral neuropathies. Ototoxic effects can be more severe in children than adults.	Ototoxicity may include tinnitus and/or hearing loss in high frequency range. Occasionally may affect ability to hear normal conversation. Peripheral neuropathies may be irreversible and can include loss of motor function.

Data from Physicians' Desk Reference. Oradell, NJ: Medical Economics, 1993.

SURGICAL OPTIONS IN THE MANAGEMENT OF ACQUIRED AND CONGENITAL LIMB DEFICIENCIES

Amputation in the Management of Traumatic Injuries and Malignant Tumors

Although most of the basic premises related to management of adults with amputations apply to children, there are important differences. First, skeletal immaturity and future growth are important factors when considering surgical alternatives. Physes should be preserved whenever possible to ensure continued growth of the limb. For the upper extremity the majority of growth occurs in physes around the shoulder and wrist, whereas in the lower extremity the physes around the knee account for most of the growth (Herzenberg, 1991).

Second, the fact that amputation through long bones may result in terminal overgrowth is an important point that should not be overlooked. Terminal overgrowth is a painful, spike-like prominence of new bone on the transected end of the residual limb. Significant pain can interfere with weight bearing and wearing of prostheses. The spike-like growth is not the result of growth from the proximal epiphysis but rather represents osteogenic activity of the periosteum (Gillespie, 1990). Terminal overgrowth occurs most frequently in the humerus, followed in order of incidence by the fibula, tibia, and femur (Herzenberg, 1991; Kruger, 1980). Surgical options include revisions and bone capping. The possibility of terminal overgrowth should not be a reason to elect higher-level amputation, such as a knee disarticulation rather than a below-knee amputation. As in adults, length of the lever arm, function of the extremity, and prosthetic fit remain important considerations when deciding on the level of amputation. Saving the child's life is, of course, the most important consideration, whether the amputation is the result of a malignancy or trauma.

Finally, wound healing in children is rarely a concern as it may be in adults with peripheral vascular disease. Skin grafts, therefore, may be used to close the amputation site in preference to performing a higher-level amputation for a child with a traumatic injury.

Acquired amputations secondary to trauma may result in a short residual limb. This is especially true of an above-knee amputation in which the distal physes have been resected. It may be possible to increase the length of a residual limb in older children by using one of the limb-lengthening techniques. Eldridge and colleagues (1990) cite a case history of a child who had a traumatic amputation at a young age that resulted in a very short below-knee residual limb. The short residual limb limited socket design and was expected to diminish the efficiency of a below-knee-amputee gait pattern. The Ilizarov technique was used to increase bone length to allow better prosthetic fit and functional gait (see Chapter 15 for a discussion of limb-lengthening techniques).

The traditional approach for malignant bone tumors has been amputation of the limb in which the tumor is found. The surgical margin for an amputation is usually 6 to 7 cm above the most proximal medullary extent of tumor as defined on computed tomography or magnetic resonance imaging. This level of surgical margin allows for removal of microscopic tumor and skip lesions while allowing for the greatest amount of residual limb length for the individual. Studies have shown only a 5% local recurrence rate using this level of surgical margin (Link & Eilber, 1988; Link et al., 1991a).

For those tumor sites that are in the proximal humerus or femur, amputation results in severe loss of function. For example, a tumor of the proximal humerus treated by amputation would leave the patient with severely diminished function as a result of loss of the hand. Most surgeons will, therefore, elect not to perform an amputation, if possible, for tumors of the upper extremity. Amputation for tumors of the pelvis or proximal femur also result in complete loss of the limb or a very short residual limb, which makes functional ambulation with a prosthesis difficult. Some limb-sparing procedures may result in a more functional extremity than an amputation without decreasing the expected rate of survival for the child. The decision regarding an amputation is based on expectations regarding control of the primary tumor and survival of the child and the functional use of the extremity.

Amputation to Revise Congenital Limb Deficiencies to Improve Function

Rarely is an amputation necessary with upper extremity limb deficiencies, but it may be indicated for some children with lower extremity limb deficiencies. A child with bilateral PFFD, however, may be more functional without any surgery. They will be of short stature but will walk quite well (Herzenberg, 1991). For cosmesis, extension prostheses may be an option.

The surgical treatment of a child with unilateral PFFD is case-specific. If the child has a stable hip and foot and a significant portion of normal femur is present, one of the limb-lengthening procedures may be appropriate. Most surgeons agree that 60% of predicted femoral length must be present for a lengthening procedure to be a viable alternative (Gillespie, 1990; Herzenberg, 1991). The more standard treatment for PFFD is a knee arthrodesis and foot amputation. Usually the Syme or Boyd amputation is recommended. A Syme amputation involves complete removal of the foot, including the calcaneus, followed by sectioning of the distal tibia perpendicular to the weight-bearing line (Tachdjian, 1990a). A Boyd amputation preserves the calcaneus, providing a more bulbous surface for weight bearing, as well as preserving leg length (Herzenberg, 1991). The knee is usually fused to form one long bone for fitting of an above-knee prosthesis (Herzenberg, 1991; Koman et al., 1982) (Fig. 14–8).

Amputation may also be an option for a child with a longitudinal tibial or fibular total deficiency in which a significant limb-length difference exists along with deformity of the foot. Frequently the foot is positioned in equinovalgus with absent lateral rays. If the leg-length difference is too significant for limb-lengthening techniques or epiphysiodesis of the uninvolved leg, or if the ankle is significantly unstable, a Syme or Boyd amputation may lead to a more functional lower extremity with the addition of a prosthesis. When considering an amputation for a child, it is important that alternatives are discussed with the family and child and that the ultimate lifestyle goals are known.

FIGURE 14–8. Child with unilateral proximal femoral focal deficiency following a Boyd amputation of his foot. Note popliteal crease near the diaper line indicating where his knee is located.

Rotationplasty

Rotationplasty, or a turnabout procedure, is a surgical option for children with congenital limb deficiencies, specifically PFFD, as well as for those with bony tumors of the proximal tibia or distal femur. This procedure involves excision of the distal femur and proximal tibia; 180° rotation of the residual lower limb, including the distal tibia, ankle joint, foot, and neurovascular supply; and reattachment to the proximal femur. The ankle then functions as a knee joint, with ankle plantar flexion used to extend the "knee" and ankle dorsiflexion to flex the "knee" (Herzenberg, 1991; Kotz & Salzer, 1982). Rotationplasty results in a functioning hip joint and ankle joint. In the case of malignant tumors, the tumor cannot have invaded the surrounding soft tissue, especially the neurovascular supply.

The advantages of a rotationplasty are the increased limb length, improved prosthetic function with the ankle serving as a knee joint, improved weight-bearing capacity, and elimination of the problems of terminal overgrowth and pain from neuromas or phantom limb sensations (Kotz & Salzer, 1982). Weight is borne through the heel, which is more suitable for weight bearing than the end of a residual limb. Rotationplasty also allows for some growth of the leg. With an appropriate prosthesis, children who have had a rotationplasty procedure can run, jump, and play with their peers.

Disadvantages are cosmesis and derotation of the foot. Critics of rotationplasty cite poor cosmesis and psychological issues as a deterrent to the procedure. In my experience with children who underwent a rotationplasty for either a tumor or congenital PFFD, cosmesis was not a complaint from the child or their parents. Krajbich and Bochmann (1992) cite their experience of 27 children with osteosarcoma who underwent a rotationplasty. Twenty-two of these children are alive with no evidence of metastatic disease. No long-term complications related to cosmesis and psychological decompensation were reported; in fact, virtually all of the children with a rotationplasty now actively participate in sports and other activities with their peers. Before a rotationplasty it may be helpful for parents and the child to meet another child who has had the rotationplasty performed. Certainly, the cosmetic disadvantages must be discussed.

When the procedure is performed on young children, derotation of the foot may occur requiring rerotation of the limb. The limb may derotate secondary to the spiral pull of the muscles proximal and distal to the osteotomy (Tachdjian, 1990a). Both Krajbich and Bochmann (1989) and Gillespie (1990) discuss surgical options to limit derotation of the limb after a rotationplasty. Derotation is more common in children younger than 10 years of age and is most frequently seen in children when a rotationplasty is performed at 3 or 4 years of age (Gillespie, 1990).

Limb-Sparing Procedures

With the use of chemotherapy, improvements in diagnostic imaging to determine tumor margins, and new techniques of reconstruction, amputation is not always the treatment of choice for children with bony malignancies. Limb-salvage or limb-sparing procedures may be an alternative to amputation for some children with malignant bone tumors. Limb-sparing procedures involve resection of the tumor and reconstruction of the limb to preserve function without amputation of the limb.

The selection of appropriate children for limb-sparing surgery is critical. The goal of saving the limb should never compromise the goal of removing all gross and microscopic tumor (Link et al., 1991a). Limb-sparing surgery is contraindicated if the tumor has invaded the surrounding soft tissue to a large extent, if it involves the neurovascular supply, or if a wide surgical margin cannot be achieved (Finn & Simon, 1991). Limb-sparing surgery for the lower extremity of a young child may also not be beneficial when the child is skeletally immature and may be left with a severe leg-length discrepancy and nonfunctional lower extremity. In these cases amputation may be a better choice than limb-sparing surgery.

The majority of limb-sparing procedures require restoration of the structural integrity of the in-volved extremity. Restoration involves use of biologic materials such as cadaver allografts or autologous grafts or nonbiologic materials such as cement and metallic endoprosthetic devices (Link & Eilber, 1988).

Autologous grafts are rarely appropriate because long segments of bone must usually be excised. Replacement of the excised bone with a near-equal length of noninvolved bone from another portion of the body is often not possible. Allografts from cadavers are another option. If a short segment of bone is replaced with an allograft, the graft provides a latticework into which normal tissue grows so that eventually the allograft is incorporated into the normal tissue. Clinical experience has shown that this bony incorporation of an allograft is unusual when larger segments are used (Link & Eilber, 1988). Bone grafting is contraindicated with the use of postoperative radiation therapy because of the possible development of pseudoarthrosis. The exact effect of chemotherapy on the incorporation of bone grafts is not known at this time (Mercuri et al., 1991).

At times a tumor may be excised without replacing the excised bone. The proximal fibula may be resected if the soft tissue involvement is minimal and the peroneal nerve is not included in the soft tissue involvement. The biceps femoris tendon and fibular collateral ligament are reattached to the lateral condyle of the tibia (Tachdjian, 1990b). After healing, full knee motion and a normal gait pattern can be expected. The Tikhoff-Linberg procedure has been successfully used for osteosarcomas involving the proximal humerus when the brachial plexus is not included in the soft tissue involvement. With this procedure the proximal humerus is excised and not replaced. The remaining muscles of the upper arm are reattached to the trapezius and pectoralis muscles to suspend the remaining portion of the humerus (Springfield, 1991). The shoulder is unstable, but the elbow and hand are functional. With the increased use of endoprosthetics, a humeral device could be implanted to provide added stability and function to the shoulder area (Link & Eilber, 1988). In either case the functional outcome is superior to that following after amputation of the entire upper extremity.

Endoprosthetic devices are ultimately an extension of joint arthroplasty procedures. These manufactured devices are implanted in the area of the excised bone and can be custom-designed for the proximal humerus, elbow, proximal and distal femur, and proximal tibia. They have the advantage of being able to provide a functional joint as well as structural integrity to replace that of excised bone (Link et al., 1991a). Problems include loosening of the prosthesis, fracture, infection, and failure of the implant. Children and adolescents may be very active and create vigorous stresses on prosthetic implants that lead to failures and the need for replacement of the devices over time (Mercuri et al., 1991). They may also not be appropriate for the young skeletally immature child since these devices may not allow for growth.

Some of the newer designs of endoprostheses incorporate a telescoping unit that can be expanded to accommodate growth. Expansion of the prosthesis involves a minor surgical procedure at periodic intervals. The expandable prosthesis may function as the permanent prosthesis after skeletal maturity has been achieved or may need to be replaced by a conventional endoprosthesis if the device provides for poor function of the limb (Finn & Simon, 1991). Clinical experience with these telescoping units is limited and the structural strength of the device when it is fully expanded needs to be determined.

Several studies have reported comparable long-term survival rates between groups undergoing amputation versus a limb-sparing procedure (Eckhardt et al., 1985; Sim et al., 1985). The data seem to point out that limb-sparing surgery is as effective in controlling the tumor as amputation when adjuvant chemotherapy is used and when particular attention is given to patient selection, surgical margins, and surgical techniques. Limb-sparing procedures for the upper extremity clearly result in improved function for the patient when compared with amputation and the use of a prosthesis. More debate centers around limb-sparing techniques of the lower extremity and their functional results for the young child (Finn & Simon, 1991; Mercuri et al., 1991; Simon, 1991). More research is needed to determine the durability of endoprosthetic devices over a long period of time and the appropriateness of expandable prostheses for young skeletally immature children.

Limb-sparing surgery is often not appropriate for the child with a congenital limb deficiency. First, most children with limb deficiencies have associated problems of the involved extremity. They may have an unstable ankle joint for weight bearing, or the length of their residual limb is too short. Finally, limb-sparing procedures, especially those involving the use of endoprosthetic devices, do not allow for the growth that these young children will experience in their uninvolved limb.

Limb Replantation

For children with traumatic amputations, limb replantation may be a surgical option. As with other surgical options, the goal of replantation is directed not only at preserving the amputated limb but also at restoring pain-free function to the extremity that is superior to the function obtained with a prosthesis. For an upper extremity, replantation entails elbow and hand function as well as distal sensation. Replantation of a lower extremity must provide a painless, sensate extremity capable of bearing weight during normal daily activities (Gayle et al., 1991).

Contraindications for replantation include warm ischemic time of more than 10 hours; severe joint destruction or crush injury resulting in an immobile extremity; peripheral nerve injury that would limit return of sensation; and substantial soft tissue damage (Axelrod & Buchler, 1991; Gayle et al., 1991). Replantation may be a surgical option for children who are skeletally immature. If epiphyseal plates are preserved and revascularized, normal bone growth can be expected (Gayle et al., 1991).

Physical therapy is indicated for these children for wound care, control of edema, joint range of motion (ROM), strengthening, ambulation, and self-care activities. Rehabilitation will include close communication with the physician and family instruction both while the child is in the hospital and as an outpatient.

Phantom Limb Sensations

Phantom limb sensations are an occurrence in many adults with amputations, but few reports are available concerning children with phantom limb sensations. Some persons may believe that if young children do not complain of phantom limb pain, they, therefore, must not have any pain. Phantom limb sensations are rarely reported before the age of 6 years (Jenson & Rasmussen, 1989; Setoguchi & Rosenfelder, 1982). Simmel (1962) reported that the incidence of phantom limb sensations increases with the age of the child so that all children older than 8 years of age reported some degree of phantom limb sensations. Mount (1989) expounds on accepted theories of pain in children and suggests that young children are more disturbed by visually painful experiences such as a cut finger or a venipuncture than by internal pain and have not yet learned the potential negative responses of internal sensations. Young children may also not be able to appropriately verbalize the sensations they may be experiencing.

The phantom limb sensations and pain of adolescents can become quite intense. If left untreated, phantom limb sensations can become debilitating and interfere with prosthetic wear and daily activities. Some teenagers are able to control the sensations through rubbing or massaging the uninvolved limb at similar points to those in which they are experiencing the phantom limb sensations of the amputated limb. Others feel more in control by keeping a daily log of their sensations and reporting the pain intensities on one of a variety of pain scales. For some adolescents the use of analgesics may be beneficial. If available, a referral to a pain management team should be instituted for children undergoing amputations.

PHYSICAL THERAPY INTERVENTION FOR THE CHILD WITH A LIMB DEFICIENCY OR ACQUIRED AMPUTATION

The parents are an integral part of the rehabilitation team for a child with an amputation or limb deficiency. The rehabilitation team should also include an orthopaedist, prosthetist, and physical therapist who are experienced in the management of children with amputations. This may often mean traveling to a major medical center for periodic assessments and prosthetic adjustments. Physical therapy can be delivered in the local community if available, but the therapist must be in communication with the managing rehabilitation team.

The overall goal of physical therapy is to facilitate as normal a sequence of development as possible for the child and to prevent the development of secondary impairments or functional limitations. These impairments can include joint contractures and weakness with resultant functional limitations of limited mobility and a lack of independence in self-care skills. Physical therapy is directed toward preventing joint contractures, minimizing muscle strength imbalances, preventing skin breakdown, and developing independence with mobility and self-care skills. Ideally these goals are accomplished through physical therapy provided directly for a child and the family, home program instruction, and follow-up of a child's progress and functional outcomes. The child's age, type of limb deficiency or level of amputation, and other medical factors will all influence the intensity of physical therapy needed.

Infancy and Toddler Period

An infant with a limb deficiency should be referred for an initial assessment by a pediatric orthopaedist and a physical therapist shortly after birth. Monitoring by the physical therapist with suggestions to parents regarding positioning and stretching may be all that is needed initially. The motor development of children with multiple limb deficiencies or upper extremity deficiencies may become delayed or impaired owing to their inability to use their arms for such activities as pushing up to sit, crawling, and pulling to stand. Physical therapy is necessary to monitor the infant's developmental progress, ROM, and strength needed for later prosthetic use and for the parents' comfort with their child's progress. This can be accomplished through periodic physical therapy consultations, optimally at 1-month intervals, with home program updates for the parents.

Generally, infants with limb deficiencies do not develop contractures after birth but ROM should be carefully monitored according to individual needs. A child with a PFFD may need a home program to decrease the hip flexion and abduction contractures that are typically noted at birth and will later interfere with prosthetic fit. Most children with upper extremity limb deficiencies will maintain ROM and strength through their developmental activities.

Careful monitoring of the developing infant is necessary to evaluate ROM, functional strength, weight-bearing capabilities, and posture while prone, sitting, and standing. Often a child with a limb deficiency will tend to bear weight asymmetrically in prone and sitting activities. Some children will take increased weight on their limb-deficient side to free their noninvolved side for reaching and movement. Other children may take more weight through their noninvolved side because of weight-shifting and balance difficulties. Either of these asymmetries can have orthopaedic consequences. Suggestions may be given to the parents and therapy provided to encourage weight-shifting activities to improve symmetry. For the child with an upper limb deficiency this will encourage the co-contraction of shoulder musculature needed later for prosthetic use. For the child with a lower limb deficiency this encourages assumption of an erect trunk with normal balance reactions. Shifting weight to the limb-deficient side is also important for pre-prosthetic training needed for standing and ambulation activities.

If an infant is not progressing developmentally, physical therapy may be warranted to provide alternative methods of achieving the normal developmental sequence. For example, a child with bilateral upper extremity limb deficiencies may need assistance to learn to stand from sitting or to safely learn to balance in standing.

A child is usually fitted with a prosthesis at a developmentally appropriate age. A child with a lower extremity deficiency will, therefore, be fitted for a prosthesis when weight bearing is appropriate and the child is beginning to pull to stand (between 8 and 10 months of age depending on the child's developmental progress). A child with a unilateral PFFD may have a Syme or Boyd amputation (usually when he or she begins to pull to stand at age 8 to 12 months) and be fitted with a prosthesis after surgery (Herzenberg, 1991; Koman et al., 1982). A child with an upper extremity limb deficiency may be fitted with a prosthesis to assist with early playing skills in sitting or even earlier to assist with weight-bearing skills while prone. A child is best fitted with an upper extremity prosthesis at between 6 and 8 months of age or when sitting can be done independently (Krebs et al., 1991; Setoguchi & Rosenfelder, 1982).

When a child first receives a prosthesis, the fit and alignment as well as the overall function of the prosthesis are assessed. The initial session is spent on instructing the parents in proper donning of the prosthesis, in checking the skin, and in developing a wearing schedule. The initial goal is to have the infant or toddler wear the prosthesis comfortably for as many hours a day as possible and for the parents to be comfortable in donning and doffing the prosthesis. The prosthesis may be removed for naps and should be removed when the child sleeps at night.

A child with an upper extremity prosthesis may initially ignore it. The focus of therapy should be on having the child wear the prosthesis while playing and to begin to use it for bimanual play such as manipulating and holding large toys and during gross motor activities such as pushing up to sitting, protective reactions, and propping in sitting.

The child's first upper extremity prosthesis may have one of several terminal device options (Fig. 14–9). A young infant may have a passive hand that is cosmetically appealing but nonfunctional. This initial prosthesis is usually passive since infants are unable to activate a terminal device. As the child begins to engage in bimanual play, either a simple split hook (Hosmer Dorrance, Campbell, CA) or a Child Amputee Prosthetics Project (CAPP) (Hosmer Dorrance, Campbell, CA) terminal device is more functional. The split hook is similar to that used with adult prosthetics except smaller. The CAPP was designed specifically for children, is cosmetically more appealing than a hook terminal device, is safer than a hook for a young child, and provides an efficient grip without requiring great operating force (Gover & McIvor, 1992). The goal for the young child at this time is to adjust to the weight of a prosthesis, to begin to use it to manipulate larger toys, and to shake or remove toys placed in the terminal device by an adult (Setoguchi & Rosenfelder, 1982) (Fig. 14–10).

FIGURE 14-9. Terminal device options: *A*, Baby Mitt (Hosmer Dorrance, Campbell, CA). *B*, Sport Mitt (Therapeutic Recreation Systems, Boulder, CO). An infant size is suitable for crawling infants. *C*, Child Amputee Prosthetics Project (CAPP) (Hosmer Dorrance) voluntary opening device. *D*, Hosmer Dorrance 12P infant voluntary opening hook. *E*, Anatomically Designed-Engineered Polymer Technology (ADEPT) (Therapeutic Recreation Systems) infant voluntary closing hook.

A child is not expected to begin to operate the terminal device until 18 months of age or later (Gover & McIvor, 1992; Patton, 1989; Setoguchi & Rosenfelder, 1982). An active terminal device and cable as needed should be added to the child's prosthesis by 18 months of age. Training to operate the terminal device is dependent on the child's developmental level. Children can be taught to release objects placed in their terminal device at 15 months of age (Patton, 1989). Generally, children are taught to open the terminal device, place objects in it, and then release them, in that order (Gover & McIvor, 1992; Setoguchi & Rosenfelder, 1982). This corresponds with the normal developmental sequence of learning to grasp before learning to release objects. The therapist must be familiar with the mechanism that controls the terminal device because it can differ from child to child, depending on the design of the device. The CAPP and Hosmer Dorrance hook are voluntary-opening terminal devices. Forward reaching of the arm pulls the cable tight and activates opening of the terminal device. Children with a transverse deficiency of the upper arm will need to use scapular abduction to activate opening of the terminal device with the elbow locked; control of the prosthetic elbow comes at a later age. The ADEPT (Therapeutic Recreation

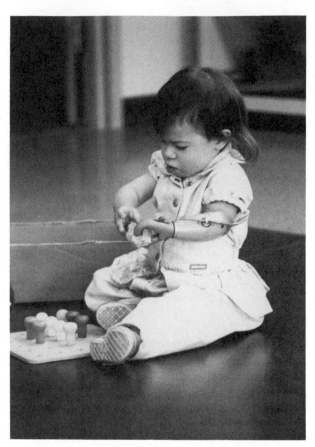

FIGURE 14–10. Child engaging in bimanual play wearing below-elbow prosthesis with an ADEPT voluntary closing hook.

Systems, Boulder, CO) hook is a voluntary-closing terminal device designed to mimic forward reaching to grasp or close on an object (Fig. 14–11). Enhanced motor development has been reported with the early fitting of a voluntary-closing terminal device (DiCowden et al., 1987).

Children younger than 2 years of age with a lower limb deficiency or above-knee amputation are often fitted with a prosthesis without a knee (Fig. 14–12). The goal is to begin weight-bearing and ambulation activities and to progress to learning control of a prosthetic knee when they are closer to 3 years of age.

When fitting a toddler with a lower extremity prosthesis, normal stance and gait patterns for their developmental age should be kept in mind. Children 1 year of age stand and walk with a wide base of support and exhibit increased hip external rotation during swing phase (Sutherland, 1984). For this reason, a toddler's prosthesis may need to be aligned with more hip abduction than that provided to an older child.

Because the goal of physical therapy is symmetry of posture and movements during developmental activities, proper alignment and controlled weight-shifting and balance activities are emphasized for children with a lower limb prosthesis. Many children with lower limb prostheses do not require an assistive device for ambulation; however, initial gait training with an assistive device promotes a reciprocal gait pattern and an erect trunk. As the child

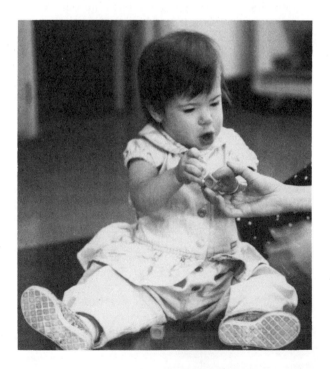

FIGURE 14–11. Therapist assisting child to operate the terminal device.

prosthesis can begin learning to control the elbow by 3 or 4 years of age. Most above-elbow prostheses will involve a dual cable system that allows the child to control both elbow flexion and extension and forearm pronation and supination. With control of the elbow and forearm the terminal device of the prosthesis becomes more functional in a variety of positions.

Emphasis should always be on assisting the child to learn skills that are appropriate for their age. Play skills involving manipulation of smaller objects, using the prosthesis to hold and turn paper for coloring and cutting activities, holding the handlebars of a tricycle, and self-dressing and feeding skills are all important. A child with a unilateral upper limb prosthesis will always use it as a helper hand and not as the dominant hand.

For those children with bilateral upper limb deficiencies the use of a prosthesis should be carefully monitored. These children should always be allowed to use their feet or mouth for play and self-care activities. A prosthesis may aid these children for only some periods of the day and may actually limit their function during some activities.

Myoelectric prostheses are an option that should be discussed with the parents of a preschool-aged child with an upper limb deficiency. These prostheses are not body-powered but are controlled by surface electrodes in the prosthetic socket that receive electrical signals from residual limb muscles to activate a motor-driven hand (Singer & Lombardo, 1992). The use of a myoelectric prosthesis is most successful when fitting occurs between 3 and 5 or 6 years of age (Gover & McIvor, 1992; Sauter, 1989). Advantages of a myoelectric prosthesis are improved cosmesis and functional use of the hand with minimal physical effort. Disadvantages include weight of the prosthesis, cost, electric components that require repair, and a lack of durability (Gover & McIvor, 1992). If a child is fitted with a myoelectric prosthesis, therapy is necessary to learn to control the hand and use the prosthesis functionally.

Children with a lower limb deficiency, including those children with unilateral PFFD, should be functional ambulators at this age. A child with a below-knee limb deficiency should be wearing a prosthesis for most of the day and engaging in normal activities with peers. The child with an above-knee limb deficiency should be ready to begin ambulation with a prosthesis with a knee joint by around age 3 years. Initially, children are usually given a constant-friction knee joint. They may need a short period of physical therapy to learn control of the knee joint and weight-shifting activities without falling.

FIGURE 14–12. Fourteen-month-old child with lower extremity prosthesis without a knee component.

develops balance and is able to control weight shifting during therapy and at home he or she will naturally discard the assistive device when he or she is comfortable with independent ambulation.

Preschool- and School-Aged Period

When a child attends a preschool or kindergarten class for the first time, many anxieties may resurface for the parents of a child with a limb deficiency. Parents will worry that their child may not fit in or will look different from his or her peers. For this reason the preschool years should emphasize development of independence in self-care skills, mobility, and acquisition of school skills such as coloring, cutting, and writing.

The child with an upper limb deficiency should be able to activate the terminal device of their prosthesis by this age. Children using an above elbow

During the preschool years some surgery is usually necessary for the child with a unilateral PFFD. Arthrodesis of the knee joint, usually performed between 2½ and 4 years of age, increases the lever arm of the thigh and decreases the hip and knee flexion contractures (Gillespie, 1990; Koman et al., 1982). Femoral and/or tibial epiphysiodesis may be performed at the time of knee arthrodesis. The ultimate goal is for limb length on the prosthetic side to be 5 cm shorter than that of the contralateral femur. This enables the prosthetic knee joint to be at approximately the same level as the contralateral knee joint at maturity (Epps, 1983). Placement of the prosthetic knee joint at the same level as the contralateral knee joint allows for improved cosmesis as well as an improved gait.

For the child with an acquired lower extremity amputation an immediate fit prosthesis is usually used. This may not be the case if significant trauma was present to the surrounding tissue or if skin grafting was necessary after the injury. Postoperative physical therapy is similar to that of an adult.

Children are more likely to move about after an amputation than an adult so contractures are less likely to occur. However, some children undergoing chemotherapy are quite ill and weak and may tend to lie in bed with their residual limb propped on pillows. They will need to be monitored for developing contractures, and parents and nursing staff will need to be instructed in ROM exercises and positioning of the residual limb.

Children are also more likely to bear weight on their immediate-fit prosthesis than adults. Gait training should begin as soon as cleared by the physician. Young children can safely learn to ambulate with an immediate-fit prosthesis using a walker or crutches. If a child has been hospitalized for a period of time, strengthening exercises of the uninvolved leg and the residual limb may be necessary.

After the removal of the immediate-fit prosthesis the child is fitted with a permanent prosthesis. The exception to this would be a child who is undergoing chemotherapy. These children tend to have weight fluctuations secondary to side effects of the medications. They are better fitted with a socket that allows for weight fluctuations, such as one with Velcro closures. Children with above-knee amputations should be fitted with a prosthesis with a knee joint. Most children with an above-knee amputation will initially require a pelvic strap to help hold the prosthesis in place. Some children may do well with a suction socket and no straps. Instruction must be given to both the parents and the child in the donning and doffing of the prosthesis and care of the prosthesis.

The child who undergoes a rotationplasty is usually casted to allow for healing of the bone. The cast may incorporate a pylon to permit the shortened leg to contact the ground for safe ambulation using a walker or crutches. After the cast is removed and the bone is healed the child with a rotationplasty must work on increasing ROM at the ankle joint, which functions as their knee. For ambulation and sitting, 0 to 20° of ankle dorsiflexion is more than adequate. Some children will be able to achieve 30° of ankle dorsiflexion, which will allow for some squatting activities and facilitate bike riding. Maximal plantar flexion will allow for greater extension of the leg in stance. Optimal plantar flexion ROM is at least 45 to 50°; the prosthetist can align the prosthesis to achieve an additional few degrees of plantar flexion for stance. Exercises should begin gently and progress to active and resistive exercises.

The child who underwent a rotationplasty is fitted with a custom-made prosthesis that incorporates the foot in a position of maximum plantar flexion and allows it to act as a knee joint. An external knee hinge joint must be used with an attached thigh cuff. The prosthesis is usually held in place with a pelvic strap.

Gait training for all children at this age will focus on symmetry and the normal characteristics of gait such as stride length, step length, and velocity, and all skills that the child needs to participate in play and games with other children.

When attending school for the first time, the child will be questioned about the prosthesis and assistive devices. This is especially true of a child with an upper limb deficiency. A meeting before the beginning of school with the child and his or her parents, the child's teacher, and perhaps the child's physical therapist may be helpful to allay any concerns and to answer or develop a way to answer the questions of the child's peers. The child with a unilateral limb deficiency or amputation should succeed in school with minimal adaptations.

The child with bilateral upper limb deficiencies may need to use a tape recorder or computer to assist with writing skills. In school, a child with bilateral upper limb deficiencies may be able to carry papers or books in the classroom between the chin and shoulder. The child also may use the mouth for manipulation and holding objects such as pencils. Whether the child uses his or her feet in school for manipulation or grasping is something that should be clearly discussed with the child, parents, and teacher before school entrance. Many children will opt not to use their feet for grasping objects in public as they get older; however, this can limit their independence, especially with toileting and feeding. If a child is adept with the use of his or her feet and is independent and chooses to use the feet, this should not be discouraged. If the teacher displays a supportive attitude toward the child's use of the feet, the child's classroom peers will soon view this as usual procedure in their classroom. The ultimate goal is for the child to be functional in our society as an adult; this may mean use of the feet or a combination of use of the feet and prostheses.

Adolescence and Transition to Adulthood

Adolescence with its hallmark concerns of appearance and acceptance by peers, relationships with the opposite sex, career decisions, and the struggle for independence can be a trying time for anyone. Teenagers with a congenital limb deficiency have been adjusting both functionally and emotionally from birth. At this point in their lives they are part of a social network of friends, realize the support of their families, and have attempted and succeeded at various activities in school and the community. They will be dealing with these adolescent issues right alongside their peers, although increased fears concerning dating and social acceptance can be typical at this time.

By contrast, an amputation of a limb during the adolescent years adds quite an emotional burden to a teenager. They have to deal with the loss of a body part and the grieving process and may be facing the possibility of death. Added to the physical appearance difficulties are the possible side effects such as hair loss from chemotherapy. A teenager who is facing a possible amputation as the result of cancer should be included, if he or she desires, in discussions of treatment options, including surgical options. Obviously, this is not possible if the amputation is the result of sudden trauma.

The immediate postoperative concerns and program for adolescents are very similar to those described for school-aged children. If an immediate-fit prosthesis is not used, teenagers are more likely to develop edema of their residual limb following surgery. In that case, wrapping of the residual limb or fitting with a shrinker sock should be instituted.

Teenagers who sustain a lower extremity amputation are fitted with a prosthesis when the residual limb has stabilized. They should be involved in the fitting of the prosthesis as well as in deciding on the design of the socket and type of knee joint and foot to be used. For most teenagers a large variety of prosthetic options are available. These should be fully discussed with the teenager and parents, and the choice should complement the lifestyle of the user. Both the teenager and his or her family should

be cautioned that the prosthesis will not function or look exactly like the contralateral limb.

Many teenagers with a high above-knee amputation will attempt to ambulate with a prosthesis but will ultimately opt for no prosthesis and crutches. A gait with crutches is faster and more energy-efficient. The decision to use or not to use a prosthesis should be the child's and not be based on society's idea of the most appropriate physical appearance. Some teenagers will use a prosthesis for certain activities and not for others. The ultimate goal is for them to be comfortable with their peers and interact with their peers in school and socially.

The use of prosthetics will vary for teenagers with upper limb deficiencies. For those who have become very adept with a prosthesis since early childhood, they likely will continue to use their prosthesis. The teenager who has an upper limb amputation may learn to operate a body-powered above- or below-elbow prosthesis. To become functional with the prosthesis requires much practice and the teenager may opt not to use one.

One major milestone for teenagers is the acquisition of a driver's license. Nearly all teenagers with a limb deficiency or amputation can learn to drive. Hand controls can be used for the teenager with bilateral PFFD or with bilateral lower extremity amputation as the result of trauma. For the teenager with a unilateral upper limb deficiency or amputation very minimal adjustments will be necessary. Driving can be done by using the sound hand, or a driving ring can be used to assist with stabilization of the steering wheel. A driving ring attaches to the steering wheel, and the terminal device, preferably a hook, is slipped into the ring. The driver can then use two extremities to control the steering wheel but can easily slip the hook out of the driving ring in case of emergencies. Driving becomes more difficult for the teenager with bilateral upper limb deficiencies or amputations. A driving ring may be used by the dominant limb. Controls on the instrument panel such as light switches may need to be moved to the dominant side and within reach of the limb. The turn signal can be extended or knee-operated. Unless specifically trained in the area of driver education, physical therapists should assist the teenager and his or her parents to seek information and driver training from a local rehabilitation center.

Career and college decisions are also made during adolescence. Some teenagers may work at a part-time job during high school. All teenagers with limb deficiencies or amputations will eventually seek employment. At times, adjustments need to be made to a prosthesis, such as a specific terminal device, to assist the young adult in his or her particular career area. Going to college is a true test of independence with self-care skills. Some individuals with bilateral upper limb deficiencies or multiple limb deficiencies will always require some degree of assistance with self-care activities. Toileting, especially wiping after defecation, and dressing, specifically managing underpants and bras, are self-care activities for which it is difficult for any one with bilateral upper limb deficiencies or short above-elbow amputations to achieve total independence. This does not preclude attending college or independent living, but an aide or other arrangements may be needed. Creativity, experimentation, and talking with other teenagers or adults with limb deficiencies can often produce strategies for accomplishing difficult tasks.

OVERVIEW OF PROSTHETICS

Upper Extremity Prosthetics

Upper extremity prosthetic components include a terminal device, a wrist unit, possibly an elbow unit, a socket, and possibly a harness and cable system. Terminal devices range from the passive baby mitten to a myoelectric hand. Terminal devices often used in pediatrics include the baby mitt, cosmetic hand, CAPP, and various hooks, including the Dorrance and ADEPT models (see Fig. 14–9). The child's age and size as well as the parents' and child's desires and functional goals determine the appropriate terminal device. The wrist unit allows forearm pronation and supination and accommodates the terminal device.

As a child's activities change, different terminal devices may be needed. Various recreational terminal devices are available to allow participation in a variety of sports activities (Krebs et al., 1991; Michael et al., 1990). Teenagers may desire a cosmetic hand for social activities and a functional terminal device for daily activities.

Most upper limb prostheses are suspended with a harness system. Two basic systems are used; the chest strap and the figure-eight. The chest strap or harness fits over the shoulder of the involved limb and around the chest to secure the prosthesis without limiting movement of the shoulders. The figure-eight harness securely anchors the prosthesis so that the child may activate the cable system of an above-elbow prosthesis (Setoguchi & Rosenfelder, 1982). Suction sockets are available for young children. A simple suction socket may be all that is necessary to suspend a below-elbow prosthesis of an infant or toddler. When the cable for the terminal device is added to the prosthesis an above-elbow pad or cuff to secure the cable can be incorporated.

A shoulder disarticulation prosthesis is secured with a chest strap and often with a thigh strap for the young child. A thigh strap can provide added power to operate the control system of a shoulder disarticulation prosthesis and may provide more excursion than the chest strap (Setoguchi & Rosenfelder, 1982).

Lower Extremity Prosthetics

Until recently few options for the foot were available in pediatric lower extremity prosthetics. The SACH (Otto Bock Orthopedic, Plymouth, MN) foot has long been the mainstay for pediatric prosthetic feet and continues to be used for young toddlers. The new designs in adult energy-storing prosthetic feet are now making their way into pediatric prosthetics. Pediatric sizes are available in the Seattle Lightfoot (Model and Instrument Development, Seattle, WA), SpringLite (SpringLite, Salt Lake City, UT), and Flex-Foot (Flex-Foot Inc., Laguna Hills, CA). Many school-aged children and adolescents may also be fitted with a STored ENergy (STEN) (Kinsley Manufacturing, Costa Mesa, CA) prosthetic foot or a College Park Foot/Ankle System (College Park, Fraser, MI) (Fig. 14–13).

The shank of a lower extremity prosthesis is either an exoskeletal or an endoskeletal design. Exoskeletal shanks are fabricated of wood covered with hard plastic, while endoskeletal shanks consist of a pylon made of ultralight materials, such as graphite, titanium, and covered with foam. Teenagers prefer endoskeletal shanks because of their cosmesis and decreased weight. The durability of exoskeletal shanks is often more appropriate for the younger child.

Knee unit availability is often limited by the child's size. Most prostheses for children utilize a constant-friction knee. A constant-friction knee is set to function at a certain walking speed. If the speed of walking increases, the prosthesis lags behind since the shank cannot swing through as quickly as the uninvolved limb. Another type of knee joint available for the pediatric population is a polycentric knee with a four-bar linkage mechanism (Fig. 14–14). A polycentric knee mimics the anatomic knee joint to increase stability. The axis of motion is posterior during stance to provide added stability and anterior during swing to shorten the shank and assist with clearance. This added stability in addition to the light weight of both the constant-friction knee and the four-bar linkage mechanism make them favored knee joints for the preschool- and school-aged child with an amputation.

Like adult sockets, pediatric socket design has changed in recent years. Movement is away from the bony weight bearing of patellar-tendon-bearing below-knee sockets and quadrilateral above-knee sockets toward more evenly distributed pressures (Michael et al., 1990). Children of all ages can be fitted with a narrowed medial-lateral ischial containment socket (Fig. 14–15). For children with an above-knee amputation the narrowed medial-lateral socket with ischial containment more evenly distributes weight-bearing pressures and allows less lateral movement of the distal femur, therefore providing more stability during stance. Some children, however, will prefer a quadrilateral socket, and some teenagers with a large fatty residual limb are more comfortable in a quadrilateral socket (Fig. 14–16).

Because teenagers and children are generally very active, a well-fitting above-knee or below-knee

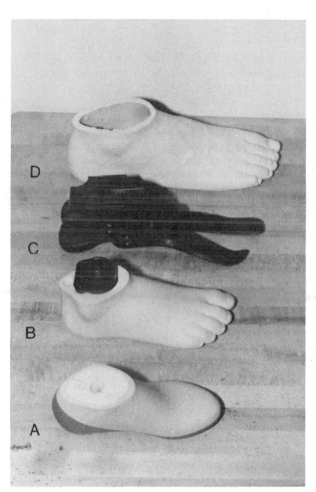

FIGURE 14–13. Prosthetic feet options. *A*, Solid-ankle cushion heel (SACH) assembly (Kinsley Manufacturing Co., Costa Mesa, CA; Otto Bock Orthopedic Industries, Inc., Minneapolis, MN). *B*, Seattle LightFoot Child's Play (Model and Instrument Development, Seattle, WA). *C*, College Park Foot/Ankle System (College Park Industries, Fraser, MI), which allows increased inversion/eversion mobility through graded ankle bushings. *D*, Cosmetic cover for College Park Foot/Ankle System.

A larger variety of knee units are available for teenagers, including hydraulic and pneumatic knees. Hydraulic and pneumatic knee units are variable-friction units that allow variable walking and running speeds. Variable-friction units are equipped with a swing control mechanism that sets the drag of the shank through swing phase and a stance control unit that permits knee flexion during stance without collapse of the leg. Swing and stance control mechanisms are excellent options for active teenagers, especially those engaged in physical activities. Drawbacks of hydraulic and pneumatic knees are the added weight to the prosthesis, cost, and intricacy of adjustments.

FIGURE 14–14 Prosthetic knee component with four-bar linkage mechanism

FIGURE 14–15. Narrowed medial-lateral ischial containment socket.

FIGURE 14–16. Quadrilateral socket.

socket is essential. During prosthetic fitting and socket design a clear plastic check socket may be used to easily identify areas of pressure and allow modification before the final socket is fabricated. Colloidal suspensions such as dental alginate can be added to a socket to fill any empty spaces during weight bearing to further distribute pressures within the prosthesis (Michael et al., 1990).

Infants and toddlers will require some type of suspension in addition to a suction socket. A Silesian belt works well for younger children with an above-knee amputation or PFFD; preschoolers can become independent in its use. By school age most children will not require this additional suspension. For active children and those participating in athletics, the newer Neoprene sleeves provide excellent suspension of the prosthesis for both below-knee and above-knee amputees.

A child with a PFFD who has not had his or her foot amputated will need a prosthesis that incorporates the foot. Usually the foot is plantar flexed in the socket to limit bulkiness (Krebs et al., 1991). The socket must be molded to fit the thigh; this is especially true if the foot has been amputated. These children often present with a bulbous upper thigh and a very thin tapered distal limb.

Children with a rotationplasty also use a prosthesis that incorporates the plantar flexed foot in the socket. The socket is essentially a below-knee socket with a thigh cuff attachment and external hinges for the knee joint. A Silesian belt may be needed for suspension.

Children of all ages with a limb deficiency or amputation should be encouraged to participate in activities with their peers. Many children may want to participate in sports at either a recreational or a competitive level (Fig. 14–17). There are many prosthetic options available that promote participation in various sports. Recreational prosthetics options are too numerous to mention for this discussion, and the reader is referred to other resources. Kegel (1986, 1992) discusses sports options in detail. Information is also available on various upper extremity terminal devices for recreational and sports activities (Michael et al., 1989; Radocy, 1992). Kegel (1992) includes a comprehensive resource list outlining sporting associations, camps for persons with amputations, and suppliers of specialized equipment and devices.

Ultimately, any prosthesis for a child must have some cosmetic appeal and be more functional than the limb without a prosthesis (Fig. 14–18). Decision-making for infants' and toddlers' prosthetic needs should include the parents, orthopaedist, prosthetist, and physical therapist. The older child

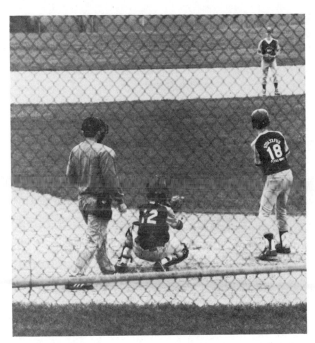

FIGURE 14-17. Catcher is an adolescent with a left below-knee amputation.

and physical therapy intervention needed to meet his or her goals.

The recent proliferation of prosthetic designs and materials available to the pediatric population has opened up many options for recreation and sports, vocation, and self-care, as well as early fitting of infants and toddlers with prostheses. Research is needed in the pediatric population to determine which surgical options, prosthetic designs, terminal devices, and materials best improve function, increase comfort, or decrease energy consumption. Physical therapists can easily contribute their expertise to the literature as well as initiate clinical research to investigate the effectiveness of various treatment options and prosthetic designs.

should be included in the decision-making process.

SUMMARY

The etiology and classification of congenital limb deficiencies and the causes of acquired amputations were reviewed in this chapter. An overview of the medical and surgical management of congenital limb deficiencies and amputations was presented. Treatment of a child with a congenital limb deficiency or amputation is complex and must involve a team of professionals who recognize the impact of various treatment options on the child's function in both the home and school environment and ultimately as an independent adult. Treatment options that involve careful planning and discussion with the family include surgical options, the use of chemotherapy and radiation therapy for those children with malignant tumors, and prosthetic options. Each child must be assessed as an individual, with consideration given to the child's age and musculoskeletal development, immediate and long-term functional abilities, family and child's activity level and lifestyle choices, and prosthetic

FIGURE 14-18. Recreational and social activities should not be limitations or obstacles for children with limb deficiencies or amputations.

Scott is a 7-year-old boy with a congenital right PFFD, Aitken type B. Aitken type B classification signifies presence of an acetabulum and femoral head, although the acetabulum may be dysplastic; ossification of the capital femoral epiphysis is delayed; the proximal portion of the femur is displaced laterally and upward, the femoral neck contains defective cartilage that fails to ossify, and the shaft of the femur is short and deformed (Tachdjian, 1990a). A radiologic assessment shortly after birth revealed an absence of the right distal femoral epiphysis, absence of right proximal tibial and fibular epiphyses, and a fibrous connection between the femoral head and proximal femur. A Boyd amputation of the right foot was performed at 8 months to allow for fitting of a lower extremity prosthesis and weight bearing. By 18 months Scott was walking independently with a prosthesis without a knee joint. He was followed every 3 to 4 months in an amputee clinic and seen by an orthopaedist, prosthetist, and physical therapist but did not receive intensive physical therapy except for a short period after receiving his first prosthesis.

A knee fusion was performed at 3 years of age to improve the lever arm length needed for an efficient gait. A metaphyseal-epiphyseal synostosis with bone grafting was also performed at that time to achieve stability in the region of the proximal femur. After cast removal, Scott was fitted with a new prosthesis with a knee joint and regular physical therapy sessions for 6 weeks were begun. Therapy was focused on strengthening of right lower extremity musculature, especially hip abduction motions, and decreasing the hip flexion contracture, along with gait training with a prosthetic knee.

Scott presently attends the first grade in his local school. He wears his prosthesis throughout the day. He ambulates independently without an assistive device, runs and climbs with his peers at recess, and is learning to ride a bicycle. He has been independent with donning and removing the prosthesis for several years. Before the start of his first year in school, Scott, his mother, and his physical therapist met with his teacher to discuss Scott's PFFD, use of a prosthesis, and his ability levels. Scott readily answers any questions his peers may ask about his prosthesis. At this time Scott requires no extra help in class or at school.

Scott will probably need to undergo a left distal femoral epiphysiodesis and right proximal tibial epiphysiodesis at age 9 or 10 years to ensure equal knee joint lengths at maturity. He continues to be followed at 6-month intervals in an amputee clinic by an orthopaedist, prosthetist, and physical therapist.

Andrew is a 6-year-old boy who was diagnosed with Ewing's sarcoma of the right distal femur at 3 years of age. He had no metastases at the time of diagnosis. Andrew underwent a course of preoperative chemotherapy to destroy any micrometastatic disease. Surgical options were discussed with the family including amputation and rotationplasty. At his young age an amputation would result in a very short above-knee residual limb. Limb-sparing procedures were not possible because of his young age and significant skeletal immaturity. For this reason also radiation therapy was not used for local tumor control. A rotationplasty was decided because it afforded a longer residual limb with more function than an above-knee amputation.

Postoperatively, Andrew was placed in a hip spica cast with his right ankle incorporated in approximately 45° of plantar flexion. A pylon was attached to the cast on the right. He received twice-daily physical therapy while an inpatient with the goals of ambulation with a walker and maintenance of upper body strength. He continued on chemotherapy postoperatively. Andrew was discharged home able to walk with a walker in the hip spica cast; the pylon attachment allowed for earlier and safer postoperative ambulation.

After cast removal Andrew received twice-weekly physical therapy to improve ROM and strength of his right ankle joint. His mother was instructed in a home program of ROM and strengthening exercises. A right ankle plantar flexion contracture was present after cast removal, but dorsiflexion to the neutral position was achieved within 1 week. Two weeks after cast removal right ankle motion was as follows: dorsiflexion 0 to 30° and plantar flexion 0 to 50°. Andrew could actively move his foot through available ranges, and resistive exercises were added. Cosmetically, Andrew exhibited no problems looking at or manipulating his foot. Both of his parents had met and spoken with a child who had had a rotationplasty before Andrew's surgery. His mother often expressed the feeling that dealing with the appearance of a "backward foot" was nothing compared with dealing with Andrew's cancer and unknown fate.

Following cast removal Andrew had been fitted with a prosthesis with external knee hinges, a thigh cuff, and a Silesian belt. He ambulated initially using a walker but quickly discarded it for independent ambulation.

Presently, Andrew attends kindergarten in his neighborhood school. He runs, climbs on playground equipment, and rides a scooter. His chemotherapy has ended, and Andrew is monitored for recurrence of his cancer. During the summer he goes to the community pool with his family and swims without the prosthesis.

So far Andrew's mother states he has not expressed any anger at the cosmesis of his leg. She has noticed stares from persons at the pool, but they quickly accept Andrew once they are aware of his medical history.

CASE HISTORY: JENNIFER

Jennifer is a 17-year-old girl who underwent a left above-knee amputation at age 14 secondary to osteosarcoma of the left distal femur. Limb-sparing procedures could not be done because the tumor encompassed both vascular and nerve supplies. Her residual limb after the amputation is very short. Before the amputation, Jennifer was a ninth grade student who actively participated on community and school sports teams. She is described by her parents as very outgoing with lots of friends.

Jennifer was fitted with an immediate-fit prosthesis in the operating room, but this had to be removed after several days when she developed open sores on her residual limb secondary to an allergic reaction. She was instructed in gait training with crutches, residual limb ROM, and wrapping to control edema and was discharged. She returned weekly to the hospital for chemotherapy and was monitored by a physical therapist at these visits. She was fitted with a temporary prosthesis with an expandable socket with Velcro closures after her wounds healed. Jennifer was very excited about receiving a prosthesis so she could run and play sports again.

Physical therapy sessions were begun three times a week when Jennifer received her prosthesis. Wearing time, skin checks, donning and removing the prosthesis, and gait training were reviewed with her and her parents. Jennifer gradually increased her prosthesis wearing time, wore it to school, and carried out her exercises. She quickly became very disenchanted with the prosthesis because she could not run and play sports as she could previously. She continued to go out socially with her friends. Gradually, Jennifer became less and less active, gained weight, and wore her prosthesis less and less. She eventually chose not to wear her prosthesis and opted for ambulation with forearm crutches. She continues to attend high school, occasionally watches her friends participate in sports, and is now working at a part-time job. Her parents sought counseling to assist Jennifer emotionally. They also enrolled her in a summer sports camp and a ski weekend for adolescents with amputations. She enjoyed those opportunities but did not use her prosthesis to participate in the activities.

In the past year, Jennifer has begun looking into getting her driver's license and has applied to work at a camp for amputees as a counselor. In conversations, she states she might like to get a new prosthesis, but at this time she appears quite content and functional without a prosthesis. Whether Jennifer goes on to further schooling, her career choice, and her use of a prosthesis are all decisions she has to make. She has a supportive family and network of friends to help her with these decisions.

References

Aitken, GT. Surgical amputation in children. Journal of Bone and Joint Surgery (American), 45:1735–1741, 1963.

Aitken, GT. Proximal femoral focal deficiency: Definition, classification, and management. In Proximal Femoral Focal Deficiency: A Congenital Anomaly. Washington, DC: National Academy of Sciences, 1969.

Austin, DF, Flannery, J, Greenberg, R, Isaacson, P, Key, C, Kolonel, LN, Platz, C, Swanson, GM, Thomas, D. West, D, & Young, JL. The SEER Program, 1973–1982. In Packin, DM, Stiller, CA, Draper, GJ, Bieber, CA, Terracini, B, & Young, JL (Eds), International Incidence of Childhood Cancer. Lyon, France: International Agency for Research on Cancer, 1988. (Distributed by Oxford University Press, New York.)

Axelrod, TS & Buchler, U. Severe complex injuries to the upper extremity: Revascularization and replantation. Journal of Hand Surgery [American], 16:574–584, 1991.

Brent, RL. Prevention of physical and mental congenital defects: The scope of the problem. In Marios, M (Ed.), Progress in Clinical and Biological Research, Vol. 163A. New York; Alan R Liss, 1985, pp. 55–68.

Butler, MS, Robertson, WW, Rate, W, D'Angio, GJ, & Drummond, DS. Skeletal sequelae of radiation therapy for malignant tumors. Clinical Orthopedics and Related Research, 251:235–239, 1990.

Challenor, Y. Limb deficiencies in children. In Molnar, GE (Ed.), Pediatric Rehabilitation (2nd ed.). Baltimore: Williams & Wilkins, 1992, pp. 400–424.

Day, HJB. The ISO/ISPO classification of congenital limb deficiency. Prosthetics and Orthotics International, 15:67–69, 1991.

Day, HJB. The ISO/ISPO classification of congenital limb deficiency. In Bowker, JH, & Michael, JW (Eds.), Atlas of Limb Prosthetics: Surgical, Prosthetic, & Rehabilitation Principles (2nd ed.). St. Louis, MO: Mosby–Year Book, 1992, pp. 743–748.

DiCowden, M, Ballard, A, Robinette, H, & Ortiz, O. Benefit of early fitting and behavior modification training with a voluntary closing terminal device. Journal of the Association of Children's Prosthetic Orthotic Clinics, 22:47–50, 1987.

Eckhardt, JJ, Eilber, FR, Grant, TT, Mirra, JM, Weisenberger, TH, & Dorey, FJ. Management of stage IIB osteogenic sarcoma: Experience at the University of California, Los Angeles. Cancer Treatment Symposia, 3:117–129, 1985.

Eldridge, JC, Armstrong, PF, & Krajbich, JI. Amputation stump lengthening with the Ilizarov technique. Clinical Orthopedics and Related Research, 256:76–79, 1990.

Epps, CH. Current concepts review proximal femoral focal deficiency. Journal of Bone and Joint Surgery (American), 65:867–870, 1983.

Finn, HA, & Simon, MA. Limb-salvage surgery in the treatment of osteosarcoma in skeletally immature individuals. Clinical Orthopedics and Related Research, 262:108–118, 1991.

Frantz, CH, & O'Rahilly, R. Congenital skeletal limb deficiencies. Journal of Bone and Joint Surgery (American), 43:1202–1204, 1961.

Gayle, LB, Lineaweaver, WC, Buncke, GM, Oliva, A, Alpert, BS, Billys, JB, & Buncke, HJ. Lower extremity replantation. Clinics in Plastic Surgery, 18:437–447, 1991.

Gillespie, R. Principles of amputation surgery in children with longitudinal deficiencies of the femur. Clinical Orthopedics and Related Research, 256:29–38, 1990.

Goldwein, JW. Effects of radiation therapy on skeletal growth in childhood. Clinical Orthopedics and Related Research, 262:101–107, 1991.

Gover, AM, & McIvor, J. Upper limb deficiencies in infants and young children. Infants and Young Children, 5:58–72, 1992.

Herzenberg, JE. Congenital limb deficiency and limb length discrepancy. In Canale, ST, & Beatty, JH (Eds), Operative Pediatric Orthopedics. St. Louis, Mosby–Year Book, 1991, pp. 187–251.

Jenson, TS, & Rasmussen, P. Phantom pain and related phenomena after amputation. In Melzack, W, & Wall, PD (Eds.), Textbook of Pain (2nd ed.). New York: Churchill Livingstone, 1989, pp. 508–519.

Kay, HW, & Fishman, S. 1018 children with skeletal limb deficiencies. New York University Post-Graduate Medical School, Prosthetics and Orthotics, 1967.

Kegel, B. Sports for the Leg Amputee. Redmond, WA: Medic Publishing, 1986, pp. 5–72.

Kegel, B. Adaptations for sports and recreation. In Bowker, JH, & Michael, JW (Eds.), Atlas of Limb Prosthetics: Surgical, Prosthetic, and Rehabilitation Principles (2nd ed.). St. Louis: Mosby–Year Book, 1992, pp. 623–654.

Koman, LA, Meyer, LC, & Warren, FH. Proximal femoral focal deficiency: Natural history and treatment. Clinical Orthopedics and Related Research, 162:135–143, 1982.

Kotz, R & Salzer, M. Rotation-plasty for childhood osteosarcoma of the distal part of the femur. Journal of Bone and Joint Surgery (American), 64:959–969, 1982.

Krajbich, JI, & Bochmann, D. Van Nes rotation-plasty in tumor surgery. In Bowker, JH, & Michael, JW (Eds.), Atlas of Limb Prosthetics: Surgical, Prosthetic, and Rehabilitation Principles (2nd ed.). St. Louis: Mosby–Year Book, 1992, pp. 885–899.

Krebs, DE, & Fishman, S. Characteristics of the child amputee population. Journal of Pediatric Orthopedics, 4:89–95, 1984.

Krebs, DE, Edelstein, JE, & Thornby, MA. Prosthetic management of children with limb deficiencies. Physical Therapy, 71:920–934, 1991.

Kruger, LM. Recent advances in surgery of lower limb deficiencies. Clinical Orthopedics and Related Research, 148:97–105, 1980.

Lamb, DW, & Law, HT. Incidence, classification, and etiology of upper limb abnormalities. In Lamb, DW, & Law, HT (Eds.), Upper Limb Deficiencies in Children. Boston: Little, Brown, & Co., 1987, pp. 7–17.

Lenz, W. Genetics and limb deficiencies. Clinical Orthopedics and Related Research, 148:9–17, 1980.

Link, MP. Cancer in Childhood: Physically Handicapped Children. New York: Grune & Stratton, 1982, pp. 43–58.

Link, MP, & Eilber, F. Osteosarcoma. In Pizzo, PA, & Poplack, DG (Eds.), Principles and Practice of Pediatric Oncology. Philadelphia: JB Lippincott, 1988, pp. 689–711.

Link, MP, Grier, HE, & Donaldson, SS. Sarcomas of bone. In Fernbach, DJ, & Vietti, TJ (Eds.), Clinical Pediatric Oncology (4th ed.). St. Louis: Mosby–Year Book, 1991a, pp. 545–575.

Link, MP, Goorin, AM, Horowitz, M, Meyer, WH, Belasco, J, Baker, A, Ayala, A, & Shuster, J. Adjuvant chemotherapy of high-grade osteosarcoma of the extremity. Clinical Orthopedics and Related Research, 270:8–14, 1991b.

Meadows, AT, Baum, E, Fossati-Bellani, F, Green, D, Jenkin, RD, Marsden, B, Nesbit, M, Newton, W, Oberlin, O, & Sallan, SG. Second malignant neoplasms in children: An update from the late effects study group. Journal of Clinical Oncology, 3:532, 1985.

Mercuri, M, Capanna, R, Manfrini, M, Bacci, G, Picci, P, Ruggieri, P, Ferruzzi, A, Ferraro, A, Donati, D, Biagini, R, DeMaio, M, Cazzola, A, & Campanacci, M. The management of malignant bone tumors in children and adolescents. Clinical Orthopedics and Related Research, 264:156–168, 1991.

Meyers, PA. Malignant bone tumors in children: Osteosarcoma. Hematology/Oncology Clinics of North America, 1:655–666, 1987a.

Meyers, PA. Malignant bone tumors in children: Ewing's sarcoma. Hematology/Oncology Clinics of North America, 1:667–673, 1987b.

Michael, JW, Gailey, RS, & Bowker, JH. New developments in recreational prostheses and adaptive devices for the amputee. Clinical Orthopedics and Related Research, 256:64–75, 1990.

Miser, JS, Triche, TJ, Pritchard, DJ, & Kinsella, T. Ewing's sarcoma and the nonrhabdomyosarcoma soft tissue sarcomas of childhood. In Pizzo, PA, & Poplack, DG (Eds.), Principles and Practice of Pediatric Oncology. Philadelphia: JB Lippincott, 1988a, pp. 659–688.

Miser, JS, Kinsella, TJ, Triche, TJ, Tsokos, M, Forquer, R, Wesley, R, Horvath, K, Belasco, J, Longo, DL, Steis, R, Glatstein, E, & Pizzo, PA. Preliminary results of treatment of Ewing's sarcoma of bone in children and young adults: Six months of intensive combined modality therapy without maintenance. Journal of Clinical Oncology, 6:484–490, 1988b.

Moore, KL. The Developing Human (3rd ed.). Philadelphia: WB Saunders, 1982, pp. 366–368.

Mount, BM. Psychological and social aspects of cancer pain. In Melzack, W, & Wall, PD (Eds.), Textbook of Pain (2nd ed.). New York: Churchill Livingstone, 1989, pp. 610–623.

Ogden, JA, Development of the lower limb. In Kalamachi, AS (Ed.), Congenital Lower Limb Deficiencies. New York: Springer-Verlag, 1989, pp. 1–45.

Patton, JG. Developmental approach to pediatric prosthetic evaluation and training. In Atkins, DJ, & Meier, RH (Eds.), Comprehensive Management of the Upper-Limb Amputee. New York: Springer-Verlag, 1989, pp. 137–149.

Radocy, B. Upper-limb prosthetic adaptations for sports and recreation. In Bowker, JH, & Michael, JW (Eds.), Atlas of Limb Prosthetics: Surgical, Prosthetic, and Rehabilitation Principles (2nd ed.). St. Louis: Mosby–Year Book, 1992, pp. 325–344.

Robison, LL, Mertens, A, & Neglia, JP. Epidemiology and etiology of childhood cancer. In Fernbach, DJ, & Vietti, TJ (Eds.), Clinical Pediatric Oncology (4th ed.). St. Louis: Mosby–Year Book, 1991, pp. 11–28.

Sauter, WF. Electric pediatric and adult prosthetic components. In Atkins, DJ, & Meier, RH (Eds.), Comprehensive Management of the Upper-Limb Amputee. New York: Springer-Verlag, 1989, pp. 121–136.

Setoguchi, Y, & Rosenfelder, R (Eds.). The Limb Deficient Child. Springfield, IL: Charles C Thomas, 1982.

Shurr, DG, & Cook, TM. Prosthetics and Orthotics. East Norwalk, CT: Appleton & Lange, 1990, pp. 183–193.

Sim, FH, Ivins, JC, Taylor, WF, & Chao, EYS. Limb-sparing surgery for osteosarcoma: Mayo Clinic experience. Cancer Treatment Symposia, 3:139–153, 1985.

Simmel, ML. Phantom experiences following amputation in childhood. Journal of Neurology, Neurosurgery, and Psychiatry, 25:69–78, 1962.

Simon, MA. Limb salvage for osteosarcoma in the 1980's. Clinical Orthopedics and Related Research, 270:264–270, 1991.

Singer, MB, & Lombardo, JR. Training can be fun at Shriner's myoelectric camp. Occupational Therapy Week, April 1992, pp. 24–25.

Springfield, DS. Musculoskeletal tumors. In Canale, ST & Beatty, JH (Eds.), Operative Pediatric Orthopedics. St. Louis: Mosby–Year Book, 1991, pp. 1073–1113.

Sutherland, DH. Gait Disorders in Childhood and Adolescence. Baltimore: Williams & Wilkins, 1984, pp. 14–27.

Swanson, AB, Barsky, AJ, & Entin, MA. Classification of limb malformations on the basis of embryological failures. Surgical Clinics of North America, 48:1169–1179, 1968.

Tachdjian, MO. Congenital deformities. In Tachdjian, MO (Ed.), Pediatric Orthopedics (2nd ed.), Vol. 1. Philadelphia: WB Saunders, 1990a, pp. 104–687.

Tachdjian, MO. Tumors and tumerous conditions of bone. In Tachdjian, MO (Ed.), Pediatric Orthopedics (2nd ed.), Vol. 1. Philadelphia: WB Saunders, 1990b, pp. 1186–1189.

Tooms, RE. The amputee. In Lovell, WW, & Winter, RB (Eds.), Pediatric Orthopedics (2nd ed.). Philadelphia: JB Lippincott. 1985, pp. 999–1053.

Tooms, RE. Acquired amputations in children. In Bowker, JH, & Michael, JW (Eds.), Atlas of Limb Prosthetics: Surgical, Prosthetic, and Rehabilitation principles (2nd ed.). St. Louis: Mosby–Year Book, 1992, pp. 735–741.

Tucker, MA, D'Angio, GJ, Boyce, JD, Strong, LC, Li, FP, Stovall, M, Stone, BJ, Green, DM, Lombardi, F, Newton, W, Hoover, RN, & Fraumeni, JF. Bone sarcomas linked to radiotherapy and chemotherapy in children. New England Journal of Medicine, 317:588, 1987.

Wright, PE, & Jobe, MT. Congenital anomalies of the hand. In Canale, ST, & Beatty, JH (Eds.), Operative Pediatric Orthopedics. St. Louis: Mosby–Year Book, 1991, pp. 253–330.

Chapter 15

Orthopaedic Conditions

JUDY LEACH, PT

In the course of their careers, physical therapists may meet patients with a wide variety of diagnoses or they may tend to specialize in one particular area. Almost without exception, however, a strong grounding in orthopaedics is a necessary part of a therapist's academic and clinical experience. For therapists specializing in the assessment and treatment of children, this orthopaedic knowledge is especially necessary and the acquisition of it particularly challenging because of one immutable fact —children grow. The human skeleton undergoes an incredible amount of growth and change in the years between birth and skeletal maturity. What may be considered "normal" at one age can be decidedly abnormal at another. For example, most infants have bowlegs (genu varum), but significant genu varum in an 8-year-old child would be cause for concern.

The rotational alignment of the lower extremity provides another example of the need for physical therapists to be familiar with the growth and development of the musculoskeletal system. Internal tibial torsion in the infant is commonly seen and considered normal for age. However, a high degree of internal tibial torsion in a 5-year-old child can result in an in-toeing gait that may produce a signifi-

icant functional deficit and require surgical correction.

In addition, as physical therapy practice becomes more autonomous, the burden and the challenge of timely identification of problems outside our scope of practice that require referral to other specialists are responsibilities we should all welcome and view as a necessary service to our patients.

In this chapter we certainly do not attempt an exhaustive review of all the orthopaedic conditions that affect children. A number of excellent texts already accomplish that (Lovell & Winter, 1978; Scoles, 1988; Tachdjian, 1990; Wenger & Rang, 1993). Instead, specific areas of concern to the physical therapist and commonly seen impairments will be highlighted in the hope that this will provide a basic framework for further independent study. Torsional conditions, angular conditions, torticollis, developmental dysplasia of the hip, causes of limp in children, back pain, and leg length inequality are discussed in this chapter.

TORSIONAL CONDITIONS

A chief complaint of either in-toeing or out-toeing is probably the most common reason for elective referral of a child to an orthopaedist. Even though these rotational conditions in the lower extremities usually do not require any treatment, they are frequently a source of significant concern to parents, grandparents, and other family members. This concern is often enhanced by the comments of neighbors, teachers, and strangers on the street— "Why does your child walk so funny?" This group has been described by Dr. Mercer Rang as "the worried well," an apt phrase that indicates the strong concern of the family and others involved with the child over alignment conditions that are often part of the spectrum of normal musculoskeletal development.

Numerous differences of opinion exist in the orthopaedic field on how to define torsional conditions, how to measure them, and especially how to treat them, or if they should be treated at all. Unfortunately the term torsional *deformities* is present throughout the literature, noted in scientific papers delivered at national meetings, and rampant in verbal discussions regarding this subject. Patients and parents hear the term *deformity*, and their worst fears regarding the condition appear validated. The term *condition* or *problem* would seem to be a less anxiety-producing and anatomically more correct description, applicable to most children. The Subcommittee on Torsional Deformity of the Pediatric Orthopaedic Society of North America has recommended a classification system in which normal limb alignment and joint range of motion (ROM) are defined as those occurring within two standard deviations of the mean. These are termed *rotational variations*. Those falling outside the two standard deviations are termed *torsional deformities* (Scoles, 1988).

Obtaining a History

A specific history provides a wealth of information regarding possible causative factors and can provide some indications of possible treatment. Specific information obtained may also direct the examiner to expand the evaluation to rule out other more severe conditions that may initially present with a chief complaint of in-toeing or out-toeing. Relevant information to be elicited from the parents includes the following:

1. *Birth history.* Was the infant full term or premature? Was it a vaginal or cesarean delivery? Was oligohydramnios (deficiency of amniotic fluid) present? How often has the mother been pregnant? What is the birth order of the patient? Many of the torsional problems seen in infants are "packaging"

defects (i.e., due to a restricted intrauterine environment). It is easy to imagine that an infant's lower limbs may "grow" into a particular position if one visualizes a full-term 9-pound fetus in the womb of a gravida 1: para 1 mother.

2. *Age when in-toeing or out-toeing was noted.* Has it improved or worsened since first noted? Has there been any prior treatment? For the walking child, at what age did the child start to walk independently? In the differential diagnosis, there should be an increased index of suspicion when a child has a history of prematurity, difficult birth, or delayed motor milestones or has significant in-toeing or out-toeing that is worsening with time or is very asymmetric. Frequently, children with mild spastic diplegia may present with a chief complaint of in-toeing. Conditions such as cerebral palsy and muscular dystrophy need to be ruled out.

3. *Family history.* In-toeing or out-toeing in the parents or other siblings should be noted, especially if these individuals required treatment for the condition. In many cases there is a positive family history for in-toeing or out-toeing.

4. *Sleeping and sitting positions.* Sleeping in the prone position with the legs internally rotated encourages the persistence of internal tibial torsion and metatarsus adductus (Staheli, 1977).

Clinical Examination: In-Toeing and Out-Toeing

Clinical assessment of the child should include documentation of the foot progression angle in standing or walking, hip rotation ROM, thigh–foot axis, and alignment of the foot. These four components form the torsional profile described by Staheli (1977). In a later study, Staheli and co-authors described means and ranges for these parameters in 1000 normal children and adults (1985).

FOOT PROGRESSION ANGLE

Foot progression angle, or "the angle of gait," is defined as the angle between the longitudinal axis of the foot and a straight line of progression of the body in walking (Staheli, 1977). The child is observed while walking, and a value is assigned to the angle of both the right and the left foot. This is of course a subjective evaluation and represents an average of the angles noted on multiple steps. It can be measured more objectively by using one of the various footprint techniques in which a permanent record of the foot progression angle is obtained, but this is time consuming and usually not practical in a clinical situation. In-toeing is expressed as a negative value (e.g., −30°), and out-toeing is expressed as a positive value (e.g., +20°). This angle gives an overall view of the degree of in-toeing or out-toeing in the walking child. The foot progression angle can also be assessed in supported stance for the younger child who is not yet walking independently. Foot progression angle is variable during infancy. During childhood and adult life, it shows little change, with a mean of +10° and a normal range of −3 to +20° (Staheli et al., 1985).

HIP ROTATION, FEMORAL ANTEVERSION, AND RETROVERSION: ASSESSMENT

Hip rotation ROM is measured most accurately in the prone position, with the hip in a position of neutral flexion or extension. (An extremely frightened, crying child can be examined more easily by having the parent stand up and hold the child against the chest, facing the parent. This allows the child's hips to hang into neutral flexion or extension, and the examiner can then bend the child's knees and evaluate the hip rotation range.) This hip rotation measurement will be a reflection of the flexibility of the soft tissues and the version of the femur.

Version is the normal angular difference between the transverse axis of each end of a long bone. The terms *femoral anteversion* and *retroversion* refer to this relationship between the neck of the femur and the femoral shaft, ending in the femoral condyles, that dictates the position of the femoral head when the knee is pointing straight ahead (Fig. 15–1). If the femoral head is directed anteriorly, the hip is in anteversion (or "anteverted") and the patient will usually have more internal than external rotation hip ROM, assuming no soft tissue tightness. In retroversion, the femoral head is directed posteriorly when the knee is aligned straight ahead and the patient will have greater external rotation ROM. It may in fact be less confusing to use the terms *medial* and *lateral rotation* rather than *internal* and *external rotation*, respectively.

Femoral and tibial torsion, or version, can be measured by computed tomography (CT). However, clinical measurements of hip medial and lateral rotation have been found accurate for diagnosing rotational abnormalities. Cahuzac and co-workers (1992) found that relationships between femoral anteversion and medial hip rotation were significant, as were relationships between the clinical and CT values of femoral and tibial torsion. Stuberg and associates (1989) found a discrepancy

FIGURE 15–1. *A*, Femoral anteversion. *B*, Femoral retroversion. In the femur, version is the angular difference between the transcondylar axis of the knee and the axis of the femoral neck (a line drawn between the center of the femoral head and the center of the base of the femoral neck). (From Salter, RB. Textbook of Disorders and Injuries of the Musculoskeletal System. Baltimore: Williams & Wilkins, 1970, p. 48. © 1970, The Williams & Wilkins Co.)

of 10 to 15° between clinical goniometric assessment and radiographic assessment by CT of femoral torsion, with the goniometric measurements lower than the amount of femoral anteversion measured by CT. Clinical examination is certainly sufficient for documentation for the vast majority of patients with what are usually very benign rotational problems.

The sum of medial and lateral rotation in a hip is usually 100° up to age 2 years, and after that 95 to 110° (Engel & Staheli, 1974). If the hip medial rotation is measured at 70° and the lateral rotation at 25°, for example, the child is said to have femoral anteversion and may in-toe when walking.

Most infants have femoral anteversion. Most infants also have contractures of the hip external rotator muscles at birth (from the intrauterine position) that mask the anteversion, and they tend to lie with their legs in an abducted and laterally rotated position. True femoral retroversion in an infant is rare; it is usually tightness in the hip lateral rotator muscles and hip capsular ligaments that is producing the laterally rotated position, masking the femoral anteversion (Pitkow, 1975). Gradually the tightness of the hip soft tissues stretches out, and the true anteversion of the hip becomes more apparent. This is often described incorrectly as "femoral anteversion increases"—the amount of femoral version is in fact decreasing, but it is more easily visualized because the muscle tightness of the lateral rotators is decreasing. The femoral anteversion becomes increasingly more apparent as the child approaches 5 to 6 years of age, as the soft tissue tightness resolves. Femoral anteversion has been measured radiologically in normal children and the average shows a gradual decrease with age: 35° at age 1 year, to 21° at age 9 years, and 15.5° in adults (Crane, 1959; Fabry et al., 1973; Shands & Steele, 1958). By mid-childhood, the femoral head and neck have usually assumed a relatively more neutral position in relationship to the femoral shaft and children typically will have approximately equal amounts of medial and lateral rotation ROM in the hip (Fig. 15–2).

FEMORAL ANTEVERSION: TREATMENT

Many types of treatment have been tried to correct femoral anteversion, including braces, twister cables, and special shoes. None of these have been proven effective in clinical trials. Anecdotal evidence of their efficacy abounds with a tendency to ignore the natural history of the condition (i.e., that spontaneous improvement will occur). One reasonable recommendation is to have the child avoid W-sitting (reverse tailor sitting) and to encourage tailor sitting in maximum external rotation (Fig. 15–3). If significant femoral anteversion is still present at age 10 to 14 years, surgical correction in the form of femoral derotation osteotomies may be considered, although the possible operative risks may outweigh the benefits of realignment.

THIGH–FOOT AXIS, TIBIAL TORSION: ASSESSMENT

The alignment of the lower leg can be measured by documenting the thigh–foot axis, which is a reflection of the version of the tibia. Tibial torsion is assessed using the thigh–foot angle, the angular difference between the longitudinal axes of the thigh and foot, measured in the prone position with the knee flexed. Some examiners measure tibial torsion with the child sitting with the knee flexed to 90°. Tibial torsion can also be described as the angle formed by a straight line axis through the knee and the axis through the medial and lateral malleoli. By convention, internal tibial torsion

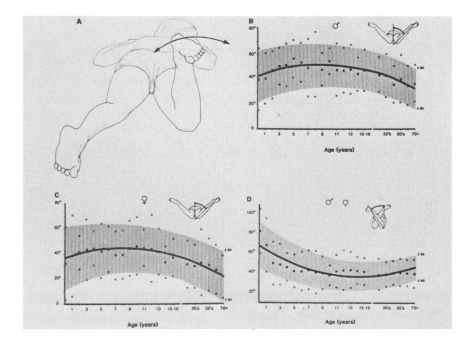

FIGURE 15–2. *A*, Hip rotation is measured with the patient prone, knee flexed to 90°.

Means for hip rotation in mid-childhood and in older subjects.

B, Medial rotation in males: 50° (range 25–65°).

C, Medial rotation in females: 40° (range 15–60°).

D, Lateral rotation: 45° (range 25–65°), with no gender difference. (From Staheli LT, Corbett, M, Wyss, C, & King, H. Lower extremity rotational problems in children. Journal of Bone and Joint Surgery [American], *67*:39–47, 1985.)

FIGURE 15–3. *A,* Children with femoral anteversion tend to "W"-sit. *B,* They should be encouraged to tailor sit.

(ITT) is expressed as a negative value, such as "tibial torsion of −30°." External tibial torsion is expressed as a positive value.

The tibia is usually medially rotated in infants as a result of intrauterine positioning (Hensinger & Jones, 1981). Spontaneous derotation on the long axis takes place during growth. The tibia gradually rotates out into external tibial torsion, especially during the first 6 months of independent walking, or by approximately 18 months of age. The normal range of thigh–foot angle is between 0 and 30° of external tibial torsion, with a mean of approximately 10° during most of childhood (Staheli & Engel, 1972). In 1988, Scoles described the following approximate thigh–foot normative angles:

Birth: −15° (normal range between −30 and +20°)

Age 3: +5° (normal range between −10 and +20°)

Mid-childhood to skeletal maturity: +10° (normal range between −5 and +30°)

ITT in infancy is often not apparent to the parents or the casual examiner because the hips have external rotation muscle contractures and the infant's legs tend to assume an abducted and laterally rotated position. The ITT may become noticeable only as the hip contractures stretch out, resulting in a more neutral position of the hip, and especially when the child begins to walk independently.

INTERNAL TIBIAL TORSION: TREATMENT

Controversy exists regarding appropriate treatment of ITT, as it does in femoral anteversion. Many orthopaedists believe that it should not be treated at all because the natural history of the condition is gradual improvement. The very small percentage of children who do not improve and who have a significant functional deficit as a result of ITT can be treated surgically at a later date with external rotational osteotomy of the tibia and fibula. A different school of thought relies on natural improvement up to about 18 months of age, and at that age advocates treating the persistent ITT with a Friedman counter splint (a flexible leather strap) or a Denis Browne bar (a metal bar) for night wear, usually for about 6 months. These devices attach to shoes and hold the feet in a laterally rotated position.

METATARSUS ADDUCTUS

Alterations in alignment of the foot can be divided into two categories: positional or "packaging" problems due to a restricted intrauterine environment and "manufacturing" defects or true congenital abnormalities such as talipes equinovarus. Metatarsus varus, also called metatarsus adductus (MTA), is one of the most commonly seen positional conditions in infants. In MTA the forefoot is curved medially, the hindfoot is in the normal slight valgus position, and there is full dorsiflexion ROM. The degree of MTA can be graded as I—mild, II—moderate, and III—severe. Having the child stand on the glass plate of a copying machine and "Xeroxing" the feet is a good way to document the amount of metarsus adductus. This is faster, easier, and less messy than the various footprint kits available. Some clinicians use grade ½ to describe dynamic MTA: the foot usually looks fairly straight at rest, but when the child walks there is a dynamic forefoot varus due to muscle action, with medial motion of the great toe, described as a "searching great toe" (Staheli, 1977). Treatment is rarely required for mild cases (grade I), which usually resolve on their own, generally by about age 4 to 6 months. Moderate cases (grade II) may be treated with stretching exercises and corrective shoes (straight-last or reverse-last shoes or both). Severe cases may be treated with progressive casting between 3 to 6 months of age, followed by use of corrective shoes. Another school of thought advocates no conservative treatment, recommending surgical correction at a later age for those feet that do not improve with time.

CLUBFOOT

A condition often confused with MTA (a positional problem) is the congenital deformity of clubfoot, or talipes equinovarus (TEV). First described by Hippocrates, the forefoot in this condition is curved in medially (adducted), the calcaneus is small, the hindfoot is in varus, and there is equinus of the ankle. The calf and the foot are generally smaller on the involved side. In some children, TEV is just one manifestation of more serious malformations such as myelomeningocele or arthrogryposis. Typical congenital clubfoot is probably the result of abnormal intrauterine restriction in a genetically predisposed individual. It occurs in 1:1000 live births, with a 2:1 male-to-female ratio (Scoles, 1988; Wynne-Davies, 1964).

Treatment consists of progressive casting, which is most effective if started immediately after birth, often followed by surgical correction at from 3 months to 1 year of age, depending on the surgeon's preference. Occasionally a positional clubfoot is seen in which the deformity is similar to that described earlier but can be treated successfully with casting alone.

CALCANEOVALGUS

Calcaneovalgus is a common positional foot problem (like MTA) in newborns. In this condition, the result of a large infant in a small space, the forefoot is curved out laterally, the hindfoot is in valgus, and there is full or excessive dorsiflexion. The dorsum of the foot may be actually touching the anterior surface of the leg at birth. The positional calcaneovalgus foot corrects spontaneously and does not require treatment. It must be distinguished from more severe conditions, such as a calcaneovalgus foot caused by a vertical talus. In this condition, the talus is vertically oriented and the navicular is displaced onto the dorsal surface of the talus. The forefoot is dorsiflexed, but the hindfoot is plantar flexed, and the foot bends at the instep. This characteristic position is described as a rocker-bottom deformity of the foot, and the foot is much more rigid than the typical calcaneovalgus foot.

FOOT ALIGNMENT PROBLEMS: SUMMARY

Table 15–1 is a decision matrix that provides a quick and easy way to categorize foot deformities (Wenger & Leach, 1986).

TORSIONAL PROFILE

The components that may contribute to in-toeing are femoral anteversion, internal tibial torsion, and metatarsus adductus. Those that may contribute to out-toeing are external rotation contractures of the hip (and, rarely, femoral retroversion), external tibial torsion, and calcaneovalgus. The foot progression angle can be viewed as the "summation" of the rotational alignment of the three segments of

TABLE 15–1. **DECISION MATRIX FOR FOOT DEFORMITY**

	Metatarsus Varus	Clubfoot	Calcaneovalgus
Side view (Can foot dorsiflex?)	Yes	No	Yes
Foot shape (viewed from bottom)	Kidney shaped (deviated medially)	Kidney shaped	Banana shaped (deviated laterally)
Heel position	Valgus	Varus	Valgus

the lower limb: the hip and femur, the lower leg, and the foot. For example, significant femoral anteversion at the hip may be balanced by external tibial torsion, with a straight foot (no MTA or calcaneovalgus). The foot progression angle would be 0°/0° (right/left) with the feet pointing straight ahead. When a child toes in or toes out, the condition is usually bilateral, but occasionally one sees "windswept" lower extremities, with one limb toeing in and the other limb toeing out.

An example of a torsional profile of a normal 8-month-old infant might be as follows:

	Right	Left
Foot progression angle	—	—(not yet standing)
Medial rotation of hip	20°	20°
Lateral rotation of hip	90°	90°
Thigh–foot angle	0°	0°
Foot	Neutral	Neutral

When supported in upright, the legs would be positioned in external rotation, the usual position for the lower extremities in infancy. The torsional profile of a 5-year-old child with in-toeing might look like this:

	Right	Left
Foot progression angle	−40°	−30°
Medial rotation of hip	70°	70°
Lateral rotation of hip	20°	20°
Thigh–foot angle	−10°	+15°
Foot	Grade I MTA	Neutral

From this discussion, it is clear that one must determine which component of the lower extremity is causing the torsional impairment and then treat that level, if treatment is indicated. For example, using heavy, high-topped orthopaedic shoes will not correct femoral anteversion. In fact, the child will probably be more clumsy and stumble more frequently. The concept of a natural history of improvement with time is also pivotal. It is important not to extoll the virtues of various treatments too vigorously, because it is quite difficult to differentiate benefits obtained from the treatment versus benefits that occurred simply with the passage of time as a result of skeletal maturation.

In children with neuromuscular diseases such as cerebral palsy, the basic assessment format described previously is very useful in helping to delineate the child's problems with gait. In addition to this assessment, which mainly addresses bony alignment, one must, of course, assess muscle tone, muscle strength, and motor control. Abnormalities in any of these areas can cause in-toeing or out-toeing, either alone or in conjunction with skeletal malalignment. An example would be a child with cerebral palsy who ambulates with a foot progression angle of −40°/−30°. This may be due to a combination of femoral anteversion, ITT, metatarsus adductus, and spasticity in the hip adductors, medial hamstrings, and posterior tibialis muscles. By contrast, a child with Duchenne's muscular dystrophy may ambulate with an in-toeing gait at age 6 because of femoral anteversion and then gradually develop an out-toeing gait by age 10, resulting from resolution of the femoral anteversion and increasing weakness of the gluteus maximus and quadriceps muscles, plus tightness in the iliotibial band.

Another area of assessment and treatment in which this multilevel concept is useful is in measurement of other gross motor activities, such as sitting. Many children with increased tone, as well as children with hypotonia, will W-sit. This postural preference is frequently ascribed to problems with spasticity, or as a compensatory mechanism to achieve better sitting balance. However, a more detailed assessment might reveal that the child has, in addition to spasticity or poor balance, significant femoral anteversion that simply does not allow comfortable sitting with the hips in external rotation.

ANGULAR CONDITIONS

Genu varum (bowlegs) and genu valgum (knock knees) are similar to torsional conditions in that they are commonly seen in normal children and a specific natural history has been described that results in normal skeletal alignment at maturity.

Moderate genu varum, often referred to as physiologic bowing (apex laterally), is normal for newborns and for infants before they are walking. This physiologic genu varum generally resolves, and the child gradually develops genu valgum between 2 and 4 years of age. By age 3 years, 80% of children have mild knock knees. This valgus angulation generally corrects by 5 to 7 years of age, and the child is left with a "normally" straight leg. The normal tibiofemoral angulation in adults is 7 to 9° of valgus in females and 4 to 6° of valgus in males (Scoles, 1988). Bowlegs and knock knees tend to run in families, however, and some children will inherit this genetic predisposition to one or the other in adulthood.

Genu Varum

ASSESSMENT

Genu varum can be documented for the medical record by having the child lie supine, approximating the medial malleoli, and then measuring the distance between the femoral condyles or at the knee joint line. The child must be undressed, with diaper removed, for this measurement to be accurate. A plastic triangle is used for this purpose with centimeters marked on both sides. This allows the examiner to more easily obtain accurate measurements than with use of a tape measure, especially when attempting assessment of a wiggling child.

Newborns and infants before they walk also usually have ITT, and the combination of ITT and genu varum tends to make the child look quite "bowlegged and pigeon-toed," causing many parents and others quite a bit of concern. Even when the genu varum has resolved and the child may actually have developed genu valgum, the presence of ITT may make the child look bowlegged.

TREATMENT

"Physiologic" (normal) genu varum does not usually require treatment unless it persists after age 2 years and either shows no tendency to correct or is actually worsening. This latter condition may require bracing in the form of hip-knee-ankle-foot orthoses (HKAFOs) or knee-ankle-foot orthoses (KAFOs) with no knee joint or a hinged knee joint that can be locked. Surgical correction is sometimes required, although this is rare.

DIFFERENTIAL DIAGNOSIS

When a child presents with severe genu varum, especially after 4 years of age or with worsening over time, systemic disorders such as vitamin D–resistant rickets must be ruled out, along with a variety of skeletal dysplasias and other conditions that cause genu varum. Radiographs may be performed to rule out idiopathic tibia vara, also known as Blount's disease. The first case of infantile tibia vara was reported in 1922, and Blount presented a complete description of the condition in 1937. In Blount's disease, increased compressive forces across the medial aspect of the knee cause growth suppression of the proximal tibia physis, resulting in a bowleg deformity (Thompson & Carter, 1990).

In Blount's disease, a characteristic beaking of the medial metaphysis is noted on radiographs, especially in younger children. In 1952, Langenskiold described six stages of infantile tibia vara based on their radiographic appearance (Langenskiold, 1989). Tibia vara is usually seen in children younger than 3 years of age, although it may be found in older children. Children with this condition may clinically resemble children with physio-

logic genu varum except that they are often obese and also have a lateral thrust to the knee during the stance phase of gait. Children with Blount's disease require aggressive treatment, with bracing in full HKAFOs worn 23 hours per day recommended for patients younger than 3 years of age (Johnson, 1990). Surgical correction by proximal tibial osteotomy is sometimes performed. To ensure a better outcome, it should be done before permanent physeal damage has occurred, as shown by Hofmann and colleagues in their series of 19 knees in 12 patients evaluated at a mean of 12 years after osteotomy (1982). Twelve of the 19 knees were symptomatic, and 8 of those had early degenerative changes. The poor results were directly correlated with the amount of physeal damage.

Physiologic genu varum must also be distinguished from anterolateral bow of the tibia, usually noted at birth (Hensinger & Jones, 1981). In this extremely serious condition, radiographs demonstrate a tibia with a narrowed, sclerotic intramedullary canal; the majority fracture in the first year of life. Both tibia and fibula fail to unite; hence the name "pseudoarthrosis of the tibia." Protective bracing and surgical treatment may be helpful, but many of these children will eventually require amputation of the affected limb because of persistent pseudarthrosis.

Genu Valgum

ASSESSMENT AND TREATMENT

Like genu varum, genu valgum can occasionally persist beyond the age range when one expects the legs to become generally straight. Children with persisting genu valgum are frequently overweight and have an out-toeing foot progression angle, an awkward gait, and flat feet. Genu valgum can be documented clinically by having the child lie supine with the medial aspect of both knees lightly touching each other and measuring the intermalleolar distance.

Children with significant femoral anteversion may often appear knock-kneed. Once again, a clear understanding of the three-level concept of torsional conditions and the differentiation of the angular conditions of genu varum and genu valgum is necessary to define the specific problem(s).

If severe, genu valgum can be corrected by stapling of the medial femoral growth plate in the teenage years. This allows the lateral femoral growth plate to continue growing and the leg gradually grows into better alignment. A second option for surgical treatment is femoral osteotomy.

FLAT FOOT

The subject of flexible flat feet is a controversial one, with a variety of players in the cast: unconcerned children, with no foot pain and no disability; concerned parents who were frequently treated in childhood for flat feet and now demand treatment for their child; physical therapists who are concerned about the abnormal appearance of the foot and ankle and the possible secondary effects on the joints above; and various other medical practitioners, some well intended and others who have made a significant profit out of providing arch supports, which frequently need to be replaced as often as once a year in a growing child.

ASSESSMENT

Children with flexible flat feet have a normal-appearing arch in sitting and when asked to walk "on their toes" in maximum plantar flexion. In standing, however, the longitudinal arch decreases or disappears. This is usually due to normal ligamentous laxity, and the child will typically demonstrate ligamentous laxity throughout the upper and lower extremities, as evidenced by hyperextension at the elbows and knees and ability to approximate the thumb to the forearm. The fat pad noted in the medial part of the foot in many infants and toddlers contributes to the flat-footed appearance. A wide variation of rate and onset of arch development was noted in the 160 children studied by Engel and Staheli (1974).

TREATMENT

A great deal of anecdotal evidence but little scientific proof exists to support the use of special shoes or arch supports for the treatment of flexible flat feet in children. In a prospective study to determine whether flexible flat foot in children can be influenced by treatment, it was concluded that wearing corrective shoes or inserts for 3 years does not alter the natural history (Wenger et al., 1989). One hundred and twenty-nine children were randomly assigned to four groups: 1) controls, 2) treatment with corrective orthopaedic shoes, 3) treatment with a Helfet heel-cup (Apex Foot Health, South Hackensack, NJ), and 4) treatment with a custom-molded plastic insert. Ninety-eight patients with documented compliance completed the minimum of 3 years of treatment. All groups showed significant improvement, including the controls, and there was no significant difference between the controls and the treated patients.

It has been widely documented that a low arch is usually less of a problem in adulthood than high-arched (cavus) feet. Most pediatric orthopaedists now counsel parents regarding the natural history of flat foot in children, which is documented as gradual improvement, and advise the use of a lightweight running shoe as the only recommendation. Using shoes with a good arch support and a strong counter will not correct the flat foot, but this type of shoe is often recommended as a help in slowing down wear on the medial border of shoes, thereby decreasing the expense of frequent shoe purchases.

DIFFERENTIAL DIAGNOSIS

A tendo Achilles contracture can produce a secondary flat foot. Examples of conditions in which this may occur are cerebral palsy, congenital or familial tight heel cords, and muscular dystrophy.

Children occasionally have an extra ossicle located at the medial border of the navicular, called an accessory navicular. This condition may become symptomatic in late childhood or early adolescence, resulting in pain over the ossicle and along the medial arch. It is frequently associated with flat feet.

A small subgroup of children with flat foot have a rigid, painful foot with limited subtalar motion. These children deserve further diagnostic scrutiny and may have a condition such as tarsal coalition that requires more definitive treatment. (See section on causes of limping later in this chapter for further information on this condition.)

DEVELOPMENTAL DYSPLASIA OF THE HIP

The term *developmental dysplasia of the hip* (DDH) is replacing the term *congenital dysplasia of the hip*. The term DDH is also used as an abbreviation for developmental dislocation of the hip. The use of this broader term *developmental dysplasia* includes hips that may have been normal, or believed to be normal, at birth but subsequently are documented to have dysplasia. Ilfeld and co-workers (1986) noted that delayed diagnosis of dislocation is not evidence that these hips were "missed" by inadequate examinations. They describe a separate entity of the delayed subluxed or dislocated hip, possibly the result of a dynamic process due to an increased acetabular index.

The term *dysplasia* describes abnormal development or growth. Normal muscle balance and a femoral head that is concentric, congruent with the acetabulum, and seated deep within the acetabulum are necessary prerequisites for normal hip development. The concave acetabulum develops in response to a spherical femoral head, and the depth normally increases with growth.

The incidence of hip dysplasia in the United States is 1:100 with dysplasia or subluxation and 1:1000 with dislocation (Mubarak et al., 1987). Prompt recognition and treatment of DDH, preferably in the newborn period, provide the best chance for subsequent optimal hip development and a normal hip at skeletal maturity.

The etiology of DDH is thought to be multifactorial. In studies of the early fetal period, measurements of femoral head coverage and acetabular anteversion do not show significant variation through the embryonic and early fetal stages (6 to 20 weeks), and the hip stays well covered (Lee et al., 1992). Dislocated fetal hips tend to appear only in the last trimester.

Factors that predispose an infant to DDH include mechanical, physiologic, and environmental factors. Mechanical factors are a small intrauterine space and tight abdominal wall of a primipara mother, breech presentation, and positioning of the fetal hip against the mother's sacrum in utero (Hensinger & Jones, 1981). Physiologic factors include maternal hormonal influence of estrogen and relaxin and the resulting ligamentous laxity of the female infant (Wynne-Davies, 1970). This is thought to account for the 6 : 1 female-to-male incidence of DDH. Environmental or cultural factors include strapping the child's lower extremities in extension, for example, on a cradle board, noted in the Eskimo and some Native American cultures. Cultures in which infants are routinely carried with their hips in flexion and wide abduction in cloth slings on the mother's back or astride her hip have a decreased incidence of DDH.

The mechanical factors listed above can act to restrict the position of the head, neck, and feet of the developing fetus, as well as the hips. Associated problems include a 20% incidence of congenital muscular torticollis (Hummer & MacEwen, 1972) and a 10% incidence of metatarsus adductus or calcaneovalgus (Dunn, 1976).

ASSESSMENT

Based on a careful clinical examination, newborn hips can be classified as follows (Mubarak et al., 1987):

1. Normal—no instability noted
2. Subluxatable (9.8/1000) (Tredwell & Bell, 1981)—the femoral head is in the hip socket but can be partially displaced out to the rim of the acetabulum
3. Dislocatable (1.3/1000)—the femoral head is reduced but can be dislocated with a Barlow maneuver

4. Dislocated but reducible (1.2/1000)—the femoral head is out of the acetabulum at rest but can be reduced with an Ortolani maneuver
5. Dislocated but not reducible—seldom encountered in the newborn to 2-month-old age group. When seen in this age group, this type of dislocation is usually teratologic, occurring before birth, usually from a neurologic or muscular abnormality such as myelomeningocele or arthrogryposis.

Clinical examination includes documentation of the ROM of hip abduction in flexion. Most infants will have between 75 and 90° of abduction. Significant limitation in this range of motion, or an asymmetry of even 5 to 10°, may be indicative of hip dysplasia and warrants further diagnostic studies. Other clinical findings may include asymmetric thigh folds, pistoning, apparent (not true) femoral shortening with uneven knee heights (positive Galeazzi sign), and positive Barlow or Ortolani signs (Fig. 15–4).

The infant must be completely relaxed for the Barlow and Ortolani maneuvers to have reliable diagnostic value. Even slight muscular contraction around the hip can obscure the instability and negate the examination. These two signs of hip instability usually gradually disappear by 2 to 3 months of age, since the hip either improves in stability and stays in the socket or becomes fixed in a dislocated position. Often limited hip abduction may be the only clinical sign of hip dysplasia in the infant older than 1 month. It continues to be the most reliable clinical finding in older infants and toddlers with dysplasia. Further diagnostic studies are warranted if the clinical examination shows positive findings and sometimes even with a normal clinical examination but a high index of suspicion due to multiple risk factors, such as a female first-born child with breech presentation and a family history of DDH.

The use of ultrasonography to examine infant hips is routine in Europe and becoming more popular in the United States (Graf, 1992). It is recognized as a more accurate and helpful test than radiographic examination in the younger age group. It is useful in the newborn and up to 3 to 6 months of age, before the femoral head starts to ossify and obscure the structures deep to it, although it may be effective in children up to 1 year of age (Harcke, 1992). The secondary ossification center is present in 80% of children at age 6 months (Scoles et al., 1987). Ultrasonography allows assessment of the cartilaginous structures not visualized on plain radiographs, allows stress testing (to document instability), and has the additional advantage of no radiation exposure. It is proving to be a useful tool not only in the diagnosis of DDH but also in the man-

FIGURE 15-4. *A* and *B*, Barlow maneuver: the hip is first flexed and abducted, then gradually adducted with pressure exerted in a posterior direction. Dislocation of the femoral head over the posterior acetabular rim indicates an unstable hip. The head may slide to the edge of the socket (subluxatable) or may dislocate out of the acetabulum (dislocatable). *C* and *D*, Ortolani test: In the Ortolani positive hip, the hip is dislocated in a position of flexion and adduction. Gentle flexion, abduction, and slight traction (the Ortolani maneuver) reduce the hip. A positive Ortolani sign indicates a more unstable hip than positive Barlow sign. (From Mubarak, SJ, Leach, J, & Wenger, DR. Management of congenital dislocation of the hip in the infant. Contemporary Orthopaedics, *15*:29-44, 1987.)

agement, providing information on the status of the hip that is helpful in deciding when to discontinue or alter treatment.

For older infants, radiography may be used in addition to, or instead of, ultrasonography. Because of the need for a radiograph of the uninvolved side for comparison, and because of the frequency of bilateral involvement, the standard radiograph is an anterior-posterior view of the pelvis. Many parameters of hip development can be measured on hip radiographs (Hensinger & Jones, 1981). Scoles and associates (1987) studied 50 boys and 50 girls at each of six age levels: 3, 6, 9, 12, 18, and 24 months. They documented a decrease in acetabular index with age and concluded that this was a helpful parameter in following hip development (Fig. 15-5). Hips can be classified radiographically as acetabular dysplasia (without subluxation or dislocation); subluxated, with associated acetabular dysplasia; and dislocated. The diagnosis of DDH be-

FIGURE 15-5. Radiographic parameters of hip development involve use of the Hilgenreiner line (H) and Perkin's line (P) to document proximal and lateral migration of the femoral head, with disruption of Shenton's line (cross-hatched line). The acetabular index (AI) is the most helpful documentation of acetabular development. (From Mubarak, SJ, Leach, J, & Wenger, DR. Management of congenital dislocation of the hip in the infant. Contemporary Orthopaedics, *15*:29-44, 1987.)

tween 18 and 24 months of age is usually made on the basis of an abnormal gait. If the dislocation is unilateral, the child will limp, demonstrating a positive Trendelenburg sign when in the stance phase of gait on the involved side. If the dislocation is bilateral, the child demonstrates a waddling gait.

TREATMENT

Birth to 9 Months

The Pavlik harness was first described by Dr. Arnold Pavlik, who originally called his treatment device "stirrups." Modifications have been made in the design of the device, but the principles of treatment and the requirements of the harness remain essentially the same as described by him over 40 years ago (Pavlik, 1950). Pavlik stressed that one of the main advantages of the harness over casts was that it allowed active motion, thereby decreasing the incidence of avascular necrosis (Pavlik, 1957).

The Pavlik harness restricts hip extension and adduction and allows the hips to be maintained in flexion and abduction, the "protective position" (Fig. 15–6). Studies with newborn pigs by Salter (1968) showed hip dislocation was precipitated by maintaining the hips in extension. The position of flexion and abduction was found to enhance normal acetabular development and the kicking motion allowed in this "human" position (not as radical as the "frog" position) stretches the contracted hip adductors and promotes spontaneous reduction of the dislocated hip. Because of the biologic plasticity of growing bone, positioning the hip in flexion and abduction can promote appropriate acetabular development.

Complications of use of the Pavlik harness include avascular necrosis of the femoral head, femoral nerve palsy, inferior dislocation, and erosion of the posterior rim of the acetabulum. Essentially all of these complications can be avoided by using a Pavlik harness of proper design, educating the caregiver to apply it correctly, and monitoring the status of the hip carefully over the entire treatment period (Mubarak et al., 1981). For infants carefully treated with the Pavlik harness, the prognosis is excellent: 90 to 95% success in cases of dysplasia and subluxation, and approximately 85% success in cases of dislocation (Fig. 15–7).

Treatment of DDH in the newborn varies in different treatment settings. A commonly used protocol is outlined here, including the use of abduction diapering and the Pavlik harness. In the lax, subluxatable hip, abduction diapers are used for 1 month and the child is then re-examined. If the hip is still unstable, treatment with a Pavlik harness is instituted. If the hip becomes stable with 1 month

FIGURE 15–6. The Pavlik harness can be used to reduce a dislocated hip, to stabilize a lax hip, and to treat acetabular dysplasia.

of abduction diapers, the child should still be evaluated at 3 and 12 months of age to document continuing hip stability and adequate acetabular development.

For the dislocatable and dislocated but reducible hip in the newborn, the Pavlik harness is used full time (24 h/d) for 2 to 3 weeks until the hip is stabilized. Its use must be carefully monitored to avoid complications, with reduction documented both clinically and by ultrasonography or radiography (Mubarak et al., 1981). Once the hip is reduced and stabilized, the harness is worn for 23 hours each day for at least 3 months. This is followed by part-time wear (12 h/d) for an additional 3 to 6 months, or until both clinical and radiographic or ultrasound examinations are normal. A shorter treatment time is advocated in some centers. Herring (1992) recommends initial Pavlik harness treatment for 6 to 8 weeks in the newborn with a Barlow or Ortolani positive hip that stabilizes well in the harness.

When diagnosis occurs after the newborn period, the Pavlik harness is generally used for infants 1 to

FIGURE 15–7. *A*, Age 4 months: right hip dislocated, severe acetabular dysplasia. *B*, Age 7 months treated with a Pavlik harness for 3 months full time. Right hip is reduced; continued acetabular dysplasia. Patient continued Pavlik harness treatment for 3 more months, part time (night and naps only). *C*, Age 15 months: both hips centered in the acetabulae with good acetabular development bilaterally.

about 9 months of age with acetabular dysplasia, with or without subluxation. For a dislocated hip in this age group, the Pavlik harness can be used to reduce the hip if a strict reduction protocol is followed and the hip is carefully monitored. It must be documented by clinical examination and ultrasonography or radiography that the femoral head is directed toward the triradiate cartilage to continue treatment with the harness.

If the Pavlik harness is not successful in reducing the hip in 3 weeks, surgical treatment is instituted. This includes a period of 2 to 3 weeks of traction, to reduce the incidence of avascular necrosis of the femoral head. Home traction has been found to be a safe, effective, and much less expensive alternative to the 2- to 3-week admission required for hospital traction (Mubarak et al., 1986). Traction is then followed by surgery. This includes arthrography, to define the anatomic landmarks of the femoral head and acetabulum and to detect the presence of soft tissue (pulvinar) interposition between the head and acetabulum; adductor tenotomy, closed or (if necessary) open reduction of the hip; and application of a spica cast. In a closed reduction, the hip can be manually reduced and the reduction maintained with a cast. In an open reduction, an incision is made, the hip joint is exposed, any pulvinar is removed, the femoral head is relocated, and often a capsulorrhaphy is performed, tightening the capsule to aid in maintaining reduction.

The spica cast is applied in the "human" position. Experimental studies have shown that immobilizing hips and knees in a forced position of maximum abduction associated with excessive pressure of the femoral head against the acetabulum causes avascular necrosis (Salter, 1966).

Indications for an open reduction include failure of closed reduction, persistent subluxation, soft tissue interposition (documented on the arthrogram), and a reducible but very unstable hip. The stability of a hip can be evaluated by documenting a "safe zone": this is defined as the range of abduction in which the hip remains located. Outside the safe zone, moving into further adduction, the hip will dislocate in the posterior direction (Fig. 15–8).

9 Months and Older

In infants more than 9 months of age, an abduction orthosis should be considered as an alternative to the Pavlik harness for treatment of acetabular dysplasia with or without subluxation. This orthosis should be designed so the child can walk in it.

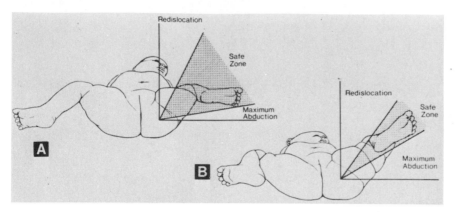

FIGURE 15–8. *A*, The femoral head is reduced in the safe zone. Adduction may cause dislocation, and further abduction may compromise circulation to the femoral head. *B*, A child with a narrow safe zone may be treated with an adductor tenotomy to increase abduction, resulting in an increased safe zone. (From Hensinger, RN, & Jones, ET. Neonatal orthopaedics. In Oliver, TK [Ed.], Monographs in Neonatalogy. New York: Grune & Stratton, 1981, p. 230.)

For dislocatable or dislocated hips diagnosed in the 6- to 18-month age group, surgical treatment is usually required with either a closed or an open reduction. Treatment falls into a gray zone in the 18- to 24-month age group. Either closed or open reduction of the hip is used.

The diagnosis of hip dislocation in the child aged 2 years or older is generally considered to mandate open reduction, since the results of closed reduction are not predictable in these older children. Instead of prior traction, femoral shortening (where a segment of the femoral shaft is removed) is often used (Galpin et al., 1989) to reduce the compressive forces on the femoral head once it is reduced back into the acetabulum. Older children with continuing acetabular dysplasia will benefit from a pelvic osteotomy, as the remodeling potential of the acetabulum decreases with age. There are a large number of different types of acetabuloplasties, which can be divided into three groups: 1) capsular arthroplasties, 2) redirectional osteotomies that change the orientation and position of the acetabulum relative to the pelvis, and 3) pericapsular osteotomies that alter the shape of the acetabulum (Staheli, 1991). The Salter innominate osteotomy is the acetabuloplasty most commonly used for DDH, providing a redirection of the acetabulum to improve hip stability when the femur is in a weight-bearing position (Salter, 1961). Varus derotation osteotomy may be used in conjunction with the acetabuloplasty and may be effective when used alone for treatment of acetabular dysplasia, with best results if the child is younger than age 4 (Kasser et al., 1985). Even with a successful reduction, there are potential problems: iatrogenic avascular necrosis, residual dysplasia, and residual subluxation (Weinstein, 1992).

In addition to the treated group, a number of children with acetabular dysplasia are never diagnosed as infants or toddlers. With mild dysplasia, they will walk without a limp, have essentially normal hip ROM, and can actively participate in all childhood activities. The hip, however, is like a tire that is out of round—you can drive on it for quite a few miles, but uneven wear will occur. The dysplastic hip, especially the one with subluxation, also demonstrates uneven wear with subsequent articular cartilage damage. The person may present as early as the late teens with degenerative arthritis, hip pain, and limp. Very mild dysplasia may go undetected for many decades but may be diagnosed later in life when the patient presents with degenerative hip joint disease. The age at symptom onset in untreated patients with subluxation is variable, with the mean in the mid 30s for women and the mid 50s for men (Weinstein, 1992). Many middle-aged adults requiring total hip replacement are patients with DDH that was never diagnosed and treated or was treated in childhood without full resolution of dysplasia and subluxation.

CAUSES OF LIMPING IN CHILDREN

The acute onset of limp in a child can present a diagnostic dilemma. In this section chronic causes of limp, such as those due to muscular weakness, are not discussed. Multiple conditions can cause a child to develop an acute limp, and a review of these will provide an overview of a wide range of orthopaedic conditions affecting children. Some are transitory and quite benign, while others can result in life-long disability, especially if not treated promptly and effectively. A clinical decision tree, as shown in Figure 15–9, is useful in identifying those problems that need immediate medical attention.

Clinical Assessment

A careful workup is required when a child presents with a limp. A detailed history must be taken, including a description of any recent illness or injury that may be related. The examiner should be

FIGURE 15-9. A clinical decision tree for children presenting with a limp (From Scoles, PV. Pediatric Orthopedics in Clinical Practice [2nd ed.]. St. Louis: Mosby-Year Book, 1988, p. 21.)

aware, however, that children do fall frequently and that parents may relate the onset of the limp to a fall or other injury that often turns out to be unrelated. Physical examination includes observational gait analysis, which usually will indicate which leg is involved and perhaps even the location within the leg. An example of an antalgic (painful) gait deviation is the Trendelenburg sign, a lean toward the involved side in the stance phase, usually due to a hip problem. A second example would be the "sore foot gait," a descriptive term used when a patient walks with decreased stance time on the involved side and decreased roll-off. This frequently will result from a problem in the foot, ankle, or lower leg, for example, a toddler's fracture of the tibia.

The physical examination should include a complete assessment of the spine, hips, thighs, knees, lower legs, ankles, and feet. The uninvolved side must be examined to provide a basis for comparison with the involved side. ROM, strength, presence of muscle atrophy, swelling, redness, increased warmth, and pain to palpation must all be assessed. The way in which a child performs functional activities, such as moving from the floor to standing, crawling, and achieving a comfortable sitting position, can provide important information. For example, a child may refuse to walk because of pain but may crawl easily, indicating that the problem is probably in the lower part of the leg rather than the hip or knee. A child may be able to walk short distances with no significant gait deviations but be reluctant to walk because of pain and may move into the seated position with difficulty and sit with a rigidly fixed spine, indicating a problem in the back, such as discitis.

Other Diagnostic Tests

In addition to a careful clinical examination, additional tests are often indicated. Radiographs can document fractures or other bony abnormalities, although there are certainly some occult fractures that are not identifiable on radiography until 10 to 14 days after onset, when a repeat radiograph may document the formation of callus. Laboratory examination of blood samples yields important information regarding the possible presence of infection or other acute processes. The erythrocyte sedimentation rate (ESR) can indicate the presence of acute inflammation. More complex diagnostic studies may also be needed to define the problem or evaluate the efficacy of treatment. These include bone scan; magnetic resonance imaging, which gives additional information on soft tissues; and CT scans, which give further information on bony structures.

Many causes of limp in children have classic presentations. Many are easily treated on a routine basis, and some require no treatment beyond observation. The two causes of limp that must definitely be recognized immediately and treated on an emergency basis are joint infections and osteomyelitis, both of which are covered in the next section. Many causes of limp are age-dependent in part, and certain common diagnoses are seen most frequently within one of three age groups of children: birth to 5 years, 5 to 10 years, and 10 to 15 years.

Obviously two very common causes of limp can occur in any age group: soft tissue injuries (e.g., contusions, ligament and tendon injuries) and fractures. Spine injury or disease may also cause a limp.

Most Common Diagnoses by Age Group

AGE BIRTH TO 5 YEARS

Osteomyelitis

In this age group, the child may present with refusal to walk, rather than a limp. One cause is osteomyelitis, an infection of a bone by bacterial organisms. In children, this infection is usually seen in the metaphyseal area. In many cases, the infection starts in the bony metaphysis (osteomyelitis) and spreads to the adjacent joint (septic arthritis). Osteomyelitis can be extremely and rapidly destructive, causing permanent damage that can have lifelong consequences for the child. The origin of the infection is usually hematogenous, or bloodborne, and the portal of entry is usually through the skin, secondary to infected scratches, boils, sore throat, and so on (Salter, 1970). Infection occasionally may result from an open fracture or a penetrating injury. The most common sites of infection are the distal femur and the proximal tibia.

The child with osteomyelitis presents with a high fever, chills, severe pain, swelling, and tenderness over the metaphysis of the involved bone. Children with osteomyelitis of the smaller bones tend to be less sick, with fewer symptoms. A newborn may also have few symptoms. The leukocyte count and ESR are usually elevated but occasionally normal; blood cultures should be done. The bone scan is positive early. Radiographs are usually normal initially, with early bone destruction not demonstrable by radiography until 7 to 14 days after onset. Subperiosteal new bone formation indicates periosteal stripping with formation of subperiosteal pus; at this stage, the cortex is already dead.

Treatment of osteomyelitis must be instituted on an emergency basis. Acute hematogenous osteomyelitis may be fatal as a result of overwhelming septicemia. Treatment consists of aspiration, antibiotics, and immobilization of the affected part. Surgical drainage is usually required when the diagnosis is delayed. Delayed treatment may be life saving by controlling the septicemia but may be ineffective in controlling progression of the pathologic process within the bone.

Septic Arthritis

Septic arthritis (pyogenic arthritis) is defined as an infection of a joint caused by bacterial organisms. This is an extremely threatening condition, because a joint may be destroyed within 48 hours of onset of symptoms. Septic arthritis causes destruction of articular cartilage and long-term growth arrest (Fig. 15–10). The resulting deformities may be permanent and have a wide-ranging, lifelong impact affecting the person's gait, participation in sports, and choice of occupation and leisure activities.

Staphylococcus aureus is the most common organism (Bennett & Namnyak, 1992), and *Haemophilus influenzae* may also be seen in children younger than 3 years of age. The organism enters the joint by hematogenous spread (e.g., from an ear

FIGURE 15–10. Septic arthritis of both hip joints in a 5-year, 9-month-old boy treated 17 days after onset of symptoms. Both capital epiphyses are destroyed, and the triradiate cartilage of both hips are sclerosed and irregular, with dysplastic acetabulae. The left hip is ankylosed. (From Bennett, OM, & Namnyak, SS. Acute septic arthritis of the hip joint in infancy and childhood. Clinical Orthopaedics and Related Research, *281*:123–132, 1992.)

infection), direct spread (from adjacent osteomyelitis), or direct inoculation (from a foreign body, needle, or surgical penetration of a joint). The hip joint is the most commonly involved in this age group, followed by the knee. Septic arthritis of the hip joint is particularly devastating in the newborn, because the femoral head is entirely cartilaginous and may be completely destroyed. Even milder cases have potentially lifelong effects because the increased intra-articular pressure can occlude the blood supply to the femoral head, causing avascular necrosis.

The child usually presents with acute onset of irritability, fever to 104°F (40.0°C), refusal to move the affected limb, and a warm, swollen joint held in flexion. Laboratory data show an elevated leukocyte count and ESR. Radiographs and ultrasound examination may show a distended joint capsule. In older children and adolescents there tends to be a more subtle clinical presentation. These patients often do walk and will allow motion. Subjective discomfort and febrile episodes can be prolonged. The incidence of avascular necrosis is higher in the older age group (Dales & Hoffinger, 1993). Interestingly, newborns may also have few clinical symptoms. Severe systemic symptoms are rarely seen in newborns. Local signs of warmth, swelling, and tenderness may be present. Usually the newborn presents with unwillingness to use an extremity, described as "pseudoparalysis of infancy" (Hensinger & Jones, 1981). Treatment of septic arthritis consists of immediate aspiration and drainage and intravenous administration of antibiotics.

Transient Synovitis

Transient synovitis (also known as toxic synovitis) is probably the most common cause of a painful hip in children younger than 10 years of age. This condition affects males more than females, in a 4:1 ratio. The child presents with the gradual or acute onset of limp. There may be occasional periods when the child refuses to walk. The child usually complains of mild to moderate hip pain but may complain of knee pain, since hip pain is often referred to the knee. Mild fever may be present, with normal leukocyte count and ESR. The cause is unclear, but often a history can be elicited of a recent upper respiratory tract infection or other illness. The treatment is symptomatic, consisting of limitation of activity, bed rest, and use of crutches if the child is old enough to manage them. Symptoms usually resolve in about 7 days. Occasionally a child will have recurrent hip synovitis. In a small percentage of these patients Legg-Perthes disease develops.

Occult Fractures

A usually benign condition causing a limp in children is an occult fracture. A commonly seen example is a toddler's fracture, a hairline fracture of the tibia. The child usually presents with refusal to walk or a limp and with no history of significant trauma. There is no fever or signs of infection. Laboratory data are normal, and radiographs of the painful area are usually normal initially. The child can be treated with a splint or cast for comfort and observed closely for signs of incipient infection. If an occult fracture is present, radiographs in 7 to 10 days show evidence of callus (new bone formation) and the diagnosis can be made in retrospect.

Kohler's Syndrome

Kohler's syndrome is an osteochondrosis affecting the navicular bone, usually occurring in children between the ages of 2 and 9 years. It was first described by Alban Kohler, a German radiologist (Wenger & Rang, 1993). The child usually presents with localized pain in the area of the navicular bone and a limp. Radiographic changes are characteristic, with the navicula being quite sclerotic and small compared with the opposite side. All of these cases resolve with time. Children with limited ambulation as a result of severe pain may be best managed with a brief period of casting.

Other orthopaedic conditions that can cause an acute limp in children from birth to 5 years include juvenile rheumatoid arthritis (see Chapter 8), non-accidental trauma (fractures or soft tissue injuries), hemophilia (Chapter 9), discitis, discoid meniscus, popliteal cysts, foreign bodies, and bone tumors.

AGE 5 TO 10 YEARS

Various types of osteochondroses are common causes of limp in the 5- to 10-year-old group as well as in the 10- to 15-year-old age group. These are idiopathic conditions (of unknown cause) characterized by a disorder of endochondral ossification. Many of these osteochondroses may be microtrauma fractures or growth plate injuries not appreciated on plain radiographs. They may be due to repetitive trauma with weight bearing (Lovell & Winter, 1978).

Perthes Disease

Legg-Calvé-Perthes disease is a condition in children who may be referred to physical therapy for treatment of the resulting muscle weakness, ROM limitations, and gait deviations. It was initially described in the early 1900s by three separate authors, Arthur T. Legg in the United States, Georg Perthes in Germany, and Jacques Calvé in France, and is defined as avascular necrosis of the ossific nucleus of the femoral head as a result of loss of blood supply. The medial femoral circumflex artery is the principal vessel in the complex vascular distribution in the neck and head of the femur.

Legg-Calvé-Perthes disease usually occurs in children between the ages of 3 and 12 and most commonly in boys aged 5 to 7 years of age (Wenger et al., 1991). The male-to-female ratio is 4:1 (Catteral, 1971). These children are frequently small for age and very active. The disease is bilateral in 20% of cases. The cause of Legg-Calvé-Perthes disease is not yet defined, but it occasionally follows repeated episodes of transient synovitis of the hip. One theory suggests that increased pressure in the joint due to synovitis blocks the blood vessels ascending the femoral neck into the femoral head. There may well be a number of pathologic processes that cause this interruption. The disease is self-limiting and always heals spontaneously in 1 to 3 years' time, as the femoral head revascularizes (Catterall, 1971). Not all patients have good outcomes, as defined by good hip ROM and no pain with activity. Prognostic factors include age at onset (younger children tend to do better), extent of the disease, the amount of femoral head deformity, and the amount of incongruity between the femoral head and acetabulum.

Patients tend to present with a limp and frequently with a positive Trendelenburg sign. This may be due to pain or hip abduction weakness. Limited hip ROM is noted, especially in hip abduction and internal rotation. The child complains of pain in the groin, hip, or knee (referred pain). Children who present with knee pain are frequently subjected to excessive radiation with multiple radiographs performed of the knee plus the opposite side for comparison. A careful clinical examination and observational gait analysis usually provide the information needed to avoid this situation, with clear indication that the problem is in the hip, not the knee. The radiographic findings reflect the temporary interruption of blood flow, with necrosis, possible subchondral fracture, collapse of the femoral head, and then regeneration of bone in the secondary ossification center.

Controversy exists regarding the appropriate treatment for Legg-Calvé-Perthes disease, or whether treatment is even necessary. Treatment methods include observation only, ROM exercises, bracing, Petrie casts (two long-leg casts with a bar between, holding the hips abducted), and surgery. Proximal varus derotation osteotomy of the femur decompresses the femoral head, centers it more deeply in the acetabulum when the limb is in the weight-bearing position, and allows long-term remodeling (Wenger et al., 1991). A pelvic osteotomy may be used alone or combined with varus derotation osteotomy for certain patients (e.g., with a femoral head so large or subluxated that femoral osteotomy alone will not contain the head).

A long-term, multicenter study is underway in the United States, coordinated by the Texas Scottish Rite Hospital. Preliminary results suggest that surgical treatment does favorably alter outcome in certain patient subgroups, but further follow-up and data analysis are needed to clarify these issues. Currently, many pediatric orthopaedists believe that treatment is required to maintain the appropriate shape of the femoral head (since it may tend to flatten if left untreated) and to prevent extrusion of the enlarged femoral head (coxa magna) from the joint, owing to poor acetabular coverage of the head. The goal of treatment is based on the theoretic principle of "containment," preserving the contour of the femoral head and keeping it centered in the acetabulum during the active phase of the disease. It is hoped that containment will prevent the development of premature degenerative arthritis. If the entire femoral head cannot be contained, it is still important to obtain and maintain hip motion, especially hip abduction.

Discoid Lateral Meniscus

The lateral meniscus can develop an abnormal discoid shape, apparently caused by hypermobility, since the more firmly attached medial meniscus rarely develops this discoid shape. A discoid lateral meniscus may become symptomatic, usually between the ages of 4 and 12 years (Scoles, 1988). It can cause pain, locking or clicking of the knee, and limp.

Sever's Disease

Sever's disease, or calcaneal apophysitis, is an osteochondrosis caused by trauma (i.e., traction of the tendo Achilles). This results in the fragmentation or avulsion of cartilage at the point of attachment, disruption of chondrogenesis, reparative callus, fibrosis, and ossification (Siffert, 1981). The child usually presents with pain in the heel area, exacerbated by sports and especially by running. The condition is usually self-limiting. It may be treated symptomatically with rest, ice, heel cups, heel lifts, reduced activity, and tendo Achilles stretching exercises. A short-leg walking cast may be used in cases with severe pain.

Growing Pains

"Growing pains" is a diagnosis frequently made by parents and probably is an entity observable in children, often during periods of rapid growth, when increased stresses occur in the musculoskeletal system. Growing pains is a diagnosis of exclusion; that is, all other more serious conditions must be ruled out. The child usually presents with aching in the legs (typically bilateral and generalized) usually at night and after high levels of activity during the day. Reassurance, symptomatic treatment such as massage and acetaminophen, and time usually resolve the symptoms. The child should be evaluated further if the pain increases or becomes localized or if other symptoms such as chronic fatigue appear.

Transient hip synovitis, described in the birth to 5 years of age section, can also be seen in this older age group.

AGE 10 TO 15 YEARS

Slipped Capital Femoral Epiphysis

Slipped capital femoral epiphysis (SCFE) is a frequent cause of limp in this older age group. It was first described by Ambroise Paré in 1572. SCFE (also called epiphysiolysis) occurs when the growth plate of the proximal femoral physis is weak and becomes displaced ("slips") from its normal position. This disorder is classified into three subtypes:

1. Acute: occurs with significant trauma and presents as immediate, severe pain, and restricted hip abduction and internal rotation.

2. Acute-on-chronic: the patient has already experienced some aching in the hip, thigh, or knee for weeks or even months as a result of a chronic slip. Then, with a significant trauma, the epiphysis suddenly slips farther and acute symptoms are noted.

3. Chronic: in this most common form the child presents with a history of limp and pain, often for weeks or months, and loss of hip motion, especially in internal rotation and abduction.

The cause of SCFE is unclear, although it is thought to involve a growth plate abnormality, probably on an endocrine basis, with or without the stress imposed by acute trauma or the chronic shearing stresses of weight bearing (Scoles, 1988). It is theorized that an imbalance exists between growth and sex hormones, causing a structural weakness in the epiphyseal plates. The incidence of SCFE is 0.71 to 3.41 per 100,000. The African-American population is more frequently affected than the white population. Males are more affected than females, with a 2 to 3:1 male-to-female ratio (Scoles, 1988). SCFE occurs about 2 years earlier in males than females and is closely related to the onset of puberty. Slips are bilateral in one fourth to one third of cases. Obesity is reported in as many as 75% of patients in some studies (Lovell & Winter, 1978).

The patient usually presents with an antalgic limp and pain in the groin, often referred to the anteromedial aspect of the thigh and knee. The leg is usually held in external rotation, both when supine and standing. Decreased hip motion is noted, especially in flexion, abduction, and internal rotation. With attempts to flex the hip, the leg tends to move into external rotation.

Radiographs demonstrate that the initial displacement is usually posteriorly and inferiorly and therefore may be missed on an anterior-posterior view. A "frog" view of both hips is needed for diagnosis. Slips are classified as grade I (displacement of the femoral head up to one third of the width of the femoral neck), grade II (more than one third but less than one half), and grade III (more than one half) (Fig. 15–11).

The goals of treatment are to keep the displacement to a minimum, to maintain motion, and to

FIGURE 15–11 Classification of the three grades of slipped capital femoral epiphysis. (From Lovell, WW & Winter, RB [Eds.], Pediatric Orthopaedics. Philadelphia. JB Lippincott, 1978, p. 767.)

FIGURE 15–12. *A*, Twelve-year-old boy with a 4-month history of hip pain, exacerbated by jumping off a picnic table 2 days ago. The slipped capital femoral epiphysis is not clearly identified on the anterior-posterior view. *B*, Frog view demonstrates a slipped capital femoral epiphysis on the left, thought to be an acute-on-chronic slip by history. *C*, Treatment with percutaneous pin fixation was successful.

delay or prevent premature degenerative arthritis. Treatment is by surgical pin fixation, usually in situ (Fig. 15–12). With higher degrees of slip, the procedure becomes more technically difficult and the incidence of pin penetration into the joint increases, leading to an increased incidence of chondrolysis (Aronson et al., 1992). There is also a significant danger of avascular necrosis with severe slips, especially if a forceful reduction is attempted, and especially if reduction is attempted with chronic slips. Most hips that have had an SCFE, even though surgically stabilized, develop some degenerative changes in later life, especially those with higher-grade slips, along with the complications of chondrolysis and avascular necrosis. These can affect the person's choice of occupation and recreational activities as an adult and cause secondary impairments, including hip pain and early degenerative arthritis.

Osgood-Schlatter Syndrome

Osgood-Schlatter disease, or syndrome, is characterized by activity-related pain and swelling at the insertion of the patellar tendon on the tibial tubercle caused by minor degrees of separation of the tibial tubercle (Salter & Harris, 1963). It may present as acute, severe pain, causing a child to limp, or be noted by the child over a period of months as low-grade discomfort, usually brought on by running or playing sports. Treatment consists of application of ice and rest, decreasing activity, and avoidance of all squatting and jumping activities. Use of a Neoprene knee brace may prove helpful. Severe cases may require cast immobilization initially. The condition is usually self-limiting and resolves when the tubercle fuses to the main body of the tibia, usually around the age of 15 years.

Osteochondritis Dissecans

Osteochondritis dissecans is a lesion affecting subchondral bone and the articular surface of a joint. The mechanism producing this disorder is believed to be ischemic necrosis, but the cause is unclear (probably trauma). It is frequently asymptomatic. Osteochondritis dissecans is most commonly noted in the distal femur, usually on the lateral surface of the medial femoral condyle. The child presents with pain, swelling around the knee, and an antalgic gait. If the fragment separates, the

FIGURE 15–13. A notch, or tunnel, view of the distal femurs demonstrates the osteochondritis dissecans lesions.

loose body may cause locking of the joint. The lesion is identified as a radiolucent area, usually on the posteromedial aspect of the distal femur, and thus often cannot be visualized on a straight anterior-posterior radiograph; a notch, or tunnel, view is needed (Fig. 15–13). In mild to moderate cases the treatment may consist of cast immobilization and then graduated activity with quadriceps strengthening exercises. If the defect has separated and an intra-articular loose fragment is present and causing symptoms, the child will need surgical treatment consisting of removal or fixation of the loose body and drilling through the cartilage into the bone in the base of the defect to stimulate healing by growth of new bone. Most cases of osteochondritis dissecans of the distal femur are self-limiting, however, and heal without surgical intervention.

Tarsal Coalition

An additional cause of limp is tarsal coalition, a failure of segmentation of the hindfoot bones. The connecting tissue may be fibrous, cartilaginous, or bony. Calcaneonavicular and talocalcaneal coalitions are the most common (Fig. 15–14). Tarsal coalition usually produces symptoms between the ages of 8 and 12 years when the abnormal cartilaginous bar begins to ossify. The child usually presents with foot pain, limp, and a rigid flat foot with decreased subtalar motion and peroneal spasm. The coalition may be defined on plain radiographs of the foot (oblique views). Often CT provides the most definitive information about the site of the fusion, especially in patients with talocalcaneal co-

FIGURE 15–14. Radiograph of a coronal section of the foot in a cadaver, demonstrating a talocalcaneal coalition affecting the middle facets of the talus and calcaneus (arrowhead) and a minimal posterior subtalar joint (arrow) (From Pineda C, et al. Diagnosis of tarsal coalition with computed tomography. Clinical Orthopaedics and Related Research, 208:282–288, 1986.)

alition (Pineda et al., 1986). Surgical excision of the coalition is usually necessary, successfully relieving symptoms.

Additional Causes of Limp

Patellofemoral pain and recurrent subluxation or dislocation of the patella are two common causes of limp in this age group (see Chapter 16 for a detailed discussion). Monoarticular arthritis and gonococcal arthritis are two other conditions that can cause a child to present acutely with a limp.

Finally, many types of neoplasms and related bone lesions can cause a child to limp. Commonly seen conditions include osteoid osteoma, unicameral bone cyst, osteochondroma (single or multiple), enchondroma, aneurysmal bone cyst, eosinophilic granuloma, and nonossifying fibroma. Presenting symptoms may include limp, pain, and pathologic fracture through the lesion.

▌ MISCELLANEOUS CONDITIONS

Several additional conditions should be briefly mentioned in a discussion of orthopaedic conditions in children.

Back Pain

Back pain in adults is frequently mechanical, but back pain in children (especially preadolescents) is often the result of organic causes (Thompson, 1993). Examples of etiology include spondylolysis and spondylolisthesis, infection (e.g., discitis or osteomyelitis), and either benign or malignant tumors. Complaints of back pain in children persisting for more than 1 to 2 weeks should be taken seriously. The child should be referred to a physician for an appropriate workup, especially if the pain is accompanied by fever, neurologic signs, or night pain.

Idiopathic Toe-Walking

A number of children tend to toe-walk some of the time when first walking independently. A smaller subset persist in toe-walking, yet have no history of prematurity or difficult delivery and no evidence of hypertonicity or abnormal developmental reflexes that might lead to a diagnosis of cerebral palsy. These children may have "soft" neurologic signs, such as a mild residual asymmetric tonic neck reflex in the quadruped position. They can be classified as "idiopathic toe-walkers" and

usually respond well to a conservative treatment program of therapeutic exercise to stretch the gastrocnemius and soleus muscles and strengthen the ankle dorsiflexors. With significant tendo Achilles contractures, they may require progressive casting, perhaps with short-leg cut-out casts to encourage active dorsiflexion.

There is also a group of idiopathic toe walkers in which a family history of toe-walking can be documented. This is an autosomal dominant pattern described by Katz and Mubarak (1984). Operative treatment is rarely required and carries the risk of overlengthening, which can cause a serious functional deficit.

Achondroplasia

Of a large group of conditions known as the osteochondroplasias, the most common is achondroplasia (dwarfism). The incidence is approximately 1:10,000 births. It is an autosomal dominant condition with about 90% of cases representing a fresh mutation (Smith & Jones, 1982). Orthopaedic manifestations of this condition include frontal bossing, cuboid-shaped vertebral bodies that may cause narrowing of the spinal canal and cord compression, with short pedicles, lumbar lordosis, short tubular bones, and short trident-shaped hands. Achondroplastic dwarfs have abnormal length ratios of limbs to trunk, with more shortening of the proximal segments, in contrast to midgets, who have proportionate limb and trunk ratios.

Congenital Muscular Torticollis

Congenital muscular torticollis is a unilateral contracture of the sternocleidomastoid muscle, first described by Hippocrates 2000 years ago. Many theories regarding its cause have been proposed; the most recent investigations suggest that this condition represents the sequela of an intrauterine or perinatal compartment syndrome (Davids et al., 1993). Congenital muscular torticollis is frequently associated with a history of difficult delivery and an increased incidence of associated conditions such as DDH and metatarsus adductus.

The child with torticollis presents with the head tilted to the side of the shortened sternocleidomastoid muscle and the chin rotated to the opposite side. Lateral neck flexion to the uninvolved side and rotation to the involved side are limited. This may be present at birth or be noted a few weeks or even months later. A firm, nontender mass in the affected sternocleidomastoid muscle may be noted. This mass may enlarge over 2 to 4 weeks and then gradually resolve over a period of months. Secondary head and facial asymmetry, termed *plagiocephaly,* may result, especially if the torticollis is not treated. The face on the side of the affected muscle will flatten as the child lies prone with the head turned to the opposite side in the position of greatest comfort.

Treatment consists of active and passive stretching exercises for the involved muscle, strengthening exercises for the contralateral sternocleidomastoid muscle, and positioning to encourage lateral bend to the opposite side and neck rotation to the involved side. Equilibrium reactions can be used in treatment for the older infant, such as using head righting to encourage lateral bend to the uninvolved side. Most cases resolve with conservative treatment and time. It is recommended that all children with persisting torticollis, and all children with concomitant DDH or metatarsus adductus, have radiography of the cervical spine to rule out congenital spine anomalies. If there is a persistent head tilt with normal passive ROM in lateral bend and rotation, an eye examination should be considered; occasionally a visual problem will cause the child to tilt the head to better focus the eyes. Only a small percentage of cases of congenital muscular torticollis require surgical correction; surgery is usually performed if significant deformity persists after 1 year of age.

LEG LENGTH INEQUALITY

A generally accepted definition of leg length inequality is 2.5 cm or greater difference in the length of the two limbs. Differences in length smaller than this tend not to cause clinical problems. The difference in leg lengths may be due to relative overgrowth of one extremity or relative shortening of one extremity.

Etiology

The etiology of leg length inequality may be divided into a number of categories: trauma, congenital, neuromuscular, acquired diseases, infections causing growth arrest of the physis, tumors, and vascular disorders. Types of trauma include epiphyseal and diaphyseal injuries. Epiphyseal injuries with growth plate closure may be asymmetric, such as a fracture involving the medial epiphysis of the distal femur. This type of injury can result in an angular deformity (varus) as well as shortening of the femur.

Congenital disorders include hemihypertrophy, in which one half of the body (the arm and leg) is larger than the other, or hemiatrophy, in which one half of the body is smaller than the other. These can sometimes be difficult to distinguish, and they often necessitate a clinical evaluation of which arm and leg best "match" the rest of the body. Proximal focal femoral deficiency, congenital coxa vara, fibular and tibial hemimelia, and other focal dysplasias are additional causes of leg length inequality (see Chapter 14). DDH can also cause a leg length discrepancy, either with an apparent femoral shortening noted when the hip is dislocated or if the femur is actually short owing to avascular necrosis of the femoral head. The femur may also be short as a result of surgical treatment of the problem (e.g., use of a varus derotation osteotomy to better center the femoral head in the acetabulum). The overall length of the leg including the hemipelvis may be actually increased as a result of surgical treatment as well. One example would be certain types of pelvic osteotomies used to create a deeper acetabulum, that may add up to 1 inch to the height of the pelvis.

Neuromuscular disorders may result in leg-length discrepancies by causing asymmetric growth of the bones in the lower extremity. Decreased growth in the affected leg may be due to decreased muscle forces in weak or paralyzed muscles. Examples of this type of condition include myelodysplasia, poliomyelitis, and hemiplegia caused by congenital or acquired cerebral palsy. Not all cases of leg length inequality should be corrected. A child with hemiplegic cerebral palsy will have a short lower limb on the affected side. Because of the weakness and spasticity in that leg, foot clearance may be difficult as a result of decreased hip and knee flexion and equinus positioning of the foot and ankle. The shortness of the leg makes foot clearance in swing easier. A similar situation may be encountered in patients with polio who may more easily advance a weakened leg if it is short.

Acquired conditions such as Legg-Calvé-Perthes disease and slipped capital femoral epiphysis can result in a shortened lower extremity, usually as a result of avascular necrosis of the femoral head or occasionally as the result of surgical treatment, as noted earlier for DDH. Fibrous dysplasia is another example of an acquired condition that can cause a leg length inequality. Finally, tumors, including benign bone cysts and malignant neoplasms, can change the length of a leg. This can occur either through interference with growth centers by the disease process or secondarily as a result of fracture or surgical treatment.

Impairments

The effects of leg length inequality vary widely among patients because of the patient's perception of the problem; the actual amount of difference; the overall picture of muscle strength, motor control, and ROM; the possibility of progression of the inequality; how well the patient physically compensates for it; and a multitude of other factors. Leg length inequality can result in poor cosmesis if the discrepancy is marked or compensation is limited; significant increase in energy expenditure required to walk; and musculoskeletal adaptations and compensations. These secondary impairments include pelvic obliquity with changes in spinal alignment that can cause low back pain and may produce a functional scoliosis. Other musculoskeletal adaptations may be required at the hip, knee, and ankle, with subsequent alterations in gait. These problems may be quite significant but, because of the inherent energy and motivation usually present in children, may be easily accommodated. In adulthood, however, the factors of increased size and weight, increased energy expenditure to walk, increased sensitivity regarding the poor cosmesis of a lurching gait, or long-term effects of an asymmetric lumbosacral spinal alignment, may combine to significantly reduce the person's ability to walk, even rendering him or her nonambulatory, resulting in significant disability.

Assessment

Assessment of leg length inequality includes obtaining a complete history, including any previous treatment; clinical analysis of gait, including observation of spine and lower extremity alignment and substitution patterns; observation of the patient with and without assistive devices and shoe lift in gait on level ground, ramps, stairs, and in functional activities, such as rising from a chair to standing and getting down to the floor and back up to standing; measurement of ROM and muscle strength of the trunk, hips, knees, ankles, and feet; body measurements including both sitting and standing height, weight, and arm span; and leg length measurements.

Two options are available for clinical measurement of leg lengths. One is to level the pelvis in standing, using blocks under the short leg. The other is to actually measure the legs using various landmarks: anterior-superior iliac spine to medial malleolus, anterior-superior iliac spine to lateral malleolus, anterior-superior iliac spine to heel pad, and umbilicus to heel pad. In a patient without significant lower extremity contractures, leveling the pelvis in standing with blocks may be the most accurate (reproducible). Radiographic measurement of leg lengths is usually done with a scanogram. In this type of radiograph, the patient is positioned on the x-ray table with a ruler alongside the legs. Three radiographs are taken on the same cassette, at the level of the hips, knees, and ankles, with the patient held motionless. These three views, with the ruler markings next to them, allow the examiner to measure the length of the femur and the tibia, and combine them for the total leg length. Landmarks commonly used are the top of the femoral head, the bottom of the medial femoral condyle, and the tibial plateau. A film of the left wrist and hand should be performed in conjunction with the scanogram. This allows determination of the skeletal age of the patient, using a reference such as Greulich and Pyle (1950).

A range of measurement error is present in the use of any of these techniques. Validity of the measurement is affected if the patient has flexion contractures of the hip or knee that "shorten" the leg and decrease the accuracy of assessing skeletal length of the leg. Determination of bone age is somewhat subjective. These and other factors make leg length determinations, both clinical and radiographic, an inexact science. The percentage of growth inhibition must also be determined because this assists in estimating the eventual discrepancy at maturity. For example, a 10% inhibition of growth in the short leg may result in a minor discrepancy when the child is quite young. When the leg is 20 cm long, a 10% shortening is 2 cm. When the leg is 70 cm long, however, a 10% inhibition of growth will result in a shortening of 7 cm, which is quite significant.

The most helpful information is gained if the patient can be followed with serial measurements over time, both clinically and by scanogram. Scanogram measurements of total length of both the long and the short leg and the skeletal age at the time of each scanogram can be plotted on the Moseley graph (Moseley, 1977) (Fig. 15–15). This graph provides not only a depiction of past growth but also a prediction of future growth. Observing the child longitudinally allows more accurate planning for treatment, avoiding errors that are possible when making decisions based on a single measurement. The leg length discrepancy at the time of skeletal maturity can be predicted to assist in the timing of surgery. The effects of surgery can also be plotted on the graph to predict the alteration in leg lengths and the eventual impact on discrepancy at skeletal maturity.

FIGURE 15-15. An example of the use of the Moseley graph to plot a patient's serial scanogram measurements and bone ages to determine the discrepancy at maturity and the possibilities for surgical intervention. Growth of the short leg is depicted by the line below the normal leg line. The increase in the length of the short leg (*arrow*) shows the effects of a leg-lengthening procedure. The two legs are approximately equal at skeletal maturity.

Treatment

Treatment of leg length inequality may be conservative or surgical. Conservative treatment consists of observation only or use of a shoe lift. Surgical treatment is directed at either shortening the long leg or lengthening the short leg. Some patients may need to have both done to achieve equality at maturity. Shortening the long leg in the growing child is usually achieved by epiphysiodesis, the surgical epiphyseal arrest of one or more growth centers in the long leg. This allows the short leg to "catch up" in length. The fastest growing growth plate in the leg is the distal femur, followed by that of the proximal tibia. The percentages of growth of the leg that occur at each center have been defined as proximal femur 30% and distal femur 70% of the total length of the femur and proximal tibia 60% and distal tibia 40% of the total length of the tibia (Moseley, 1977). The percentages of growth for the entire leg are proximal femur, 15%; distal femur,

35%; proximal tibia, 30%; and distal tibia, 20%. Timing of the epiphysiodesis is obviously crucial. Future growth of each leg must be predicted and the surgery performed at a time when the amount of growth denied the long leg will match the amount of growth still available in the short leg, allowing them to be approximately equal in length at skeletal maturity. If epiphysiodesis is performed too early, the long leg may actually become the short leg, with an obviously less than optimal surgical result. One other option for shortening the long leg is a shortening osteotomy. This is usually considered in a patient who has already reached skeletal maturity and is not a candidate for epiphysiodesis.

Epiphysiodesis may also be performed on only the medial or lateral part of the growth plate to correct varus or valgus problems. For example, a fracture of the distal femur may cause damage to the medial aspect of the distal femoral growth plate. The lateral part of the growth plate then continues to function normally and the leg grows into varus, which also produces a functional shortening. If the medial portion of the growth plate is still open, stapling of the lateral portion can allow the femur to gradually grow out of varus. This type of surgery may also include resection of a bony bar on the involved side of the growth plate.

LIMB LENGTHENING

Surgical lengthening of the short leg has appeal as a treatment alternative because the surgery is performed on the affected leg, not the "normal" leg, and the opportunity exists for correction of discrepancies of much greater magnitude. Leg lengthening may be indicated when the discrepancy is greater than 4 to 6 cm; adequate soft tissue mobility is available to allow correction; and there is a stable joint above and below, although unstable joints can be protected with an external frame. A decision must be made whether to lengthen the femur or the tibia or both. Ideally the final result will be fairly equal leg lengths and equal knee heights in standing. If the discrepancy is too large to be amenable to these procedures, as in some cases of proximal focal femoral deficiency, then amputation of the distal segment to allow the use of a prosthesis would be considered to be the most practical alternative (see Chapter 14). Another option is a rotationplasty of the affected limb (Torode & Gillespie, 1983).

Limb lengthening was first reported in the literature by Codivilla in Italy in 1905 (Coleman & Scott, 1991), and the field has expanded significantly since that time. Two biologic approaches to lengthening exist: 1) lengthening through bone and

2) lengthening by physeal distraction. Physeal distraction includes the option of subacute epiphysiolysis, initially described by Monticelli and Spinelli and called chondrodiatasis (Coleman & Scott, 1991). It consists of gradual distraction of the growth plate using a circular fixator, leading to a sudden rupture of the growth plate 3 to 4 days after the procedure begins. This is rarely used except for adolescent limb lengthening near the end of the patient's growth, since it may lead to premature closure of the growth plate.

A number of devices have been developed for lengthening bone, including diaphyseal lengthening devices (Wagner, unilateral frame) and metaphyseal lengthening devices, such as the Ilizarov (circular frame), Monticelli-Spinelli (circular frame and half ring), and DeBastiani (Orthofix unilateral frame) devices (Coleman & Scott, 1991). The Wagner technique for lengthening through bone involves an osteotomy of the bone followed by rapid distraction, with cancellous bone grafting and plating of the distraction gap (Wagner, 1978).

The Ilizarov technique of slow distraction does not use bone grafting of the distraction gap. The circular design and the custom fitting of the external fixator allows simultaneous correction of rotational and angular deformities, as well as achieving the lengthening. The standard rate of distraction is 1 mm/d, but this may vary with the individual case. The frequency of distraction is usually four times per day (0.25 mm each time). After the desired correction has been achieved, the fixator is left in place to allow consolidation of new bone. Dr. Gavriil Abramovich Ilizarov first developed his technique and device to treat World War II veterans in Russia, many of whom had osteomyelitis and other complications of gunshot-related fractures (Golykhovsky, 1992, in the introduction to Ilizarov & Ledyaev, 1969). In the 1950s he improved his apparatus and widened the application of his techniques to treat a variety of orthopaedic problems. At that time, all parts of the apparatus were fabricated by patients and their relatives in a factory that made bus parts and smuggled out. He continued with his pioneering work in using the plasticity of bone for clinical benefit, such as lengthening, and healing nonunions and pseudarthroses with distraction and fixation. His successful treatment of Valery Brumel, the famous Soviet high jumper who sustained an open fracture of the tibia, led to long overdue national and international prominence and expansion of his services to an 800-bed institute with 24 operating rooms; 350 orthopaedic surgeons; 1500 nurses, physical therapists, and other medical personnel; and 26 research and clinical laboratories.

Many applications of the Ilizarov technique are currently in use for both adult and pediatric disorders, including limb length discrepancy, angular deformities such as adolescent Blount's disease, congenital tibial pseudarthrosis, resistant or recurrent clubfeet, correction of forearm or humeral shortening and deformity due to trauma or infection, and others (Rajacich et al., 1992). Another more controversial indication for leg lengthening is its bilateral use in patients with achondroplasia to achieve a more normal height (Paley, 1988).

Complications of lengthening procedures can be divided into five categories: bone, joint, nerve, muscle, and vascular complications. Bone complications include angulation, delayed union or nonunion, fractures, pin tract infections, and osteomyelitis. Joint complications include cartilage degeneration, stiffness, subluxation, or dislocation. Nerves can suffer stretch paralysis that may be transient or permanent. Complications of muscle include weakness, contracture, and ischemia. There may also be vascular complications, such as a transient hypertension, probably due to stretching of the sciatic nerve, although this has not been well documented. As defined by Paley (1990), "problems" following lengthening procedures represent difficulties that do not require operative intervention, "obstacles" require operative intervention, and true "complications" include all problems that do not resolve by the end of treatment.

Children undergoing leg lengthening must adjust to the discomfort and temporary loss of independence inherent in the procedure and may experience frustration, anger, and fear. Difficult behavior may require intervention by a psychologist to assist the child and family in developing appropriate strategies for coping with all of the ramifications of this undertaking. Candidates for surgical lengthening must be extremely motivated, with a supportive and committed family. Successful undertaking of surgical lengthening also mandates a comprehensive medical care system, with knowledgeable, experienced physicians, nurses, and therapists to guide the patient and family through the process.

ROLE OF PHYSICAL THERAPY IN LIMB LENGTHENING

Physical therapy involvement with the child undergoing limb lengthening may vary with the patient and the institution in which the procedure is performed. An excellent description of the physical therapy goals and program for these patients is provided by Simard and colleagues (1992). They describe the phases of intervention in patients undergoing leg lengthening by the Ilizarov technique.

The preoperative phase includes assessment of muscle strength, passive ROM, sensation, girth of thighs and calves, leg length discrepancy, and joint stability; description of bony deformities; evaluation of posture and gait; functional mobility skills assessment; crutch-fitting and instruction in ambulation; and instruction in a home exercise program and postoperative positioning and splinting as well as stretching and strengthening exercises to use in preparation for surgery.

The greatest challenges for the physical therapist treating children in the postoperative phase include promoting weight bearing in the presence of significant pain, maintaining the child's ROM, and motivating the patient to continue with the program both in the hospital and at home over the long period of treatment. There can also be significant difficulty in obtaining funding for physical therapy because insurance carriers usually want documentation of improved function during the treatment period. For the patient undergoing leg lengthening by the Ilizarov technique, the goal is to maintain ambulation, joint ROM, and strength while undergoing the lengthening, with a long-term goal of improved function after the device is removed.

The postoperative phase includes instruction in functional activities, active assistive and isometric exercise, proper positioning of the extremity, gait training with progressive weight bearing as tolerated, and sterile pin care. Modalities such as ice or transcutaneous electrical nerve stimulation may be useful for pain management. Dynamic splinting may be used in the limb-lengthening stage to provide low-intensity, prolonged stretch to joints with significantly limited ROM. Exercise techniques useful throughout the Ilizarov lengthening include both closed- and open-chain exercise for strengthening and active assistive or passive exercise for ROM. A stationary bicycle and treadmill may be used. After removal of the fixator, the patient may require additional gait training, monitoring and adjusting of the exercise program, and possibly refitting and retraining with orthotic or prosthetic devices worn preoperatively. Throughout the course of treatment, children are encouraged to participate in their usual school and leisure activities to the fullest extent possible.

CASE HISTORY: AMY

Amy was referred for orthopaedic consultation at 1 day of age, and the following clinical findings were documented: positive Galeazzi sign on the left with the femur approximately 2 cm short, anterior bow and asymmetric shape of the left thigh, hip abduction right/left 70°/40°, shortening of the left tibia measured clinically at 2 cm, a band in the area of the left fibula, calcaneovalgus of the left foot with the fibula not palpable at the ankle; the ankle could be moved into 30° of plantar flexion and varus. Radiographs showed both hips located, with decreased distance between the femur and acetabulum suggestive of both coxa vara and decreased femoral neck length, and slight bow of the left femur; shortening of the left femur by 2 cm compared with the right, with the tibia 1 cm short; and complete absence of the fibula. The diagnosis was made of left proximal focal femoral deficiency and absent left fibula.

The following summary documents the progression of Amy's limb-length discrepancy as she grew older and the treatment for it:

1 month:	physical therapy—home exercise program
3 months:	30° knee flexion contracture, valgus foot
10 months:	excision of fibular anlage, peroneus longus muscle lengthening; scanogram showed 5.6 cm of shortening
13 months:	fitted with a step-in prosthesis, follow-up physical therapy. Options for treatment: 1) knee fusion and Syme's amputation, followed by fitting with an above-knee prosthesis; 2) maintain use of her step-in prosthesis; 3) modified Van Nes rotationplasty
2 years:	using step-in prosthesis, able to run and jump; left leg 7.3 cm short by scanogram
3 years:	left leg 9.2 cm short, continuing with the 20% inhibition of growth noted earlier
8 years:	left leg 12.7 cm short; able to ski with step-in prosthesis
9 years, 9 months:	left Salter pelvic osteotomy to correct her mild acetabular dysplasia

At age 10 years, Amy had the following problems in her left leg: significant shortening of the femur and tibia requiring the use of a prosthesis to equalize her leg lengths, external rotational deformity of the femur, genu valgum secondary to a hypoplastic lateral femoral condyle, an apex medial bow in the tibia, and equinus of the ankle. Her projected leg length inequality at skeletal maturity was 18 cm. This combination of problems resulted in an awkward gait, decreased abilities in sports, and poor cosmesis. At this time a limb-lengthening procedure was recommended and agreed to by the child and family, who were very much against amputation, the only other alternative. Surgery consisted of application of Ilizarov frames to the left femur, tibia, and foot to accomplish femoral lengthening, rotational and angular correction, and tibial lengthening and angular correction. She also underwent a tendo Achilles lengthening.

Lengthening in the Ilizarov frame can be varied in amount and frequency, depending on patient status. Amy's initial lengthening was 0.25 mm 4 times a day, in both the femur and tibia. This rate will provide 1 mm of lengthening each 24 hours in each bone.

The following summary documents her progress during the course of postoperative treatment:

3 weeks:	attending school part time. Knee extension − 15°; continued on a regular physical therapy program of active and active-assistive ROM and strengthening exercises
4 weeks:	left tibia subluxating posteriorly on femur; rate of lengthening decreased temporarily
3 months:	foot frame removed; weight bearing as tolerated; ongoing exercise program of ROM exercises of left knee and ankle, strengthening exercises for quadriceps, hip abductor, and hip extensor muscles; able to exercise in pool
7 months:	tibial frame removed with 3 cm of tibial lengthening achieved; knee passively taken through ROM, to aid in ROM exercises postoperatively
8 months:	resumed an aggressive knee ROM exercise program; care was taken to hold the tibia just distal to the knee, avoiding a long lever arm across the regenerate bone site
9 months:	losing knee ROM; continuous passive motion machine instituted 4 hours per day; dynamic splint also used
10 months:	femoral frame removed with 13 cm of femoral lengthening achieved
10½ months:	5-day history of deformity of the proximal femur and increased pain; diagnosis of femoral fracture through one of the half-pin sites; closed reduction, insertion of distal femoral traction pin, and application of Neufeld traction
11 months:	further closed reduction, removal of traction pin and application of a spica cast
12 months:	total contact HKAFO, with free hip, knee, and ankle joints; worn full time, with time out for bathing; ROM exercise (active only)
13 months:	radiographs showed evidence of an additional, healing pathologic stress fracture of the femur
14½ months:	able to walk well with HKAFO and one crutch, no pain; extensive stretching and strengthening program through physical therapy, physical education at school, and home exercise program.

Of her original projected discrepancy of 18 cm, a total of 16 cm was gained through the femoral and tibial lengthenings. Amy's knees were essentially level when the procedure was completed. Goals at this time include independent ambulation without bracing or assistive devices, a smoother gait with decreased energy expenditure, increased agility in sports, and improved cosmesis. The abbreviated documentation of the process noted earlier can only hint at the incredible amount of work, time, and commitment required by this type of treatment on the part of everyone involved.

Acknowledgments

I would like to thank Scott J. Mubarak, MD, Director of the Orthopaedic Institute, Children's Hospital, San Diego, for his review and helpful comments for this chapter, and Patricia Silva, PT, Children's Hospital, San Diego, for her contributions to the section on the role of physical therapy in limb lengthening.

References

Aronson, DD, Peterson, DA, & Miller, DV. Slipped capital femoral epiphysis: The case for internal fixation in situ. Clinical Orthopaedics and Related Research, 281:115–122, 1992.

Bennett, OM, & Namnyak, SS. Acute septic arthritis of the hip joint in infancy and childhood. Clinical Orthopaedics and Related Research, 281:123–132, 1992.

Cahuzac, JP, Hobatho, MC, Baunin, C, Boulot, J, Darmana, R, & Autefage, A. Classification of 125 children with rotational abnormalities. Journal of Pediatric Orthopaedics, Part B, 1:59–66, 1992.

Catteral, A. The natural history of Perthes' disease. Journal of Bone and Joint Surgery (British), 53:37–53, 1971.

Coleman, SS, & Scott, SM. The present attitude toward the biology and technology of limb lengthening. Clinical Orthopaedics and Related Research, 264:76–83, 1991.

Crane, L. Femoral torsion and its relation to toeing-in and toeing-out. Journal of Bone and Joint Surgery (American), 41:421–428, 1959.

Dales, MC, & Hoffinger, SA. Septic hip in older children and adolescents (Abstract). Proceedings of the American Academy of Orthopaedic Surgeons Annual Meeting, San Francisco. American Academy of Orthopaedic Surgeons, 1993.

Davids, JR, Wenger, DR, & Mubarak, SJ. Congenital muscular torticollis: Sequela of intrauterine or perinatal compartment syndrome. Journal of Pediatric Orthopaedics, 13:1–7, 1993.

Dunn, PM. Perinatal observations of the etiology of congenital dislocation of the hip. Clinical Orthopaedics and Related Research, 119:11–22, 1976.

Engel, GM, & Staheli, LT. The natural history of torsion and other factors influencing gait in childhood. Clinical Orthopaedics and Related Research, 99:12–17, 1974.

Fabry, G, MacEwen, D, & Shands, AR. Torsion of the femur: A follow-up study in normal and abnormal conditions. Journal of Bone and Joint Surgery (American), 55:1726–1738, 1973.

Galpin, RD, Roach, JW, Wenger, DR, Herring, JA, & Birch, JG. One-stage treatment of congenital dislocation of the hip in older children, including femoral shortening. Journal of Bone and Joint Surgery (American), 71:734–741, 1989.

Graf, R. Hip sonography—how reliable? Sector scanning versus linear scanning? Dynamic versus static examination? Clinical Orthopaedics and Related Research, 281:18–21, 1992.

Greulich, WW, & Pyle, SI. Radiographic Atlas of Skeletal Development of the Hand and Wrist. Stanford, CA: Stanford University Press, 1950.

Harcke, HT. Imaging in congenital dislocation and dysplasia of the hip. Clinical Orthopaedics and Related Research, 281:22–28, 1992.

Hensinger, RH, & Jones, ET. Neonatal orthopaedics. In Oliver, TK (Ed.), Monographs in Neonatalogy. New York: Grune & Stratton, 1981.

Herring, JA. Conservative treatment of congenital dislocation of the hip in the newborn and infant. Clinical Orthopaedics and Related Research, 281:41–47, 1992.

Hofmann, A, Jones, RE, & Herring, JA. Blount's disease after skeletal maturity. Journal of Bone and Joint Surgery (American), 64:1004–1009, 1982.

Hummer, CD, & MacEwen, GD. The coexistence of torticollis and congenital dysplasia of the hip. Journal of Bone and Joint Surgery (American), 54:1255–1256, 1972.

Ilfeld, FW, Westin, GW, & Makin, M. Missed or developmental dislocation of the hip. Clinical Orthopaedics and Related Research, 203:276–281, 1986.

Ilizarov, GA, & Ledyaev, VI. The replacement of long tubular bone defects by lengthening distraction osteotomy of one of the fragments. Vestnik. Khururgii, 6:78, 1969. Translated by Schwartzman, V. in Clinical Orthopaedics and Related Research, 280:7–10, 1992.

Johnson, CE. Infantile tibia vara. Clinical Orthopaedics and Related Research, 255:13–23, 1990.

Kasser, JR, Bowen, JR, & MacEwen, GD. Varus derotation osteotomy in the treatment of persistent dysplasia due to congenital dislocation of the hip. Journal of Bone and Joint Surgery (American), 67:195, 1985.

Katz, MM, & Mubarak, SJ, Hereditary tendo Achillis contractures. Journal of Pediatric Orthopedics, 4:711–714, 1984.

Langenskiold, A. Tibia vara: A critical review. Clinical Orthopaedics and Related Research, 246:195–206, 1989.

Lee, J, Jarvis, J, Uhthoff, HK, & Avruch, L. The fetal acetabulum. Clinical Orthopaedics and Related Research, 281:48–55, 1992.

Lovell, WW, & Winter, RB. Pediatric Orthopaedics. Vols. I and II. Philadelphia: JB Lippincott, 1978.

Moseley, CF. A straight-line graph for leg-length discrepancies. Journal of Bone and Joint Surgery (American), 59:174–179, 1977.

Mubarak, SJ, Beck, L, & Sutherland, D. Home traction in the management of congenital dislocation of the hips. Journal of Pediatric Orthopaedics, 6:721–723, 1986.

Mubarak, SJ, Garfin, SR, Vance, R, McKinnon, B, & Suther-

land, D. Pitfalls in the use of the Pavlik harness for treatment of congenital dysplasia, subluxation, and dislocation of the hip. Journal of Bone and Joint Surgery (American), 63:1239–1248, 1981.

Mubarak, SJ, Leach, JL, & Wenger, DR. Management of congenital dislocation of the hip in the infant. Contemporary Orthopaedics, 15:29–44, 1987.

Paley, D. Current techniques of limb lengthening. Journal of Pediatric Orthopaedics, 8:73–92, 1988.

Paley, D. Problems, obstacles, and complications of limb lengthening by the Ilizarov technique. Clinical Orthopaedics and Related Research, 250:81–104, 1990.

Pavlik, A. Stirrups as an aid in the treatment of congenital dysplasias of the hip in children. LeKarskeListy 5(3–4):81–85, 1950. Translated by Bialik, V, & Reis, ND in Journal of Pediatric Orthopaedics, 9:157–159, 1989.

Pavlik, A. The functional method of treatment using a harness with stirrups as the primary method of conservative therapy for infants with congenital dislocation of the hip. Zeitschrift fur Orthopadie und Ihre Grenzgebeit 89:341, 1957. Translated by Peltier, L.F. in Clinical Orthopaedics and Related Research, 281:4–10, 1992.

Pineda, C, Resnick, D, & Greenway, G. Diagnosis of tarsal coalition with computed tomography. Clinical Orthopaedics and Related Research, 208:282–288, 1986.

Pitkow, RB. External rotation contracture of the extended hip. Clinical Orthopaedics and Related Research, 110:139–144, 1975.

Rajacich, N, Bell, DF, & Armstrong, PF. Pediatric applications of the Ilizarov method. Clinical Orthopaedics and Related Research, 280:72–80, 1992.

Salter, RB. Innominate osteotomy in the treatment of congenital dislocation and subluxation of the hip. Journal of Bone and Joint Surgery (British), 43:518, 1961.

Salter, RB. Role of innominate osteotomy in the treatment of congenital dislocation and subluxation of the hip in the older child. Journal of Bone and Joint Surgery (American), 48:1413–1439, 1966.

Salter, RB. Etiology, pathogenesis and possible prevention of congenital dislocation of the hip. Canadian Medical Association Journal, 98:933–945, 1968.

Salter, RB. Textbook of Disorders and Injuries of the Musculoskeletal System. Baltimore: Williams & Wilkins, 1970.

Salter, RB, & Harris, WR. Injuries involving the epiphyseal plate. Journal of Bone and Joint Surgery (American), 45:587–622, 1963.

Scoles, PV. Pediatric Orthopaedics in Clinical Practice (2nd ed). Chicago: Year Book Medical Publishers, 1988.

Scoles, PV, Boyd, A, & Jones, PK. Roentgenographic parameters of the normal infant hip. Journal of Pediatric Orthopaedics, 7:656–663, 1987.

Shands, AR, & Steele, MK. Torsion of the femur: A follow-up report on the use of the Dunlap method for its determination. Journal of Bone and Joint Surgery (American), 40:803–816, 1958.

Siffert, RS. Classification of the osteochondroses. Clinical Orthopaedics and Related Research, 158:10–18, 1981.

Simard, S, Marchant, M, & Mencio, G. The Ilizarov procedure: Limb lengthening and its implications. Physical Therapy, 72:25–34, 1992.

Smith, DW, & Jones, KL. Recognizable Patterns of Human Malformation, Vol. VII. Major Problems in Clinical Pediatrics. Philadelphia: WB Saunders, 1982.

Staheli, LT. Torsional deformity. Pediatric Clinics of North America, 24:799–811, 1977.

Staheli, LT. Surgical management of acetabular dysplasia. Clinical Orthopaedics and Related Research, 264:111–121, 1991.

Staheli, LT, Corbett, M, Wyss, C, & King, H. Lower extremity rotational problems in children. Journal of Bone and Joint Surgery (American), *67*:39–47, 1985.

Staheli, LT, Engel, GM. Tibial torsion: A method of assessment and a study of normal children. Clinical Orthopaedics and Related Research, *86*:183–186, 1972.

Stuberg, WA, Koehler, A, Wichita, M, Temme, J, & Kaplan, P. A comparison of femoral torsion assessment using goniometry and computerized tomography. Pediatric Physical Therapy, *1*:115–118, 1989.

Tachdjian, MO. Pediatric Orthopaedics, (2nd ed.), Vols. 1–4. Philadelphia: WB Saunders, 1990.

Thompson, GH. Back pain in children: An instructional course lecture. Journal of Bone and Joint Surgery (American), *75*:928–938, 1993.

Thompson, GH, & Carter, JR. Late onset tibia vara (Blount's disease). Clinical Orthopaedics and Related Research, *255*:24–35, 1990.

Torode, IP, & Gillespie, R. Rotationplasty of the lower limb for congenital defects of the femur. Journal of Bone and Joint Surgery (British), *65*:569–573, 1983.

Tredwell, SJ, & Bell, HM. Efficacy of neonatal hip examination. Journal of Pediatric Orthopaedics, *1*:61–65, 1981.

Wagner, H. Operative lengthening of the femur. Clinical Orthopaedics and Related Research, *136*:125–142, 1978.

Weinstein, SL. Congenital hip dislocation: Long range problems, residual signs and symptoms after successful treatment. Clinical Orthopaedics and Related Research, *281*:69–74, 1992.

Wenger, DR, & Leach, J. Foot deformities in infants and children. Pediatric Clinics of North America, *33*:1411–1427, 1986.

Wenger, DR, Mauldin, D, Speck, G, Morgan, D, & Lieber, RL. Corrective shoes and inserts as treatment for flexible flatfoot in infants and children. Journal of Bone and Joint Surgery (American), *71*:800–810, 1989.

Wenger, DR, & Rang, M. The Art of Pediatric Orthopaedics. New York: Raven Press, 1993.

Wenger, DR, Ward, WT, & Herring, JA. Current concepts review: Legg-Calvé-Perthes disease. Journal of Bone and Joint Surgery (American), *73*:778–788, 1991.

Wynne-Davies, R. Family studies and the cause of congenital clubfoot: Talipes equinovarus, talipes calcaneovalgus and metatarsus varus. Journal of Bone and Joint Surgery (British), *46*:445–463, 1964.

Wynne-Davies, R. Acetabular dysplasia and familial joint laxity: Two etiological factors in congenital dislocation of the hip. Journal of Bone and Joint Surgery (British), *52*:704–716, 1970.

Bibliography

Bucholz, RB, Lippert, FG, Wenger, DR, & Ezaki, M. Orthopaedic Decision Making. Philadelphia: BC Decker, 1984.

Coleman, SS. Complex Foot Deformities in Children. Philadelphia: Lea & Febiger, 1983.

Greene, WB, & Jones, ET (Eds.). Selected Bibliography of Pediatric Orthopaedics with Commentary. Park Ridge, IL: American Academy of Orthopaedic Surgeons, 1990.

Hensinger, RN. Congenital Dislocation of the Hip. Ciba Clinical Symposia, Vol 31, no. 1. Summit, NJ: Ciba Pharmaceutical, 1979.

Orthopaedic Knowledge Update: Home Study Syllabus, Vols. 1–3. Park Ridge, IL: American Academy of Orthopaedic Surgeons, 1984, 1987, 1990.

Ramsey, PL, Lasser S, & MacEwen, GD. Congenital dislocation of the hip: Use of the Pavlik harness in the child during the first six months of life. Journal of Bone and Joint Surgery (American), *58*:1000–1004, 1976.

Rang, M. Children's Fractures. Philadelphia: JB Lippincott, 1974.

Tachdjian, MO (Ed.). Congenital Dislocation of the Hip. New York: Churchill Livingstone, 1982.

Chapter 16

Sports Injuries in Children

DONNA BERNHARDT-BAINBRIDGE, PT, ATC, EdD

On playgrounds, on fields, in gyms, on courts, and in pools, more children than ever before are playing and competing in sports. No fewer than 50 million children and adolescents take part in school-sponsored or extracurricular athletics. Seventy-five percent of American middle and junior high schools had significant competitive sports programs by 1981 (Stanitski, 1989). More than 1.85 million girls and 3.5 million boys participated in varsity athletics in 1980 to 1981, a gain of 5.9% in girls' participation and a decline of 0.4% in boys' participation over previous years. Thirty million youngsters aged 6 to 21 years were involved in out-of-school programs. Football was the most popular sport for boys, while basketball was number one for girls. The largest increases in participation were noted in baseball and volleyball (Mueller & Blythe, 1982). Six and one-half million teenagers regularly participated in competitive high school team sports by 1987 (Birrer & Brecher, 1987). In 1989, half of all males and one fourth of all females aged 8 to 16 years (approximately 7 million) were engaged in competitive, organized school sports (Stanitski, 1989).

The incidence of injury has also escalated as participation has increased. Although broad epidemiologic information is lacking because of varying methodologies and definitions of injury, many studies have documented risk in sports participation (DeHaven & Lintner, 1986; Sheps & Evans, 1987). One of the earliest studies, completed over a 2-year period (1973–1975) in four Seattle high schools, demonstrated 1181 injuries in 3049 students who participated in 19 different sports (Garrick, 1982). Sprains and strains accounted for 60.5% of all injuries. The sports that placed boys most at risk were football, which accounted for 50% of total injuries, followed by wrestling (17.3%) and track (10%). Injuries in girls occurred largely in tennis (38%), gymnastics (20%), and basketball

(15%). The highest proportion of fractures, contusions, and strains occurred in boys, while a greater percentage of overuse injuries were noted in girls. Sprains were documented equally in both groups.

When Garrick (1982) related the total number of injuries to total participants, he noted boys to have an 85% injury rate while girls had only a 22% rate of injury. If, however, injuries received in football and wrestling were not included, the injury rate for the genders was similar (27% for boys, 22% for girls). Snively and co-workers (1981) compared boys and girls who participated in eight similar sports and reported no difference in overall injury rate. Other researchers concurred with these findings (Backx et al., 1989; Kvist et al., 1989; Lodge et al., 1990; McLain & Reynolds, 1989; Mueller & Blythe, 1982).

A Dutch study further suggested that sports characterized by contact, repetitive jumping, and indoor activities create the most risk (Backx et al., 1991). Athletic trainers in four high schools (Whieldon & Cerny, 1990) reported that collision sports such as football and wrestling generated the highest injury rates, followed by contact sports such as baseball and basketball. Boys had higher injury rates than girls only in contact sports.

Many studies have documented injury rates in specific sports. Youth football (played by children aged 8 to 15 years) was shown to cause an overall injury rate of 5%, with 61% classified as moderate and 39% as major injuries, although permanent disability was rare. Fractures of the upper extremity were the most common injury. Both the injury rate and the site of injury change with age (Goldberg et al., 1988; Halpern et al., 1987). Injuries in high school athletes occurred primarily in the lower extremity and especially affected the knee. Forty percent of injuries were sprains and strains, 25% were contusions, and only 10% were fractures (Halpern et al., 1987).

Injuries related to soccer occur with an incidence of 10.6 injuries per 1000 hours of play in girls and of 7.3 injuries per 1000 hours of play in boys (Backous et al., 1988). The incidence of injury in both groups increased at 14 years of age and continued at a higher rate as the participants became older. The authors noted that 70% of the injuries were to the lower extremities, with a total of 84.2% represented by contusions, sprains, and strains (Backous et al., 1988). Keller and colleagues (1987) postulated that ball and body momentum increased with age and affected injury rates. They suggested that the greater incidence of head and upper extremity injuries in young soccer players could be related to lack of technical expertise, weakness of dental tissues, and increased ball-to-head weight ratios. Overall injury rates were higher in outdoor than in indoor soccer (Hoff & Martin, 1986; Keller et al., 1987). Players of outdoor soccer experienced more strains, fractures, cuts, and infections, while dental and upper extremity injuries and tendinitis occurred more frequently in players of indoor soccer. The cleanliness, traction, and shock absorption of the playing surface, the weather, the perimeter boards, and the pace of play were all postulated to influence injury characteristics.

A study that evaluated track and field athletes from 17 teams found one injury for every 5.8 males and every 7.5 females. The majority of injuries (83%) involved the lower extremities, with sprinting responsible for 46% of all injuries (Watson & DiMartino, 1987). Another research group evaluated the members of 12 high school ice hockey teams (Gerberich et al., 1987). Seventy-five injuries in 100 players were documented, with 22% of these injuries to the head and neck. Patterns of ski injuries were assessed in Australia, where children were found to be less prone to injury than adults but more likely to sustain serious injuries, particularly tibial fractures (Sherry et al., 1987).

Several studies have assessed injuries in recreational sports. Retsky and associates (1991) assessed the U.S. Consumer Product Safety Commission injury frequency estimates for skateboarding. A marked increase in injuries was noted: 19,182 injuries were reported in 1984, with 37,180 in 1985. Injuries occurred with greater frequency in children aged 10 to 14 years. More frequent head and neck trauma occurred in children younger than 5 years of age, while more severe head and neck injuries were reported in older children. Older children experienced more injuries to the extremities than younger children. Nakayama and associates (1990) examined hospital records and interviewed parents of 372 children aged 2 to 15 years who had been admitted with cycling-related injuries in 1979 through 1986. Head injury was the most common complaint (69.1% of all cases). Twelve children (3.2%) died of head injury; 4 suffered permanent impairment and were institutionalized. One third of those children with head injuries had persistent disability, and cognitive or behavioral changes were noted in 31.9%. Many other recreational activities such as dancing, riding a dirt bike, and playing tag football cause injury, but no data on the types or incidence of injury have been collected in children.

The incidence of catastrophic injuries and fatalities in high school and college athletes has been documented for the years 1982 through 1988 (Mueller & Cantu, 1990). A total of 218 injuries, including 44 fatalities, 74 nonfatal but permanent injuries resulting in severe functional neurologic disability, and 100 serious injuries with no permanent functional neurologic disability, were reported in high school athletes. During the same period 76 indirect deaths caused by heart failure, heat stroke, sickle cell crisis, or asthma occurred in the following sports, which are listed in decreasing order of number of deaths: football, wrestling, basketball, track, and baseball. Even lower in incidence of injury or death were cross-country, soccer, gymnastics, ice hockey, and swimming. Attention to the causes of severe injuries or deaths, such as overaggression in hockey, grading of risk in gymnastics, improper padding of landing pits, insufficient clearance at field events, and takeoff dives into shallow water, will assist in their elimination.

Lack of fitness has been associated with injury in both children and adults (Birrer & Levine, 1987; Macera et al., 1989). Fitness levels have declined for boys older than age 14 and for girls older than age 12. One third of American children younger than age 8 are overweight. Fifty percent of children in grades 5 through 12 do not get the vigorous activity necessary to maintain or improve cardiovascular status. Forty percent of children between 5 and 8 years of age show at least one risk factor for heart disease (President's Council on Physical Fitness and Sports, 1986).

The issue of sports injury in children can no longer be ignored. The child, however, is not just a small adult. Children have different structural and physiologic components that must be specifically addressed. The purpose of this chapter is to review the unique sports injuries that occur in children who are either able-bodied or disabled. The prevention, risk factors, types, and sites of injury and the management and rehabilitation of injuries in children are discussed.

▌ PREVENTION OF INJURIES

The key to management of sports injuries in children is prevention. As discussed in Chapter 5, children need proper physiologic conditioning, strength, and flexibility to participate safely in an organized or recreational athletic endeavor. Although lack of fitness, strength, and flexibility does not preclude participation, remediation must be built into conditioning and training programs to decrease the risk of injury. The major elements in this process of injury risk management are preparticipation examination, conditioning and training, proper supervision, protection of the body, and environmental control.

Preparticipation Examination

The preparticipation examination is the initial step in the process of injury prevention. The American Medical Association Committee on Medical Aspects of Sports constructed a Bill of Rights for the Athlete, one part of which is a thorough preseason history and medical examination. The purposes are fivefold: 1) to determine the general health of the athlete and detect conditions that place the participant at additional risk; 2) to identify relative or absolute medical contraindications to participation; 3) to identify sports that may be played safely; 4) to assess maturity and overall fitness; and 5) to educate the athlete. These examinations are also necessary to meet legal and insurance requirements in many states (Bar-Or et al., 1988).

The usefulness of these assessments in identifying children at risk has been demonstrated. In one study, 15% of participants had conditions requiring further evaluation, although only 9 of 701 were excluded. One third of the musculoskeletal problems identified were previously unknown to the primary care physician (Goldberg et al., 1980). In another study it was noted that in 1977–1978 and 1978–1979, respectively, 3.2% and 6.5% of athletes had abnormalities severe enough to require further evaluation. Only 0.3% were excluded from participation (Linder et al., 1981). In a study to assess utilization of preseason assessment, questionnaires were mailed to 300 secondary schools. Seventy-one percent of schools used a health history form, while 94.2% administered preseason physical examinations to all interscholastic athletes. It was noted, however, that the health forms were not specific to sports, were evaluated by individuals who were not competent for the task, were not available during the season, and were not followed by appropriate student counseling (Harvey, 1982).

Most states require either an individual examination or a multistation screening. The merits and disadvantages of these methods have been evaluated. The primary physician performing an individual examination knows or has access to the athlete's health records, can discuss sensitive health or personal issues, and may be most qualified to oversee any necessary follow-up care. The time and cost are a disadvantage of the individual examination. Additionally, disparate knowledge and interest among physicians regarding sports and the requirements to participate may hinder effective evaluation for all participants. The multistation examination is more cost and time efficient and provides a thorough and appropriate screening for all potential participants. Professional experts assess each athlete in the area of their specialization (Table 16–1), increasing

TABLE 16–1. **STATIONS AND PERSONNEL FOR MULTISTATION PREPARTICIPATION EVALUATION**

Station	Personnel
Sign-in	Ancillary personnel/volunteers
Height/weight	Nurse or coach
Vital signs	Nurse, exercise physiologist, athletic trainer, physical therapist
Visual examination	Nurse or physician
Medical examination	Internist or family practitioner
Orthopaedic evaluation	Physician or physical therapist
Flexibility assessment	Physical therapist or athletic trainer
Strength evaluation	Physical therapist, athletic trainer, or exercise physiologist
Body composition	Exercise physiologist, physical therapist, or athletic trainer
Speed, agility, power, balance, endurance	Exercise physiologist, physical therapist, or athletic trainer
Assessment/clearance	Physician

From Cantu, RC, & Micheli, LJ. ACSM's Guidelines for the Team Physician. Philadelphia: Lea & Febiger, 1991.

the probability of detection of abnormalities (Bar-Or et al., 1988; Harvey, 1982).

The frequency of the preparticipation examination is being debated. Although annual evaluations are most traditional (American Academy of Family Physicians et al., in press; McKeag, 1985), many clinicians advocate evaluation before each season (Micheli & Stone, 1984). The American Academy of Pediatrics (1989) recommends a biannual complete evaluation followed by an interim history before each season. The schedule that meets the primary objectives of the academy, however, is a complete entry-level evaluation followed by a limited annual reevaluation that includes a brief physical examination (to evaluate height, weight, blood pressure and pulse, perform auscultation, examine the skin, and test visual acuity), a physical maturity assessment if previous level was less than Tanner stage IV, and an evaluation of all new problems (American Academy of Family Physicians et al., 1992).

The components of the preparticipation examination are the medical history; the physical examination, including cardiovascular and eye examinations; musculoskeletal assessment; body composition and height and weight determination; specific field testing; and readiness, both physical and psychologic. The examination should be completed 6 weeks before the practice season to allow adequate time for further evaluation or for correction of any problems (Bar-Or et al., 1988; Goldberg et al., 1980; Harvey, 1982; Lehman, 1988; Linder et al., 1981; Lombardo, 1991; McKeag, 1985; Rooks & Micheli, 1988; Smilkstein, 1981). The components of the examination should be tailored to the specific demands of the sport.

HISTORY

The medical history is the cornerstone of the medical evaluation (Bar-Or et al., 1988; Lombardo,

1991; McKeag, 1985) and will identify 63 to 74% of problems affecting athletes (Goldberg et al., 1980). Forms that are short, easy to complete, and written in lay terms are preferable (Fig. 16–1). Forms should be completed by the athlete and parent or legal guardian and then signed by the parent or legal guardian. Content areas that should be particularly noted include exercise-induced syncope or asthma; family history of heart disease or sudden death; history of loss of consciousness, concussion, or neurologic conditions; history of heat stroke; medications; allergies; history of musculoskeletal dysfunction; dates of hospitalizations or surgery; absence or loss of a paired organ; and immunizations.

PHYSICAL EXAMINATION

The physical examination is used to evaluate areas of concern identified by the history. The minimally sufficient examination includes cardiovascular and eye examinations, a maturity assessment, and a review of all body systems. Blood pressure should be measured using appropriately sized sphygmomanometer cuffs for accuracy (Lombardo, 1991; McKeag, 1985). The 95th percentile upper limit values for normal blood pressure are 120/80 mm Hg for 8-year-olds, 135/85 mm Hg for 12-year-olds, and 145/90 mm Hg for 16-year-olds (Bar-Or et al., 1988). A diagnosis of hypertension requires three abnormal readings. If blood pressure is elevated, repeat measures should be taken later in the examination or the next day. High blood pressure requires further evaluation by the personal physician for clearance to participate in sports (Lombardo, 1991). The remainder of the cardiovascular screening evaluation assesses peripheral pulses and heart beat for symmetry and rate. Auscultation of the heart should be performed with the young person both seated and supine (Lombardo,

Name _____   Date of Birth _____
Address_____   Class _____
Parents _____   Phone # _____
Physician _____
Sports _____   _____

Fill in details of "YES" answers in space below:

	Yes	No
1. Have you ever been hospitalized?	___	___
Have you ever had surgery?	___	___
2. Are you currently taking medication?	___	___
3. Do you have any allergies (medicines, bees)?	___	___
4. Have you ever passed out during exercise?	___	___
Have you ever been dizzy during exercise?	___	___
Have you ever had chest pain?	___	___
Do you tire more quickly than your friends during exercise?	___	___
Have you ever had high blood pressure?	___	___
Have you ever been told you have a heart murmur?	___	___
Have you ever had racing of your heart or skipped beats?	___	
Has anyone in your family died of heart problems or a sudden death before age 40?	___	___
5. Do you have any skin problems? (itching, moles, breaking out)	___	___
6. Have you ever had a head injury?	___	___
Have you ever been knocked out?	___	___
Have you ever had a seizure?	___	___
Have you ever had a stinger or burner?	___	___

7. Have you ever injured (sprained, dislocated, fractured, etc.):

_____ Hand	_____ Shoulder	_____ Thigh
_____ Wrist	_____ Neck	_____ Knee
_____ Forearm	_____ Chest	_____ Shin/Calf
_____ Elbow	_____ Back	_____ Ankle
_____ Arm	_____ Hip	_____ Foot

	Yes	No
8. Have you ever had heat cramps?	___	___
Have you ever been dizzy or passed out in the heat?	___	___

9. Have you ever had:

_____ Mononucleosis	_____ Diabetes
_____ Hepatitis	_____ Headaches (frequent)
_____ Asthma	_____ Eye injuries
_____ Tuberculosis	_____ Stomach ulcer

10. Do you use special pads or braces?	___	___
11. When was your last tetanus shot?	_____	
12. When was your first period?	_____	
When was your last period?	_____	

Explain YES answers here:

_____
_____
_____
_____
_____
_____
_____
_____

Parent's signature: _____

FIGURE 16–1. Medical questionnaire. (From Lombardo, J. Preparticipation examination. In Cantu, R., & Micheli, L [Eds.], ACSM's Guidelines for the Team Physician. Philadelphia: Lea & Febiger, 1991.)

1991). As many as 85% of youths have benign heart murmurs. Various maneuvers such as squat to stand, Valsalva, and deep inspiration can differentiate functional from pathologic murmurs (Bar-Or et al., 1988). Arrhythmias are not abnormal in children, but increases in premature ventricular con-

tractions with exercise require further assessment. Paroxysmal supraventricular tachycardia, once evaluated, is not a reason for disqualification (American Academy of Family Physicians et al., 1992; Bar-Or et al., 1988).

Visual acuity is tested using a Snelling chart and

should be correctable to 20/200. Any inequality of pupil diameter or reactivity should be noted so responses after potential injury can be compared with this baseline value. Uncorrectable legal blindness (acuity less than 20/200 or absence of an eye) requires counseling regarding participation in collision or contact sports. The importance of protective eyewear for athletes who wear glasses or have unilateral vision should be stressed (Bar-Or et al., 1988; Lombardo, 1991).

Pulmonary status is determined by symmetry of diaphragmatic excursion and breath sounds. Children with asthma, including exercise-induced asthma, should be allowed to participate in activities if the condition is properly controlled with medication (Bar-Or et al., 1988; Lombardo, 1991). Abdominal assessment determines rigidity, tenderness, organomegaly, or the presence of masses. Participation by any athlete with organomegaly is restricted until further tests determine the cause of the enlarged organ (American Academy of Family Physicians et al., 1992; Bar-Or et al., 1988; McKeag, 1985).

Careful examination of the skin is vital in examination of all persons, but it is particularly important for those who will participate in contact sports. Participation in these sports should be deferred for children with evidence of any communicable skin disease, such as impetigo, carbuncles, herpes, scabies, and louse or fungal infections (Bar-Or et al., 1988; Lombardo, 1991; McKeag, 1985).

Genitourinary examination of males is used to assess the child for testicular presence, descended testicles, and possible inguinal hernia. The genital examination is deferred in girls unless a history of amenorrhea or menstrual irregularity warrants referral. A maturational index should be determined for all athletes so that appropriate matching of age and sport can occur (McKeag, 1985). Guidelines for staging of secondary sexual characteristics are reliable, proven, and practical (Table 16–2).

The musculoskeletal screening examination should include assessment of posture with particular attention to atrophy, spinal asymmetry, pelvic level, discrepancy of leg lengths, and lower extremity deformities such as genu valgus or varus, patellar deformities, and pes planus. Gait should be examined with the child walking and running, as well as walking on toes and heels. Passive range of motion and two-joint musculotendinous flexibility should be screened, using the Thomas, Ober, and Ely tests. Muscle strength can be assessed using a manual muscle test, hand-held dynamometer, or isokinetic device. Special stability testing of the shoulders, knees, and ankles should be conducted if the child has had a previous injury or if the current assessment indicates that instability may be present (American Academy of Family Physicians et al., 1992) (Appendix I).

BODY COMPOSITION

Height and weight should be assessed and results compared with standard growth charts. Weight, however, gives no specific assessment of the percentage of lean mass and fat tissue. Assessment

TABLE 16–2. **MATURITY STAGING GUIDELINES (TANNER, 1962)**

Male		
PUBIC HAIR	**PENIS**	**TESTIS**
None	Preadolescent	
Slight, long, slight pigmentation	Slight enlargement	Enlarged scrotum, pink slight ruga
Darker, starts to curl, small amount	Longer	Larger
Coarse, curly, adult type, but less quantity	Increase in glans size and breadth of penis	Larger, scrotum darker
Adult—spread to inner thighs	Adult	Adult

Female	
PUBIC HAIR	**BREASTS**
Preadolescent (none)	Preadolescent (no germinal button)
Sparse, lightly pigmented, straight medial border of labia	Breast and papilla elevated as small mound; areolar diameter increased
Darker, beginning to curl, increased	Breast and areola enlarged; no contour separation
Coarse, curly, abundant, but less than adult	Areola and papilla form secondary mound
Adult female triangle and spread to medial surface	Mature, nipple projects, areola part of general breast contour

From McKeag, D. Preseason physical examination for the prevention of sports injuries. Sports Medicine, 2:425, 1985.

of subcutaneous body fat provides a more specific evaluation of body composition, although fat thickness varies from birth to adolescence (see Chapter 5). The most practical method for screening is skinfold measurement. This method has demonstrated correlations of .70 to .85 with hydrostatic weighing if performed by an experienced examiner (Going, 1988). Although the criterion ranges for body fatness related to optimal health are 15 to 25% for girls and 10 to 25% for boys (Lohman, 1992), 20% for girls and 12% for boys are ideal for most activities (Bar-Or et al., 1988). Elevated body fat levels may indicate the need for weight reduction. Low weight or low body fat warrants a thorough evaluation of eating habits, weight loss, and body image to rule out the possibility of an eating disorder. High weight and very low body fat could signal use of anabolic steroids, growth hormone, or other performance-enhancing drugs (Lombardo, 1991; McKeag, 1985).

The physical examination would be incomplete without a thorough evaluation for possible use of pharmacologic ergogenic aids. Observation for physical symptoms and signs as well as careful examination can reveal potential abuse. The most frequently used drugs, particularly in sports requiring muscle power, are anabolic steroids. Although reliably reported data are difficult to obtain, probably over 1 million individuals in the United States use steroids (Yesalis et al., 1989). The most compelling reasons for taking steroids are to increase body weight and muscle mass, decrease fatigue, and increase aggressive behavior. The side effects, including hypertension, hepatitis, testicular atrophy, loss of libido, hepatic carcinoma, and premature epiphyseal closure, far outweigh the benefits of these drugs (Birrer & Brecher, 1987; Costill et al., 1984; Council on Scientific Affairs, 1988; Haupt & Rovere, 1984; Hickson & Kurowski, 1986; Rogozin, 1979). Warning signs of steroid abuse might include irritability; sudden mood swings; puffiness in face, upper arms, and chest; sudden increases in blood pressure and weight; yellowish coloration around the fingernails and eyes; hirsutism; and deepening of voice and acne in girls (Haupt & Rovere, 1984; Nevole & Prentice, 1987; Perry, 1985; Yesalis et al., 1989).

Diuretics are frequently used to "make weight" for an event or to mask drug usage (Grana & Kalenak, 1991). Performance may, however, be decreased as a result of dehydration or electrolyte losses (Birrer & Brecher, 1987; Grana & Kalenak, 1989). Likewise, stimulants are commonly abused in an effort to increase performance in sports. They serve only to mask normal fatigue and to increase aggression, hostility, and uncooperativeness and

can lead to addiction and death (Birrer & Brecher, 1987).

SPECIFIC FIELD TESTS

Field testing is done to assess specific athletic potential in a specific sport. The components assessed are muscle strength, muscle power, endurance, speed, agility and flexibility, and cardiovascular performance (Bar-Or et al., 1988).

General muscle strength can be assessed with a maximal activity pertinent to the sport, such as a bench press, pull-ups or push-ups for the upper extremities, and leg press or sit-ups for the lower extremities. Endurance can be assessed by performing as many repetitions of the task as possible. Muscle power can be evaluated with vertical jumping, performing a standing long jump, or throwing a medicine ball, as appropriate.

Speed is evaluated using a 40- or 50-yard dash, while agility can be assessed with Vodak's agility test (Gaillard et al., 1978) or a similar battery of tests. The most common, standardized methods of assessing flexibility are the sit and reach test, which has norms for children, and active knee extension performed in a supine position with the hips flexed to 90° (Hunter et al., 1985). Cardiovascular performance is most easily assessed using a submaximal test on an appropriate device, such as a cycle ergometer, treadmill, or upper-body ergometer. A field test for cardiovascular performance is the 12-minute run or the timed 1.5-mile run (Bar-Or et al., 1988).

The outcome of the preparticipation examination is a definition of clearance to participate in sports. Clearance can be unrestricted for any sport or restricted to specific types of sports in the following manner: 1) no collision or contact; 2) limited contact or impact; or 3) noncontact only. The American Academy of Pediatrics has developed a classification system for sports activities (Table 16–3) as well as recommendations for restriction of participation (Table 16–4) that are excellent guides in making decisions for individual athletes. All decisions or recommendations for further evaluation should be thoroughly discussed with the athletes and their parents (American Academy of Family Physicians et al., 1992; Bar-Or et al., 1988).

Training Program

The preseason examination provides a clear definition of the individual athlete's areas of strength and limitations (Fig. 16–2). The next appropriate step in prevention is the development of an *individ*

TABLE 16–3. **SPORTS CLASSIFICATION SYSTEM**

Contact Collision	Limited Contact Impact	Noncontact		
		STRENUOUS	MODERATELY STRENUOUS	NONSTRENUOUS
Boxing	Baseball	Aerobic dancing	Badminton	Archery
Field hockey	Basketball	Crew	Curling	Golf
Football	Bicycling	Fencing	Table tennis	Riflery
Ice hockey	Diving	Field		
Lacrosse	Field	Discus		
Martial arts	High jump	Javelin		
Rodeo	Pole vault	Shot put		
Soccer	Gymnastics	Running		
Wrestling	Horseback riding	Swimming		
	Skating	Tennis		
	Ice	Track		
	Roller	Weight lifting		
	Skiing			
	Cross-country			
	Downhill			
	Water			
	Softball			
	Squash, handball			
	Volleyball			

From American Academy of Pediatrics Committee on Sports Medicine. Recommendations for participation in competitive sports. Pediatrics *81*:737, 1988.

From Lombardo, J. Preparticipation examination. In Cantu, R, & Micheli, L (Eds.), ACSM's Guidelines for the Team Physician. Philadelphia: Lea & Febiger, 1991, p. 74.

ualized training plan designed to address the particular problems of the athlete as they relate to the requirements of the sport(s). This program could be developed by a sports physical therapist, athletic trainer, or exercise physiologist involved in the preseason screening. Once developed, it should be taught to the athlete, the parent, and the coach.

The training program should be a systematic, progressive plan to address the athlete's weaknesses and to maximally condition the athlete for participation. Training consists of off-season, preseason, in-season, and postseason programs for year-round conditioning and for development of appropriate peak performance. Components should include energy training (aerobic foundation and anaerobic training), muscle training (strength, endurance, flexibility, and power), speed, and proper nutrition. A well-developed, variable, and well-paced program will avoid boredom and potential overuse injury. The psychologic effects of year-round training, or exercise in general, are controversial and not well documented. The risk–benefit ratio, however, tends to favor exercise for improvement of mood, self-concept, and work behavior when competition is sensibly controlled (Brown, 1982).

ENERGY TRAINING

The basis of energy training, a strong aerobic base, should be developed during the off-season.

Good training consists of low-intensity, long-duration activity with natural intervals of low- and moderate-intensity work that is sport-specific. Swimming would be a good choice for the field athlete, while cycling or running is appropriate for those in track, soccer, and football. Training on hills or performance of similar resistance efforts should be done once weekly. Children exhibit less efficient movement patterns and a lower maximal acidosis level. They are less able to withstand high temperatures secondary to a greater rate of heat exchange and less sweat production (Ilmarinen & Valimaki, 1984). Consequently, intense training in the extreme heat and hard training involving long durations should be minimized until puberty. This avoidance of excessive exercise also helps avert early burnout (Sharkey, 1991).

Anaerobic training programs consist of exertion at 85 to 90% of maximal heart rate for short periods. Anaerobic drills develop a person's ability to tolerate the production of excess lactic acid. Twice-weekly anaerobic training should be performed for maximal benefit. Methods including interval training, fartlek (speed play), or pace training are variations of the anaerobic method. Sports-specific anaerobic skills should be developed during preseason and early season activities (Sharkey, 1991). Young children are less able to use muscle glycogen and produce lactic acid, so this training is difficult for young athletes and has only minor fitness benefits

TABLE 16-4. RECOMMENDATIONS FOR PARTICIPATION

	Contact/ Collision	Limited Contact/Impact	Noncontact		
			STRENUOUS	MODERATELY STRENUOUS	NONSTRENUOUS
Atlantoaxial instability *Swimming: no butterfly, breast stroke, or diving starts	No	No	Yes*	Yes	Yes
Acute illnesses *Needs individual assessment, e.g., contagiousness to others, risk of worsening illness	*	*	*	*	*
Cardiovascular					
Carditis*	No	No	No	No	No
Hypertension					
Mild	Yes	Yes	Yes	Yes	Yes
Moderate	*	*	*	*	*
Severe	*	*	*	*	*
Congenital heart disease	†	†	†	†	†
*Needs individual assessment †Patients with mild forms can be allowed a full range of physical activities; patients with moderate or severe forms, or who are postoperative, should be evaluated by a cardiologist before athletic participation.					
Eyes					
Absence or loss of function of one eye	*	*	*	*	*
Detached retina	†	†	†	†	†
*Availability of American Society for Testing and Materials (ASTM)-approved eye guards may allow competitor to participate in most sports, but this must be judged on an individual basis. †Consult ophthalmologist					
Inguinal hernia	Yes	Yes	Yes	Yes	Yes
Kidney: absence of one	No	Yes	Yes	Yes	Yes
Liver: enlarged	No	No	Yes	Yes	Yes
Musculoskeletal disorders	*	*	*	*	*
*Needs individual assessment					
Neurologic					
History of serious head or spine trauma, repeated concussions, or craniotomy	*	*	Yes	Yes	Yes
Convulsive disorder					
Well controlled	Yes	Yes	Yes	Yes	Yes
Poorly controlled	No	No	Yes†	Yes	Yes‡
*Needs individual assessment †No swimming or weight lifting ‡No archery or riflery					
Ovary: absence of one	Yes	Yes	Yes	Yes	Yes
Respiratory					
Pulmonary insufficiency	*	*	*	*	Yes
Asthma	Yes	Yes	Yes	Yes	Yes
*May be allowed to compete if oxygenation remains satisfactory during a graded stress test					
Sickle cell trait	Yes	Yes	Yes	Yes	Yes
Skin: Boils, herpes, impetigo, scabies	*	*	Yes	Yes	Yes
*No gymnastics with mats, martial arts, wrestling, or contact sports until not contagious					
Spleen: Enlarged	No	No	No	Yes	Yes
Testicle: Absent or undescended	Yes*	Yes*	Yes	Yes	Yes
*Certain sports may require protective cup					

From Lombardo, J. Preparticipation examination. In Cantu, R., & Micheli, L (Eds.), ACSM's Guidelines for the Team Physician, Philadelphia: Lea & Febiger, 1991, p. 74.

Athletic fitness scorecard for boys

Test	0 Below average	1 Above average	2 Good	3 Very good	4 Excellent
Strength Pull-ups (no)	Fewer than 7	7 to 9	10 to 12	13 to 14	15 or more
Power Long jump (in)	Fewer than 85	85 to 88	89 to 91	92 to 94	95 or more
Speed 50-yd dash (sec)	Slower than 6.7	6.7 to 6.4	6.3 to 6.0	5.9 to 5.6	5.5 or less
Agility 6-c agility (c)	Fewer than 5-5	5-5 to 6-3	6-4 to 7-2	7-3 to 8-1	8-2 or more
Flexibility Forward flexion (in)	Not reach ruler	1 to 2	3 to 5	6 to 8	9 or more
Muscular endurance Sit-ups (no)	Fewer than 38	38 to 45	46 to 52	53 to 59	60 or more
Cardiorespiratory endurance 12-min run (mi)	Fewer than 1½	1½	1¾	2	2¼ or more

YOUR SCORE

	Strength	Power	Speed	Agility	Flexibility	Muscular endurance	Cardiorespiratory endurance
Your Score							
Rating (0–4)							

Athletic fitness scorecard for girls

Test	0 Below average	1 Above average	2 Good	3 Very good	4 Excellent
Strength Pull-ups (no)	Fewer than 2	2 to 3	4 to 5	6 to 7	8 or more
Power Long jump (in)	Fewer than 63	63 to 65	66 to 68	69 to 71	72 or more
Speed 50-yd dash (sec)	Slower than 8.2	8.2 to 7.9	7.8 to 7.1	6.9 to 6.0	5.9 or less
Agility 6-c agility (c)	Fewer than 3-5	3-5 to 4-3	4-4 to 5-2	5-3 to 6-2	6-3 or more
Flexibility Forward flexion (in)	Fewer than 3	3 to 5	6 to 8	9 to 11	12 or more
Muscular endurance Sit-ups (no)	Fewer than 26	26 to 31	32 to 38	39 to 45	46 or more
Cardiorespiratory endurance 12-min run (mi)	Fewer than 1¼	1¼	1½	1¾	2 or more

YOUR SCORE

	Strength	Power	Speed	Agility	Flexibility	Muscular endurance	Cardiorespiratory endurance
Your Score							
Rating (0–4)							

FIGURE 16-2. Athletic fitness scorecards. (Reproduced with permission from Patient Care, October 30, 1988, Copyright © Medical Economics Publishing, Montvale, NJ 07645. All rights reserved.)

TABLE 16-5. **GUIDELINES FOR PEDIATRIC WEIGHT TRAINING**

Ages	9-11	12-14	15-16	17+
Exercises per Body Part	1	1	2	>2
Sets	2	3	3-4	4-6
Repetitions	12-15	10-12	7-11	6-10
Maximum Weight (Resistance)	Very light	Light	Moderate	Heavy

From Rooks, D., & Micheli, L. Musculoskeletal assessment and training: The young athlete. Clinics in Sports Medicine, 7(3):663, 1988.

until they mature. Some training should be used, however, to achieve relaxation and mechanical efficiency at these levels.

STRENGTH TRAINING

Weight training in children has been controversial because of concerns regarding injury to growing bones and the questionable efficacy of this type of training to increase strength. Several research studies have demonstrated that strength can be improved by systematic overload of muscle in postpubescent athletes with similar results as in adults (Blanksby & Gregor, 1981; Ekblom, 1969; Pfeiffer & Francis, 1986; Sailors & Berg, 1987; Sewall & Micheli, 1986; Wilmore, 1974).

The area of greatest debate in strength training is how it affects the prepubescent athlete. Since the levels of circulating androgens are low, questions of efficacy have been raised. Several studies have demonstrated that, although little increase in muscle bulk occurs, definite changes in strength can be achieved through controlled weight training in this group (Ramsey et al., 1990; Servedio et al., 1985; Sharkey, 1991; Weltman et al., 1986). The trends documenting increased twitch torque and motor unit activation suggest neuromuscular changes, including motor learning and reduction of inhibition (Ramsey et al., 1990; Sharkey, 1991). All authors firmly state, however, that weight lifting in the prepubescent athlete should follow a thorough preparticipation screening for constitutional or anatomic abnormalities (Sewall & Micheli, 1986; Sharkey, 1991). The program should be closely monitored by an adult with emphasis on form and technique and with careful spotting. Movements should be nonballistic, with avoidance of extremely heavy weights. The training apparatus should be scaled to fit the athlete.

Guidelines for strength training are provided in Table 16-5. Athletes will increase strength at a rate of 1 to 3% per week with strength training routines (Sharkey, 1991). Most strength training occurs during the late off-season and preseason periods. Pro-

grams should be sports-specific both for the muscles used and the rests between sets. For example, a wrestler, gymnast, or sprinter may have 60- to 90-second rests between exercise bursts while a distance runner may move slowly and continuously through all exercises with little rest (Rooks & Micheli, 1988). When athletes have achieved the adequate level for their sport, they should work on the appropriate type of muscle endurance (Table 16-6) with one set of higher resistance training per week to maintain strength. Endurance work begins in late preseason and continues during the early in-season period.

Power is the ability to do work over a given period of time. As such, it involves both strength and speed in a sports-specific movement. Power is usually developed by performing 15 to 25 repetitions of three sets at 30 to 60% maximal effort as fast as possible. Although power develops slowly in children, some training can help a child develop the neuromuscular skill of quick movement against low resistance (Sharkey, 1991). Because of the requirements of power training, variable-resistance devices that allow control of speed or resistance are

TABLE 16-6. **THE STRENGTH-ENDURANCE CONTINUUM**

Strength	Short-Term Endurance	Intermediate Endurance
Maximum force	Persistence with heavy load	Persistence with intermediate load
6-10 RM	15-25 RM	30-50 RM
3 sets	3 sets	2 sets
3 times/week	3 times/week	3 times/week
Contractile protein (actin and myosin)	Some strength and anaerobic metabolism (glycolysis)	Some endurance and anaerobic metabolism
Connective tissue		Slight strength improvement
Oxygen intake Endurance	Oxygen intake	

From Sharkey, B. Training for sport. In Cantu, R., & Micheli, L (Eds.), ACSM's Guidelines for the Team Physician, Philadelphia: Lea & Febiger, 1991.

the best approach. Plyometrics, or muscle stretch followed by a burst of contraction, is another available form of power training. Since body weight is approximately 33% of maximal leg strength, these exercises fit the power prescription. An example of a plyometric exercise is step jumping.

Power training can cause muscle soreness and potential injury if conducted improperly. Proper technique includes adequate warm-up; slowly increased intensity; performance of jumping activities on dirt, grass, or soft surfaces; and thoroughly stretching after each session.

Achieving joint and musculotendinous flexibility is an essential part of any training program. Although the effects of flexibility on injury prevention are unclear, enhanced joint mobility, improved comfort of the muscle crossing the joint, and increased blood supply have been documented (Rooks & Micheli, 1990). Stretching is most effective if nonballistic. Effective methods include static or proprioceptive neuromuscular stretching. The young athlete should be placed on a daily program that stretches all areas of the extremities and trunk with emphasis on the body parts to be used in the sport. Stretches should be easy and simple and demand appropriate levels of neuromuscular control for the age of the child (Rooks & Micheli, 1990).

SPEED

Because the proportion of fast twitch fibers in muscle is inherited, speed is "born" in the child (Sharkey, 1991; Smith, MJ, 1983). All athletes, however, can train the intermediate fibers and improve the components of reaction and movement time. Faster reactions are taught in sports-specific practice drills such as starts, acceleration drills, or play drills that gradually narrow choice. Movement time is enhanced from a base of flexibility and strength with ballistic motions, sprint loading (explosive jump or throw), overspeed, or resisted sprinting (Sharkey, 1991).

NUTRITION

Many general articles have been written on nutritional requirements for athletes (Bauman, 1986; Clark, 1990) with recent revisions for pediatric and adolescent athletes (Heim, 1965; Peterson & Peterson, 1988; Ziegler, 1982). The preparticipation screening includes components of a nutritional assessment: skinfold measurements, height, and weight. Skinfold standards for the triceps in children allow one to determine if the child is overfat (Table 16–7). The ideal range for adolescent males is 10 to 12% total body fat, while in females the range is 20 to 22% body fat (Bar-Or et al., 1988; Ziegler, 1982). The body fat percentage can be matched to the approximated body fat values developed for various sports, although standards do not yet exist for younger athletes (Haskell et al., 1982).

Caloric requirements for children are age-dependent and vary directly with body weight and surface area. Generally, a young child requires more calories than an adolescent or adult—36 to 40 calories/lb/day (Peterson & Peterson, 1988; Ziegler, 1982). An additional caloric load is necessary depending on the level of energy output. An approximation for energy expenditure, based on a child weighing 100 lb, is 4 kcal/min for low-intensity activities, 4 to 7 kcal/min for moderate-intensity activities, and greater than 7 kcal/min for high-intensity activities (Peterson & Peterson, 1988). A

TABLE 16–7. **STANDARDS FOR TRICEPS FATFOLD (MM): TRICEPS SKINFOLD PERCENTILES**

Age	Male					Female				
	5TH	15TH	50TH	85TH	95TH	5TH	15TH	50TH	85TH	95TH
4½–5½	5	6	8	12	16	6	7	10	13	16
5½–6½	5	6	8	11	15	6	7	10	12	15
6½–7½	4	6	8	11	14	6	7	10	13	17
7½–8½	5	6	8	12	17	6	7	10	15	19
8½–9½	5	6	9	14	19	6	7	11	17	21
9½–10½	5	6	10	16	22	6	8	12	19	24
10½–11½	6	7	10	17	25	7	8	12	20	29
11½–12½	5	7	11	19	26	6	9	13	20	25
12½–13½	5	6	10	18	25	7	9	14	23	30
13½–14½	5	6	10	17	22	8	10	15	22	28
14½–15½	4	6	9	19	26	8	11	16	24	30
15½–16½	4	5	9	20	27	8	10	15	23	27
16½–17½	4	5	8	14	20	9	12	16	26	31

From Ziegler, M. Nutritional card of the pediatric athlete. Clinics in Sports Medicine, 1(3):376, 1982.

more complex, but also more accurate, method is to multiply ideal weight in pounds times 10 for basal calories. Basal activity calories are then calculated by multiplying weight in pounds times 3 for sedentary activity, times 5 for moderate activity, and times 10 for vigorous activity. The additional requirements of the sports activity are determined by adding 10 to 14 calories per minute for boys and 9 to 12 calories per minute for girls. For example, an active female gymnast who weighs 92 pounds requires 920 basal calories plus 920 basal activity calories. Her daily 2-hour workout requires another 1200 calories (10 calories times 120 minutes). Her total caloric need is 3040 calories (Birrer & Brecher, 1987).

Protein requirements of the preadolescent and adolescent athlete approximate those of the adult, but younger athletes have increased protein needs for growth. Small children have special iron needs, as do females after menarche (Peterson & Peterson, 1988; Smith, NJ, 1983). Recommended dietary allowances for children are presented in Table 16–8.

The child needs more fluid per proportional weight than the adult. A useful formula for daily water requirements of children is 100 ml/kg/day for the first 10 kg of weight, 50 ml/kg additional for the next 10 kg of weight, and 25 ml/kg additional for the next 10 kg of weight. Above 30 kg of weight the requirements should approximate adult values (64 oz of liquid daily) (Ziegler, 1982).

The training diet of the young athlete should routinely consist of 50 to 55% carbohydrate, 15% protein, and 30 to 35% fat, of which only 10% is saturated. Smaller, growing muscles cannot store glycogen as efficiently as larger, strong muscles so more complex carbohydrates may be necessary if the child complains of fatigue (Peterson & Peterson, 1988). The basic food groups should be included in these plans with attention to total caloric intake (Food Guide Pyramid, 1992; Smith, NJ, 1983). Additional supplements are not necessary if the diet is adequate and may even be dangerous in the growing child (Ziegler, 1982). Glycogen loading, or increased amounts of glycogen to increase muscle stores to two to three times their normal levels, is not recommended in young children or in early adolescence because of the side effects of muscle stiffness and water retention. Glycogen loading can be used with caution by teenagers (Birrer & Brecher, 1987).

Dietary recommendations differ during the four phases of training and competition. In the postseason and off-season periods, the athlete should receive all nutritional and caloric needs for optimal weight, while during preseason and in-season optimal weight and performance should guide the nutritional balance and caloric load. The pregame meal should be eaten 2 to 3 hours before competition to guarantee digestion in the stomach and upper intestine. The meal should be easy to digest;

TABLE 16–8. **RECOMMENDED DAILY DIETARY ALLOWANCES FOR THE GROWING CHILD**

Age (yr):	Males				Females			
	4–6	7–10	11–14	15–18	4–6	7–10	11–14	15–18
Calories	1800	2100	2800	3000	1800	2100	2100	2100
Protein (g)	30	36	44	54	30	36	44	48
Fat-soluble vitamins								
A (IU)	2000	2500	3300	5000	2000	2500	4000	4000
D (IU)	100	100	100	100	100	100	100	100
E (IU)	9	10	12	15	9	10	12	12
Water-soluble vitamins								
Ascorbic acid (mg)	40	40	45	45	40	40	45	45
Folacin (μg)	200	300	400	400	200	300	400	400
Niacin (mg)	12	16	18	20	12	16	16	14
Riboflavin (mg)	1.1	1.2	1.5	1.8	1.1	1.2	1.3	1.4
Thiamin (mg)	0.9	1.2	1.4	1.5	0.9	1.2	1.2	1.1
B_6 (mg)	0.9	1.2	1.5	2.0	0.9	1.2	1.6	2.0
B_{12} (μg)	1.5	2.0	3.0	3.0	1.5	2.0	3.0	3.0
Minerals								
Calcium (mg)	800	800	1200	1200	800	800	1200	1200
Phosphorus (mg)	800	800	1200	1200	800	800	1200	1200
Iron (mg)	10	10	18	18	10	10	18	18
Magnesium (mg)	200	250	350	400	200	250	300	300
Trace elements								
Iodine (μg)	30	110	130	150	80	110	115	115
Zinc (mg)	10	10	15	15	10	10	15	15

From Ziegler, M. Nutritional care of the pediatric athlete. Clinics in Sports Medicine, 1(3):375, 1982. Adapted from Food and Nutrition Board, National Academy of Sciences–National Research Council, 1974.

be low in fat, protein, salt, and bulk; and have abundant liquid content and complex carbohydrates for adequate energy and hydration. Examples are waffles, pasta, sandwiches, or liquid meals. The goal during competition is maintenance of adequate hydration (and glycogen for endurance events). Postcompetition meals should immediately replenish glycogen stores and restore fluid balance. Two cups of water should be consumed for each pound lost (Clark, 1991; Grana & Kalenak, 1991; Peterson & Peterson, 1988; Ziegler, 1982).

Alterations in weight can and should be made carefully. Weight gain diets should have a similar composition to the training diet but include additional calories. An added 1000 calories a day will result in a gain of 2 lb weekly. This gain will occur in lean body tissue if the child is moderately active. Determination of whether an athlete is overfat or overweight must be made before recommendation of a diet for weight loss. If the athlete is excessively fat or has too great a percentage of body fat in relation to total body composition, careful structure of a training plan can convert fat to lean muscle mass. If an athlete is also overweight, a weight loss diet of composition similar to that of the normal athlete but with 1000 less calories per day should be constructed. This will result in a safe loss of 2 lb weekly. Additional exercise will hasten weight loss and maintain firmness of body tissue (Peterson & Peterson, 1988; Smith, NJ, 1983).

Proper Supervision

The first in the series of supervisors is the coach, the key to a successful sports program. Approximately 20 million children, however, are coached by 2.5 million adult volunteers with varying levels of expertise. The American Academy of Pediatrics has stated that coaches should encourage preparticipation screenings every 1 to 2 years; enforce use of warm-up procedures, require suitable protective equipment, and enforce rules concerning safety. In addition, it recommends completion of a certification program that covers teaching techniques, basic sports skills, fitness, first aid, sportsmanship, enhancement of self-image, and motivational skills (American Academy of Pediatrics, 1989).

Qualified officials and professional medical personnel at games and practices are the second level of supervision. These individuals provide game control and immediate injury containment on site. Medical personnel could include physicians, physical therapists, or athletic trainers who have certification in basic first aid and cardiopulmonary resuscitation techniques in addition to their medical skills (American Academy of Pediatrics, 1989; Puffer, 1991).

Protection

Outfitting the child athlete with proper equipment should be mandated and enforced for the protection of the participants. Equipment must be appropriate for the sport. High quality and proper fit are essential to correct function (Stanitski, 1989). Proper footwear with adequate cushioning, rearfoot control, and sole flexibility for the sport should be required (Trepman & Micheli, 1988). Protective padding in contact or kicking sports, such as shoulder and shin pads, should be recommended.

Protective headgear for contact and collision in football, baseball, and hockey is necessary to limit the number of head and neck injuries. Schuller and colleagues (1989) have demonstrated a lower risk of auricular damage in wrestlers wearing headgear (26% incidence) versus those with no headgear (52% incidence). Helmets should be approved by the National Operating Committee on Standards for Athletic Equipment and the American National Safety Institute (Grana & Kalenak, 1991; Occupational Health and Safety, 1988).

Eye injuries have been on the increase in recent years, particularly in racquet sports, baseball, and basketball (Jones, 1989; Stock & Cornell, 1991). An estimated 100,000 sports-related eye injuries occur yearly and are the most common cause of eye trauma in children younger than the age of 15 years (Stock & Cornell, 1991) (Table 16–9). Eye protec-

TABLE 16–9. **SPORTS ASSOCIATED WITH EYE INJURY AT VARIOUS AGES**

Children (5 to 12 years of age)
  Baseball
  Basketball
  Soccer
  BB gun injuries
Adolescents (13 to 21 years of age)
  Basketball
  Football
  Ice hockey
  Soccer
Adults (21 years of age and older)
  Racquetball
  Squash
  Tennis
  Badminton

From Stock, J, & Cornell, M. Prevention of sports-related eye injury. American Family Practice, 44:516, 1991; published by the American Academy of Family Physicians.

tors that dissipate injury to a wider area without reducing visual field should be required in the following sports: racquet sports, ice hockey, baseball, basketball, use of air-powered weapons, and football. They should be cosmetically and functionally acceptable as well as made of impact-resistant material. Polycarbonate is the most impact- and scratch-resistant material. A list of high-risk sports and recommended protection is given in Table 16–10. All eye protectors should be approved by either the Canadian Standards Association or the American Society for Testing and Materials.

Studies have highlighted the incidence of oral

TABLE 16 10. RISK LEVEL FOR EYE INJURY WITH RECOMMENDATIONS FOR PROTECTIVE EYEWEAR

Risk	Sport	Protective Wear
Unacceptable	Boxing	Not applicable
Very high	Ice hockey	Helmet with full visor
	Squash	Polycarbonate sports protector
	Badminton	Polycarbonate sports protector
	Basketball	Polycarbonate sports protector
	Men's lacrosse	Helmet with full visor
High	Racquetball	Polycarbonate sports protector
	Baseball	Polycarbonate sports protector
	Cricket	Helmet with full visor
	Field hockey	Helmet with full visor
	Rugby football	Debatable
	Soccer	Debatable
	Water polo	Polycarbonate goggles
	Shooting	Polycarbonate sports protector
	Women's lacrosse	Helmet with full visor
Moderate	Tennis	Plastic lens spectacles
	American football	Helmet with polycarbonate visor
Low	Golf	Sports protector if one-eyed
	Volleyball	Sports protector if one-eyed
	Skiing	UV filter goggles ± helmet
	Cycling	Sports protector ± helmet
	Fishing	Polycarbonate protector if one-eyed
	Swimming	Goggles if in water for long periods
	High diving	Not feasible
	Track & field	None required

From Jones, N. Eye injury in sport, Sports Medicine, 7;178, 1989.

and facial injuries in many sports, particularly football, hockey, baseball, basketball, wrestling, and boxing. Youth baseball generated the greatest number of head and face injuries in 1980 (Castaldi, 1986). Before mandatory use of mouthguards, oral trauma constituted 50% of all football injuries (McNutt et al., 1989). The mandatory use of mouthguards has cut the injury rate in football alone to less than 1% of all injuries (Kerr, 1986). The mouth protector serves to prevent injury to the teeth and lacerations of the mouth. Because it absorbs blows to the oral and facial structures, it also prevents fractures, dislocations, and concussions. It should position the bite so the condyles of the mandible do not contact the fossae of the joints. These mouthguards should be inexpensive, strong, and easy to clean and should not interfere with speech or breathing. They should be used alone in field hockey, rugby, wrestling, basketball, and other field events and used in conjunction with face protectors in football, ice hockey, baseball, and lacrosse (Grana & Kalenak, 1991; Kerr, 1986).

Environmental Control

Assessment and control of the environment is also vital to the safety of the child athlete. The playing area should be well lighted and maintained for safety. Surfaces should be free from obstacles and smooth and even, with good shock-absorbing qualities (wood as opposed to concrete). Modifications of equipment that have been shown to decrease injury (e.g., breakaway bases) should be installed. Sports equipment and playing environments should be scaled down to the size of the athlete (Stanitski, 1989).

Ambient temperature and humidity should be carefully monitored. Children have a greater surface area per body weight so their rate of heat exchange is greater with lower ability to endure exercise in climatic extremes. They also have a distinctly deficient ability to perspire so they carry a larger heat load. They acclimatize less efficiently and require more "exposures" for acclimatization to occur (Ilmarinen & Valimaki, 1984). Exercise should be modified if the temperature is above 80°F or if relative humidity is above 95% (Peterson & Peterson, 1988). The recommendations for exercise and hydration in relation to the environment are noted in Table 16–11.

Dehydration can be avoided by drinking plenty of liquid before, during, and after play. Thirst is not a valid indicator of the amount of water needed, so every pound lost should be replaced with 2 cups of water (Peterson & Peterson, 1988). The American

TABLE 16–11. WET-BULB TEMPERATURE AND FIELD PRECAUTIONS

Temperature	Precaution
Under 68°	No precautions necessary except close observation of those squad members most susceptible to heat illness (those who lose over 3% of their body weight as determined from weight chart).
69°–79°	Insist that unlimited amounts of drinking water be given on the field. Ice water is preferable.
Over 80°	Lighten the practice routine or practice in shorts. Withhold susceptible players from participation. Whenever the humidity is over 95%, alter practice as described for "Over 80°."

From Murphy, R. Heat illness in the athlete. In Athletic Training, Schering Symposium, Nashville, 1984, p. 2.

College of Sports Medicine recommends that 400 to 500 ml of water be ingested before distance running. They further recommend water intake every 35 to 45 minutes of football practice and nude weighing before and after practice. If residual weight loss from day to day exceeds 2 to 3 pounds, practice is restricted until water is replenished (Ziegler, 1982). Table 16–12 outlines the recommended amount and time of fluid breaks for degree of weight loss.

TABLE 16–12. RECOMMENDED FLUID INTAKE AND AVAILABILITY FOR A 90-MINUTE PRACTICE

Weight Loss LB	Weight Loss KG	Minutes Between Water Break	Fluid per Break OZ	Fluid per Break ML
8	3.6	*		
7.5	3.4	*		
7	3.2	10	8–10	266
6.5	3.0	10	8–9	251
6	2.7	10	8–9	251
5.5	2.5	15	10–12	325
5	2.3	15	10–11	311
4.5	2.1	15	9–10	281
4	1.8	15	8–9	251
3.5	1.6	20	10–11	311
3	1.4	20	9–10	281
2.5	1.1	20	7–8	222
2	0.9	30	8	237
1.5	0.7	30	6	177
1	0.5	45	6	177
0.5	0.2	60	6	177

*No practice recommended.
From Peterson, M, & Peterson, K. Eat to Compete: A Guide to Sports Nutrition. Chicago: Year Book Medical Publishers, 1988, p. 182.

The American Academy of Pediatrics has established guidelines on dangerous sports. It does not recommend boxing or trampoline jumping for any growing child (Mellion, 1988). One pediatric sports orthopaedist recommends that children younger than the age of 14 not be allowed to run distances greater than 10 km secondary to the effects of repetitive trauma on growing bone (Physician and Sports Medicine, 1982).

RISK FACTORS FOR INJURY

Injury can be the result of a single macrotrauma or of repetitive microtrauma (Micheli, 1991). Seven risk factors for repetitive trauma, or "overuse," have been identified. These include 1) training errors; 2) musculotendinous imbalances of strength, flexibility, or bulk; 3) anatomic malalignment of the lower extremity; 4) improper footwear; 5) faulty playing surface; 6) associated disease states of the lower extremity such as old injury or arthritis; and 7) growth factors (Maffulli, 1990; Micheli, 1983; Taimela et al., 1990).

Training Error

Training error is frequently the cause of overuse injuries in children, as it is in adults. The evolution of sports-specific camps from the generalized summer camp experience has dramatically increased the daily level of participation. The sudden transition from casual play to 6 or 8 hours of intense participation has contributed to the incidence of overuse injury in children.

Muscle–Tendon Imbalance

Muscle–tendon imbalance can occur in strength, flexibility, or bulk. Until recently, little attention was paid to conditioning in children. This attitude may have been appropriate for free play activities but not for organized sport. The repetitive, often predictable, demands of a sport may result in imbalances of muscle and tendon unless the child is on a well-designed training plan. For example, a baseball pitcher or swimmer who does the breast stroke might develop a loose anterior capsule and a tight posterior capsule, a situation that could lead to impingement or anterior shoulder subluxation. Repetitive running creates strength and tightness in the quadriceps femoris and triceps surae muscles with relatively weaker hamstrings. This could be problematic if pace and hence stride length are increased.

Anatomic Malalignment

Anatomic malalignment can be a factor in the occurrence of injury since the body may not be able to compensate for the malalignment under the demands of a sport. Femoral anteversion in a young dancer can cause excessive tibial external rotation and ankle pronation as substitutes for natural hip external rotation. Hyperlordosis of the spine or hyperextension of the knee creates abnormal loading on portions of the joint, leading to pain. Pes planus can increase the valgus moment at the knee as well as allowing the weight of the body to land on a flexible foot. This malalignment can cause pain and abnormal wear on the medial knee joint and foot.

Footwear

Well-fitting shoes with a firm heel counter, slight heel lift, and flexible toe box are essential for the young athlete. Inadequate footwear that does not support the structures of the foot while playing can lead to a number of foot and lower extremity problems. The shoe should compensate for changes in alignment and shock absorption. Likewise, improper playing surfaces can predispose the child to knee pain, shin splints, or stress fractures. These symptoms have been associated with playing on hard, banked surfaces or synthetic courts, as opposed to clay and hardwood surfaces (O'Neill & Micheli, 1988).

Associated Disease States

Associated disease is occasionally an issue, as in the child with previous Legg-Calvé-Perthes disease who has limited hip rotation. Likewise, a child with juvenile rheumatoid arthritis or hemophilia may have exacerbations of joint pain or synovitis with participation in sports.

Growth

The first aspect of growth that is a factor in overuse injuries is the articular cartilage (Fig. 16–3). Clinical and biomechanical evidence suggests that growing cartilage has low resistance to repetitive loading, resulting in microtrauma to either the cartilage or the underlying growth plate. Damage may result in osteoarthritis or growth asymmetry (Micheli, 1983).

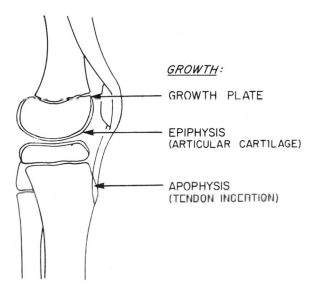

FIGURE 16–3. Sites of susceptibility of the growth cartilage. (From Micheli, L. Overuse injuries in children's sports: The growth factor. Orthopedic Clinics of North America, *14*[2]:341, 1983.)

The growing articular cartilage is also less resistant to shear, particularly at the elbow, knee, and ankle. Repetitive shear has been implicated in osteochondritis dissecans of the capitellum in Little League pitchers and of the proximal and distal femur and talus in runners. Studies postulate that a segment of subchondral bone becomes avascular and separates with its articular cartilage from the surrounding bone to become a loose body (Maffulli, 1990). Shear stress has further been implicated in epiphyseal displacement (Micheli, 1983).

The final site of growth cartilage weakness is the apophysis. Increasing evidence suggests that traction apophysitis, such as Osgood-Schlatter disease, Sever's disease, and irritation of the rectus femoris or sartorius muscle origins, is the result of degeneration of the growth center with tiny avulsion fractures and associated healing (Maffulli, 1990; Micheli, 1983; O'Neill & Micheli, 1988).

The second element of growth involved in overuse injury is the process itself. Longitudinal growth occurs in the bones, with secondary elongation of the soft tissues. During periods of rapid bone growth ("growth spurts") the musculotendinous structures tighten and cause loss of flexibility. A coincidence of overuse injury and growth spurt has been noted (Micheli, 1983).

TYPES OF INJURIES

Although injuries in children have some similarity to those in adults, several are peculiar to the growing child. These specific injuries fall into three categories: 1) fractures, 2) joint injuries, and 3) muscle–tendon unit injuries (Micheli, 1983; O'Neill & Micheli, 1988).

Fractures

A relatively new injury in children is the stress fracture, which usually results from repetitive microtrauma or poor training. Repetition causes cancellous bone fractures as opposed to cortical bone fatigue in adults (Maffulli, 1990). These cancellous bone fractures are often imperceptible on radiographs until 6 to 8 weeks after the onset of pain. Stress fractures cause persistent, activity-related pain that can be reproduced by indirect force to the bone. Suspicion based on clinical signs and symptoms can be reinforced by bone scans if diagnostic uncertainty exists.

Growth plate or epiphyseal fractures are peculiar to the child. The cartilaginous growth plate is less resistant to shear or tensile-deforming force than either the ligament or bony cortex, so mechanical disruption frequently occurs through the plate itself, usually in the zone of hypertrophy (Maffulli, 1990). This disruption can be caused by a single macrotrauma, such as jumping, or by repetitive microtrauma as in distance running. The potential for problems from epiphyseal fracture depends on the specific plate involved and on the extent of the injury. Decreased limb length, angular deformity, joint incongruity, and premature closure are frequent sequelae (Maffulli, 1990; Micheli, 1984). Shaft fractures are usually noted in the older child who is approaching adult status.

Joint Injuries

Joint injuries in the young athlete include ligamentous sprains, internal derangement, and musculotendinous insertional injuries. These can result from a single discrete injury or from repetitive trauma. The diagnosis of sprain must be made carefully in the child. During a growth spurt, ligaments may be stronger than the growth plate so excessive bending or twisting forces cause the plate rather than the ligament to yield. Severe ligamentous injuries can occur, however, so careful examination is necessary to differentiate among these injuries (Micheli, 1983; Trepman & Micheli, 1988).

Repetitive microtrauma of the joint articular cartilage often results in softening, followed by frank shredding and thinning of the surface. Compression to the joint causes exacerbation of the symptoms, such as pain, edema, and decreased functional use of the joint (Trepman & Micheli, 1988).

Muscle–Tendon Unit Injuries

Another area at particular risk of injury in the growing child is the insertion of the musculotendinous unit into the bone through the epiphyseal cartilage. Growth occurs at the apophyseal growth plate, where tendons and ligaments are attached. During growth spurts the increased tension on the attachments often leads to detachment of the structure at the apophysis (avulsion fracture). Tendonitis occurs much less frequently in the child than in the adult since the insertion becomes symptomatic before the tendon (Micheli, 1983, 1984; Trepman & Micheli, 1988).

Irritation of the insertional area of the musculotendinous unit, the enthesis, can cause pain and inflammation. This area is highly vascular and metabolically active. During exercise, when blood is diverted to the active muscle, these areas may suffer periods of ischemia (Maffulli, 1990). The symptoms cause inhibition of muscle activity with resultant weakness and loss of flexibility. The weakness and tightness then lead to greater irritation and pain (O'Neill & Micheli, 1988).

Children can overuse muscles, resulting in strain, just like adults. The increase in muscle volume during exercise may cause exertional compartment syndromes. Muscle hernias, however, occur in children secondary to tight fascial or musculotendinous structures (Trepman & Micheli, 1988).

▌ SITES OF INJURY

The anatomy and the factor of growth combine to make certain injuries more likely and more serious in the various segments of the child's body.

Brain and Cervical Injuries

The incidence of central nervous system injury in children is low, varying from 1 to 5% of sport-related injuries, but these cases constitute 50 to 100% of the deaths from injury. Cervical spine injuries result in 30 to 50% of cases of childhood quadriplegia (Bruce et al., 1982). The rate of spinal cord injuries in children younger than the age of 11 years is low but it escalates dramatically in the 15- to 18-year-old age bracket. Since the brain and spinal cord are largely incapable of regeneration, these injuries take on a singular importance (Cantu, 1988).

Participation in several sports carries a particularly high risk for head and neck injuries. Football accounts for 40% of all concussion injuries in school sports. The incidence of serious head injuries has decreased by 60% over the past 20 years, probably because of use of better equipment. Fatalities in children younger than the age of 12 have not been reported, but the mortality rate is .44 per 100,000 participants in tackle football. The incidence of serious head injury is still .75 to 1.5 per 100,000 participants per season, with a mortality rate of .5 to 1.09 per season (Bruce et al., 1982). Severe injuries, however, often result in quadriplegia and total disability. Rugby, a popular collision sport outside the United States, has head and neck injury rates similar to those of American football. Wrestling has the second highest injury rate of all high school sports, although the central nervous system injury rate is low. The rate of concussion is 1.7% of all wrestling injuries as a result of direct blows or falls (Bruce et al., 1982). Baseball accounts for a large number of concussions secondary to collision with the bat, other players, or the ball, although exact incidence figures have not been reported. Diving accounts for 3 to 18% of all cervical spine injuries in young people (Bruce et al., 1982).

Concussion, or temporary disturbance of brain function, results from a traumatic blow to the head. Symptoms are caused by biomechanical or physiologic aberrations, but no permanent pathologic process occurs (Birrer & Brecher, 1987). Concussions are graded according to duration of unconsciousness (Table 16–13). Because of the occurrence of second impact syndrome in which a series of insults can lead to cerebral damage when one impact would not, decisions regarding return to

TABLE 16–13. GRADING OF SEVERITY OF CONCUSSION

Grade	Severity
1 (mild)	No loss of consciousness; post-traumatic amnesia 30 minutes
2 (moderate)	Loss of consciousness < 5 minutes or post-traumatic amnesia > 30 minutes
3 (severe)	Loss of consciousness ≥ 5 minutes or post-traumatic amnesia ≥ 24 hours

Adapted from Cantu, R. Guidelines to return to contact sports after a cerebral concussion. Phys Sportsmed 14:76, 1986. Reproduced with permission of McGraw-Hill, Inc.

play are critical. No universally accepted criteria for return to play exist, but Table 16–14 contains recommendations based on the severity and incidence of prior concussion (Birrer & Brecher, 1987; Bruce et al., 1982; Cantu, 1988). Postconcussion syndrome, which is characterized by headache, irritability, labyrinthine disturbance, and impaired memory and concentration, is rare but suggests altered neurotransmitter function. Further evaluation is warranted before clearance to play is granted (Cantu, 1988).

The leading cause of death from head injury is intracranial hemorrhage. The most rapidly progressing and universally fatal disorder if missed is the epidural hematoma. Symptoms include initial preservation of consciousness with increasingly severe headache, lethargy, and focal neurologic signs. It is frequently associated with temporal bone fracture. An acute subdural hematoma is the most common fatal head injury and should always be considered as a possible diagnosis in the athlete who loses and does not regain consciousness. A chronic subdural hematoma should be suspected in

TABLE 16–14. GUIDELINES FOR RETURN TO PLAY AFTER CONCUSSION

Grade	First Concussion	Second Concussion	Third Concussion
1 (mild)	May return to play if asymptomatic* for 1 week	Return to play in 2 weeks if asymptomatic at that time for 1 week	Terminate season; may return to play next season if asymptomatic
2 (moderate)	Return to play after asymptomatic for 1 week	Minimum of 1 month; may return to play then if asymptomatic for 1 week; consider terminating season	Terminate season; may return to play next season if asymptomatic
3 (severe)	Minimum of 1 month; may then return to play if asymptomatic for 1 week	Terminate season; may return to play next season if asymptomatic	

*No headache, dizziness, or impaired orientation, concentration, or memory during rest.
Adapted from Cantu, R. Guidelines to return to contact sports after a cerebral concussion. Physician and Sports Medicine 14:79, 1986.

the athlete who is not quite the same for days or weeks after a head injury. Signs may include headache or mild mental, motor, or sensory signs and symptoms (Cantu, 1988).

The intracerebral hemorrhage is also rapidly progressive since the bleeding is into the brain itself. No lucid interval is noted, and death often occurs before arrival at a hospital. The subarachnoid hemorrhage is a brain contusion that causes headache and associated neurologic deficits that are dependent on the area of the brain involved. All injured athletes with potential intracranial hemorrhages should be transported to a hospital for further evaluation and medical or surgical management (Bruce et al., 1982).

Most neck injuries are caused by hyperflexion or hyperextension. Hyperflexion injuries, the most common, result from spearing or butt blocking (Fig. 16–4). Because of the poorly developed musculature in youngsters and the commonly associated fracture, hyperflexion injury can be serious. Hyperextension injuries often occur even in the absence of severe force because the anterior neck musculature is weaker than the posterior musculature. Common causes are face or head tackling (Fig. 16–5). Hyperextension injury with a rotatory component is the most common cause of nerve root damage (Birrer & Brecher, 1987). Evaluation of these injuries should always include radiographs of the cervical spine. In the adolescent the second cervical vertebra is normally displaced posteriorly over the third secondary to hypermobility. This pseudosubluxation is normal and not the result of injury (Cantu, 1988) but should be referred for assessment.

FIGURE 16–4. Hyperflexion damage from head butting. (From Birrer, R, & Brecher, D. Common Sports Injuries in Youngsters. Oradell, NJ: Medical Economics, 1987, p. 36.)

FIGURE 16–5. Hyperextension injury from face blocking. (From Birrer, R, & Brecher, D. Common Sports Injuries in Youngsters. Oradell, NJ: Medical Economics, 1987, p. 38.)

Another common injury is a "burner," which is a traction injury to the brachial plexus. It is caused by a forceful blow to the head from the side or from depression of the shoulder while the head and neck are fixed. Repeated injuries may cause weakness of the deltoid, biceps, and teres major muscles, which should be resolved with strengthening exercises. If the use of a collar or a change in technique or neck strength does not solve the problem, cessation of participation is warranted (Cantu, 1988).

Thoracic and Lumbar Spinal Injuries

Spinal injuries can occur in both the thoracic and the lumbar areas, although thoracic injuries are rare. Costovertebral injury secondary to compression of the rib cage in a pileup in football or from a forceful takedown in wrestling can injure the costovertebral articulations. Complaints include pain and muscle spasm along the associated rib. Axial compression forces on a preflexed spine, as in sledding or tobogganing, can fracture the vertebrae, particularly at the vulnerable T-12–L-1 level. These injuries can cause pain but are frequently asymptomatic (Birrer & Brecher, 1987).

The most common injuries in the lumbar spine are spondylolysis and spondylolisthesis. One study of 3132 competitive athletes aged 15 to 27 years noted an incidence of spondylolysis of 12.5% (Rossi & Dragoni, 1990). Repeated hyperflexion and hyperextension in football blocking, clean and jerk lift, diving, pole vaulting, wrestling, high jump, or gymnastic maneuvers can place excessive forces on the pars interarticularis and cause a stress fracture. Spondylolisthesis, or fracture and slippage of one vertebra on another, usually L-5 over S-1, is most common at ages 9 to 14 years. Loading of a bilateral spondylolysis, in which there is a defect in the bony connection of the posterior arch with the vertebral body, can cause a spondylolisthesis, as can traumatic or repetitive bilateral loading of a normal spine. The slippage is graded from 1 to 4, depending on the degree of slippage. Athletes with grade 2 or greater slippage should be counseled against participation in weight lifting, baseball, diving, gymnastics, or wrestling. Participation in basketball or football is permissible with use of a brace (Birrer & Brecher, 1987). The growth spurt in the spine causes lumbar lordosis secondary to the enhanced anterior growth with posterior tethering by the heavy lumbodorsal fascia. This biomechanical situation increases the tendency of posterior element failure at the pars and perhaps at the disc (Micheli, 1983). Athletes with spondylolysis are managed in a brace until healing occurs. Physical therapy is indicated to maintain flexibility in the lumbosacral spine and the spinal and hip musculature and to improve trunk and abdominal muscle strength while braced. Surgery is only indicated in cases of unstable lesions or nerve root compression (Birrer & Brecher, 1987).

The true incidence of disc lesions in young athletes is unclear, but several studies have demonstrated disturbing data. Although acute trauma has a role in this condition, degenerative changes of the vertebral bodies and intervertebral joints may be the leading factor, with trauma only as the precipitating incident (Maffulli, 1990).

Shoulder Injuries

Specific shoulder injuries can be predicted based on the biomechanics of the sport and the age of the athlete. Football, wrestling, and ice hockey cause upper extremity fractures and dislocations, while sports with repeated overhead activities contribute to overuse injuries. The hyperelasticity of juvenile joints, particularly the shoulder, makes them vulnerable to passive and dynamic instability patterns that can predispose the shoulder to injury (Ireland & Andrews, 1988).

Acromioclavicular sprains may occur in the immature athlete without clavicular fracture. The most common mechanism is direct force from a fall or blow to the lateral aspect of the shoulder or a fall on an outstretched arm (Birrer & Brecher, 1987; Micheli, 1984; Micheli & Smith, 1982; Nevaiser, 1986). Grade I and II sprains are more common in the athlete whose skeleton is immature. Grade III sprains commonly rupture the dorsal clavicular periosteum, but the acromioclavicular and coracoclavicular ligaments remain intact (Ireland & Andrews, 1988). These lesions are treated symptomatically with rest, ice, compression, and elevation in a sling (RICE). Exercises are often necessary to increase scapulothoracic and glenohumeral mobility and strength (see Rehabilitation source material in Appendix II).

Fractures are most common in the middle third of the clavicle from a direct blow. These can be actual fractures in the older child or greenstick fractures in the youngster. They are managed with a figure-of-eight strap until healed.

Because the proximal humerus is an area of bone growth, fractures are more common in children than in adults, who are more prone to dislocation. Epiphyseal displacements occur in the younger child, while metaphyseal fractures are more common in the older child or adolescent (Micheli, 1984). After healing, therapeutic intervention to normalize mobility and strength of the scapular, shoulder, and elbow muscles is frequently indicated.

Little League shoulder, a relatively common injury in young pitchers and catchers, involves a fracture of the proximal humeral growth plate secondary to rotatory torque. Any athlete who complains of proximal shoulder pain in the absence of trauma should be suspected of having an epiphyseal fracture until proven otherwise. The athlete should not do any throwing until the pain subsides (Ireland & Andrews, 1988).

Frank anterior subluxation and dislocation of the glenohumeral joint is rare in children but common in adolescents. Because of the laxity of juvenile joints, a blow or forceful maneuver in abduction, external rotation, or extension can dislodge the head of the humerus (Birrer & Brecher, 1987; Ireland & Andrews, 1988; Nevaiser, 1986). This condition is common in throwing or racquet sports, gymnastics, and swimming. Clients with posterior glenohumeral instability respond better to conservative strengthening of appropriate musculature than those with anterior instability, although a program of scapular and shoulder muscle strengthening in a biomechanically correct range of motion should be attempted. Motion should be limited to ranges that prevent chronic subluxation. Surgery is more often an option with anterior or multidirectional instability than in posterior instability (Ireland & Andrews, 1988).

Rotator cuff tears are not as common in the skeletally immature athlete as in the older athlete. They do occur in throwing and racquet sports, as well as from direct contact blows in collision sports. These tears can be treated successfully with arthroscopic surgery and rehabilitation that includes strength and endurance training for all scapular and shoulder muscles as well as training with

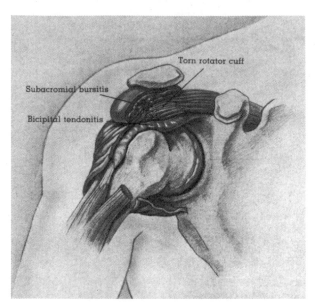

FIGURE 16–6. Common causes of impingement. (From Birrer, R, & Brecher, D. Common Sports Injuries in Youngsters. Oradell, NJ: Medical Economics, 1987, p. 61.)

correct biomechanical movements of the shoulder complex (Ireland & Andrews, 1988; Nevaiser, 1986).

Rotator cuff impingement syndrome (Fig. 16–6) is a frequent injury in athletes younger than 25 years of age. More than 50% of swimmers aged 12 to 18 years complain of shoulder pain (Birrer & Brecher, 1987). One hypothesis is that these athletes develop a characteristic contracture around the shoulder with loss of internal rotation at 90° of abduction and with increased external rotation in all positions of abduction. This might reflect a tightened posterior and a loosened anterior capsule, suggesting a tendency to subluxate anteriorly. Conservative physical therapy with normalization of mobility and strength has been successful in resolving the primary instability (Micheli, 1983). All positions of impingement (anterior, lateral, or overhead) should be avoided until the child is free of pain.

Elbow Injuries

Supracondylar fracture of the humerus is the second most common fracture in the skeletally immature client. Most of these fractures occur in the age group of 5 to 10 years. They are the result of significant forces into extension. Avulsion fractures of the medial epicondyle are not uncommon and are associated with elbow dislocations or throwing injuries. Anatomic reduction usually requires internal

fixation with early protected range of motion to avoid loss of extension (Ireland & Andrews, 1988). Subsequent to healing, normalization of mobility and strength of the elbow and forearm are necessary for full function.

Repetitive microtrauma from pitching may result in epiphyseal fracture of the radial head. Loss of extension and supination with a history of repetitive loading of the radiocapitellar joint indicates fracture. A radial head fracture is treated with rest (Ireland & Andrews, 1988). Jerking of the elbow in the child younger than 7 years old can subluxate the radial head because of the poor development of the annular ligament. The child positions the injured arm in flexion and pronation, dangling it at the side of the body (Birrer & Brecher, 1987; Micheli et al., 1980).

Elbow dislocation is seen in contact sports secondary to a fall on an abducted, extended arm. Early reduction will avoid neurovascular damage, and further evaluation and radiographs are necessary to assess the presence of associated fracture. Early protected mobility is necessary to preserve normal elbow motion (Birrer & Brecher, 1987; Ireland & Andrews, 1988). Physical therapy to normalize elbow and forearm mobility and to improve strength at the elbow, forearm, and hand is appropriate.

Little League elbow commonly results from the extreme valgus stress placed on the epicondyles during the acceleration phase of pitching (Fig. 16–7). If this is not recognized and regular throwing

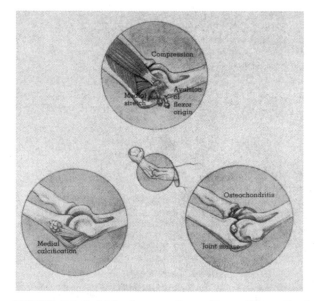

FIGURE 16–7. Little League elbow. (From Birrer, R, & Brecher, D. Common Sports Injuries in Youngsters. Oradell, NJ: Medical Economics, 1987, p. 74.)

continues, mild separation of the medial epicondyle with hypertrophy, irregularity, fragmentation, and avulsion can occur. The most serious damage is the jamming of the radial head against the capitellum on the lateral side, a finding that occurs in 8 to 10% of young pitchers. The results of this jamming can be osteochondritis of the capitellum, avascular necrosis of the radial head, and loose bodies within the joint. Treatment is RICE and rest from throwing (Birrer & Brecher, 1987). Eventual alteration of throwing technique may be necessary.

Tennis elbow is seen in a variety of racquet sports as a result of repeated injury to the lateral epicondyle. A faulty stroke initiates the process. The resulting friction between the extensor muscles, the lateral epicondyle, and the radial head causes irritation, microtears in the extensor muscle origin, and adhesions between the annular ligament and the joint capsule. Using tightly strung racquets, racquets with small handles, and old tennis balls will aggravate the situation. Rehabilitation to decrease irritation, reduce adhesions, and strengthen the forearm and hand musculature is required. Alteration of technique and equipment, such as enlargement of the racquet grip area or reduction of string tension, is helpful (Birrer & Brecher, 1987; Knowles et al., 1987).

Wrist and Hand Injuries

Because of the inherent complexity of the anatomy of the wrist joint, potentially serious injuries may be missed or underdiagnosed. Careful diagnosis using knowledge of biomechanics of the wrist and hand is crucial (Birrer & Brecher, 1987; Micheli, 1984).

Fractures about the wrist follow an age-related pattern. In the young child a torus, or buckle fracture, of the distal radial epiphysis is common after a fall. Clinical signs are minimal pain and tenderness, so careful radiologic examination is necessary. Simple splinting is adequate for healing (Birrer & Brecher, 1987; Micheli, 1984). Metaphyseal fractures of the distal radius and ulna are more common in the child. Often displaced, they require reduction with the use of anesthesia. In the younger adolescent, fractures through the growth plate are common, again from falls, and require operative reduction to minimize trauma to the growth plate (Micheli, 1984). Rehabilitation to regain normal forearm and wrist mobility as well as wrist and grip strength is desirable. Stress injuries to the distal radial epiphysis have been noted in athletes such as gymnasts who bear weight on their hands. Complaints of pain with wrist dorsiflexion and of wrist

stiffness are common. Radiographs demonstrate a widened epiphysis, cystic changes, and breaking of the distal metaphysis. Management consists of cessation of gymnastics with or without casting (Simmons & Lovallo, 1988).

Although fracture of most carpal bones is rare, fracture of the navicular or scaphoid bone is common in children from 12 to 15 years of age. This fracture results from a fall on the dorsiflexed hand of an outstretched arm. Although the fracture is not readily visible on a radiograph, early diagnosis is important because of the high incidence of avascular necrosis and nonunion. If tenderness in the anatomical snuffbox occurs with a high degree of suspicion of fracture, use of a short-arm spica cast will be adequate management (Birrer & Brecher, 1987; Micheli, 1984; Simmons & Lovallo, 1988).

Because the hand and fingers are so essential in most sports, the small structures absorb tremendous forces of initial contact (Birrer & Brecher, 1987). Injuries are therefore common. Dislocations are uncommon in the child's hand because the forces necessary to produce these injuries are usually dissipated by producing a fracture. If dislocations do occur, it is usually in the adolescent and in patterns similar to those in an adult. Thus, the most common dislocation occurs at the carpometacarpal joint of the thumb, usually secondary to axial compression forces on the thumb tip in contact sports. Although reduction is easy, maintenance is not, and chronic instability can result. The thumb is put in a short-arm thumb spica, and participation in sports should be avoided for 6 weeks. A short opponens splint is advisable for the initial 6 weeks of re-entry to play (Simmons & Lovallo, 1988).

Dorsal dislocation of the thumb metacarpophalangeal joint is the most common dislocation in the hand of a child. A fall or forceful contact hyperextends the metacarpophalangeal joint. If the proximal phalanx is parallel to the metacarpal, the volar plate has been avulsed and surgical reduction is necessary. Cast immobilization for 3 weeks with sports participation permitted is adequate for healing. Physical therapy may be indicated to normalize thumb mobility and strength following casting. Metacarpophalangeal dislocations in the fingers are rare except for those that affect the index finger. After this injury is reduced, splinting in flexion for 3 weeks with immediate mobilization after splint removal is the treatment of choice (Birrer & Brecher, 1987; Simmons & Lovallo, 1988).

Joint injuries are common in ball sports and skiing. The metacarpophalangeal joint of the thumb is the most commonly injured joint in skiers. The majority of these injuries in youth are bony gamekeeper's thumb in which the ulnar collateral ligament avulses a segment of bone, as compared with the purely ligamentous injury in adults. If the bony fragment lies close to its origin, good results are obtained with use of a short-arm thumb spica for 6 weeks, followed by exercises to normalize mobility and strength. Athletic participation, even molding the cast to fit the ski pole, can be allowed. If the radiograph is negative, integrity of the ulnar collateral ligament must be established by assessing radial deviation in extension and 30° of flexion. Deviation of greater than 30° indicates at least a partial tear. No firm end point in full extension or greater than 45° of deviation in flexion indicates full ligamentous tear with volar plate injury, which will require surgical repair (Birrer & Brecher, 1987; Simmons & Lovallo, 1988). Hand therapy is necessary to regain normal mobility, strength, and pinch.

Jammed fingers are common injuries in all age groups. Axial compression force to the fingertips causes distal interphalangeal flexion with proximal interphalangeal hyperextension. Reduction is easily accomplished by distal traction. Buddy taping will allow the athlete to return to play (Birrer & Brecher, 1987; Simmons & Lovallo, 1988). Caution should be exhibited, however, since fractures through the growth plate of the phalanx are common. These intra-articular, or neck, fractures have a great tendency to displace and then require open reduction with internal fixation (Micheli, 1984). In the absence of a fracture or dislocation, damage to the collateral ligaments can occur and is managed in similar fashion. Jamming at the distal interphalangeal joint can result in "mallet finger," or tearing of the terminal extensor tendon with or without a bony fragment. This injury is easily managed with use of a dorsal extension splint for 6 to 8 weeks. If active and passive extension ranges are equal at 6 weeks, then active flexion can be initiated. If not, splinting is continued for another month. Participation is allowed with the splint in place (Birrer & Brecher, 1987; Simmons & Lovallo, 1988).

Pelvis and Hip Injuries

Because the hip and pelvis have complex ossification patterns and fuse late in childhood, the possibility for injury is high. The acetabulum has three sections joined by triradiate cartilage. Likewise, three ossification centers exist on the femoral head: the capital femoral epiphysis, the greater trochanter, and the lesser trochanter. The circular vascularity of the femoral head and neck also creates risk for injury in the growing child (Waters & Millis, 1988).

Fractures are uncommon but can occur in the epiphyseal plate, the femoral neck, or the subtrochanteric area. Slipped capital femoral epiphysis is not caused by sports but must be suspected in any athlete with persistent hip or knee pain and a limp. It occurs during the rapid growth in adolescence in either obese or very thin males. Surgical reduction with internal fixation is necessary (see Chapter 15).

Fractures of the neck or subtrochanteric area are rare but can be the result of severe trauma, usually incurred during contact sports such as football and rugby. Surgical reduction is necessary to maintain position (Waters & Millis, 1988). More common are avulsion fractures from a sudden violent muscular contraction or excessive muscle stretch. The most common sites are the anterior-superior iliac spine (origin of the sartorius), the ischium (hamstring origin) (Fig. 16–8), the lesser trochanter (insertion of the iliopsoas), the anterior-inferior iliac spine (rectus femoris origin), and iliac crest (abdominal insertion). These injuries are classic in sprinting, jumping, soccer, football, and weight lifting. Rest with gradual increase of excursion to full mobility followed by progressive resistance exercise and reintegration to play is the treatment sequence (Birrer & Brecher, 1987; Micheli & Smith, 1982; Waters & Millis, 1988). One less traumatic overuse parallel of avulsion is iliac apophysitis, which usually affects adolescent track, field, or cross-country athletes or dancers. Repeated contraction of the tensor fascia lata, rectus femoris, sartorius, gluteus medius, and oblique abdominal muscles causes nonspecific pain and tenderness over the iliac crest.

FIGURE 16–8. Avulsion of the ischial tuberosity. (From Birrer, R, & Brecher, D. Common Sports Injuries in Youngsters. Oradell, NJ: Medical Economics, 1987, p. 101.)

Rest helps this problem (Birrer & Brecher, 1987), but often exercises to increase strength and normalize two-joint muscle flexibility are required.

Stress fractures and osteitis pubis are being diagnosed more frequently as a result of repetitive microtrauma in runners or athletes who have suddenly increased their involvement in jumping or kicking activities. Persistent pain and tenderness in the groin with limited mobility and activity-related increases in pain could signal either of these conditions. Radiographs showing inflammation, demineralization, and sclerosis confirm the diagnosis of osteitis pubis, but a bone scan is necessary to diagnose a stress fracture. Stress fractures have been seen in the pelvis at the junction of the ischium and pubic ramus and in the femoral neck and shaft (Birrer & Brecher, 1987; Waters & Millis, 1988). Relative rest, use of crutches, and restriction from percussive activities (running and jumping) are required for resolution of these disorders.

Snapping hip syndrome is an overuse problem noted in gymnasts, dancers, and sprinters. This term can refer to either irritation of the iliotibial band over the greater trochanter with hip motion or to tenosynovitis of the iliopsoas tendon near its femoral insertion. Usually, relative rest, use of appropriate modalities, stretching, and improved muscle strength overcome these symptoms (Micheli, 1983; Waters & Millis, 1988).

A serious condition seen in the young athlete aged 5 to 12 years is avascular necrosis of the femoral head. Activity can irritate the synovium, leading to joint effusion and reduction of the blood supply to the femoral head. The initial complaint is nonspecific hip pain, but radiographs demonstrate periosteal rarefaction followed by sclerosis and irregular collapse of the humeral head. Bracing or surgery may be required, depending on the degree of progression of the problem (Birrer & Brecher, 1987; Micheli, 1983) (see Chapter 15).

Contusions are common, but the most frequent is the hip pointer. This iliac crest contusion is caused by a driving blow by a helmet, occurring typically in football or hockey. The overlying muscle is damaged with a resultant subperiosteal hematoma. RICE and padding will resolve this problem with time (Birrer & Brecher, 1987). Occasionally, use of ultrasound evaluation and soft tissue mobilization along with stretching may be necessary.

Knee Injuries

As the largest joint in the body and one with minimal anatomic protection, the knee is the focal point of stress forces applied along the tibia and femur. Consequently, it is not only the site of macrotrauma but also the most frequent site of overuse injury (Birrer & Brecher, 1987; Micheli, 1983).

Fractures about the knee, although not frequent, are significant for their possible influences on growth. Distal femoral epiphyseal fractures occur in the young athlete as a consequence of twisting injuries. Careful open anatomic reduction with internal fixation is necessary to avoid subsequent growth disturbances (Steiner & Grana, 1988). Physical therapy is usually necessary for children who sustain distal femoral or proximal tibial epiphyseal fractures. Either open reduction with internal fixation or casting causes loss of knee and ankle mobility as well as decreased thigh and calf muscle strength. Rehabilitation to reverse these effects as well as retrain the youngster in balance and agility skills is necessary.

Fractures of the proximal tibial epiphysis are rare but treacherous because of associated popliteal artery damage and compartment syndrome. More common is fracture of the tibial tuberosity alone or in association with the proximal tibia. These are most common at the end of adolescence in jumping sports such as basketball and track. These fractures can be managed with extension casting if minimal displacement has occurred or with internal fixation if displaced. Growth disturbances are rare because of the late occurrence of the fracture (Mirby et al., 1988; Steiner & Grana, 1988). Stress fractures were rare but are being reported more commonly in the tibias of runners and swimmers. Reduction of the loading stress of running or of turns in swimming is suggested until healing occurs (Steiner & Grana, 1988). Ligament injuries are becoming more common in the young athlete, with one study reporting medial collateral ligament injury in children as young as 4 years of age (Steiner & Grana, 1988). All ligament injuries should be assessed for coincident physis fractures (Steiner & Grana, 1988). Medial collateral ligament tears in youth can include both the superficial and the capsular components of the ligament. Nonoperative treatment with splinting and avoidance of valgus stress has been successful in adolescents, so it may be possible to obtain equally good results in younger children (Steiner & Grana, 1988). Physical therapy to retain or improve lower extremity strength and coordination, especially in the thigh and calf, is often needed.

Most anterior cruciate ligament tears in the preteen group are in fact avulsion fractures at the tibial insertion. The fracture of the tibial spine usually occurs through the cancellous bone, demonstrating avulsion of the tibial spine on a radiograph. The mechanism of injury is typically a bicycle accident or a fall in preteens and a contact sport in adolescents. Casting in 30° of knee flexion is accepted practice for minimally displaced fractures, but internal fixation is needed for full displacement of the fragment. Midsubstance tears of the anterior cruciate ligament are most common in the adolescent. Traditional reconstructive procedures are avoided because of fear of injury to the growth plate with the proximal tibial drill hole. Classic management is functional bracing and development of muscular strength and balance for knee stability (Steiner & Grana, 1988; Zarins, 1982).

Internal derangement of the knee joint can be either juvenile osteochondritis dissecans or meniscal injury. The etiology of juvenile osteochondritis dissecans is still an enigma. Compression of the tibial spine against the medial femoral condyle, interruption of the vascularity, anatomic variations in the knee, and abnormal subchondral bone are all viable possibilities. Athletic children do not seem to be at greater risk for this injury than more sedentary children. The most common sites of involvement are the lateral side of the medial femoral condyle or the lateral femoral condyle in the weight-bearing region or posteriorly. The condition usually presents as pain, recurrent swelling, or catching in the knee. Pain is usually evident as the tibia rotates internally and the knee extends from a flexed position (Birrer & Brecher, 1987). Because these lesions have a poor prognosis after skeletal maturity, every attempt should be made to gain healing before growth plate closure. In the child younger than 15 years of age, diminished activity to the point of not bearing weight is suggested. Drilling of the condyles with removal of fragments is recommended in children older than 15 years of age. This procedure usually necessitates restriction of running and jumping for at least 6 weeks with concomitant intensive rehabilitation to regain strength, balance, and agility in the lower extremity (Grana & Kalenak, 1990; Steiner & Grana, 1988).

The challenge of meniscal injuries in the young athlete is accurate diagnosis. Often the initial incident is forgotten and clinical testing is less diagnostic than in the adult. Arthroscopic excision or repair is the treatment of choice if conservative management fails. Excision necessitates physical therapy to regain mobility and strength deficits. Meniscal repair further requires limitations of knee mobility and weight bearing while healing occurs. Discoid lateral meniscus, which is particularly common in the Japanese, can create joint line tenderness, decreased joint mobility, effusion, and, most notably, a prominent snap in the lateral compartment as the knee is extended (Steiner & Grana, 1988). Normal menisci do not go through a discoid

stage during development. The complete type of discoid meniscus, producing symptoms in late adolescence, is distinguished by intact peripheral attachments. Good results are obtained with saucerization of the meniscus. The Wrisberg type of discoid meniscus, which is more common in the pediatric group, has an attachment only through the ligament of Wrisberg and can be resolved by cutting the ligament and removing the portions with no peripheral attachments (Steiner & Grana, 1988).

The majority of problems at the knee in children are disorders of the patellar mechanism (Birrer & Brecher, 1987; Micheli, 1983; Steiner & Grana, 1988). Macrotrauma, repetitive microtrauma, and growth all can contribute to the disorders of the patellofemoral joint. Patellofemoral pain is the most frequent problem in the young athlete. Malalignment of the patellofemoral joint is the major cause of this pain. Several factors can cause or contribute to this malalignment. Anatomic factors such as patella alta, large Q angle, hip anteversion, flattened lateral femoral condyle, shallow femoral groove, or pes planus and hyperpronation can cause abnormal tracking of the patella during knee motion. Acquired factors such as weakness of the medial quadriceps, tension in the lateral retinaculum and lateral soft tissues, or ligamentous laxity can affect patellar alignment and tracking (Fig. 16–9). The malalignment can assume one of three dif-

FIGURE 16–9. Tension resulting from growth. Pain may occur at the patella (*A*), lower pole of the patella (*B*), or patellar tendon insertion on the tibia (*C*). (From Micheli, L. Overuse injuries in children's sports: The growth factor. Orthopedic Clinics of North America, *14*[2]:353, 1983.)

ferent patterns: 1) lateral subluxation and tilting, 2) lateral subluxation alone, or 3) isolated tilting. The source of pain has been postulated to be the increased stress on the subchondral bone from abnormal patellar stresses, increased tension in the lateral retinaculum, or formation of synovitis from articular cartilage degeneration (Steiner & Grana, 1988). Management of patellofemoral pain can be conservative or surgical. Conservative management consists of relative rest, balancing of muscle strength and length, and correction of abnormal biomechanics with patellar taping or orthotics. Surgical options include arthroscopic shaving, lateral retinacular release, or patellar realignment (Micheli, 1983; Steiner & Grana, 1988).

Apophysitis, or degeneration of the ossification centers where tendons attach with chronic inflammation and microavulsion, is common in the knee in girls between the ages of 8 and 13 years and in boys between 10 and 15 years. These can result from longitudinal traction with bone growth or from repetitive activity of sports participation. The most common apophysitides are Osgood-Schlatter disease of the tibial tubercle, and Sinding-Larsen-Johansson disease at the inferior pole of the patella. Careful differential diagnosis is necessary to correctly identify these disorders (see Chapter 15). Relative rest, maintenance of quadriceps muscle strength with pain-free exercise, and possible extension splinting are treatment options (Birrer & Brecher, 1987; Maffulli, 1990; Micheli, 1983; Steiner & Grana, 1988).

Infrapatellar tendinitis or traction irritation at the inferior pole, otherwise known as jumper's knee, is noted most frequently in the older adolescent. The etiology includes involvement in sports that require running, jumping, climbing, or kicking. RICE with subsequent strengthening of the knee musculature is important in treatment. Assessment of two-joint muscle length is vital because tightness of the hamstrings muscles or iliotibial band may increase the flexion moment at the knee (Birrer & Brecher, 1987; Micheli, 1983; Steiner & Grana, 1988).

Patellar subluxation or dislocation can be seen in young athletes secondary to the stresses of sports requiring cutting and twisting such as soccer, dancing, cheerleading, gymnastics, and track jumping events or as a result of a direct blow to the knee. Imbalance of the length or strength of the extensor muscles, the hamstrings, the retinaculum, or the iliotibial band as well as anatomic malalignments such as genu valgus, patella alta, or shallow condylar cup can be etiologic factors. Management of patellar instability may include bracing in conjunction with physical therapy to normalize length-

strength relationships. Failure of conservative management, although the exception, may necessitate surgical intervention to realign the patella by release of the tight structures or by alteration of the line of pull of the infrapatellar tendon (Grana & Kavenak, 1990; Micheli, 1983).

Ankle and Foot Injuries

Because of the peculiarities of their growing skeleton and their penchant for ingenious physical activity, children suffer from foot and ankle problems that may not have counterparts in the adult (Gregg & Das, 1982; McManama, 1988). Injuries to the distal tibial and fibular growth plates are common in the young athlete. Gregg and Das (1982) have classified growth plate injuries into a clinically useful system (Fig. 16–10). The most common fractures to the ankle in the skeletally immature athlete are the Salter-Harris type 1 and 2 injuries to the distal fibula. Although these fractures can occur with adduction and abduction injury to the distal tibia, they frequently occur alone as a result of inversion injury. Treatment with immobilization in a short-leg cast for 4 to 6 weeks is suggested, although the fracture will usually heal even if untreated (Gregg & Das, 1982; McManama, 1988). Physical therapy after casting to increase ankle and foot mobility and strength and to improve balance may be indicated.

Type 2 injury of the distal tibia is a result of ankle pronation and eversion. Common in football and soccer players, this injury is frequently associated with greenstick fracture of the distal fibula. Care must be taken to reduce these fractures and immobilize them in a long-leg cast with knee flexion to prevent impaction of the tibial metaphysis into the growth plate. The results of this type of fracture are unpredictable; occasionally angulation or premature closure of the plate occurs (Gregg & Das, 1982; McManama, 1988). The most common mechanism of injury in type 3 and 4 fractures of the medial malleolus is ankle supination or inversion. Adduction injuries appear in approximately 15% of these injuries and are characterized by medial displacement of part or all of the distal tibial epiphysis. The affected children are usually young, so the incidence of growth disturbance is higher. Internal fixation with restoration of ankle joint congruity is critical (Gregg & Das, 1982; McManama, 1988).

Because of the porosity of the bones of the foot in a child, stress fractures are common in the metatarsals in all jumping and distance running activities. If suspected by local tenderness that is aggravated with activity, these injuries should be casted for 3

FIGURE 16–10. Modified Salter-Harris classification of growth plate injuries: *1*. Disruption entirely confined to the growth plate; distraction or slip injury. *2*. Fracture line runs partially through the growth plate, then extends through the metaphysis. *3*. Fracture line runs partially through the growth plate, then extends through the epiphysis. *4*. Combined disruption of metaphysis, growth plate, and epiphysis. *5*. Crush or compression injury of growth plate. *6*. Abrasion, avulsion, or burn of the perichondrial ring of the growth plate. (From Gregg, J, & Das, M. Foot and ankle problems in the preadolescent and adolescent athlete. Clinics in Sports Medicine, *1*[1]:133, 1982.)

weeks. After casting, one can progressively and slowly increase activities to former levels over 3 more weeks (McManama, 1988).

Several types of ischemia can occur in the bones of the child's foot. Freiberg infarction, or avascular necrosis of the metatarsal epiphysis, occurs in those who walk or perform on their toes. Initial synovitis is followed by sclerosis, resorption, plate fracture and collapse, and bone re-formation. It does not affect children younger than the age of 12 years. Most commonly affected is the second metatarsal head. Treatment consists of cessation of toe-walking, use of high-heeled shoes, and jumping. A negative-heel shoe is fitted. Kohler disease is seen in active boys aged 3 to 7 years who have a tendency to cavus feet. Focal tenderness and swelling around the navicular bone are noted clinically. The radiograph reveals sclerosis and irregular rarefaction indicative of ischemia. Conservative treatment calls for use of a walking cast for 6 to 8 weeks followed by use of an arch support and limitation of activity for another 6 weeks (McManama, 1988).

Although ankle sprains can occur in the young athlete, epiphyseal fractures are more common. Sprains occur in the older adolescent near the end of growth. The common cause of injury is landing on the lateral border of a plantar flexed foot (Fig. 16–11). Management is similar to that in adults. Surgery is only indicated in multiple sprains with gross instability.

Apophysitis of the calcaneus is an Osgood-Schlatter syndrome of the foot (Fig. 16–12). It is seen most frequently in basketball and soccer players with complaint of heel pain on running. The usual age of occurrence is 8 to 13 years. Frequently, tight heel cords, a tendency toward in-toe-

FIGURE 16–11. Plantarflexion-inversion injury. (From Birrer, R, & Brecher, D. Common Sports Injuries in Youngsters. Oradell, NJ: Medical Economics, 1987, p. 120.)

FIGURE 16–12. Insertion of Sharpey's fibers from the Achilles tendon into the calcaneal apophysis. (From Gregg, J, & Das, M. Foot and ankle problems in the preadolescent and adolescent athlete. Clinics in Sports Medicine, *1*[1]:140, 1982.)

ing, and forefoot varus are noted. Treatment consists of heel cord stretching and initial use of a heel lift in well-constructed shoes (Doxey, 1987; Gregg & Das, 1982).

REHABILITATION AND RETURN TO PLAY

Contrary to some opinions, the young athlete will not return to normal function spontaneously. Children and adolescents require supervised rehabilitation programs that begin with first aid on the field of play (Davis, 1986; Stanitski, 1989). The goal of first aid is to contain the extent of injury and reduce any possibility of further harm. The long-term goal of rehabilitation is return to play in a safe manner. Short term goals should include the accomplishment of the component skills needed to reach the long-term goal. The general process of rehabilitation should emphasize maintenance of cardiovascular skills while normalizing mobility and flexibility. Emphasis then shifts to normalization of muscular endurance and strength, or both the injured area and the entire extremity. Eventually attention is directed toward resumption of purposeful controlled movements at the appropriate

speed (Davis, 1986). Utilization of the "10% rule" —no weekly increase greater than 10% of the previous—is a safe progression for training (Trepman & Micheli, 1988).

Complete rehabilitation is synonymous with return to play. Premature return to activity courts reinjury and the development of chronic problems (Stanitski, 1989). The criteria for return include no edema; full, pain-free, biomechanically normal mobility; normal strength by objective testing; and normal completion of appropriate functional tests such as vertical leap, hopping, running, or cutting activities (Davis, 1986). Supportive or protective devices such as orthoses or braces may be used to supplement rehabilitation and to provide stability and anatomic alignment (Trepman & Micheli, 1988).

THE YOUNG ATHLETE WITH A PHYSICAL DISABILITY

Children with a disability have the same basic needs as their able-bodied peers. With the approval in the United States of Public Law 94-142, the Rehabilitation Act of 1973, and the Americans with Disabilities Act in 1991, a variety of physical activity and sports programs are now available to those with impairments (Bernhardt, 1985b; Birrer & Brecher, 1987; McCormick, 1985). Several studies have demonstrated that those with physical disabilities do indeed participate in sports. In a survey of 100 persons with lower extremity amputations, 60% were active in sports. Younger persons of both genders were most active (Kegel et al., 1980). Of a group of 67 individuals with spinal cord injury, 72% participated in sports at least once weekly. These sports included basketball, swimming, weight lifting, road racing, and boating. The group included 19 athletes currently involved in competition (Curtis et al., 1986).

Both psychological and physiologic benefits of sports participation have been demonstrated in individuals with disabilities. Self-concept and self-acceptance were shown to be equal or greater in athletes of various ages with disabilities when compared with control subjects who were able-bodied (Jackson & Davis, 1983; Patrick, 1984; Sherrill et al., 1990). Wheelchair basketball players had significantly better mental profiles than players who were able-bodied and nonathletes (Paulsen et al., 1991). When novice and veteran wheelchair athletes were compared, the novice group had lower perceived social adequacy and lower self-perception, suggesting that sports participation might change these perceptions in a positive way (Patrick, 1984). Among children with limb deficiencies, athletic competence was one predictor of higher perceived physical appearance and, in turn, lower levels of depression and higher self-esteem (Varni & Setoguchi, 1991).

Disability often causes some reduction of fitness relative to the general population (Jackson & Davis, 1983). Several research studies have demonstrated, however, that fitness training in those with disabilities can reverse this reduction of physiologic status. In classic studies by Zwiren and Bar-Or (1975) and others, the physiologic capabilities of athletes who played in wheelchairs were shown to be only 9% lower than athletes without disabilities and fully 50% greater than sedentary individuals who used wheelchairs. Other studies have confirmed these findings (Jackson & Davis, 1983; Bernhardt, 1985a). Decreases in body fat as well as increases in muscle strength and endurance, often beyond that of individuals without disabilities, have also been documented (Jackson & Davis, 1983). In a comparison of the health and functional status of athletes and nonathletes with spinal cord injuries, the athletes had only 2.4 physician visits per year compared with 6.7 physician visits for the nonathletes. Although they were involved in sports significantly more hours per week (10.2 ± 9.6 hours for athletes; 4.9 ± 4.1 hours for nonathletes), the athletes on average had fewer hospitalizations, decubitus ulcers, medical complications, and hours of required attendant care. The researchers concluded that the medical risks associated with intense sports activity for those with spinal cord injuries are minimal (Curtis et al., 1986).

Preparticipation Examination

Preparticipation assessment of a young person with a disability is similar to that of someone who is able-bodied, and can be conducted in a multistation fashion. Several areas, however, need to be more thoroughly addressed. The personnel performing the assessment must understand not only the physical, physiologic, and psychological requirements of the sport but also the potential medical risks of participation. The physically challenged athlete may be prone to additional injury or illness secondary to the disability. In addition, the physician may be involved in classification of the athlete depending on the type and severity of the disability and needs to be aware of international and national classification systems (Bernhardt, 1991; Jackson & Davis, 1983).

The history should include the date of the onset of disability. Description and dates of all medical problems, hospitalizations, and operations before and after the onset of disability should be included. Releases for participation from all attending physicians are required. Thorough documentation of medications for comparison with lists of permissible drugs is necessary (Bernhardt, 1991).

Physical examination must include documentation of level of understanding, vocalization, communication abilities, and hearing. Flexibility should be evaluated because greater than normal muscle length may be required for certain activities (e.g., flexible hips for positioning in sports wheelchair). Special consideration should be given to instability in specific disability groups, such as the propensity for cervical instability and subluxation in Down syndrome (Cantu, 1988). Complete assessment of all sensory systems is required for classification and safety. Documentation of the presence of abnormal muscle tone and primitive, protective, or pathologic reflexes is critical for participation in sports such as archery, horseback riding, and swimming. Assessment of integrity and toughness of the skin and documentation of any history of skin problems are vital in any athlete with sensory impairment (Bernhardt, 1991).

The level of sitting and standing posture and balance as it pertains to the sport is critical for effective and safe participation. The athlete who skis while seated or rides horseback must have adequate balance to perform. The athlete can be placed in a mock-up situation for assessment if necessary. Assessment of gait is mandatory in all clients who are ambulatory. The pattern and efficacy as well as assistive devices needed must be reviewed. Estimation of locomotor endurance is helpful.

The assessment of gross and fine motor skills should be performed in tasks similar to those required by the sport. Bilateral comparisons as well as timing and quality should be noted (Bernhardt, 1991). Muscle strength and endurance should be assessed, if possible, with either manual or mechanical methods. Although this area has received little attention, dominant hand grip force can be used as a partial predictor of upper body strength (Jackson et al., 1981; Jackson & Davis, 1983). Davis and associates (1981) have also shown that a good relationship exists between upper body isokinetic strength and habitual activity.

Physiologic assessment should include nutritional analysis, body composition measurement, and exercise testing. Exercise testing may be advisable for assessment of cardiopulmonary functional capacity or the efficacy of medications. Testing must often be adjusted for the disability, such as armcrank, wheelchair, or single leg ergometry

(Bernhardt, 1985a, 1991; Jackson & Davis, 1983). Field testing can be completed as long as standard testing principles are followed (Crews, 1982; Kofsky et al., 1983). Although maximal oxygen consumption is the best single indicator of cardiovascular fitness, submaximal testing can be performed as an estimation of maximal capacity.

For many athletes with a disability, equipment is part of their participation. Specially designed wheelchairs, skiing outriggers, ergonomic racquet handles, rotation platforms for field events, and custom prostheses are but a few of the technologic advances that have made sports more assessible. The assessor should check the equipment for function and fit as well as safety and conformity to rules of competition or participation (Bernhardt, 1991).

Training Programs

Persons with disabilities should be placed on training programs in a manner similar to those who are able-bodied (Bernhardt, 1985a and b; Curtis, 1981a) (Fig. 16–13). Several studies have evaluated the efficacy of these training programs in various disability groups. Research on wheelchair training demonstrated increases in maximal oxygen uptake, decreases in exercise and resting heart rate, and increases in maximal work capacity. Documented increases in muscle force and endurance as well as peak force have been noted after strength training (Davis, 1981; Jackson & Davis, 1983).

Injury Data

Little information has been gathered on the incidence and type of sports injuries that occur in persons who are disabled. Although several studies have appeared in the literature, they have had small sample sizes and select groups of individuals with specific disabilities. An exception was a survey distributed to 1200 athletes in regional wheelchair competition during 1981. One hundred two male and 27 female athletes responded. Thirty-two different sports were represented by the group. Seventy-two percent of all athletes had sustained at least 1 injury, with some reporting as many as 14 injuries. The most prevalent injuries were soft tissue trauma (33%), blisters (18%), and lacerations or abrasions (17%). The majority of the injuries occurred in the upper extremity. Most of the injuries were associated with track (26%), basketball (24%), and road racing (22%) (Curtis, 1982).

A study of the injuries at the Special Olympic games demonstrated that 3.3% of the athletes re-

quired care for an injury or illness. Track and field events consumed the least time but had the greatest injury rate (McCormick et al., 1990). Data from the International Flower Marathon showed that 19 athletes experienced 20 medical problems, many caused by climate and spills. Problems were more frequent in groups with disabilities caused by paraplegia and polio. Thirteen medical problems were classified as injuries: five were ulcers and abrasions and eight were soft tissue injuries (Hoeberigs et al., 1990).

The largest study, a retrospective survey of 426 athletes participating in the 1989 competitions of the National Wheelchair Athletic Association (NWAA), the United States Association for Blind Athletes (USABA), and the United States Cerebral Palsy Association (USCPA), demonstrated that 32% of the respondents had at least one time-loss injury. Twenty-six percent of all injuries were from the NWAA, with 57% of this total at the shoulder and elbow. Fifty-three percent of all USABA athletes' injuries were in the lower extremity, while the injuries in the USCPA athletes were noted in all areas. Injury rates were the same for athletes with or without disabilities (Ferrara et al., 1992). Thus, very limited data are available that document the occurrence or management of injuries in the athlete with a disability. Research is needed to address these issues before further conclusions can be drawn.

▌CONCLUSIONS

Young athletes, whether able-bodied or disabled, are not just small adults. They have unique issues in sports participation that must be specifically addressed. Recognition of these unusual qualities is necessary for effective prevention and management of sports-related injuries.

Physical therapists should play a significant role in the total management of the child athlete. The broad-based and eclectic medical background of physical therapists makes them ideal professionals for the assessment and rehabilitation of sports injuries in athletes with full or altered physical capabilities. Depending on advanced experience or certification in sports physical therapy, athletic training, or exercise physiology, they may be the primary medical professional to administer total management from prevention to return to participation after injury.

If lacking in expertise or time, a physical therapist may alternatively work with a certified athletic trainer and an exercise physiologist to provide comprehensive sports safety management. The ser

FIGURE 16–13. Stretching exercises for the athlete in a wheelchair. *A*, Exhale; lean forward to touch ground. *B*, Lift one arm over head and lean to side. Repeat with opposite side. *C*, Exhale, clasp hands, lean forward, and lift arms high in back. *D*, Pull arms to side with palms facing forward. Pull back with elbows straight. *E*, Bend arm across chest. Reach for opposite blade. Push on elbow. Repeat. *F*, Straighten elbow. Push wrist and fingers back. Repeat with opposite side.

tified trainer is appropriately skilled to assist with preparticipation screenings and to provide on-site coverage of practices and games with immediate triage and injury management. The exercise physiologist plays an integral part in the preseason screening and in conditioning and training programs. The physical therapist can provide assessment and total rehabilitation of sports injuries as well as aid in phasing the athlete back to play with appropriate progression, supportive devices, or medical limitations. The certified trainer or the exercise physiologist often works with the physical therapist in the return-to-play planning and follow-up.

The goal of these programs is to promote the health and safety of the young athlete. All those involved should work in a manner appropriate to their education, skills, and practice statutes as members of a team, including coaches and parents, toward the goal of safe, rewarding, and successful participation in sport and recreation.

CASE HISTORY: CB

CB was a 15-year-old high school basketball player who was scheduled for a preparticipation assessment in September. Her medical history was normal except for vague musculoskeletal complaints. She reported that in the past year she had been plagued by pain in her hips during vigorous activities. The pain was occasionally so severe that she could not play pick-up basketball.

She demonstrated no abnormalities on her medical examination with no report of menstrual irregularities. Further questioning revealed that she had grown 2 inches in the past year. She also reported that she did very minimal routine stretching.

Her orthopaedic examination revealed extreme tenderness over the crest of the ilia bilaterally, both over and under the lip. She complained of no pain with either palpation or motion of either hip. Flexibility evaluation demonstrated positive bilateral results on the following tests: Ely, Ober, Active Knee Extension, Thomas, and Thomas modified for the rectus femoris and sartorius muscles. Her straight-leg raising was only 50° bilaterally. She further demonstrated a sensation of "pulling" with lateral flexion to either side. A diagnosis of inflexibility with bilateral iliac crest apophysitis was made by her orthopaedist.

The physical therapist designed a home program to increase CB's flexibility and decrease her pain. CB warmed up for 10 minutes on an exercycle before stretching and was given stretching exercises to address her particular tightness. These exercises included partner Thomas test stretch; partner Thomas test stretch with knee flexion; partner Thomas test stretch in hip adduction and internal rotation; standing sidebend; standing iliotibial band stretch; active hamstring stretch; seated hamstring stretch; standing Achilles muscle group stretch in knee extension and flexion; and seated counter rotation stretch for the piriformis muscle and iliotibial band.

CB was noted to have only good strength on manual muscle testing, so a program was developed to increase endurance and then strength of her hip musculature. She was shown standing hip exercises using an exercise band to develop both endurance and balance. These exercises included hip and knee flexion (march in place); standing hip and knee extension (straight-leg raising); hip adduction and abduction; hip extension; and hip flexion, abduction, and external rotation. She was instructed to work on these exercises daily following her stretching. She was to perform one set × 12 repetitions, one set × 10 repetitions, and one set × 8 repetitions every other day with heavy resistance. On alternate days she performed three sets × 15 repetitions with minimal resistance for muscle endurance. She was instructed to stretch following her exercises and then use ice packs on her iliac crests.

CB performed this program consistently for 2 weeks. She then reported a decrease of pain with vigorous activity. She was reassessed after 1 month. At this time she demonstrated straight-leg raising of 65° bilaterally. Her special tests for flexibility, although still positive, were less tight. Her strength on manual muscle testing was good/good +. After continuing the program for 2 months, she was free of pain during all activities, including basketball. She continues on her daily program.

CASE HISTORY: TJ

TJ is a 12-year-old member of the local ski team who sustained a severe contusion and strain of the back muscles during a jump. He was referred to physical therapy for assessment and management of his back pain in addition to appropriate reconditioning for skiing.

TJ was a slight young man who weighed 85 pounds. He reported back pain with all activities. He was uncomfortable at night in any sleeping position. He stated that he had stopped all activities since his injury. He demonstrated little muscle bulk, indicative of a prepubescent status.

Initial assessment revealed moderate tenderness to palpation in the thoracolumbar erector spinae and scapular muscles (lower and middle trapezius, rhomboids, and latissimus dorsi). Spinal alignment was normal with no rotation or lateral shift. The radiograph was negative for fracture or facet joint abnormality. Passive intervertebral movement was painless and normal. He could forward bend only to fingertips 3 inches above the midpatellar area. Lateral trunk flexion was limited to fingertips to the knee joint line. Any extension caused pain, level 8. Straight-leg raising was 45° bilaterally. Active knee extension was −50°. Ankle dorsiflexion was 90° in knee flexion and extension. Manual muscle testing revealed only good strength throughout selected upper and lower extremity muscles. Strength in the trunk and scapular musculature could not be assessed secondary to pain.

A diagnosis of deconditioning and muscle strain was confirmed. A program to decrease his pain, improve his flexibility, and recondition him for skiing was designed after thorough discussion with TJ and his parents. He was to be treated in the clinic twice weekly and performed a home program on 4 other days. His program consisted of moist heat while cycling for 10 minutes as a warmup. He was positioned on the cycle in an upright position to relax his back and scapular muscles. He then received pulsed ultrasound at 1.2 W/cm² to the involved muscles, followed by soft tissue mobilization and stretching. He was shown stretches for his thoracolumbar and scapular muscles, as well as his hamstrings, iliotibial band, gastrocnemius-soleus, and rectus femoris muscles. Initially, he was placed on a strength program for his lower extremities with good stabilization of his back. He performed one set × 12 repetitions, one set × 10 repetitions, and one set × 8 repetitions on the following exercises: leg press; calf raise with knee extended; straight-leg raise; seated knee extension; and standing knee flexion. He was also taught step-ups on a 4-inch block, wall squats, and freestanding quarter squats. Following these exercises, an ice pack was applied to his back. He performed this program at home with alternation of strength and endurance (three sets × 15 repetitions) regimens.

After five treatments, TJ's back pain began to resolve so he was begun on an advanced program of conditioning. He was instructed in a dumbbell weight program for all upper extremity, chest, and scapular muscles with 3 pounds. He was also taught to use the leg press as if he was skiing turns. Stretching was continued vigorously.

After 3 weeks TJ's back pain had resolved completely so ultrasound and soft tissue mobilization were discontinued. His program was accelerated to include trunk flexor muscle strengthening, seated push-ups, and modified tabletop push-ups. His exercise cord program was advanced to jumping activities. Step-ups were advanced to a 6-, then an 8-inch level. Dumbbell weights were increased by 1-lb increments as he demonstrated good control and no fatigue.

The family purchased an exercise cord so the clinic program was altered to include hip exercises using a weighted pulley system, a pyramid training program for the quadriceps and hamstrings muscles, push-pull activities for the upper extremities, and lateral slides for the lower extremities. Plyometric jumping was advanced from the minitrampoline to an angled trampoline.

A home training program was developed for continued improvement in endurance, strength, agility, and balance. TJ continued diligent training for 6 weeks before return to skiing. He continued dry land ski training after consultation with his coach. He was placed on novice slopes for two half-day periods with no jumping or moguls at the termination of the 6-week training period. If he succeeds with this level, he will be permitted to ski full slopes and finally race.

References

American Academy of Pediatrics. Organized athletics for pre-adolescent children. Pediatrics 84:583–584, 1989.

American Academy of Family Physicians, American Academy of Pediatrics, American Medical Society of Sports Medicine, & American Osteopathic Academy of Sports Medicine. Preparticipation physical evaluation. In press.

Backous, DD, Triedl, KE, Smith, NJ, Parr, TJ, & Carpine, WD. Soccer injuries and their relation to physical maturity. American Journal of Diseases in Children, 148:839–842, 1988.

Backx, FJ, Beijer, HJ, Bol, E, & Erich, WB. Injuries in high-risk persons and high-risk sports: A longitudinal study of 1818 school children. American Journal of Sports Medicine, 19:124–130, 1991.

Backx, FJ, Erich, WB, Kemper, AB, & Verbeek, AL. Sports injuries in school-aged children: An epidemiological study. American Journal of Sports Medicine, 17:234–240, 1989.

Bar-Or, O, Lombardo, JA, & Rowland, TW. The preparticipation sports exam. Patient Care, October 1988, pp. 75–102.

Bauman, M. Nutritional requirements for athletes. In Bernhardt, DB (Ed.), Sports Physical Therapy. New York: Churchill Livingstone, 1986, pp. 89–105.

Bernhardt, DB. Exercise testing and training for disabled populations: The state of the art. In Bernhardt, DB (Ed.), Recreation for the Disabled Child. New York: Haworth Press, 1985a, pp. 3–25.

Bernhardt, DB. The competitive spirit. In Bernhardt, DB (Ed.), Recreation for the Disabled Child. New York: Haworth Press, 1985b, pp. 77–86.

Bernhardt, DB. The physically challenged athlete. In Cantu, RC, & Micheli, LJ (Eds.), ACSM's Guidelines for the Team Physician. Philadelphia: Lea & Febiger, 1991, pp. 242–251.

Birrer, RB, & Brecher, DB. Common Sports Injuries in Youngsters. Los Angeles, CA: PMIC, 1987.

Birrer, RB, & Levine, R. Performance parameters in children and adolescent athletes. Sports Medicine, 4:211–237, 1987.

Blanksby, B, & Gregor, J. Anthropometric strength and physical changes in male and female swimmers with progressive resistive training. Australian Journal of Sports Science, 1:3–6, 1981.

Brown, RS. Exercise and mental health in the pediatric population. Clinics in Sports Medicine, 1:515–527, 1982.

Bruce, DA, Schut, L, & Sutton, LN. Brain and cervical spine injuries occurring during organized sports activities in children and adolescents. Clinics in Sports Medicine, 1:495–514, 1982.

Cantu, R. Head and spine injuries in the young athlete. Clinics in Sports Medicine, 7:459–472, 1988.

Castaldi, CR. Sports related oral and facial injuries in the young athlete: A new challenge for the pediatric dentist. Pediatric Dentistry, 8:311–316, 1986.

Clark, N. Nutrition: Pre-, intra-, and postcompetition. In Cantu, RC, & Micheli, LJ (Eds.), ACSM's Guidelines for the Team Physician. Philadelphia: Lea & Febiger, 1991, pp. 58–65.

Costill, D, Pearson, DR, & Fink, WJ. Anabolic steroid use among athletes: Changes in HDL-C levels. Physician and Sports Medicine, 12(6):113–117, 1984.

Council on Scientific Affairs. Drug abuse in athletes. Journal of the American Medical Association, 259:1703–1705, 1988.

Crews, D. Field testing the wheelchair athlete. Sports n' Spokes, March/April 1982, p. 37.

Curtis, KA. Wheelchair sportsmedicine: II. Training. Sports n' Spokes, July/August 1981a, pp. 16–19.

Curtis, KA. Wheelchair sportsmedicine: III. Stretching. Sports n' Spokes, September/October 1981b, pp. 16–18.

Curtis, KA. Wheelchair sportsmedicine: IV. Athletic injuries. Sports n' Spokes, January/February 1982, pp. 20–24.

Curtis, KA, McClanahan, S, Hail, KM, Dillon, D, & Brown, KF. Health, vocational and functional status in spinal cord injured athletes and nonathletes. Archives of Physical Medicine and Rehabilitation, 67:862–865, 1986.

Davis, GM. Cardiorespiratory fitness and muscle strength in lower-limb disability. Canadian Journal of Applied Sports Science, 6:159–165, 1981.

Davis, JM. Rehabilitation of sports injuries: A practical approach. In Bernhardt, DB (Ed.), Sports Physical Therapy. New York: Churchill Livingstone, 1986, pp. 155–171.

DeHaven, KE, & Lintner, DM. Athletic injuries: Comparison by age, sport and gender. American Journal of Sports Medicine, 14:218–224, 1986.

Doxey, GE. Calcaneal pain: A review of various disorders. Journal of Orthopedic and Sport Physical Therapy, 9:25–32, 1987.

Ekblom, B. Effects of physical training in adolescent boys. Journal of Applied Physiology, 17:350–355, 1969.

Ferrara, MS, Buckley, WE, McCann, BC, Limbird, TJ, Powell, JW, & Robl, R. The injury experience of a competitive athlete with a disability: Prevention implications. Medicine and Science in Sports and Exercise, 24:184–188, 1992.

Food Guide Pyramid. US Department of Agriculture, 1992.

Gaillard, B, Haskell, W, Smith, N, Ogilvie, B. Handbook for the Young Athlete. Palo Alto, CA: Bull Publishing, 1978, pp. 32–33.

Garrick, JG. Epidemiological perspective. Clinics in Sports Medicine, 1:13–18, 1982.

Gerberich, SG, Finke, R, Madden, M, Priest, JD, Aamoth, G, & Murray, K. An epidemiological study of high school ice hockey injuries. Childs Nervous System, 3:59–64, 1987.

Going, S. Physical best: Body composition in the assessment of youth fitness. Journal of Physical Education, Recreation and Dance, 59(9):32–36, 1988.

Goldberg, B, Rosenthal, PP, Robertson, LS, & Nicholas, JA. Injuries in youth football. Pediatrics, 81:255–261, 1988.

Goldberg, B, Saranti, A, Witman, P, Gavin, M, & Nicholas, J. Preparticipation sports assessment: An objective evaluation. Pediatrics 66:736–745, 1980.

Grana, WA, & Kalenak, A. Clinical Sports Medicine. Philadelphia: WB Saunders, 1991.

Gregg, JR, & Das, M. Foot and ankle problems in the preadolescent and adolescent athlete. Clinics in Sports Medicine, 1:131–147, 1982.

Halpern, B, Thompson, N, Curl, WW, Andrews, J, Hunter, SC, & Boring, JR. High school football injuries: Identifying the risk factors. American Journal of Sports Medicine, 15:316–320, 1987.

Harvey, J. The preparticipation examination of the child athlete. Clinics in Sports Medicine, 1:353–369, 1982.

Haskell, W, Scala, J, & Whittam, J (Eds.). Nutrition and Athletic Performance. Palo Alto, CA: Bull Publishing, 1982.

Haupt, HA, & Rovere, GD. Anabolic steroids: A review of the literature. American Journal of Sports Medicine, 12:169–191, 1984.

Heim, K. Basic sports nutrition for the young athlete. National Strength and Conditioning Association Journal, 7:60, 1985.

Hickson, RC, & Kurowski, TG. Anabolic steroids and training. Clinics in Sports Medicine, 5:461–469, 1986.

Hoeberigs, JH, Deberts-Eggen, HB, & Debets, PM. Sports medical experience from the International Flower Marathon for disabled wheelers. American Journal of Sports Medicine, 18:418–421, 1990.

Hoff, GL, & Martin, TA. Outdoor and indoor soccer: Injuries among youth players. American Journal of Sports Medicine, 14:231–233, 1986.

Hunter, SC, Etchison, WC, & Halpern, B. Standards and norms of fitness and flexibility in the high school athlete. Athletic Training, Fall 1985, pp. 210–212.

Ilmarinen, J, & Valimaki, I (Eds.). Children and Sport. New York: Springer-Verlag, 1984, pp. 1–17.

Ireland, ML, & Andrews, JR. Shoulder and elbow injuries in the young athlete. Clinics in Sports Medicine, 7:473–494, 1988.

Jackson, RW, & Davis, GM. The value of sports and recreation for the physically disabled. Orthopedic Clinics of North America, 14:301–315, 1983.

Jackson, RW, Davis, GM, Kofsky, PR, Shepard, RJ, Keene, GCR. Fitness levels in the lower-limb disabled. In Transactions of the 27th Annual Meeting of the Orthopedic Research Society (Vol. 6). Rosemont, IL: Orthopedic Research Society, 1981.

Jones, NP. Eye injury in sport. Sports Medicine, 7:163–181, 1989.

Kegel, B, Webster, JC, & Burgess, EM. Recreational activities of lower extremity amputees. Archives of Physical Medicine and Rehabilitation, 61:258–264, 1980.

Keller, CS, Noyes, FR, & Buncher, CR. The medical aspects of soccer injury epidemiology. American Journal of Sports Medicine, 15:230–236, 1987.

Kerr, IL. Mouth guards for the prevention of injuries in contact sports. Sports Medicine, 5:415–427, 1986.

Knowles, KG, Yakavonis, VJ, & George, F. Overuse syndromes about the elbow. Postgraduate Advances in Sports Medicine II–VIII, 1987, pp. 3–17.

Kofsky, PR, Davis, GM, Shepard, RJ, Jackson, RW, & Keene, GC. Field testing: Assessment of physical fitness of disabled youth. Journal of Applied Physiology, 51:109–120, 1983.

Kvist, M, Kujala, UM, Heinonen, OJ, Vuori, IV, Aho, AJ, Pajulo, O, Huintsa, A, & Parvinen, T. Sports-related injuries in children. International Journal of Sports Medicine, April 1989, pp. 81–86.

Lehman, L. The preseason athletic screening examination. Medical Times, 116(8):29–31, 1988.

Linder, CW, DuRant, RH, Seklecki, RM, & Strong, WB. Preparticipation health screening of young athletes. American Journal of Sports Medicine, 9:187–193, 1981.

Lodge, JF, Langley, JD, & Begg, DJ. Injuries in the 14th and 15th years of life. Journal of Paediatric and Child Health, 26:316–322, 1990.

Lohman, TG. Advances in Body Composition Assessment. Champaign, IL: Human Kinetics Publishers, 1992.

Lombardo, JA. Preparticipation examination. In Cantu, RC, & Micheli, LJ (Eds.), ACSM's Guidelines for the Team Physician. Philadelphia: Lea & Febiger, 1991, pp. 71–94.

Macera, CA, Jackson, KL, Hagenmaier, GW, & Kronenfeld, JJ. Age, physical activity, physical fitness, body composition, and incidence of orthopedic problems. Research Quarterly for Exercise and Sport, 60:225–233, 1989.

McCormick, D. Handicapped skiing. In Bernhardt, DB (Ed.), Recreation for the Disabled Child. New York: Haworth Press, 1985, pp. 27–44.

McCormick, DP, Niebiehr, VN, & Risser, WL. Injury and illness surveillance at local Special Olympic Games. British Journal of Sports Medicine, 24:221–224, 1990.

McKeag, D. Preseason physical examination for prevention of sports injuries. Sports Medicine, 2:413–431, 1985.

McLain, LG, & Reynolds, S. Sports injuries in a high school. Pediatrics, 84:446–450, 1989.

McManama, GB. Ankle injuries in the young athlete. Clinics in Sports Medicine, 7:547–562, 1988.

McNutt, T, Shannon, SW, Wright, JT, & Feinstein, RA. Oral trauma in adolescent athletes: A study of mouth protectors. Pediatric Dentistry, 11:209–213, 1989.

Maffulli, N. Intensive training in young athletes. Sports Medicine, 9:229–243, 1990.

Mellion, MB (Ed.). Office Management of Sports Injuries and Athletic Problems. Philadelphia: Hanley & Belfus, 1988.

Micheli, LJ. Overuse injuries in children's sports: The growth factor. Orthopedic Clinics of North America, 14:337–360, 1983.

Micheli, LJ. Musculoskeletal trauma in children. In Green, M, & Haggerty, RJ (Eds.), Ambulatory Pediatrics III. Philadelphia: WB Saunders, 1984, pp. 95–208.

Micheli, LJ. The child athlete. In Cantu, RC, & Micheli, LJ (Eds.), ACSM's Guidelines for the Team Physician. Philadelphia: Lea & Febiger, 1991, pp. 228–241.

Micheli, LJ, Santore, R, & Stanitski, CL. Epiphyseal fractures of the elbow in children. American Family Physician, November 1980, pp. 107–116.

Micheli, LJ, & Smith, AD. Sports injuries in children. Current Problems in Pediatrics, 12:1–54, 1982.

Micheli, LJ, & Stone, KR. The pre-sports physical: Only the first step. Journal of Musculoskeletal Medicine, May 1984, pp. 56–60.

Mirby, J, Besancenot, J, Chambers, RT, Durey, A, & Vichard, P. Avulsion fractures of the tibial tuberosity in the adolescent athlete. American Journal of Sports Medicine, 16:336–340, 1988.

Mueller, F, & Blythe, C. Epidemiology of sports injuries in children. Clinics in Sports Medicine, 1(3):343–352, 1982.

Mueller, FD, & Cantu, RC. Catastrophic injuries and fatalities in high school and college sports, Fall 1982–Spring 1988. Medicine and Science in Sports and Exercise, 22:737–741, 1990.

Nakayama, DK, Gardner, MJ, & Rogers, KD. Disability from bicycle-related injuries in children. Journal of Trauma, 30:1390–1394, 1990.

Nevaiser, RJ: Injuries to and developmental deformities of the shoulder. In Bora, FW (Ed.), The Pediatric Upper Extremity. Philadelphia: WB Saunders, 1986, pp. 235–246.

Nevole, GJ, & Prentice, WJ. The effect of anabolic steroids on female athletes. Athletic Training, 22:297–299, 1987.

Objective testing group certifies head protection. Occupational Health and Safety, March 1988, pp. 18–20.

O'Neill, DB, & Micheli, LJ. Overuse injuries in the young athlete. Clinics in Sports Medicine, 7:591–610, 1988.

Patrick, GD. Comparison of novice and veteran wheelchair athletes' self-concept and acceptance of disability. Rehabilitation Counseling Bulletin, 27:186–188, 1984.

Paulsen, P, French, R, & Sherrill, C. Comparison of mood states of college able-bodies and wheelchair basketball players. Perceptual Motor Skills, 73:396–398, 1991.

Perry, A. Distinction between drug use and abuse. Athletic Training, Summer 1985, pp. 114–116.

Peterson, M, & Peterson, K. Eat to Compete: A Guide to Sports Nutrition. Chicago: Year Book Medical Publishers, 1988.

Pfeiffer, RD, & Francis, RS. Effects of strength training on muscle development in prepubescent, pubescent and postpubescent males. Physician and Sports Medicine, 14:134–143, 1986.

Physician urges caution for child marathoners. Physician and Sports Medicine, 10:26, 1982.

President's Council on Physical Fitness and Sports, Washington, DC, 1986.

Puffer, JC. Organizational aspects. In Cantu, RC, & Micheli, LJ (Eds.), ACSM's Guidelines for the Team Physician. Philadelphia: Lea & Febiger, 1991, pp. 95–100.

Ramsey, JA, Blunkie, C, Smith, K, Garner, S, MacDougall, JD, & Digby, GS. Strength training effects in prepubescent boys. Medicine and Science in Sports and Exercise, 22:605–614, 1990.

Retsky, J, Jaffe, D, & Christoffel, K. Skateboarding injuries in children: A second wave. American Journal of Disease in Children, 145:188–192, 1991.

Rogozin, V. Metabolic effects of anabolic steroid on skeletal muscle. Medicine and Science in Sports, 11:160–163, 1979.

Rooks, DS, & Micheli, LJ. Musculoskeletal assessment and training: The young athlete. Clinics in Sports Medicine, 7:641–677, 1988.

Rossi, F, & Dragoni, S. Lumbar spondylolisthesis: Occurrence in competitive athletes. Journal of Sports Medicine and Physical Fitness, 30:450–452, 1990.

Sailors, M, & Berg, K. Comparison of responses to weight training in pubescent boys and men. Journal of Sports Medicine, 27:30–37, 1987.

Schuller, DE, Dankle, SK, Martin, M, & Strauss, RH. Auricular injury and the use of headgear in wrestlers. Archives Otolaryngology and Head/Neck Surgery, 115:714–717, 1989.

Servedio, FJ, Bartels, RL, Hamlin, D, Teske, T, Schaffer, T, & Servedio, A. The effect of weight training using Olympic style lifts on various physiological variables in prepubescent boys. Medicine and Science in Sports and Exercise, 17:228, 1985.

Sewall, L, & Micheli, LJ. Strength training for children. Journal of Pediatric Orthopedics, 6:143–146, 1986.

Sharkey, B. Training for sports. In Cantu, RC, & Micheli, LJ. (Eds.), ACSM's Guidelines for the Team Physician. Philadelphia: Lea & Febiger, 1991, pp. 34–47.

Sheps, SB, & Evans, GD. Epidemiology of school injuries: A 2-year experience in a municipal health department. Pediatrics, 79:69–75, 1987.

Sherrill, C, Hinson, M, Gench, B, Kennedy, SO, & Low, L. Self-concepts of disabled youth athletes. Perceptual Motor Skills, 70:1093–1098, 1990.

Sherry, E, Korbel, P, & Henderson, A. Children's skiing injuries in Australia. Medical Journal of Australia, 146:193–195, 1987.

Simmons, BP, & Lovallo, JL. Hand and wrist injuries in children. Clinics in Sports Medicine, 7:493–512, 1988.

Smilkstein, G. Health examination of high school athletes. Physician and Sports Medicine, 9(8):73–80, 1981.

Smith, MJ. Muscle fiber types. Orthopedic Clinics of North America, 14:403–412, 1983.

Smith, NJ. Nutrition and the athlete. Orthopedic Clinics of North America, 14:387–396, 1983.

Snively, RA, Grove, WA, & Ellis, D. High school sports injuries. Physician and Sports Medicine, 9(8):46–55, 1981.

Stanitski, C. Common injuries in preadolescent athletes. Sports Medicine, 7:32–41, 1989.

Steiner, ME, & Grana, WA. The young athlete's knee: Recent advances. Clinics in Sports Medicine, 7:527–546, 1988.

Stock, JG, & Cornell, FM. Prevention of sports-related eye injuries. American Family Practice, 44:515–520, 1991.

Taimela, S, Kujala, UM, & Osterman, K. Intrinsic risk factors and athletic injuries. Sports Medicine, 9:205–215, 1990.

Trepman, E, & Micheli, LJ. Overuse injuries in sports. Seminars in Orthopedics, 3:217–222, 1988.

Varni, JW, & Setoguchi, Y. Correlates of perceived physical appearance in children with congenital/acquired limb deficiencies. Journal of Development and Behavior in Pediatrics, 12:171–176, 1991.

Waters, PM, & Millis, MB. Hip and pelvic injuries in the young athlete. Clinics in Sports Medicine, 7:513–526, 1988.

Watson, MD, & DiMartino, PP. Incidence of injuries in high school track and field athletes and its relation to performance ability. American Journal of Sports Medicine, 15:251–254, 1987.

Weltman, AC, Janney, CB, Rains, CB, Strand, K, Berg, B, Tippitt, S, Wise, J, Cahill, BR, & Katch, FI. The effects of hydraulic resistance strength training in pre-pubescent males. Medicine and Science in Sports and Exercise, *18*:629–638, 1986.

Whieldon, TJ, & Cerny, FJ. Incidence and severity of high school athletic injuries. Athletic Training, *25*:344–350, 1990.

Wilmore, JH. Alterations in strength, body composition and anthropometric measurements consequent to a 10 week training program. Medicine and Science in Sports, *6*:1333–1338, 1974.

Yesalis, CE, Wright, JE, & Bahrke, MS. Epidemiological and policy issues in the measurement of long term health effects and anabolic-androgenic steroids. Sports Medicine, *8*:129–138, 1989.

Zarins, B. Knee injuries in sports. New England Journal of Medicine, *318*:950–961, 1982.

Ziegler, MM. Nutritional care of the pediatric athlete. Clinics in Sports Medicine, *1*:371–381, 1982.

Zwiren, L, & Bar-Or, O. Response to exercise of paraplegics who differ in conditioning level. Medicine and Science in Sports, *7*:94–98, 1975.

Appendix I

Selected Special Musculoskeletal Tests

Differential Diagnosis	Test Performed	Differential Diagnosis	Test Performed
Acromioclavicular separation	Horizontal adduction in flexion and internal rotation Step deformity Stress test with hand weight		Static/dynamic medial-lateral position Patellar motion in knee flexion-extension
Shoulder impingement	Neer impingement test Painful arc	Patellar dysfunction	Crepitus Patellar compression test Patellar grind test
Shoulder instability	Anterior-posterior translation Inferior glide in abduction Apprehension test Sulcus test		Anterior-posterior tilt Patellar rotation Ballotable patella Q angle
Rotator cuff injury	Clunk test Drop arm test Impingement tests Instability tests	Ligamentous laxity (knee)	Lachman test Losee test Posterior drawer/drop Valgus/varus stress tests
Patellar instability	Apprehension test Glide test	Ankle instability	Talar tilt (medial-lateral) Anterior drawer Single limb balance

Appendix II

Resource List

ORGANIZATIONS

Accessibility Information Center, National Center for a Barrier Free Environment, 1140 Connecticut Avenue, NW, Washington, DC 20036

American Academy of Pediatrics, 141 Northwest Point Blvd., Elk Grove, IL 60009-0927

American Academy of Orthopaedic Surgeons, 222 South Prospect Avenue, Park Ridge, IL 60068

American Wheelchair Pilots Association, 1621 East 2nd Avenue, Mesa, AZ 85204

Breckenridge Outdoor Recreation Center, P.O. Box 697, Breckenridge, CO 80424

Bureau of Outdoor Recreation, Department of the Interior, Washington, DC 20240

Courage Center, 3915 Golden Valley Road, Golden Valley, MN 55422

Drug Hotline, 800-223-0393, U.S.O.C. Sports Medicine and Science Division.

Handicapped Scuba Association, 1104 El Prado, San Clemente, CA 92672

National Archery Association, 1750 East Boulder Street, Colorado Springs, CO 80909

National Foundation for Horsemanship for the Handicapped, Box 462, Malvern, PA 19355

National Handicapped Sports and Recreation Association, P.O. Box 18664, Capitol Hill Station, Denver, CO 80218

National Information Center for Handicapped Children and Youth, P.O. Box 492, Washington, DC 20013

National Wheelchair Athletic Association, 2107 Templeton Gap Road, Colorado Springs, CO 80907

National Wheelchair Basketball Association, 110 Seaton Bldg., University of Kentucky, Lexington, KY 40506

National Wheelchair Marathon, 15 Marlborough Street, Belmont, MA 02178

National Wheelchair Racquetball Association, c/o American Amateur Racquetball Association, 815 North Weber, Colorado Springs, CO 80903

National Youth Sports Foundation, 10 Meredith Circle, Needham, MA 02192

North American Riding for the Handicapped Association, Box 100, Ashburn, VA 22011

Recreation and Athletic Rehabilitation-Education Center, University of Illinois, 1207 South Oak Street, Champaign, IL 61820

Skating Association for the Blind and Handicapped, 3236 Main Street, Buffalo, NY 14214

Vinland National Center, 3675 Ihduhapi Road, Loretto, MN 55347

Voyageur Outward Bound, Box 250, Long Lake, MN 55356

Wilderness Inquiry II, 1313 Fifth Street, SE, Minneapolis, MN 55414

BIBLIOGRAPHY

Rehabilitation

Albert, M. Eccentric Muscle Training in Sports and Orthopaedics. New York: Churchill Livingstone, 1991.

Andrews, J, & Harrelson, GL. Physical Rehabilitation of the Injured Athlete. Philadelphia: WB Saunders, 1992.

Arnheim, D. Modern Principles of Athletic Training (7th ed.). St. Louis: CV Mosby, 1989.

Booher, J, & Thibodeau, G. Athletic Injury Assessment. St. Louis: CV Mosby, 1985.

Chu, D. Jumping into Plyometrics. Champaign, IL: Human Kinetics Publishers, 1992.

Coaches' and Trainer's Guide to Nonprescription Medications. Upjohn, Box 307, Coventry, CT 06238.

DeValentine, SJ (Ed.). Foot and Ankle Disorders in Children. New York: Churchill Livingstone, 1992.

Donatelli, R, & Wooden, MJ (Eds.) Orthopaedic Physical Therapy. New York: Churchill Livingstone, 1989.

Garrick, JG, & Webb, DR. Sports Injuries: Diagnosis and Management. Philadelphia: WB Saunders, 1990.

Gould, J, & Davis, G (Eds.). Orthopaedic and Sports Physical Therapy. St Louis: CV Mosby, 1985.

Hoppenfeld, S. Physical Examination of the Spine and Extremities. New York: Appleton-Century-Crofts, 1976.

Kessler, R, & Hertling, D. Management of Common Musculoskeletal Disorders. Philadelphia: Harper & Row, 1983.

Kibler, WB. The Sport Preparticipation Fitness Examination. Champaign, IL: Human Kinetics Publishers, 1990. ·

Kraemer, W, & Fleck, S. Strength Training for Young Athletes. Champaign, IL: Human Kinetics Publishers, 1993.

Kuprian, W (Ed.). Physical Therapy for Sports. Philadelphia: WB Saunders, 1982.

Magee, DJ. Orthopedic Physical Assessment (2nd ed.). Philadelphia: WB Saunders, 1992.

McLaren, DS, Burman, D, Belton, NR, & Williams, AF (Eds.). Textbook of Paediatric Nutrition (3rd ed.). New York: Churchill Livingstone, 1992.

McLatchie, GR (Ed.). Essentials of Sports Medicine. New York: Churchill Livingstone, 1986.

Nickel, VL, & Botte, MJ (Eds.). Orthopaedic Rehabilitation (2nd ed.). New York: Churchill Livingstone, 1992.

O'Donoghue, DH (Ed.). Treatment of Injuries to Athletes (4th ed.). Philadelphia: WB Saunders, 1984.

Orthopedic Clinics of North America. Philadelphia: WB Saunders, 1992.

Perrin, D (Ed.). Journal of Sports Rehabilitation. Champaign, IL: Human Kinetics Publishers, 1992.

Reid, DC. Sports Injury Assessment and Rehabilitation. New York: Churchill Livingstone, 1992.

Reider, B (Ed.). Sports Medicine: The School Age Athlete. Philadelphia: WB Saunders, 1991.

Rowland, TW (Ed.). Exercise and Children's Health. Champaign, IL: Human Kinetics Publishers, 1990.

Rowland, TW (Ed.). Pediatric Exercise Science. Champaign, IL: Human Kinetics Publishers, 1992.

Rowland, TW (Ed.). Pediatric Laboratory Exercise Testing. Champaign, IL: Human Kinetics Publishers, 1993.

Roy, W, & Irwin, R. Sports Medicine: Prevention, Evaluation, Management, and Rehabilitation. Englewood Cliffs, NJ: Prentice-Hall, 1983.

Sportsmediscope. U.S.O.C. Sports Medicine and Science Division Newsletter.

Strauss, RH (Ed.). Sports Medicine (2nd ed.). Philadelphia: WB Saunders, 1991.

Stretching Charts, P.O. Box 44646, Tacoma, WA 98444.

Strickland, JW. Hand Injuries in Athletes. Philadelphia: WB Saunders, 1992.

Subotnick, SI (Ed.). Sports Medicine of the Lower Extremity. New York: Churchill Livingstone, 1989.

Parental and Coaching Information

Access National Park: A Guide for Handicapped Visitors. U.S. Government Printing Office, Washington, DC 20402.

Exceptional Parent, 605 Commonwealth Avenue, Boston, MA 02215.

Facile Fashions, Irwin/Taylor, 80 Superior Road, Rochester, NY 14625.

Human Kinetics Publishers, Box 5076, Champaign, IL 61825-5076.

Sports and Physical Education Videos and Books, The Athletic Institute, 200 Castlewood Drive, North Palm Beach, FL 33408-5697.

Sports n' Spokes, Paralyzed Veterans of America, 5201 North 19th Avenue, Phoenix, AZ 85015.

U.S. Department of Health and Human Services, Alcohol, Drug Abuse and Mental Health Administration, Washington, DC.

Section Three

Management of Neurologic Impairment

DARL W. VANDER LINDEN, PT, PhD
Section Editor

Chapter 17

Developmental Coordination Disorders

KATHRYN STEYER DAVID, PT, PCS, MS

Why are some children considered to be born athletes or graceful dancers? Why do other children always seem to be falling over their feet or bumping into walls? When is clumsiness considered a normal part of growing up and when is it abnormal? What can physical therapists do to help children with a developmental coordination disorder (DCD)?

Physical therapists have a unique service to offer individuals with DCD. Their background in normal as well as abnormal motor control, motor learning, and motor development can be used to individually assess, plan programs for, treat, and educate children with DCD as well as consult with their families. As members of a collaborative team, physical therapists can influence functional outcomes for a group of individuals with very real problems that are often overlooked by members of the medical and educational community.

DEFINITIONS

Many professionals have attempted to identify and define variables related to incoordination. Different terms have been used in different professions, and the resulting confusion has often inhibited dialogue and limited the generalization of research. The disorder currently identified in the third revised edition of the *Diagnostic and Statistical Manual of Mental Disorders (DSM-III-R)* (American Psychiatric Association, 1987) is *development coordination disorder.* DCD is diagnosed when motor coordination is markedly below expected levels, significantly interferes with academic achievement or activities of daily living, and is not due to known physical disorders. I have chosen to use this term because it highlights movement as the primary focus of the nonprogressive motor abnormalities seen initially in childhood, but often identified throughout an individual's life-span, and measured on standardized, norm-referenced tests of motor skills. This term is meant to be closely synonymous with the terms *developmental clumsiness, clumsy child,* and *developmental apraxia* (Gubbay, 1975). The word *developmental* is used because the problem is related to age. An awkward gait pattern with frequent falling is normal for a 12-month-old child but abnormal for an 8-year-old child. However, whether an awkward gait pattern in an 8-year-old child is simply a delay in maturation or a sign of abnormal functioning is still being debated (Losse et al., 1991).

Clumsiness has been associated with the medical term *minimal brain dysfunction* (MBD). The definition of MBD has changed over time (Shaywitz & Shaywitz, 1988). The term was created in the early 1960s when the term *minimal brain damage* and the concept of a learning disability were combined. The presence of soft neurologic signs was used to infer brain dysfunction as opposed to requiring the documentation of specific brain damage. Although the term *MBD* was used by the medical community, the term *specific learning disability* was retained by educators. Clumsiness is considered one of the many possible characteristics seen in children with either MBD or learning disability.

The American Psychiatric Association changed its terminology in 1968 from MBD to *hyperkinetic syndrome of childhood.* In 1980 the *DSM-III* of the American Psychiatric Association identified two subcategories: attention deficit disorder with hyperactivity and without hyperactivity. Further evolution in terminology occurred in 1987 when the *DSM-III-R* listed only one term, *attention deficit hyperactivity disorder* (ADHD) and added the term *developmental coordination disorder.* The criteria for diagnosing ADHD include whether the child has difficulty remaining seated, fidgets with hands or feet, squirms in seat, shifts from one uncompleted activity to another, has difficulty following through on instructions, and often loses things needed for tasks. Children with ADHD are more likely to have had developmental problems including clumsiness and delayed walking than other children (Conte, 1991). In Scandinavian countries, however, the term *MBD* continues to be used as an umbrella term applied to nonretarded children without cerebral palsy who show signs of attentional deficits or hyperactivity in combination with either problems of motor control or perceptual difficulties (Gillberg et al., 1982). A link may exist between DCD, MBD, and ADHD, but the definitions are far from synonymous.

Although the term *learning disability* has remained constant in its use by the educational community, its definition varies and it is sometimes divided into subcategories of developmental and academic learning disability (Kirk & Gallagher, 1989). Learning disability as defined by the U.S. federal government in the 1975 Education for All Handicapped Children Act is different from that adopted by the National Joint Committee for Learning Disabilities in 1981 and modified by the U.S. Interagency Committee on Learning Disabilities in 1988 (Kavanagh & Truss, 1988). There is still considerable controversy over whether learning disability inherently implies any neurologic dysfunction.

Incoordination has also been associated with a variety of other terms such as *visuomotor problems, dyspraxia,* and *somatodyspraxia.* The last two terms are used most frequently by occupational therapists when they discuss sensory integration theory and practice (Cermak, 1991).

By definition, motor incoordination caused by or closely associated with mental retardation, genetic disorders (e.g., Down syndrome), neurologic disorders (e.g., cerebral palsy, traumatic brain damage, Friedreich's ataxia), brain tumors, or loss of sensory function (e.g., visual, auditory) is not discussed in this chapter. However, one should always consider the possibility that DCD can occur along with any of these problems. It has long been recognized that children with cerebral palsy often exhibit agnosic and apraxic defects that compound the problem of integration of movement (Gubbay, 1975). Deciding when motor incoordination is caused by or closely associated with another disorder such as cerebral palsy rather than occurring along with, but not caused by, that disorder is an important program planning decision. The specific combination of DCD, learning disability, prematurity, and spastic diplegia is further explored in this chapter because it is a combination of which physical therapists need to be especially aware.

INCIDENCE

Just as the term *DCD* and associated terms of *MBD, ADHD,* and *learning disability* are difficult to define, the incidence of each is equally unclear. Gubbay (1975) believed that at least 5% of the school-aged population displayed clumsiness or DCD. Other estimates project that 5 to 10% of the school-aged population display MBD with soft neurologic signs (Gaddes, 1985; Gillberg et al., 1982) and that 98% of children with MBD have motor problems, as evidenced by poor, slow, labored handwriting (Clements et al., 1971). Other attempts to identify the incidence of MBD have been unsuccessful. Schmidt and colleagues (1987) concluded that MBD is not a homogeneous syndrome. Four to 6% of the school-aged population are believed to have ADHD (Conte, 1991). Reports indicate that children with educationally identified learning disability are 4 to 5% of the school-aged population (U.S. Department of Education, 1990), and it is estimated that 90% of children with learning disability have motor coordination or visuomotor problems (Tarnopol & Tarnopol, 1977). Obviously the problem of motor incoordination exists whether or not it can be consistently categorized and quantified.

Gubbay (1975) believed so strongly that clumsiness should be studied by the medical community as an entity separate from MBD or learning disability that he created a standardized battery of eight tests for physicians to use. A survey was conducted on 992 children and normative data were collected on 919 children aged 8 to 12 years. Children were identified as clumsy based on the number of failures for their age. For example, an 8-year-old was identified as clumsy when there were six or more failures while a 12-year-old was identified when there were two or more failures. On this basis, Gubbay identified 32 children as clumsy and 14 children as borderline clumsy, resulting in a sample of 56 children who were matched to a control group of children of the same sex, age, and classroom. Most of Gubbay's conclusions regarding clumsiness are based on this descriptive study.

PATHOPHYSIOLOGY

No specific pathologic process or single neuroanatomic site has been associated with DCD (Table 17–1). Gaddes (1985) believed that motor clumsiness may find its origin in dysfunction of the cerebellum, of one of the two cerebral motor strips, or of the efferent motor pathways or in some imbalance in one or more of the sensory neural mechanisms. From a systems perspective, smooth motor functioning depends not only on an intact central nervous system but also on use of appropriate, environmentally referenced inputs. Roy and Square (1985) argue that control of praxis involves both top-down and bottom-up influences that operate in parallel. According to Gubbay (1975), clumsiness could be regarded as an all-inclusive end-product of differing etiologies, implying a heterogeneous pathophysiology.

By definition, DCD is not related to muscle pathology, peripheral sensory abnormality, or central nervous system damage that causes spasticity, athetosis, or ataxia. Hypotonia, however, is sometimes associated with motor clumsiness as a neurologic soft sign (Ayres, 1974). Among infants with low birth weight but no major congenital problems, infants with truncal or lower extremity hypotonia had the worst developmental outcome (Georgieff et al., 1986). Gubbay (1975) found, however, that hypotonia was not more prevalent in children with clumsiness than in a control group. The exact cause

Table 17–1. **The Disabling Process in Children with Developmental Coordination Disorders**

Pathophysiology	Impairments	Functional Limitations	Disability	Societal Limitation
Heterogeneous central nervous system sites	Soft signs: Poor strength	Awkward gait	Dependent self-help skills	Limited indoor and outdoor play with peers
Prenatal, perinatal, and neonatal insults	Poor coordination Jerky movements	Delayed and poor quality of fine and gross motor skills, such as hopping, jumping, ball skills, and threading beads	Limited participation in physical education	Strained child–parent relationships
	Poor visual perception		Poor written communication	Social isolation
	Joint laxity			
	Poor spatial organization	Delayed oral-motor skills	Poor language skills and social interaction	Limited vocational success
	Inadequate information processing	Low self-esteem	Depression	Design of objects such as tamper-proof packaging
	Poor sequencing	Distractibility	Low academic achievement	
	Poor feedback			
	Poor short- and long-term memory			

of excessive hypotonia and its specific relationship to DCD is not clear and warrants further study.

Studies have been inconclusive in correlating abnormal electroencephalographic findings (Gubbay, 1975) or abnormal results of computed tomographic scans (Knuckey et al., 1983) with clumsiness in children. Either the abnormal findings were not of sufficient magnitude to account for the clumsiness or were not directly related to one anatomic site or pathologic process.

The extent to which research with adults can be applied to children is unclear. The similarities between children with developmental dyspraxia and adults with apraxia have not been thoroughly researched (Cermak, 1985). Some studies with adults have searched for an anatomic site to explain apraxia (Geshwind, 1975; Volpe et al., 1982; Watson et al., 1986), while other theories support a concept of apraxia as an integration problem involving the entire brain (Faglioni & Basso, 1985; Luria, 1966; Roy & Square, 1985). Current theories suggest that multiple mechanisms are involved with praxis and that lesions at any of the multiple pathways can result in one of the many forms of apraxia (Kertesz, 1985) (Fig. 17–1). Kertesz believes that the anterior half of the periventricular white matter

and the frontal lobe are the most frequent location of lesions resulting in apraxia. Interestingly, spastic diplegia is the most common form of cerebral palsy likely to result from damage to the periventricular white matter in premature infants (Soltesz & Brockway, 1989). This may be the link between the observed simultaneous occurrence of prematurity, spastic diplegia, and DCD in some children.

Although no certain way of preventing DCD is known, some hypotheses can be made about the causes of DCD. DCD has been associated with perinatal abnormalities of anoxia at birth (Gubbay, 1975). In a later study (Gubbay, 1978) it was found that 50% of children identified as clumsy had prenatal, perinatal, or neonatal risk factors. Infants with low birth weight, especially those with increasing grades of intracranial hemorrhage, score lower on motor development during infancy and preschool years (Cohen, 1983; Leonard et al., 1990; Williams et al., 1987) and at 5 years of age (Levene et al., 1992). A longitudinal study of 66 premature infants and infants with low birth weight found that, at the average age of 8 years, 20 of the children had two or more soft neurologic signs, including problems related to balance, coordination, choreiform movements, muscle tone, speech, gait, sequential finger–thumb opposition, graphesthesia, and stereognosis (Hertzig, 1981). Nineteen of these 20 children had histories of perinatal complications.

Vohr and Coll (1985) studied the neurologic and developmental functioning of infants weighing less than or equal to 1500 g at birth up to age 7. Forty-two infants were classified at 1 year old as either neurologically normal (n = 22), suspect (n = 12), or abnormal (n = 8). At 7 years of age, 45% of the normal group, 75% of the suspect group, and 100% of the abnormal group had poor visuomotor integration as measured on the Beery Visual-Motor Integration Test (Beery & Buktenica, 1967). At age 7, of the 34 children who had been classified as either normal or suspect, 11 had soft neurologic findings. Als (1986) has suggested that better prenatal care, perinatal monitoring, and newborn care may decrease the occurrence of developmental motor incoordination problems.

MECHANISMS OF PRAXIS

FIGURE 17–1. Diagrammatic representation of the neural mechanisms of praxis. Interruption of this network at any point may result in apraxia. Small lesions may affect the system most consistently where convergence of pathways occur. Dotted lines represent alternate routes that may become active with recovery. (From Roy, EA [Ed.], Neuropsychological Studies of Apraxia and Related Disorders. Amsterdam: North-Holland, 1985, p 175.)

| ASSOCIATED IMPAIRMENTS

Referral

Primary impairments are the first signs of problems that result from the primary pathophysiology and that assist in making an eventual diagnosis or identification of dysfunction (see Table 17–1). The first signs of DCD are often not identified until the child reaches school age. Gubbay (1975) stated that clumsiness is usually only a problem between the ages of 6 and 12 years when functional limitations appear. Gubbay reported that in the younger age groups the environment tends to be less reactive and generally kinder because of the wider range of normal variation. The early signs of clumsiness are often viewed as part of normal developmental awkwardness or normal delay for premature infants. Parents often report that their children were overly messy when eating and dressing, started walking later than other children and are still awkward, were late talkers, had excessive levels of frustration and crying, and demanded continual adult attention. Laszlo and colleagues (1988) concluded that parents were poor judges of motor competence because although many described their child as "messy," "slow," and "uncoordinated" they were certain that this was "normal."

Parents, preschool teachers, or early elementary school teachers are usually the first to raise a concern related to impairments associated with DCD. If the concern is taken to a pediatrician or family doctor, a preliminary neurologic examination might reveal soft neurologic signs, such as muscle weakness, especially of the hands; poor coordination, especially in finger-to-nose movement and finger–thumb opposition; and possible choreiform movements seen as small jerky twitches of the upper extremities. But not all children with DCD have detectable soft signs, and initially these impairments may not be identified. In fact, there are some who believe that neurologic soft signs are an assortment of poorly related behaviors with poor reliability as an assessment of the impairments related to DCD (Henderson, 1987). In spite of these criticisms, a neurologic evaluation serves the important function of ruling out the existence of more serious neurologic causes of motor incoordination.

As children with DCD reach school age, a set of behavioral and emotional limitations can become apparent and warrant another referral to a physician. Problems with distractibility have been identified in children with DCD (Hulme & Lord, 1986). Gubbay (1975) cited temper tantrums, frustration, poor self-esteem, depression, and rejection as possible problems. Shaw and colleagues (1982) concluded that children with learning disability and clumsiness had significantly lowered self-esteem and were less happy than other children. If depression is serious, psychiatric intervention or counseling might be needed. These emotional symptoms might also be signs of ADHD because clumsiness is an overlapping characteristic. A diagnosis of ADHD would influence future medical and educational programming decisions. Additional physical symptoms of abdominal pain, loss of bowel or bladder control unrelated to any physical problems, or headaches are often seen as children with DCD grow older (Levine, 1987). These complaints should be taken seriously, and previously unidentified medical conditions should be ruled out before other approaches to deal with the symptoms are tried.

Physical Therapy Assessment Findings

Significant delays on standardized gross and fine motor evaluations may or may not be present when a physical therapist assesses a young child for the first time. Immature movement patterns and inconsistent motor responses are often noted. Postural reactions can be delayed or absent in some positions. It is not uncommon to find an absent or poorly elicited backward protective extension in ambulatory children with DCD. Joint laxity with scapular winging, elbow hyperextension, hypermobile fingers, and poor trunk extension, especially in sitting, can sometimes be identified. Static balance tasks are often difficult. By carefully observing associated areas of performance, the therapist may be able to relate the most striking impairments to difficulties in following directions when asked to perform a motor task or to poor attention-to-task. Children with DCD often cannot imitate body postures or follow two- or three-step motor commands. Frequent demonstration and actual physical assistance may be needed to accomplish items on standardized tests. Physical therapists must make assessment hypotheses regarding the origin of a child's impairments.

As Roy and Square (1985) point out, apraxia can involve dysfunction of either the cognitive-linguistic (information processing) system or the motor-production system. Others have concluded that children with verbal sequencing deficits also have difficulty with sequential limb and oral gestures, suggesting an underlying motor disorder (Dewey et al., 1988). As experts in the motor-production system, physical therapists need to distinguish the motor-production component of DCD from other sources of dysfunction. Referral to other team members with expertise in cognitive-linguistic functioning (e.g., psychologist, speech and language pathologist) should be made when deficits in these areas are hypothesized to be associated with a child's motor functioning problems.

Problem Definition

An information processing model has been used to explain some of the possible impairments of DCD. Schmidt (1988) describes the three stages of information processing as stimulus identification, response selection, and response programming. The systems that presumably hold the information for future processing and that are the location of the actual processing are collectively called *memory* (Schmidt, 1988). Various abnormalities within and among these processing stages and within motor memory have been examined with respect to DCD.

While applying this information processing model to learning disabilities, Silver (1988) formed hypotheses regarding how different types of processing problems might result in motor incoordination. Using visual perception as an example of stimulus identification, Silver hypothesized that when children are impaired in judging distances, they will exhibit functional limitations such as bumping into things, falling off chairs, or knocking over drinks. Children with DCD also can be functionally limited by becoming disoriented on the playground or during physical education class because they have impairments related to organization of their position in space in relation to other persons and objects. Any activity that requires the eyes to tell the hands what to do (such as ball catching, rope jumping, completing puzzles) will be a functional limitation for these children. O'Brien and colleagues (1988) studied the relationship between visuoperceptual motor abilities and clumsiness in children 5 to 8 years old. They concluded that the degree of clumsiness was significantly related to the degree of visuoperceptual and visuomotor impairment.

Response selection is the next step in the information processing model. Van Dellan and Geuze (1988) screened 1443 children, aged 6 to 13 years, using a motor observation scale and identified 111 as having "suspected" clumsiness. These children were further tested with the Henderson Revision of the Test of Motor Impairment (Stott et al., 1984) and 31 children were classified as clumsy. Twelve of the 31 were then randomly selected, and a fine motor task was used to compare reaction time and movement time to those of a control group of children. Van Dellen and Geuze (1988) concluded that the impaired cognitive decision process of response selection contributed to the functional limitation of slow performance in the children identified as clumsy.

Henderson and colleagues (1992) also found prolonged simple reaction time and movement time in 12 children (aged 7.8 to 11.6 years) identified as having a DCD when compared with 12 age-matched control children. A simple aiming task on a computer screen was used to measure movement latency and duration. It was concluded that the principal source of prolonged response latency in children with DCD is within the process of searching for and retrieval of the correct response from memory. Timing and force are two parameters often requiring selection during information processing before a motor response. Using the same groups of children described earlier and a second computer task requiring coincidence timing, Henderson and colleagues (1992) concluded that some of the problems children with DCD have are related to difficulties generating responses with reliable timing and not with the cognitive process of timing estimation.

Lundy-Ekman and colleagues (1991) also concluded that one of the mechanisms underlying clumsiness in some children is an inability to control temporal parameters of movements. Through a process of selective testing, two groups of children with DCD aged 7 and 8 years were identified and compared with a control group (n = 10). Children with clumsiness and soft signs of cerebellar dysfunction (n = 14) were more variable on a tapping task requiring timing control. The children with clumsiness and soft signs of basal ganglia dysfunction (n = 11) were similar to the control group on the timing task but were more variable on tasks requiring force control. Timing and force control were identified as separate response components associated with poor motor skills in children with DCD.

Response selection requires memory skills. Forgetting which way to stand when preparing to hit a baseball and how to hold your hands on the bat can result in the appearance of clumsiness. Knowing how to cross your legs to assume a sitting posture is something parents, therapists, and teachers take for granted (Fig. 17–2). Children who have DCD and have an impairment related to response selection can be functionally limited because they have to figure out how to position their body every time they are asked to sit on the floor for group activities.

Considerable research exists regarding young children's use of memory strategies, especially for cognitive tasks. Memory strategies are intentionally used for cognitive sequencing tasks beginning around 7 years of age (Flavel et al., 1966). I (1985) have shown that even though 76% of normal 8-year-old children used verbal rehearsal to remember a cognitive sequencing task only 33% used the same strategy to help them remember a motor sequencing task. Dewey (1991) found that children between 5 and 8 years of age performed motor sequences better to verbal command than to gestures. She also found that children between 5 and 8

FIGURE 17–2. *A*, After many therapy sessions with verbal and physical prompts, this child is still unable to sit on the floor and cross his legs independently. *B*, After being reminded of the verbal cues he needs to say to himself, he now successfully crosses his legs.

years of age with sensorimotor dysfunction had a greater impairment in their ability to perform limb gestures and motor sequences both to verbal command and by imitation than their normal peers. In a similar study, Murphy and Gliner (1988) found that children designated as clumsy and aged 6 to 9 years have even more trouble than their peers with visual and motor sequencing tasks requiring short- and long-term recall. Poor use of mnemonic aids including verbal rehearsal is one of the impairments seen in children with learning disability (Sattler, 1988).

Response programming requires sequencing of movement parameters. Children with impairments in sequencing skills cannot correctly sequence the steps in shoe-tying even though they have practiced it many times before. When children with DCD make a mistake in one step of the sequence, they have to start over again rather than simply redo the last step. Or, they will omit a different step in the sequence each time they try to tie their shoes (Fig. 17–3). This results in functional limitations related to slow and laborious movements and sometimes messy outcomes for certain tasks.

FIGURE 17–3. This 8-year-old boy still cannot independently tie his shoes. His verbal cues were "loop around and go through." He forgot to "loop around" and forgot to make a second loop.

Smyth (1991) used Gubbay's Test of Motor Proficiency (1975) to identify 12 children with an average age of 8 years, 7 months as clumsy. Using a simple and a complex fine motor task to measure reaction and movement times, he compared the responses of the children identified as clumsy to nondisabled peers. The simple task consisted of lifting the dominant hand vertically through a wooden maze to a predetermined position. During the complex task, the children were asked to raise their hands first vertically, then toward their dominant side through the maze to a predetermined point, and then reverse direction to a third predetermined point. Because the reaction time of the children with clumsiness was longer on both tasks but their movement time was longer only on the complex task, Smyth concluded that the children with clumsiness had impaired ability to program the movement and, therefore, depended on feedback more than the normal peers did.

An information processing framework also includes the concept of feedback loops regarding knowledge of performance or knowledge of results. The use of kinesthetic feedback is one way learners receive information about their performance. The role of kinesthetic impairments in the performance of motor skills by children with DCD has been questioned. Hoare and Larkin (1991) have attempted to clarify this issue. They studied 80 children with DCD and 80 children without clumsiness between the ages of 6 and 9. Of the seven kinesthetic tasks performed, children with DCD demonstrated impaired performance compared with their peers on only three: kinesthetic acuity, linear positioning, and weight discrimination. Hoare and Larkin concluded that caution should be used when labeling children as kinesthetically impaired on the basis of their performance on only a few tasks. Kinesthetic intervention must be individual- and task-specific to improve motor performance for children with developmental clumsiness.

Other methods of performance feedback were studied by Lord and Hulme (1987), who found that children with motor clumsiness demonstrated impairments of size-constancy judgments, spatial position, and visual discrimination tasks. Visual acuity differences were not responsible for their impaired performance. Lord and Hulme concluded that these impairments will affect decisions relating to error detection and correction during motor tasks. Impaired use of visual feedback by children with motor clumsiness rather than impaired ability to develop motor programs has been cited as the reason for inferior performance on a rotary pursuit task (Lord & Hulme, 1988). Inefficient use of visual feedback was also cited as a possible cause for poor performance by children identified as clumsy when they attempted a fast, goal-directed arm movement (van der Meulen et al., 1991a), but visual feedback was not a discriminating factor when an arm-tracking task was used (van der Meulen et al., 1991b).

Although the recent research from an information processing framework adds to the knowledge base about children with DCD, physical therapists should remember that most of these studies have used experimental, motor learning tasks that are nonfunctional and performed outside of everyday environmental contexts. Exactly how performance on these types of tasks is related to functional motor tasks in natural environments is unclear. Future research should focus on measurements of movement times when completing a writing sample, reaction times when asked to stand up from a classroom desk, or sequencing errors when tying shoes after physical education class.

As stated earlier, unless a child is receiving physical therapy for some other problem or being closely followed by a high-risk infant program, referral due to processing impairments such as diminished visual perception, limited motor memory, poor motor sequencing, excessive use of feedback, or poor spatial organization is often not made before kindergarten or early elementary school. Even when referred, standardized evaluations that assess information processing impairments are not currently available, except as part of some neuropsychological assessments (Kaufman & Kaufman, 1983; Reitan & Wolfson, 1985; Rourke et al., 1986).

Prevention

Prevention of the impairments related to DCD has not been well addressed. General early intervention programs for infants at risk are becoming more common in the United States, especially as a result of the legislative mandates associated with Part H of the Individuals with Disabilities Education Act (previously PL 99-457). To date, most studies on the effects of early intervention have focused on improvements in cognitive development but not specifically on motor development (Mastropieri, 1988). Interestingly, some of the characteristics described by parents of children with DCD are similar to those used by Als and colleagues (1986, 1988) to describe preterm infants who display state disorganization.

Als's model of synactive organization, as applied to preterm infants, describes a behavioral interaction among the autonomic system, the motor system, the state organizational system, the attention and interacting system, and a self-regulatory balancing system (Als, 1986). Some premature infants demonstrate disorganized behavior shortly after birth. Als has shown that these clusters of disorganized behaviors do not disappear with development and that behavioral differences between the healthy preterm infants and healthy full-term infants were still recognizable at 2 weeks post term (Als et al., 1988). The greatest differences were in autonomic and motoric functioning. When these children were grouped according to their level of behavioral organization, differences were still discernible at 9 months of age (Als & Brazelton, 1981) and at 5 years of age (Als et al., 1989). Als (1986) has suggested the use of specific positioning and handling techniques to improve state regulation and diminish disorganized behavior to encourage more normal development in infants, toddlers, and preschoolers. This can be a significant contribution that physical therapists make to prevent or minimize future motor problems. Physical therapists must take advantage of single-subject research designs and systematic case studies with data-based progress monitoring to determine the efficacy of early intervention for at-risk infants and young children in reducing the impairments associated with DCD.

Referral to Other Disciplines

There is another group of young children seen by physical therapists who should be considered at risk for DCD. These are the children who were premature and were subsequently diagnosed with spastic diplegic cerebral palsy. Some of these children enter school and have increasing academic difficulties that eventually lead to an educational diagnosis of learning disability. When treating a preschool child with spastic diplegia and a birth history of prematurity and perinatal complications, physical therapists need to be aware of early signs of motor incoordination.

The physical therapist can be the first to identify DCD and is, therefore, responsible for making appropriate referrals to other disciplines. Inconsistencies and abnormal functioning may be noticed in fine motor areas that are unrelated to impairments from cerebral palsy, such as abnormal muscle tone, postural control, muscle strength, and endurance. These findings may suggest that problems are not due to a motor-production component of the incoordination, leading the therapist to suspect a cognitive-linguistic component. For example, an 18-month-old child's poor visuomotor perception can be the reason the child cannot remove large pegs from a pegboard when other fine motor skills are

age-appropriate, visual acuity is normal, and abnormal muscle tone or strength are not interfering. Or, motor memory problems might explain why movement patterns that have been practiced repeatedly during past therapy sessions seem totally unfamiliar at the beginning of a subsequent session and have to be retaught each time with extensive verbal, visual, and physical cues. An observant physical therapist may notice that auditory memory is highly developed, especially for television commercials and songs, but conversational language is stereotypical and eye contact is difficult to achieve.

Research has found an increased incidence of DCD in combination with ocular motor and oral motor apraxia (Dewey et al., 1988; Rappaport et al., 1987). A follow-up study of adolescents who had been identified as having DCD when they were in elementary school documented associated problems of lower academic attainment, fewer social contacts, and poorer classroom concentration and behavior than other children (Geuze & Börger, 1993). It should not be assumed that DCD is an isolated motor problem. If a child's overall developmental profile is age-appropriate but unexplained gaps in performance or atypical behaviors unrelated to motor-production problems are present, physical therapists need to consider the possibility of cognitive-linguistic components of DCD. Referrals to other disciplines (e.g., occupational therapy, speech and language pathology, early childhood education) should be made. If a child with spastic diplegia has academic problems, the physical therapist, as a member of the educational team, can help distinguish motor production problems from other possible learning problems. Additional special or general education services may need to be recommended.

Summary

In conclusion, physical therapists have typically not treated the underlying impairments of DCD. However, when young children are referred to physical therapy for assessment and movement dysfunction is identified as a possible impairment associated with DCD, intervention with progress monitoring techniques using objective outcome measures should be initiated. Often consultative services in conjunction with day care or preschool gross motor play programs are the most appropriate recommendation. Physical therapists can help to educate parents and teachers concerning the progression of normal motor milestones and assist in the development of motor curricula for preschools, day care settings, and community recreation programs. Continued research to identify additional motor-production impairments using a motor control perspective may lead to new implications for physical therapy for the impairments related to developmental clumsiness.

TEAM ASSESSMENT AND MANAGEMENT OF DISABILITY

School-Aged Period

PERFORMANCE IN NATURAL ENVIRONMENTS AND TYPICAL DISABILITIES

Parents know their child's developmental history and have observed his or her functioning in multiple environments. They have the best composite of diagnostic information. A thorough parental interview is, therefore, essential to any understanding of DCD. Parents identify disabilities that include ongoing problems with everyday activities of dressing, eating, grooming, and speech (see Table 17-1). When their children were preschoolers, these disabilities were excused as "slow development" or temperamental differences. Poor performance on everyday activities is tolerated less and less as children with DCD reach school age. Impairments mentioned earlier, including slow movement times, poor motor sequencing, poor motor memory and perceptual problems, and resulting functional limitations of delayed motor skills make dressing, eating, and grooming painfully slow, messy, and dependent skills.

Teachers are the next most likely individuals to identify disabilities related to DCD. Often the structured demands of the classroom with expectations of increasingly precise motor skills and shorter time frames for performance stress a child with DCD to his or her limit. Teachers are able to compare the performance of children with incoordination to their peers, something parents do not have as many opportunities to do.

Poor written communication is frequently the first disability educators identify (Fig. 17-4). There are many reasons for poor written communication, and the functional limitation of poor handwriting associated with DCD is only one of them. According to Gaddes (1985), handwriting is not a simple learning task. As well as being essentially related to cerebral dominance, many other functions must be sequentially integrated with handwriting, such as visual scanning, right-left orientation, sequencing, motor development, spatial imagery, visuomotor coordination, visual form recognition, and all or most of the complexities of speech and language development. Treating handwriting as a motor production problem when the real issue is poor visual form recognition will only frustrate the child and the teacher. Whether the underlying processing impairments or the functional motor limitation should be treated is a question the family and the entire educational team should address.

Another common disability identified in early elementary school is poor performance in physical education class. Simple delayed maturation, limited gross motor play experience, poor motivation, or significant health or medical disorders, as well as DCD, need to be considered as possible reasons for problems in physical education class.

FUNCTIONAL LIMITATIONS

Functional limitations associated with the disabilities related to DCD (see Table 17-1) are typically assessed by administering standardized and norm-referenced tests composed of discrete items of motor performance. One example of a test battery designed to identify children with DCD is the Gubbay Tests of Motor Proficiency (Gubbay, 1975), which is reproduced in Appendix II at the end of this chapter. The test items Gubbay found to discriminate between children with and without clumsiness include whistling, skipping, rolling a ball with their foot, clapping while throwing a ball in the air, shoe-tying, threading beads, piercing holes in paper, and placing shapes in a form board. Normative data were collected on 922 children aged 8 to 12 years. Scores on the test battery are compared with norms for each age level, and specific cutoff scores exist for each of the eight items. A score below the 10th percentile in each age category is considered a failure. The number of failures for each age group identifying dysfunction varies. A child is considered below the 5th percentile for his or her age when three or more of the eight scores are below the 10th percentile. No specific reliability data were reported; however, Gubbay (1975) stated that it was axiomatic that a highly significant difference between the results in the clumsy children and all the other children would occur but that these analyses were helpful in indicating the degree of reliability of the individual tests. The timed tests were clearly more reliable than the untimed tests.

In a later study of 39 children with clumsiness, Gubbay (1978) found that the battery could be shortened to four items when one score below the 5th percentile on any of the four items was used as the criterion level. The four items on the shortened test battery are throwing a ball in the air and clapping before it is caught, using a foot to roll a ball

We did math.
We did spening.
We bot a pumpkin.
tow weeks faum toda
we're going to carve
it.

A

We did math
We did seplling

We bought a pumpkin

2 week from today

We're going to carve it

B

10-19-92

Handwriting Cassidy

aa bb oo dd ee ff gg hh ii jj
kk ll mm nn oo pp gg rr
ss tt uu vv ww xx yy zz
0123456789 10 PP BB RR Kk
Hh Happy Halloween scared
Kind kids trick-or-treat haunted
house jack olanterns mom off...

C

FIGURE 17–4. *A,* Handwriting sample of a third-grade child with a developmental coordination disorder and a learning disability. *B,* Handwriting sample obtained for comparison from a randomly selected third grade peer without motor dysfunction. *C,* Sample of cursive writing from another peer without motor dysfunction demonstrates an even more advanced expectation of third graders.

along a path, threading beads, and inserting shapes in slots. However, the 5th percentiles were only normed on this small sample of 39 children between 6 and 12 years of age.

Ehrhardt and colleagues (1987) used a modified version of the shortened Gubbay Tests of Motor Proficiency with 885 children, aged 6 years to 11 years, 11 months. A test-retest reliability study was performed using 78 ten-year-old children. Product moment correlation coefficients for the four test items were 0.41 for ball rolling, 0.48 for shape sorting, 0.58 for clap and catch, and 0.76 for bead threading. No explanation was offered for this poor reliability.

In addition to his Tests of Motor Proficiency, Gubbay believed that a full assessment for DCD should include eight items related to the general history of the child; six items related to a physical examination; a supplementary neurologic examination; academic testing in the areas of reading, writing, and drawing; an electroencephalogram; a skull radiograph; and psychological testing.

Other researchers have also screened a large number of elementary school–aged children to determine discriminating motor tasks. The Henderson Revision of the Test of Motor Impairment is another test designed to discriminate children with motor impairment from their peers (Stott et al., 1984). It has three parts: a norm-referenced test battery, the Concurrent Observations Checklist to identify behavioral sources of poor performance, and a Faults of Motor Control Checklist for a task-by-task analysis of motor faults. The test battery is divided into four age groupings (5 and 6 years, 7 and 8 years, 9 and 10 years, and 11 years and older) with one test item for each age group in each of eight categories. The categories include manual dexterity, ball skills, static balance, and dynamic balance. A 3-point scale is used, and different criteria exist to identify failure at each age level. A total score of 6 or more relates to performance at the 15% range or below and indicates an impairment. The Henderson Revision of the Test of Motor Impairment was standardized on approximately 1000 children, 5 to 12 years old, in Canada and the United Kingdom. A test-retest reliability of 0.71 is reported (Stott et al., 1984).

Ball catching and throwing, hopping, dribbling, and using a yo-yo are some of the items found on the Hughes Basic Gross Motor Assessment, which was created to assess children aged 6 to 12 years believed to have minor motor dysfunction (Hughes, 1979). It was normed on 1260 children in the Denver, Colorado, school system. Quality of movement is assessed on 36 observational deviations. A 4-point scoring system is related to the number of deviation observed per test item. A test-retest reliability coefficient of 0.97 and an inter-rater reliability score of 0.996 are reported (Hughes, 1979).

Roussounis and colleagues (1987) wanted a test to screen kindergarten children. They tested 210 five- to six-year-olds before creating their Standardized Motor Test Battery (SMTB). The SMTB has six items (standing on one leg, hopping, walking, finger tapping, peg moving, and bead threading) and can be completed in 5 minutes.

Standardized tests of developmentally sequenced gross and fine motor items can be used to identify the motor delay associated with DCD. The Bayley Scales of Infant Development (Bayley, 1993), Peabody Developmental Motor Scales (Folio & Fewell, 1983), and Miller Assessment for Preschoolers (Miller, 1982) are examples of developmental motor assessments used to identify motor delay in infants and preschool children. The Bruininks-Oseretsky Test of Motor Proficiency is designed to identify motor delay in older children (Bruininks, 1978). These are examples of tests to determine developmental motor delay, and they are *not* designed to be used for the identification of DCD.

SOCIETAL LIMITATIONS

When peers, parents, teachers, or communities place unwarranted restrictions, artificial barriers, or rigid expectations on individuals with DCD, then a functional limitation or disability becomes a societal limitation. This can happen at any age. Rules may prevent a child from playing with his or her friends, restaurants may prevent families from eating out together, and police departments may prevent adolescents or adults from driving a car.

Poor gross motor skills of running, skipping, hopping, or jumping may create a functional limitation or disability for a child with DCD. But, if a physical education class or community recreation program strictly adheres to performance criteria for group activities such as baseball, basketball, or dance class, then a child with DCD has been artificially prevented from participating with peers. If parents prevent their child from going down the street to play at a neighborhood park because they are unduly afraid the child will be hurt or will get lost, then a barrier has been established and peer relationships have been limited.

Indoor manipulative play can pose just as much of a problem. When functional limitations exist in fine motor skills of coloring, cutting, and stacking objects, imaginative play with paper, small toy people, or building blocks is very difficult. Again, this becomes a societal limitation when materials and play expectations are not modified. By not allowing children to play with modified toys or when individualized expectations are not permitted, a child's experiences are artificially limited and the lack of practice prevents ongoing skill development. Manipulative games are soon avoided, and random, nonconstructive activities may take their place (Fig. 17–5). Isolation imposed by society becomes a

self-perpetuating cycle of poor skill development, limited skill practice, poor performance, and further isolation. This cycle and its many negative consequences may all be due to an initial limitation created by teachers, parents, or peers.

If a community police department refuses to recognize that an adolescent or adult cannot pass a field sobriety test owing to inherent coordination problems, the individual with DCD may be mistak-

FIGURE 17–5. *A*, Arrangement of toys by a 4-year-old, who was later identified as having a developmental coordination disorder and a learning disability, after he was told to "show me what you can do with these toys." *B*, A 4-year-old with normal development and given the same instructions arranged the toys like this.

enly arrested for drunken driving. In this case, society may unnecessarily limit the person's freedom to drive and restrict community mobility and vocational options.

If a restaurant makes a family feel uncomfortable or asks them to leave because their child spills drinks or drops food on the floor, then eating out will occur less often or may be limited to certain environments. When excessive cultural expectations related to independence or proper manners are not met and restrictions are created, then a disability has become a societal limitation (see Table 17–1). Helping families and individuals with DCD to know their rights and identify compensatory means for full participation in meaningful activities is one of the physical therapist's most significant roles.

PHYSICAL THERAPY REFERRAL AND ASSESSMENT

With the passage of the Education of the Handicapped Act in 1975 (amended in 1990 and titled Individuals with Disabilities Education Act), physical therapists working in educational environments in the United States are often asked to assess children demonstrating problems with motor skills at school. Some of these children display the impairments and functional limitations described previously. The physical therapist in educational environments has the advantage of observing and assessing children in their natural environments while the children participate in everyday, functional activities. Immediate collaborative consultation can occur with the classroom or physical education teacher to problem solve some of the concerns. Often an initial collection of specific data can solve the problem without a complete physical therapy assessment. Perhaps data collected during recess would reveal that the child in question really does not fall more frequently than two randomly chosen peers. The child may just come to the teacher more often for help. In this case the problem is not motoric, but behavioral, and an assessment by physical therapy is not needed. When data reveal that the child does indeed fall three times more often than other children during recess, an appropriate physical therapy assessment can begin with already collected baseline data related to function. When children with possible DCD are assessed in a clinic setting, in-depth interviewing of the parents and teachers and simulation of functional activities are needed to accurately identify true functional limitations and disabilities.

A physical therapist should avoid repeating assessments already performed by other disciplines.

When possible, an arena or transdisciplinary assessment should be considered. After initially collecting information related to birth history, medical history, parent and teacher concerns, and motor developmental milestones, a physical therapy assessment can begin with the same areas identified previously for the younger child. If not already completed, standardized tests of motor development are performed to obtain a current level of motor functioning. Depending on the age of the child, the Peabody Developmental Motor Scales (Folio & Fewell, 1983) or the Bruininks-Oseretsky Test of Motor Proficiency (Bruininks, 1978) are possible choices. The Hughes Basic Gross Motor Assessment (Hughes, 1979) can be administered as a more direct assessment of developmental clumsiness. To rule out abnormal movement patterns and motor control problems (related to neuromuscular or musculoskeletal disorders such as cerebral palsy, polyneuropathies, or muscular dystrophy), typical screening procedures or assessments are administered, including muscle strength and endurance; muscle tone; joint mobility and spinal alignment; postural control and balance; righting, protective, and equilibrium responses; quality of movement during postural transitions; and gait analysis.

Throughout the assessment, the physical therapist should note possible signs of related processing and planning problems that might be contributing to motor incoordination. If the functional motor skills of dressing, eating, grooming, drawing, writing, or cutting have not been directly observed in their natural environments, then simulations of these natural environmental conditions need to be evaluated. Putting a coat on surrounded by 25 other 7-year-old children, all struggling in a small space to get dressed and get outside first, is much different than putting on a coat in a quiet room with one adult giving positive encouragement. If assessments must be performed in a hospital or clinic setting, then behavior might need to be observed in a noisy, distracting, fast-paced environment such as a busy waiting room or children's play area.

With all this information, the physical therapist must decide whether further assessment is needed by any of the following individuals: 1) a family physician or neurologist when neuromuscular or musculoskeletal concerns are identified; 2) an occupational therapist when fine motor, self-help, or motor planning areas need further assessment; 3) a speech and language pathologist when speech, oral-motor dysfunction, or possible cognitive-linguistic problems are observed; 4) a psychologist when intellectual or behavioral issues have surfaced; or 5) an adapted physical education teacher when more thorough gross motor skill training is needed.

Decisions related to the need for physical therapy intervention must then be made. When an assessment is performed by a physical therapist in an educational setting, the results are shared with the parents and other educational team members at a school conference or an individualized education program (IEP) meeting for a student in special education. When an assessment is performed in a clinic, the proposed therapy needs are discussed with the family and appropriate medical staff. In both instances, the need to share information with other service agencies is considered. If indicated, parental permission to release reports is obtained. Interagency service coordination is extremely important.

PHYSICAL THERAPY

Physical therapy goals to improve motor functioning can be related to the functional limitations of walking, running, ball handling, poor handwriting, and so on, or the typical disabilities of poor performance in physical education activities, poor written communication, or poor self-help skills. Specific measurable outcome objectives should be identified because very little research evidence exists that substantiates the successful remediation of developmental incoordination. A few studies have shown that children with DCD improve in motor skills even without intervention (Knuckey & Gubbay, 1983; Roussounis et al., 1987). However, these studies have been short term or have used only isolated tasks normed for younger children, or the children have improved but still demonstrate deficits compared with their peers. Losse and colleagues (1991) found that even with a year of intervention at the age of 6, children with DCD still had significant motor problems when they were 16 years old. Some believe that an important (Fisher & Murray, 1991) or even the primary (Gubbay, 1978) benefit of an assessment for DCD is not subsequent intervention but rather the follow-up consultation that provides an explanation of the dysfunction to the child, the parents, and school personnel. Appendix I contains some resources for parents that may be useful in planning a program for family education.

In those cases in which a decision is made to proceed with physical therapy, the therapist must determine the content of the intervention. Controversy exists regarding whether intervention should be directed toward the underlying impairments, toward the functional limitations, or toward the actual disability or encompass a combination of all of these areas. Motor learning research would suggest that to decrease the functional limitation associated with DCD, the specific functional task or motor skill needs to be practiced in its appropriate functional environment (Gentile, 1987; Schmidt, 1988).

For example, to improve functional limitations related to static balance (standing on one foot to put on a boot, or kicking a ball, or standing in line without touching the people or objects around you), the skills have to be practiced repeatedly with slight variation so that underlying motor and cognitive strategies are learned. These skills also need to be practiced in an environment complete with multiple distractions and simultaneous activities occurring. The same is true for practicing handwriting or self-help skills such as putting on a jacket.

When underlying impairments are the target of remediation, treatment activities such as the following need to be emphasized: 1) increasing muscle strength in hand muscles needed for handwriting; 2) verbally identifying and remembering sequences for a task such as shoe-tying; 3) improving visual perception used for cutting skills; and 4) practicing attending to visual, auditory, or kinesthetic performance feedback information, such as watching in a mirror or trying to listen to the sounds generated when skipping and using this information to make a different response next time.

One can easily see how these approaches can be combined, especially when consultative physical therapy services are integrated with more direct intervention and a variety of natural environments are used. If, for example, the problem is the inability to quickly and safely climb stairs between classes at school, isolated time with the physical therapist can initially be used to improve strength and endurance of hip and knee extensor muscles by repeatedly practicing going up and down stairs. The therapist can assist the student to verbally identify and rehearse the motor sequence needed to reciprocally climb up a flight of stairs and then practice the timing and order of the sequence in isolation until stair climbing can be performed faster and safely (Fig. 17–6A). Then, the physical therapist would instruct others so that the task can be repeated during the school day, but with extra time allowances, modified disturbances from other students, and prompted feedback by an educational associate or teacher (see Fig. 17–6B). This can be combined with additional practice at home in a quieter environment and with prompting from a parent. Finally, reciprocal stair climbing would be performed during normal transition times between classes with typical numbers of other students, without prompts, and without adult guidance (see Fig. 17–6C).

Whatever treatment approach is used, careful monitoring of progress toward remediation of the identified functional limitation or disability is im-

FIGURE 17–6. *A*, During the first stages of learning, natural environments are used with direct instruction from the physical therapist. *B*, During later stages of learning, natural environments and modified distractions are used with faded feedback from the classroom associate. *C*, Stair climbing is now performed in its natural environment with typical environmental distractions. The child is expected to monitor his own performance and make corrections as needed.

perative to be sure that the child is benefiting from the service. There are very few standardized assessment instruments that are useful to monitor and document change in performance of functional skills in children. Haley and colleagues (1991) describe six different pediatric functional outcome measures, including the Gross Motor Function Measure (Russell et al., 1989), the Wee-Functional Independence Measure (Granger et al., 1989), and the Pediatric Evaluation of Disability (Haley et al., 1989). Unfortunately these instruments were designed for use in clinical settings and, therefore, are not individualized to a specific environmental context for a specific student.

IEPs, with goals and short-term objectives written in behavioral terms with specific performance criteria and assessment schedules, can be used to monitor individual function within a school setting. Another alternative is the use of goal attainment scaling (Palisano et al., 1992). Five possible levels of specific functional attainment are individualized for a child to create a criterion-referenced measurement. (See Chapter 18 for additional information on goal attainment scaling.)

If theories that propose that DCD is related to MBD are correct, one can assume that the primary neurologic problem is still present in older children

and adults, even though compensatory mechanisms have developed. Studies of some children with learning disabilities suggest that learning disability persists through one's lifetime (Johnson, 1988). The identification of ways to prevent functional limitations from becoming disabilities can be one of the most important outcomes of physical therapy intervention.

Continued physical therapy screening or assessment throughout the elementary school years can help the educational team identify changes in motor development related to the child with DCD and to his or her peers. Environmental demands are always changing, and levels of peer performance are continuing to improve typically at a faster rate than that of the child with a DCD. Physical therapy consultative services can help the educational team, which includes the parents, identify the appropriate balance between interventions to improve underlying motor impairments and appropriate functional compensations. Physical therapists can analyze movements required for play during recess and suggest ways to include children with DCD in group play or suggest alternative equipment for safer play so that accidents are prevented. Promoting peer interactions during motor play or altering play settings to lessen the motor demands of an activity can break the avoidance cycles that may have begun.

Helping parents to understand their child's motor limitations is an important outcome of physical therapy. Family and cultural expectations can be inconsistent with a child's motor abilities. Expecting proficiency in competitive sports or dance or valuing perfect penmanship can lead to frustration and unhappiness for everyone. Therapists can help families and children match interests and skills with expectations that lead to success. When parents can analyze a play situation in their neighborhood or community recreation program to determine which motor skills are interfering with their child's ability to participate, the play situation can be adapted to minimize their child's disability and help prevent the imposition of societal limitations on full participation in community activities.

MANAGEMENT OF DEVELOPMENTAL COORDINATION DISORDERS BY OTHER DISCIPLINES AND FAMILY MEMBERS

If delays in speech and poor social language skills are functional limitations and disabilities associated with developmental incoordination, intervention by speech and language pathologists is appropriate. As mentioned earlier, DCD is hypothesized to be related to processing problems that can be cognitive or linguistic as well as, or instead of, motor production problems. If linguistic concerns are identified, goals related to improved word recall and retrieval or verbal sequencing of multiple-step instructions are appropriate. If oral-motor impairments are related to motor production, goals are directed at improving articulation and fluency of speech.

Occupational therapists often use sensory integrative therapy to treat sensory impairments associated with motor incoordination. According to Fisher and Murray (1991), sensory integration theory is intended to explain mild-to-moderate problems in learning and behavior in children, especially those problems associated with motor incoordination and poor sensory processing that cannot be attributed to frank central nervous system damage or abnormalities. They also state that sensory integration intervention is hypothesized to improve the ability of the central nervous system to process and integrate sensory inputs and, through this process, to enhance conceptual and motor learning. However, Ottenbacher (1991) believes that clear empiric consensus does not exist regarding the validity of sensory integration theory or the effectiveness of sensory integration practice.

Adapted physical education teachers can consult with regular physical education teachers to help modify the curriculum so that the child with DCD can participate and be successful. If the child cannot run fast enough or safely without falling, then games such as baseball can be modified so that a designated runner is used or players are grouped in teams for all activities with one person hitting and one person running or one person catching and one person throwing. In addition, peer helpers can be identified to help the child with DCD practice basic motor skills such as hopping, jumping, or skipping.

If distractibility and organizational problems are identified, a school psychologist might consult with the classroom teacher to identify ways that classroom materials can be modified to minimize the number of separate pieces of paper, books, and pencils needed to complete a project. Or, a behavior modification program might be started to reinforce classwork that is turned in on time and completed consistent with the instructions given. The psychologist can also assist the physical therapist in managing disruptive or otherwise negative behaviors that interfere with therapy.

When concerns regarding distractibility and hyperactivity arise, a referral to a physician should be considered for assessment of possible attention deficit disorder or ADHD and to consider the appropriateness of stimulant medication. Although there is not evidence that drug therapy is indicated for motor production components of DCD (Gubbay, 1975), when children who attend poorly bump into and trip over objects in their environment, medication might have the secondary effect of decreasing clumsiness (Conte, 1991). A physician can also determine if medication is indicated when prolonged unhappiness or depression is suspected.

When a child is receiving services from many disciplines, professionals must work with the family to jointly identify priority problems and to set mutual goals and objectives. When using handwriting as an example of a functional limitation identified as a priority for intervention, a number of cooperative activities might take place. The physical therapist determines that proper positioning in the classroom can be facilitated by changing the height of the chair and position of the desk. The occupational therapist chooses the appropriate writing utensil and paper modifications so that the teacher can expect some written penmanship during selected school activities. At the same time, the occupational therapist has identified an appropriate computer program and keyboard modifications so that word processing skills can be taught and used for other written assignments during the class day. The parents may decide that they will devote time at home to practice the keyboarding skills in a nondistracting, low-demand environment.

Classroom activities that cannot be accomplished quickly enough with penmanship or keyboarding are adapted by the teacher to minimize written demands. Tests are given with multiple choice answers or lines connecting the matching pairs. Some assignments can be dictated and retained as an audio response, or an educational associate can transcribe the assignment, including mistakes, so that the student can practice proofreading skills. With a team effort, the child with DCD can become an adolescent who is better able to cope with environmental demands at home and at school.

Adolescence and Transition to Adulthood

TYPICAL DISABILITIES

Although Gubbay (1975) believed that clumsiness was usually not a problem after the age of 12 years because intellectually the older child usually has matured sufficiently to compensate for these problems either by avoidance or concealment, many parents report that adolescence is especially difficult for children with DCD. Teenagers can be verbally and emotionally unaccepting of differences. Even though general motor clumsiness is a developmental characteristic for many adolescents as their body proportions change, motor proficiency is valued because competitive sports play an important role in peer interactions and expectations of some families. Academic demands increase in middle school and high school, and poor written communication skills can seriously interfere with academic achievement.

Although the research results are few and mixed, some studies do support the existence of ongoing motor disability in adolescents (Cermak et al., 1990; Geuze & Börger, 1993; Losse et al., 1991). Losse and colleagues (1991) conducted a 10-year follow-up study of 32 children, including 16 who had been identified as clumsy when they were around 6 years old. Although the 6-year-olds who had been identified as clumsy participated in 1 year of intervention (the specific type and amount of intervention were not identified) to promote learning of motor skills, the gains that were made were not maintained. After extensive retesting, Losse and colleagues concluded that the children with DCD continued to have significant motor difficulties at 16 years of age, with qualitative differences greater than quantitative measures indicated. These children also demonstrated significantly lower academic scores and handwriting problems and had difficulty organizing materials. The teenagers with continued DCD had more behavior problems, including being bullied, poor school attendance, and

easy distractibility. Emotional problems such as low self-esteem, depression, and being shy or timid were also found. Losse and colleagues concluded that other studies reporting that some children apparently "outgrew" their clumsiness had used clinical or laboratory-based tests that underestimated qualitative problems and did not reflect competence in natural environments. Not all of the children identified as clumsy at age 6 were having problems at age 16, however. Losse and colleagues found that some bright and well-adjusted children seemed to have come to terms with their ineptitude and appeared to cope well with their school experiences, were able to talk freely about their problems, and evidently enjoyed other aspects of life.

PHYSICAL THERAPY ASSESSMENT

Adolescents with DCD would not typically reach middle school without previous identification of impairments, functional limitations, and disabilities. However, these problems could have been misinterpreted or misidentified in the past and assessment from a physical therapist at this time can still help to clarify the problem. An initial assessment or reassessment would include the same areas mentioned for the younger school-aged child. The use of standardized tests is limited by the lack of norms for teenagers. The Bruininks-Oseretsky Test of Motor Proficiency (Bruininks, 1978) is one of the few developmental tests normed for adolescents up to 14 years, 6 months. Beyond this age the best alternative is to use criterion-referenced functional outcome measures (Haley et al., 1991) or ecologic, data-based, direct observation of individual function.

PHYSICAL THERAPY

Direct intervention would probably not be indicated except on a trial basis because compensatory skills are usually well established by now. Physical therapy consultation can provide information to school personnel and help establish a new set of expectations and accommodations to a new school environment. If avoidance tactics have been used in early years, these tactics can be interpreted by a new set of middle school teachers as laziness or low motivation. Demands on written communication increase, and new strategies and advanced keyboarding skills may be needed. If DCD is interfering with physical organizational skills needed to move from class to class without losing books and papers, physical therapists can analyze the environmental demands placed on changing postures and mobility. Suggestions can be made to strategically place a student's desk or books or shorten the distance between classes so that functional limitations related to impairments of poor spatial orientation or motor sequencing do not become an educational disability. Physical therapists can consult with families and physical educators to jointly identify leisure activities that promote fitness and lifelong skills rather than competitive sports that might lower self-esteem and risk injury.

High school classes, learning to drive a car, and vocational exploration present new challenges for the student with DCD. The need for new strategies again arises. Physical therapy rescreening or re-evaluation can help determine whether basic motor skill development is still changing or has reached a plateau. Ehrhardt and colleagues (1987), using modified Gubbay tests, found that children without learning difficulties stopped showing improvement on test items around the age of 9 or 10 years while children with moderate learning disabilities continued to improve and did not reach a ceiling score until 14 years of age. High schools have to provide individualized assessment and modifications in driver education instruction for students with DCD when driver's education is offered as part of the general high school curriculum. Referral to the state vocational rehabilitation agency for assessment and future service provision can also be pursued before graduation from high school.

Although very little research exists on adult outcomes for children with DCD, some inferences can be drawn from follow-up studies with adults who have a learning disability. Spreen (1988) followed 303 eight- to 12-year-old students with learning disability until they were in their 20s. A subset of these children had soft neurologic signs. This long-term follow-up study revealed that the learning problems did not disappear and that the learning problems put these adults at a disadvantage for advanced education and vocational opportunities. In addition, the subset of students with neurologic soft signs still had soft neurologic signs as adults. There was a strong direct relationship between overall achievement and integrity of motor skills. Spreen (1988) concluded that "soft" neurologic signs were not maturational inconsistencies or due to inattention but represented a persistent, probably lifelong impairment. The following quote from a 26-year-old woman with a learning disability supports this conclusion (Cermak & Henderson, 1985, p. 235).

Motor activities are also a problem; my muscles don't seem to remember past motions. Despite the many times I've walked down steps and through doors, I still have to think about how high to lift my foot and about planning my movements . . . I'm physically inept; I can bump into the same table ten times running. I'm always bruised and as a child people constantly labeled me as clumsy. Physical education courses were hell as a child, especially gymnastics . . . I cannot begin to explain the terror or disorientation.

For individuals with DCD, developing ongoing compensatory strategies for activities requiring motor skills is a life-long endeavor.

CASE HISTORY: EVAN

Evan is currently 12 years old. At the adjusted age of 19 months, Evan's pediatrician referred him to a developmental disabilities clinic at a university-affiliated facility. As a part of this evaluation, Evan was seen by a physical therapist who reviewed Evan's medical history and interviewed his parents to gather the following information. Evan was born at 32 weeks' gestation and was treated at a neonatal intensive care unit for respiratory distress syndrome and cardiac enlargement. At the adjusted age of 16 months, eye surgery was performed to correct a persistent strabismus on the left. Evan lives with his parents and was enrolled in a community day care program. Evan sat alone at 7 months, creeped on hands and knees at 10 months, and started walking at 16 months (all ages adjusted for prematurity).

The physical therapy assessment results included the following: joint range of motion within normal limits, posture normal except for a slightly rounded back in sitting, and low muscle tone in Evan's trunk, but slightly increased muscle tone in the lower extremities on physical exertion, especially when Evan tried to move from back-lying to sitting. Backward protective extension response in sitting could not be elicited, and asymmetric weight bearing was present in standing with the right leg internally rotated and the pelvis retracted on the right. Gross motor skills on the Motor Scale of the Bayley Scales of Infant Development (Bayley, 1969) were around the 13-month level (a raw score of 48 and a Psychomotor Developmental Index of 66). Evan could throw a ball but could not walk sideways or backward. Speech and language and cognitive scores were also around the 13 to 15-month level. A diagnosis of developmental delay was made, and a referral to the local early childhood special education program was suggested.

This assessment represented a crucial point in decision making for the physical therapist. Are Evan's slightly abnormal physical findings and motor delay significant enough to warrant 1) outpatient physical therapy, 2) physical therapy consultation with the family and day care personnel, or 3) recommendations for regular gross motor experiences through the day care? In this case, this decision was left up to the local physical therapist employed by the early childhood special education program.* A follow-up evaluation appointment at the clinic (including physical therapy) was made for 1 year later.

The local physical therapist evaluated Evan at his day care setting and interviewed the day care personnel and Evan's parents. Procedures performed at the developmental disabilities clinic 2 months previously were not repeated. Some gains in gross motor skills were noted. Evan could now walk sideways and backward and up and down stairs with help but still could not stand on one foot alone or jump. Gross motor scores were scattered from 18 to 21 months (chronologic age = 23 months, adjusted to 21 months) on the Early Learning Accomplishment Profile for Young Children (Glover et al., 1978), which was administered by the early intervention preschool teacher.†

Movement quality remained a concern, however. During play, Evan was observed to prefer to "W-sit" and would "bunny-hop" at times rather than crawling reciprocally. Movements lacked trunk rotation, and his gait still had awkward characteristics that included a wide base, low arm guard, and slightly bent hips and knees. No asymmetries were noted during the observation, but day care staff confirmed that asymmetries were sometimes present. Consultative physical therapy services were recommended. Evan's IEP objectives included the following:

1. When playing spontaneously at day care, Evan will use three different sitting positions during a 20-minute free-play session on three consecutive observations. Day care staff will observe play and record the number and type of sitting positions used during three randomly chosen times per week.

2. When participating in structured gross motor play experiences, Evan will use a walking pattern that includes reciprocal arm swing when observed on three of four occasions per play session. Day care staff will observe and record data once a week.

3. Evan will be able to walk up and down his stairs at home without assistance. His parents will observe this once a week and record Evan's stair climbing pattern on data sheets provided by the physical therapist.‡

A home and day care program stressing positioning during play, games to promote trunk rotation, smooth transitions between postures, and general gross motor skills for 2-year-old children was written. Progress monitoring procedures were initiated; a sample is illustrated in Figure 17–7. The preschool teachers collected periodic data, the early childhood special education teacher monitored the program every week during her visits, and the physical therapist planned to return every 3 months or sooner if requested. The return visit to the developmental disabilities clinic was eventually canceled because Evan's parents did not believe that another evaluation was necessary and did not want to take the extra time off work.

After 9 months of service (when Evan was 32 months old) the physical therapist employed by the early childhood education program noted that backward protective extension was observed spontaneously during play and movements with trunk rotation were seen more frequently. "W-sitting" was still occasionally observed, but so were other types of sitting postures. Evan's gross motor skills as measured on the Brigance Diagnostic Inventory of Early Development (Brigance, 1978) were scattered from a 2-year (jumping off floor) to a 3-year age-level (alternated feet going up stairs with railing).§

Evan's gait pattern still reflected some internal rotation on the right and some toe dragging. Asymmetries inconsistently appeared and then disappeared but were never significant enough to warrant consideration of other diagnoses, such as hemiplegia from cerebral palsy. Day care staff reported that Evan disliked walking outside in the sand and strongly disliked having his socks removed. The day care and home programs were modified to reflect Evan's new skills and to include activities that encouraged sensory experiences, especially involving Evan's hands and feet.

When Evan was 3 years, 6 months old, an educational staffing was held and consultative physical therapy services were discontinued because Evan had met all of his IEP objectives requiring physical therapy and no new functional motor goals requiring physical therapy services were identified.

This is a critical point in the decision-making process

---

*In the state that Evan lived, special education programs were available to all eligible children beginning at birth.

†It is not uncommon to see a significant change in gross motor scores in a short time especially when different assessment tools are used or when only a few items per age level appear on a test. The achievement of only a few new skills can move a motor score to a higher developmental-age level. For example, within a short time span of a few weeks, a 24-month-old child successfully passes items 56 and 57 on the Motor Scale of the Bayley Scales of Infant Development, "Walks with one foot on walking board" and "Stands up: II" (Bayley, 1969). The Psychomotor Developmental Index then changes from 77 to 87 with age placement changing from 17.8 months to 21.9 months.

---

‡These objectives would now appear as outcomes in Evan's Individualized Family Service Plan, but, when written, Part H of the Individuals with Disabilities Education Act was not in effect.

§This may seem like a large range in developmental levels, but it is very common, especially between 2 and 3 years of age when there are, again, very few items on most motor scales. In addition to wide ranges in motor levels due to test characteristics, clinical experience would support the finding that children with developmental clumsiness often display scattered motor skill profiles.

Week	Date	Type of sitting	Total positions used
1	9-10	w-sit	1
	9-12	w-sit, ring sit	2
	9-13	w-sit	1
2	9-17	w-sit	1
	9-18	w-sit, long sit	2
	9-21	w-sit, ring sit	2
3	9-25	w-sit	1
	9-27	w-sit, ring sit	2
	9-28	w-sit, modified ring	2
4	10-1	w-sit, modified ring	2
	10-4	w-sit, long sit, ring	3
	10-5	w-sit	1
5	10-9	w-sit, cross-leg	2
	10-10	w-sit, long, ring	3
	10-12	w-sit, cross-leg, long	3

FIGURE 17–7. Progress monitoring chart and graph for Evan.

for the physical therapist and the IEP team. Continuing physical therapy services beyond a beneficial level would be an overutilization of service and a violation of some state licensure laws and the American Physical Therapy Association Guide for Professional Conduct (American Physical Therapy Association, 1991). Physical therapy should only continue when the skilled expertise of a physical therapist is needed. In this case, the IEP team including the physical therapist determined that the early childhood special education teacher had the skills needed to monitor Evan's motor behaviors.

Some concerns still existed because Evan would occasionally bump into objects and at times seemed oblivious to his surroundings. He was starting to avoid some gross motor play experiences, but day care staff believed that this was not yet a significant problem and were aware that the physical therapist could always be asked to consult again, if needed. Other areas of development continued to be slightly delayed and inconsistencies in performance were increasing. For example, with a chronologic age of 3 years, 6 months, Evan's intelligence quotient (IQ) score on the Stanford-Binet Intelligence Scale — Form L-M (Terman & Merrill, 1973) was 91 plus or minus 3. Four subtests from the Illinois Test of Psycholinguistic Abilities (Kirk et al., 1968) indicated that Evan's auditory reception and association were at or slightly above age level, but his scores for visual reception and association were delayed 1 to 1½ years. The occupational therapist reported that Evan could not imitate block designs but when given verbal guidance, he repeated the directions to himself and successfully completed the design. The team decided that Evan would benefit from a half-day preschool special education program. He returned to the day care program in the afternoon.

Evan's educational program was reviewed when he was 4 years old and referrals for an occupational therapy and adapted physical education evaluation were made. The occupational therapy assessment revealed joint laxity, especially in Evan's fingers and hands. His fine motor scores were around the 3-year level on the Peabody Developmental Motor Scales (Folio & Fewell, 1983). Dressing skills, as measured by a few items on the Peabody Fine Motor Scales, were also delayed. He was able to remove socks and a cap and lace a shoe through three holes but could not unbutton buttons. Functionally, Evan could not put on his jacket or a pullover shirt. A 6-month trial period of occupational therapy service was recommended. Individual weekly sessions with the physical education teacher were offered in addition to the group gross motor experience he was already receiving.

Evan's parents and preschool teacher were especially concerned about his poor visual skills. An assessment was requested at the vision clinic at the university-affiliated facility where he was initially evaluated. A computed tomographic scan and electroretinogram were performed with normal results. Slightly decreased visual acuity was identified as well as persistent "lazy eye" syndrome. Eye patching was recommended. Problems with visual perception were noted, and the ophthalmologist anticipated that Evan would have difficulty with depth perception.

After 6 months of occupational therapy, Evan's IEP objectives related to dressing and fine motor skills were implemented by the teacher of the preschool special education class. Occupational therapy was discontinued because the IEP team decided that the early childhood special education teacher could appropriately meet Evan's short-term objectives without the additional expertise of the occupational therapist. The logic behind this decision was similar to the decision to discontinue physical therapy when Evan was 3½ years old.

When Evan turned 6 years old, a re-evaluation by special education personnel identified him as learning disabled and a special class with integration into first grade was recommended for the next school year. Adapted physical education services were continued, and new occupational and physical therapy assessments were recommended for the following fall.

Shortly after beginning first grade (at age 6½), Evan was re-evaluated by the physical therapist employed by the educational system. Evan's mother, his kindergarten teacher, and his special education consulting teacher were interviewed, and past medical and educational evaluations were read. Evan's teacher was especially concerned about his walking pattern. When walking

down the hall, he often "bounced" from step-to-step, landing on his toes. He could walk appropriately on command but soon returned to this atypical pattern. A screening of gross motor skills using the Brigance Diagnostic Inventory of Early Development (Brigance, 1978) was performed by the adapted physical education teacher and revealed that Evan's skills were generally around the 5-year level, but some skills were scattered up to his age level (Fig. 17–8). Evan's mother was pleased with the progress he had made over the years and had no concerns related to his walking or outdoor play.

The physical therapist observed Evan in the classroom, walking down the school hallway, at recess, and in physical education class. Playground skills were observed to be safe and generally consistent with Evan's peer group. Evan's mother was asked to send summer shorts and a tank top to school, and an individual evaluation was performed in the school gymnasium. A postural assessment revealed scapular winging (right greater than left), a functional kyphosis, and diminished lordosis when standing. Subjectively, muscle tone appeared to be slightly low with elbow and knee hyperextension bilaterally. The Hughes Basic Gross Motor Assessment (Hughes, 1979) was administered, and Evan's overall score was 12 of an expected score of 33 for 6-year-old boys (Fig. 17–9). Considerable difficulties were noted with any skill requiring motor planning. Movement quality was questionable with awkward, slow, and sometimes jerky responses in attempts at new skills and skills requiring dynamic balance (especially heel-to-toe walking, skipping, hopping, or ball-handling skills). The physical therapist noticed that Evan had difficulty imitating postures and following verbal directions.*

Because Evan had safe and functional mobility skills at school, the educational team decided to not include physical therapy services on his IEP, but consultation to the adapted and regular physical education teachers was offered. Their collaboration led to the identification of appropriate activities to promote static balance, improve erect postures, and increase shoulder girdle sta-

---

*The apparent discrepancy between Evan's score of approximately 5 years on the Brigance Inventory (Brigance, 1978) and the low score on the Hughes Basic Gross Motor Assessment (Hughes, 1979) is not surprising. These two tests are designed for different purposes. The Brigance (Brigance, 1978) is a criterion-referenced, developmental inventory sequenced for task analysis of motor behaviors without rigid administration procedures. The Hughes Gross Motor Assessment (Hughes, 1979) is a test designed specifically to identify minor motor dysfunction in children who appear to perform motor skills reasonably well. Children with DCD would be expected to perform better on a general inventory of skills than on a test with items specifically designed to identify the qualitative factors of performance.

B. GROSS MOTOR SKILLS AND BEHAVIORS   EVAN CA=6½yrs

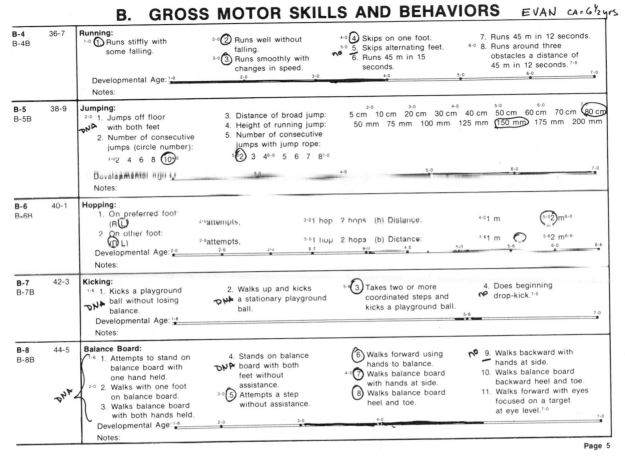

FIGURE 17–8. One page of the gross motor section of the Brigance Diagnostic Inventory of Early Development completed for Evan. (From Brigance, AH. BRIGANCE® Diagnostic Inventory of Early Development. North Billerica, MA: Curriculum Associates, 1978. © 1978, Curriculum Associates, Inc. Reprinted by permission.)

bility and general upper extremity and hand strength. The physical education class was already participating in a unit on general fitness, so the physical education teacher added wheelbarrow walking, crab-walking, and modified push-ups to the other activities the entire class performed. During their next unit on ball skills, the physical education teacher planned to use a variety of different sizes and weights of balls to increase grip strength and two-handed throwing. Students in a fifth grade peer-helper program helped Evan practice balance skills such as one-foot standing, "Simon-says" games, and "stop and go" movements to music to encourage static posture imitation. Strategies to improve motor planning such as verbal labeling and rehearsing of motor sequences before skill performance were also implemented.

The classroom teacher was asked to monitor Evan's walking pattern and to notify the physical therapist if there was an increase in the number of times Evan fell

or tripped. Evan's teacher, with the assistance of the school psychologist, also decided to try a behavior modification system of verbal or visual prompts to change Evan's walking pattern if it did not improve with the added emphasis on motor skills in physical education class. Suggestions were also given to the classroom teacher to modify Evan's desk and chair height to improve his sitting posture in class, especially for written work. A straight wooden chair was found that allowed Evan's feet to rest flat on the floor. Nonslip material was added to his chair to prevent him from slipping forward. (Evan's previous chair was molded plastic and was very slippery.) These changes also helped to promote an anterior pelvic tilt and back extension (Fig. 17–10).

Evan's fine motor skills in the classroom were becoming more of a concern and, following a reevaluation by occupational therapy, an IEP meeting was held to add occupational therapy consultation. IEP objectives were identified for Evan to promote the use of new

HUGHES BASIC GROSS MOTOR ASSESSMENT

Copyright 1975
Jeanne E. Hughes

NAME: Evan   SCHOOL: BIRTHDATE: AGE AT TIME OF TEST: 6yr 5 mo

TESTING DATE: 9-12   REFERRED BY: IEP team   TOTAL SCORE: 12

(1) STATIC BALANCE			(2) STRIDE JUMP	(3) TANDEM WALK	(4) HOPPING	(5) SKIPPING	(6) TARGET	(7) YO-YO	(8) BALL HANDLING SKILLS		
									CATCH	THROW	DRIBBLE
a. Leans flexed leg against supporting leg			a. Hits ankles together	a. Turns feet out	a. Shuffle hops	a. Shuffle skips	a. Poor adjustment	a. Lacks rhythm	a. Stiffly extends arms & catches on chest	a. poor coordination	a. Uneven push on ball
b. Excessive arm movement			b. Jumps stiffly uneven rhythm	b. Turns feet in	b. Poor rhythm	b. Poor rhythm	b. Lacks ease & coordination	b. Lacks coordination	b. Poor position of fingers	b. Lacks strength	b. Poor timing or rhythm problems
c. Excessive body sway			c. Uneven strides	c. Large steps	c. Excessive arm movement	c. Excessive arm movement	c. Uses two hands	c. Hits self with ball	c. Eyes do not follow ball	c. Poor aim	c. Unable to coordinate hands
d. Shifts to maintain balance by jumping on supporting leg			d. Pushes off more on one leg	d. Excessive arm movement	d. Cannot stay between lines	d. Hops with one leg held behind	d. Hurls overhand	d. Wraps string around arm	d. One side catch only		
				e. Looks back							
				f. Moves fast							
				g. Can't stay on line							
ARMS DOWN		ARMS CROSS									
L	R	L	R	FWD BKWD	L R		H # F	H # F			
0 a c	0 a b	-	-	-	2 c 1 a g	3 1 a b	0	R 0 a d	—	1 a c	2 a	2 a

OBSERVATIONS:

GAIT: bounces on toes

PREFERRED HAND FOR FINE MOTOR ACTIVITIES: R

MIDLINE: yes

POSTURE: kyphosis scap. wing

OTHER OBSERVATIONS:
- Ill-fitting clothing
- Unusual size for age
- Temporary injury
- Appears weak
- (Hyperextends joints)
- Moves total body
- Very right or left handed
- Switches hands

(Tremor-like movements)
Tongue out excessively when working
Tense or rigid movements
(Associated movements)
Spatial Orientation problems
(Motor planning problems)
Eye problems
Overtries
Distractible or poor attention
Delayed response
Giggly or covers up with silliness
Lacks visual fixation
Refuses to try or resentful when failed

(Can't follow directions)
Talks incessantly
Seems pressured or anxious
Says I can't
Immature responses
Touches everything or everybody
Perfectionistic
Improves with practice
Erratic
Seems shy

SCORING
3 = no difficulty
2 = one observed difficulty
1 = two observed difficulties
0 = three observed difficulties or unable to perform task

COMMENTS
Great difficulty imitating underhand beanbag toss

FIGURE 17-9. Hughes Basic Gross Motor Assessment completed for Evan. (From Hughes, JE. Hughes Basic Gross Motor Assessment. Yonkers, NY: GE Miller, 1979.)

learning strategies when writing and when using scissors, and to improve Evan's ability to button, snap, and zip clothing. The entire IEP team including Evan's parents identified strategies to improve visual and motor sequencing during classroom activities and agreed to use the same strategies when Evan dressed at school or home.

At the end of first grade, the occupational therapist reported that Evan could button and unbutton medium-sized buttons on a "dressing vest" he used for practice. He was able to unbutton his own shirt that had small buttons, but he still needed assistance with the two upper buttons. Evan now understood the placement of each of his hands for buttoning and how the button must be manipulated. The occupational therapist reported that much of Evan's improvement was related to his increased attention span and concentration skills. Evan's mother was asked if she could come to school to observe these new dressing skills so that they could be practiced over the summer.

When Evan was in second grade, occupational therapy was discontinued because Evan's dressing skills were functional. Consultation to the classroom teacher

was offered to assist with ongoing visuoperceptual problems during academic tasks such as writing. Evan continued to receive instruction in a special class with other students also identified as learning disabled, but he spent 2 hours a day in regular second grade and attended music, art, physical education, lunch, and recess with his second-grade peers. Adapted physical education collaborative consultation with the regular physical education teacher was continued.

Throughout elementary school Evan's parents and his educational team knew that a physical therapist was available to answer questions, but no new concerns arose. Evan's ongoing problems related to DCD (difficulty planning and sequencing new motor activities, poor balance in environments with changing surfaces and many obstacles, and occasional falls) were managed by other members of his educational team.

Evan is now in seventh grade at a middle school. He continues to receive resource instructional assistance and consultative adapted physical education. Evan still stands with his knees slightly bent (right more than left) and demonstrates a "bouncy" gait without a heelstrike. However, he has no difficulty moving around the

FIGURE 17–10. *A*, This child demonstrates poor posture that interferes with fine motor classroom activities. *B*, A different desk and chair improve this child's posture and improve the precision of his fine motor activities.

larger school building. He attends physical education class with other seventh graders (Fig. 17–11). His physical education teacher reports that Evan is weak and small compared with his peers. He participates in all the activities but performs them at his own rate and performance level. Evan is on task 80 to 90% of the time during warm-up activities. The only difficulties so far are frequent conflicts with the other boys. The physical education teacher believes that sometimes Evan solicits the conflict but that other times Evan is "picked on" by the other boys.

The adapted physical education teacher repeated an assessment using the Bruininks-Oseretsky Test of Motor Proficiency (Bruininks, 1978) (Fig. 17–12). Evan's composite gross motor score yielded an age equivalency of 5 years, 4 months (standard score of 16), and his composite fine motor score age equivalency was 6 years, 8 months (standard score of 7). Although this test identifies Evan's developmental motor level, it is inappropriate for Evan to engage in 5- to 6-year-old gross

motor activities when he is 12 years old. This information is used, instead, to modify regular middle school physical education activities.

No new motor concerns are expected to arise while Evan is attending middle school. Before the beginning of high school when Evan will move to an even larger building, the physical therapist, the special education consultant, and the adapted physical education teacher will discuss the transition issues that are related to Evan's DCD.

SUMMARY

DCD represents a cluster of characteristics affecting around 5% of the regular school-aged population. The exact etiology is unknown, but DCD appears to have both motor production and cognitive-linguistic components. Physical therapists play

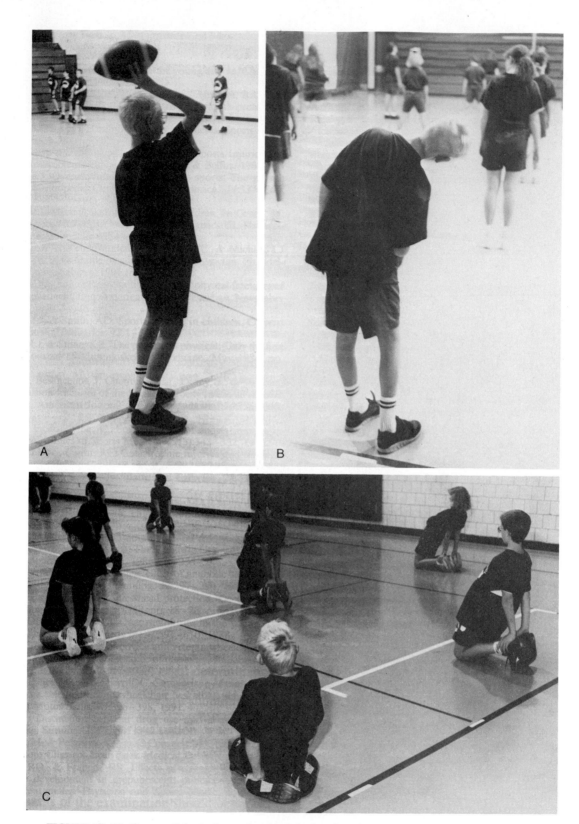

FIGURE 17–11. Evan participates in regular physical education classes, but his motor performance is still qualitatively and quantitatively below his peers. *A,* Evan and his peers are throwing footballs. His poor form contributes to decreased distance and accuracy. *B,* During warm-up exercises, Evan moves his entire body instead of isolating "neck circles." *C,* Evan has difficulty following instructions for a stretching exercise.

BRUININKS-OSERETSKY TEST OF MOTOR PROFICIENCY / Robert H. Bruininks, Ph.D.

INDIVIDUAL RECORD FORM
COMPLETE BATTERY AND SHORT FORM

NAME __Evan__ SEX: Boy ☒ Girl ☐ GRADE __7__

SCHOOL/AGENCY __Middle School__ CITY _____ STATE _____

EXAMINER _____ REFERRED BY _____

PURPOSE OF TESTING __re-evaluation__

Arm Preference: (circle one)
(RIGHT) LEFT MIXED

Leg Preference: (circle one)
RIGHT (LEFT) MIXED

	Year	Month	Day
Date Tested			
Date of Birth			
Chronological Age	12	9	9

Complete Battery:

SUBTEST	POINT SCORE Maximum	Subject's	STANDARD SCORE Test (Table 23)	Composite (Table 24)	PERCENTILE RANK (Table 25)	STANINE (Table 25)	OTHER Age equiv.
GROSS MOTOR SUBTESTS:							
1. Running Speed and Agility	15	6	2				5-11
2. Balance	32	19	3				5-8
3. Bilateral Coordination	20	9	6				7-11
4. Strength	42	16	5				4-11
GROSS MOTOR COMPOSITE			*16 SUM	20-	1-	1	59
5. Upper-Limb Coordination	21	7	*1				5-2
FINE MOTOR SUBTESTS:							
6. Response Speed	17	6	5				6-11
7. Visual-Motor Control	24	11	1				5-8
8. Upper-Limb Speed and Dexterity	72	21	1				5-8
FINE MOTOR COMPOSITE			*7 SUM	20-	1-	1	58
BATTERY COMPOSITE			*24 SUM	20-	1-	1	58

*To obtain Battery Composite: Add Gross Motor Composite, Subtest 5 Standard Score, and Fine Motor Composite. Check result by adding Standard Scores on Subtests 1-8.

Short Form:

	POINT SCORE Maximum	Subject's	STANDARD SCORE (Table 27)	PERCENTILE RANK (Table 27)	STANINE (Table 27)
SHORT FORM	98				

DIRECTIONS

Complete Battery:

1. During test administration, record subject's response for each trial.

2. After test administration, convert performance on each item (item raw score) to a point score, using scale provided. For an item with more than one trial, choose best performance. Record item point score in circle to right of scale.

3. For each subtest, add item point scores; record total in circle provided at end of each subtest and in Test Score Summary section. Consult Examiner's Manual for norms tables.

Short Form:

1. Follow Steps 1 and 2 for Complete Battery, except record each point score in box to right of scale.

2. Add point scores for all 14 Short Form items and record total in Test Score Summary section. Consult Examiner's Manual for norms tables.

FIGURE 17–12. Cover page from Evan's current Bruininks-Oseretsky Test of Motor Proficiency. (From Bruininks Oseretsky Test of Motor Proficiency: Individual Record Form by Robert H. Bruininks © 1978 American Guidance Service, Inc., 4201 Woodland Road, Circle Pines, Minnesota 55014-1796. All rights reserved.)

a role both in identifying the motor impairments and functional limitations associated with DCD and in providing intervention to prevent or minimize the disabilities and societal limitations that might otherwise occur. Physical therapists function as members of the comprehensive team needed to manage the multiple ramifications of DCD and its many associated learning and medical problems. DCD is a life-long impairment that presents challenges for adults as well as children.

References

Als, H. A synactive model of neonatal behavioral organization: Framework for the assessment of neurobehavioral development in the premature infant and for support of infants and parents in the neonatal intensive care environment. In Sweeney, J (Ed.), The High-Risk Neonate: Developmental Therapy Perspectives. New York: Haworth Press, 1986, pp. 3–55.

Als, H, & Brazelton, TB. A new model of assessing the behavioral organization in preterm and full-term infants. Journal of the American Academy of Child Psychiatry, 20:239–263, 1981.

Als, H, Duffy, FH, & McAnulty, G. Behavioral differences between preterm and full-term newborns as measured with the APIB system scores: I. Infant Behavior and Development, 11:305–318, 1988.

Als, H, Duffy, FH, McAnulty, G, & Badian, N. Continuity of neurobehavioral functioning in preterm and full-term newborns. In Bornstein, M, & Krasnegor, N (Eds.), Stability and Continuity in Mental Development. Hillsdale, NJ: Lawrence Erlbaum, 1989, pp. 3–28.

American Physical Therapy Association. Guide for Professional Conduct (Amended). Alexandria, VA: American Physical Therapy Association, 1991.

American Psychiatric Association. Diagnostic and Statistical Manual of Mental Disorders—DSM III. Washington, DC: American Psychiatric Association, 1980.

American Psychiatric Association. Diagnostic and Statistical Manual of Mental Disorders—DSM-III-R (3rd ed., rev.). Washington, DC: American Psychiatric Association, 1987.

Ayres, JA. Sensory Integration and Learning Disorders. Los Angeles: Western Psychological Services, 1974.

Bayley, N. Bayley Scales of Infant Development. San Antonio, TX: Psychological Corporation, 1969.

Bayley, N. Bayley Scales of Infant Development (2nd ed.). San Antonio, TX: Psychological Corporation, 1993.

Beery, KE, & Buktenica, NA. Developmental Test of Visual-Motor Integration. Chicago: Follett, 1967.

Brigance, AH. Inventory of Early Development. North Billerica, MA: Curriculum Associates, 1978.

Bruininks, R. Bruininks-Oseretsky Test of Motor Proficiency. Circle Pines, MN: American Guidance Services, 1978.

Cermak, S. Developmental dyspraxia. In Roy, EA (Ed.), Neuropsychologic Studies of Apraxia and Related Disorders. Amsterdam: North-Holland, 1985, pp. 225–250.

Cermak, S. Somatodyspraxia. In Fisher, A, Murray, E, & Bundy, A (Eds.), Sensory Integration: Theory and Practice. Philadelphia: FA Davis, 1991, pp. 72–108.

Cermak, S, & Henderson, A. Learning disabilities. In Umphred, D (Ed.), Neurological Rehabilitation. St. Louis: CV Mosby, 1985, pp. 207–249.

Cermak, S, Trimble, J, Coryell, J, & Drake, C. Bilateral motor coordination in adolescents with and without learning disabilities. Physical and Occupational Therapy in Pediatrics, 10(1):5–17, 1990.

Clements, SD, David, JS, Edgington, R, Goolsby, CM, & Peters, JE. Two cases of learning disabilities. In Tarnopol, L (Ed.), Learning Disorders in Children: Diagnosis, Medication, Education. Boston: Little, Brown, 1971.

Cohen, S. Low birthweight. In Brown, D (Ed.), Childhood Learning Disabilities and Prenatal Risk: An Interdisciplinary Data Review for Health Care Professionals and Parents. Skillman, NJ: Johnson & Johnson, 1983, pp. 70–78.

Conte, R. Attention disorders. In Wong, B (Ed.), Learning About Learning Disorders. San Diego: Academic Press, 1991, pp. 60–103.

David, KS. Motor sequencing strategies in school-aged children. Physical Therapy, 65:883–889, 1985.

Dewey, D. Praxis and sequencing skills in children with sensori-motor dysfunction. Developmental Neuropsychology, 7:197–206, 1991.

Dewey, D, Roy, E, Square-Storer, PA, & Hayden, D. Limb and oral praxic abilities of children with verbal sequencing deficits. Developmental Medicine and Child Neurology, 30:743–751, 1988.

Ehrhardt, P, McKinlay, I, & Bradley, G. Co-ordination screening for learning difficulties: Further experience with Gubbay's tests. Developmental Medicine and Child Neurology, 29:666–673, 1987.

Faglioni, P, & Basso, A. Historical perspectives on neuroanatomical correlates of limb apraxia. In Roy, E (Ed.), Neuropsychological Studies of Apraxia and Related Disorders. Amsterdam: North-Holland, 1985, pp. 3–44.

Fisher, A, & Murray, E. Introduction to sensory integration theory. In Fisher, A, Murray, E, & Bundy A. (Eds.), Sensory Integration: Theory and Practice. Philadelphia: FA Davis, 1991, pp. 3–26.

Flavel, J, Beach, D, & Chinsky, J. Spontaneous verbal rehearsal in a memory task as a function of age. Child Development, 37:283–299, 1966.

Folio, MR, & Fewell, RR. Peabody Developmental Motor Scales and Activity Cards Manual. Allen, TX: DLM Teaching Resources, 1983.

Gaddes, W. Learning Disabilities and Brain Function: A Neuropsychological Approach. New York: Springer-Verlag, 1985.

Gentile, AM. Skill acquisition: Action, movement, and neuromotor processes. In Carr, JH, & Shepherd, RB (Eds.), Movement Science: Foundations for Physical Therapy in Rehabilitation. Rockville, MD: Aspen Publishers, 1987, pp. 93–154.

Georgieff, MK, Bernbaum, JC, Hoffman-Williamson, M, & Daft, A. Abnormal truncal muscle tone as a useful early marker for developmental delay in low birth weight infants. Pediatrics, 77:659–663, 1986.

Geschwind, N. The apraxias: Neural mechanisms of disorder of learned movements. American Scientist, 63:188–195, 1975.

Geuze, R, & Börger, H. Children who are clumsy: Five years later. Adapted Physical Activity Quarterly, 10:10–21, 1993.

Gillberg, C, Rasmussen, P, Carlstrom, G, Svenson, B, & Waldenstrom, E. Perceptual, motor and attentional deficits in six-year-old children: Epidemiological aspects. Journal of Child Psychology and Psychiatry, 23:131–144, 1982.

Glover, ME, Preminger, JL, & Sanford, AR. The Early Learning Accomplishment Profile for Young Children: Birth to 36 Months. Chapel Hill, NC, Chapel Hill Training-Outreach Project, 1978.

Granger, CV, Hamilton BB, & Kayton, R. Guide for the use of the functional independence measure (WeeFIM) of the Uniform Data Set for Medical Rehabilitation. Buffalo: Research Foundation, State University of New York, 1989.

Gubbay, SS. The Clumsy Child: A Study of Developmental Apraxic and Agnosic Ataxia. London: WB Saunders, 1975.

Gubbay, SS. The management of developmental apraxia. Developmental Medicine and Child Neurology, 20:643–646, 1978.

Haley, SM, Faas, RM, Coster, WJ, Gans, BM, & Webster, HM. Pediatric Evaluation of Disability Inventory (PEDI). Boston: New England Medical Center, 1989.

Haley, SM, Coster, WJ, & Ludlow, LH. Pediatric functional outcome measures. Physical Medicine and Rehabilitation Clinics of North America, 2(4), 1991.

Henderson, L, Rose, P, & Henderson, S. Reaction time and movement time in children with a developmental coordination disorder. Journal of Child Psychology and Psychiatry, 33:895–905, 1992.

Henderson, SE. The assessment of "clumsy" children: Old and new approaches. Journal of Child Psychology and Psychiatry and Allied Disciplines, 28:511–527, 1987.

Hertzig, ME. Neurological soft signs in low birthweight children.

Developmental Medicine and Child Neurology, 23:778–791, 1981.

Hoare, D, & Larkin, D. Kinaesthetic abilities of clumsy children. Developmental Medicine and Child Neurology, 33: 671–678, 1991.

Hughes, J. Hughes Basic Gross Motor Assessment. Yonkers, NY: GE Miller, 1979.

Hulme, C, & Lord, R. Clumsy children: A review of recent research. Child: Care, Health & Development, 12(4):257–269, 1986.

Johnson, D. Review of research on specific reading, writing, and mathematics disorder. In Kavanagh, J, & Truss, T (Eds.), Learning Disabilities: Proceedings of the National Conference. Parkton, MD: York Press, 1988, pp. 79–163.

Kaufman, AS, & Kaufman, NL. Kaufman Assessment Battery for Children! Interpretive Manual. Circle Pines, MN. American Guidance Service, 1993.

Kavanagh, J, & Truss, T. Learning Disabilities: Proceedings of the National Conference. Parkton, MD: York Press, 1988.

Kertesz, A. Apraxia and aphasia: Anatomical and clinical relationship. In Roy, EA (Ed.), Neuropsychological Studies of Apraxia and Related Disorders. Amsterdam: North-Holland, 1985, pp. 163–178.

Kirk, SA, McCarthy, JJ, & Kirk, WD. Illinois Test of Psycholinguistic Abilities (rev. ed.). Urbana, IL: University of Illinois Press, 1968.

Kirk, SA, & Gallagher, J. Educating Exceptional Children. Boston: Houghton Mifflin, 1989.

Knuckey, N, & Gubbay, S. Clumsy children: A prognostic study. Australian Pediatric Journal, 19:9–13, 1983.

Knuckey, N, Apsimon, T, & Gubbay, S. Computerized axial tomography in clumsy children with developmental apraxia and agnosia. Brain and Development, 5:14–20, 1983.

Laszlo, JI, Bairstow, PJ, Bartrip, J, & Rolfe, UT. Clumsiness or perceptuo-motor dysfunction? In Colley, AM, & Beech, JR (Eds.), Cognition and Action in Skilled Behavior. Amsterdam: North-Holland, 1988, pp. 293–310.

Leonard, CH, Clyman, RI, Piecuch, RE, Juster, RP, Ballard, RA, & Behle, MB. Effect of medical and social risk factors on outcome of prematurity and very low birth weight. Journal of Pediatrics, 116:620–626, 1990.

Levene, M, Dowling, S, Graham, M, Fogellman, K, Galton, M, & Phillips, M. Impaired motor function (clumsiness) in 5 year old children: Correlation with neonatal ultrasound scans. Archives of Disease in Childhood, 67:687–690, 1992.

Levine, M. Developmental pediatrics: Developmental dysfunction in the school-age child. In Behrman, R, & Vaughen, V (Eds.), Nelson Textbook of Pediatrics (13th ed.). Philadelphia: WB Saunders, 1987, pp. 84–95.

Lord, R, & Hulme, C. Kinesthetic sensitivity of normal and clumsy children. Developmental Medicine & Child Neurology, 29:720–725, 1987.

Lord, R, & Hulme, C. Patterns of rotary pursuit performance in clumsy and normal children. Journal of Child Psychology & Psychiatry & Allied Disciplines, 29:691–701, 1988.

Losse, A, Henderson, SE, Elliman, D, Hall, D, Knight, E, & Jongmans, M. Clumsiness in children—Do they grow out of it? A 10-year follow-up study. Developmental Medicine and Child Neurology, 33:55–68, 1991.

Lundy-Ekman, L, Ivry, R, Keele, S, & Woollacott, M. Timing and force control deficits in clumsy children. Journal of Cognitive Neuroscience, 3:367–376, 1991.

Luria, AR. Higher Cortical Functions in Man. New York: Basic Books, 1966.

Mastropieri, M. Learning disabilities in early childhood. In Kavale, K (Ed.), Learning Disabilities: State of the Art and Practice. Boston: College-Hill Publication, 1988, pp. 161–179.

Miller, LJ. Miller Assessment for Preschoolers. Littleton, CO: Foundation for Knowledge in Development, 1982.

Murphy, J, & Gliner, J. Visual and motor sequencing in normal and clumsy children. Occupational Therapy Journal, 8:89–103, 1988.

O'Brien, V, Cermak, S, & Murray, E. The relationship between visual-perceptual motor abilities and clumsiness in children with and without learning disabilities. American Journal of Occupational Therapy, 42:359–363, 1988.

Ottenbacher, KJ. Research in sensory integration: Empirical perceptions. In Fisher, A, Murray, E, & Bundy, A (Eds.), Sensory Integration: Theory and Practice. Philadelphia: FA Davis, 1991, pp. 387–401.

Palisano, RJ, Haley, SM, & Brown, DA. Goal attainment scaling as a measure of change in infants with motor delays. Physical Therapy, 72:432–448, 1992.

Rappaport, L, Urion, D, Strand, K, & Fulton, A. Concurrence of congenital ocular motor apraxia and motor problems: An expanded syndrome. Developmental Medicine and Child Neurology, 29:85–90, 1987.

Reitan, RM, & Wolfson, D. The Hallstead-Reitan Neuropsychological Test Battery: Theory and Clinical Interpretation. Tucson, AZ: Neuropsychology Press, 1985.

Rourke, BP, Bakker, D, Fisk, JL, & Strang, JD. The Neuropsychological Assessment of Children: A Treatment-Oriented Approach. New York: Guilford Press, 1986.

Roussounis, S, Gaussen, T, & Stratton, P. A 2-year follow-up study of children with motor coordination problems identified at school entry age. Child: Care, Health & Development, 13:77–391, 1987.

Roy, EA, & Square, P. Common considerations in the study of limb, verbal and oral apraxia. In Roy, EA (Ed.), Neuropsychological Studies of Apraxia and Related Disorders. New York: North-Holland, 1985, pp. 111–162.

Russell DJ, Rosenbaum PL, Cadman DT, Gowland C, Hardy S, & Jarvis, S. The Gross Motor Function Measure: Reliability, validity and responsiveness of an evaluative instrument. Developmental Medicine and Child Neurology, 31:341–352, 1989.

Sattler, J. Assessment of Children (3rd ed.). San Diego: J Sattler, 1988.

Schmidt, MH, Esser, G, Allehoff, W, Geisel, B, Laucht, M, & Woerner W. Evaluating the significance of minimal brain dysfunction: Results of an epidemiological study. Journal of Child Psychology and Psychiatry and Allied Disciplines, 28:803–821, 1987.

Schmidt, R. Motor Control and Learning: A Behavioral Emphasis. Champaign, IL: Human Kinetics, 1988.

Shaw, L, Levine, MD, & Belfer, M. Developmental double jeopardy: A study of clumsiness and self-esteem in children with learning problems. Developmental and Behavioral Pediatrics, 3:191–196, 1982.

Shaywitz, S, & Shaywitz, B. Attention deficit disorder: Current perspectives. In Kavanagh, J, & Truss, T (Eds.), Learning Disabilities: Proceedings of the National Conference. Parkton, MD: York Press, 1988, pp. 369–524.

Silver, L. The Misunderstood Child: A Guide for Parents of Learning Disabled Children. New York: McGraw-Hill, 1988.

Smyth, TR. Abnormal clumsiness in children: A defect of motor programming? Child: Care, Health & Development, 17:283–294, 1991.

Soltesz, M, & Brockway, N. The high-risk infant. In Tecklin, J (Ed.), Pediatric Physical Therapy. Philadelphia: JB Lippincott, 1989, pp. 40–67.

Spreen, O. Learning Disabled Children Growing Up: A Follow-up into Adulthood. New York: Oxford University Press, 1988.

Stott, DH, Moyes, FA, & Henderson, SE. The Henderson Revision of The Test of Motor Impairment. San Antonio: Psychological Corporation, 1984.

Tarnopol, L, & Tarnopol, M. Brain Function and Reading Disabilities. Baltimore: University Park Press, 1977.

Terman, LM, & Merrill, MA. Stanford-Binet Intelligence Scale: Form L-M. Chicago: Riverside Publishing, 1973.

U.S. Department of Education. Twelfth annual report to Congress on the implementation of the Education of the Handicapped Act, Washington, DC, US Government Printing Office, 1990.

Van Dellen, T, & Geuze, R. Motor response processing in clumsy children. Journal of Child Psychology and Psychiatry and Allied Disciplines, 29:489–500, 1988.

van der Meulen, JHP, Denier van der Gon, JJ, Gielen, CCAM, Gooskens, RHJM, & Willemse, J. Visuomotor performance of normal and clumsy children: I. Fast goal-directed arm movements with and without visual feedback. Developmental Medicine and Child Neurology, 33:40–54, 1991a.

van der Meulen, JHP, Denier van der Gon, JJ, Gielen, CCAM, Gooskens, RHJM, & Willemse, J. Visuomotor performance of normal and clumsy children: II. Arm-tracking with and without visual feedback. Developmental Medicine and Child Neurology, 33:118–129, 1991b.

Vohr, BR, & Coll, CG. Neurodevelopmental and school performance of very low-birth-weight infants: A seven-year longitudinal study. Pediatrics, 76:345–350, 1985.

Volpe, B, Sidtis, J, Holtzman, J, Wilson, D, & Gazzaniga, M. Cortical mechanisms involved in praxis: Observations following partial and complete section of the corpus callosum in man. Neurology, 32:645–650, 1982.

Watson, R, Fleet, W, Gonzalez-Rothi, L, & Heilman, K. Apraxia and the supplemental motor area. Archives of Neurology, 43:787–792, 1986.

Williams, ML, Lewandowski, LJ, Coplan, J, & D'Eugenio, DB. Neurodevelopmental outcome of preschool children born preterm with and without intracranial hemorrhage. Developmental Medicine and Child Neurology, 29:243–249, 1987.

Appendix I

Resources for Parents of Children with Developmental Coordination Disorders

None of the following resources were written specifically for parents of children with developmental coordination disorders. There is a significant void in this area. The following resources contain information that can be adapted to specific children especially if parents have the ability to consult with professionals who know their child's strengths and needs.

Barlin, AL, & Kalev, N. Hello Toes! Movement Games for Children. Pennington, NJ: Princeton Book Co, 1989.

Activities that parents can do with children 2 to 5 years old to enhance physical development are discussed in this book. It is a book of movement and dance games for adults and children to perform together.

Bossenmeyer, M. Perceptual-Motor Development Guide: Skill Development Movement Program for Preschool and Elementary Teachers. Byron, CA: Front Row Experience, 1988.

This is a skill-based guide designed for quick reference and contains many motor activities in the areas of balance, body and space awareness, eye foot coordination, hand eye coordination, jumping, social skill development, and fine motor coordination.

Evans, JR. They Have to Be Carefully Taught: A Handbook for Parents and Teachers of Young Children with Handicapping Conditions. Reston, VA: The American Alliance for Health, Physical Education, Recreation and Dance, 1980.

The purpose of this book is to present physical activities appropriate for children between 2 and 5 years of age with disabling conditions.

Fish, HT, Fish, RB, & Golding, LA. Starting Out Well: A Parents' Approach to Physical Activity and Nutrition. Champaign, IL: Leisure Press, 1989.

Part I of this book is designed to give parents and educators concrete ways to enhance physical activity from birth through kindergarten age. Part II discusses nutritional choices for children.

Fowler, MC. Maybe You Know My Kid: A Parent's Guide to Identifying, Understanding, and Helping Your Child with ADHD. New York: Birch Lane Press, 1990.

Gordon, M. ADHD/Hyperactivity: A Consumer's Guide. DeWitt, NY: GSI Publications, 1990.

Morris, LR, & Schulz, L. Creative Play Activities for Children with Disabilities: A Resource Book for Teachers and Parents (2nd ed.). Champaign, IL: Human Kinetics Books, 1989.

Included are 250 games and activities to help infants to 8-year-olds with all types of disabilities grow.

Osman, B. No One to Play With: The Social Side of Learning Disabilities. New York: Random House, 1982.

Silver, L. The Misunderstood Child: A Guide for Parents of Learning Disabled Children. New York: McGraw-Hill, 1988.

Stillwell, J. Perceptual-Motor Activities for Preschool and Elementary Children. Durham, NC: Great Activities Publishing Co., 1990.

This book is designed for early childhood educators and physical educators to enhance group cooperation skills, improve student self-esteem, and help master basic movement and general coordination skills.

Stinson, B. To Move, to Learn, to Grow: Movement Experiences for Young Children (2nd ed.). Emporia, KS: W & W Press, 1989.

Movement experiences for 3- to 8-year-old children are described. The chapters include topics on physical fitness, perceptual-motor development, movement, education, challenging and cooperative activities, inexpensive play equipment, and games for big spaces.

Wender, PH. The Hyperactive Child, Adolescent, and Adult. New York: Oxford University Press, 1987.

Appendix II

Gubbay Tests of Motor Proficiency (Standardized for children between the ages of 8 and 12 years)

THE ASSESSMENT OF THE CLUMSY CHILD

Test 1

Whistle through pouted lips.
The child is required to make a musical note of any pitch and intensity by blowing air through pouted lips.
Score: Pass or fail.

Test 2

Skip forward five steps.
Three attempts are allowed after demonstration of the test by the examiner (i.e., single hop on left leg, step, single hop on right leg, etc.—without skipping rope).
Score: Pass or fail.

Test 3

Roll ball with foot.
The child is required to roll a tennis ball under the sole of the preferred foot (with or without footwear) in spiral fashion around 6 matchboxes placed 30 cm apart. The ball is permitted to touch a maximum of 3 matchboxes before disqualification. Three attempts are allowed before failure.
Score: Expressed in seconds' time or as failure.

Gubbay, SS. The Clumsy Child: A Study of Developmental Apraxic and Agnosic Ataxia. London: WB Saunders, 1975, pp. 155–156.

Test 4

Throw, clap hands, then catch tennis ball.
The child is required to clap his or her hands to a maximum of 4 times after throwing a tennis ball upward and catching the ball with both hands. If able to catch the ball after 4 claps, the child is then required to catch the ball with one (either) hand after 4 claps. Three attempts are allowed before failure at any point.
Score: Expressed in one of the following seven categories:

1. Cannot catch the ball with both hands.
2. Can catch the ball with both hands after 0 claps.
3. Can catch the ball with both hands after 1 clap.
4. Can catch the ball with both hands after 2 claps.
5. Can catch the ball with both hands after 3 claps.
6. Can catch the ball with both hands after 4 claps.
7. Can catch the ball with preferred hand after 4 claps.

Test 5

Tie one shoelace with double bow (single knot).
The examiner's right shoelace with approximately 10 cm lengths protruding from the shoe is offered.
Score: Expressed in seconds' time or failure if greater than 60 seconds.

Test 6

Thread 10 beads.

The wooden beads are 3 cm in diameter with a bore of 0.8 cm and the terminal 6 cm of the string is stiffened. (The beads are patented Kiddicraft toys that can be readily purchased.)

Score: Expressed in seconds' time.

Test 7

Pierce 20 pinholes.

The child is supplied with a stylus (long hatpin) and asked to pierce two successive rows of 0.1 inch × 0.1 inch (2.5 mm × 2.5 mm) squares on graph paper.

Score: Expressed in seconds' time.

Test 8

Posting box.

The child is required to fit six different plastic shapes in appropriate slots. (The posting box is a patented Kiddicraft toy that can be readily purchased.)

Score: Expressed in seconds' time or failure if greater than 60 seconds.

Chapter 18

Mental Retardation

IRENE McEWEN, PT, PCS, PhD

Children with mental retardation often have secondary or associated delays in motor development and may have problems with motor learning and motor control. This is especially true of children with greater than mild mental retardation. Some children's motor problems are minimal, requiring little, if any, physical therapy. Other children have cerebral palsy and other neurologic, musculoskeletal, and cardiopulmonary impairments that require considerable attention by physical therapists and other members of service delivery teams.

Many of the physical therapy assessment and intervention strategies used with children who have mental retardation differ little from approaches employed with any child who has similar motor characteristics, as described in other chapters of this volume. However, the learning characteristics of children with mental retardation can make it necessary to modify or supplement these approaches. These aspects of intervention are the focus of this chapter.

DEFINITION OF MENTAL RETARDATION

The definition of mental retardation and the means by which children are identified as having mental retardation are, and have been, highly controversial (Evans, 1991; Zucker & Polloway, 1987). Much of the controversy surrounds the risk of inappropriately classifying children of cultural and linguistic minorities as having mental retardation. The validity of this concern is supported by over-representation of children from cultural and linguistic minorities among children who have been labeled as mentally retarded and children placed in special education (Jones & Payne, 1986).

Children with motor and sensory impairments are also at risk for being labeled mentally retarded when they are not or for being classified as having a greater degree of mental retardation than actually exists (Chinitz & Feder, 1992). This is especially true if the evaluator has neither experience nor skill in examining children who require alternative input modes, such as manual signs, or alternate response modes, such as a communication board.

The definition of mental retardation has evolved over the years from primary emphasis on intelligence test scores to an emphasis on functional abilities within natural environments. The most widely accepted definitions of mental retardation have been proposed by the American Association on Mental Retardation (AAMR), formerly the American Association on Mental Deficiency (AAMD), which have served as a basis for many other definitions, including those used by school districts for placement of students in special education (Evans, 1991; Jones & Payne, 1986; Zucker & Polloway, 1987).

In 1992, the AAMR board of directors adopted a new definition of mental retardation, one that is intended to help change the way people with mental retardation are viewed and is based on the supports needed by individuals within their own environments, rather than on an intelligence quotient (IQ) derived level of retardation.

Mental Retardation refers to substantial limitations in present functioning. It is characterized by significantly subaverage intellectual functioning, existing concurrently with related limitations in two or more of the following applicable adaptive skills areas: communication, self-care, home living, social skills, community use, self-direction, health and safety, functional academics, leisure, and work. Mental retardation manifests before age 18 (American Association on Mental Retardation, 1992, p. 1).

Although an IQ of 70 to 75 or below is still required for a diagnosis of mental retardation, the new definition emphasizes identification of the changing supports one needs over a lifetime to live successfully in the community, rather than simply on classification of the individual.

Other definitions of mental retardation and classification systems have coexisted with the AAMR definition, including those used in the United States by states to qualify students for special education and for services for individuals with developmental disabilities. In the United States, Public Law 98–527, the Developmental Disabilities Act of 1984, authorized states to provide habilitation, medical, and social services for children and adults with mental retardation and, in some states, for people with other disabilities.

Because of the varying definitions of mental retardation and eligibility criteria, there can be confusing differences both within and between states as to who is considered to have mental retardation and who qualifies for which services. For this rea-son, physical therapists often need to seek information about programs for children with mental retardation in their own areas, the criteria for eligibility, and who is qualified to classify a child as mentally retarded. Some programs will provide wheelchairs, splints, and other equipment; other programs will pay for services, such as physical therapy, respite care, and recreational activities.

For any child, the mental retardation label is primarily useful as a "passport" to early intervention, special education, and other education, social, and medical programs. Such a label provides little, if any, insight into the strengths of the individual or the services that are needed (Evans, 1991; Grossman, 1983; McCall, 1982) and may limit a child's opportunities if the label causes others to have inappropriate or inadequate expectations of the child's capabilities.

Assessment of Intellectual Functioning

Assessment of intellectual functioning requires a standardized, norm-referenced measure of intelligence, which is usually administered by a psychologist or psychometrist. Even though most physical therapists do not administer intelligence tests, they are often able to promote an environment in which children with motor impairments can perform optimally, such as by providing positioning to enhance a child's communication and eye and hand use (Sents & Marks, 1989) or by assisting the examiner to determine alternative response modes for use by children who have motor impairments.

ASSESSMENT OF INFANTS

Physical therapists may be involved in the administration of tests designed to assess the mental abilities of infants, because many of these tests focus on an infant's sensorimotor development, such as accomplishment of motor developmental milestones or coordination of vision and hearing with body movement (Chinitz & Feder, 1992; Gibbs, 1990). These tests include instruments described by Campbell in Chapter 1 of this volume, such as the Gesell Developmental Schedules (Gesell, 1940), the Bayley Scales of Infant Development (Bayley, 1993), and the Battelle Developmental Inventory (Newborg et al., 1984).

Unfortunately, these and other sensorimotor-based infant assessments are poor predictors of mental ability at later ages, with little, if any, relationship found between scores on infant tests and children's subsequent scores on intelligence tests for preschool or school-aged children (Gibbs, 1990,

Zelazo & Weiss, 1990). The most common error is identification of infants as mentally retarded who later demonstrate normal intelligence (McCall, 1982). Better predictability has been found with children who have severe mental delays and multiple disabilities (Kopp & McCall, 1982), with most children who have severe mental delays being identified before they are a year old (Jones & Payne, 1989). Gibbs (1990) proposed that this is a result of the limited capacity of infants with severe impairments to be influenced by positive environmental circumstances; thus their range of possible outcomes is more restricted and their test scores are more stable over time.

Some recent tests of infant mental abilities have attempted to determine infants' intellectual functioning through assessment of their information processing capacity rather than their sensorimotor skills. These tests utilize infants' behavioral responses to novel and previously presented stimuli to assess their visual or auditory memory and their ability to discriminate among stimuli (Chinitz & Feder, 1992; Zelazo & Weiss, 1990). These tests are based on the tendency of infants, almost from birth, to respond for shorter periods of time to stimuli to which they have been previously exposed. Thus, if an infant has a longer response to a new stimulus than to one presented previously, memory for the familiar stimulus and discrimination of the two stimuli are demonstrated. Visual attention to stimuli is often assessed, as with the Fagan Test of Infant Intelligence (FTII) (Fagan & Shepherd, 1987), but changes in heart rate, smiling, and other responses can also indicate an infant's processing of information (Zelazo & Weiss, 1990).

One advantage of information processing tests for infants is that they are essentially motor and language free, making them more appropriate for infants with motor and hearing impairments than many other tests (Drotar et al., 1989). Another advantage is that their predictive validity is much better than that of the tests that focus on sensorimotor behaviors (Rose & Wallace, 1988; Slater et al., 1989; Zelazo & Weiss, 1990). This is probably because they tap information processing capacities that are more similar to requirements of intelligence tests for older children than are the qualities assessed by sensorimotor-based tests (Chinitz & Feder, 1992; Gibbs, 1990).

ASSESSMENT OF CHILDREN

According to Zucker and Polloway (1987), the most widely used IQ tests for children are the Stanford-Binet Intelligence Scale (Terman & Merrill, 1973), the Wechsler Intelligence Scale for Children,

Revised (WISC-R) (Wechsler, 1974), and the Kaufman Assessment Battery for Children (Kaufman & Kaufman, 1983). Standardized administration of these and most other intelligence tests requires spoken and motor responses that seriously limit their usefulness with children who have communication and motor impairments.

A few intelligence tests have been developed that require children only to indicate a choice from among an array of alternatives. The Columbia Mental Maturity Scale (Burgemeister et al., 1972) is one such test, which was developed specifically to assess the intelligence of children with cerebral palsy and requires only that a child be capable of indicating which pictures are unrelated to others.

Raven's Progressive Matrices (Raven, 1958), requiring selection of missing elements of abstract designs, and the Leiter International Performance Scale (Leiter, 1969) are other non–language-based tests with minimal motor requirements. They may, however, suggest spuriously low cognitive abilities in children who have visual-perceptual deficits or visual impairments. It is also important to be aware that all of the tests with limited motor and language requirements sample only a narrow range of abilities compared with more traditional tests of intelligence, so may either overestimate or underestimate more global aspects of a child's intelligence (Chinitz & Feder, 1992). For children with profound multiple disabilities, whose cognitive abilities are the most difficult to assess, tests of visual memory, similar to those developed for assessment of infants, could provide some of the elusive information about their capacities to store and process information (Switzky et al., 1979).

Assessment of Adaptive Behaviors

Although emphasis is often placed on intelligence test scores in the diagnosis of mental retardation (Evans, 1991), adaptive behaviors play an equal role. Assessment of adaptive behavior relies heavily on professional judgment, in both the selection of means to assess adaptive behaviors and in their interpretation. Physical therapists can often provide information about a child's adaptive behaviors, such as self-help and mobility skills, and may also be instrumental in provision of assistive devices that can help improve a child's adaptive skills.

Instruments to measure adaptive behaviors have been developed, but they are of more recent vintage than many of the intelligence tests and there are fewer of them. Tests that are commonly used include the AAMD Adaptive Behavior Scales (Nihira et al., 1974) and the Vineland Adaptive Behavior Scales (Sparrow et al., 1984).

Classification of Mental Retardation

Although the 1992 AAMR definition of mental retardation no longer uses subcategories of mental retardation, four levels of retardation were included in the 1983 AAMD definition (Grossman, 1983) and are still used in many programs. Mild, moderate, severe, and profound levels of retardation are based on intelligence test scores, even though deficits in adaptive behaviors are also required for a diagnosis of mental retardation. School districts in many states also use intelligence test scores to categorize students for special education services (Zucker & Polloway, 1987). Table 18–1 compares the 1983 AAMD classification by intelligence test score with the classifications often used by school districts to categorize students for special education purposes.

INCIDENCE AND PREVALENCE OF MENTAL RETARDATION

Reported estimates of incidence and prevalence of mental retardation vary widely. The differences are thought to be due to a number of factors, including variations in the definition of mental retardation; the methodologies employed; the sex, age, and communities of the samples; and the sociopolitical factors affecting the design and interpretation of the studies (Jones & Payne, 1986).

The President's Committee on Mental Retardation estimated that 3% of the population has mental retardation, an estimate that some have challenged as being too high (Mercer, 1973; Tarjan et al., 1973). They believe not only that members of cultural and ethnic minorities have been inaccurately classified as mentally retarded but also that schools tend to identify students as mentally retarded who were not considered to have mental retardation before starting school and are not so identified as adults. Children who are classified as having mild mental retardation are often not identified until age 6 or older (Jones & Payne, 1986).

It has been estimated that among those with mental retardation, from 70 to 89% have mild retardation, 20% have moderate retardation, 5% have severe retardation, and 1% have profound mental retardation (Jones & Payne, 1989). Approximately 2% of all school-aged children have been identified for educational purposes as having a severe disability (Evans, 1991).

ETIOLOGY AND PATHOPHYSIOLOGY OF MENTAL RETARDATION

There are multiple causes of mental retardation, many of which have been identified and many that have not. McLaren and Bryson (1987) reviewed 13 epidemiologic studies of mental retardation and concluded that causes could be identified for approximately 70% of those with severe mental retardation and 50% of those with mild retardation.

Over 350 etiologies for mental retardation have been identified that can be broadly categorized into prenatal, perinatal, and postnatal causes. Prenatal etiologies have been further classified as chromosomal disorders, syndromes, inborn errors of metabolism, developmental disorders of brain formation, and environmental influences. Perinatal causes include intrauterine disorders and neonatal disorders. Classifications of postnatal causes include head injuries, infections, demyelinating disorders, degenerative disorders, seizure disorders, toxic-metabolic disorders, malnutrition, environmental deprivation, and hypoconnection syndrome (American Association on Mental Retardation, 1992).

Movement dysfunction is more often associated with some etiologies than with others, and, in general, children with more severe mental retardation are likely to have more severe motor delays and impairments (Anwar, 1986; Chinitz & Feder, 1992). Ellis (1963) proposed that the relatively poor motor performance of people with mental retardation is the result of their limited capacity to process information and the rapid decay of that information over time. Such cognitive deficits impede motor learning (Anwar, 1986), leading to the slow and clumsy movements that children with mental retardation often have, even when they do not have

TABLE 18–1. **COMPARISON OF 1983 AMERICAN ASSOCIATION ON MENTAL DEFICIENCY (AAMD) LEVELS OF RETARDATION AND TRADITIONAL SPECIAL EDUCATION CATEGORIES**

AAMD Level of Retardation	Intelligence Test Score	Educational Category	Intelligence Test Score
Mild	55 to 70		
		Educable	50 to 75
Moderate	40 to 55		
		Trainable	25 to 50
Severe	25 to 40		
Profound	below 25		

cerebral palsy or another movement-related diagnosis. Many children also have associated problems, such as vision and hearing impairments, cerebral palsy, low levels of arousal, seizure disorders, cardiopulmonary dysfunction, and various other medical problems that can further influence motor development, motor learning, and motor performance (Anwar, 1986; Molnar, 1992).

Prevention

Some forms of mental retardation and associated disorders can now be prevented, such as those resulting from phenylketonuria, rubella, and lead poisoning. In addition, amniocentesis, ultrasound, and other techniques have enabled prenatal diagnosis of many conditions, which may help to decrease morbidity, such as through delivery of a child with myelodysplasia by caesarean section. Results of such tests can also offer parents an opportunity to terminate a pregnancy, if they wish (Badell, 1992). Genetic counseling can also be offered.

Although the etiologic factors known to cause mental retardation may be present in a given child, complex and powerful interactions between those factors and later environmental events can alter the actuality or the severity of mental retardation and associated impairments. Some infants, for example, who have severe medical problems during the postnatal course, with documented neuroanatomic pathology during this period, have little, if any, sequelae (see Chapter 7). On the other hand, children with no known pathology but who experience one or more environmental risk factors may eventually be classified as having mental retardation, usually mild mental retardation (Campbell & Ramey, 1985).

Campbell and Ramey (1985) identified four important environmental factors in mental retardation: 1) malnutrition, 2) teratogens, 3) accidents, and injuries, and 4) a poor psychological environment. These environmental factors are likely to be related to socioeconomic status, which has been found to be one of the most powerful predictors of childhood intellectual functioning (Gibbs, 1990). Kochanek and colleagues (1990) found that, in children aged birth to 3 years, characteristics of their parents, such as the mother's education, more accurately predict whether a child will have a disability as an adolescent than the child's own characteristics.

In the United States, the family-centered services directed by Part H of the Individuals with Disabilities Education Act (IDEA), described in Chapters 30 and 33 of this volume, reflect a belief in the power of early social and physical environments to influence a child's development. It also implies confidence in the capability of physical therapists and other service providers to assist families to provide environments that both prevent unnecessary disability and promote the achievement of a child's potential. Ramey & Ramey (1992) found six components of early intervention programs to be the most critical for children's intellectual development and learning: 1) encouragement to explore and learn from the environment; 2) mentoring by trusted adults in basic cognitive skills; 3) celebration of the child's developmental accomplishments by others; 4) guided rehearsal and elaboration of new skills; 5) protection from inappropriate disapproval, teasing, and punishment; and 6) provision of a rich and responsive language environment.

▌ PRIMARY IMPAIRMENT

Diagnosis/Problem Identification

The time at which impairments in intellectual functioning and movement become recognized varies widely, both within and between medical diagnoses. In some cases, prenatal or neonatal diagnosis can predict impairments that may not yet be apparent, such as with Down syndrome or myelodysplasia. In other cases, a medical diagnosis will not be made until after impaired functioning is noted, perhaps not until months or years after birth.

Delay in achievement of developmental motor milestones is often the first indication of mental retardation that was present prenatally or perinatally (Chinitz & Feder, 1992). This is particularly true for children with greater than mild mental retardation. Some children will develop normally for a period of time and then regress, such as those with Rett syndrome or Tay-Sachs disease. In these cases, too, motor manifestations of the condition are often the first indication of a more global developmental problem (Nomura & Segawa, 1990).

NEUROMOTOR IMPAIRMENTS OF CHILDREN WITH MENTAL RETARDATION

The movement impairments of children with mental retardation are as diverse as the pathophysiology of their primary and associated conditions. Most of the movement problems, however, have their bases in central nervous system pathology that most often leads to impairments in flexibility, force production, coordination, postural control, balance, endurance, and efficiency (Campbell, S. K., 1991). Cardiopulmonary and musculoskeletal impairments may also contribute to the movement problems.

Although the type and degree of movement and related problems vary greatly, certain medical diagnoses are likely to be associated with specific constellations of neuromuscular, musculoskeletal, and cardiopulmonary impairments. Table 18–2 summarizes impairments that are common among children with selected diagnoses who are often seen by physical therapists.

Physical therapy assessment of the movement impairments of children who have mental retardation is similar to that of other children who have problems addressed by physical therapists. Observation, criterion-referenced instruments, norm-referenced tests, and other formats are used, depending on the age of the child, the problem being assessed, and the purpose of the assessment (see other chapters of this volume).

Although the same assessment methods and tools may be used for children with and without mental retardation, it is important to recognize that a

TABLE 18–2. NEUROMUSCULAR, MUSCULOSKELETAL, AND CARDIOPULMONARY IMPAIRMENTS DESCRIBED IN CHILDREN WITH MENTAL RETARDATION CAUSED BY SELECTED CONDITIONS*

Condition (Source)	Neuromuscular	Musculoskeletal	Cardiopulmonary
Cri-du-chat syndrome (Nyhan & Sakati, 1976)	Hypotonia in early childhood, sometimes hypertonia later	Minor upper extremity anomalies, scoliosis	Congenital heart disease is common
Cytomegalovirus infection (prenatal) (Bergsma, 1973)	Hypertonia, seizure disorder, microcephaly	Secondary to neuromuscular problems	Pulmonary valvular stenosis, mitral stenosis, atrial septal defect
de Lange syndrome (Berg et al., 1970; Smith, 1976)	Spasticity, intention tremor, seizure disorder (10–20%), microcephaly	Decreased bone age, small stature, small hands and feet, short digits, proximal thumb placement, clinodactyly of fifth fingers, other arm and hand defects, limited elbow extension	Neonatal respiratory problems, cardiac malformations, recurrent upper respiratory tract infections
Down syndrome (Harris & Shea, 1991; Shumway-Cook & Woollacott, 1985)	Hypotonia, low muscle force production, slow automatic postural reactions, slow reaction time, motor delays increase with age	Joint hyperflexibility, ligamentous laxity, foot deformities, scoliosis, atlantoaxial instability (20%)	Congenital heart disease (40%), lung hypoplasia with pulmonary hypertension
Fetal alcohol syndrome (Bloom et al., 1985; Smith, 1976)	Fine motor dysfunction, weak grasp, visual motor deficits, ptosis	Joint anomalies with abnormal position or function, maxillary hypoplasia	Heart murmur, often disappears after the first year
Fragile X syndrome (Keenan et al., 1992; Rinck, 1992)	Hypotonia, poor coordination and motor planning, seizures	Hyperextensible finger joints, prominent jaw, scoliosis	Mitral valve prolapse
Hurler's syndrome (Carter, 1970; Smith, 1976)	Hydrocephalus	Joint contractures, claw-like deformities of hands, short fingers, thoracolumbar kyphosis, shallow acetabular and glenoid fossae, irregularly shaped bones	Cardiac deformities, including cardiac enlargement because of right ventricular hypertension; death frequently due to cardiac failure
Lesch-Nyhan syndrome (Jankovic et al., 1988)	Hypotonia followed by spasticity and chorea, athetosis, and/or dystonia; compulsive self-injurious behavior	Secondary to neuromuscular problems	
Prader-Willi syndrome (Aughton & Cassidy, 1990; Laurance, 1981)	Severe hypotonia and feeding problems in infancy, excessive eating and obesity in childhood; poor fine and gross motor coordination	Short stature, small hands and feet	May be associated with cor pulmonale (most common cause of death)

TABLE 18-2. **NEUROMUSCULAR, MUSCULOSKELETAL, AND CARDIOPULMONARY IMPAIRMENTS DESCRIBED IN CHILDREN WITH MENTAL RETARDATION CAUSED BY SELECTED CONDITIONS*** *Continued*

Condition (Source)	Neuromuscular	Musculoskeletal	Cardiopulmonary
Rett syndrome (Guidera et al., 1991; Holm & King, 1990; Nomura & Segawa, 1990; Stewart et al., 1989)	Hypotonia in infancy, then gradually increasing hypertonia and loss of acquired skills; ataxia, apraxia, choreothestosis and/or dystonia; progression from hyperkinesia to bradykinesia with age; slow reaction time; stereotypical hand movements (clapping, wringing, clenching); drooling, involuntary, rhythmic tongue movement and deviation; seizure disorder	Scoliosis, kyphosis, joint contractures, hip subluxation or dislocation, equinovarus deformities	Immature respiratory patterns; breathing irregularities, such as hyperventilation and apnea
Williams (elfin facies) syndrome (Bloom et al., 1985; Smith, 1976)	Mild neurologic dysfunction; poor motor coordination	Hallux valgus	Variable congenital heart disease

*Some impairments are not exhibited by all children with the condition.

child's intellectual impairment may affect performance of motor activities. This is especially the case when a child has to follow directions or perform motor tasks that have major cognitive components. Assessment of infants and young children may be less affected by intellectual abilities than that of older children and adolescents, and cognitive function will probably affect assessment at the impairment level less than at the disability level, which reflects a child's ability to perform age- and socially appropriate functional skills in daily life.

LEARNING IMPAIRMENTS OF CHILDREN WITH MENTAL RETARDATION

By definition, impaired learning is what distinguishes children with mental retardation from other children. Although their motor problems are often similar to those of children without mental retardation and they respond to intervention based on the same physical therapy principles, the application of those principles needs to be sensitive to the children's learning characteristics. Research demonstrating that physical therapy is less effective with children who have mental retardation (Parette & Hourcade, 1984) may at least partially relate to inadequate modification of therapeutic approaches to enhance the learning of children with mental retardation.

The degree and types of learning impairments of children with mental retardation vary considerably, but several common learning characteristics have been identified. Compared with normally developing children, children with mental retardation have been found 1) to be capable of learning a fewer number of things; 2) to need a greater number of repetitions to learn; 3) to have greater difficulty generalizing skills; 4) to have greater difficulty maintaining skills that are not practiced regularly; 5) to have slower response times; and 6) to have a more limited repertoire of responses (Brown et al., 1979; Falvey, 1989; Orelove & Sobsey, 1991). Implications of these learning characteristics for physical therapy intervention are described in later sections of this chapter.

Intervention to Limit Impairments and Functional Limitations and Prevent Secondary Impairment

Pediatric physical therapists have traditionally focused their efforts on interventions designed to limit musculoskeletal, neuromuscular, and cardiopulmonary impairments, reduce functional limitations, and prevent secondary impairments. Less emphasis has been placed on the potentially important role of physical therapy in limiting or preventing secondary cognitive, communication, and social-emotional impairments, which may result from motor disorders and restrictions.

LIMITING PHYSICAL IMPAIRMENTS AND FUNCTIONAL LIMITATIONS OF CHILDREN WITH MENTAL RETARDATION

Early identification of neuromuscular, musculoskeletal, and cardiopulmonary problems, at whatever age they occur, allows for intervention designed to limit the impairments, thus restricting the development of secondary impairments and functional limitations. Specific intervention will depend on the identified problems and on consequences that can be predicted to follow from the natural history of the condition. Children with Down syndrome and other relatively mild movement impairments, for example, often benefit from activities designed to enhance postural control and force production and accomplishment of motor milestones (Harris & Shay, 1991). Other children with more severe impairments may benefit from positioning and handling designed to maintain flexibility, prevent musculoskeletal malalignments and deformities, and enhance motor development and control (Fraser et al., 1990). Such intervention is described in other chapters of this volume.

LIMITING COGNITIVE, COMMUNICATION, AND PSYCHOSOCIAL IMPAIRMENTS AND FUNCTIONAL LIMITATIONS

Children who have motor impairments that restrict or prevent exploration of their environments may be at risk for secondary delays in domains that are not primarily affected (Campbell, SK, 1991; Hays, 1987), especially cognition, communication, and psychosocial development (Affolter, 1991; Kermoian & Campos, 1988; Rosenberg & Robinson, 1990; Telzrow et al., 1987).

Children's need to act is impressive! They never get tired of touching and exploring neighboring relationships of things in their environment. They search for problems and try to solve them. They hunt for new events and make use of familiar objects in unusual ways. They perceive and they act upon them. They change actions serving as causes and observe the effects (Affolter, 1991, p. 55).

Campos and Bertenthal (1987) believe that independent mobility is an organizer of psychological changes in normally developing infants, especially developmental changes in social understanding, spatial cognition, and emotions. They also propose theoretical links between independent mobility and the growth of brain structures, self-awareness, attachment to others, and ability to cope with the environment.

Most of the theoretical links have not been examined empirically, but relations between mobility and spatial cognition have received considerable research attention. Several studies have demonstrated that locomotion, not age per se, is related to changes in such spatial cognitive tasks as recognition of heights (Bertenthal et al., 1984), retrieving hidden toys (Acredolo et al., 1984; Benson & Uzgiris, 1985), and performance on Piagetian spatial search tasks by typical infants and infants with meningomyelocele (Kermonian & Campos, 1988; Telzrow et al., 1987). Self-produced locomotion has also been shown to influence social-communicative behaviors of infants (Gustafson, 1984), and the proposed theoretical link between mobility and development of brain structures was supported by a study in which kittens' sensory and motor experiences affected synaptic development in the frontal lobes (Greenough et al., 1987).

Although much of the research has demonstrated an association between motor and cognitive development, other research suggests that the links are indirect, with motor and cognitive abilities facilitating each other but capable of relatively independent development (Chinitz & Feder, 1992). One study, for example, found that the object permanence task performance of children with cerebral palsy was more closely related to their mental age than to the severity of their motor impairments (Eagle, 1985). This finding is consistent with the well-known capacity for some people to develop average or superior mental abilities in spite of severe motor impairments.

Further research is needed to determine the relative contributions of innate mental capability and sensorimotor experiences on various aspects of cognitive development. It may be that the inborn intelligence of some children enables them to compensate for their motor limitations, thus making them less vulnerable to effects of sensorimotor deprivation than children whose intellectual capacities are more limited.

Assuming that exploration and manipulation of the environment do influence cognitive, communication, and social-emotional development, physical therapy has an obvious role in the development of these nonmotor domains of children who have motor impairments. One means is through treatment strategies designed to improve motor performance, as described in other chapters of this volume. Two other potentially important means are providing alternative means of mobility when children's motor impairments prevent exploration of the environment at an age when other children are crawling and walking and the use of postural support systems to promote interaction with the environment.

Use of Power Mobility to Prevent Secondary Impairments

Butler (1991) asserts that self-produced locomotion can have such a powerful impact on development that functional means of mobility should be provided for all young children who have mobility restrictions, regardless of whether or not the child is expected to walk eventually. She proposes the concept of augmentative mobility, which, like augmentative communication, supports a child's own capabilities, allowing the child to select a means of mobility that is most convenient and efficient for a particular situation. Aided mobility is not seen as "giving up" on walking for young children, but as providing critical assistance at a time it is needed for optimal development.

Several studies have demonstrated that very young children can learn to use power mobility devices. Zazula and Foulds (1983) reported that an 11-month-old child with congenital limb deformities learned to activate the controls of a motorized cart within 4 hours and controlled all aspects of the cart by 17 months. In another study, 12 of 13 children between the ages of 20 to 37 months, with various disabilities, became competent motorized wheelchair drivers within their homes after an average of 16.4 days (Butler et al., 1983).

Although these young children were believed to have normal intelligence, other studies have demonstrated that older children with mental retardation can also become independent users of power mobility devices (Verburg et al., 1990). It is reasonable to assume that certain cognitive abilities are necessary to achieve independent aided mobility, but the specific abilities that are necessary and the means to assess them have not been determined. Because normally developing children learn to crawl and become independently mobile well before their first birthday, and because children have become independently mobile using power mobility devices before the age of 2, children with mental retardation who have adequate vision and the cognitive skills typical of a 18-month-old (or, perhaps, younger) are likely to be capable of learning to use powered means of mobility, given appropriate equipment and opportunities.

Use of Assistive Positioning to Promote Environmental Interaction

Seating and other assistive positioning devices, as described in Chapter 23, can also influence children's interactions with their physical and social environments through their effects on such variables as hand function (Nwaobi, 1987), switch activation (McEwen & Karlan, 1989), respiration (Nwaobi & Smith, 1986), and head position (Hulme et al., 1987). One of the most important environmental interactions is communication with others, because it affects not only a child's own communication development but also cognitive and social-emotional development (Campbell, PH, 1989; Siegel-Causey & Downing, 1987).

To learn to communicate, children must have opportunities to communicate. One study found that teachers initiated interactions at higher rates when children were positioned in wheelchairs than when they were in sidelyers or supine on a mat (McEwen, 1992). Observations suggested that wheelchairs promoted interaction by placing students nearer the normal interaction level of adults than positioning on the floor. The adults who participated in the study rarely sat on the floor to interact with children, unless they were involved in structured programming, a finding that is consistent with other investigations (Houghton et al., 1987).

In addition to providing opportunities for interaction with other persons in the environment, research suggests that positioning can also influence children's own communicative behaviors. Normally developing 3- to 6-month-old infants looked at their mothers for longer periods of time when they were supine, than when reclined 45° or seated upright (Fogel et al., 1992). Similarly, children with profound mental retardation and physical disabilities interacted with attentive teachers and classroom assistants for longer periods of time when they were in the supine position than when they were seated in their wheelchairs or in a sidelyer (McEwen, 1992).

Positioning may also influence children's interactions with their environments through the effect of position on their behavioral state or arousal. Low levels of arousal and behavioral states that interfere with attention to environmental stimuli are common among children with the most severe multiple cognitive and motor impairments (Guess et al., 1988; Rainforth, 1982). Guess and colleagues (1991) found that when children with multiple disabilities were positioned upright their behavioral states were more compatible with learning than when they were placed in recumbent positions. Similarly, Landesman-Dwyer and Sackett (1978) found that children's activity levels and receptivity to environmental stimuli were improved when intervention included an upright position. Other studies suggest that oxygenation is improved in the upright position (Navajas et al, 1988; Thoresen et al., 1988), and inadequate oxygenation has been proposed as a factor contributing to the lethargy of children with profound multiple disabilities (Guess, 1989; Guess et al., 1988).

Although research concerning effects of positioning with children who have multiple disabilities is limited, it does suggest that positioning may influence children's interactions with their environments through a variety of mechanisms. The upright position is more likely to enhance children's receptivity to, and opportunities for interaction with the environment than recumbent positions (Campbell, PH, 1989; McEwen & Lloyd, 1990) and thus may help to limit or prevent secondary cognitive, emotional, and communication impairments and functional limitations. There are some children, however, especially those functioning at very low levels of communication development, whose own communication may be facilitated by the supine position. Because supine may be socially isolating and physically detrimental, it should be monitored carefully and used only while the child is actively engaged in social interaction.

Role of Other Disciplines

The number of disciplines represented in the care of a child with mental retardation is often directly proportional to the severity of the retardation and to the number and severity of any associated disorders. All of a child's problems are usually not identified at the same time, so increasing numbers of disciplines may become involved as a child grows older. Because motor delays and movement disorders are often recognized relatively early, a physical therapist is likely to be one of the first members of an intervention team and so be in a position to recognize the need for input by other disciplines and refer the family to physicians and other service providers.

It has been estimated that nearly 50% of people with mental retardation have at least one other impairment (Kelleher & Mulcahy, 1985), each of which is likely to require the services of several different service providers. The prevalence of additional impairments is positively related to the severity of the cognitive impairment, with many children with mental retardation and motor dysfunction having such problems as impaired hearing and vision, seizure disorders, and cardiopulmonary dysfunction (Kelleher & Mulcahy, 1985; Molnar, 1992).

Some of the service providers who may need to be involved with children who have mental retardation and motor impairments are suggested by the 14 early intervention services named in Public Law 99-457: audiology, case management services; family training, counseling, and home visits; health service; medical services for diagnostic or evaluation purposes; nursing; nutrition services; occupational

therapy; physical therapy; psychological services; social work; special instruction; speech-language pathology; and transportation. Many children also require the services of several physicians and surgeons, orthotists, and vendors of assistive technology.

As children with mental retardation grow older and their impairments lead to functional limitations and disabilities, the number of involved disciplines often expands to include a variety of teachers, vocational counselors, and personnel of health and social service agencies. Young adults may need job coaches, group home supervisors, personal care assistants, and others who can provide the supports necessary to enable them to live as independently and successfully as possible in their communities.

Determinants of Outcomes

The determinants of outcomes for children with mental retardation or who are at risk for mental retardation are usually numerous and complex. From a dynamical systems point of view, described by Campbell in Chapter 1, the internal capacity of the child and the virtually unlimited environmental influences are logically equivalent and capable of affecting outcomes (Fogel & Thelen, 1987; McEwen, 1992). The natural history of mental retardation and associated problems resulting from some etiologies, particularly those that are progressive, are relatively well described. Scoliosis, for example, nearly always develops in children with Rett syndrome (Holm & King, 1990). For others, especially infants and very young children, many complex endogenous and exogenous factors contribute to the ultimate impact of the initial insult and resulting pathophysiology, which makes prediction of outcome difficult. As discussed previously in this chapter, family environment has been found to be the best predictor of outcome, especially with children who have mild mental retardation (Gibbs, 1990: Ramey & Ramey, 1992).

▌TEAM ASSESSMENT OF DISABILITY

The complex problems of children with mental retardation and motor impairments usually require a team approach for assessment of disability and for planning, implementation, and evaluation of intervention (Foley, 1990; Orelove & Sobsey, 1991; Rainforth et al., 1992b). The team will always include the child's family or other caregiver, with other team members as required by the nature and severity of the child's problems, the child's age, and the service delivery setting. Many children need the services of two or more teams at the same time, such as a clinically based health care team and an early intervention or public school team. Usually, the health care team is primarily responsible for assessment of the child's impairment-level needs, with the early intervention or school-based team responsible for limiting impairments and ongoing efforts to promote the highest possible level of functioning in the community. When the teams have mutual responsibilities and concerns, overlapping or conflicting services can result, with confusion for the family and unnecessary expenditure of limited resources. To avoid such problems, it is essential that the teams communicate well and that the roles and responsibilities of the members of each team are clear to all (Rainforth et al., 1992b).

Because the nature and severity of a child's impairments often play a greater role in the foci of assessment and intervention than a child's age, this chapter is not organized chronologically, as are several other chapters of this volume that describe conditions in which age-related progressions can be identified. Age-related needs that occur during the transition to adulthood and are common to most children with mental retardation are discussed separately. The case histories at the end of the chapter describe application of assessment and intervention principles for children with mental retardation of different ages with various mental and motor characteristics.

Models of Team Functioning

Each team must decide on a model of service delivery that will enable comprehensive evaluation of a child's disabilities and provide the most effective intervention. The transdisciplinary model of service delivery, developed in the mid 1970s by the United Cerebral Palsy National Collaborative Infant Project (1976), is increasingly being recommended as "best practice" in early intervention programs and in special education programs for children with severe and multiple disabilities (Foley, 1990; Giangreco, 1986; Orelove & Sobsey, 1991; Rainforth et al., 1992b).

The transdisciplinary model permits greater coordination of comprehensive services for individuals with complex health, educational, and social needs than most other approaches. Two of the distinguishing features of the model are that assessments are conducted collaboratively by team members and a single, discipline-free service plan is

developed to meet the highest priority needs of the child and family. This mode of operation contrasts with other service delivery models in which service providers conduct separate assessments and develop separate, discipline-referenced intervention plans (Woodruff & McGonigel, 1988).

Another distinguishing feature of the transdisciplinary model is that one team member is designated as the primary service provider, who is usually the person who spends the greatest amount of time with the child or the person who has the skills necessary to address the child's greatest areas of need (Orelove & Sobsey, 1991; Woodruff & McGonigel, 1988). The primary service provider will change as the child's needs and environments change over time. A parent or physical therapist may be the primary service provider for an infant or young child, a teacher the primary service provider for an older child, and a personal care assistant the primary service provider for a young adult.

When employing a transdisciplinary approach, team members are responsible for determining which of their own disciplinary knowledge and skills are needed by the child, for consulting with and teaching the necessary knowledge and skills to the primary service provider and for monitoring outcomes. The primary service provider incorporates the knowledge and strategies of other disciplines into ongoing intervention with the child. In effect, team members "release" part of their roles to the primary service provider (Orelove & Sobsey, 1991; Woodruff & McGonigel, 1988).

Assessment of Disability

Assessment of a child's disability is best conducted in the environments in which the child actually participates or environments in which children of similar age and social background participate. Assessment in natural environments is increasingly advocated for all children who have disabilities, but especially for children with mental retardation who have difficulty generalizing skills from one setting to another. Such environmentally based assessment is also far more likely to lead to intervention that results in age-appropriate, functional outcomes than assessment that takes place in isolated or clinical settings, assessments that are based on a normal developmental sequence, or assessments that focus primarily on identification of impairments, such as range of motion, postural responses, or retention of primitive reflexes (Brown et al., 1979; Orelove & Sobsey, 1991; Rainforth et al., 1992b).

ECOLOGICAL OR ENVIRONMENTAL ASSESSMENTS

Brown and associates (1979) described an ecological or environmental approach to assessment that has subsequently been promoted by many others as a means to determine functional outcomes and plan programs for people who have mental retardation and, more recently, for children in early intervention programs (Falvey, 1989; Orelove & Sobsey, 1991; Rainforth et al., 1992a; Thurman & Widerstrom, 1990). Functional outcomes have been emphasized in special education for a number of years and are increasingly being supported by pediatric physical therapists and therapists in other areas of practice (Harris, 1991; McEwen, 1992; Rainforth et al., 1992a). Functional skills have been defined as those activities or tasks that someone else will have to do if the child does not (Brown et al., 1979), are age appropriate (Falvey, 1989), and reflect the needs and interests of the child and family (Orelove & Sobsey, 1991). Some children can learn to complete a task or activity, others will be capable of learning to carry out only a part of it. Partial participation, or completion of only part of a task, is a legitimate outcome for some children who have severe disabilities (Ferguson & Baumgart, 1991). A child may, for example, be unable to transfer independently but can learn to unbuckle a seat belt and support his or her weight in standing. Another child may be unable to put a tape into a tape recorder but can learn to turn it on using a switch.

An ecological assessment is an approach or format, rather than a specific assessment instrument. There are four major steps in an ecological assessment, as described by Orelove and Sobsey (1991):

1. *Determine the domains to be included in the child's program.* Four domains are considered to be primary: home, community (e.g., school, stores, and church), vocational, and recreation-leisure. Certain critical skills, such as mobility, communication, and hand use are required for functioning in all domains.

2. *Determine the environments and subenvironments within each domain in which the child currently functions or could function in the future.* A child's team might identify the home, school, and restaurant as especially important. Subenvironments could be the bedroom at home, the cafeteria at school, and the restroom in a restaurant.

3. *Determine the activities the child needs to function in each of the subenvironments.* Activities could include getting out of bed at home, obtaining and eating lunch at school, and using the toilet in a restaurant.

4. *Determine the skills the child needs for each activity.* Skills are determined through task analysis of the activities and identifying the components the child needs to be able to do to accomplish each of them. To get out of bed, for example, one child may need to respond to the alarm, remove the covers, assume a sitting position, and transfer to a wheelchair. A child with less ability could learn to do other components of the task, such as rolling over to sit up after the covers have been removed and assisting with the transfer.

An example of an ecological assessment is included in the case history of Jeff at the end of the chapter.

ARENA ASSESSMENT

An arena assessment is another type of assessment format that has been recommended for children with severe disabilities (Wolery & Dyk, 1984) and is widely used by transdisciplinary teams in early intervention programs (Foley, 1990; Woodruff & McGonigel, 1988). In an arena assessment, all team members observe the child at the same time and write an integrated report of their observations. This approach not only provides a more holistic and focused picture of the child than occurs when each discipline assesses the child separately, but both parents and professional team members have perceived the arena approach to give a truer picture of the child's abilities, lead to more parent involvement, and promote greater team interaction and consensus (Wolery & Dyk, 1984).

During an arena assessment, one family member or professional interacts with the child and directs preplanned activities, while the other team members sit at the periphery of the interaction and record their observations of the child's behaviors. These observations often focus on discipline-specific concerns, including discipline-related portions of comprehensive developmental tests, but observations are made within the context of the overall flow of behaviors exhibited as the child and facilitator interact. Team members are encouraged to record observations that may not be considered part of their disciplinary expertise.

Following the assessment, the team meets to discuss their observations, consider other available information, and collaboratively plan the intervention. In this way each team member can gain an understanding of the child's overall capabilities and limitations, and recognize relationships among motor, communication, cognitive, social-emotional, and other behaviors. One criticism of the arena assessment is that it is conducted under artificial conditions using contrived tasks, so does not provide as accurate a picture of a child's functional capabilities and limitations within the natural environment as does an ecological assessment (Rainforth et al., 1992a).

Determining Intervention Goals

Goals of intervention to reduce a child's disability need to represent specific functional skills that the child will acquire. Team members cannot assume that goals directed toward remediation of impairments, such as improving postural responses, range of motion, or strength, or toward reducing the degree of functional limitations indicated by failed items on a developmental test, will necessarily lead to meaningful outcomes (Harris, 1991; McEwen, 1992; Rainforth et al., 1992a). This is especially true of children with mental retardation who need many repetitions to learn, forget easily, and generalize poorly. This makes it unlikely that a child with mental retardation will be able to synthesize isolated activities or components of movement into meaningful skills (Orelove & Sobsey, 1991; Rainforth et al., 1992a).

PH Campbell (1991) proposed a "top-down" approach to determining goals, in which the desired functional outcomes or goals are determined first, then obstacles to their accomplishment are identified, and then intervention to overcome the obstacles is planned and implemented (Fig. 18-1). As described earlier as a component of an ecological assessment, functional outcomes can be anything that are high priority and meaningful to the child and family, are age appropriate, and are, or could be, a home, community, recreation-leisure, or vocational activity (Brown et al., 1979; Falvey, 1989; Orelove & Sobsey, 1991). Five valued life outcomes for all children, including those with severe disabilities have been proposed (Giangreco et al., 1993, p. 4):

1. Having a safe, stable home in which to live now and/or in the future
2. Having access to a variety of places and engaging in meaningful activities
3. Having a social network of personally meaningful relationships
4. Having a level of personal choice and control that matches one's age
5. Being safe and healthy

Obstacles to accomplishment of functional skills

TOP-DOWN APPROACH

A

BOTTOM-UP APPROACH

B

FIGURE 18-1. Comparison of a top-down approach (A), in which assessments identify means to achieve desired outcomes, and a bottom-up approach (B), in which assessment results determine outcomes. (From Campbell, PH: Evaluation and assessment in early intervention for infants and toddlers. Journal of Early Intervention, 15:42, 1991. Copyright 1991 by Division for Early Childhood, the Council for Exceptional Children.)

are often impairments associated with the child's condition, such as poor postural control or inadequate force production. These obstacles can either be overcome by intervention designed to reduce the impairments and develop skilled movement or bypassed through use of assistive technology or other compensatory strategies. An ecological assessment is a useful tool for identifying obstacles to be overcome and skills that the child needs to acquire to accomplish a desired outcome.

Teams usually have the most difficulty determining meaningful outcomes for children with profound multiple disabilities who often have extremely limited repertoires of behavior. Evans and Scotti (1989) maintain that even these children can accomplish goals that require active behavioral changes, such as indicating a choice of food or activity or increasing body movements used to activate switches. Such active goals lead to acquisition of skills that reduce disability and are in contrast to passive activities that are done to the child, such as sensory stimulation, range of motion exercises, and positioning (often stated as something the child will "tolerate"). Passive activities may be part of the intervention to help a child accomplish active goals, but only the child's active behavior can reduce disability (Downing, 1988).

When desired outcomes are determined first, goals are discipline free; that is, they describe the skills the child will accomplish without regard for discipline-related concerns. Only after team members identify the highest priority goals do they decide which disciplines will be needed to help the child accomplish each one (Rainforth et al., 1992a). Amy's case history at the end of this chapter provides an example of functional outcomes and the physical therapist's role.

INTERVENTION

During planning and implementation of intervention for children with mental retardation, it is important to keep in mind what are widely regarded as "best practices" for working with children who have cognitive disabilities. Some of these practices have been discussed previously and include: families and children as full and equal team members; assessment in natural environments; and an emphasis on functional outcomes with active participation by children.

Other considerations that influence if and how intervention is provided for children with mental retardation involve full inclusion of children with mental retardation in least restrictive environ-

ments; use of cognitive referencing as a means to determine who will receive physical therapy services; use of teaching methods that are most likely to result in acquisition of motor skills by children with mental retardation; and the role of physical therapists in promoting development in nonmotor domains. These issues are discussed in the following sections.

Inclusion of Children with Mental Retardation

The concept of least restrictive environments has its roots in the United States constitution, which affirms that the government shall intrude into peoples' lives in the least restrictive manner possible (Witkin & Fox, 1992). Since the 1960s, this concept has been incorporated into state and federal laws affecting services for people with mental retardation, mandating that, to the extent possible, people with disabilities will go to school, live, and work in environments with people who do not have disabilities (Taylor, 1988).

The definition of the least restrictive environment for people with mental retardation has been moving steadily away from segregated services and toward full inclusion in community-based settings, as evidenced by closure of many institutions for people with mental retardation and court-ordered inclusion of children with mental retardation in general education classrooms. In 1992, for example, a judge of the U.S. Court for the District of New Jersey ordered a New Jersey school district to develop a plan to include an 8-year-old boy with Down syndrome in his neighborhood elementary school, with any needed supplementary aids and services. One of the court's findings was that "School districts . . . must consider placing children with disabilities in regular classroom settings, with the use of supplementary aids and services . . ., before exploring other, more restrictive, alternatives." ("The TASH Force," 1992, p. 2).

Physical therapy is one of the services that must follow children with mental retardation as they move into their communities and neighborhood schools. Not only must physical therapy be provided in these settings, but it must promote children's accomplishment of functional outcomes that will enable them to participate as successfully as possible in inclusive environments (Rainforth et al., 1992a). Giangreco and colleagues (1993) have written a helpful "how to" manual for inclusion of children with severe disabilities in general education classrooms that addresses provision of physical therapy and other related services.

Cognitive Referencing

Cognitive referencing is an approach that has been used to determine whether children are eligible for services, especially for physical therapy, occupational therapy, and speech pathology in public schools (Carr, 1989). The approach is based on an assumption that children's potentials for gains in motor and communication development are related to their cognitive abilities and that children whose cognitive abilities are lower than or equal to their motor or communication abilities cannot benefit from services, so are not eligible for them.

Obviously, many children with mental retardation could be declared "ineligible" for physical therapy services under such an assumption, so the use of cognitive referencing has been highly controversial (Giangreco, 1990; Notari et al., 1992; Rainforth, 1991). Critics have been supported by at least one retrospective study that cast doubt on the validity of cognitive referencing as a means to predict which children will make gains in motor development (Cole et al., 1991) and by the U.S. Department of Education, Office of Special Programs (OSEP), which declared cognitive referencing to be an unlawful means to determine whether a child should receive related services in public schools (Rainforth, 1991). The OSEP statement reiterated the authority of each child's educational team to decide on the services necessary for that child to meet individualized educational goals. When goals of children with mental retardation and neuromotor impairments focus on functional outcomes, some type of physical therapy is often needed.

Teaching and Learning Considerations

Much of what physical therapists do is teach children to move more effectively and efficiently. A number of teaching strategies have been identified by educational researchers that optimize the learning of students with mental retardation and can be helpful to physical therapists when designing and implementing intervention plans. Although most of the strategies were designed for educational programming of students with mental retardation, they have also been recommended for infants and toddlers participating in early intervention (Hanson & Lynch 1989), and they can be applied to motor learning as well as academic learning. Many

of the strategies are closely related to current motor learning principles (see Chapter 6).

INSTRUCTION IN NATURAL ENVIRONMENTS

One strategy that has received considerable attention in recent years and is intended to address several of the learning problems of students with mental retardation, especially severe mental retardation, is a focus on teaching functional skills in natural environments (Brown et al., 1979; Falvey, 1989). Because it takes students with mental retardation a long time to learn a few things, and because they have difficulty generalizing and maintaining skills, traditional curricula that build sequentially on fundamental, nonfunctional skills have not generally led to meaningful gains. Children are often unable to generalize such nonfunctional activities as putting pegs in pegboards, for example, to functional activities such as putting coins in a machine to get a soft drink. Practicing "prerequisite" skills, such as writing the letters of the alphabet, also often fails to result in such functional outcomes as the ability to sign one's name or select the correct restroom in a public place.

Similar difficulties are often encountered by children with severe motor impairments when nonfunctional or presumed prerequisite skills are the focus of physical therapy. Research has largely failed to support children's generalization (carryover) of skills demonstrated during physical therapy sessions to other settings or synthesis of presumed components and prerequisites of movement into measurable functional motor activities (Horn, 1991).

When the emphasis is on acquisition of specific functional skills in natural environments, generalization is unnecessary or less difficult and skills are likely to be maintained by natural reinforcers and ongoing occasions for practice (Orelove & Sobsey, 1991). If several people work with the child on the same skills, learning may be enhanced by providing more opportunities to learn (repetitions) and by varying the stimulus conditions under which the skill is practiced, thus promoting generalization. These principles serve as a basis for integrated models of service delivery that have been advocated for physical therapists and occupational therapists working in early intervention and public school programs (Giangreco, 1986; Orelove & Sobsey, 1991; Rainforth et al., 1992a). Although there is limited research to support the effectiveness of teaching motor skills in natural environments, research in other areas, such as life skills, language, and social interaction, suggests that such an approach would be valuable.

BEHAVIORAL PROGRAMMING INTERVENTION

Behavioral programming is based on the assumption that behaviors are learned through interactions with the social, physical, and biological environments, so, by manipulating the environment, behaviors can be taught (Bijou, 1966). Following a review of research on the effectiveness of motor skills instruction for children with neuromotor impairments, Horn (1991) concluded that physical therapists and occupational therapists should develop procedures to incorporate behavioral techniques into their intervention programs. She made this recommendation because of the relative success of interventions using behavioral techniques compared with the neuromotor and sensory stimulation techniques commonly used by occupational therapists and physical therapists. By incorporating behavioral techniques into other intervention strategies, physical therapists may not only be able to increase the rate at which children with mental retardation acquire motor skills and the number of skills they acquire but may also promote generalization and maintenance of motor behaviors.

Positive Reinforcement. A child is positively reinforced by a stimulus if a behavior that preceded the stimulus increases (Lutzker et al., 1983). Possible reinforcing stimuli are unlimited, ranging from tangible items, such as food and stickers, to social reinforcers, such as attention or praise, and abstract reinforcers, such as self-approval (Snell & Zirpoli, 1987). With children who have mental retardation, especially severe or profound retardation, common reinforcers such as praise, access to activities, and food often fail to lead to increases in behaviors, and identification of reinforcers can be a challenge (Orelove & Sobsey, 1991). To identify potential reinforcers, Haney and Falvey (1989) suggest 1) identifying natural consequences of the behavior, such as playing in water as a consequence of walking to the sink; 2) surveying the child's likes and dislikes by observing the child, or asking the child, parents, or teachers; and 3) offering paired choices to determine which of several potential reinforcers the child considers to be the most desirable. It is important that reinforcers not be overused, because children can become satiated and the stimuli will no longer have reinforcement value (Snell & Zirpoli, 1987).

Reinforcers have been effective in increasing motor behaviors, such as use of music as biofeedback to increase an erect head position (Maloney &

Kurtz, 1982), and a combination of music and food to increase the distance that a child walked independently (Chandler & Adams, 1972). A common limitation of such studies, however, is that few have examined generalization to nonexperimental settings or maintenance of the behaviors beyond the period of intervention. Also, reinforcement has not been shown to result in acquisition of behaviors not previously in the child's repertoire. A combination of reinforcement with antecedent techniques and modification of consequences have, however, resulted in new behavioral responses (Horn, 1991; Reid et al., 1991).

Antecedent Techniques. The first step in shaping a new behavior is to prompt the desired behavior or an approximation by providing instructions, models, cues, or physical prompts (Snell & Zirpoli, 1987). *Instructions* can take a variety of forms, such as verbal or gestural instructions (e.g., "reach for the toy") or verbal instructions paired with models, cues, or physical prompts (e.g., "reach for the toy," paired with facilitation of movement at the shoulder). *Modeling* provides a demonstration of a behavior that the child attempts to imitate. *Cues* direct a child's attention to a task that can result in the desired behavior, without a physical prompt. To cue the child to reach for the toy, the toy could be tapped on the table or held above the child to encourage an erect posture, reaching, and/or assuming a standing position. Many of the handling techniques used by physical therapists provide *physical prompts* for motor behaviors.

For optimal learning to occur, the type and amount of prompting needs to be matched to the skills of the child, with the least amount of help necessary being the most conducive to the child's learning (Snell & Zirpoli, 1987). Prompting should be faded as the child responds, so that natural cues eventually provide the stimulus for response. A natural cue is the least intrusive prompt (e.g., the presence of a friend serving as a cue for a child to lift the head) and is the level of prompt required for independent behaviors. Physical prompts, often used by physical therapists, are the most intrusive.

Providing Consequences. Once a behavior has been prompted, it can be improved or expanded through shaping or chaining techniques. Shaping and chaining can also be used to build new behaviors (Snell & Zirpoli, 1987) through reinforcement of behaviors that successively approximate the desired behavior.

New behaviors can be *shaped* by reinforcing behaviors that are increasingly similar to the target behavior, such as reinforcing components of standing up from a chair, or *chaining* to link standing, walking, opening doors, and other behaviors necessary to accomplish a goal of walking to lunch. Backward chaining, in which the last step in the sequence is learned first, is often a useful technique because children receive the reward of task completion, often a natural reinforcer, throughout the process of learning the skill (Lutzker et al., 1983; Snell & Zirpoli, 1987).

Behavioral intervention is one of the areas in which physical therapists should take advantage of the expertise of other members of service delivery teams, such as teachers and psychologists. Physical therapy educational prerequisites and curricula rarely provide more than superficial information about behavioral strategies, which limits the extent to which many physical therapists can use them effectively to promote the development of motor skills by children with mental retardation.

Promoting Children's Communication Development

When working with children who have mental retardation, all team members are responsible for promoting development in areas often not considered part of their disciplinary domains. One of the most effective ways physical therapists can contribute to the overall development of children with mental retardation is to assist efforts to improve their communicative competence. At its most basic, communication enables children to influence their social and physical environments to control what happens to themselves. All children, even those with the most profound multiple disabilities, can communicate. Some communicate in many of the same ways as infants, such as looking at a person, crying, or smiling; others can learn to communicate using signs, communication boards, or electronic voice-output communication aids (Siegel-Causey & Downing; 1987; see also Chapter 23). Ability to control what happens to themselves is often said to be the key to prevention or reduction of these children's pervasive passivity or "learned helplessness," a condition that can effectively block educational efforts and be extremely resistant to change (Campbell, PH, 1989).

The critical importance of communication and the need for all team members to participate in communication development was recognized by creation in the United States of the National Joint Committee for the Communicative Needs of Persons with Severe Disabilities in 1986. Representatives of seven organizations, including the American Physical Therapy Association, served on the joint committee and developed guidelines that crossed traditional disciplinary boundaries and re-flect a "shared commitment to promoting effective communication by persons with severe disabilities thus providing a common ground on which the disciplines of the member organizations can unite their efforts to improve the quality of life of such persons" (National Joint Committee for the Communicative Needs of Persons with Severe Disabilities, 1992, pp. 1–2). This means that physical therapists are responsible for promoting effective communication, not only through such traditional means as positioning and improving motor skills to enable access to communication aids but also through provision of environments that acknowledge and address the Communication Bill of Rights (Fig. 18–2) of children who have communication impairments (National Joint Committee for the Communicative Needs of Persons with Severe Disabilities, 1992).

Assessment of Outcomes for All Age Groups

Because children and young adults with mental retardation often progress slowly, particularly those with severe disabilities, it is important to use assessment methods that can be sensitive to small changes. This is necessary not only to document progress but also to prevent expenditure of time and effort on intervention strategies that are not leading to meaningful outcomes. Three related methods that are especially useful for assessing outcomes of physical therapy intervention for children with mental retardation are 1) accomplishment of behavioral objectives, 2) goal attainment scaling, and 3) single-subject research methodologies.

USE OF BEHAVIORAL OBJECTIVES

Assessment of outcomes can be relatively straightforward if functional goals and behavioral objectives leading to them are identified before intervention. As described by O'Neill and Harris (1982), the components of a behavioral objective enable therapists to monitor a child's progress toward accomplishment of a goal, to determine if it is necessary to modify an intervention, and to establish that goals have been met. Once a goal has been identified, such as "David will go to the kitchen and make himself a peanut butter sandwich," behavioral objectives leading to achievement of the goal can be developed by comparing David's abilities with the goal's requirements. There are five components of a behavioral objective: *Who* will do *what*, under what *conditions*, *how*

All persons, regardless of the extent or severity of their disabilities, have a basic right to affect, through communication, the conditions of their own existence. Beyond this general right, a number of specific communication rights should be ensured in all daily interactions and interventions involving persons who have severe disabilities. These basic communication rights are as follows:

1. The right to request desired objects, actions, events, and persons and to express personal preferences or feelings.

2. The right to be offered choices and alternatives.

3. The right to reject or refuse undesired objects, events, or actions, including the right to decline or reject all proffered choices.

4. The right to request, and be given, attention from and interaction with another person.

5. The right to request feedback or information about a state, an object, a person, or an event of interest.

6. The right to active treatment and intervention efforts to enable people with severe disabilities to communicate messages in whatever modes and as effectively and efficiently as their specific abilities will allow.

7. The right to have communication acts acknowledged and responded to, even when the intent of these acts cannot be fulfilled by the responder.

8. The right to have access at all times to any needed augmentative and alternative communication devices and other assistive devices and to have those devices in good working order.

9. The right to environmental contexts, interactions, and opportunities that expect and encourage persons with disabilities to participate as full communicative partners with other people, including peers.

10. The right to be informed about the people, things, and events in one's immediate environment.

11. The right to be communicated with in a manner that recognizes and acknowledges the inherent dignity of the person being addressed, including the right to be part of communication exchanges about individuals that are conducted in his or her presence.

12. The right to be communicated with in ways that are meaningful, understandable, and culturally and linguistically appropriate.

FIGURE 18-2. Communication bill of rights. (From Guidelines for Meeting the Communication Needs of Persons with Severe Disabilities by the National Joint Committee for the Communication Needs of Persons with Severe Disabilities, 1992.)

well, by *when*. These components permit an objective assessment of whether the goal is being met within the projected time frame. One of David's behavioral objectives, leading to the sandwich-making goal, may be to move himself from the living room to the kitchen, which could be written, "David will walk using his reverse walker from the living room to the kitchen in less than 2 minutes on four of five consecutive days after school by December 14, 199—." It should not be difficult to assess whether this objective, or part of it, is accomplished, regardless of the intervention methods used.

GOAL ATTAINMENT SCALING

Goal attainment scaling is a measure that is similar to a behavioral objective, but it permits more finely tuned assessment of outcomes. A change score can also be calculated, which provides a useful measure to examine the effectiveness of interventions across children or to assess change across all goals of one child (Palisano et al., 1992).

For goal attainment scaling, goals are first identified that have all of the components of behavioral objectives, described above. Then two levels of attainment that exceed the goal and two levels of attainment that do not meet the goal are written. This provides five possible outcomes that relate specifically to a child's individual needs and abilities. By specifying goals both above and below a child's expected achievement, it is possible to assess a range of outcomes directed toward the same general goal (Palisano et al., 1992).

SINGLE-SUBJECT RESEARCH METHODOLOGIES

Single-subject research methodologies are another useful means to objectively assess intervention outcomes in clinical, educational, and other service settings. As described in Chapter 7 of this volume, these methodologies can be used to assess the outcomes for a single child or can assess effects of intervention across several children (Harris, 1991). McEwen and Karlan (1989) used an alternating treatment single-subject design to compare the effect of positioning in a chair, stander, prone wedge, and sidelyer on the ability of two preschool children to access a switch placed in several locations on a communication board–like grid. As shown in Figure 18–3, the data revealed that it took longer for both of the children to press the switch when they were in the sidelyer than when in the other three positions.

TRANSITION TO ADULTHOOD

Some children with mental retardation, especially those with severe and profound multiple disabilities, have need for physical therapy throughout their childhood years and during their transition to adulthood. The type of services provided will change with the needs of the child, as will the intensity of services and the service delivery model employed. Therapists working in public schools are especially likely to be involved in the transition to adulthood because Part B of the Individuals with Disabilities Education Act now requires that transi-

tion planning begin by at least age 16 for all students in special education.

The transition to adulthood is difficult for many young people, regardless of their abilities or disabilities. Until relatively recently, most young adults with mental retardation had few options available to them and the greater their cognitive impairments, the fewer options they had. Employment options either did not exist or were limited to sheltered workshops or activity centers. Residential options usually included staying at home with aging parents or moving into a large residential facility. They also had few choices about how they spent their time, with whom they spent time, or where they could go.

In recent years more employment and community life options have become available for people with mental retardation, including those with the most severe multiple disabilities. To be able to take full advantage of these options, young people need to prepare for transition to adult life throughout their years in school and then continue to receive support as the transition takes place and the new life begins. Physical therapy services can often make a critical difference in the options available to young people with mental retardation and neuromotor impairments as they make the transition to adult life and in the success of their transitions. Employment and residential options are especially important for most young people.

FIGURE 18-3. A single-subject alternating treatment design assessing means and ranges of switch-activation latency when two children were positioned in a chair, stander, pronewedge, and sidelyer. (From McEwen, IR, & Karlan, GR. Assessment of the effects of position on communication board access by individuals with cerebral palsy. Augmentative and Alternative Communication, 5:238–239, 1989. Copyright 1989 by the International Society for Augmentative and Alternative Communication.)

Employment

Employment options in the United States for people with mental retardation and multiple disabilities have expanded greatly over the past several years, particularly in some parts of the country. There are still many places in which sheltered workshops, activity centers, or unemployment are the only alternatives, but progress is being made nationwide as federal, state, and other public and private initiatives support development and expansion of employment opportunities for people with disabilities (Bates, 1989; Rusch et al., 1991).

Supported employment, one model of employment services, has been responsible for increasing the employment options for those who have severe disabilities. Supported employment not only provides assistance to identify and acquire a job but also provides a person with ongoing support to learn how to do the job and to keep the job. There is no need to wait until a person is "ready" to do a job through sheltered training or "prevocational" activities, which usually fail to lead to meaningful, integrated employment even after long periods of time.

Since the early 1980s, supported employment has been gaining credibility as a viable employment option and received significant support from the Vocational Rehabilitation Act Amendments of 1986 (PL 99-506), which authorized new funds for states to provide supported employment services to people with severe disabilities. Few communities, as yet, however, offer a supported employment alternative to sheltered workshops and day activity centers for those with the most severe disabilities (Black & Meyer, 1992; Rusch et al., 1991). The value of supported employment was indicated by Rusch and his colleagues (1991), who reviewed reports of supported employment programs from around the United States. They concluded that 1) people with any type of disability can earn significantly more money in supported employment than in sheltered programs; 2) employers have shown strong commitments to the integration of employees with disabilities; and 3) supported employment programs are more cost effective than activity and workshop programs.

Physical therapy can often have a pivotal role in the successful employment of individuals who have both mental retardation and limited motor skills. Physical therapists can assist employment specialists to assess an individual's abilities to perform job-related motor skills and to identify jobs that are compatible with those skills. They can also identify assistive technology and environmental modifications that may enable the person to perform a job that might not be possible otherwise. Physical ther-apists can also help to develop training for job-related motor skills and for self-care and mobility during working hours.

Residential Options

Most children with mental retardation live with their birth parents or with foster families. Some live in congregate residential facilities, such as state institutions for people with mental retardation, but many states have limited admission of children to such facilities in recent years (Willer & Intagliata, 1984). Although it was once believed that placement outside the home was the best alternative for children with mental retardation, public policy, education, and professional opinion now promote inclusion of most children in their natural homes (Blacher et al., 1992; Brown et al., 1989).

The factors associated with out-of-home placement of children with disabilities have been of concern to a number of researchers in recent years. Level of retardation, maladaptive behaviors, and physical disability are variables that have been shown to predict whether children with mental retardation will be placed out of their homes (Eyman et al., 1972; Meyers et al., 1985; Sherman, 1988). A more recent study suggests that ethnic background may also play a role in placement decisions, with more Anglo children being placed than African-American, Hispanic, or other ethnic groups (Blacher et al., 1992). Family characteristics, such as needs and resources, are also likely to influence whether a child is placed out of the home (Cole & Meyer, 1989).

With the current emphasis on deinstitutionalization and providing supports needed by families to keep their children with disabilities at home, planning for residential transitions has become an important part of their service programs as children with disabilities approach adulthood. The available residential options depend largely on the philosophies of those providing residential services, funding from state, federal, and other agencies, and the needs of the individual (Brown et al., 1989).

Large institutions are rarely considered a viable residential option today. Group homes for 3 to 6 people, located among other homes in residential neighborhoods, are about as large as facilities can be and still provide opportunities for integration into the neighborhood and community (Brown et al., 1989). Such living arrangements in the United States can be designated as an intermediate care facility for the mentally retarded, thus qualifying for Medicaid funds to provide the necessary staff and services. Residential options can also include living alone, or with one to three others in a house, apartment, or duplex, with the necessary support services.

Although community-living options for people with severe disabilities have increased steadily over the past decade, they are still limited in most communities, and necessary support services are often not available, either because of lack of funds or personnel shortages (Smull & Bellamy, 1991). Whatever the residential future of children with mental retardation and neuromotor impairments, physical therapy services can often help to expand the options, ease the transition, and promote independence within the residential environment.

CASE HISTORY: ALISE

Alise is 32 months old and has received home-based early intervention services since the age of 8 months. She has lissencephaly (also known as smooth brain syndrome), which was identified when she was 5 months old and had a seizure. Alise lives with her parents and 12-year-old brother in a suburb of a large city.

When Alise was 8 months old she did very little. She had great difficulty moving against the force of gravity, did not have head control, and could not roll over, sit, reach for objects, or grasp objects placed in her hands. She did not appear to make eye contact with people or objects and had difficulty sucking from a bottle and swallowing. The evaluation team conducted an arena assessment to document Alise's eligibility for early intervention services, with team members using the tests or parts of tests that they thought would be the most appropriate. The physical therapist and occupational

therapist used the Peabody Developmental Motor Scales (PDMS) (Folio & Fewell, 1983) to assess gross and fine motor development; the speech-language pathologist used the Early Learning Accomplishment Profile for Young Children (ELAP) (Glover et al., 1988) to evaluate Alise's communication; the child development specialist used the ELAP to evaluate cognitive and social/emotional development; and the occupational therapist used the Hawaii Early Learning Profile (HELP) (Furuno et al., 1988) to evaluate self-help skills. At the age of 8 months, Alise's age-equivalent scores were in the birth to 2-month range on all measures.

During the meeting to develop the Individualized Family Service Plan (IFSP), a top-down approach was used to first identify outcomes of intervention and then the strategies to achieve them. Alise's parents said that what they wanted most for Alise was for her to be able to roll over and sit by herself. They were also concerned about her vision and the difficulty she had swallowing without choking while drinking from her bottle.

A transdisciplinary model of service delivery was used by the early intervention program, and the team selected the physical therapist to be the primary service provider because Alise's parents were primarily concerned about her motor problems. The occupational therapist and a vision specialist would consult with the physical therapist to address the feeding and vision concerns, and other team members would be available for consultation as other needs were identified.

The physical therapist made weekly visits to Alise's home, working with Alise, her parents, and her brother to promote Alise's ability to move in opposition to the force of gravity, to eat more effectively, and to attend visually to people and objects in her environment (Figs. 18–4 and 18–5). A plastic booster chair with a tray,

FIGURE 18-4. Physical therapist showing Alise's mother how to help her to learn to move from a sitting position.

FIGURE 18-5. Physical therapist doing an ecological assessment of Alise's mealtime in her home.

which is widely available for typical infants, was modified to enable Alise to maintain a seated position while on the floor or at the table. A stroller was also adapted for her.

Two years later, at 2 years, 8 months, Alise can now maintain a sitting position when placed on the floor, drink liquids and eat ground foods without difficulty, and easily focus on and track objects and people. She is still unable to assume a sitting position, roll or move about on the floor. She has particular difficulty using her hands and holds only her bottle, if it is placed in her hands, and will occasionally reach for her favorite fuzzy rubber ball. She sometimes uses her mouth to get things that she wants and will raise her legs when she is on her back in bed and wants to be picked up. She says about 10 words, including "no," "ahm" (mom), "da" (dad), and an approximation of her brother's name. Assistive equipment she now uses includes an adapted highchair, booster chair, and stroller, a prone stander, a walker with a tray, and a bath seat.

Two months ago, when Alise was 30 months old, she was reevaluated and the IFSP was revised. Her age equivalent scores on the following tests were

Gross motor: 4 months (PDMS)
Fine motor: 2 months (PDMS)
Cognition: 9–10 months (ELAP)
Communication: 10–12 months (ELAP)
Social-emotional: 11–12 months (ELAP)
Self-help: 10–12 months (HELP)

When the IFSP was revised, the desired outcomes identified by her parents were 1) that Alise would learn to get into and out of sitting by herself, 2) that she would learn to move around on the floor, and 3) that she would be able to play with toys with her hands. Because Alise's family continued to be primarily concerned about her motor development, the physical therapist remained the primary service provider. The IFSP also included a plan to prepare for Alise's transition from the early intervention program when she turns 3. Her mother wants Alise to stay at home until she is 5, so the early intervention team must identify the services that Alise and her family will need and determine how they can be obtained through other community agencies, such as the local education agency or developmental disabilities services.

CASE HISTORY: AMY

Amy is an 8-year-old who is in a third-grade class in her neighborhood elementary school where her favorite subjects are music and science. Until the beginning of the current school year, she was in a self-contained special education class with seven other children with severe and profound disabilities. The Battelle Developmental Inventory (Newborg et al., 1984) was administered to document her continuing eligibility for special education services and her age-equivalent scores were personal-social, 7 months; adaptive, 5 months; motor, 4 months; communication, 6 months; and cognitive, 5 months. For special education purposes, she is classified as having profound mental retardation with multiple disabilities.

During a meeting last spring to develop her Individualized Education Program (IEP), Amy's parents said they were concerned because Amy was so passive, did so little, and seemed interested in so few things. They had three priorities for her education: 1) that she learn to choose things, people, and activities that she wants; 2) that she become someone that other people like to be with because one of the things she seems to enjoy is being with other children; and 3) that she learn to help more during caregiving activities because she is becoming heavier and more difficult to handle and move. After some discussion and clarification, her parents and educational team developed the following long-term goals to address these priorities:

1. Amy will indicate her choice of a person, activity, or object at least 10 times each day at school and 10 times at home for 5 consecutive days by May, 199—.

2. When engaged in an activity with her classmates, Amy will interact with them by such means as looking at them, smiling, reaching, or vocalizing for at least 3 of 10 minutes during two activities on 5 consecutive school days by May, 199—.

3. Amy will assist in transferring from her wheelchair by leaning forward when touched on the shoulder and asked to stand up and then bear her full weight after being assisted to a standing position during 10 consecutive transfers from her wheelchair by May, 199—.

The team then wrote a sequence of short-term behavioral objectives leading to each goal and decided which team members would be necessary to help Amy to achieve them and what each would contribute. The team also identified the general supports that Amy needs to attend school and to achieve her goals. Giangreco and associates (1993) described five categories of general supports, including supports needed to meet personal, physical, and sensory needs, to teach others about the student, and to provide the student with access and opportunities. The supports identified for Amy were

1. Personal: feeding, diaper changing, and other self-care

2. Physical: positioning and mobility

3. Sensory: avoiding intense stimuli, which cause Amy to withdraw

4. Teaching: teaching other children about Amy, her means of communication, and how to help her participate in activities

5. Access: promoting hand use during classroom activities

Given the educational program they had developed for Amy, her parents and the rest of the educational team decided that her educational needs could be met in a general education classroom, with supplemental aids and services. They agreed that a congregated special

education setting was not only unnecessarily restrictive but that a general education classroom was more likely to provide the social and educational environment necessary to help Amy accomplish her goals. Supplemental aids and services in the general education classroom include a half-time assistant assigned to the classroom and ongoing consultation between Amy's classroom teacher and her special education team (a resource teacher, occupational therapist, physical therapist, and speech-language pathologist).

Amy's physical therapist is primarily involved with her third goal, involving transfers, and with the physical supports of positioning and mobility. She also assists, when necessary, with aspects of other goals and consults with the physical education teacher about how to include Amy in activities that are meaningful for her.

To provide the necessary positioning and mobility supports, the physical therapist first determined that Amy's wheelchair was adequate for her needs. She also consulted with Amy's classroom teacher to determine which alternatives to wheelchair positioning would be used during which activities and who would be responsible for position changes. Positions and activities were matched to enable Amy to function as well as possible throughout the day. She uses a supine stander, for example, during a morning science class, which usually involves groups of students standing around tables as they work on a project together. She also stands in the afternoon during art class because her hand use seems to be better when she is standing.

The therapist taught the teacher and assistant how to place Amy in her wheelchair and other positioning devices, about some of the basic mechanics of the wheelchair, and how to push the chair safely. She also taught Amy's classmates how to push Amy safely and issued wheelchair pushing licenses to those who demonstrated safe pushing techniques. Other supports provided by the physical therapist were to teach Amy's teacher, the assistant, and her classmates some ways to encourage Amy to raise her head and use her hands during classroom activities, and teaching the assistant methods to use caregiving activities, especially diaper changing, to help maintain Amy's joint flexibility. The assistant also used diaper changing, when Amy was supine, as an opportunity to teach basic social interaction skills.

To help Amy achieve the goal of assisting with transfers, the physical therapist first worked with Amy to identify how best to help her to learn. She found that, although Amy could perform some aspects of a transfer, such as lean forward to prepare to stand, she usually would not, either spontaneously or when asked. She also did not place her feet on the floor as she was moved toward a standing position and did not bear her weight when placed on her feet. To teach Amy to assist with these components of the transfer, the physical therapist consulted with the special education resource teacher to develop a behavioral program. The program included 1) providing verbal and natural cues for a transfer (such as the presence of the supine stander), physical prompts, and reinforcement for leaning forward in her wheelchair, a motor behavior that was already within Amy's repertoire; 2) providing cues, physical prompts, and reinforcement during practice to learn to place her feet on the floor and bear increasing amounts of weight, during transfers and other activities, to shape these skills, which were not yet within Amy's repertoire; 3) chaining the various components of the transfer, as Amy began to learn each one; and 4) eventually fading the verbal cues and physical prompts to permit the natural cues surrounding transfers to prompt Amy's participation.

After she was reasonably sure that the program developed to teach Amy to lean forward was effective, the physical therapist taught Amy's teacher, the classroom assistant, and her parents to implement the techniques whenever Amy transferred. Because Amy had not demonstrated the ability to place her feet on the floor and bear her weight in standing, the physical therapist worked with Amy several days a week for 2 weeks during transfers and other classroom activities to determine how best to provide physical prompts and other cues and to teach Amy to begin to learn to stand. She then taught Amy's teacher, the assistant, and her parents how to help Amy continue to develop this skill.

CASE HISTORY: JEFF

Jeff is a 20-year-old who recently moved from Sunnyvale, a state residential facility for people with mental retardation, to a boarding house in the small town where his parents live. Three other young adults with disabilities live at the boarding house and they invited Jeff to live with them after he visited with them several months ago.

Jeff has spastic quadriplegic cerebral palsy and moderate mental retardation and lived at Sunnyvale since he was 7 years old. For the first 9 years he spent most of his time in bed, receiving basic care but little education or habilitative services other than passive range of motion exercises.

When Jeff was 18, physical therapy and other services were expanded as a result of a court order. Since then, Jeff acquired and learned to use an electronic communication aid and an electric wheelchair. The chair has a custom-contoured seat and back to accommodate his moderate scoliosis, pelvic asymmetry with windswept hips, and lower extremity flexion contrac-

tures, which developed in spite of the passive range of motion exercises. He also learned to assume a standing position and bear much of his weight during assisted transfers. Bilateral ankle-foot orthoses, improved positioning in bed and wheelchair, active participation during all transfers, and use of good alternative positioning appear to have helped to limit progression of his musculoskeletal deformities.

In preparation for Jeff's transition to the boarding house, his physical therapist, occupational therapist, and mother took him there for an ecological assessment to determine what skills Jeff needed to live there successfully. He can get help with dressing, bathing, and laundry, if necessary, but he has to be able to use the toilet independently and transfer to and from his bed without assistance. He also has to be able to use the telephone, make his own breakfast and lunch, and go shopping in a nearby grocery-variety store (see ecological assessment in Table 18–3, format from Baumgart et al., 1982).

To prepare for his move, Jeff's physical therapist worked with him on the aspects of toilet transfers and shopping identified by the ecological assessment, simulating what he will encounter in the community. Before Jeff actually moved, he, his therapists, and his mother spent several days at the boarding house going through a typical day to help Jeff generalize skills he learned at Sunnyvale to the boarding house and to identify problems and the means to overcome them.

When he moved to the community, Jeff enrolled in the local high school and a new IEP was written. Two of Jeff's educational goals relate to improving his independence at home and obtaining, learning, and keeping a job. His school physical therapist works with Jeff and his personal care assistant to increase his independence in his home and is working with his job coach to identify a job that Jeff can learn. Once a job is found, his physical therapist will also help Jeff learn to use public transportation and to use the toilet at work and will provide ongoing consultation with the job coach to solve problems as they arise.

The physical therapist's involvement to help Jeff become more independent in his home and work environments is directed toward reducing his disabilities. Positioning and orthoses are used to reduce functional limitations and prevent the development of additional musculoskeletal impairments. For Jeff, it is also important that he maintain or increase his flexibility and endurance. For this reason, the physical therapist helped Jeff find a YMCA in his community that has an accessible swimming pool and a gym in which he can work out. In collaboration with YMCA staff, the therapist and Jeff developed an exercise program appropriate for Jeff's needs and that he can carry out with the assistance of YMCA personnel. The physical therapist is available to serve as a consultant as needed.

TABLE 18-3 EXAMPLE OF AN ECOLOGICAL ASSESSMENT

Name: Jeff
Activity: Shopping
Environment: Dan's One-Stop

Steps Required	Jeff's Current Performance	Steps Can Acquire	Steps May Not Acquire	Compensatory Strategies	Intervention
1. Go from home to Dan's and back using electric wheelchair	Can open front door (outward), go down ramp and drive to the corner. Cannot go down curb (no curb cut), cross street safely, or go up curb. Once on the sidewalk, can drive to Dan's. Cannot open door from outside. Can maneuver inside store and open door when leaving (outward). Cannot open door of home when returning.	1. Open doors of home and store when the door opens toward him; 2. go down curb 3. ask for assistance and tell someone how to help him up a curb; and 4. cross the street safely.	Go up a curb without assistance	Curb cut	1. Teach Jeff to open doors, go down curbs, and cross streets safely (PT, PCA). 2. Talk with city about making curb cuts and with store and house manager about modifying doors (Jeff, CM). 3. Program communication aid to request help with curbs and give instructions (mother, PT).
2. Select items in the store	Does not always remember what he needs to get and cannot make or read a shopping list. Can get items that are at hand level, cannot shift weight or extend arm to reach low or high items.	1. Make and use shopping list; 2. improve ability to reach high and low items; and 3. ask for assistance to get out-of-reach items.	Reach items that are very high or very low	A reacher	1. Teach Jeff to make and use a shopping list (OT, PCA). 2. to use a reacher, if it seems feasible (OT, PCA); and 3. to reach to higher and lower shelves (PT, PCA).
3. Carry items to checkout stand	Cannot maneuver shopping cart. Items slide off lap, does not want to use tray.	Carry items in a bag or other container on lap or chair	Push a grocery cart without endangering store and other people	Bag or other container that is accessible to Jeff	Find container and teach Jeff to use it (OT and PCA).
4. Put items on counter	Can put items on counter, but is very slow, which annoys people in line behind him.	1. Put container on counter so clerk can remove items; or 2. ask for assistance	1. Increase speed sufficiently; or 2. lift full container to counter.	None	1. Try to improve speed and lifting of container (PT, PCA); and 2. program communication aid and teach Jeff to ask for assistance (mother and PCA).

Table continued on following page

483

TABLE 18–3. **EXAMPLE OF AN ECOLOGICAL ASSESSMENT** *Continued*

Steps Required	Jeff's Current Performance	Steps Can Acquire	Steps May Not Acquire	Compensatory Strategies	Intervention
5. Pay for purchases	Cannot get wallet out of pocket, cannot get money out of wallet. Does not recognize denominations of bills or coins, cannot pay correct amount or check change.	1. Get money out of suitable container; 2. recognize bills and coins; and 3. give sufficient money to cover the purchase.	1. Get wallet out of pocket or money out of wallet; and 2. determine if change is accurate.	1. Use an accessible container for money; and 2. ask personal care assistant to compare bill and change occasionally.	1. Find accessible container for money and teach Jeff to use it (OT, PCA); and 2. teach Jeff to use money (OT, mother, PCA).
6. Carry purchases home	Can carry small bag on lap, cannot carry large bag(s)	Carry purchases in container attached to chair	Carry large or multiple bags on lap	Alternate container (probably the same as in 3, above)	Find appropriate container for purchases (OT, PCA).
7. Put purchases away	Can open cupboards with flat surfaces or knobs, drawers with knobs, and the refrigerator. Cannot open high or low cupboards or drawers with flat surfaces. Can put purchases away in places he can open and reach.	1. Open all drawers he can reach; and 2. put items away in higher and lower places.	Put items in very high or low places.	1. Make adaptations to allow Jeff to open kitchen drawers he can reach. 2. Rearrange cupboards and drawers so items Jeff uses are accessible.	1. Discuss adaptations and rearrangement with house manager (OT); and 2. improve Jeff's reach (also in 2, above) (PT, PCA).

*Note: Those involved with each intervention are determined after the intervention is identified. At this time, Jeff has the assistance of his personal care assistant (PCA), case manager (CM), mother, occupational therapist (OT), and physical therapist (PT).

References

Acredolo, LP, Adams, A, & Goodwyn, SW. The role of self-produced movement and visual tracking in infant spatial orientation. Journal of Experimental Child Psychology, 38:312–327, 1984.

Affolter, FD. Perception, Interaction and Language: Interaction of Daily Living: The Root of Development. New York: Springer-Verlag, 1991.

American Association on Mental Retardation. Mental Retardation: Definition, Classification, and Systems of Supports (9th ed.). Washington, DC: American Association on Mental Retardation, 1992.

Anwar, F. Cognitive deficit and motor skill. In Ellis, D (Ed.), Sensory Impairments in Mentally Handicapped People. San Diego: College Hill Press, 1986, pp. 169–183.

Aughton, DJ, & Cassidy, SB. Physical features of Prader-Willi syndrome in neonates. American Journal of Diseases of Children, 144:1251–1254, 1990.

Badell, A. Myelodysplasia. In Molnar, GE (Ed.), Pediatric Rehabilitation. Baltimore: Williams & Wilkins, 1992, pp. 222–253.

Bates, P. Vocational training for persons with profound disabilities. In Brown, F, & Lehr, DH (Eds.), Persons with Profound Disabilities: Issues and Practices. Baltimore: Paul H Brookes, 1989, pp. 265–293.

Baumgart, D, Brown, L, Pumpian, I, Nisbet, J, Ford, A, Sweet, M, Messina, R, & Schroeder, J. Principle of partial participation and individualized adaptations in educational programs for severely handicapped students. The Journal of the Association for the Severely Handicapped, 7(2):17–27, 1982.

Bayley, N. Bayley II (2nd ed.). San Antonio: Psychological Corporation, 1993.

Benson, JB, & Uzgiris, IC. Effect of self-initiated locomotion on infant search activity. Developmental Psychology, 21:923–931, 1985.

Berg, JM, McCreary, BD, Ridler, MAC, & Smith, GF. The de Lange Syndrome. New York: Pergamon Press, 1970.

Bergsma, D. Birth Defects: Atlas and Compendium. Baltimore: Williams & Wilkins, 1973.

Bertenthal, BI, Campos, JJ, & Barrett, KC. Self-produced locomotion: An organizer of emotional, cognitive, and social development in infancy. In Emde, RN, & Harmon, RJ (Eds.), Continuities and Discontinuities in Development. New York: Plenum, 1984.

Bijou, SW. A functional analysis of retarded development. In Ellis, NR (Ed.), International Review of Research in Mental Retardation, Vol. 1. New York: Academic Press, 1966, pp. 1–19.

Blacher, JB, Hanneman, RA, & Rousey, AB. Out-of-home placement of children with severe handicaps: A comparison of approaches. American Journal of Mental Retardation, 96:607–616, 1992.

Black, JW, & Meyer, LH. But . . . is it really work? Social validity of employment training for persons with very severe disabilities. American Journal on Mental Retardation, 96:463–474, 1992.

Bloom, AS, Hersh, JH, Podruch, PE, Weisskopf, B, Topinka, CW, & Reese, A. Developmental characteristics of recognizable patterns of human malformation. In Berg, JM (Ed.), Science and Service in Mental Retardation: Proceedings of the Seventh Congress of the International Association for the Scientific Study of Mental Deficiency (IASSMD). New York: Methuen, 1985, pp. 34–55.

Brown, L, Branston, MB, Hamre-Nietupski, S, Pumpian, I, Certo, N, & Gruenewald, L. A strategy for developing chronological age appropriate and functional curricular content for severely handicapped adolescents and young adults. Journal of Special Education, 13:81–90, 1979.

Brown, F, Davis, R, Richards, M, & Kelly, K. Residential services for adults with profound disabilities. In Brown, F, & Lehr, DH (Eds.), Persons with Profound Disabilities: Issues and Practices. Baltimore: Paul H Brookes, 1989, pp. 295–331.

Burgemeister, BB, Blum, LH, & Lorge, I. Manual: Columbia Mental Maturity Scale (3rd ed.). New York: Psychological Corporation, 1972.

Butler, C. Augmentative mobility: Why do it? Physical Medicine and Rehabilitation Clinics of North America, 2:801–815, 1991.

Butler, C, Okamoto, GA, & McKay, TM. Powered mobility for very young disabled children. Developmental Medicine and Child Neurology, 25:472–474, 1983.

Campbell, FA, & Ramey, CT. High risk infants: Environmental risk factors. In Berg, JM (Ed.), Science and Service in Mental Retardation: Proceedings of the Seventh Congress of the International Association for the Scientific Study of Mental Deficiency (IASSMD). New York: Methuen, 1985, pp. 23–33.

Campbell, PH. Dysfunction in posture and movement with individuals with profound disabilities. In Brown, F, and Lehr, DH (Eds.), Persons with Profound Disabilities: Issues and Practices. Baltimore: Paul H. Brookes, 1989, pp. 163–189.

Campbell, PH. Evaluation and assessment in early intervention for infants and toddlers. Journal of Early Intervention, 15:36–45, 1991.

Campbell, SK. Central nervous system dysfunction in children. In Campbell, SK (Ed.), Pediatric Neurologic Physical Therapy (2nd ed.) New York: Churchill Livingstone, 1991, pp. 1–17.

Campos, JJ, & Bertenthal, BI. Locomotion and psychological development in infancy. In Jaffe, KM (Ed.), Childhood Powered Mobility: Developmental, Technical and Clinical Perspectives: Proceedings of the RESNA First Northwest Regional Conference. Washington, DC: RESNA, 1987, pp 11–42.

Carr, SH. Louisiana's criteria of eligibility for occupational therapy services in the public school system. American Journal of Occupational Therapy, 43:503–506, 1989.

Carter, CH. Handbook of Mental Retardation Syndromes (2nd ed.). Springfield, IL: Charles C. Thomas, 1970.

Chandler, LS, & Adams, MA. Multiply handicapped child motivated for ambulation through behavior modification. Physical Therapy, 52:339–401, 1972.

Chinitz, SP, & Feder, CZ. Psychological assessment. In Molnar, GE (Ed.), Pediatric Rehabilitation (2nd ed.). Baltimore: Williams & Wilkins, 1992, pp. 48–87.

Cole, DA, & Meyer, LH. Impact of needs and resources on family plans to seek out-of-home placement. American Journal on Mental Retardation, 93:380–387, 1989.

Cole, KN, Mills, PE, & Harris, SR. Retrospective analysis of physical and occupational therapy progress in young children: An examination of cognitive referencing. Pediatric Physical Therapy, 3:185–189, 1991.

Downing, J. Active versus passive programming: A critique of IEP objectives for students with the most severe disabilities. Journal of the Association for Persons with Severe Handicaps, 13:197–201, 1988.

Drotar, D, Mortimer, J, Shepherd, PA, & Fagan, JF. Recognition memory as a method of assessing intelligence of an infant with quadriplegia. Developmental Medicine and Child Neurology, 31:391–394, 1989.

Eagle, RS. Deprivation of early sensorimotor experience and cognition in the severely involved cerebral-palsied child. Journal of Autism and Developmental Disabilities, 15:269–283, 1985.

Ellis, NR. Handbook of Mental Deficiency: Psychological Theory and Research. London: McGraw Hill, 1963.

Evans, IM. Testing and diagnosis: A review and evaluation. In

Meyer, LH, Peck, CA, & Brown, L (Eds.), Critical Issues in the Lives of People with Severe Disabilities. Baltimore: Paul H Brookes, 1991, pp. 25–43.

Evans, IM, & Scotti, JR. Defining meaningful outcomes for persons with profound disabilities. In Brown, F, & Lehr, DH (Eds.), Persons with Profound Disabilities: Issues and Practices. Baltimore: Paul H Brookes, 1989, pp. 83–107.

Eyman, RK, O'Connor, G, Tarjan, G, & Justice, RS. Factors determining residential placement of mentally retarded children. American Journal on Mental Deficiency, 76:692–698, 1972.

Fagan, JF, & Shepherd, PA. The Fagan Test of Infant Intelligence Training Manual. Cleveland: Infatest Corporation, 1987.

Falvey, MA. Introduction. In Falvey, MA (Ed.), Community-Based Curriculum: Instructional Strategies for Students with Severe Handicaps. Baltimore: Paul H Brookes, 1989, pp. 1–13.

Ferguson, DL, & Baumgart, D. Partial participation revisited. Journal of the Association for Persons with Severe Handicaps, 16:218–227, 1991.

Fogel, A, Dedo, JY, & McEwen, IR. Effect of postural position and reaching on gaze during mother-infant face-to-face interaction. Infant Behavior and Development, 15:231–244, 1992.

Fogel, A, & Thelen, E. The development of early expressive and communicative action: Reinterpreting the evidence from a dynamic systems perspective. Child Development, 23:747–761, 1987.

Foley, GM. Arena evaluation: Assessment in the transdisciplinary approach. In Gibbs, ED, & Teti, DM (Eds.), Interdisciplinary Assessment of Infants: A Guide for Early Intervention Professionals. Baltimore: Paul H Brookes, 1990, pp 271–286.

Folio, MR, & Fewell, RR. Peabody Developmental Motor Scales and Activity Cards. Chicago: Riverside Publishing, 1983.

Fraser, BA, Hensinger, RN, & Phelps, JA. Physical Management of Multiple Handicaps: A Professional's Guide (2nd ed.). Baltimore: Paul H Brookes, 1990.

Furuno, S, O'Reilly, KA, Hosaka, CM, Inatsuka, TT, Zeisloft-Falbey, B, & Allman, T. Hawaii Early Learning Profile. Palo Alto, CA: VORT Corporation, 1988.

Gesell, A. Gesell Development Schedules. New York: Psychological Corporation, 1940.

Giangreco, MF. Delivery of therapeutic services in special education programs for learners with severe handicaps. Physical and Occupational Therapy in Pediatrics, 6(2):5–15, 1986.

Giangreco, MF. Letter to the editor. American Journal of Occupational Therapy, 44:470, 1990.

Giangreco, MF, Cloninger, CH, & Iverson, VS. Choosing Options and Accommodations for Children: A Guide to Planning Inclusive Education. Baltimore: Paul H Brookes, 1993.

Gibbs, ED. Assessment of infant mental ability: Conventional tests and issues of prediction. In Gibbs, ED, & Teti, DM (Eds.), Interdisciplinary Assessment of Infants: A Guide for Early Intervention Professionals. Baltimore: Paul H Brookes, 1990, pp. 77–89.

Glover, ME, Preminger, JL, & Sandford, AR. The Early Learning Accomplishment Profile for Young Children. Chapel Hill, NC: Chapel Hill Training-Outreach Project, 1988.

Greenough, WT, Black, JE, & Wallace, CS. Experience and brain development. Child Development, 58:539–559, 1987.

Grossman, HJ. Classification in Mental Retardation. Washington, DC: American Association on Mental Retardation, 1983.

Guess, D. Forward. In Brown, F, & Lehr, DH (Eds.), Persons with Profound Disabilities: Issues and Practices. Baltimore: Paul H Brookes, 1989, pp. ix–xi.

Guess, D, Mulligan-Ault, M, Roberts, S, Struth, J, Siegel-Causey, E, Thompson, B, Bronicki, GJB, & Guy, B. Implications of biobehavioral states for the education and treatment of students with the most profoundly handicapping conditions. Journal of the Association for Persons with Severe Handicaps, 13:163–174, 1988.

Guidera, KJ, Borrelli, J, Jr, Raney, E, Thompson-Rangel, T, & Ogden, JA. Orthopaedic manifestations of Rett syndrome. Journal of Pediatric Orthopaedics, 11:204–208, 1991.

Gustafson, GE. Effects of the ability to locomote on infants' social and exploratory behaviors: An experimental study. Developmental Psychology, 20:397–405, 1984.

Haney, M, & Falvey, MA. Instructional strategies. In Falvey, MA (Ed.), Community-Based Curriculum: Instructional Strategies for Students with Severe Handicaps. Baltimore: Paul H Brookes, 1989, pp. 63–90.

Hanson, MJ, & Lynch, EW. Early Intervention: Implementing Child and Family Services for Infants and Toddlers Who Are At-Risk or Disabled. Austin, TX: PRO-ED, 1989.

Harris, SR. Functional abilities in context. In Lister, MJ (Ed.), Contemporary Management of Motor Control Problems: Proceedings of the II Step Conference. Alexandria, VA: Foundation for Physical Therapy, 1991, pp. 253–259.

Harris, SR, & Shea, AM. Down syndrome. In Campbell, SK (Ed.), Pediatric Neurologic Physical Therapy (2nd ed.). New York: Churchill Livingstone, 1991, pp. 131–168.

Hays, RM. Childhood motor impairments: Clinical overview and scope of the problem. In Jaffe, KM (Ed.), Childhood Powered Mobility: Developmental, Technical and Clinical Perspectives: Proceedings of the RESNA First Northwest Regional Conference. Washington, DC: RESNA, 1987, pp. 1–10.

Holm, VA, & King, HA. Scoliosis in the Rett syndrome. Brain Development, 12:151–153, 1990.

Horn, EM. Basic motor skills instruction for children with neuromotor delays: A critical review. Journal of Special Education, 25:168–197, 1991.

Houghton, J, Bronicki, GJB, & Guess, D. Opportunities to express preferences and make choices among students with severe disabilities in classroom settings. Journal of the Association for Persons with Severe Handicaps, 12:18–27, 1987.

Hulme, JB, Gallacher, K, Walsh, J, Niesen, S, & Waldron, D. Behavioral and postural changes observed with use of adaptive seating by clients with multiple handicaps. Physical Therapy, 67:1060–1067, 1987.

Jankovic, J, Caskey, TC, Stout, JT, & Butler, IJ. Lesch-Nyhan syndrome: A study of motor behavior and cerebrospinal fluid neurotransmitters. Annals of Neurology, 23:466–469, 1988.

Jones, ED, & Payne, JS. Definition and prevalence. In Patton, JR, Payne, JS, & Beirne-Smith, M (Eds.), Mental Retardation (2nd ed.). Columbus, OH: Charles E Merrill, 1986, pp. 33–75.

Kaufman, A, & Kaufman, N. Kaufman Assessment Battery for Children. Circle Pines, MN: American Guidance Service, 1983.

Kelleher, A, & Mulcahy, M. Patterns of disability in the mentally handicapped. In Berg, JM (Ed.), Science and Service in Mental Retardation: Proceedings of the Seventh Congress of the International Association for the Scientific Study of Mental Deficiency (IASSMD). New York: Methuen, 1985, pp. 15–22.

Keenan, J, Kastner, T, Nathanson, R, Richardson, N, Hinton, J, & Cress, DA. A statewide public and professional education program on fragile X syndrome. Mental Retardation, 30:355–361, 1992.

Kermonian, R, & Campos, JJ. Locomotor experience: A facilitator of spatial cognitive development. Child Development, 59:908–917, 1988.

Kochanek, TT, Kabacoff, RI, & Lipsitt, LP. Early identification of developmentally disabled and at-risk preschool children. Exceptional Children, 56:528–538, 1990.

Kopp, CB, & McCall, RB. Predicting later mental performance for normal at-risk, and handicapped infants. In Baltes, PB, & Brim, OG (Eds.), Life-Span Development and Behavior. New York: Academic Press, 1982, pp. 33–61.

Landesman-Dwyer, S, & Sackett, GP. Behavioral changes in nonambulatory, profoundly mentally retarded individuals. In Meyers, CE (Ed.), Quality of Life in Severely and Profoundly Mentally Retarded People: Research Foundations for Improvement. Washington, DC: American Association on Mental Deficiency, 1978, pp. 55–144.

Laurance, BM, Brito, A, & Wilkinson, J. Prader-Willi syndrome after age 15 years. Archives of Disease in Childhood, 56:181–186, 1981.

Leiter, R. The Leiter International Performance Scale. Chicago: Stoelting, 1969.

Lutzker, JR, McClinsey-McRae, S, & McClinsey, JP. General description of behavioral approaches. In Hersen, M, Van Hasselt, VB, & Matson, JL (Eds.), Behavior Therapy for the Developmentally and Physically Disabled. New York: Academic Press, 1983, pp. 25–56.

Maloney, FP, & Kurtz, PA. The use of a mercury switch head control device in profoundly retarded, multiply handicapped children. Physical and Occupational Therapy in Pediatrics, 2(4):11–17, 1982.

McCall, RB. Issues in the early development of intelligence and its assessment. In Lewis, M, & Taft, L (Eds.), Developmental Disabilities: Theory, Assessment and Intervention. New York: SP Medical and Scientific Books, 1982, pp. 177–184.

McEwen, IR. Assistive positioning as a control parameter of social-communicative interactions between students with profound multiple disabilities and classroom staff. Physical Therapy, 72:634–647.

McEwen, IR, & Karlan, GR. Assessment of effects of position on communication board access by individuals with cerebral palsy. Augmentative and Alternative Communication, 5:235–242, 1989.

McEwen, IR & Lloyd, LL. Positioning children with cerebral palsy to use augmentative and alternative communication. Language, Speech, and Hearing Services in Schools, 21:15–21, 1990.

McLaren, J, & Bryson, SE. Review of recent epidemiological studies of mental retardation: Prevalence, associated disorders, and etiology. American Journal on Mental Retardation, 92:243–254, 1987.

Mercer, JR. Labeling the Mentally Retarded. Berkeley: University of California Press, 1973.

Meyers, CE, Borthwick, SA, & Eyman, RK. Place of residency by age, ethnicity, and level of retardation of the mentally retarded/developmentally disabled population of California. American Journal on Mental Deficiency, 90:266–270, 1985.

Molnar, GE. Cerebral palsy. In Molnar, GE (Ed.), Pediatric Rehabilitation. Baltimore: Williams & Wilkins, 1992, pp. 481–533.

National Joint Committee for the Communicative Needs of Persons with Severe Disabilities. Guidelines for meeting the communication needs of persons with severe disabilities. ASHA, 34 (suppl 7).1–8, 1992.

Navajas, D, Farre, R, Mar Rotger, M, Milic-Emili, J, & Sanchis, J. Effect of body posture on respiratory impedance. Journal of Applied Physiology, 64:194–199, 1988.

Newborg, J, Stock, JR, Wnek, L, Guidubaldi, J, & Svinicki, J. Battelle Developmental Inventory. Chicago: Riverside Publishing, 1984.

Nihira, K, Foster, R, Shellhaas, M, & Leland, H. AAMD Adaptive Behavior Scale (rev. ed.). Washington, DC: American Association on Mental Deficiency, 1974.

Nomura, Y, & Segawa, Y. Characteristics of motor disturbance in Rett syndrome. Brain Development, 12:27–30, 1990.

Notari, AR, Cole, KN, & Mills, PE. Cognitive referencing: The (non)relationship between theory and application. Topics in Early Childhood Special Education, 11(4):22–38, 1992.

Nwaobi, OM. Seating orientations and upper extremity function in children with cerebral palsy. Physical Therapy, 67:1209–1212, 1987.

Nwaobi, OM, & Smith, PD. Effect of adaptive seating on pulmonary function of children with cerebral palsy. Developmental Medicine and Child Neurology, 28:351–354, 1986.

Nyhan, WL, & Sakati, NO. Genetic and Malformation Syndromes in Clinical Medicine. Chicago: Year Book Medical Publishers, 1976.

O'Neill, DL, & Harris, SR. Developing goals and objectives for handicapped children. Physical Therapy, 62:295–298, 1982.

Orelove, FP, & Sobsey, D. Designing transdisciplinary services. In Orelove, FP, & Sobsey, D (Eds.), Educating Children with Multiple Disabilities. A Transdisciplinary Approach (2nd ed.). Baltimore: Paul H Brookes, 1991, pp. 1–31.

Palisano, RJ, Halcy, SM, & Brown, DA. Goal attainment scaling as a measure of change in infants with motor delays. Physical Therapy, 72:432–437, 1992.

Parette, HP, Jr, & Hourcade, JJ. How effective are physiotherapeutic programmes with young mentally retarded children who have cerebral palsy? Journal of Mental Deficiency Research, 28:167–175, 1984.

Rainforth B. Biobehavioral state and orienting: Implications for educating profoundly retarded students. Journal of the Association for the Severely Handicapped, 6:33–37, 1982.

Rainforth, B. OSERS clarifies legality of related services eligibility criteria. TASH Newsletter, April 1991, p. 8.

Rainforth, B, Macdonald, C, York, J, & Dunn, W. Collaborative assessment. In Rainforth, B, York, J, & Macdonald, C (Eds.), Collaborative Teams for Students with Severe Disabilities: Integrating Therapy and Educational Services. Baltimore: Paul H Brookes, 1992a, pp. 105–155.

Rainforth, B, York, J, & Macdonald, C. Foundations of collaborative teamwork. In Rainforth, B, York, J, & Macdonald, C (Eds.), Collaborative Teams for Students with Severe Disabilities: Integrating Therapy and Educational Services. Baltimore: Paul H Brookes, 1992b, pp. 9–41.

Ramey, CT, & Ramey, SL. Effective early intervention. Mental Retardation, 30:337–345, 1992.

Raven, J. Raven's Progressive Matrices. Dumfries, Scotland: Crichton Royal, 1958.

Reid, DH, Phillips, JF, & Green, CW. Teaching persons with profound multiple handicaps: A review of the effects of behavioral research. Journal of Applied Behavior Analysis, 24:319–336, 1991.

Rinck, C. Fragile X syndrome. Dialogue on Drugs, Behavior and Developmental Disabilities (University of Missouri), 4(3):1–4, 1992.

Rosenberg, SA, & Robinson, CC. Assessment of the infant with multiple handicaps. In Gibbs, ED, & Teti, DM (Eds.), Interdisciplinary Assessment of Infants: A Guide for Early Intervention Professionals. Baltimore: Paul H Brookes, 1990, pp. 177–188.

Rose, SA, & Wallace, IF. Individual differences in infants' information processing. Reliability, stability, and prediction. Child Development, 59:1177–1197, 1988.

Rusch, FR, Chadsey-Rusch, J, & Johnson, JR. Supported employment: Emerging opportunities for employment integration. In Meyer, LH, Peck, CA, & Brown, L (Eds.), Critical Issues in the Lives of People with Severe Disabilities. Baltimore: Paul H Brookes, 1991, pp. 145–169.

Sents, B, & Marks, H. Changes in preschool children's IQ scores as a function of positioning. American Journal of Occupational Therapy, 43:685–687, 1989.

Sherman, BR. Predictors of the decision to place developmentally disabled family members in residential care. American Journal on Mental Retardation, 92:344–351, 1988.

Shumway-Cook, A, & Woollacott, MH. Dynamics of postural control in the child with Down syndrome. Physical Therapy, 65:1315–1322, 1985.

Siegel-Causey, E, Downing, J. Nonsymbolic communication development: Theoretical concepts and educational strategies. In Goetz, L, Guess, D, Stremel-Campbell, K (Eds.), Innovative Program Design for Individuals with Dual Sensory Impairments. Baltimore: Paul H Brookes, 1987, pp. 15–48.

Slater, A, Cooper, R, Rose, D, & Morrison, V. Prediction of cognitive performance from infancy to early childhood. Human Development, 32:137–147, 1989.

Smith, DW. Recognizable Patterns of Human Malformation (2nd ed.). Philadelphia: WB Saunders, 1976.

Smull, MW, & Bellamy, GT. Community services for adults with disabilities: Policy challenges in the emerging support paradigm. In Meyer, LH, Peck, CA, & Brown, L (Eds.), Critical Issues in the Lives of People with Severe Disabilities. Baltimore: Paul H Brookes, 1991, pp. 527–536.

Snell, ME, & Zirpoli, TJ. Intervention strategies. In Snell, ME (Ed.), Systematic Instruction of Persons with Severe Handicaps (3rd ed.). Columbus, OH: Charles E Merrill, 1987, pp. 110–149.

Sparrow, SS, Balla, DA, & Cichetti, CV. Vineland Adaptive Behavior Scales. Circle Pines, MN: American Guidance Service, 1984.

Stewart, KB, Brady, DK, Crowe, TK, & Naganuma, GM. Rett syndrome: A literature review and survey of parents and therapists. Physical and Occupational Therapy in Pediatrics, 9(3):35–55, 1989.

Switzky, HN, Woolsey-Hill, J, & Quoss, T. Habituation of visual fixation responses: An assessment tool to measure visual sensory-perceptual cognitive processes in nonverbal profoundly handicapped children in the classroom. AAESPH Review, 4:136–147, 1979.

Tarjan, G, Wright, SW, Eyman, RK, & Keeran, DV. Natural history of mental retardation: Some aspects of epidemiology. American Journal on Mental Deficiency, 77:369–379, 1973.

TASH force strikes again: Laski and Boyd win Oberti case in New Jersey. TASH Newsletter, November 1992, pp. 1–2.

Taylor, SJ. Caught in the continuum: A critical analysis of the principle of the least restrictive environment. Journal of the Association for Persons with Severe Handicaps, 13:41–53, 1988.

Telzrow, RW, Campos, JJ, Shepherd, A, Bertenthal, BI, & Atwater, S. Spatial understanding in infants with motor handicaps. In Jaffe, KM (Ed.), Childhood Powered Mobility: Developmental, Technical and Clinical Perspectives: Proceedings of the RESNA first Northwest Regional Conference. Washington, DC: RESNA, 1987, pp. 62–69.

Terman, LM, & Merrill, MA. Stanford-Binet Intelligence Scales (3rd rev.). Boston: Houghton Mifflin, 1973.

Thoresen, M, Cowan, F, & Whitelaw, A. Effect of tilting on oxygenation in newborn infants. Archives of Disease in Childhood, 63:315–317, 1988.

Thurman, SK, & Widerstrom, AH. Infants and Young Children with Special Needs: A Developmental and Ecological Approach. Baltimore: Paul H Brookes, 1990.

United Cerebral Palsy National Infant Collaborative Project. Staff Development Handbook: A Resource for the Transdisciplinary Process. New York: United Cerebral Palsy Association, 1976.

Verburg, G, Naumann, S, Balfour, L, & Snell, E. Remote training of mobility skills in persons who are physically and developmentally disabled. Proceedings of the RESNA 13th Annual Conference. Washington, DC: RESNA, 1990, pp. 195–196.

Verburg, G, Snell, E, Pilkington, M, & Milner, M. Effects of powered mobility on young handicapped children and their families. Proceedings of the 2nd International Conference on Rehabilitation Engineering. Washington, DC: RESNA, 1984, pp. 172–173.

Wechsler, D. Wechsler Intelligence Scale for Children—Revised. New York: Psychological Corporation, 1974.

Willer, B, & Intagliata, J. An overview of the social policy of deinstitutionalization. In Ellis, N, & Bray, N (Eds.), International Review of Research in Mental Retardation, Vol. 12. New York: Academic Press, 1984.

Witkin, SL, & Fox, L. Beyond the least restrictive environment. In Villa, RA, Thousand, JS, Stainback, W, & Stainback, S (Eds.), Restructuring for Caring and Effective Education. Baltimore: Paul H Brookes, 1992, pp. 325–334.

Wolery, M, & Dyk, L. Arena assessment: Description and preliminary social validity data. Journal of the Association for Persons with Severe Handicaps, 9:231–234, 1984.

Woodruff, G, & McGonigel, MJ. Early intervention team approaches: The transdisciplinary model. In Jordan, JB, Gallagher, JJ, Huntinger, PL, & Karnes, MB (Eds.), Early Childhood Special Education: Birth to Three. Reston, VA: The Council for Exceptional Children and its Division for Early Childhood, 1988, pp. 163–181.

Zazula, JL, & Foulds, RA. Mobility device for a child with phocomelia. Archives of Physical Medicine and Rehabilitation, 64:137–139, 1983.

Zelazo, PR, & Weiss, MJ. Infant information processing: An alternative approach. In Gibbs, ED, & Teti, DM (Eds.), Interdisciplinary Assessment of Infants: A Guide for Early Intervention Professionals. Baltimore: Paul H Brookes, 1990, pp. 129–143.

Zucker, SH, & Polloway, EA. Issues in identification and assessment in mental retardation. Education and Training in Mental Retardation, 22:69–76, 1987.

Chapter 19

Cerebral Palsy

SANDRA J. OLNEY, BSc(P&OT), MEd, PhD
MARILYN J. WRIGHT, BScPT, MEd

INTRODUCTION

Cerebral palsy (CP) is a neurodevelopmental impairment caused by a nonprogressive defect or lesion in single or multiple locations in the immature brain. The defect or lesion can occur in utero or during or shortly after birth and produces motor impairment and possible sensory deficits that are usually evident in early infancy (Scherzer & Tscharnuter, 1990). CP involves one or more limbs and frequently the trunk. It causes disturbances of voluntary motor function and produces a variety of symptoms. Nevertheless, CP is itself an artificial concept, comprising several causes and clinical syndromes that have been lumped together because of a commonality of management. The impaired control and coordination of voluntary muscles is accompanied by mental retardation or learning disabilities in 50 to 75% of children and by disorders of speech (25%), auditory impairments (25%), seizure disorders (25–35%), or abnormalities of vision (40–50%) (Batshaw & Perret, 1992; Ndlazalaukaa, 1992). Social and family problems may occur secondary to the presence of primary deficits.

CP has been classified in a number of ways. A classification based on the area of the body showing impairment yields the designations monoplegia (one limb), diplegia (lower limbs), hemiplegia (upper and lower limbs on one side of the body), and quadriplegia (all limbs). Another classification, based on the most obvious impairment resulting from common brain lesions, yields spastic, dyskinetic, and ataxic types. The spastic type, in which the muscles are perceived as excessively stiff and taut, especially during attempted movement, results from involvement of the motor cortex or white matter projections to and from cortical sensorimotor areas of the brain. Involvement of the basal ganglia is reflected in dyskinesia or athetosis and sometimes in intermittent muscular tension of the extremities or trunk and involuntary movement patterns. A cerebellar lesion produces ataxia, or general instability of movement. A hypotonic classification, not known to be related to a particular lesion, is characterized by diminished resting tension and decreased ability to generate voluntary muscle force. Symptoms of spasticity and dyskinesia may both be present in a child, with the type of CP referred to as mixed. The degree of severity of CP varies greatly, and the designations mild, moderate, and severe are often applied within types. Although the proportions of the various subtypes of CP vary with the reporting source, a series from Sweden noted that hemiplegia accounted for 36.4%; diplegia, 41.5%, quadriplegia, 7.3%; dyskinesia or athetosis, 10%; and ataxic forms, 5% (Hagberg et al., 1989a).

CP is a condition with multiple causes leading to damage within the central nervous system. Although the causes are not completely understood, certain prenatal, perinatal, and postnatal factors have been associated with CP (Torfs et al., 1990). There is general agreement that the majority of cases of CP in term infants are due to prenatal or unknown causes, whereas in the vast majority of preterm infants the lesion causing CP develops during the perinatal period. Preterm birth, although not believed to be causative, is associated with up to 33% of all cases, including more than 50% of diplegia (Pharoah et al., 1990), 25% of hemiplegia, (Uvebrandt, 1988), and 5% of quadriplegia (Edebol-Tysk, 1989). Prenatal malnutrition, intrinsic developmental problems of the fetus, poor maternal prenatal condition, and maternal infection are also associated with CP (Menkes, 1990). Intracranial hemorrhage, especially among premature infants, is a well-established causal factor. Neonatal asphyxia is a significant perinatal event, but only a small minority of cases result from such events (Nelson & Ellenberg, 1986). Infection in the perinatal period is also important. The effects of hyperbilirubinemia and other blood incompatibilities, frequently resulting in athetoid CP, have been virtually eliminated in developed countries but remain an important concern in developing countries.

The statistics from developing countries are in sharp contrast to those of developed countries. Studies have suggested that up to 63% of cases in the former have preventable causes associated with shortage of care personnel and inadequate financing for effective services (Karumuna & Mgone, 1990; Nottidge & Okogbo, 1991).

The dramatic decrease in perinatal mortality in developed countries during the 1980s, largely a result of improved survival rates for low birth weight infants, has given rise to the fear of increased numbers of children with neurodevelopmental impairments. In fact, there was a steady-state incidence of CP of about 2.5 per 1000 live births until about the mid-1950s (Little, 1958), which was followed by a decrease in incidence to about 1.5 per 1000 for about 15 years. Since then, the incidence has increased to near mid-1950s levels, if Swedish statistics are typical (Hagberg et al., 1989b). The change in trend mainly reflects changes in the live birth rate of preterm infants, especially in those with spastic diplegia. The risk of CP increases sharply with decreasing birth weight (Atkinson & Stanley, 1983; Hagberg et al., 1989a, Pharoah et al., 1987) and has been reported to be as much as 40 times

higher in infants weighing less than 1000 g (Hagberg et al., 1989b).

The increased risk of CP in preterm infants must be put in perspective, however. Reports of long-term outcome of extremely premature infants, that is, infants born between 24 and 28 weeks of gestational age, suggest about a 75% survival rate, with more than 50% of those who survive free of major neurodevelopmental impairments, about 25% with major impairments, and about 11% with CP (Msall et al., 1991).

Pathophysiology

The autopsy of infants has revealed three types of neuropathic lesions (Weinstein & Tharp, 1989): neuropathy resulting from hemorrhage below the lining of the ventricles (subependymal), encephalopathy caused by anoxia or hypoxia, and neuropathy resulting from malformations of the central nervous system.

Most subependymal hemorrhages occur in infants of less than 28 weeks of gestational age and those with low birth weight. Intraventricular hemorrhages, present in up to 46% of infants weighing less than 1500 g (Papile et al., 1978), are thought to develop secondary to lesions of ischemic origin. In most cases, blood ruptures into the lateral ventricle and the ensuing connective tissue blocks the cerebrospinal fluid flow, frequently resulting in hydrocephalus. Anoxic or hypoxic encephalopathy results in gray matter and white matter lesions. Gray-matter lesions are diffusely present throughout the cortex, basal ganglia and thalamus, brain stem, and spinal cord, whereas lesions in the white matter are frequently in the periventricular zone. Periventricular atrophy has been identified as the most common abnormality found in preterm infants who developed hemiplegic CP, occurring in 50% of cases (Wiklund et al., 1991b). It is unclear, however, whether the lesions occur before, during, or after birth. Although periventricular atrophy is a bilateral lesion thought to be responsible for most cases of preterm spastic diplegia, it has also been reported as an asymmetric or unilateral lesion or one with bilateral lesions expressing only unilateral clinical symptoms (Wiklund et al., 1991b).

Malformations of the central nervous system may generate hemorrhagic and anoxic lesions. Many factors may be responsible, including drug ingestion, radiation, and infection by viruses such as herpes simplex and rubella.

Attempts to relate cerebral lesions to the extent of disability have had only limited success. With respect to the side of expression, in the small percentage of hemiplegic children with bilateral morphologic findings, subtle physical abnormalities were sometimes seen on the nonhemiplegic side (Wiklund & Uvebrant, 1991a). Results suggest the existence of a continuum between hemiplegia and diplegia resulting from periventricular lesions. Magnetic resonance imaging showed that, of several measures, only the amount of white matter correlated with the severity of disability (Yokochi et al., 1991). In children with hemiplegia, no significant correlations between size of lesion and severity of impairment have been found, although trends toward the association of less impairment with smaller lesions have been reported (Molteni et al., 1987; Wiklund & Uvebrant, 1991a). Quadriplegia has been associated with brain stem and basal nuclei damage in addition to cortical and subcortical lesions (Wilson et al., 1982). Further discussion of the causes of the various types of CP can be found in works by Menkes (1990) and Weinstein and Tharp (1989).

Progress in Primary Prevention

The primary way to reduce the incidence of CP is through good socioeconomic health of the population coupled with maternal education. The role of poverty and low socioeconomic status in the prevalence of CP (Dowding & Barry, 1990) and in determining the need for special educational resources (Msall et al., 1991) has frequently been overlooked, yet there is empirical evidence of its importance.

Certain maternal prepregnancy and pregnancy-related risk factors are associated with delivery of a child with a disability (Holst et al., 1989). Studies have suggested that improved intrapartum diagnosis of risk factors, prevention of asphyxia, and medical treatment of children with low Apgar scores would reduce the incidence of disabilities, as would intervention to prevent premature rupture of membranes. However reasonable these hypotheses may seem, no studies are known to have tested them.

The role of the obstetrician in preventing CP before birth occurs is limited (Weinstein & Tharp, 1989). Attention is directed toward developing effective preventions of and interventions for premature delivery, fetal distress, neonatal asphyxia, and mechanical birth trauma. Methods of inhibiting labor have met with much success, although the effects on incidence of CP remain unclear. Methods of antepartum fetal evaluation, including sonographic measurement, electronic fetal monitoring, fetal pH monitoring, and intrauterine pressure monitoring, have provided the obstetrician with powerful tools for assessing the need for active intervention in the labor process. Delivery procedures using high forceps and certain presentations of breech deliveries that were found to be associated with increased perinatal morbidity have dramatically decreased in favor of cesarean section. This is partly due to the increased safety of cesarean birth for both the mother and the fetus.

Impairment

MEDICAL DIAGNOSIS

Early detection of CP facilitates optimal management by the family and the health care and educational community. Complicating the picture is the instability of diagnosis; CP is reported to disappear over time in many low birth weight infants (Kitchen et al., 1987). In a study designed to determine the accuracy of diagnosis of CP at 2 years of age (Kitchen et al., 1987), only 55% of those so diagnosed at age 2 were deemed to have CP at age 5, but the diagnosis of those with moderate or severe involvement did not change. Only 1% of children not diagnosed at age 2 were identified at age 5 to have CP. Of those children in whom the diagnosis was no longer accurate at age 5, most had minor neurologic abnormalities and left-hand preference, but their psychologic test scores were no different from those of children who had never been diagnosed as having CP.

Tests of neurologic status, motor function, primitive reflexes, and posture have been assessed for their ability to identify CP (Burns et al., 1989). Although assessments performed at the age of 1 month failed to identify several of the infants who later showed CP, assessments made at 4 months of age resulted in some overidentification. At 8 months of age, the presence of three or more abnormal signs was highly predictive of CP, and the authors concluded that all but the mildest cases of CP can be identified by that age. Formal tests have varying abilities to detect motor abnormalities (Harris, 1989). The sensitivity of the Movement Assessment of Infants (MAI) has been calculated to be 73.5% in a high-risk population (Harris, 1987). When compared with the Bayley motor scale (Bayley, 1993), the MAI identified more than 3 times as many children with diplegia at 4 months of age, more than 2 times as many children with hemiplegia, and about 1.5 times as many children with quadriplegia (Harris, 1989). In children at 1 year corrected age, however, the Bayley motor scale demonstrated sensitivities of 100% for both spastic diplegia and quadriplegia and 75% for spastic hemiplegia. Furthermore, the MAI has a lower rate of specificity than does the Bayley motor scale, that is, a greater percentage of children with normal outcomes are identified as being at risk.

PHYSICAL THERAPY – RELATED IMPAIRMENTS

Impairments in CP are problems with the neuro-muscular and skeletal systems that are either an immediate result of the existing pathophysiologic process or an indirect consequence that has developed over time. Impairments can be sorted, somewhat artificially, into single-system impairments and multisystem impairments.

Single-System Impairments

Single-system impairments are expressed in the muscular system and the skeletal system, even though the pathophysiologic damage occurred in the central nervous system. Primary impairments such as insufficient force generation, spasticity, abnormal extensibility, and exaggerated or hyperactive reflexes are evident in the muscular system; malalignments such as femoral anteversion and femoral and tibial torsion (Cusick & Stuberg, 1992) are secondary impairments evident in the skeletal system.

CP is characterized by insufficient force generation by affected muscle groups, which is consistent with low levels of electromyographic (EMG) activity and decreased moment of force output (Berger et al., 1982). When an activity leads to an active contraction, this impairment may be expressed as a deficiency in power (Olney et al., 1990), or when considered over time, in work. The term *strength* may refer to any of these measurable factors. Strength measurement in neurologic conditions is problematic, but when measured, strength has frequently been intimately linked with functional capabilities such as speed of walking (Bohannon, 1989).

The clinical term *tone* is used to describe the impairments of spasticity and abnormal extensibility. A sensation of abnormally high tone may be caused by spasticity, a velocity-dependent overactivity that is proportional to the imposed velocity of limb movement. Spasticity is especially evident in children with clonus but is frequently mistaken for problems of extensibility. It was once thought that human spasticity of supraspinal origin resulted from unbalanced facilitation and inhibition descending to the spinal cord from damaged cortical areas by descending fiber tracts, probably by disinhibition of the lateral vestibulospinal tract. Attention is now also focusing on the spinal interneuronal level (Harrison, 1988), where abnormal interneuronal function could cause hyperreflexia, reciprocal excitation, and excessive responsiveness to stimuli that do not cause reactions in the normal system. Studies in stroke subjects suggest that the stretch reflex is activated at a shorter muscle length in spastic muscles than in normal muscles but that the "gain," or force output, is not increased (Katz & Rymer, 1989). The specific neural causes of spasticity have not been clearly identified and may be different for adult and pediatric patients.

The sense of abnormally high tone can also result from hypoextensibility of the muscle because of abnormal mechanical characteristics. Comparing normal children with children with CP, Berger and colleagues (1982) found that the EMG activity of leg muscles in nearly all children with CP was reduced in affected limbs and that there were no indications of pathologic reflex effects on muscle activity. A force transducer on the tendo Achillis indicated tension that was disproportionate to muscle activity and could best be attributed to mechanical changes in the muscle rather than to increased stretch reflexes from spasticity. These muscles were also seen to be abnormally stiff; that is, they produced more force for a given length change than did muscles in nondisabled children (Tardieu, C, et al., 1982). The most accurate term for this impairment is hypoextensibility. The muscle offers resistance to passive stretching at a shorter length than that expected in a normal muscle. In addition, if greater than normal amounts of force are required to produce a change in length, the muscle is said to have increased stiffness. This is represented as the passive tension curve for CP (p,CP) in Figure 19–1*A*, in contrast to the normal passive tension curve (p,N) in Figure 19–1*D*, when one moves the ankle from a position of plantar flexion to one of dorsiflexion. When a clinician finds that it is not possible to manually stretch the muscle through a normal range using reasonable amounts of manual force, the muscle group is deemed to have a contracture, represented in Figure 19–2 as "contracture," the difference between the joint angle at which this extreme resistance is encountered in the CP muscle and that of the normal muscle.

Figure 19–1 shows hypothetic active force-length characteristics of spastic plantar flexors (a, CP, see Fig. 19–1*B*) and normal plantar flexors (a, N, see Fig. 19–1*E*), that is, the force generated by the contractile elements of the muscle over the range of muscle lengths from a shortened position (plantar flexed) to a longer position (dorsiflexed). Note that the maximal force is lower for the CP muscle and also that the peak force occurs at a more plantar flexed position in the CP muscle than in the normal muscle. The sum of the combined

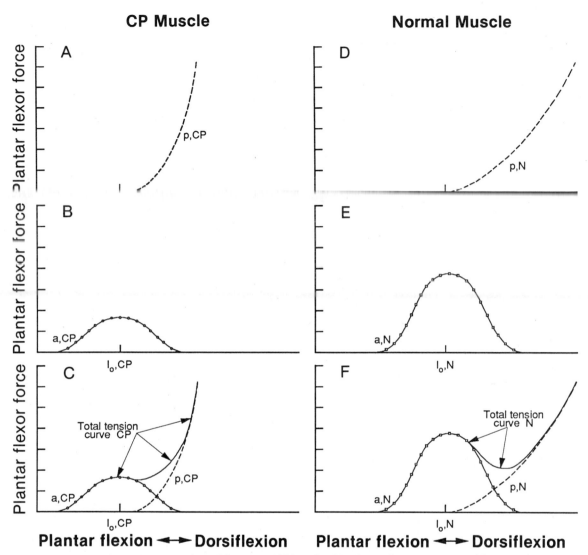

FIGURE 19-1. Representation of force capabilities of ankle plantar flexor muscle at different joint angles in normal muscle (N) and spastic muscle (CP). *A,* Resistance to passive stretch of spastic muscle (p,CP) increasing with more dorsiflexion. *B,* The force of active contraction (a,CP) varying with the joint angle, l_o denoting resting length. *C,* The sum of the passive and active effects in spastic muscle. *D,* Resistance to passive stretch in normal muscle (p,N). *E,* Force of active contraction in normal muscle (a,N). *F,* The total tension curve comprising the sum of the passive and active effects in normal muscle. Note that 1) the slope, i.e., the stiffness, of p,CP in *A* is greater for the spastic muscle than for the normal muscles (p,N) in *D,* 2) the maximal active force achieved by the spastic muscle (a,CP) in *B* is less than the maximal active force of normal muscle (a,N) in *E,* and 3) the maximal active force for spastic muscle (a,CP) shown in *B* occurs at a more plantar flexed position than that of the normal muscle (a,N) shown in *E.*

effects of active force output and passive stiffness for the CP muscle is shown as the total tension curve CP, and the corresponding curve for the normal muscle is shown as total tension curve N (see Fig. 19-2). The complexity of the representation in Figure 19-2 underlines the difficulty faced by a

physical therapist or physician in correctly assessing the cause of increased tone through clinical methods such as passive manipulation of the limb and clinical assessment of muscle strength.

If a muscle complex has become overlengthened, which is usually a secondary impairment resulting

FIGURE 19–2. Complete representation of force capabilities of ankle plantar flexor muscle at different joint angles in normal muscle (N) and spastic muscle (CP) shown in Figure 19–1. a,CP = force of active contraction of spastic muscle; l_o,CP = resting length of spastic muscle; l_o,N = resting length of normal muscle; a,N = force of active contraction of normal muscle; p,CP = resistance to passive stretch of spastic muscle; p,N = resistance to passive stretch of normal muscle.

from repeated mechanical stretch, it is referred to as hyperextensible. The muscle complex may also have decreased force-generating capabilities.

Few studies of the histology and morphology of spastic muscle have been reported, but they have shown that differences are present when spastic muscle is compared with normal muscle (Romanini et al., 1989). The slowly contracting fibers of the spastic adductor muscles demonstrate hypertrophy, whereas the fast fibers show atrophy. Surprisingly, there has been no evidence of increase in endomysial or perimysial connective tissue at any age of child, regardless of the clinical picture. The authors concluded that joint restrictions are attributable to the atrophy of muscle fibers, which makes the muscle less elastic and extensible, and possibly to an increase of fibrous tissue in the periarticular structures, although the latter was not verified.

There are no universally accepted methods of measuring spasticity (Katz & Rymer, 1989), although techniques include measurement of forces in response to standard passive stretches (tonic) or standard hammer stimuli (phasic), Hoffmann's re-

flex recording (Jones, EW, & Mulley, 1982), and measurement of responses to sinusoidal cycling (Price et al., 1991). The modified Ashworth scale has been shown to have reliability in adults with neurologic conditions, although reliability has not been established for children (Bohannon & Smith, 1987).

Multisystem Impairments

In the second group of impairments are three multisystem impairments expressed in the neuromuscular system: poor selective control of muscle activity, poor regulation of activity in muscle groups in anticipation of postural changes and body movement (referred to as anticipatory regulation), and decreased ability to learn unique movements.

In CP there is poor selective control of muscle activity. Normal movement is characterized by orderly phasing in and out of muscle activation, coactivation of muscles with similar biomechanical functions, and limited coactivation of antagonists during phasic or free movement. In CP there is abundant evidence of inappropriate sequencing (Nashner et al., 1983) and coactivation of synergists and antagonists (Knutsson & Martensson, 1980).

The reasons for poor selective control of muscle activity are unknown. Failure of the normal reciprocal relationship of activity between agonist and antagonist muscles during voluntary movements has been observed (Berger et al., 1982; Hallett & Alvarez, 1983; Leonard et al., 1990), but whether segmental or supraspinal mechanisms or both are involved is unclear. Although Berbrayer and Ashby (1990) clearly demonstrated the presence of reciprocal inhibition in CP, it is not possible to exclude the possibility that other spinal mechanisms may be impaired (Harrison, 1988). Direct evidence for a supraspinal origin is scant; however, researchers have concluded that in CP, the corticospinal projections are directed equally to the motoneurons of agonist and antagonist muscles of the ankle (Brouwer & Ashby, 1991). Reflex overflow to antagonist muscles in children with CP (Leonard et al., 1991) has been attributed either to exuberant motoneuronal projections or to exuberant projections that extend to motoneurons innervating muscles other than the one being stimulated. It appears certain that the neuronal "wiring" in CP is not normal.

Poor anticipatory regulation of muscle sequencing when postural correction is attempted has been reported by Nashner and colleagues (1983). In normal individuals, changes in posture are preceded by preparatory muscle contractions that stabilize the body. In people with CP, the contraction that is needed to produce stability is frequently interrupted by destabilizing synergistic or antagonistic muscle activity.

There is some evidence that motor memory in children with CP is frequently impaired (Lesny et al., 1990). This finding is important in considering strategies for teaching movement, but it has received little attention to date.

Assessment of multisystem impairments usually involves measurement of a closely associated variable or number of variables and frequently involves different dimensions of the disabling process. Assessment of the impairments of poor selective control of muscle activity, poor anticipatory regulation of muscle groups, and decreased ability to learn unique movements includes use of measures of balance, coordination, and motor control. Most are not in general clinical use. Two approaches to assessing balance have been taken: one is to disturb the supporting surface in a variety of ways (Nashner et al., 1983); the other is to perturb the subject or environment (Patla et al., 1989). In each

case, kinematic, kinetic, and EMG responses are measured. Coordination has been documented with EMG records, which makes it possible to detect differences from normal records in timing of muscle activity onset and duration, in sequencing of agonists, and in cocontraction of antagonists. Gait has been the most commonly observed activity used to evaluate specific impairments of CP (Perry et al., 1976), and the potential for its wide clinical application has increased with the advent of fast and efficient computer systems.

Models of Treatment

Three models of multidisciplinary professional involvement are common in management of CP. In one, professionals, usually those representing pediatrics, physical therapy, occupational therapy, infant development or education, speech therapy, social work, and psychology, ensure that all areas are covered in an initial assessment. Although this approach is comprehensive, overlap, superfluity, and differences of opinion can cause difficulties. A second model is use of a flexible team that plans for a minimum of pertinent professional involvement at the assessment stage and recruits the involvement of others as needed. Generally a more economic model, it requires more formal communication to ensure smooth operation. In a third model, parents seek whatever professional advice they wish and make management decisions themselves. The notion of empowerment of informed health care consumers is expected to make this a more commonly employed model in the future, although integration of the various components of the child's life can be difficult.

Determinants of Prognosis or Outcome

Although about 90% of children with CP in developed countries survive to adulthood (Evans et al., 1990), predictions of lifetime outcomes in CP are rare. A California study (Residential arrangements for adults with cerebral palsy—California, 1988, 1991) reported that only 12 to 17% of people with CP registered with developmental services were competitively employed. Positive prognostic factors for employment included mild physical involvement, good family support, vocational training, and having good employment contacts. Mental retardation, seizures, and wheelchair dependency were factors reducing the likelihood of living independently. Senft and colleagues (1990) reported that more than 60% of registrants in a neuromuscular disability program were dependent on aging parents. In a review of the literature, Bleck (1987) included the following positive predictors of independence and employment of a person with CP: regular schooling, completion of secondary schooling, independence in mobility with the ability to travel beyond the home, good hand skills, living in a small rather than a large community, and having a diagnosis of spasticity rather than one of involuntary movements. Preliminary studies of life satisfaction suggest more positive outcomes, but few studies have included this important variable (Wacker et al., 1983).

Certain factors assist in predicting the ambulation potential of children with CP. Children with the hemiplegic type of CP usually have a good prognosis for ambulation, whereas the prognosis is less favorable for those with rigid or hypotonic types of CP (Crothers & Paine, 1988). Persistent tonic neck reflexes are associated with decreased likelihood of walking (Crothers & Paine, 1988). Some studies have reported that a remarkably large percentage of children who are able to sit independently by the age of 24 months eventually walk (Crothers & Paine, 1988) and that nearly all children with CP who eventually walk do so before 8 years of age (Bleck, 1975). Watt and colleagues (1989), examining all survivors of neonatal intensive care, have reported that nearly all who sat by 24 months of age walked 15 meters or more with or without assistive devices or orthoses by the age of 8 years. Independent sitting by 24 months remains the best predictor of ambulation, despite inclusion of neonatal variables, clinical types, primitive reflexes, and reactions (Watt et al., 1989).

ASSESSMENT AND INTERVENTION

Infancy

The life role of an infant is to grow and develop in response to being loved and nurtured by parents and caregivers in a home environment. Despite being dependent in most aspects of life, infants interact with, and develop an understanding of, the people in their lives, their surroundings, and themselves. From the time of birth, a child with CP may not experience the normal activities associated with infancy. As a result, the parents of an infant with CP may not receive the positive feedback of a normal nurturing experience and the satisfaction of observing the development of motor and social skills, that is, the normal rewards of caring for an infant.

The parents have many other concerns. They must cope with the impact of the diagnosis and the grieving process that accompanies the awareness that their expectations of having a normal child will not be realized. They may be overwhelmed with the uncertainty that the future holds for them, their child, and their family. Many parents are also concerned with the immediate issues of providing basic infant care and are apprehensive about incorporating the specialized care necessary for their child's optimal development.

Movement is an important component in the learning and interactive processes of infancy. In infants who have CP, the nature and extent of their impairments affect their potential to develop and learn through movement. This may result in functional limitations in the development of gross motor skills and may affect their ability to interact with their parents, themselves, and their environment.

PHYSICAL THERAPY ASSESSMENT

Infant assessment provides a base line for the monitoring of improvement or deterioration, growth, maturation, and treatment effects in children with CP. Assessment of impairment involves qualitative and, when possible, quantitative evaluation of the single-system and multisystem impairments. Observation of active range of motion (ROM) provides indirect assessment of the force-generating ability of muscle groups as well as some information about muscle extensibility. In an infant, this is assessed by observing movement. Determination of the passive ROM, using a slow, maintained stretch in a position that promotes relaxation, assesses muscle group extensibility and provides information about joints, such as the presence of dislocation. Quantitative measures of joint ROM and skeletal alignment, including the rotational and torsional alignment of the pelvis and lower extremities (Cusick & Stuberg, 1992; see Chapter 15), should be documented using consistent and standardized procedures. Variations of 10 to 15° occur in intrarater goniometric measurement in children with CP (Stuberg et al., 1988), and caution must be used to avoid misinterpreting small changes. Normal maturational changes in joint range and alignment must be considered in interpreting the significance of measures.

Passive movement performed with greater velocity is used to assess spasticity and the sensitivity of the stretch reflex. Spasticity can be documented descriptively on the basis of resistance to movement and observations of spontaneous active movement and posturing. The severity of spasticity—whether it is mild, moderate, or severe

—its distribution over the body and limbs, and its variations under different conditions should be noted. Frequently, there are variations in spasticity associated with positioning and the infant's effort and behavior. The modified Ashworth scale (Bohannon & Smith, 1987) or the muscle tone section of the MAI can be used (Chandler et al., 1980).

The presence or persistence of primitive reflexes and the development of the postural reactions of equilibrium, righting, and protective extension are assessed to determine their influence on selective control and anticipatory regulation of muscle group activity. The effects these reflexes and postural reactions have on positioning, handling, and the facilitation or inhibition of functional movement also need to be evaluated (Bly, 1991). The primitive reflex and the automatic reaction sections of the MAI (Chandler et al., 1980) are appropriate to use when evaluating infants with CP.

Selective control and anticipatory regulation of muscle groups are assessed in the context of functional evaluation: for the infant, this is indicated by the assessment of gross motor skills. Standardized instruments used by physical therapists when assessing infant movement include the MAI, the Gross Motor Function Measure (Russell et al., 1989), the Peabody Developmental Motor Scales (Hinderer et al., 1989), the Bayley Scales of Infant Development (Bayley, 1993), and the Alberta Infant Motor Scale (Piper & Daviah, 1994). Various elements of movements and posture combine to produce functional gross motor skills. These include the ability to align one part of the body on another; to bear weight through different parts of the body; to shift weight; to move against gravity; to assume, maintain, and move into and out of different positions; and to perform graded, isolated, and variable movements with an appropriate degree of effort. When assessing functional motor skills, proficiency in incorporating these elements into the achievement of purposeful and efficient movement must be analyzed.

Specific functional assessments of seating, feeding (Evans Morris & Dunn Klein, 1987), or respiratory problems may be necessary for infants with problems in these areas. Growth is often affected in children with CP; therefore, anthropometric measures, including head circumference, weight, and length, should be documented. Growth may influence, or be influenced by, feeding, exercise, and energy efficiency (Campbell et al., 1989). Other factors to be considered during assessment include the influence of an infant's temperament and behavior on performance; sensory, social, communication, and cognitive abilities; and support from the environment.

PHYSICAL THERAPY GOALS AND TREATMENT

From infancy to adulthood, physical therapy goals for clients with CP should focus on the prevention of disability by minimizing the effects of impairments, preventing or limiting secondary impairments, and maximizing the gross motor functions allowed by the organic deficits. Achieving these goals involves the promotion and maintenance of musculoskeletal integrity, the prevention of deformity, and the enhancement of optimal postures and movement to promote functional independence. Furthermore, the physical therapist attempts to prevent environmental deprivation that could increase existing disabilities and attempts to provide support, guidance, and education for the child, the family, and the community. Goals are individualized for the particular child; are based on the needs of the whole child; and take into consideration the needs, expectations, and values of the family (Bailey, 1987) and community. Goal attainment should be regularly reassessed so that the therapy plan is adapted to reflect changes in the child's progress and the family's needs.

The presence of impairments such as low levels of force generation, spasticity, abnormal extensibility, disturbed reflexes, and skeletal malalignments can result in abnormal weight bearing, alignment, and soft tissue extensibility, which can, in turn, affect the orthopaedic development of the spine and the extremities. The application of correct forces is required for optimal skeletal modeling before the skeleton ossifies (LeVeau & Bernhardt, 1984), although the research reported to date has offered little specific guidance. Of particular concern is the effect of increased hip flexion and adduction in acetabular development and hip joint stability. Neck and trunk asymmetry can result in torticollis or spinal deformities. Infants with hypoextensibility and spasticity are prone to developing contractures. Although patterns of tightness vary, commonly at risk for contractures are the shoulder adductors; the elbow, wrist, and finger flexors; the hip flexors and adductors; the knee flexors; and the ankle plantar flexors (Massagli, 1991). The abnormal postures and movements resulting from impairments also make an infant difficult to handle and position. These difficulties can affect an infant's interaction with the environment, reaction to caregiving activities, and development of gross motor skills.

Physical therapy in infancy is focused on facilitating caregiving, promoting optimal sensorimotor experiences and skills, and educating the family. Early treatment for children with CP has been advocated to help the infants organize potential abilities in the most normal way for them, although there is no definitive support for its efficacy (Campbell, 1990).

Handling and Care

The first physical therapy goal is to promote the parents' skill, ease, and confidence in handling and caring for their infant. These skills alleviate unnecessary stress for parents and child and also help to reduce the influence of the impairments, thereby preventing unnecessary secondary impairments and limitations. Parents are taught positioning, carrying, feeding, and dressing techniques that promote symmetry, limit abnormal posturing and movement, and facilitate functional motor activity. The principles guiding these methods are 1) to use a variety of movements and postures to promote sensory variety, 2) to frequently include positions that promote the full lengthening of spastic or hypoextensible muscles, and 3) to use positions that promote functional voluntary movement of limbs.

Facilitating Optimal Sensorimotor Development

The second physical therapy goal in infancy is to facilitate optimal sensorimotor experiences and skills, thereby reducing functional limitations and disabilities. Therapy should focus on the development of well-aligned postural stability coupled with smooth mobility to allow the emergence of motor skills such as reaching, rolling, sitting, crawling, transitional movements, standing, and prewalking skills. These skills promote the development of spatial perception, body awareness, and mobility to facilitate play, social interaction, and exploration of the environment. Movements that include trunk rotation, dissociation of body segments, weight shifting, weight bearing, and isolated movements should be incorporated into gross motor exercises and activities. These movement components, if experienced with proper alignment, can give the sensory feedback of normal movement patterns and activities. Good sources for the handling and treatment of infants and children of other ages include the works of Finnie (1975), Jaeger (1987, 1989), Scherzer and Tscharnuter (1990), and Wilson (1991). A practical reference for parents is *Children with Cerebral Palsy* (Geralis, 1991). Careful instruction of the family in specific techniques and activities, ongoing reinforcement, encouragement, and support are essential. Clearly written, illustrated, and updated home programs can be beneficial.

The normal motor developmental sequence may assist in guiding the progression of motor activities, although current research indicates that motor milestones and their components develop in over-lapping sequences, with spurts of development interspersed with some plateaus and even regressions (Atwater, 1991). The child with CP is not always able to proceed along the normal developmental sequence, and therapy becomes more functionally oriented within the scope of the child's physical capabilities (Bly, 1991). The stage at which this happens depends on the severity of the impairments; in some children, it may occur early in life.

Activities or equipment may be used to allow attainment of functional skills when impairments otherwise prevent the development of certain skills. For example, the sitting position promotes visual attending, upper extremity use, and social interaction. Infants with CP may be unable to sit independently, may sit statically only with precarious balance, or may not even be able to be seated in normal infant equipment. Customized seating or adaptations to regular infant seats may be necessary to allow function in other areas of development to progress. Infants with limited upper extremity movement may be unable to bring their hands or toys to their mouths to provide normal oral-motor sensory input. In these cases, mouthing activities should be incorporated into therapy. Toys may need to be adapted to facilitate developmental activities.

The care of an infant exhibiting asymmetry, extensor posturing, and shoulder retraction illustrates these approaches. Such an infant should be carried, seated, and fed in a symmetric position that does not allow axial hyperextension and keeps the hips and knees flexed. Positioning of or playing with the upper extremities to allow the infant to see his or her hands, practice midline play, reach for his or her feet, or suck on fingers can promote sensorimotor awareness. Active movements, such as the handling of toys that require two hands and that encourage the infant to develop flexor control and symmetry, are incorporated into daily activities. These activities facilitate the use of the neck and trunk muscles, promoting anterior and posterior control. The introduction of lateral control is the next step in achieving functional head and trunk control. In some severely affected children, slight gains in head control may be a goal, whereas in minimally affected children a fairly normal progression of motor development is expected, even without intervention.

Some physical therapists may adhere to specific treatment philosophies and approaches, two of which are described here. Neurodevelopmental treatment (NDT) is an approach widely used throughout North America and other parts of the world as a basis for the treatment of infants with CP. NDT is based on the theory that inhibiting or modifying impairments of spasticity and abnormal reflex patterns can improve movement. Handling techniques encourage the infant to move actively and experience the sensations of normal movement patterns. The ultimate aim of the treatment is the acquisition of functional movements that permit children the greatest degree of independence possible to prepare them for as normal an adolescence and adult life as can be achieved (Bobath & Bobath, 1984). The Vojta approach, which is practiced in parts of Europe, is another example of a treatment method that can be used for infants. Proprioceptive information from the trunk and extremities is believed to activate the central nervous system and guide it toward normal motor ontogenesis by eliciting appropriate movement patterns (Vojta, 1984).

Family Education

A third group of goals is to educate families about CP, to provide support in their acceptance of their child's problems, and to be of assistance when parents make decisions about managing both their own and their child's lives. Infancy is an important time to foster collaborative goal-setting and programming strategies with the parents. These skills empower them to make decisions, solve problems, and set priorities as well as to become effective advocates for their children and themselves. At this stage, the parents' goals may be overly optimistic and hopeful. Therapists need to be realistic about the prognosis and the efficacy of physical therapy while remaining hopeful. They can break down overall goals into objectives that are meaningful, obtainable, sequential, observable, and measurable (Kolobe, 1992).

The involvement of other health care professionals in the treatment of the infant with CP depends on the child's needs and the practices of the institution where the program occurs. Some facilities may have professionals from several disciplines working with the family, whereas at others it may be thought better to have a primary therapist initially, bringing in others for assessment or treatment as necessary.

Occupational therapists may be involved in upper extremity function, particularly as it relates to play. Speech and language pathologists may be involved if there are oral-motor problems interfering with feeding or early language development. Community infant development workers may be involved in home-based programs. Social workers may help the parents through the grieving process, explain programs, and direct them to appropriate resources. Parent support groups or individual meetings with parents who have been through similar experiences may be helpful.

Preschool Period

During the preschool years, locomotor, cognitive, communication, fine motor, self-care, and social abilities develop to promote functional independence in children. The process is a dynamic one in which all these areas constantly interact with one another. The child's environment remains oriented toward the parents, family, and home during this period, but he or she begins to interact with the outside world. Child care centers, babysitters, nursery schools, and playmates thus become part of a preschooler's world.

For children with CP, the limitations in motor functioning may create disabilities in learning, socialization, and attainment of independence (Butler, 1991). Concerns of the parents include the impact of impaired performance on all areas of development: for example, their child's ability to participate in and become integrated into normal preschool activities, the development of cognition and language, and the long-term effect of disabilities on future life and independence.

During these years, the child's attainable level of motor skills can be predicted with a greater degree of accuracy as the influences of motor impairments on functioning become apparent. A major area of concern for physical therapists is the child's ability to achieve independent mobility. In addition, skills in overall gross motor development continue to be a focus of physical therapy to minimize disabilities, such as the inability to learn and perform the self-care skills of toileting, dressing, grooming, and feeding, and the limitations in play, communication, social skills, and problem-solving behavior.

PHYSICAL THERAPY ASSESSMENT

Assessment of disability assumes a primary focus, but it is important to determine the role of function and impairment in the production of disability. Within the dimension of impairment, direct testing of the force-generating ability of muscle groups is not always appropriate because spasticity, abnormal extensibility, hyperactive reflexes, and poor selective control affect the assessment. In such cases, muscle strength should continue to be considered in a functional context. Both concentric and eccentric power should be assessed by observing activities such as moving between sitting and standing positions or ascending and descending stairs. Endurance should be evaluated by observing the ability to walk age-appropriate distances or propel a wheelchair a comparable span.

Evaluation of function and disability are frequently included in the same assessments. The

Gross Motor Function Measure (Russell et al., 1989) and the Peabody Developmental Motor Scales (Hinderer et al., 1989) can continue to be used to monitor the child's motor progress. When assessing motor skills, the use of equipment to achieve an activity should be taken into consideration. For example, the use of orthoses in ambulation may substantially affect walking abilities.

Function and disability assessment should also include mobility and transfers, communication, social function, bowel and bladder control, self-care and the degree of reliance on caregivers, adaptive equipment, and environmental modifications in the performance of activities of daily living (ADL). The Pediatric Evaluation of Disability Inventory (Feldman et al., 1990) assesses many of these functional skills in the preschooler. The Functional Independence Measure for Children (WeeFIM), a pediatric version of the Functional Independence Measure (Msall et al., 1990), measures disability as quantified by burden of care. Other measures of ADL (Gowland et al., 1991) include the Canadian Occupational Performance Measure (Law et al., 1990), the Vulpe Assessment Battery (Vulpe, 1982), the Klein-Bell ADL Scale (Klein & Bell, 1982), and the Vineland Adaptive Behavior Scales (Sparrow et al., 1984). Disability measures also include attempts to assess health-related quality of life. There has been increased interest in developing these measures for children, taking into account age, specific disability, and the factors and values believed to be important by health care professionals, parents, and children themselves (Rosenbaum et al., 1990).

Assessments specific to certain activities may be indicated. These include evaluations of gait (Olney et al., 1990), augmentative communication, and mobility. Gait assessment measures ambulatory function, and if kinetic and EMG analyses are included, certain impairments are also evaluated (Fig. 19–3). The ROM of the hips, knees, and ankles in each phase of gait can be observed using a videotape. Particular attention should be paid to the propulsive movement of ankle plantar flexion during push-off and to the concurrent hip flexion. These two events are responsible for much of the forward movement of the body and are indirect measures of force generation of muscle groups. EMG recordings during walking show the general level of activation of each muscle group, the degree of cocontraction, and the selectivity and degree of sequencing of muscle-group activity—all indicators of impairment. Upper extremity activities such as reaching (Kluzik et al., 1990) have also been studied using videotaping and other sensing systems.

When assessing children in this age group, it is

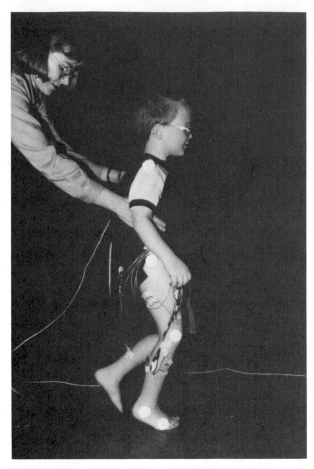

FIGURE 19–3. Child taking part in gait analysis. Electromyography shows patterns of muscle activities and aids identification of the presence of cocontraction of muscle groups. Markers at joints allow computer calculation of joint movements; force platforms embedded in floor permit measurement of individual muscle group contributions to the work of walking. (Courtesy of Human Motion Laboratory at School of Rehabilitation Therapy at Queen's University, Kingston, Ontario.)

necessary to be aware of the effects of attention, cooperation, and the children's reaction to being assessed on the evaluation process. Parents or other caregivers can provide information on whether a child's performance is characteristic of his or her abilities.

PHYSICAL THERAPY GOALS AND TREATMENT

The impact and extent of the child's impairments become more established during the preschool years. Treatment focused specifically on reducing impairments and preventing secondary effects of impairment provides a backdrop for interventions aimed at higher levels of the disabling process to prevent isolation from the typical experiences of early childhood and family life. Optimal postural alignment and movements of the body that are conducive to musculoskeletal development, neurophysiologic control, and function, through exercise, positioning, and equipment are the aims of many interventions. In many cases, physical therapy goals may serve as the building blocks for global interdisciplinary goals in communication, play, social interaction, and self-care activities. Therapists must be willing to respect the priorities of parents and other professionals when determining goals, since it may not be possible to work on all areas at once.

Reducing Primary Impairment and Preventing Secondary Impairment

Increasing Force Generation. Treatment to improve force generation of muscles in this age group is achieved through performing activities that create increased demands for production of both concentric and eccentric muscle force. Such activities include transitional movements, ball gymnastics, and practice of functional skills such as using stairs.

Spasticity. It was once thought that individuals had no control of their spasticity. Subjects with CP, however, have been able to reduce their responsiveness to a stretch reflex stimulus imposed during an upper arm activity (Harrison & Kruze, 1987) and a lower limb activity (Nash et al., 1989). These findings encourage further exploration of the possibilities of reducing spastic responses.

Selective posterior rhizotomy is a surgical procedure directed toward decreasing the impairment of spasticity with the goal of improving functional movement. The posterior nerve rootlets supplying the lower extremity muscles are selectively cut. Surgery is not performed if a child appears dependent on spasticity for function. Ideal candidates have fair to good trunk control and selective muscle control and cognitive abilities, motivation, and parental support that are conducive to intensive postoperative therapy programs. Severely affected patients, such as children with spastic quadriplegia, may be appropriate rhizotomy candidates; however, in these cases the goals are improved positioning, care, and comfort (Cahan et al., 1990; McDonald, 1991).

Muscle strengthening is emphasized postoperatively because the children are weakened without their spasticity (Fig. 19-4). Results in noncontrolled studies appear promising and complications usually minimal. Parents and children have been

FIGURE 19-4. Exercises after rhizotomy are frequently directed toward increasing force generation of extensor muscles

pleased with the results. Reduction of spasticity and improvements in ROM and function have been documented, and studies have shown the results lasting for as long as 7 years (Arens et al., 1989). Gait analysis has shown improved sagittal motion at the hip, knee, and ankle; however, abnormalities in patterns of muscle activation have persisted. This is attributed to continuing problems with motor control, which prohibit the proper sequencing of muscle action (Cahan et al., 1990; Giuliani, 1991). Positive changes in upper extremity function, particularly in play and ADL skills, have been found (Kinghorn, 1992), but changes were not evident in isolated finger movement. Other positive effects that have been noted include improved oral-motor control, increased voice volume and endurance, improved temperament and concentration, improved bowel and bladder control, and improvement in growth parameters (McDonald, 1991).

Reported negative side effects of dorsal rhizotomy include decreased muscle force production, bladder dysfunction, and sensory changes. The latter two are rarely lasting. The risk of developing spinal deformity after laminectomy is a concern, but reports of the rate of its occurring after rhizotomy have been no greater than is generally seen in patients with CP (McDonald, 1991). In conclusion, the procedure appears to be beneficial in children who are carefully selected. Studies are under way to investigate further the effects of this surgery while controlling for such factors as the increased therapy that these children usually receive. Long-term follow-up studies are also necessary.

Hypoextensibility. Various approaches are used to maintain muscle extensibility and joint mobility.

Manual stretching programs are used by some therapists. The usefulness of these passive ROM maneuvers is difficult to assess because active exercises, positioning programs, and equipment are usually used simultaneously. Research on the effectiveness of manual stretching on extensibility is inconclusive (Miedaner & Renander, 1987). Tremblay and colleagues (1990) found that a prolonged stretch of 30 minutes to the plantar flexors of children with CP reduced the impairment of spasticity and improved the voluntary activation of the plantar flexors but not the dorsiflexors. The effect lasted for as long as 35 minutes. In a parallel study, the stretching session did not produce a functional improvement in gait (Richards et al., 1991).

The effects of prolonged stretching programs have been studied (Tardieu, C, et al., 1988), and it was found that contractures were prevented if the plantar flexor muscles were stretched beyond a minimum threshold length for at least 6 hours during daily activity. The threshold length was the length at which the muscle began to resist a stretch. The data prompting this statement are suggestive rather than conclusive, however.

Casting and Orthoses. Standard plaster casting has been used as an economic method of providing stretch and is commonly used in serial casting to lengthen hypoextensible calf muscles. Casting for a 3-week period was shown to be effective if the hypoextensibility was due to imbalance between the triceps surae and dorsiflexor muscles but not if the primary impairment was lack of appropriate muscle growth in response to bone growth (Tardieu, G, et al., 1982). Serial casting has also been used for other muscle groups, such as the hamstrings and elbow flexors.

Lower extremity orthoses are used to reduce impairment, to prevent secondary impairment, and to facilitate function. The specific goals are prevention of contracture and deformity, provision of optimal joint alignment, provision of selective motion restriction, protection of weak muscles, control of tone and tonus-related deviations, enhancement of function, and postoperative protection of tissues (Cusick, 1990).

There has been an evolution in the use of orthoses in children with CP. Presently, ankle-foot orthoses (AFOs) are used extensively. Many variations are available, depending on the biomechanical and functional needs of the individual child (Knutsson & Clark, 1991). Solid AFOs are used if restriction of ankle movement is desired. Children who would benefit from freedom of movement at the joint can be fitted with hinged AFOs. Hinged AFOs frequently prevent plantar flexion but permit dorsiflexion, which allows stretching of the plantar

flexor muscle group during walking. Hinged AFOs have been found to promote a more normal and efficient gait pattern than do rigid braces (Middleton et al., 1988). Foot orthoses may be used for children with pronation who do not require the ankle stabilization of an AFO (Knutsson & Clark, 1991).

Bivalved casts or therapist-fabricated splints have been used in place of AFOs as a less expensive alternative for children who are growing quickly, do not have access to funding, or require a period of evaluation. The bivalved casts, popular during the 1980s, incorporate design features such as toe extension support, which is purported to inhibit abnormal tone or reflex activity. Although clinicians have claimed that the splints reduce abnormal tone, improve positioning, and reduce unwanted reflexes, research has not substantiated the claims (Carlson, 1984). Although the bivalved casts have been replaced by AFOs in many instances, they may be used for young children, since the circumferential support and stable base are effective when children are first learning to stand and walk.

Orthoses have also been used during sleep to prevent the secondary impairment of hypoextensibility, or contracture. Baumann and Zumstein (1985) found that the use of double-shell foot orthoses as night splints from the age of 3 years to the end of the skeletal growth period prevented calf muscle contractures from developing and made the need for surgery rare.

Orthopaedic Surgery. Orthopaedic surgery in preschoolers is usually performed to prevent secondary impairment by limiting the effects of hypoextensibility and spasticity. For example, the lengthening of hypoextensible or spastic hip adductors or both may be performed to prevent subluxation or dislocation of the hip joint. Sometimes, however, surgery such as tendo Achillis lengthening is delayed because of the tendency for recurrence necessitating repeated surgery (Tardieu, G, et al., 1982). Massagli (1991) has emphasized that musculoskeletal surgery does not alter the neurologically driven patterns of muscle activity, although lengthening, releasing, or transferring a muscle can alter its influence. Orthopaedic surgery is sometimes combined with neurectomy if tonic activity of the muscle is present as a result of spasticity or other neurologic causes. A full discussion of the role of orthopaedic surgery in CP can be found in the work of Rang (1990). Physical therapists play important roles in surgical decision-making. They are also involved in the care of the child who is immobilized and in providing postoperative therapy (Harryman, 1992). Frequently forgotten is the importance of transporting children safely in motor vehicles when they are in casts, an activity for which various devices are available (Bull et al., 1989).

Skeletal Alignment. Alignment of the body as a whole is important. Children should have a variety of positions in which they can function, travel, and rest. Varying the positions of children who are limited in movement also helps to prevent the secondary impairments of positional contractures and deformity. Adaptive seating has also been shown to improve pulmonary functioning (Nwaobi & Smith, 1986). For the preschooler, sitting, standing, lying, and a position suitable for playing on the floor are all important. When prescribing seating systems, it is necessary to be aware of not only the child's comfort and functional abilities but also the caregivers' concerns and needs and the child's environment. Seating inserts can be used in a variety of situations and with equipment such as strollers and wheelchairs, which are often needed to enable parents to transport their child easily. Specific suggestions are included in Chapter 23. Approved car seats and restraints are necessary for safe and comfortable vehicular transportation (Shaw, 1987).

Positioning in standing is thought to reduce or prevent secondary impairments by maintaining lower extremity muscle extensibility, by maintaining or increasing bone mineral density, and by promoting optimal musculoskeletal development (Stuberg, 1992), including acetabular development. Optimally, standing involves movement and activity to provide intermittent loading and muscle strain. More affected children require special equipment. Force gauges can be used to measure weight bearing (Stuberg, 1992).

Standing programs are often started at 1 year of age if children are not able to bear their weight effectively on their own. Stuberg (1992) recommended positioning in standing for 45 minutes 2 or 3 times a day to control lower extremity flexor contractures, and for 60 minutes 4 or 5 times per week to facilitate bone development. Maintenance of the child's ability to bear full weight through the legs reduces the need to be lifted by caregivers.

Treatment of Functional Limitations

Physical therapy for treatment of functional limitations is often intensive during the preschool years. The frequency of treatment varies, depending on the resources available, complementary programming, client goals, parental needs and desires, and the child's response to treatment. Optimal treatment frequency is unknown, but periods of increased frequencies have shown improvements in attainment of specific treatment goals at levels that were maintained when frequency decreased, provided the skills were incorporated into daily functional activities. Improvements in nonspecified areas were not consistently affected (Bower & McLellan, 1992).

Strategies incorporated into treatment approaches such as NDT have been shown to improve control of functional movements. Kluzik and colleagues (1990) found that the speed and smoothness of movement of upper extremity reaching improved after a treatment session of NDT. Upper extremity weight bearing has been shown to improve hand opening and prehension patterns (Chakerian & Larson, 1993). It is difficult, however, to determine whether the changes were directly related to treatment effects on single-system or multisystem impairments.

Therapy should be challenging and meaningful to the child and progress to integrating the skills learned into functional and cognitively directed skills for carryover. Movement tasks should be goal oriented and interesting to maintain motivation and arousal. For example, kicking a soccer ball may be a more functional and motivating method of developing balance skills than practicing standing on one foot. Children with CP are able to perform concrete perceptuomotor tasks much more readily than abstract ones, even if the same movements are involved (van der Weel et al., 1991), because more information is available from the environment to direct the task.

Motor-learning principles (see Chapter 6) can be used to develop treatment strategies for reducing functional limitations. Feedback is important in the process of learning skilled movement. Feedback through the child's sensory receptors provides intrinsic information, whereas extrinsic feedback through various forms of biofeedback provides information from external sources. Knowledge of results contributes information about movement outcome, and knowledge of performance supplies feedback about the nature of the movement (Poole, 1991).

Feedforward mechanisms must also be considered, since there is a cognitive component to movement skills. In some instances, cognitive strategies may be able to compensate for some of the inherent motor limitations.

Many children with CP do not have normal cognition and behavior, and activities must be adapted accordingly. If a child is unable to learn, training using memorization of solutions may be necessary, although limited transfer to novel situations will occur (Higgins, 1991). If behavioral factors are negatively affecting treatment, a behavioral approach using appropriate motivators may encourage children to work on certain skills (Horton & Taylor, 1989).

Example of Teaching to Improve Function. Improvements in function of the preschool-aged child are made by reducing the effects on functional movement of the multisystem impairments of selective control, anticipatory regulation, and learning of unique movements. Although there is a growing literature on motor learning (see Chapter 6), on motor control in skill acquisition (see Chapter 2), and on the biomechanics of movement, the profession is still far from being able to provide optimal strategies for treatment that are known to be effective (Fetters, 1991). The therapist who treats children with CP constantly modifies approaches as research produces new insights.

The following partial example of a child's learning to climb a set of stairs illustrates an approach to the learning of a functional activity. The approach involves the therapist's planning of the movement, evaluation, adaptation, and repetition.

The plan for the target function is based on the goal, which must be a relevant and purposeful task for the child: in this case, to climb a set of stairs to reach a parent. The therapist first analyzes the movement and the potential strategies for accomplishing it, knowing the child's impairments, the environmental demands, the preparatory postural changes needed, the demands on the musculoskeletal system, and the sensorimotor strategies that the child may be able to use.

Environmental requirements dictate the height the foot must be raised to clear the stair. An anticipatory strategy is needed to shift the center of mass of the body, first sideways onto the supporting limb, then forward in preparation for transfer up to the next stair. As the child's anticipatory regulation is likely to be deficient, the therapist may help the child to develop anticipatory strategies by using similar movements, such as standing on one foot to kick a ball or squeezing a squeaky toy with the foot. The instructions and the methods for training strategies should be kept as similar as possible to those of the functional activity, however, since transfer is impaired even when differences between tasks are small (Ashby et al., 1988). Manual guidance of postural shift, often referred to as facilitation, can be used for its positive effect on the acquisition phase of learning a movement, although it is less useful in the later learning stages (see Chapter 6). Directing attention to sensory input may facilitate anticipatory regulation of body position. The therapist may say, "Make your foot feel really light when you are going to step up on the red stair." Motor memory, known to be deficient in those with CP, is also likely to be assisted by the attention the child pays to sensory information.

The child's musculoskeletal system is required to generate extensor moments on the supporting limb that are adequate for supporting the weight of the body. This skill may also require prior development. First, the flexor muscle activity on the climbing limb is needed to generate flexor power to lift the limb, and then knee extensor activity is needed to extend and place the foot on the stair. Poor selective control and timing of these muscles is likely to be present. The therapist helps the child to select wanted muscle activity and minimize unwanted muscle activity by weight shifting that will make the child most stable, thereby minimizing cocontraction. Also, the child's attention is directed to the sequence of movements that are to be performed: "Gently bring your knee up to touch my finger" (to encourage selection of hip flexors without knee extensors), and then, "Put your foot on the red stair" (to activate knee extensors). Augmented sensory information, such as EMG biofeedback, can be used to assist in the selecting and sequencing of muscle activation at this stage of stair climbing. For example, with auditory EMG feedback of ankle dorsiflexor activity, the child can be asked to make a beep when lifting the foot to the stair.

This plan and approach to the child's learning of stair climbing are evaluated by the therapist with close observation of the child's ability to 1) shift weight to prepare the appropriate posture, 2) generate the musculoskeletal requirements, and 3) use the available sensorimotor strategies to meet the environmental demands. The plan or the environmental demand of the task or both are adapted, if necessary, to achieve successful performance. The activity requires a great deal of practice to facilitate learning, since motor memory can be expected to be impaired.

During the later learning stages, hands-on facilitation is minimized to allow the child to be a fully active participant in the process and to develop a motor program to accomplish the task without the guidance of the therapist. To maximize learning, the practice of stair climbing includes variability in the task, the degree of difficulty, and the environment (see Chapter 6).

Feeding, Drooling, and Toileting. Some children with CP, particularly those who are severely affected, may have oral-motor problems, such as poor mouth closure, retraction or thrusting of the tongue, poor tongue movements, and poor coordination in swallowing, which can make speech and feeding difficult. Feeding problems can be aggravated by other problems such as impaired self-feeding and difficulties in expressing hunger or food preferences that may result in inadequate nutritional intake and poor growth (Gisel & Patrick,

1988; Reilly & Skuse, 1992). Gastroesophageal reflux and aspiration also occur in children with severe CP. Oral-motor programs, proper positioning, and parent education and support are important issues to address (Evans Morris & Dunn Klein, 1987). In extreme cases, gastrostomy and antireflux procedures may be necessary to improve growth and enhance the quality of life for the child and the family (Rempel, 1988).

Drooling, a significant problem in about 10% of children with CP, can cause social embarrassment and affect the quality of social integration (Blasco et al., 1992). It can result from dysfunctional oral-motor activity, oral sensory problems, or inefficient and infrequent swallowing. Management may include waiting for further neurologic maturation, feeding and oral stimulation programs, behavior modification programs, medications, or surgery.

Failure to develop an appropriate toileting routine during the preschool years can result in an ongoing disability, since incontinence can provoke negative reactions from caregivers and peers. Expectations of toileting in children with CP should be similar to those for children of comparable cognitive abilities, and therapists should encourage training at a comparable age and recommend appropriate adaptive equipment as necessary (Shaw, 1990).

Mobility

Ambulation is a major concern of physical therapists during these years. Emphasis in treatment is initially on prewalking skills, such as attaining effective and well-aligned weight bearing, promoting dissociation and weight shifting, and improving balance. Ambulatory aids, such as walkers and crutches, may be used, either temporarily while the child is progressing to more advanced gait skills or as long-term aids for independent mobility. The use of posterior walkers has been found to encourage a more upright posture during gait and to promote better gait characteristics than does the use of anterior walkers (Fig. 19–5) (Logan et al., 1990).

Children in this age group are becoming aware of the concept of achievement, and although ambulation is a coveted skill, it should not become an all-consuming goal, particularly if it may not be attainable. When interviewing adults with significant impairment, Kibele (1989) found that they remembered walking as the most important goal set for them by their parents and therapists. This resulted in feelings of failure from an early age and also in a loss of faith in rehabilitation professionals.

The provision of alternative means to allow children functional, independent mobility when ambulation is impossible or inefficient is recommended. Sometimes, this need is met with an

FIGURE 19–5. Child using a posterior walker, reported to promote upright posture and higher walking speeds than an anterior walker.

adapted tricycle (Fig. 19–6) or manual wheelchair; other children require one of a wide variety of power mobility devices available (Jones, CK, 1990) and may need special controls (Fig. 19–7). These enable children with CP to explore their environment and achieve a sense of independence and competence. Power mobility may also promote the development of initiative (Butler, 1991) and the acquisition of spatial concepts. The lack of self-propelled locomotion can result in apathy, withdrawal, passivity, and dependent behavior that can persist into later life (Butler, 1991).

If power mobility is being considered, fine motor control, cognitive abilities, behavior, environment, visual and auditory abilities, and financial resources must all be taken into account. Children with motor limitations have become safely and effectively mobile in power wheelchairs at as young as 17 months of age (Butler, 1991). Parents may initially be hesitant about introducing power mobility to young children, fearing that it signifies giving up on walking. Power mobility does not pre-

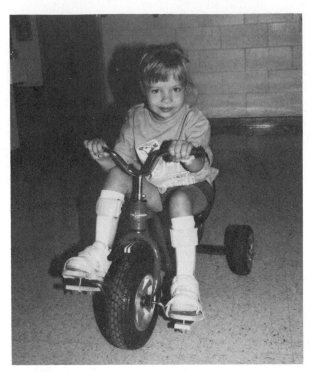

FIGURE 19-6. An adapted tricycle may meet a child's needs for mobility.

transportation needs. For more information, see Chapter 23.

Play

Play, the primary productive activity for children, is intrinsically motivating and pleasurable. The benefits of play include the childrens' discovering the effects they can have on objects and people in their environment, cultivating and testing social roles, and promoting the development of perceptual, conceptual, intellectual, and language skills (Missiuna & Pollock, 1991). Limitations in the play of children with physical disabilities may affect their experiential learning derived from play and result in decreased independence, motivation, imagination, creativity, assertiveness, social skills, and self-esteem (Missiuna & Pollock, 1991). Therapy should provide and demonstrate play opportunities (Fig. 19-8). Appropriate toys and play methods should be suggested to parents and caregivers. If children are physically unable to play with regular toys, a variety of adaptations, such as switch accessing, can make their toys usable (Langley, 1990). Environmental control equipment also can be introduced to preschoolers.

clude ambulation-oriented therapy but provides the child with a method of moving about independently in the meantime. For children who will continue to be wholly dependent on power mobility for independence, it provides mobility at an appropriate age and gives the families an indication of the implications of power mobility on housing and

FIGURE 19-7. Single-switch scanning computer controller for power wheelchair permits independent mobility for children with very limited motor control. Developed at Hugh MacMillan Rehabilitation Centre, Toronto, Ontario.

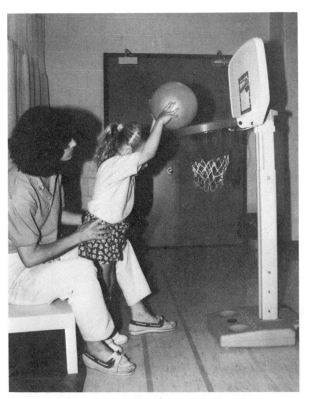

FIGURE 19-8. Therapeutic exercise programs can include highly motivating play activities. Throwing a basketball may be more motivating than trunk extension exercises.

It is important that children are not overprotected in their attempts to play. Parents should be encouraged to let their children enjoy typical play activities, such as rolling down hills and getting dirty in the mud. Therapists must ensure that home programs promote, rather than interfere with, the normal play experiences parents have with their children.

Specialized Treatment

Various therapy approaches may be initiated during the preschool years. One approach sometimes used, often in conjunction with NDT, is sensory integration (Degangi, 1990). The theory suggests that children with CP may have sensory integrative dysfunction as a result of either neurologic dysfunction within the central nervous system or limitation in sensory experiences resulting from the lack of normal motor control. Rather than work directly on a functional motor skill, sensory integrative therapy proposes to facilitate the child's organization and processing of proprioceptive, tactile, and vestibular input in the central nervous system to influence postural responses, environmental awareness, and motor planning (White, 1984).

"Conductive" education, an educational approach originated by Andras Peto in Hungary, is based on the theory that the difficulties of the child with motor dysfunction are problems of learning. The goal of treatment is the ability to function independently in the world without aids, an important objective in Hungary, where schools are not adapted for children with disabilities. Participants, selected for their ability to learn, are usually treated in group settings that provide the incentive of competition and allow more intensive therapy than does individual treatment. They are instructed by "conductors" who are trained in all facets of rehabilitation. Functional goals are broken down into small steps. Children initiate the activities on their own, with direct conscious action aided by mental preparation (Hari & Tillemans, 1984).

The preschool period is a time when parents may consider alternative treatments that are not accepted by some professionals. If parents choose to take an approach other than the one offered by the therapist, it is necessary to respect their choice. Their reasons for seeking alternatives may include both their feeling that they must try everything and their hostility toward those who initially diagnosed the disability without offering a cure or without providing what they consider to be enough therapy. Therapists should not react defensively but should provide impartial information about the therapies

in question and assure parents that they can resume their child's usual treatment if they choose.

Family Involvement

Family involvement remains crucial for integrating treatment into everyday life. It is necessary to find a balance between providing parents with home programs that make them an integral part of their child's therapy and burdening them with activities they cannot realistically be expected to carry out because of constraints on time, energy, skills, or resources or because of negative effects on the parent-child relationship. Hinojosa and Anderson (1991) found that although mothers of preschoolers with CP did not carry out specific home programs designed by therapists, they did activities that could be integrated into their daily routines and interactions and that were not stressful for the child or the caregiver.

Siblings can be included in home programs. Craft and colleagues (1990) studied a group of children with CP whose siblings had been educated about the condition and ways in which they could encourage their brother or sister to be more independent. As a result of this, the children with CP showed increases in ROM and in functional independence.

There is currently an emphasis on defining strategies to make the management of children with disabilities more family centered. Planning of interventions should take into account the child within the context of the family. Therapists should be sensitive to the family's stresses, dynamics, child-rearing practices, coping mechanisms, privacy, values, and cultural variations. Therapists should be flexible in their approach and programming (Kolobe, 1992). Special efforts must be made to deal with the effects of a child with CP on the siblings (Powell, 1985).

Role of Other Disciplines

Occupational therapists work closely with the children at this age to develop independence in activities such as dressing, feeding, toileting, and playing. Speech and language pathologists continue to develop efficient methods of communication in children with CP. Psychologists assess cognitive skills and advise on the interaction of intellectual abilities with the other areas of development. Social workers and behavior therapists continue to provide ongoing support to the families, since the stresses involved in parenting a child with a disability persist (Sternisha et al., 1992). Team assessment and intervention are imperative for addressing issues such as feeding problems, augmentative communication, and transition into school.

School-Aged and Adolescent Period

During the school-aged and adolescent years, children typically become more involved in school and community life while remaining dependent on their families and living in their parental homes. They refine and augment the basic functional skills they have learned and develop life skills that will enable them to cope effectively with the demands of daily living and, it is hoped, independent adult life.

These can be difficult years for children with CP. They become more aware of the reality, extent, and impact of their disabilities on themselves and their families. As they strive to contend with the normal stresses of growing up, particularly those of adolescence, they must also cope with being different, acknowledge the potential obstacles to attaining independence, and work to overcome them.

Parents remain anxious about how their child's disabilities will affect their participation in educational environments and in social situations. They may worry about their child's future as an adult. While continuing to be naturally attentive, they have to avoid being overprotective and begin to allow their child to take risks and become independent in the outside world. In some cases, there may be financial concerns regarding the need for special equipment, transportation, and home renovations. Parents of children who are dependent in ADL and transfers may suffer from physical stresses, such as back problems.

Typical disabilities encountered during these years include a lack of independent mobility, poor endurance in performing routine activities, and continued difficulty and slowness with self-care and hygiene skills at a time when privacy is becoming increasingly important. Adolescents may also not have the opportunity to develop socially and sexually and may lack the ability to acquire age-appropriate levels of independence from the family. Societal barriers may reduce access to community and school facilities, thus limiting opportunities for participation in social, cultural, and athletic activities.

PHYSICAL THERAPY ASSESSMENT

The privacy of individuals at all ages should be respected, but it is particularly important during these years when children are becoming more aware of their bodies and their sexuality. Children should be appropriately dressed when attending therapy sessions and clinics, particularly if they are being seen by unfamiliar people or are being photographed or videotaped. If it is necessary to remove their clothing, their permission should be asked and a reason given for doing so. It is important to include the clients in conversations that involve them and not to converse only with caregivers or other professional staff.

Assessment of impairments that could interfere with function, or lead to further secondary impairment, such as scoliosis, continues to be important. Assessment of gross motor function is appropriate, since children may still be making some gross motor progress during their school years. They may also change as a result of interventions such as surgery, the use of orthoses, and periods of intensive therapy. The development of the Gross Motor Performance Measure (Boyce et al., 1992) may help in detecting the fine increments of motor skill gains that are characteristic of children who are severely affected. For children with mild degrees of involvement, the Bruininks-Oseretsky Test of Motor Proficiency (Bruininks, 1978) may be useful in measuring specific components of higher levels of motor function.

Gait analysis continues to be helpful in assessing ambulatory children, particularly when decisions about surgery are being made (Lee et al., 1992). Endurance and efficiency of movement become increasingly important during these years as the children venture into the community on their own or with their peers. Mechanical energy costs can be assessed with motion analysis equipment (Olney et al., 1987). In the clinical setting, physiologic measures such as the physiologic cost index for activities such as ambulation can give useful information for optimizing function (Butler, 1991; Mossberg et al., 1990) or selecting assistive devices (Rose et al., 1985). In a laboratory setting, ergometer assessment can analyze other aspects of endurance (Parker et al., 1992). An important consideration in maximizing endurance for daily activities is the effect of excessive weight gain, since it can compromise optimal function and efficiency.

PHYSICAL THERAPY GOALS AND TREATMENT

As goals become oriented toward the child's or adolescent's lifestyle, emphasis is on maintaining or improving the level of function while considering the stresses of growth, maturation, and the increasing demands in life skills. Although the pathophysiologic impairment of CP is nonprogressive, there are changes related to the stresses of increasing size and a more competitive lifestyle. For example, as children advance to higher grades in school, there may be longer distances to walk between classes. Contractures may rapidly develop during periods when bones are growing faster than muscles (Tardieu, G, et al., 1982). Secondary orthopaedic and functional problems must be anticipated and avoided. The maintenance of muscle extensibility and force generation, joint integrity, and fitness is important in preventing secondary impairments that can result from the stresses of aging. This age group also needs to develop strategies to overcome environmental and societal barriers to become as independent and active as possible in home, school, recreational or social, and community life.

In many cases, adolescents can and should be involved in setting goals and determining programming. It is important during these years to encourage them to take responsibility for their own health, care, and decision-making so that they are prepared to assume these responsibilities in adulthood (Fox et al., 1992). It is also important to look ahead and set goals that are appropriate for their later life situations and independence. Therapists should strive to foster self-esteem and assertiveness in children and adolescents by emphasizing their abilities, finding areas and activities in which they can excel, and helping them to acknowledge their difficulties with a view toward identifying appropriate compensations. In the case of children with severe disorder, goals are oriented toward minimizing impairments to facilitate caregiving and comfort.

Reducing Primary Impairment and Preventing Secondary Impairment

The impairment of deficient muscle force generation that may result in functional limitations and disabilities is important to confront in this age group. McCubbin and Shasby (1985) found that isokinetic resistance exercise improved movement time and torque development in adolescents with CP and concluded that the exercise had affected neuromuscular performance in a manner similar to that in the nondisabled population. An isokinetic training program for mildly affected adolescents effected strength gains of 12 to 30% in knee extensors and flexors (MacPhail & Kramer, 1993). Although isokinetic strength was related to a measure of energy cost of walking, it is not clear at this time whether increasing strength alters efficiency.

Electrical stimulation has been used as an adjunct to the treatment of CP to reduce spasticity, to increase force production and extensibility, and to improve function. It is particularly useful in postoperative muscle training and strengthening. Bowser and colleagues (1985) treated children with plantar flexor contractures by stimulating the peroneal nerve or tibialis anterior muscle. This improved dorsiflexion during the swing phase of gait as well as during the active range of dorsiflexion. In a similar experiment, Dubowitz and colleagues (1988) found that electrical stimulation improved the voluntary contraction of tibialis anterior, and they observed less muscle fatigue with improved motor performance in standing and gait.

Pharmacologic intervention can be used to control the impairment of spasticity. Baclofen, a synthetic agonist of aminobutyric acid, has an inhibitory effect on the presynaptic excitatory neurotransmitter release. It has been shown to reduce spasticity in individuals with CP (Armstrong, 1992). If taken orally, doses high enough to give the proper concentration in the cerebrospinal fluid can cause side effects such as drowsiness. To circumvent this problem, baclofen is most effective if given intrathecally by a continuous infusion pump implanted in the abdomen that releases the drug at a slow, constant rate into the subarachnoid space.

Biofeedback is a useful tool in addressing single-system and multisystem impairments during these years (Fig. 19–9) because by this time children have usually developed abstract thinking and sufficient cognitive ability to use it optimally. Positive results have been reported (Kassover et al., 1986), but carryover is often limited.

The secondary impairment of joint or muscle contracture may occur in this age group, particularly in the more severely affected patients. This can be a result of chronic muscle imbalance, abnormal posturing, or static positioning. Casting may be used to increase the range of joint movement by lengthening muscles or tendons or both (O'Dwyer et al., 1989; Tardieu, G, et al., 1982). Anderson and colleagues (1988) found that soft splints made of polyurethane foam were effective in reducing severe knee flexor contractures; this

FIGURE 19–9. Biofeedback is a useful treatment tool when precise objectives can be identified.

may be an attractive alternative for low-income families.

Orthopaedic surgery continues to be used to reduce the effects of primary and secondary impairment on mobility, posture, cosmesis, and hygiene and to prevent further secondary impairment. Possible surgical procedures include muscle lengthenings or transfers, tenotomies, neurectomies, osteotomies, and fusions. As children get older, they should be active participants in surgical decision-making that may be influenced by their interests, priorities, and concerns about interruptions in their lives as a result of hospitalizations, immobilizations, and recovery periods.

Some physical therapists are treating the secondary impairment of joint hypomobility resulting from capsular or ligamentous tightness with manual therapy techniques. Joint mobilizations may be used to regain joint mobility, particularly after immobilization. Therapists must ascertain whether joint structures are causing movement restriction and must also be aware of the contraindications and precautions relevant to using mobilizations in growing and neurologically involved patients (Harris & Lundgren, 1991).

Spasticity, abnormal extensibility of muscles, muscular imbalance, and decreased force generation can result in scoliosis, which, in turn, can affect positioning and respiratory status. Spinal deformity can be a particularly difficult problem in the severely affected patient. Rigid orthoses can result in skin breakdown and patient intolerance; by contrast, the use of a soft orthosis has been found to be beneficial in the management of scoliosis in patients with CP (Letts et al., 1992). In some cases, surgical intervention may be necessary (see Chapter 10).

Mobility and Endurance

Many compensatory strategies can be implemented to promote function and circumvent disability during the school years. The continued use of power mobility devices is important for independent mobility. Often children who are able to walk independently need an alternative form of mobility, such as a manual wheelchair or a power scooter, as they become larger and need to travel greater distances to meet their social and educational objectives. Availability of power mobility should not preclude activity to the point of decreased musculoskeletal integrity or physical fitness. The use of mobility devices may require modifications, such as ramps to buildings or washroom renovations, for accessibility. Driver training offers the freedom to travel independently. For those unable to drive, instruction in the use of public or special transportation should be provided.

The functional limitation of low endurance levels, frequently related to inefficiency of movement, has been identified in children with CP. Rose and colleagues (1990) found that energy expenditure indices based on oxygen uptake and heart rate measured at a given walking speed were 3 times higher in children with CP than in normal control children. Findings that were similar, but based on mechanical energy analyses, were reported for children with hemiplegia (Olney et al., 1987). Rose and colleagues (1985) also found that children who were ambulatory with wheeled walkers or quadripod canes had high physiologic workloads when walking for 5 minutes, suggesting that it is impractical for such children to walk long distances. Orthoses may also influence energy expenditure. Mossberg and colleagues (1990) showed that the use of AFOs significantly reduced the energy demands of walking in children with spastic diplegia.

School and Community

Many children are involved in school-based programs, particularly with continuing application of the Education for all Handicapped Children Act in 1975 in the United States (Poirier et al., 1988) and the Charter of Rights and Freedoms in Canada in 1982 (Poirier et al., 1988). In most jurisdictions, the educational program must be implemented in the least restrictive environment for that child, and "the child . . . mainstreamed to the fullest possible extent" (Clune & Van Pelt, 1985). Facilities and resources such as support personnel, equipment for accessibility, and computer-based systems (Fig. 19–10) are necessary to meet the physical needs of children in the school system. Therapists working

FIGURE 19–10. Computer-based communication system with visual keyboard on computer screen and head pointer acting as controller. Developed at Hugh MacMillan Rehabilitation Centre, Toronto, Ontario.

with school personnel may instruct assistants and teachers in positioning, lifting, and transferring the children; carrying out exercise programs; and adapting and developing physical education programs (Wilcox, 1988). Therapists may also be involved in accessibility, transportation, evacuation, and other safety issues. Therapists working in school settings must be sensitive to the physical and scheduling constraints of the educational environment and be willing to compromise to meet the educational priorities of the students. For example, ambulation and climbing stairs may be excellent fitness activities, but the resulting fatigue could affect classroom performance. Therefore, fitness may have to be addressed in other ways. Therapy may range from consultation and monitoring, for students who are thought to have reached their maximal level of physical functioning, to active therapy, for children who have specific treatment goals. When children are primarily seen through the educational system, effort must be made to keep the family involved in all aspects of care and treatment. See Chapter 31 for further information on this subject based on experiences in the United States.

In addition to educating school staff about children with CP, therapists can help to educate the other children in the classroom. Knowledge about, and positive interactions with, people with disabilities can create positive attitudes, particularly when children are between 7 and 9 years of age, because their attitudes about people with disabilities are flexible at this age (Morrison & Ursprung, 1987).

It is important for children with disabilities to be involved in community and recreational activities that provide social as well as therapeutic opportunities. Many adapted or integrated sports activities are suitable for people with CP, including horseback riding (Bertoti, 1988), swimming, skiing, sailing, canoeing, camping, kayaking, fishing, bungee jumping, yoga, and tai chi. Adapted games can provide athletic competition and participation in team experiences and can facilitate the social aspects of sports (Jones, JA, 1988).

All athletes are at risk for sports-related injuries, but relatively minor injuries can incapacitate people with CP. They should be encouraged to be responsible for their bodies during sports activities by following appropriate conditioning and warm-up and cool-down routines, and observing the guidelines of regular exercise prescriptions (Jones, JA, 1988). For more information, see Chapter 16.

During these years, children learn about their bodies, their sexuality, and appropriate interactions with other people. Children and adults with disabilities have an increased risk of suffering abuse, including sexual abuse, which can result in physical, social, emotional, and behavioral consequences

(Sobsey & Doe, 1991). Many of the perpetrators have relationships with the victims that are similar to those commonly found among non-disabled victims; however, some abusers have relationships specifically related to the victim's disability. These people can be personal care attendants, transportation providers, residential care staff, and other disabled individuals. Abuse is a serious matter that must be guarded against at all times. Physical therapists must know how to detect the signs of abuse, be sensitive and receptive to clients who may choose to confide in them, and know the proper procedures to follow if they suspect abuse. They must work with other professionals to promote assertiveness and positive self-esteem in their clients.

All professionals involved with patients who have CP must educate them in being streetwise. Their physical and sometimes cognitive limitations can make them particularly vulnerable to crime. Children and adolescents with disabilities should be taught to avoid threatening situations. They should be warned about carrying valuables (large sums of money or important medications) with them, particularly in a purse that attracts attention and is easy to grab, such as one slung over a wheelchair handle. Attendance at self-defense courses should be encouraged; some that are specifically designed for people with disabilities are becoming available.

Health care professionals must realize that although parents have been coping with their children's needs for a number of years, parent education is still important: their children and their needs are constantly changing. Continued attention to education in lifting and transferring is necessary to prevent injury to caregivers as their children grow larger and heavier.

Role of Other Disciplines

Occupational therapists may be involved in promoting independence in ADL. Multidisciplinary life-skills training may be offered to focus on self-care, community living, and interpersonal relationships. Prevocational training and related activities, such as money management and employment searching, may be necessary. Psychologists or social workers may be involved in social and sexual counseling.

Transition into Adulthood

The life role of an adult is to be an independently functioning and self-sufficient individual who has a satisfying social and emotional life and is a contributing member of society. The natural environment for adults is living independently in the community, alone or with others, with employment to support themselves.

The extent to which people with CP can realize these goals depends on factors such as level of cognition, available resources and support, and independence in self-care activities and mobility. Many adults with CP continue to live with their families, in group homes, or in institutions, and a small proportion of them are employed. In Finland, a study of young adults who had been followed since childhood revealed that 31% of those older than 19 years were competitively employed, but an additional 21% who were judged to be employable were unemployed (Sillanpaa et al., 1982). Finding employment can be particularly difficult when there is considerable unemployment in the able-bodied population.

At a time when most parents are experiencing freedom from caregiving responsibilities, many parents of children with CP continue to have these obligations and have to cope with many anxieties (Hallum & Krumboltz, 1993). Their concerns focus on how their child can function as an independent adult, how they can continue to care for their child as they themselves age, and who will care for the child when they are unable to do so. They, and their child, may also be coping with a decrease in the number of relatively organized and available programs that were available for the younger child.

Physical therapy involvement continues to address all levels of the disabling process; however, there is an emphasis on working together with the individual, the family, and the health care team to provide comprehensive planning to ease the transition to adulthood.

PHYSICAL THERAPY ASSESSMENT

Although there is a continuing need to assess impairment, adult assessments focus on function and disability, particularly on the level of independent functioning. A variety of functional disability scales, such as the Barthel Index, have been developed for adults in general rather than for adults with a particular disability (Mahoney & Barthel, 1965). These measure performance in various self-care, independence, and mobility functions (Spector, 1990).

PHYSICAL THERAPY GOALS AND TREATMENT

The major goal during this period of transition is to maximize the client's capabilities to achieve optimal independence and happiness as an adult. Ideally, the medical, therapeutic, and educational

goals of childhood have had this as a long-term goal in earlier intervention. In many situations, professionals, the client, and the family are dealing with external environmental forces that make it difficult for a person to overcome disabilities (Kibele, 1989).

Reducing Primary Impairment and Preventing Secondary Impairment

Although there is a focus on overall disability, therapists must still be cognizant of the impact of impairment on function. The impairments of insufficient force generation and hypoextensibility can still respond to therapy. In a single-subject study of an adult with CP, Horvat (1987) found improvements in strength, endurance, and ROM after an 8-week training program involving the use of free weights and training machines. He noted that training procedures and resistance in the exercise activities must be designed to improve ROM and not contribute to shortening of muscle groups.

Although secondary impairments such as contracture may appear to be static, there can still be deterioration, so monitoring and treatment, if necessary, should be available. If significant deformity occurs, aggressive salvage surgery in adulthood may be necessary for comfort and ease of care. One example is proximal femoral resection if a hip is painful or if hip mobility is limited to the extent that sitting and perineal care are affected (McCarthy et al., 1988).

Of particular importance is the prevention of overuse syndromes, joint degeneration, osteoporosis, and pathologic fractures. Nerve entrapment syndromes or tendinitis can occur as a result of excessive and repetitive physical stresses. Such injuries should be treated with orthopaedic therapy techniques as they would be in the general population. Preventive treatment to minimize the long-term effects of the neuromuscular dysfunction may be beneficial. This may include use of additional mobility aids or devices, orthoses, or surgery.

Life Skills

Ongoing involvement in fitness and recreational activities should be planned. This will provide social opportunities as well as maintain or improve cardiovascular fitness, weight control, and integrity of joints and muscles; help to prevent osteoporosis; and generally promote the optimal health that contributes to independent functioning. Fitness clubs, swimming, wheelchair aerobics, and adapted sports are options. Endurance continues to be an important concern. Fernandez and Pitetti (1993) found that the values for physical work capacity of ambulatory adults with CP were significantly lower than normal values and concluded that adults with CP would possibly experience fatigue before completing a normal workday. However, physical work capacity and work-related activities improved with training.

Technology is providing adults with CP many options that were not previously available. These include computers for communication, artificial speech devices, environmental control devices, and mobility devices. For more information, see Chapter 23.

Society is becoming more conscious of the rights and needs of the disabled (Bickenbach, 1993). Human rights legislation now exists to accommodate people with disabilities and to prevent discrimination against them in areas such as employment, accessibility, the legal system, and education. Government programs and services are available to people with disabilities. Theaters, restaurants, libraries, museums, government buildings, educational facilities, shopping areas, parks, campground facilities, and parking lots are becoming accessible, where possible, through the provision of ramps, appropriate washroom facilities, and other modifications. Air and rail travel is also becoming more accessible to people with special mobility needs, and there are now travel organizations that cater to people with disabilities. In some situations, funding for assistive devices, living allowances, and housing and tax exemptions help prevent undue hardship. Therapists should be aware of the facilities available to the disabled and the political policies and issues concerning the disabled and should advocate their advancement.

Transition Planning

Ideally, the planning for the transition to adult services and lifestyle takes place before the actual major life changes. Areas to be addressed when planning for the transition include vocational training or postsecondary educational placement, which may range from higher education to supported work models; living arrangements (independent, with family, institutional, or with other supportive care); leisure and recreation (religious groups, community programs, and recreational centers); personal management, including birth control; social skills; and household management. The continuation of professional health services must also be dealt with (Fox et al, 1992) This includes the provision of therapy when needed, medical consultation, primary care, and equipment needs and maintenance. Financial planning and education about budgeting, tax and other governmental benefits, advocacy and legal services, guardianship, conservatorship, wills, and trusts must be addressed.

RESEARCH NEEDS

Research in CP is urgently needed. The selection of treatment for an individual with CP requires predictive information about the effects of interventions, if any, on the pathophysiology, impairments, functional limitations, and disabilities of the person throughout the life span, yet even descriptive information is limited. To take a simple example, to decide whether orthoses are appropriate for a particular child, we should know whether the impairment of hypoextensibility is preventable by orthoses, as some studies suggest (Tardieu, C, et al., 1988), and, if so, under what conditions. Further, we should know if force generation capability is changed with orthotic wear, how force output changes with growth, and what conditions favor successful long-term outcomes. These relationships are virtually unreported. The multisystem impairments of poor selective control of muscles, poor anticipatory regulation of movement, and decreased ability to learn unique movements have received little attention, yet their exploration is mandatory if we are to determine how these components of movement are affected by physical therapy.

We need better information concerning the influence of interventions that are primarily directed toward one dimension of the disabling process on other dimensions of the disabling process. For example, we need to be able to predict the effects of orthoses, which are directed toward the impairment of hypoextensibility, on the functional activity of stair climbing and on the disability of being unable to go on a school excursion. Many questions must be addressed, for example, the degree to which the impairment of low force generation affects specific functions and produces disability, whether it is possible to increase force production as some studies suggest (MacPhail, 1993), and, if so, whether these changes affect function or disabilities. Further, it is important to understand how function and disability affect the overall quality of life.

There is a need for research that permits long-term predictions. Information related to the effects of interventions over many years is virtually nonexistent. Finally, there are needs for specific and sensitive measurements of all dimensions of the disabling process to be developed within a focused research program.

GLOBAL ISSUES

The treatment of children with CP varies throughout the world. Physical therapists use many different approaches and combinations of approaches, depending on the facilities available, the child's and the family's needs, and the therapist's training and background. Many of the treatments and technologies discussed are practiced in developed countries, where services, although variable in their extent, quality, and funding, are available and accessible. However, much of the world's population lives in underserviced areas, particularly in the Third World, developing nations or in remote areas. Often, many of the principles and equipment ideas developed elsewhere can be adapted to the various situations (Werner, 1987). Using indigenous materials to fabricate effective and affordable equipment, recycling used equipment, and training local personnel or fostering exchange programs can help provide resources to underserviced areas.

It is important to be sensitive to local customs, cultures, and environmental situations when adapting programs for different settings. Often, the direct application of a certain method is impractical or inappropriate because of economic, geographic, or cultural differences. There is an increasing emphasis on community-based rehabilitation, which promotes interventions that are practical and functional for the particular settings, lifestyles, and cultures.

PROFESSIONAL ISSUES

Therapists who care for children with CP must realize that the work can be physically demanding. They must practice appropriate lifting and handling precautions and should maintain a suitable level of fitness if they are actively treating patients. Working with children and their families can also be emotionally stressful. Therapists may often be challenged with ethical issues, unrealistic expectations and demands, limited resources, and the pressures of dealing with families during the grieving period and other times of crisis. Therapists need to concentrate on what is positive and realize that they cannot control all the variables in their patients' conditions and lives. Professionals must acknowledge their own needs and reactions and feel comfortable in seeking assistance and support from others.

This chapter concludes with two case histories that illustrate some of the management principles discussed in this chapter.

CASE HISTORY: JAMIE

Jamie is an 8-year-old boy with spastic diplegia and microcephaly. After a pregnancy complicated by pre-

eclamptic toxemia, labor began at 37 weeks of gestation, and an emergency cesarean section became necessary when fetal distress occurred. Treatment was begun in the hospital. On returning home with their child, the parents performed routine stretches daily, and a therapist visited every other week. A mothers' support group met every 2 weeks, which provided general information and guidance as well as support.

When Jamie was about 1.5 years of age, the family moved to a town in another province where coordinated services were provided. Jamie took part in physical therapy, occupational therapy, and speech therapy and was assessed routinely by the psychologic services. When he began attending day care, he received services from the same therapists, and the parents, teachers, and therapists worked together on his treatment.

When Jamie was 3.5 years old, the impairment of hypoextensibility of the hamstrings and heel cords was present. Functionally, he was able to walk independently, although he fatigued easily. Toe-walking was common and accompanied by slight knee flexion and adduction and internal rotation of the hips. His right limb showed more impairment than his left. Bivalved short-leg casts were worn for 2 hours 3 times a day in an attempt to prevent further hypoextensibility of the ankle plantar flexors.

At the age of 4.5 years, Jamie's gait was assessed in the Motion Analysis Laboratory at the School of Rehabilitation Therapy at Queen's University in Kingston, Ontario. He walked at an average of 0.71 m/s, compared with the normal value for his age of about 1.00 m/s (Sutherland et al., 1980). Joint excursions were reduced (Fig. 19–11). He walked with marked plantar flexion of the right foot and with slight flexion and reduced excursion of both knees, and he had reduced power generation of the ankle plantar flexors on both sides (A2-PF, Fig. 19–12), which was evidence of low force-generating capability or hypoextensibility or both. He was compensating for these deficiencies with larger than normal pull-off by hip flexors on the left side (H3-F, in Fig. 19–12). The family engaged Jamie in an electrostimulation program from an outside clinic in which the quadriceps and ankle dorsiflexors were stimulated overnight at a level below that required to produce muscle contraction. During the next few months, while electrostimulation and weekly therapy were continued but the use of casts was not, Jamie's ankle plantar flexors became much more hypoextensible. The use of bivalved casts was reintroduced, and the previous range was regained rapidly.

Clinical examination when Jamie was 5.5 years old revealed that his hip adductors, knee flexors, and ankle plantar flexors were more hypoextensible; functionally, he was walking on his toes with reduced excursions of his ankles. Although a number of surgical alternatives were considered, including rhizotomy, the family de-

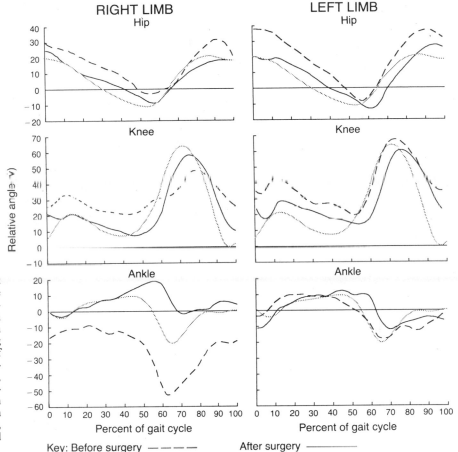

RIGHT LIMB

LEFT LIMB

Relative angle (°v)

Percent of gait cycle

Percent of gait cycle

Key: Before surgery — — — —   After surgery ————

FIGURE 19–11. Plots of joint angles from gait analysis of one stride for Jamie, shown presurgically and postsurgically and with normal values (dotted line). Each plot represents one stride beginning and ending with initial contact of the foot on the floor. Plotted upward (positively) are hip flexion, knee flexion, and ankle dorsiflexion. Note limited knee extension on both sides, extreme limitation of ankle dorsiflexion on the right, and normalization of postsurgical values.

cided on a heel cord lengthening on the right side. Gait re-education was directed toward attaining initial contact with the heel and an extended knee and achieving effective push-off with the ankle plantar flexors. His electrical stimulator was used in treatment postoperatively to strengthen the ankle dorsiflexors and the surgically weakened plantar flexors. Other treatment goals and activities included climbing and descending stairs with one foot per stair and stepping off a stair or curb without hand support. Since Jamie had a keen interest in sports, movement components such as weight shifting, balancing, and eye-hand-foot coordination and skills such as running, starting and stopping, changing direction, and throwing were incorporated into sports activities such as baseball, soccer, and badminton. The improvement noted at a 6-month postsurgical gait analysis (see Fig. 19–11) was more marked on the right side, but several improvements were noted on the left. On the right side, initial contact was made with the heel, and ankle dorsiflexion during late stance reached about 15°. The knees on both sides were more extended at initial contact and extended more in late

stance than was the case before surgery. The push-off power of the right ankle was greater after surgery (A2-PF, in Fig. 19–12) than before surgery, and right hip power was more effective (H1-E, hip extensors in early stance; and H3-F, hip flexors at pull-off; in Fig. 19–12). Average walking velocity was 0.82 m/s. Jamie was able to join the community soccer league the following summer.

Jamie attends school in a regular classroom, although he has some cognitive limitations. He is visited by a familiar therapist from the treatment center every 2 or 3 weeks and attends speech therapy weekly. The main problem the parents have encountered within the school system is a practice of inflexibly classifying the children according to their chronologic age only. Although Jamie is cognitively young and physically small for his age, there has been considerable reluctance to permit him to join younger groups, even for sports. Outside of school, Jamie takes part in a number of athletic activities. He is interested in team sports, and the family has been pleased with the efforts of coaches and managers to include him in organized teams.

FIGURE 19–12. Plots of joint power from gait analysis of one stride for Jamie, shown presurgically and postsurgically and with normal values (dotted line). Each plot represents one stride beginning and ending with initial contact of the foot on the floor. Plotted upward (positively) are muscle power generations (concentric contractions), and downward (negatively) are muscle power absorptions (eccentric contractions). Plots of Jamie's right side show low force generation of right hip extensors in early stance (H1-E) and hip flexors at pull-off (H3-F) and ankle plantar flexors (A2-PF) presurgically, and increases in all of these after surgery. Plots of Jamie's left side show compensatory increase in H3-F (pull-off of hip flexors) presurgically, and normalization after surgery.

CASE HISTORY: NICOLE

Nicole is a 6-year-old girl with moderate to severe spastic diplegia. She was born at 29.5 weeks of gestation after placental separation. She weighed 1300 g and had Apgar scores of 5 at 1 minute, 8 at 5 minutes, and 9 at 10 minutes. She was treated with ventilation for 8 hours and then was weaned off the ventilator onto continuous positive airway pressure, and then to oxygen. She received phototherapy for 3 days for an increased bilirubin level and was administered theophylline for apnea. Nicole remained in the neonatal intensive care unit for 6 weeks and then went home to live with her parents and 3-year-old sister.

Nicole was followed up at the screening clinic for high-risk infants. At 3 months of age corrected for prematurity, she exhibited extensor positioning of her neck and trunk, and hypertonicity was emerging in her lower extremities. At 4 months of corrected age, these findings were discussed with her mother, and positioning and handling recommendations were made. At 5 months of corrected age, the diagnosis of CP was made

on the basis of hypertonicity in her extremities, affecting lower extremities more than upper; strong, persisting primitive reflex activity; and delayed development of head and trunk control. An ultrasound scan at this time showed the left lateral ventricle to be slightly enlarged and the right lateral ventricle to be at the upper limits of normal in size. The periventricular brain parenchyma appeared normal.

Management by a developmental pediatrician, a social worker, an orthopaedic surgeon, a physical therapist, and later an occupational therapist was coordinated at the local children's treatment center. Nicole attended physical therapy sessions weekly. The basic therapy was based on NDT and encouraged active control of movement and play. Positions that reduced the influence of her extensor posturing were used to encourage active control of movements and functional skills. Bivalved casts were introduced early to maintain muscle extensibility and provide optimal alignment of her feet when she was working on standing activities. The casts also reduced some of the extensor posturing in her lower extremities, resulting in improvements in her alignment in sitting and standing and improvements in the quality of functional activities in these positions. These casts were later replaced with solid AFOs when growth slowed down, and Nicole was eager to wear regular shoes. Customized seating and a standing frame gave her a variety of positions that offered opportunities to interact with others and use her hands and provided some weight bearing with her body optimally aligned.

At 2 years of age, the impairments of adductor hypoexensibility and spasticity were treated surgically with bilateral adductor muscle releases and anterior obturator neurectomies. The purpose of the surgery was to give her more functional motion at her hips and to put her hip joints in an optimal position for acetabular development; it was also intended to avoid the potential secondary impairment of hip subluxation or dislocation.

During her preschool years, Nicole attended an integrated child care program with government-subsidized funding for children with special needs. This setting allowed for integration with able-bodied children and also gave Nicole and her family opportunities to meet other children with special needs and their families. Nicole's physical and occupational therapists visited the center regularly to discuss Nicole's abilities, programs, handling, and equipment. Her resource teacher was invaluable in coordinating care, supporting the family, and adapting or acquiring equipment.

When Nicole was 5 years of age, she was progressing slowly in her gross and fine motor skills. However, spasticity in her lower extremities that was clinically apparent was affecting her ability to maintain well-aligned postural stability, and she could not move easily using optimal patterns of movement. These restrictions resulted in functional limitations in sitting, standing, transitional movements, fine motor activities, and ADL and limited her potential for independence. Ambulation was not functional, but she could move about independently in a power chair and had some limited mobility in a manual wheelchair. The prominence of spasticity and the generally good force-generating capabilities of her musculature prompted the decision to have a selective dorsal rhizotomy.

After the rhizotomy, Nicole's lower extremity tone was greatly reduced, and Nicole participated in daily in patient physical therapy and occupational therapy sessions for 8 weeks postoperatively and then had sessions twice a week for the next year (Figs. 19-13 and 19-14).

A Gross Motor Function Measure evaluation was done preoperatively and 1 year after the surgery. Her scores improved from 88% to 96% in lying and rolling, from 70% to 87% in sitting, from 19% to 57% in crawling and kneeling, from 13% to 32% in standing (with AFOs), and from 7% to 10% in walking, running, and jumping (with AFOs). She had been able to walk 10 m

FIGURE 19-13. Mother and therapist with Nicole, encouraging force generation of trunk and hip extensors.

at 0.04 m/s preoperatively but could walk 30 m at 0.15 m/sec at her 1-year follow-up. Although these findings indicated that there had been improvements in her gait, the distance and velocity of her walking were still much below age norms and did not result in functional ambulation. She had improved isolated muscle control, which was demonstrated by improved active ROM of

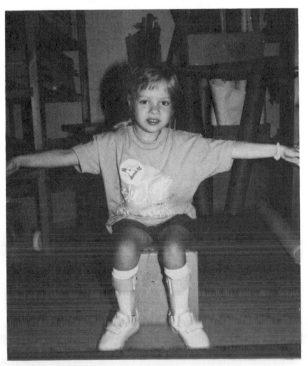

FIGURE 19-14. Nicole, wearing ankle-foot orthoses, doing exercises at school.

FIGURE 19–15. Despite many improvements after posterior rhizotomy, Nicole still shows diminished force-generating ability in hip and knee muscles.

her quadriceps, dorsiflexors, and plantar flexors. Her passive ROM improved in her hips, knees, and ankles, particularly in motions involving the hamstring muscles. Nicole continues to have decreased muscle force production, particularly in her hip and knee extensor muscles (Fig. 19–15).

Nicole showed improvements in her self-care skills, particularly in dressing her lower extremities, because she was able to move one leg independently of the other. On a modified Klein-Bell test of ADL, she achieved 9/33 before surgery and 19/33 when tested 1 year later. She was able to function better with her hands in activities such as opening jars, printing, and propelling her manual wheelchair. The improvements were believed to be the result of better trunk control and cocontraction in the shoulder musculature rather than of changes in the intrinsic muscles of her hands, motor planning, or visuoperceptual skills—areas that continue to be problems for Nicole. The Beery Developmental Test of visuomotor integration score was at an age-equivalency of 4.1 both pre- and postoperatively.

Nicole now attends first grade at her neighborhood school. Transportation in a taxi is provided by the school board, and next year, the regular school bus will have a wheelchair lift installed so that she can travel to school with her peers. The educational system also provides a full-time educational assistant to help Nicole with transfers, toileting, schoolwork, and exercise and sports programs. She plays with her friends on the playground at lunch and recess in her power chair. She is beginning to use a typewriter to increase the speed at which she can put information down on paper.

Nicole's family has worked with medical, educational, governmental, and community organizations to gain access to services and programs that provide her with normal childhood experiences and minimize disabilities. Nicole has been involved with horseback riding, swimming programs, and adapted games. She rides in her family's boat using a Tumble Form seat, goes on an annual vacation to Florida, and recently traveled to England to be a flower girl at her aunt's wedding. She attends her peers' birthday parties, where her friends or their parents help her as necessary. She has modeled in fashion shows in her wheelchair. Nicole attends the community day camp, Brownies, and the Easter Seals family camp in the summer.

Resources her family has found useful include the Easter Seals Society; the Ontario government's Assistive Devices Program; parent support groups; and the Community and Social Services Respite Care Program, which provides funds for students to work with Nicole and provide parent relief. The Canadian railroad, VIA Rail, which allows wheelchair escorts to ride free and offers reduced rates for Nicole, is useful for traveling to out-of-town appointments.

Nicole and her family still face some barriers. The family home is in the country and has a gravel driveway. The house is not wheelchair-accessible since there are stairs into the house, stairs inside, and narrow doorways. Thick carpeting makes manual wheelchair pushing and walker maneuvering difficult. Renovations are possible but costly. When Nicole visits friends, their homes have similar obstacles. Renovations have been made to the school washroom, and equipment has been provided, but the entrance doors are too heavy to open, playground equipment is inaccessible, and classroom door handles are difficult to turn. There is no public wheelchair transportation in their township community. Although obstacles are becoming less common as society becomes more aware of accommodations necessary for people with disabilities, barriers such as buildings without ramps, inadequate parking, and inaccessible washrooms still exist.

Nicole's parents have found regular family conferences invaluable in helping to facilitate effective family and school involvement in therapy programs. In these conferences, all the team members meet to discuss short- and long-term goals. Agendas and minutes clarify the objectives of the meetings and document the decisions that are made. Such conferences help to empower parents and allow them to become effective advocates for their children. They also reinforce the philosophy of teamwork and partnership with the therapists and the treatment center.

Nicole's parents have found Craig Shield's book *Strategies: A Practical Guide for Dealing with Professionals and Human Service Systems* to be helpful (Shields, 1987). They believe that home visits designed to deal with issues of daily routines, integrate treatment goals into home life, and involve all family members are important. Similarly, school visits are important. Nicole's parents believe that it is particularly important not to withhold any information from the family. They also emphasize the need for feedback and encouragement to the family, especially to the primary caregiver.

Acknowledgments

Acknowledgments are extended to the Child Development Centre of the Hôtel Dieu Hospital, Kingston, Ontario; the Motion Analysis Laboratory at the School of Rehabilitation Therapy at Queen's University, Kingston, Ontario; the Hugh MacMillan Rehabilitation Centre, Toronto, Ontario, for assistance in providing data and photographs; and to the parents of Jamie and Nicole for their support of and contributions to the case histories.

References

Anderson, JP, Snow, B, Dorey, FJ, & Kabo, JM. Efficacy of soft splints in reducing severe knee-flexion contractures. Developmental Medicine and Child Neurology, 30:502–508, 1988.

Arens, LJ, Peacock, WJ, & Peter, J. Selective posterior rhizotomy: A long-term follow-up study. Child's Nervous System, 5:148–152, 1989.

Armstrong, RW. Intrathecal baclofen and spasticity: What do we know and what do we need to know? Developmental Medicine and Child Neurology, 34:739–745, 1992.

Ashby, MH, Lee, AM, & Landin, DK. Relationship of practice using correct technique to achievement in a motor skill. Journal of Teaching in Physical Education, 7:115–120, 1988.

Atkinson, S, & Stanley, FJ. Spastic diplegia among children of low and normal birthweight. Developmental Medicine and Child Neurology, 25:693–708, 1983.

Atwater, SW. Should the normal motor developmental sequence be used as a theoretical model in pediatric physical therapy? In Lister, MJ (Ed.), Contemporary Management of Motor Control Problems: Proceedings of the II STEP Conference. Alexandria, VA: Foundation for Physical Therapy, 1991, pp 89–93.

Bailey, DB. Collaborative goal setting with families: Resolving differences in values and priorities for services. Topics in Early Childhood Special Education, 7(2):59–71, 1987.

Batshaw, MI, & Perret, YM. Children with Disabilities: A Medical Primer (3rd ed.). Toronto: Paul H. Brookes, 1992.

Baumann, JU, & Zumstein, M. Experience with a plastic ankle-foot orthosis for prevention of muscle contracture. Developmental Medicine and Child Neurology, 27:83, 1985.

Bayley, N. Bayley II. San Antonio: Psychological Corporation, 1993.

Berbrayer, D, & Ashby, P. Reciprocal inhibition in cerebral palsy. Neurology, 40:653–656, 1990.

Berger, W, Quintern, J, & Deitz, V. Pathophysiology of gait in children with cerebral palsy. Electroencephalography and Clinical Neurophysiology, 53:538–548, 1982.

Bertoti, DB. Effect of therapeutic horseback riding on posture in children with cerebral palsy. Physical Therapy, 68:1505–1512, 1988.

Bickenbach, J. Physical Disability and Social Policy. Toronto: University of Toronto Press, 1993.

Blasco, PA, Allaire, JH, and participants of the Consortium on Drooling. Drooling in the developmentally disabled: Management practices and recommendations. Developmental Medicine and Child Neurology, 34:849–862, 1992.

Bleck, EE. Locomotor prognosis in cerebral palsy. Developmental Medicine and Child Neurology, 17:18–25, 1975.

Bleck, EE. Orthopedic Management in Cerebral Palsy. Philadelphia: JB Lippincott, 1987.

Bly, L. A historical and current view of the basis of NDT. Pediatric Physical Therapy, 3:131–135, 1991.

Bobath, K, & Bobath, B. The neuro-developmental treatment. In Scrutton, D (Ed.), Management of the Motor Disorders of Children with Cerebral Palsy. Clinics in Developmental Medicine (No. 90). Philadelphia: JB Lippincott, 1984, pp. 6–18.

Bohannon, RW. Is the measurement of muscle strength appropriate in patients with brain lesions? Physical Therapy, 69:225–236, 1989.

Bohannon, RW, & Smith, MB. Interrater reliability of a modified Ashworth scale of muscle spasticity. Physical Therapy, 67:206–207, 1987.

Bower, E, & McLellan, DL. Effect of increased exposure to physiotherapy on skill acquisition of children with cerebral palsy. Developmental Medicine and Child Neurology, 34:25–39, 1992.

Bowser, BL, Dimitrijevic, MM, Erdmann, M, & Solis, IS. Effects of neuromuscular stimulation on passive ankle dorsiflexion in children with cerebral palsy: Preliminary report. Developmental Medicine and Child Neurology, 27:116–117, 1985.

Boyce, W, Gowland, C, Rosenbaum, P, Lane, M, Plews, N, Goldsmith, C, Russell, D, Wright, V, Zdrobov, S, & Harding, D. Gross motor performance measure for children with cerebral palsy: Study design and preliminary findings. Canadian Journal of Public Health, 83(suppl 2):S34–S40, 1992.

Brouwer, B, & Ashby, P. Altered corticospinal projections to lower limb motoneurons in subjects with cerebral palsy. Brain, 114:1395–1407, 1991.

Bruininks, RH. Bruininks-Oseretsky Test of Motor Proficiency: Examiner's Manual. Circle Pines, MN: American Guidance Service, 1978.

Bull, MJ, Weber, KL, DeRosa, GP, & Bruner Stroup, K. Transporting children in body casts. Journal of Pediatric Orthopedics, 9:280–284, 1989.

Burns, YR, O'Callaghan, M, & Tudehope, DI. Early identification of cerebral palsy in high risk infants. Australian Paediatric Journal, 25:215–219, 1989.

Butler, C. Augmentative mobility, why do it? Physical Medicine and Rehabilitation Clinics of North America, 2(4):801–815, 1991.

Cahan, LD, Adams, JM, Perry, J, & Beeler, LM. Instrumented gait analysis after selective dorsal rhizotomy. Developmental Medicine and Child Neurology, 32:1037–1043, 1990.

Campbell, SK. Introduction to the special issue. Pediatric Physical Therapy, 2:123–125, 1990.

Campbell, SK, Wilhelm, IJ, & Slaton, DS. Anthropometric characteristics of young children with cerebral palsy. Pediatric Physical Therapy, 1:105–108, 1989.

Carlson, SJ. A neurophysiological analysis of inhibitive casting. Physical and Occupational Therapy in Pediatrics, 4(4):31–42, 1984.

Chakerian, DL, & Larson, MA. Effects of upper-extremity weight-bearing on hand-opening and prehension patterns in children with cerebral palsy. Developmental Medicine and Child Neurology, 35:216–229, 1993.

Chandler, L, & Harris, S. Movement assessment of infants. Workshop Presentation, Northeastern District of the Section on Pediatrics of the American Physical Therapy Association, Amherst, MA. Cited in Campbell, SK. Assessment of the child with CNS dysfunction. In Rothstein, JM (Ed.), Measurement in Physical Therapy. New York: Churchill Livingstone, 1985.

Chandler, LS, Andrew, MS, & Swanson, MW. Movement Assessment of Infants: A Manual. Rolling Bay, WA: Infant Movement Research, 1980.

Clune, WH, & Van Pelt, MH. A political method of evaluating the Education for All Handicapped Children Act of 1975. Law and Contemporary Problems, 48(1):7–62, 1985.

Craft, MJ, Lakin, JA, Oppliger, RA, Clancy, GM, & Vanderlinden, DW. Siblings as change agents for promoting the functional status of children with cerebral palsy. Developmental Medicine and Child Neurology, 32, 1049–1057, 1990.

Crothers, B, & Paine, RS. The Natural History of Cerebral Palsy. Cambridge, MA: Harvard University Press, 1959.

Cusick, BD. Progressive Casting and Splinting for Lower Extremity Deformities in Children with Neuromotor Dysfunction. Tucson, AZ: Therapy Skill Builders, 1990.

Cusick, BD, & Stuberg, WA. Assessment of lower extremity alignment in the transverse plane: Implications for management of children with neuromotor dysfunction. Physical Therapy, 72:3–15, 1992.

Degangi, G. Perspectives on the integration of neurodevelopmental treatment and sensory integrative therapy. NDTA newsletter, 1990, January:1–4, March:1–6, May:1–5.

Dowding, VM, & Barry, C. Cerebral palsy: Social class differences in prevalence in relation to birthweight and severity of disability. Journal of Epidemiology and Community Health, 44:191–195, 1990.

Dubowitz, L, Finnie, N, Hyde, SA, Scott, OM, & Vrbova, G. Improvement in muscle performance by chronic electrical stimulation in children with cerebral palsy. Lancet, 12(1):587–588, 1988. Letter.

Edebol-Tysk, K. Epidemiology of spastic tetraplegic cerebral palsy in Sweden. I: Impairments and disabilities. Neuropediatrics, 20:41–45, 1989.

Evans Morris, S, & Dunn Klein, M. Pre-feeding Skills: A Comprehensive Resource for Feeding Development. Tucson, Az: Therapy Skill Builders, 1987.

Evans, PM, Evans, SJW, & Alberman, E. Cerebral palsy: Why we must plan for survival. Archives of Disease in Childhood, 65:1329–1333, 1990.

Feldman, AB, Haley, SM, & Coryell, J. Concurrent and construct validity of the Pediatric Evaluation of Disability Inventory. Physical Therapy, 70:602–610, 1990.

Fernandez, JE, & Pitetti, KH. Training of ambulatory individuals with cerebral palsy. Archives of Physical Medicine and Rehabilitation, 74:468–472, 1993.

Fetters, L. Measurement and treatment in cerebral palsy: An argument for a new approach. Physical Therapy, 71:244–247, 1991.

Finnie, NR. Handling the Young Cerebral Palsied Child at Home (2nd ed.). New York: EP Dutton, 1975.

Fox, AM, Gillett, JM, & Goldberg, B. Adults with cerebral palsy: Who provides medical care? Annals of the Royal College of Physicians and Surgeons of Canada, 25:206–209, 1992.

Geralis, E (Ed.). Children with Cerebral Palsy. Rockville, MD: Woodbine House, 1991. (Available from Ingram, 1125 Heilquaker Boulevard, Leverane, TN 37086–1986.)

Gisel, EG, & Patrick, J. Identification of children with cerebral palsy unable to maintain a normal nutritional state. Lancet 1:283–286, 1988.

Giuliani, CA. Dorsal rhizotomy for children with cerebral palsy: Support for concepts of motor control. Physical Therapy, 71:248–259, 1991.

Gowland, C, King, G, King, S, Law, M, Letts, L, MacKinnon, L, Rosenbaum, P, & Russell, D. Review of Selected Measures in Neurodevelopmental Rehabilitation. Research Report 91–2, Neurodevelopmental Clinical Research Unit, Chedoke-McMaster Hospitals, 1991. (Available from Chedoke-McMaster Hospitals, PO Box 2000, Station A, Hamilton, Ontario, Canada, L8N 3Z5.)

Hagberg, B, Hagberg, G, Olow, I, & vonWendt, L. The changing panorama of cerebral palsy in Sweden. V. The birth year period 1979–82. Acta Paediatrica Scandinavica, 78:283–290, 1989a.

Hagberg, B, Hagberg, G, & Zetterstrom, R. Decreasing perinatal mortality—Increase in cerebral palsy morbidity? Acta Paediatrica Scandinavica, 78:664–670, 1989b.

Hallett, M, & Alvarez, N. Attempted rapid elbow flexion movements in patients with athetosis. Journal of Neurology, Neurosurgery and Psychiatry, 46:745–750, 1983.

Hallum, A, & Krumboltz, JD. Parents caring for young adults with severe physical disabilities: Psychological issues. Developmental Medicine and Child Neurology, 35:24–32, 1993.

Hari, M, & Tillemans, T. Conductive education. In Scrutton, D (Ed.), Management of the Motor Disorders of Children with Cerebral Palsy. Clinics in Developmental Medicine (No. 90). Philadelphia: JB Lippincott, 1984, pp. 19–35.

Harris, SR. Early detection of cerebral palsy: Sensitivity and specificity of two motor assessment tools. Journal of Perinatology, 7:11–15, 1987.

Harris, SR. Early diagnosis of spastic diplegia, spastic hemiplegia, and quadriplegia. American Journal of Diseases of Children, 143:1356–1360, 1989.

Harris, SR, & Lundgren, BD. Joint mobilization for children with central nervous system disorders: Indications and precautions. Physical Therapy, 71:890–896, 1991.

Harrison, A. Spastic cerebral palsy: Possible spinal interneuronal contributions. Developmental Medicine and Child Neurology, 30:769–780, 1988.

Harrison, A, & Kruze, R. Perturbation of a skilled action. The responsiveness of neurologically normal and cerebral palsied individuals. Human Movement Science, 6:37–65, 1987.

Harryman, SE. Lower-extremity surgery for children with cerebral palsy: Physical therapy management. Physical Therapy, 72:16–24, 1992.

Higgins, S. Motor skill acquisition. Physical Therapy, 71:123–139, 1991.

Hinderer, KA, Richardson, PK, & Atwater, SW. Clinical implications of the Peabody Developmental Motor Scales: A constructive review. Physical and Occupational Therapy in Pediatrics, 9(2):81–106, 1989.

Hinojosa, J, & Anderson, J. Mothers' perceptions of home treatment programs for their preschool children with cerebral palsy. The American Journal of Occupational Therapy, 45:273–279, 1991.

Holst, K, Andersen, E, Philip, J, & Henningsen, I. Antenatal and perinatal conditions correlated to handicap among 4-year-old children. American Journal of Perinatology, 6:258–267, 1989.

Horton, SV, & Taylor, DC. The use of behavior therapy and physical therapy to promote independent ambulation in a preschooler with mental retardation and cerebral palsy. Research in Developmental Disabilities, 10(4):363–375, 1989.

Horvat, M. Effects of a progressive resistance training program on an individual with spastic cerebral palsy. American Corrective Therapy Journal, 41:7–11, 1987.

Jaeger, DL. Transferring and lifting children and adolescents: Home instruction sheets. 1989. (Available from Therapy Skill Builders, 3830 East Bellevue, PO Box 42050, Tucson, AZ, 85733.)

Jaeger, L. Home program instruction sheets for infants and young children. 1987. (Available from Therapy Skill Builders, 3830 East Bellevue, PO Box 42050, Tucson, AZ, 85733.)

Jones, CK. In search of power for the pediatric client. Physical and Occupational Therapy in Pediatrics, 10(2):47–68, 1990.

Jones, EW, & Mulley, GP. The measurement of spasticity. In Rose, FC (Ed.), Advances in Stroke Therapy. New York: Raven Press, 1982.

Jones, JA (Ed.). Training Guide to Cerebral Palsy Sports. Champaign, IL: Human Kinetics Books, 1988.

Karumuna, JMS, & Mgone, CS. Cerebral palsy in Dar es Salaam. Central African Journal of Medicine, 36(1):8–10, 1990.

Kassover, M, Tauber, C, Au, J, & Pugh, J. Auditory biofeedback in spastic diplegia. Journal of Orthopaedic Research, 4:246–249, 1986.

Katz, RT, & Rymer, WZ. Spastic hypertonia: Mechanisms and measurement. Archives of Physical Medicine and Rehabilitation, 70:144–155, 1989.

Kibele, A. Occupational therapy's role in improving the quality of life for persons with cerebral palsy. American Journal of Occupational Therapy, 43:371–377, 1989.

Kinghorn, J. Upper extremity functional changes following selective posterior rhizotomy in children with cerebral palsy. American Journal of Occupational Therapy, 46:502–507, 1992.

Kitchen, WH, Ford, GW, Rickards, AL, Lissenden, JV, & Ryan, MM. Children of birth weight < 1000 g: Changing outcome between ages 2 and 5 years. Journal of Pediatrics, 110:283–288, 1987.

Klein, RM, & Bell, B. Self-care skills: Behavioral measurement with Klein-Bell ADL Scale. Archives of Physical Medicine and Rehabilitation, 63:335–338, 1982.

Kluzik, J, Fetters, L, & Coryell, J. Quantification of control: A preliminary study of effects of neurodevelopmental treatment on reaching in children with spastic cerebral palsy. Physical Therapy, 70:65–78, 1990.

Knutsson, LM, & Clark, DE. Orthotic devices for ambulation in children with cerebral palsy and myelomeningocele. Physical Therapy, 71:947–960, 1991.

Knutsson, LM, & Martensson, A. Dynamic motor capacity in spastic paresis and its relation to prime mover dysfunction, spastic reflexes and antagonist co-activation. Scandinavian Journal of Rehabilitation Medicine, 12:93–106, 1980.

Kolobe, THA. Working with families of children with disabilities. Pediatric Physical Therapy, 4:57–60, 1992.

Langley, MB. A developmental approach to the use of toys for facilitation of environmental control. Physical and Occupational Therapy in Pediatrics, 10(2):69–91, 1990.

Law, M, Baptiste, S, McColl, MA, Opzoomer, A, Polatajko, H,
& Pollock, N. The Canadian Occupational Performance Measure: An outcome measure for occupational therapy. Canadian Journal of Occupational Therapy, 57:82–87, 1990.

Lee, EH, Goh, JCH, & Bose, K. Value of gait analysis in the assessment of surgery in cerebral palsy. Archives of Physical Medicine and Rehabilitation, 73:642–646, 1992.

Leonard, CT, Hirschfeld, H, Moritani, T, & Forssberg, H. Myotatic reflex development in normal children and children with cerebral palsy. Experimental Neurology, 111:379–382, 1991.

Leonard, CT, Moritani, T, Hirschfeld, H, & Forssberg, H. Deficits in reciprocal inhibition of children with cerebral palsy as revealed by H reflex testing. Developmental Medicine and Child Neurology, 32,974–984, 1990.

Lesny, I, Nachtmann, M, Stehlik, A, Tomankova, A, & Zajidkova, J. Disorders of memory of motor sequences in cerebral palsied children. Brain and Development, 12:339–341, 1990.

Letts, M, Rathbone, D, Yamashita, T, Nichol, B, & Keeler, A. Soft Boston orthosis in management of neuromuscular scoliosis: A preliminary report. Journal of Pediatric Orthopedics, 12:470–474, 1992.

LeVeau, BF, & Bernhardt, DB. Developmental biomechanics: Effects of forces on the growth, development and maintenance of the human body. Physical Therapy, 64:1874–1882, 1984.

Little, WJ. On the influence of abnormal parturition, difficult labours, premature births and asphyxia neonatorum on the mental and physical condition of the child, especially in relation to deformities. Transactions of the Obstetrical Society of London 1862. Cerebral Palsy Bulletin, 1:5–34, 1958.

Logan, L, Byers-Hinkley, K, & Ciccone, CD. Anterior versus posterior walkers: A gait analysis study. Developmental Medicine and Child Neurology, 32:1044–1048, 1990.

MacPhail, HEA, & Kramer, J. Personal Communication, June 10, 1993.

Mahoney, FI, & Barthel, DW. Functional evaluation: The Barthel Index. Maryland Medical Journal, 14:61–65, 1965.

Massagli, TL. Spasticity and its management in children. Physical Medicine and Rehabilitation Clinics of North America, 2:867–889, 1991.

McCarthy, RE, Simon, S, Douglas, B, Zawacki, R, & Resse, N. Proximal femoral resection to allow adults who have severe cerebral palsy to sit. Journal of Bone and Joint Surgery (American), 70:1011–1016, 1988.

McCubbin, JA, & Shasby, GB. Effects of isokinetic exercise on adolescents with cerebral palsy. Adapted Physical Activity Quarterly, 2:56–64, 1985.

McDonald, CM. Selective dorsal rhizotomy: A critical review. Physical Medicine and Rehabilitation Clinics of North America, 2:891–915, 1991.

Menkes, JH. Textbook of Child Neurology (4th ed.). Philadelphia: Lea & Febiger, 1990.

Middleton, EA, Hurley, GRB, & McIlwain, JS. The role of rigid and hinged polypropylene ankle-foot-orthoses in the management of cerebral palsy: A case study. Prosthetics and Orthotics International, 12:129–135, 1988.

Miedaner, JA, & Renander, J. The effectiveness of classroom passive stretching programs for increasing or maintaining passive range of motion in non-ambulatory children: An evaluation of frequency. Physical & Occupational Therapy in Pediatrics, 7(3):35–43, 1987.

Missiuna, C, & Pollock, N. Play deprivation in children with physical disabilities: The role of the occupational therapist in preventing secondary disability. American Journal of Occupational Therapy, 45:882–888, 1991.

Molteni, B, Oleari, G, Fedrizzi, E, & Bracchi, M. Relation between CT patterns, clinical findings and etiology in children born at term, affected by congenital hemiparesis. Neuropediatrics, *18*:75–80, 1987.

Morrison, JM, & Ursprung, AW. Children's attitudes toward people with disabilities: A review of the literature. Journal of Rehabilitation, *53*(1):45–49, 1987.

Mossberg, KA, Linton, KA, & Friske, K. Ankle-foot orthoses: Effect on energy expenditure of gait in spastic diplegic children. Archives of Physical Medicine and Rehabilitation, *71*:490–494, 1990.

Msall, ME, Buck, GM, Rogers, BT, Merke, D, Catanzaro, NL, & Zorn, WA. Risk factors for major neurodevelopmental impairments and need for special education resources in extremely premature infants. Journal of Pediatrics, *119*:606–614, 1991.

Msall, ME, Roseberg, S, DiGuadio, KM, Braun, SL, Duffy, L, & Granger, CV. Pilot test for the WeeFIM for children with motor impairments (Abstract). Developmental Medicine and Child Neurology, *32*(9)(suppl. 62):41, 1990.

Nash, J, Neilson, PD, & O'Dwyer, NJ. Reducing spasticity to control muscle contracture of children with cerebral palsy. Developmental Medicine and Child Neurology, *31*:471–480, 1989.

Nashner, L, Shumway-Cooke, A, & Marin, O. Stance posture control in select groups of children with cerebal palsy: Deficits in sensory organization and muscular coordination. Experimental Brain Research, *49*:393–409, 1983.

Nelson, KB, & Ellenberg, J. Antecedents of cerebral palsy. Multivariate analysis of risk. New England Journal of Medicine, *315*:81–86, 1986.

Nottidge, VD, & Okogbo, ME. Cerebral palsy in Ibadan, Nigeria. Developmental Medicine and Child Neurology, *33*:241–245, 1991.

Nwaobi, OM, & Smith, PD. Effect of adaptive seating on pulmonary function of children with cerebral palsy. Developmental Medicine and Child Neurology, *28*:351–354, 1986.

O'Dwyer, NJ, Neilson, PD, & Nash, J. Mechanisms of muscle growth related to muscle contracture in cerebral palsy. Developmental Medicine and Child Neurology, *31*:543–552, 1989.

Olney, SJ, Costigan, PA, & Hedden, DM. Mechanical energy patterns in gait of cerebral palsied children. Physical Therapy, *67*:1348–1354, 1987.

Olney, SJ, MacPhail, HEA, Hedden, DM, & Boyce, WF. Work and power in hemiplegic cerebral palsy gait. Physical Therapy, *70*:431–438, 1990.

Papile, L, Burstein, J, Burstein, R, & Koffler, H. Incidence and evolution of subependymal and intraventricular hemorrhage: A study of infants with birthweight of less than 1500 gms. Journal of Pediatrics, *92*:529–534, 1978.

Parker, DF, Carriere, L, Hebestreit, H, & Bar-Or, O. Anaerobic endurance and peak muscle power in children with spastic cerebral palsy. American Journal of Diseases of Children, *146*:1069–1073, 1992.

Patla, AE, Winter, DA, Frank, JS, Walt, JS, & Prasad, S. Identification of age-related changes in the balance control system. Proceedings of the APTA Forum on Balance. Nashville, TN: American Physical Therapy Association, 1989.

Perry, J, Hoffer, M, Antonelli, D, Plut, J, Lewis, G, & Greenberg, R. Electromyography before and after surgery for hip deformity in children with cerebral palsy. Journal of Bone and Joint Surgery (American), *58*:201–208, 1976.

Pharoah, POD, Cooke, T, Cooke, RWI, & Rosenbloom, L. Birthweight specific trends in cerebral palsy. Archives of Disease in Childhood, *65*:602–606, 1990.

Pharoah, POD, Cooke, T, Rosenbloom, L, & Cooke, RWI. Trends in birth prevalence of cerebral palsy. Archives of Disease in Childhood, *62*:379–384, 1987.

Piper, MC, Darrah, J. Motor Assessment of the Developing Infant. Philadelphia: WB Saunders, 1994.

Poirier, D, Goguen, L, & Leslie, P. Educational Rights of Exceptional Children. Toronto: Carswell, 1988.

Poole, JL. Application of motor learning principles in occupational therapy. American Journal of Occupational Therapy, *45*:531–537, 1991.

Powell, TH, & Ogle, PA. Brothers and Sisters—a Special Part of Exceptional Families. Baltimore, MD: Paul H Brookes, 1985.

Price, R, Bjornson, KF, Lehmann, JF, McLaughlin, JF, & Hays, RM. Quantitative measurement of spasticity in children with cerebral palsy. Developmental Medicine and Child Neurology, *33*:585–595, 1991.

Rang, M. Cerebral palsy. In Morrissy, RT (Ed.), Lovell and Winter's Paediatric Orthopedics (3rd ed.). Philadelphia: JB Lippincott, 1990, pp. 465–506.

Reilly, S, & Skuse, D. Characteristics and management of feeding problems of young children with cerebral palsy. Developmental Medicine and Child Neurology, *34*:379–388, 1992.

Rempel, GR, Colwell, SO, & Nelson, RP. Growth in children with cerebral palsy fed via gastrostomy. Pediatrics, *82*:857–862, 1988.

Richards, CL, Malouin, F, & Dumas, F. Effects of a single session of prolonged stretch on muscle activations during gait in spastic cerebral palsy. Scandinavian Journal of Rehabilitation Medicine, *23*:103–111, 1991.

Romanini, L, Villani, C, Meloni, C, & Calvisi, V. Histological and morphological aspects of muscle in infantile cerebral palsy. Italian Journal of Orthopaedics and Traumatology, *15*:87–93, 1989.

Rose, J, Gamble, JG, Burgos, A, Medeiros, J, & Haskell, WL. Energy expenditure index of walking for normal children and for children with cerebral palsy. Developmental Medicine and Child Neurology, *32*:333–340, 1990.

Rose, J, Medeiros, JM, & Parker, R. Energy cost index as an estimate of energy expenditure of cerebral-palsied children during assisted ambulation. Developmental Medicine and Child Neurology, *27*:485–490, 1985.

Rosenbaum, P, Cadman, D, & Kirpalani, H. Pediatrics: Assessing quality of life. In Spilker, B (Ed.), Quality of Life Assessment in Clinical Trials. New York: Raven Press, 1990, pp. 205–215.

Russell, D, Rosenbaum, P, Cadman, D, Gowland, C, Hardy, S, & Jarvis, S. The Gross Motor Function Measure: A means to evaluate the effects of physical therapy. Developmental Medicine and Child Neurology, *31*:341–352, 1989.

Schanzenbacher, KE. Diagnostic problems in pediatrics. In Pratt, PN, & Allen, AS (Eds.), Occupational Therapy for Children. Toronto: Mosby, 1989, p. 97.

Scherzer, AL, & Tscharnuter, I. Early Diagnosis and Therapy in Cerebral Palsy: A Primer on Infant Developmental Problems (2nd ed.). New York: Marcel Dekker, 1990.

Senft, KE, Pueschel, SM, Robison, NA, & Kiessling, LS. Level of function of young adults with cerebral palsy. Physical and Occupational Therapy in Pediatrics, *10*(1):19–25, 1990.

Shaw, G. Vehicular transport safety for the child with disabilities. American Journal of Occupational Therapy, *41*:35–42, 1987.

Shaw, J. Continence in cerebral palsy. Health Visitor, *63*:301–302, 1990.

Shields, CV. Strategies: A Practical Guide for Dealing with Professionals and Human Service Systems. Richmond Hill, Ontario: Human Services Press, 1987.

Sillanpaa, M, Piekkala, P, & Pisirici, H. The young adult with cerebral palsy and his chances of employment. International Journal of Rehabilitation Research, *5*:467–476, 1982.

Sobsey, D, & Doe, T. Patterns of sexual abuse and assault. Sexuality and Disability, *9*:243–259, 1991.

Sparrow, SS, Balla, DA, & Ciccetti, DV. Vineland Adaptive

Behavior Scales (survey form). Circle Pines, MN: American Guidance Service, 1984.

Spector, RC. Functional Disability Scales. In Spilker, B (Ed.), Quality of Life Assessments in Clinical Trials. New York: Raven Press, 1990, pp. 115–129.

Sternisha, C, Cays, M, & Campbell, L. Stress responses in families with handicapped children: An annotated bibliography. Physical & Occupational Therapy in Pediatrics, 12(1):89–103, 1992.

Stuberg, WA. Considerations related to weight-bearing programs in children with developmental disabilities. Physical Therapy, 72:35–40, 1992.

Stuberg, WA, Fuchs, RH, & Miedaner, JA. Reliability of goniometric measurements of children with cerebral palsy. Developmental Medicine and Child Neurology, 30:657–666, 1988.

Sutherland, DH, Olshen, R, Cooper, L, & Woo, S-Y. The development of mature gait. Journal of Bone and Joint Surgery (American), 62:336–353, 1980.

Tardieu, C, Huet de la Tour, E, Bret, MD, & Tardieu, G. Muscle hypoextensibility in children with cerebral palsy: I. Clinical and experimental observations. Archives of Physical Medicine and Rehabilitation, 63:97–102, 1982.

Tardieu, C, Lespargot, A, Tabary, C, & Bret, MD. For how long must the soleus muscle be stretched each day to prevent contracture? Developmental Medicine and Child Neurology, 30:3–10, 1988.

Tardieu, G, Tardieu, C, Colbeau-Justin, P, & Lespargot, A. Muscle hypoextensibility in children with cerebral palsy: II. Therapeutic implications. Archives of Physical Medicine and Rehabilitation, 63:103–107, 1982.

Torfs, CP, van den Berg, BJ, & Oechsli, FW. Prenatal and perinatal factors in the etiology of cerebral palsy. Journal of Pediatrics, 116:615–619, 1990.

Tremblay, F, Malouin, F, Richards, CL, & Dumas, F. Effects of prolonged muscle stretch on reflex and voluntary muscle activations in children with spastic cerebral palsy. Scandinavian Journal of Rehabilitation Medicine, 22:171–180, 1990.

Uvebrandt, P. Hemiplegic cerebral palsy. Aetiology and outcome. Acta Paediatrica Scandinavica. Supplement, 345:5–100, 1988.

van der Weel, FR, van der Meer, ALH, & Lee, DN. Effect of task on movement control in cerebral palsy: Implications for assessment and therapy. Developmental Medicine and Child Neurology, 33:419–426, 1991.

Vojta, V. The basic elements of treatment according to Vojta. In Scrutton, D (Ed.), Management of the Motor Disorders of Children with Cerebral Palsy. Philadelphia: JB Lippincott, 1984, pp. 75–85.

Vulpe, SG. Vulpe Assessment Battery. Toronto: National Institute on Mental Retardation, 1982.

Wacker, DP, Harper, DC, Powell, WJ, & Healy, A. Life outcomes and satisfaction ratings of multihandicapped adults. Developmental Medicine and Child Neurology, 25:625–631, 1983.

Watt, JM, Robertson, CMT, & Grace, MGA. Early prognosis for ambulation of neonatal intensive care survivors with cerebral palsy. Developmental Medicine and Child Neurology, 31:766–773, 1989.

Weinstein, SL, & Tharp, BR. Etiology and timing of static encephalopathies of childhood (cerebral palsy). In Stevenson, DK, & Sunshine, P (Eds.), Fetal and Neonatal Brain Injury. Toronto: BC Decker, 1989.

Werner, D. Disabled Village Children: A Guide for Community Health Workers, Rehabilitation Workers, and Families. Palo Alto, CA: Hesperian Foundation, 1987.

White, R. Sensory integrative therapy for the cerebral-palsied child. In Scrutton, D (Ed.), Management of the Motor Disorders of Children with Cerebral Palsy. Clinics in Developmental Medicine (No. 90). Philadelphia: JB Lippincott, 1984, pp. 86–95.

Wiklund, LM, & Uvebrant, P. Hemiplegic cerebral palsy: Correlation between CT morphology and clinical findings. Developmental Medicine and Child Neurology, 33:512–523, 1991a.

Wiklund, LM, Uvebrant, P, & Flodmark, O. Computed tomography as an adjunct in etiological analysis of hemiplegic cerebral palsy. I: Children born preterm. Neuropediatrics, 22:50–56, 1991b.

Wilcox, C. Hey, What About Me!: Activities for Disabled Children. Toronto: Doubleday Canada, 1988. (Available from Doubleday, 105 Bond Street, Toronto, Ontario, Canada, M5B 1Y3.)

Wilson, ER, Mirra, S, & Schwartz, JF. Congenital diencephalic and brain stem damage: Neuropathologic study of three cases. Acta Neuropathologica, 57:70–74, 1982.

Wilson, JM. Cerebral palsy. In Campbell, S (Ed.), Pediatric Neurologic Physical Therapy (2nd ed.). New York: Churchill Livingston, 1991, pp. 301–360.

Yokochi, K, Aiba, K, Horie, M, Inukai, K, Fujimoto, S, Kodama, M, & Kodama, K. Magnetic resonance imaging in children with spastic diplegia: Correlation with severity of their motor and mental abnormality. Developmental Medicine and Child Neurology, 33:18–25, 1991.

Chapter 20

Spinal Cord Injury

TERESA L. SOUTHARD, PT
TERESA L. MASSAGLI, MD

INTRODUCTION

Acquired lesions of the spinal cord occur far less commonly in children than in adults, but the unique aspects of growth and development can make treatment of the rare child with spinal cord injury (SCI) a challenge for pediatric physical therapists. This chapter describes the pathophysiology and resulting neurologic impairments of SCI in children and uses the conceptual model of the disabling process to outline assessment, treatment goals, and intervention for the pediatric physical therapist.

The most common cause of SCI for all ages is trauma. The overall incidence is estimated to be 28 to 50 injuries per million persons per year, or 6000 to 10,000 new cases each year in the United States, but children younger than 16 years of age account for less than 5% of these cases (Centers for Disease Control, 1987; Stover & Fine, 1986). Motor vehicle accidents, sports, violence, and falls are the leading causes, and traumatic SCI more frequently occurs in boys, during the summer, and on weekends (Stover & Fine, 1986). Traumatic SCI is more common in children 10 to 15 years old and birth to 5 years old than in children who are 5 to 9 years old (Kewalramani et al., 1980). Violence as a cause of SCI is increasing in frequency, particularly in older teenagers. Owing to the more "mature" behavior patterns of such victims, they are often sent to facilities that treat adults, but in many cities, pedi-atric physical therapists encounter such patients. Child abuse may account for some instances of SCI, particularly in younger children, but its frequency as a cause of SCI is unknown. Developmental anomalies of the cervical vertebrae can place the spinal cord at increased risk of injury. These anomalies include instability of the atlantoaxial joint, as seen in Down syndrome or juvenile rheumatoid arthritis, and dysplasia of the base of the skull or upper cervical vertebrae, as seen in achondroplasia.

Nontraumatic causes of SCI in children often have an insidious onset and can be difficult to diagnose. Specific incidence data are not available for such causes, which include tumor, transverse myelitis, epidural abscess, arteriovenous malformation, and multiple sclerosis. Treating the child with SCI resulting from the presence of a tumor is especially challenging because the child's overall medical condition and the progression of disease dramatically influence the formulation or attainment of goals.

PATHOPHYSIOLOGY

The site or level at which SCI occurs is often related to the cause of injury and the child's age. Most of the nontraumatic causes of SCI occur in the thoracic spinal cord. By contrast, vertebral dysplasias place the upper cervical spinal cord or lower brain stem at risk. Birth trauma due to traction and angulation of the spine at delivery most commonly causes SCI at the cervicothoracic junction. In the child younger than 8 to 10 years old, the cervical spine has greater mobility than it does in adults because of ligamentous laxity, shallow angulation of the facets, incomplete ossification of vertebrae, and relative underdevelopment of the neck muscles for the size of the head (Wilberger, 1986). Young children are therefore more likely to experience injury at the upper cervical spine than are adults (Bohn et al., 1990), and SCI may occur without any signs of bone damage by radiography, a finding referred to as spinal cord injury without radiographic abnormality, or SCIWORA (Pang & Wilberger, 1982). In children, 56% of cases of traumatic SCI result in quadriplegia owing to injury between the first cervical and first thoracic root levels, and 44% result in paraplegia from injury below the first thoracic level (Stover & Fine, 1986).

Most cases of traumatic SCI are caused by a blunt, nonpenetrating injury to the spinal cord in which the cord is not lacerated or transected. The direct effect of the trauma is immediate disruption of neural transmission in the gray and white matter of the spinal cord at and below the injury site, resulting in spinal shock. Reactive physiologic events evolve over a period of hours and induce secondary injury to the spinal cord (Faden, 1983). The exact sequence of events between transfer of kinetic energy to the cord and subsequent neuronal death is unknown. Animal models have shown that ischemia, hemorrhage, edema, calcium influx into cells, and generation of free radicals contribute to cell membrane degradation and death of neurons (Janssen & Hansebout, 1989). In gray matter, neurons that die are not replaced. In white matter, axonal segments distal to the injury degenerate and synapses no longer function. Although axonal sprouting does occur to a limited degree in the central nervous system, it appears to be functionally insignificant, and most of the recovery observed in patients with incomplete lesions is probably due to resolution of neurapraxic injury.

The zone of injury within the spinal cord is usually large enough to cause a transition in neurologic function from normal to abnormal or to absent over several spinal root levels. Soon after SCI, the level of injury may appear to move cephalad as the secondary or indirect processes set in. Later, the level of injury may move caudally as these factors resolve, as sprouting develops (either within the spinal cord or peripherally to denervated muscles), or as hypertrophy of weak muscles occurs. Research has shown that the extent of injury may

diminish for as long as 1 year (Wu et al., 1992), and it is obvious that until the natural history of SCI and recovery is delineated, experimental treatments may be inappropriately credited with enhancing recovery.

If some function below the zone of the spinal cord injury remains, the child has an incomplete SCI. After traumatic SCI, incomplete lesions are found in 41% of children with paraplegia and in 53% of those with quadriplegia (Stover & Fine, 1986). Several distinct patterns of clinical syndromes have been described. Injury to the anterior spinal cord produces motor paralysis, with reduced sensation of pain and temperature but with preserved dorsal column function. Hemorrhage in the central part of the cervical spinal cord produces flaccid weakness of the arms and strong but spastic legs, with preservation of bladder and bowel function. Posterior cord lesions are rare and produce selective loss of proprioception. Stab wounds may produce a Brown-Séquard lesion with ipsilateral paralysis and contralateral loss of pain and temperature sensation. Injury to the lumbosacral nerve roots results in cauda equina syndrome, with lower extremity weakness and hypotonia of the legs and bladder.

Delayed cavitation (syringomyelia) within the damaged spinal cord can occur in patients with complete or incomplete lesions. The occurrence of a cystic cavitation, or syrinx, appears to be common after SCI, but in a small number of such patients the cyst may progressively enlarge, resulting in further loss of neurologic function months to years after SCI (LaHaye & Batzdorf, 1988). Signs and symptoms that may herald presence of a syrinx include loss of motor function, ascending sensory level, increased spasticity or sweating, and new onset of pain or dysesthesia.

▌PREVENTION

The traumatic causes of SCI are the best targets for efforts at prevention. The Committee on Sports Medicine of the American Academy of Pediatrics (1984) has recommended screening programs to assess cervical spine stability for children known to be at risk of atlantoaxial instability (e.g., Down syndrome). Pediatric health professionals play important roles in educating children regarding proper seat belt and car seat use. Lap seat belts must be placed across the pelvis, not across the waist, and shoulder harnesses should cross the clavicle, not the neck, to avoid lumbar or cervical spine injury in the event of a collision. Health care professionals and schools have supported cooperative programs to reduce diving injuries (the most common sports-related cause of SCI) and other high-risk activities (Richards et al., 1991). Scientists at the Centers for Disease Control have recommended that SCI become the first injury condition reportable to state health agencies and the Centers for Disease Control (1987). Reporting would assist in identifying high-risk groups and would guide development of prevention programs.

MEDICAL DIAGNOSIS AND MANAGEMENT

The early management of a child with SCI is focused on stabilization of the spine to prevent further damage to the intact but injured spinal cord. The spine is immobilized during transport and throughout all assessments and procedures. At the hospital, a thorough neurologic examination is performed to determine the motor and sensory level of SCI and the completeness of injury. Spinal shock is usually present, although occasionally it has resolved by the time of presentation to the emergency room. In spinal shock, the muscles are flaccid below the SCI and all cutaneous and deep tendon reflexes are absent. This state persists for hours to weeks and is said to be over when sacral reflexes, including the bulbocavernous and anal reflexes, are present.

Further evaluation is undertaken with plain radiographs of the whole spine from the first cervical to the sacral vertebrae to identify any fractures, facet subluxations, or dislocations. A small but significant number of patients may have more than one site of injury to the spine and spinal cord. Computed tomography and magnetic resonance imaging are used to diagnose root impingement, presence of bone fragments in the spinal canal, cord compression, and spinal cord hemorrhage.

Research has failed to identify any pharmacologic intervention that can halt the chain of secondary events producing neural damage. Antioxidants, free radical scavengers, opiate antagonists, and calcium channel blockers are a few of the agents that have been tested (Faden, 1983). High doses of corticosteroids (methylprednisolone) administered within the first 36 hours have been shown to slightly enhance motor recovery in humans, and further clinical trials are under way (Bracken et al., 1990).

Trauma to the spinal cord provokes the development of scar tissue, which includes both connective tissue elements and glial hyperplasia. Scientists have not yet determined why axons are unable to grow across this scar tissue area. Some researchers have proposed that the glial cells act as a surrogate target for the regrowing axons, whereas others have argued that the glial cells engender a nonpermissive substrate for axonal growth. Strategies to promote spinal cord regeneration have included use of neurotrophic factors, monoclonal antibodies directed against glial cells, and intraspinal transplants of peripheral nerve or fetal spinal cord tissue. Both in vitro techniques and animal models have been used to demonstrate that injured axons can survive and grow under certain environmental conditions, but the feat of effecting axonal growth across scar tissue and through appropriate myelin sheaths to reach and innervate appropriate muscles remains elusive (Kliot & Lustgarten, 1990; Tessler, 1991). Significant progress has occurred in the last 5 to 10 years in understanding the inhibitory factors as well as those promoting axonal sprouting, but it is likely that a number of years will pass before clinical applications are available.

Whether immediate surgical intervention to correct bone injury and decompress the spinal cord is effective in reducing paralysis is unknown because the numerous surgical procedures have never been subjected to randomized clinical trials. Surgery often allows a patient to be mobilized more quickly, but ultimate levels of independence or recovery do not appear to be altered (Murphy et al., 1990). The main goal of surgery is to prevent later deformity, pain, or loss of neurologic function. Surgery may not be necessary if spinal alignment can be achieved with traction and maintained with an orthosis. Surgery is indicated if there is a penetrating injury, if traction has failed to reduce a dislocation, if nerve root impingement exists, or if bone fragments are compressing the cauda equina. Regardless of whether surgery is performed, if bone injury has occurred patients usually wear an external orthosis until bone fusion is complete, often 3 or more months. Even with the use of an orthosis, pull of adjacent muscles may place undue torque on the immature fusion mass, and the surgeon may restrict the patient from performing certain activities, such as asymmetric weight lifting in the patient with thoracic SCI and hip flexion beyond 90° in the patient with lumbar injury. Newer surgical techniques using segmental wiring may make these precautions less necessary.

With ongoing appropriate medical care, long-term survival after traumatic SCI is not only possible but likely. More than 90% of children younger than 19 years of age survive 10 years beyond discharge (Stover & Fine, 1986). A nearly normal life expectancy can be anticipated for those with paraplegia and incomplete quadriplegia, and life expectancy is about 85% of average for those with quadriplegia (Flett, 1992).

IMPAIRMENTS AND FUNCTIONAL LIMITATIONS

Diagnosis and Problem Identification

MEDICAL MANAGEMENT

A host of medical complications ensue after SCI and may affect a child's ability to participate in physical therapy and rehabilitation (Massagli & Jaffe, 1990). With lesions of the cervical or thoracic spinal cord, altered respiratory function may occur, ranging from total paralysis of the diaphragm to diminished vital capacity or weakened forced expiration during coughing. Midthoracic SCI can interrupt sympathetic outflow, leading to orthostatic hypotension, impaired ability to sweat or shiver, and autonomic dysreflexia. Autonomic dysreflexia is a massive reflex sympathetic discharge that occurs after SCI above midthoracic levels in response to noxious stimuli. Clinical features include headache, flushing, sweating, pilomotor activity, rapid or reduced heart rate, and hypertension. The hypertensive crisis poses a danger to patients and can cause hemorrhages, seizures, or even death. School-aged children and adolescents are capable of reporting headaches, but younger children may have difficulty in verbalizing symptoms, and autonomic dysreflexia is often overlooked in these youngsters. Paralyzed and dependent lower extremities can develop edema and deep vein thromboses. In the first weeks after SCI, gastrointestinal bleeding from stress ulcers may occur but the frequency (20%) is no greater than that in patients with other acute serious medical conditions (Sugarman, 1985). Deep vein thrombosis occurs as frequently in children with SCI as it does in adults, or in about 13% of cases (Waring & Karunas, 1991). Neurogenic pain can occur after SCI at, above, or below the level of injury and is relatively more common with cauda equina lesions. Loss of descending input to the sacral spinal cord or damage to the sacral nerve roots leads to impairment of bladder and bowel emptying, sexual response, and male fertility.

Almost unique to children is the problem of immobilization hypercalcemia. Although immobiliza-tion from any cause produces increased urinary calcium excretion within a few days, this process is of greater magnitude after SCI and can produce increased serum levels of calcium at 1 to 3 months after injury. Nonspecific symptoms include lethargy, nausea, altered mood, and anorexia. Remobilization is an important aspect of treatment in persons without SCI, but it is not known if this is effective in reducing hypercalcemia after SCI. The mainstays of treatment are primarily medical and aimed at reducing calcium loss from bones or at enhancing urinary excretion. Osteopenia (loss of bone mineral density) develops in paralyzed extremities and increases the risk of osteoporosis (pathologic fractures). Deposition of new bone in periarticular soft tissue can also occur in paralyzed extremities. This heterotopic ossification can be asymptomatic, or it may interfere with range of motion (ROM) around a joint or even cause bone ankylosis. The most commonly affected joints are hips, knees, shoulders, and elbows.

Spasticity is a frequent occurrence after SCI and usually evolves within a period of 1 to 2 years. Although initially the patient is flaccid, hypertonus gradually appears, and in the first 3 to 6 months after SCI the patient develops hyperreflexia, clonus, and flexor spasms. Later, extensor spasms usually predominate. Some researchers have suggested that the passive positioning of extremities during the period when spasticity develops can influence its ultimate manifestations (Guttmann, 1976), but this is unproved. Evolution of spasticity after central nervous system insult is common and is seen in other conditions such as cerebral palsy and stroke. In SCI, the immediate effects of loss of supraspinal inhibition and the later developing effects of denervation supersensitivity and sprouting by afferent and collateral neurons likely all contribute to the development of spasticity, but the sequence of events behind the evolution of clinical manifestations of spasticity is not known.

A pediatric physiatrist provides medical management of the complications noted earlier and serves as a team leader. In some centers, this role may be filled by an orthopaedist, a neurologist, or even a pediatrician. Researchers, however, have shown that referral of patients with SCI to comprehensive, multidisciplinary SCI centers is more cost-effective, with improved patient outcomes, reduced hospital and long-term nursing care charges, and improved prospect for long-term patient earnings, compared with unspecialized care for SCI patients (Johnston & Keith, 1983). The lead physician may also request consultation by other physicians such as an orthopaedic surgeon or neurosurgeon to monitor spine stability and alignment, a urologist to monitor urinary tract function, and a pulmonologist for ventilator management.

A clinical psychologist may monitor and facilitate adaptation by the child and family. As described by Fordyce (1981), the forced and involuntary acquisition of SCI—accompanied by pain, medical complications, and altered cosmesis and body image—and the forced practice of new and challenging rehabilitation procedures can be expected to have a significant impact on the patient's affect, self-esteem, and behavior. The child's adjustment to SCI does not necessarily follow predictable stages of crisis response such as shock, denial, depression, and adaptation. Adjustment to SCI probably occurs over several years. The verbal or attitudinal expressions of children with new SCI are less predictive of outcome than are their behaviors. Physical therapists can facilitate adjustment by actively engaging the child in acquiring the skills needed to deal with the new impairments.

MANAGEMENT BY OTHER DISCIPLINES

The acute rehabilitation and long-term treatment of children with SCI require a comprehensive interdisciplinary approach involving both hospital and school-based personnel. Team members typically include physicians, nurses, a dietitian, occupational therapists, recreation therapists, a social worker, an orthotist, a clinical psychologist, and teachers, as well as physical therapists, the child, and the family. For the younger child, much of the training is provided for the parents.

Rehabilitation nurses manage bladder and bowel care, monitor skin for pressure ulcers, provide emotional support to patients, and train the patient and family to carry out these tasks at home. Children can be taught self-management of bladder and bowel emptying at about age 5 years but may need reminders or supervision for many more years. The dietitian educates the child and family in meal selection to avoid protein catabolism or, conversely, obesity and to choose high-fiber foods to facilitate bowel management. Occupational therapists provide training in self-care management, in use of orthoses to aid hand function in quadriplegia, and in use of adaptive writing equipment; they often assist physical therapists with upper extremity strengthening and wheelchair prescription. Goals for self-care management need to be set according to usual expectations for age. For the older teenager, the occupational therapist may also provide training in home and money management, prevocational skills, travel within the community, and use of adaptive equipment for driving. An orthotist is needed if either functional hand orthoses or

lower extremity orthoses are necessary. Recreation therapists find leisure activities, including sports, in which the child can be independent and explore function in the community.

Social workers are indispensable for working with funding agencies, assisting with discharge planning, and providing support to the patient and family. A team member skilled in mental health should monitor the child's adaptation to disability and be available to help the child verbally process the injury and rehabilitation process. This could be a skilled social worker, but if a behavior management program using reinforcers is needed, a clinical psychologist should be consulted. In some rare cases, the child may truly be clinically depressed, and a psychiatrist can be consulted if a medication trial is contemplated. The psychologist or psychiatrist may also need to deal with issues of premorbid risk-taking behavior or even substance abuse. Psychologists, nurses, and pediatric physiatrists collaborate in discussing sexuality and changes in sexual functioning with teenagers who have had SCI.

Teachers are particularly important during the acute rehabilitation phase because the length of hospitalization after SCI is often 2 to 4 months and the child needs to keep up with his or her curriculum. The teacher can be instrumental in assisting the receiving school to prepare for the child's return. For teenagers, schools and state agencies should be asked to participate in vocational planning and counseling.

MANAGEMENT BY PHYSICAL THERAPISTS

The impairments resulting from SCI that are addressed by a physical therapist include muscle weakness or paralysis, sensory loss or impairment, altered muscle tone and ROM, diminished endurane, poor postural control, and altered cardiovascular responses, producing autonomic dysreflexia or orthostatic hypotension.

A common terminology should be used by all professionals when describing the motor or sensory level of SCI. The most widely used standards are those published by the American Spinal Injury Association (ASIA) (1992). These standards have been developed by consensus of a multidisciplinary group of clinical experts and have been revised three times since their initial publication in 1982. Inter-rater reliability for the 1989 version was acceptable, but further revisions were made owing to shortcomings in describing very incomplete lesions (Ditunno, 1992a; Priebe & Waring, 1991). The ASIA standards define right and left motor levels, right and left sensory levels, and incomplete and complete injuries.

The ASIA standards accept the widely used system of muscle grading: 0 = absence, total paralysis; 1 = trace, palpable or visible contraction; 2 = poor, active movement through full ROM with gravity eliminated; 3 = fair, active movement through full ROM against gravity; 4 = good, active movement through full ROM against resistance; and 5 = normal. The ASIA-defined motor level is the most caudal root level in which muscle strength is grade 3 or more. Motor levels may differ for right and left sides of the body. The key muscles for determination of motor level are listed in Table 20–1. Since all muscles have innervation from more than one root level, the presence of innervation by one root level and the absence by the next lower level results in a weakened muscle. By convention, if a muscle has grade 3 strength, it is considered to have full innervation by the higher root level, for which it is named.

The sensory level may not correspond exactly to the motor level. Determining the sensory level is especially helpful in injuries above C-5, or to the thoracic spinal cord, where there are no key muscles to define the level of SCI. Rather than relying on dermatome charts, which vary from one text to another, the ASIA standards rely on the presence of normal light touch and pinprick sensation at a key point in each of the 28 dermatomes on the right and left sides of the body (Fig. 20–1 & Table 20–2). Proprioception should also be assessed below the level of injury in patients with incomplete SCI to determine integrity of dorsal column function.

A patient is said to have an incomplete SCI only if motor or sensory function is present in the lowest sacral segment, implying voluntary control of the external anal sphincter or sensation at the mucocutaneous junction or both. Incomplete lesions are referred to in two ways: by the ASIA Impairment Scale and by neuroanatomic description. The ASIA Impairment Scale is given in Table 20–3 and is an adaptation of the Frankel scale (Frankel, 1969). Distinct neuroanatomic patterns of incomplete lesions include the central cord syndrome, Brown-Séquard syndrome, anterior cord syndrome, and posterior cord syndrome previously described in the section on pathophysiology. The cauda equina syndrome may be complete or incomplete.

Precise description of the motor and sensory loss after SCI is important for two reasons. First, it helps predict the likelihood of further neurologic recovery in both complete and incomplete syndromes. For instance, in motor complete C-5 quadriplegia, most if not all patients gain one full motor level, achieving grade 3 wrist extensor movement (a C-6 muscle) during the first 8 months after injury (Ditunno et al., 1987). By analyzing data from a national database, researchers are currently attempting to see if this recovery of one motor level in complete SCI is true for all neurologic levels of injury. Researchers have also determined that in SCI above T-11, preservation of pinprick sensation has predictive value for return of motor function and independent ambulation, probably due to the proximity of the ascending pain fibers and descending motor fibers in the spinal cord (Crozier et al., 1991). Lesions of the cauda equina are essentially lesions of the peripheral nerve or lower motoneuron and may show recovery over several years owing to resolution of neurapraxia or to regrowth of damaged axons as well as to peripheral sprouting.

Prognostic information is also available for the neuroanatomic incomplete syndromes. Anterior cord syndrome is usually due to damage to the anterior spinal artery, causing infarction in the spinal cord. Prognosis for return of function is poor. In posterior cord syndrome, motor function is preserved but the loss of proprioception means ambulation is unlikely. In Brown-Séquard and central cord syndromes, prognosis for ambulation and bladder and bowel control is very good but hand function may be impaired, depending on the level of injury.

The second reason for the importance of precise definition of the level of SCI is that it helps to predict the ultimate level of independence a patient can expect to achieve in the areas of mobility, self-care, and even communication. Tables 20–4 and 20–5 delineate the optimal functional abilities for each level of motor complete SCI. Patients with incomplete SCI may exceed the expectations for any given level of injury. Such expectations for independence must also be tempered by considera-

TABLE 20–1. **KEY MUSCLES FOR MOTOR LEVEL CLASSIFICATION**

C-5	Elbow flexors (biceps, brachialis)
C-6	Wrist extensors (extensor carpi radialis longus and brevis)
C-7	Elbow extensors (triceps)
C-8	Finger flexors to the middle finger (flexor digitorum profundus)
T-1	Small finger abductors (aductor digiti minimi manus)
L-2	Hip flexors (iliopsoas)
L-3	Knee extensors (quadriceps)
L-4	Ankle dorsiflexors (tibialis anterior)
L-5	Long toe extensors (extensor hallucis longus)
S-1	Ankle plantar flexors (gastrocnemius, soleus)

From American Spinal Injury Association. International Standards for Neurological and Functional Classification of Spinal Cord Injury. Chicago: American Spinal Injury Association, 1992. Endorsed by the International Medical Society of Paraplegia and supported by the American Paralysis Association.

FIGURE 20–1. *A*, Anterior view of key sensory areas by dermatome; *B*, posterior view of key sensory areas by dermatome. (From American Spinal Injury Association. International Standards for Neurological and Functional Classification of Spinal Cord Injury, Revised 1992. Chicago: American Spinal Injury Association, 1992. Endorsed by the International Medical Society of Paraplegia and supported by the American Paralysis Association.)

tion of the child's age, which influences developmental expectations, as well as upper body strength.

The Young Child with Spinal Cord Injury

ASSESSMENT OF PERFORMANCE

Infants, toddlers, and preschoolers can incur SCI as a result of birth trauma, child abuse, motor vehi

cle crashes, tumor, or even transverse myelitis. In infants, determination of the motor and sensory levels of SCI can be challenging and may require multiple assessments to determine what is voluntary and what is reflex mediated. Assessment of passive ROM should be performed, as for any infant. Determination of functional limitations is less informative, as infants are expected to be dependent. Very young children with SCI require careful follow-up over time to be sure they meet functional expectations and are not infantilized by caregivers

TABLE 20-2. **KEY SENSORY AREAS**

C-2	Occipital protuberance
C-3	Supraclavicular fossa
C-4	Top of the acromioclavicular joint
C-5	Lateral side of the antecubital fossa
C-6	Thumb
C-7	Middle finger
C-8	Little finger
T-1	Medial (ulnar) side of the antecubital fossa
T-2	Apex of the axilla
T-3	3rd intercostal space
T-4	4th intercostal space (nipple line)
T-5	5th intercostal space (midway between T-4 and T-6)
T-6	6th intercostal space (level of xiphisternum)
T-7	7th intercostal space (midway between T-6 and T-8)
T-8	8th intercostal space (midway between T-6 and T-10)
T-9	9th intercostal space (midway between T-8 and T-10)
T-10	10th intercostal space (umbilicus)
T-11	11th intercostal space (midway between T-10 and T-12)
T-12	Inguinal ligament at midpoint
L-1	Half the distance between T-12 and L-2
L-2	Midanterior thigh
L-3	Medial femoral condyle
L-4	Medial malleolus
L-5	Dorsum of the foot at the 3rd metatarsal phalangeal joint
S-1	Lateral heel
S-2	Popliteal fossa in the midline
S-3	Ischial tuberosity
S-4-5	Perianal area (taken as one level)

From American Spinal Injury Association. International Standards for Neurological and Functional Classification of Spinal Cord Injury. Chicago: American Spinal Injury Association, 1992. Endorsed by the International Medical Society of Paraplegia and supported by the American Paralysis Association.

Assessing the performance of preschool children with a recent SCI is rarely completed in one session. These children are commonly and appropriately anxious in the presence of health care professionals. In order to gather the most accurate information about the child's level of function, trust must be established in the child and the parents. As with any young child, this means taking extra time to play and talk with the child and to interact with the parents. Some children are initially fearful of movement, whereas others act fearlessly. In the former case, it will take time to build their confidence. In the latter case, the child may attempt to remove the cervical collar or body jacket or they may assume body positions that stress the healing fusion. Thus, additional adult supervision may be necessary to comply with precautions during the healing phase.

Quantification of impairments in the young child is often unreliable because young children are unable to cooperate consistently with formal testing. Passive ROM measurement is possibly an exception to this, but its reliability in children with SCI has not been established. In normal children and in children with myelodysplasia, manual mus-

TABLE 20-3. **ASIA IMPAIRMENT SCALE**

A   Complete—No sensory or motor function in the sacral segments S4-5.

B   Incomplete—Sensory but not motor function is preserved below the neurological level and extends through the sacral segments S4-5.

C   Incomplete—Motor function is preserved below the neurological level, and the majority of key muscles below the neurologic level have a muscle grade less than 3.

D   Incomplete—Motor function is preserved below the neurologic level, and the majority of key muscles below the neurologic level have a muscle grade greater than or equal to 3.

E   Normal—Sensory and motor function is normal.

From American Spinal Injury Association. International Standards for Neurological and Functional Classification of Spinal Cord Injury. Chicago: American Spinal Injury Association, 1992. Endorsed by the International Medical Society of Paraplegia and supported by the American Paralysis Association.

TABLE 20-4. **MOBILITY IN COMPLETE QUADRIPLEGIA: EXPECTED FUNCTION AND NECESSARY EQUIPMENT**

Functional Skill	Mobility for Level of Injury			
	C-1 to C-4	C-5	C-6	C-7 to T-1
Bed mobility	D	A: Even with electric bed	I: With equipment; electric bed helpful	I: Electric bed helpful
Transfers	D	D	Some I with sliding board	I: May need sliding board
Wheelchair	I: PWC, chin or mouth control	I: PWC, hand control with splint	I: MWC, adapted rims	I: MWC
Pressure relief	D: Bed, MWC I: Power recline WC	D: Bed, MWC I: Power recline WC	I: Leaning to side	I: Push-up on open hands
Transportation	U: Driving; van with lift needed	U: Driving; van with lift needed	I: Hand controls A: Load WC	I: Hand controls I: Load WC

Key: A = assistance required, D = dependent, I = independent, MWC = manual wheelchair, PWC = power wheelchair, U = unable, WC = wheelchair.

Adapted from Massagli, TL, & Jaffe, KM. Pediatric spinal cord injury: Treatment and outcome. Pediatrician, 17:244–254, 1990. Reprinted with permission of S. Karger, Basel.

TABLE 20-5. **MOBILITY IN COMPLETE PARAPLEGIA: EXPECTED FUNCTION AND NECESSARY EQUIPMENT**

Functional Skill	Level of Injury		
	T-2 to T-10	T-11 to L-2	L-3 to S-2
Manual wheelchair	I: Indoors	I: Indoors	May not need MWC except long distances, recreation
Ambulation	SBA: Exercise only; need KAFOs or RGOs and forearm crutches or walker; not practical for T2–T6	I: Indoors with KAFOs or RGOs, and forearm crutches; some can do stairs with railing	I: Indoors and community with AFOs; may need forearm crutches or cane
Driving	I: Hand controls II: Load WC	I: Hand controls II: Load WC	Can drive automatic transmission; may prefer hand controls

Key: AFOS = ankle-foot orthoses, KAFOs = knee-ankle-foot orthoses, RGOs = reciprocating gait orthoses, I = independent, SBA = standby assistance, MWC = manual wheelchair; WC = wheelchair.
Adapted from Massagli TL, & Jaffe, KM. Pediatric spinal cord injury: Treatment and outcome. Pediatrician, 17:244–254, 1990. Reprinted with permission of S. Karger, Basel

cle testing is generally unreliable if the child is younger than 5 years old (McDonald et al., 1986; Molnar & Kaminer, 1992). In young children, strength testing is often estimated by encouraging and observing movement. Ideally, the therapist places the child in various positions and encourages him or her to reach for targets (toys) with a single extremity. This allows manipulation of gravity-eliminated and antigravity movements as well as comparison of left and right extremities. Resistance can be provided with small wrap weights (0.25 lb) or the weight of hand-held toys. In reality, the physical therapist is often forced to observe spontaneous play and record descriptions of available movements. This may also include facilitating the child's basic postural responses, such as positive support of the lower extremities or protective extension of the upper extremities. Ruling out substitutions can be challenging. Through playful formats, the therapist may be able to position and stabilize the child to isolate muscle groups. Muscle strength is recorded as 0 through 5, as with adults (rarely with the finer + or − gradations). Scores of 4 and 5 are subjective measures, particularly in growing children, but with experience, the therapist can become a more accurate evaluator.

Cardiorespiratory endurance is commonly diminished in children with recent SCI but difficult to quantify because they cannot complete the available standardized tests requiring walking or running (see Chapter 5). Therapists can make clinical estimates of endurance by recording the length of time a child can engage in an activity or the number of repetitions of a movement completed before the child needs to rest. Accurate recording of these data can be used to document changes in endurance over time. When respiratory status is compromised, the physical therapist must coordinate efforts with the respiratory therapist and the nurses to ensure that the child maintains adequate ventilation. In some settings, the physical therapist may take a more primary role by providing chest physical therapy.

Both the Functional Independence Measure for Children (WeeFIM) (Granger et al., 1988) and the Pediatric Evaluation of Disability Inventory (PEDI) (Haley et al., 1989) are used as measures of functional skills for patients with SCI, and both are currently undergoing reliability testing. Regardless of which assessment tools are preferred, the physical therapist must establish a complete baseline of the child's abilities and determine whether limitations are due to the child's age, the neurologic impairment, the need to wear a spinal orthosis, or other causes. Any standard physical therapy assessment includes testing of the child's ability to reach, roll and position in bed, come to sitting, balance in sitting, scoot, crawl, transfer, come to kneel, stand, and ambulate. Obviously, some or all of these may not be possible, so the type and amount of assistance needed are carefully recorded. For some skills, such as ambulation, the therapist may simply record "unable." Length of sitting tolerance is also recorded.

Physical therapists should include parents as active participants during the assessment phase. Parents need to receive accurate, understandable information about their child's condition. Because they are trying to adapt to the sudden change in their child's health, they often are unable to generate therapy goals for their child beyond the obvious one of "to walk again." The therapist and management team must assist the family and child in establishing realistic goals. One must consider the child's level of injury (see Tables 20–4 & 20–5), the completeness of injury, the age of the child, and the family's expectations for the child. The therapist must also take into consideration that the wearing of a spinal orthosis restricts some movements. If the child needs to wear the orthosis beyond the predicted acute rehabilitation hospitalization, then some goals for independence may need to be postponed until it is removed.

IMPAIRMENTS AND FUNCTIONAL LIMITATIONS

The child's anxiety with strangers, fear of hospital personnel, and fear of movement often persist beyond the assessment phase and affect treatment sessions. These problems are best addressed by starting with brief sessions that have low demand and high success. Gradually increasing the time and difficulty can be facilitated by providing predictability and promoting trust. The therapist can establish routines for scheduling, treatment session locations, and safe play space, and whenever possible, should give the child choices.

Parents should be included in treatment sessions whenever possible. Although many children work better in therapy sessions in the absence of parents, parents should be regularly included to see the new skills their child can independently accomplish and the emerging skills that require assistance. Parents need to become experts in all aspects of their child's mobility and use of adaptive equipment and need to understand the information taught by other team members. Parent education and training should be an ongoing process that begins soon after the initial evaluation and is completed in time for practice on day or overnight outings.

During physical therapy sessions with the child, it is nearly impossible to do isolated treatment of impairments, with the exception of ROM activities. The child's motivation for play gives overall structure for the sessions. Within that, the therapist designs activities that encourage strengthening, reaching, rolling, transitions, and mobility in various combinations.

Sitting balance is often one of the major goals of therapy. Balance is impaired by altered strength and sensation and often by the presence of a spinal orthosis. The seated child is encouraged to progress from therapist support to self-support at a table top or on a mat and to independent sitting if this is realistic given the level and completeness of injury. These goals may be achieved by distracting the child or engaging the child in play activities. If the child has a lumbar SCI and the orthopaedist has recommended precautions, such as no hip flexion

past 90° to avoid stressing the fusion, it can be challenging to help the young child comply. The child may be tempted to long-sit or ring-sit and to prop forward on the hands to scoot or drag himself or herself.

If some lower extremity function has been preserved, the therapist helps children progress to crawling, kneeling, and standing activities when the functioning lower extremity muscles can be appropriately strengthened. Some children require orthoses for distal weakness in the lower extremities. Table 20–5 outlines the expected functional ambulation by level of SCI. Preschool-aged children can learn to use reciprocating gait orthoses and knee-ankle-foot orthoses (KAFOs), but they generally rely on a front-wheeled walker, as opposed to crutches, until the age of 7 to 8 years. Further discussion of gait training and use of orthoses will be presented in the section on school-aged and adolescent children.

Orthoses may also be needed by children with absent muscle function for maintaining ROM, for instance at the ankle or in the hands. As with any insensate area, the skin must be regularly examined to avoid pressure ulcers.

If long-distance ambulation is not a goal, the child needs a wheelchair for mobility. For children with SCI at or above C-5, a power wheelchair is needed for independent mobility. In addition, a manual wheelchair is necessary to provide these children with a substitute when the power chair needs repairs. The manual wheelchair is also useful for transport and in places where the larger, heavier power chair is impractical. Many families do not have a home with hallways or doors large enough to accommodate a power wheelchair, so this wheelchair may be used primarily in public and school settings and the manual wheelchair used in the home. A child as young as 18 to 24 months may be trained to use a power wheelchair but requires adult supervision for safety. Some young children with lower levels of SCI, for example, C-6, C-7, C-8, or even lower thoracic injuries, may be able to propel a manual wheelchair for only limited distances on smooth, level surfaces owing to lack of upper body strength and endurance. For these children to be exposed to a broader range of environments, such as preschool playgrounds or uneven or steep terrain around the family home, prescription of a power wheelchair is justifiable to promote age-appropriate functional mobility.

The seating components of either a power or manual wheelchair are prescribed with skin protection and spinal alignment in mind. A level pelvis avoids undue pressure over the ischial tuberosities and facilitates a straight spine (Hobson & Tooms,

1992). A solid seat and solid back are preferred to sling upholstery in this age group. Several types of wheelchair cushions are available, but none is universally effective for all persons with SCI, and individual assessment and reassessment are required to prevent pressure ulcers (Garber & Dylerly, 1991). If the level of SCI permits self-propulsion of the manual wheelchair, light-weight frame construction has been shown to be preferable for initiating rolling and for maintaining a higher velocity (Parziale, 1991).

Children who use a wheelchair and their parents must be trained to complete transfers. Children younger than 4 years often lack the upper body strength to transfer independently and typically require a one-person lift transfer. Use of a sliding board or pivot transfer is appropriate for older children of 5 to 7 years. Pressure relief techniques must also be taught. Younger children often rely on caregivers for a recline relief. Older children may be able to complete one of the techniques independently, depending on the level and completeness of injury (see Table 20–4).

PREVENTION OF SECONDARY IMPAIRMENTS

As discussed in the section on medical management, a number of secondary impairments can arise after SCI. Many of these can lead to functional limitations and disability. Physical therapists contribute to prevention, treatment, and monitoring of pressure ulcers, contractures, edema, spasticity, pathologic fractures, and scoliosis. Pressure ulcers occur as a result of improper positioning or inadequate pressure relief and can limit ability to sit. Very young children may not need frequent pressure relief because body weight is not great enough to impair tissue blood flow and they are often held and handled frequently enough that they do not remain in one position too long. As children grow older, it is often difficult for them to understand the imperativeness of incorporating pressure relief into their self-care routines.

Contractures can arise as a result of static positioning, spasticity, or heterotopic bone formation and may interfere with positioning or voluntary movement. Dependent edema is more common in children with flaccid lower extremities. When it develops, it predisposes skin to breakdown by increasing fragility and by altering the fit of garments and braces. Spasticity may be present and cause no functional limitations, or it may impair positioning, transfers, or other voluntary movements. Conversely, spasticity may be helpful for those with incomplete SCI who use it to achieve or maintain

standing. Pathologic fractures can occur to osteopenic extremities with improper transfers, falls, or forceful ROM exercises. Scoliosis occurs in virtually all children with SCI in this age group and can affect comfortable seating and respiratory function. Although family training and positioning needs are initially managed or determined by inpatient physical therapists, outpatient and school physical therapists have an important role in monitoring and maintaining ROM and in using stretching and positioning to minimize spasticity. They monitor the upper body strength that allows the growing child to perform independent pressure relief. They also monitor positioning in seating devices and the fit of adaptive equipment, including wheelchairs and orthoses.

No treatment, including passive standing and electrical stimulation, has yet been found to prevent or reverse osteopenia in paralyzed extremities, so the presence of osteopenia and the risk of pathologic fractures should be assumed for all children with SCI, even for those with spasticity. Although it is important to provide proper pelvic alignment and trunk support in wheelchairs, external devices do not prevent the ultimate development of scoliosis, and many children require treatment with bracing and then spinal fusion after they have achieved the majority of their expected height.

MINIMIZING DISABILITY AND DISADVANTAGE

While hospitalized, the child must practice mobility skills outside of structured therapy sessions. Thus, children must be encouraged to self-propel part or all the way to various activities during the day. Family and other team members need to be familiar with each child's skills and routines to maximize the child's independence across settings and activities. For instance, nurses should be updated on progress in mobility skills so that the child can be encouraged to incorporate these abilities into play activities or getting to meals.

The child must eventually be trained in using these new skills out in the community. Community reentry activities are often the combined responsibility of physical therapists, occupational therapists, and recreational therapists. Children must become familiar with common architectural barriers such as curbs, heavy doors, and high shelves and learn how to negotiate them or ask for help. Caregivers need to be trained in the type and amount of assistance to provide and cautioned against being overly helpful. Discharge planning and long-term management should address mobility issues in the child's home, school, and community. Whenever possible, a home evaluation should be conducted early in the child's hospital stay. If home modifications are necessary for wheelchair accessibility or safety, the family needs time to gather financial resources and complete modifications. These modifications can be tested during weekend passes. School accessibility may also be an issue. Some schools have therapists who can provide the needed information and assist with the return to school. For children living great distances from the hospital, other community therapists can provide a local perspective and become a resource to the family. Another area of concern in community reentry is safe transportation. The physical therapist can assist the family with evaluating safe transportation of their child and identifying any equipment needs. If a van will be used, then wheelchair tie downs will be necessary. If the child can sit in a vehicle seat, then appropriate car seats, booster seats, or restraints are needed, depending on the child's age.

ONGOING MONITORING

The key to ensuring maximal function in young children with SCI is to provide ongoing assessment of impairments and function and to regularly reestablish goals appropriate for the child's age. At least two mechanisms are available to accomplish this objective. Children who are discharged from rehabilitation centers are routinely seen in follow-up visits two or more times each year. These reevaluations include medical follow-up to reassess the level and completeness of injury, to evaluate changes in bladder function or skin integrity, to monitor the spine for development of scoliosis, and to determine the need for medications to treat spasticity or bladder or bowel incontinence. At about age 5 years, children with adequate hand function should learn self-management of bladder and bowel care. They will likely need adult supervision and assistance with caring for adaptive equipment such as catheters for many years but should be able to carry out most of their bladder management. At about this age, they should also begin to take responsibility for checking skin integrity each day but again will need reminders or supervision for a number of years.

Reassessment by physical therapists is an important part of these follow-up visits. For children who have developed sufficient upper extremity strength, a standard push-up for pressure relief in the wheelchair may be taught. These children are often gaining more independence in self-propelling outdoors and on inclines. They may need instruction and training to participate more in transfers. The child's wheelchair should be reassessed and adapted as needed to accommodate the child's growth and to ensure that any modifications enhance independence.

The physical therapy reassessments at the rehabilitation facility follow a consultative model. The ongoing progress toward age-appropriate goals may occur in a hospital-based outpatient therapy program, but it is more typically accomplished through therapy services offered in early intervention programs or in publicly funded developmental preschools. Therapists in these programs ideally are in contact with the rehabilitation centers on a regular basis to update progress and goals and to identify new concerns and equipment needs.

A small number of children with SCI may actually experience progressive decline in function over time. These are usually children with SCI due to progressive or metastatic tumor. It can be unsettling and challenging for rehabilitation professionals to care for such patients, but it is an important aspect of their work. Often such children need more equipment over time, such as more bracing or a wheelchair with more supportive seating. These children can often be very ill from ongoing chemotherapy or radiation treatments, and it may be more practical to rent equipment than to purchase it. Coordination of efforts among oncology and rehabilitation staff, the patient, and the family is crucial.

The School-Aged Child and Adolescent with Spinal Cord Injury

ASSESSMENT OF PERFORMANCE

Assessing older children is generally more straightforward than assessing preschoolers, toddlers, or infants. The therapist must nevertheless keep in mind that these children may be confronting the potential permanence of their condition. The therapist may notice the adolescent being withdrawn or angry or in denial or even enthusiastic to begin therapy. These behaviors may fluctuate and change rapidly. The therapist and team can help the child develop realistic expectations of the rehabilitation process.

The evaluation can be conducted as for an adult. ROM measurements and manual muscle testing are completed. As previously noted, endurance testing is limited because standardized assessments require lower extremity function. Much research is needed in this area, particularly in standardization of upper extremity ergometry. The same basic mobility skills must be assessed as with younger children, that is, rolling, coming to sit, sitting balance, transfers, and locomotion. Functional assessment may include the PEDI or Functional Independence Measure (FIM) (Hamilton et al., 1987). The FIM is a measure of functional limitations or disability for those older than 7 years. It can be used to assess the same categories of function (using the same 7-level scale) as the WeeFIM. The FIM is widely used in national databases of persons with SCI, but unanswered questions related to its use with SCI patients remain. Reliability for relating functional change to neurologic recovery has not been established for the FIM, nor has its precision in correlating levels of quadriplegia with self-care capability (Ditunno, 1992b). The social cognition and communication subscales may have too low a ceiling to reliably indicate cognitive deficits in SCI patients with brain injuries or with a history of substance abuse (Davidoff et al., 1990).

Parents may or may not be present during the actual assessment. Nevertheless, they should be provided with accurate, understandable information, and as previously noted, families and children in their early crisis phase often need the rehabilitation team to assist them with realistic goal setting. Children who have returned to school may be better able to identify personal goals. Although age plays a smaller role in goal development, level and completeness of injury must be taken into account.

IMPAIRMENTS AND FUNCTIONAL LIMITATIONS

When designing physical therapy sessions, it is important to be sensitive to the child's current emotional status. Treatment session demands can be modified to most appropriately challenge the child. An issue commonly expressed by teenagers is that of not being able to trust their bodies. The altered motor and sensory processes and potential changes in bowel and bladder function can make their bodies feel foreign to them. In addition, teenagers are accustomed to privacy and independence in their lives. Both their injury and subsequent reliance on a hospital environment and adaptive equipment can disrupt their sense of control. The rehabilitation team should respect their privacy and allow them to participate in scheduling therapy, nursing care, and free time.

Parents still need to be included regularly in sessions to observe their child's progress and receive updated training for transfers, wheelchair mobility, pressure relief, use of orthoses, and ambulation. It can be helpful to allow close friends to observe therapy and attend outings. If friends feel comfort-able with the injured adolescent, their presence may help to lessen social isolation.

Treatment sessions are more structured with older than with younger children. The first step is to get the child upright and out of bed. If orthostatic hypotension is a problem, this process may require several sessions and use of a wheelchair with a reclinable back to allow the child to gradually assume a fully upright posture. Protocols for remobilizing the newly injured older child or teenager with SCI often use a tilt table to gradually elevate the child's head, although use of this tactic has not yet been proved to hasten resolution of orthostatic hypotension. In addition, the therapist should be alert for any complaints of headaches that may signal autonomic dysreflexia, a problem described in the section on medical management. The therapist should monitor heart rate and blood pressure and, when appropriate, alert the medical staff.

Teenagers are familiar with the concept of exercise, so they can participate in progressive resistive exercises beginning with powder board and progressing to weight lifting. Depending on the level of SCI, the orthopaedist may restrict upper extremity exercises to those performed symmetrically to avoid torque on the spinal fusion. Teenagers can also concentrate on specific sitting activities as well. Activities should be alternated to such an extent that the child moves among balance, strength, endurance, and functional skills. Too often, training sessions are conducted that do not simulate real-life situations.

For children with paraplegia, transfer training initially includes sliding board transfers. As upper extremity strength increases, the child may be able to transfer without a sliding board. Older children must also practice car transfers and how to get up from and down to the floor with and without assistance. Wheelchair mobility must be practiced on even and uneven terrain and up and down ramps and curbs. Wheelies can be taught about the age of 8 years to facilitate managing curbs. Various pressure relief techniques must also be taught, depending on the level and completeness of SCI (see Table 20–4). Those with limited upper extremity strength and trunk control are able to shift their weight to the side. At lower levels of paraplegia, the child can lift the buttocks off the seat for 20 to 60 seconds, 2 or 3 times an hour. If the child with paraplegia is not able to ambulate long distances, a manual wheelchair should be prescribed. Lightweight components should be used, but if it is anticipated that the child will be very active or frequently traverse rough terrain, then a rigid frame, as opposed to a folding frame, should be considered. If the teenager has completed most of his or her growth and has a low thoracic or lumbar level SCI, then a low sling back with a taut sling seat may be used in place of the solid seat and back.

For teenagers with preserved or recovered lower extremity function, ambulation may be a realistic goal. Often, some sort of orthosis is needed, and general guidelines are presented in Table 20–5. Donning and doffing of orthoses must be practiced as well as controlled sit-to-stand maneuvers and finding the balance point in standing. As with most ambulation training, practice begins in the parallel bars and progresses to use of other assistive devices when the child gains enough control. Ambulation is most practical for those who have at least anti-gravity strength (grade 3) in one set of quadriceps muscles. At higher injury levels, the child requires KAFOs and some type of upper extremity assistive device. A four-point gait is possible for those with strong hip flexors or with the use of reciprocating gait orthoses. The swing-through gait pattern is, however, much more efficient. Five to 12 times as much energy is expended walking with KAFOs compared with that required for normal gait on even terrain (Jaeger et al., 1989). Numerous follow-up studies of adults have found that more than half of patients who have KAFOs prescribed do not use them at all in the long term, and the majority of the rest of patients use them only for standing or exercise (Jaeger et al., 1989; Subbarao, 1991). The most common reasons for discontinuing use of the braces are the excessive energy costs and the need for assistance to wear and use them. Given the significant expense of brace manufacture and ambulation training, it is often best to complete initial rehabilitation goals, mastering independent wheelchair mobility, and periodically reassess the child's physical abilities and goals as an outpatient. Many patients become less interested in the use of KAFOs over time as the permanence of the injury becomes more apparent, and those who remain interested may have more specific needs for standing or limited walking that increase the likelihood of long-term use.

For children and teenagers with quadriplegia, the focus of physical therapy is on maintaining ROM, transfer training, and the ordering and training in use of adaptive equipment. Wheelchairs need to be ordered as soon as possible to allow for training time in the hospital and to coordinate with the patient's discharge, but ordering the appropriate wheelchair can be challenging because approximately half these children have incomplete injuries and the extent of their recovery may not be clear for months. Those with quadriplegia at C-5 or above (and some at C-6, depending on terrain)

need a power wheelchair as well as a manual wheelchair for the reasons previously described. Pressure relief may be accomplished by weight shift or may require mechanical recline. If the child has no trunk control, a power recline mechanism should be used. Shearing of skin over the low back and buttocks is avoided by using a wheelchair with a tilt-in-space option in which the back and seat tilt together. The wheelchair as well as environmental control systems should be chosen by the rehabilitation team, child, and family in consultation with a knowledgeable vendor.

A small number of children with quadriplegia have upper cervical injuries that necessitate mechanical ventilation (see Chapter 24). Physical therapy goals remain much the same as for other children with quadriplegia, but wheelchair prescription must take into account a safe platform for transport of a portable ventilator. The joystick is replaced with a tongue switch or sip and puff controls, and the power recline must allow for ventilator placement.

Those with quadriplegia above C-7 need assistance for transfers. Caregivers need to learn pivot transfers and use of a mechanical lift. The family must be thoroughly trained in all aspects of the child's mobility and care, and the child must be trained to instruct others in his or her care, including use and maintenance of the wheelchair and any other equipment.

FUNCTIONAL ELECTRICAL STIMULATION

Functional electrical stimulation (FES) has been applied in several problems in SCI. Present technology is useful only in cases of upper motoneuron paralysis where the intact peripheral nerve is stimulated, causing muscle contraction. In lower motorneuron injuries to the cauda equina, the peripheral nerve and its muscular branches undergo Wallerian degeneration, so the muscle must be stimulated directly and larger pulse widths and current amplitudes are necessary to produce contractions. The whole muscle must be flooded with current, and the contraction response is often inadequate. The stimulation parameters can be painful in those who have some preservation of sensation.

FES has been used as a strengthening modality for partially paralyzed muscles. In crossover studies of FES-assisted exercise versus conventional exercise, no significant increases in maximal strength have been found with use of FES (Seeger et al., 1989). FES does improve both strength and endurance of totally paralyzed muscles, and aerobic training programs have been found to reverse myocardial atrophy as a result of the pressure and volume challenge to the heart (Nash et al., 1991; Ragnarsson et al., 1988). The peak levels of cardiorespiratory performance achievable with FES are, however, similar to those attained by persons with SCI performing maximal voluntary upper extremity exercises (Pollack et al., 1989). Because degenerative joint disease of the shoulder is a significant problem for aging persons with SCI, one advantage of FES over conventional exercise as an aerobic training strategy is that more muscle groups are exercising, placing less stress on the upper extremities.

Obviously, exercise must be performed regularly to maintain any effect. Home bicycle ergometer units are now available, but follow-up studies have shown that patients with SCI are often too busy to use this expensive equipment on a regular and long-term basis (Sipski et al., 1991). In patients who do exercise consistently, increase of muscle bulk occurs concomitantly with increase of strength in paralyzed muscles. In addition, blood flow to muscles is increased during stimulation, and the combination of increased bulk and improved circulatory flow may help to prevent pressure ulcers (Levine et al., 1990). Researchers and clinicians had hoped that FES could help to reverse osteopenia after SCI, but to date, none of the protocols used has been able to increase bone mass, and FES may actually be dangerous in those with the most severe osteopenia because it may cause pathologic fractures (Phillips, 1987).

FES has also been applied to facilitate standing and walking after SCI. Surface, percutaneous, or implanted electrodes are used to deliver current to lower extremity nerves innervating muscles such as the quadriceps and gluteals. The development of sensors to determine leg position, force, acceleration, and muscle fatigue has lagged behind progress in stimulation but is necessary to improve the quality and efficiency of movement. None of the currently available technologic methods permits standing or walking without upper extremity assistive devices. Hybrid systems using FES and orthoses have also been developed, and less expensive garments with surface electrodes sewn into them for easier application are available. The energy costs of walking with FES are comparable to those of using KAFOs but may be slightly reduced when FES is combined with reciprocating gait orthoses (Hirokawa et al., 1990; Yarkony et al., 1992). At present, this technology remains imperfect, expensive, and not widely available. Data on long-term use other than in a limited number of research subjects have not been published.

PREVENTION OF SECONDARY IMPAIRMENTS

The secondary impairments facing older children and adolescents with SCI are similar to those for younger children, with a few additions. In this older age group, cardiovascular fitness and overuse syndromes are important to consider. Studies of adults with chronic SCI have shown that physical work capacity inversely correlates with lesion level and that cardiovascular responses to exercise are abnormal due to a deficient sympathetic nervous system (Drory et al., 1990). Such persons may be at increased risk for cardiovascular compromise and disease. Clinicians are prudent to encourage regular aerobic exercise in older children and young adults with SCI to help them develop lifelong habits of health promotion. School therapists can facilitate participation in an adaptive physical education program or in competitive wheelchair sports. Stotts (1986) found that athletes with paraplegia were less likely to incur avoidable medical complications than nonathletes with paraplegia. Consideration of such participation must be balanced against the recently recognized propensity for overuse syndromes in these athletes, including such problems as carpal tunnel syndrome, tendonitis, and degenerative disease of shoulder joints.

Substance abuse after SCI is a problem that is only beginning to receive attention in adults with SCI, and its prevalence in teenagers is not known. In adults with SCI, those who abuse alcohol are likely to have done so before their injury. Screening programs have found that the frequency of abuse of other substances is relatively low (13%) in inner city adult patients with SCI (Rothstein et al., 1992). Cigarette smoking should be discouraged for all the obvious reasons in addition to the risk of burns to insensate skin.

MINIMIZING DISABILITY AND DISADVANTAGE

In addition to the aforementioned need for children to practice skills across settings, teenagers can take on responsibility for transporting themselves to appointments and activities within the hospital. As is the case with younger children, outings are practice sessions for return to the community. In addition to the usual home and school assessments, the complex issue of transportation must be addressed. The teenager's friends may need to be trained in car transfers so that he or she can stay socially active. The teenager returning to driving needs to be independent with transfers and with loading and unloading the wheelchair. How the wheelchair can be loaded into the car influences decisions about prescribing a rigid or folding frame wheelchair. Above all, teenagers should be encouraged to problem solve the management of architectural barriers and ask for assistance if safety is jeopardized. Upon return to the community, the teenager's primary resource for mobility and seating issues is the school therapist. Some teenagers, especially those with higher levels of injury, may benefit from use of animal aids, such as dogs trained by the program Canine Companions for Independence (PO Box 446, Santa Rosa, CA 95402).

ONGOING MONITORING AND TRANSITION TO ADULTHOOD

Unlike younger children, school-aged children and adolescents with SCI are usually closer to their predicted function for level of injury by the time of discharge from the rehabilitation unit. As mentioned previously, however, neurologic changes may continue for some months; for example, children with C-5 complete quadriplegia may develop antigravity wrist extension during the first 8 months after injury, and outpatient or school therapists may need to formulate new goals. In many children, upper body strength of intact muscles continues to improve, enabling smoother transfers or easier wheelchair propulsion up inclines. In general, however, the majority of physical therapy involvement after discharge eventually entails a monitoring role, for example, making sure that mobility skills learned in the hospital environment are generalized to the real world, monitoring ROM or spasticity, and updating equipment. Any deterioration in motor strength should be referred for medical evaluation since it may signify development of a syrinx.

Older children and adolescents require reevaluation similar to that of younger children in a rehabilitation center once or twice a year. The focus of these assessments is on medical issues, equipment needs, and efficacy of home or outpatient stretching or exercise programs. For teenagers, such visits should include discussions related to sexuality and reproduction (Haseltine et al., 1990). Young women need to know that their fertility is not impaired by spinal cord injury but that sexual response and orgasm may be. Pregnant women with SCI should be managed at high-risk centers to avoid respiratory and urinary tract complications, detect threatened preterm births, and prevent autonomic dysreflexia during delivery. Although the majority of males with SCI can have erections,

these are often fleeting and not adequate for vaginal penetration. Few men with SCI have ejaculations, and sperm quality decreases over time for reasons that are not entirely clear. New techniques for retrieval of sperm and for artificial insemination have helped some men with SCI to father children. In addition to this physiologic information, it is important to include issues of intimacy and relationships in discussions of sexuality.

We have found that although the majority of young school-aged children with SCI receive physical and occupational therapy services in school, few adolescents receive such services. A survey of adolescents revealed that many face problems of accessibility at school and have no physical education program and that breakdown of wheelchairs, both power and manual, contributes to absences at school. The fact that the number of years of education after injury is more significant than absolute amount of education in predicting employment after SCI (El Ghahit & Hanson, 1979) speaks to the importance of ensuring success in school for such children. Unfortunately, only 50% of teenagers with a 9th- to 11th-grade education at the time of their SCI finish high school (DeVivo et al., 1991).

We and others have found that few adolescents with SCI receive educational or vocational counseling beyond selection of classes each term (Graham et al., 1991). Such students may qualify for transition planning under the Individuals with Disabilities Education Act, Public Law 101–476, enacted in 1990. School physical therapists might participate in a transition program by assessing functional mobility skills in the community or work-study setting. When the teenager with SCI becomes 18 years of age, she or he is eligible for state vocational counseling services. Such services are often important sources of funding for vocationally related education or even equipment.

Three case histories illustrate the application of the principles discussed in this chapter. The first describes the experiences of a very young child; the second, those of a preschooler; and third, those of a teenager.

CASE HISTORY: STACY

The following case demonstrates the physical therapy management of a very young child with incomplete quadriplegia. Stacy was injured at 9 months of age in January 1991. She was an unrestrained passenger in a motor vehicle crash. Although she did not sustain bone injury to the spine, magnetic resonance imaging revealed a C-6 to T-1 intracord hemorrhage. She was diagnosed with C-7 quadriplegia, ASIA Impairment Scale level B. Lower extremity movements were noted, but it was unclear if they were reflex mediated or voluntary. Stacy also sustained a right frontoparietal contusion of the brain. She was intubated for 1 to 2 weeks to assist with respiratory function. At her initial physical therapy examination, Stacy showed passive ROM throughout the trunk and extremities within normal limits. Tightness was noted at the end range of shoulder flexion and abduction as well as elbow extension. Although formal manual muscle testing could not be conducted with a child her age, gross estimates of muscle strength were made. Right shoulder flexion was estimated at grade 3, left shoulder flexion and abduction grade 2, and elbow motions grade 3. Wrist extension was estimated at grade 3, with movements of the fingers graded at trace. Functionally, Stacy was unable to roll but when placed in prone-on-elbows could sustain the position very briefly. When placed in sitting with full trunk support, she could raise her head to within about 20° of vertical.

After approximately 2 weeks of acute medical care, Stacy was transferred to an inpatient pediatric rehabilitation facility. At that time, physical therapy goals were targeted at three major areas. The first area was ROM. Stacy underwent daily ROM therapy and was provided with bilateral hand and ankle splints for night wear. Her caregivers were instructed in the donning and doffing of the splints as well as carrying out ROM activities. The second area of goals was seating and positioning. The family was provided with a standard stroller with a foam insert that could be used in both the stroller and a highchair. Stacy was also provided with a car seat for safe transportation. The third area of focus was facilitation of active movement, sitting balance, and general mobility. These areas of function were affected by the SCI and possibly by the brain injury as well. Treatment sessions focused on increasing sitting balance and tolerance for a variety of positions, including long-sitting, ring-sitting, side-lying, and prone on elbows. Heavy emphasis was placed on training the caregivers regarding safe and therapeutic play activities.

Within approximately 2 weeks, Stacy's caregivers had learned and demonstrated competence in all aspects of her care, and she was discharged to home. At that time, she continued to show good ROM and some increase in using her upper torso musculature. She was showing some movement in the lower extremities, but it was difficult to discern whether it was reflexive or voluntary. Her shoulder strength was generally grade 4 and elbow strength grades 3 to 4 bilaterally. Wrist extensors continued to be in the 3 range bilaterally, with noted weakness in the finger flexors. Finger extensor strength was only trace in the radial digits and completely absent in the ulnar digits. Strength of the intrinsics appeared absent. From a functional standpoint, Stacy was able to reach antigravity when lying supine and to assist minimally in rolling herself to the side. In prone, once she was positioned on elbows, she was able to maintain her head upright intermittently for 1 to 2 minutes. She was unable to roll out of prone into supine. When in sitting, she was able to prop herself on the upper extremities with some success. Stacy was showing more visual tracking, better head control, and more upper extremity reaching for toys. Approximately half of the time she required assistance when reaching for toys. Stacy was discharged to home with the equipment described. A MacLaren stroller (KidCo Company, Mundelein, IL) with a Carrie seat (Tumble Forms, Clifton, NJ) was also ordered for her permanent use in the home and community. Caregivers were given a thorough home program and care manual before Stacy's discharge. Stacy was scheduled for follow up at the clinic 8 weeks after discharge. At the time of that clinic visit, caregivers reported that the home program and plans were going well. Stacy was receiving physical therapy and occupational therapy 2 times per week through a community Birth to Three program.

Stacy was then seen approximately 1 year later through the SCI clinic. She did not show substantial changes in ROM, tone, or general strength, but was showing continued improvement in her functional skills. She was able to move from prone to supine independently. When placed in sitting she could play in short-, long-, and side-sitting independently. Stacy was able to move from sitting to prone by moving onto her forearms over her legs. She was able to "commando crawl" 5 to 10 feet by pulling with the upper extremities. With minimal facilitation she could also assume a quadruped position and show some forward movement if assisted with the lower extremities.

Her family reported two major concerns. The first was whether Stacy would eventually be able to walk with braces. Her prognosis was discussed and the concept of the use of a wheelchair was introduced. Benefits of increasing her strength and increasing her independence in mobility were emphasized. It was also emphasized that the use of the wheelchair would in no way hinder her potential ability to walk someday if she were to have neurologic return of function. The other concern was that of headaches and flushing of the face that the family had noted. This raised the question of autonomic dysreflexia. The family was instructed in taking Stacy's blood pressure when these episodes occurred. The visiting home nurse was also contacted in order to be a resource to the family in this regard. Stacy was continuing to receive physical and occupational therapy services 2 times per week through the school district. The focus was on her trunk control, upper extremity weight bearing, and facilitation of developmental milestones. The school occupational therapist had decided to discontinue the use of hand splints because Stacy's ROM had been good and she was doing a significant amount of weight bearing on the arms and hands.

The next follow-up visit to the SCI clinic was approximately 6 months later when Stacy was 2.5 years old. In addition to monitoring her physical skills, evaluations were conducted by an occupational therapist and a speech and language therapist to assess her cognitive and language development after brain injury. The physical therapy assessment revealed continued gains in physical function. Stacy was demonstrating independent commando crawling and the ability to sit up from prone without difficulty. Her sitting balance had improved. In ring-sitting or cross-legged sitting, her balance was good and she could turn her head and reach for toys. In short-sitting she could maintain a static posture for brief periods of up to 30 seconds. She was having much more success with transitional postures. She was beginning to scoot in sitting and pivot in prone. Her hand strength was notably improved, and overall hand function was better. She had nearly full active extension of the fingers on the left hand and of some on the right. Voluntary movement of the lower extremities was still absent and increased tone was still evident but not impinging on full ROM. Some reflexive movements were still noted in the lower extremities; ankle clonus was evident bilaterally. Stacy was continuing to use the MacLaren stroller with the Carrie seat for mobility in the community. Owing to her growth and improvements in upper extremity function, a trial use of a manual wheelchair was conducted. Stacy was able to sit well with hip pads and a hip belt on a solid seat with a solid back. She was able to propel only minimally during the initial trial. A wheelchair prescription was provided, with recommendations for a solid seat and back, and hip pads and belt, as well as headrest and knee adductor. The wheelchair was provided through a local vendor. Stacy was then scheduled for a return visit for a power wheelchair mobility trial. Although the family had a very small home making use of the large power wheelchair difficult, it was anticipated that Stacy would enroll in a public preschool at age 3. Although Stacy exhibited improving upper extremity function, it was unlikely that she would attain enough strength in the upper extremities to keep up with her peers at school or in her rural home setting, so a power wheelchair would be necessary.

CASE HISTORY: MEGAN

This case demonstrates the ongoing need to monitor acquisition of skills in a young child who had sustained complete paraplegia at age 5 years when she was injured in a motor vehicle accident in Texas in April 1985. Megan was initially seen in our facility as an outpatient in November 1990 after moving to Seattle from Texas. She was 11 years old at the time. Megan was diagnosed with T-4 paraplegia, ASIA Impairment Scale level A. Review of her medical records showed that in addition to her SCI, Megan suffered a fracture to her left femur as well as internal injuries. At the time of her discharge from her initial rehabilitation stay, she had no volitional movement in her lower extremities. Her sensation was absent below a point approximately 2.5 cm above the nipple line. Megan had minimal lower extremity spasticity, with more on the right side than the left. She had full passive ROM in her lower extremities with the exception of ankle dorsiflexion, which was to neutral. Megan's upper extremities were within normal limits for active ROM. From a functional standpoint, Megan was able to transfer herself with standby assistance from her bed to a wheelchair. She was independent with basic wheelchair mobility on level surfaces. Megan was able to roll in bed with minimal assistance and move from supine to sitting with moderate assistance. Bilateral KAFOs with a pelvic band were fitted. Using these, she could come to standing in the parallel bars with maximal assistance. She was able to tolerate standing in the bars for approximately 10 minutes. Megan was discharged from inpatient rehabilitation in July 1985, 4 months after her initial injury.

Megan was then followed through the rehabilitation clinic and continued daily outpatient physical therapy. Treatment focused on improving transfer skills and on ambulation with a walker and KAFOs. During the next 6 to 9 months, Megan was able to ambulate with the KAFOs with a swing-through pattern, leading with the left foot. She did this, however, only during therapy sessions, which had decreased to 3 times per week. She required numerous adjustments of her KAFOs for growth. She also needed a lift in the left shoe to compensate for a leg length discrepancy after the left femur fracture. During the next 18 months, Megan had problems with curvature of the spine, talipes equinus in the feet, and decreasing ROM in the lower extremities. She was reporting increased difficulty with spasticity and muscle spasms in the lower extremities. A body jacket was prescribed to slow the progression of scoliosis, and antispasticity medication was initiated.

By early 1988, Megan was no longer ambulating with her braces. She continued to struggle with increasing tightness in the hamstrings as well as increasing curvature of the spine. Medical records did not indicate the status of her wheelchair mobility or transfer skills. In April 1989, she received casts for use during the nighttime to control her spasms. Later that summer, Megan and her family relocated to Washington.

When we first evaluated Megan in November 1990, she was 11 years of age. She reported that she was able to dress and feed herself independently. She required some assistance during bathing in order to wash her hair. Her transportation was by means of a van with a lift and tie downs. Megan was attending the sixth grade in regular education classes and attending adaptive physical education, but was receiving no physical therapy. Megan reported that she had limited access to student desks and was unable to get to many bookshelves or have access to bathrooms. Otherwise, she had no significant difficulties in the school setting. She reported that it was no longer a priority to ambulate, but that she wanted assistance with controlling the spasticity in her lower extremities. She had stopped the medication due to the side effect of diarrhea. She and her caregiver also requested some type of ankle foot orthosis (AFO) to protect her ankle dorsiflexion range. Megan used a light-weight wheelchair with solid seat and back. Megan requested a change in the foot plates on her wheelchair so that she could use a power add-on device to assist with navigating inclines in her community. On examination, there was notable clonus in both ankles and 10° hip flexion and knee flexion contractures. Ankles could be stretched to neutral with knees extended.

Her FIM scores indicated complete independence (7) in communication and social cognition. In self-care, she was completely independent (7) in eating, grooming, and upper extremity dressing; had modified independence (6) for lower body dressing, toileting, and bladder and bowel management; and needed minimal assistance (4) for bathing. She was completely independent (7) for transfers to bed, chair, wheelchair, and toilet, but needed maximal assistance (2) to get in and out of the bathtub. Wheelchair skills were at the level of modified independence (6), and she needed total assistance for stairs. Better scores would have been predicted for bathtub transfers (either 6 or 7) based on the level of injury, and the FIM score for mobility does not characterize her problems in managing the wheelchair on inclines and outdoors.

Orthotic resting splints were provided as well as an updated home program for ROM exercises. She was instructed to do ROM exercises twice a day to see if this alleviated her spasticity. Wheelchair adjustments were made for growth, and new foot plates were ordered. A school physical therapist was enlisted to observe access in the school building and to see if the power add-on was really necessary. She determined that Megan's upper body strength and endurance were inadequate to allow her to use the ramp between buildings and change classes in a timely fashion. The therapist also remained available for monitoring problems with the wheelchair. Ongoing therapy at school did not occur owing to the lack of personnel and funding in the district as well as to the fact that no further disabilities affecting her ability to be educated were identified.

Megan returned for SCI clinic and therapy reevaluations in May 1991. She was nearly 12 years old and

continuing to be successful in the sixth grade. She was receiving no school physical therapy. She used the power add-on daily at school. She was not involved in any activities after school and did not often go outside. She found that self-directed ROM exercising did provide her with several hours of relief from spasticity after each stretching session. Her caregiver was concerned about the wheelchair fit as well as Megan's ongoing need for assistance when transferring to different heights from her wheelchair, such as when getting into the bathtub or when moving up from the floor into the wheelchair. Assessment revealed hip flexion contractures of 10 to 15°, knee flexion contractures of 20 to 25°, and ankle dorsiflexion to approximately neutral. These findings suggested that although resting AFOs were adequate to maintain ankle ROM, her home stretching program was not preventing slow progression of hip and knee contractures.

Manual muscle testing of the upper extremities revealed strength in the 4 to 4 + range. Megan's sitting balance was found to be functional only when she was using unilateral upper extremity support. She was unable to maintain her sitting balance while using her upper extremities for basic activities of daily living. Even without having to use her upper extremities for a functional task, maintaining static sitting balance was possible only for approximately 20 seconds.

Although Megan continued to be successful with basic level transfers, she was unable to move from the floor up into the chair or from the chair to another surface of significantly different height. She could not do wheelies or manage curbs independently. Despite the expectation that a preteenager with T-4 paraplegia should be able to do independent transfers and possess advanced wheelchair mobility skills, Megan lacked the upper extremity strength to do these activities. She did little self-propulsion of her wheelchair except on flat indoor surfaces. Megan still had difficulties with curvature of the spine when seated in her chair.

Therapy recommendations included an updated home program for lower extremity stretching; modifications to the wheelchair, including the use of a Jay cushion (Jay Medical, Boulder, CO) to position the pelvis with more support; and a referral to outpatient therapy with focus on improving her transfer skills, sitting balance, and upper extremity strength. She also had new orthoses made for nighttime wear that extended above the knees. She was referred to and participated in an adapted skiing program for children and adults with disabilities.

A major portion of the clinic visit was devoted to discussing the need for Megan to assume more self-reliance. It was explained that as she grew and became heavier, it would be more difficult for her caregivers to lift her for transfers, and the need to have someone with her would impede her ability to travel in the community independently. We agreed that if the outpatient treatment program did not result in significant increases in strength and mobility within 8 to 12 weeks, that a 2- to 4-week inpatient rehabilitation program would be undertaken during the summer. Before further assessment occurred, the family returned to Texas.

CASE HISTORY: ADAM

The following case demonstrates the long-term physical therapy management of a teenager with incomplete paraplegia due to cauda equina injury. This teenager continued to experience long-term functional improvements owing to a combination of neurologic recovery as well as active strengthening programs. More than 3 years of treatment and follow-up were needed before he reached a stable pattern of function.

Adam was injured at age 14 in October 1988 when he fell from a tree. He sustained a burst fracture of the L-3 vertebra and a complete anterior dislocation of L-3 on the L-4 vertebra. On the day after his injury, he underwent surgery to reduce the dislocation, and instrumentation was placed across the two vertebrae for stabilization. Postoperatively, Adam was given a thoracolumbosacral orthosis (TLSO) to wear 24 hours a day for the next 3 to 4 months until fusion was complete. Owing to the instability of the initial injury and the short segment of fusion and instrumentation, he was restricted from activities that flexed his hips beyond 90°.

Eight days after his injury, Adam was admitted to a pediatric rehabilitation program. His cauda equina spinal cord injury was classified as L-3 paraplegia, ASIA Impairment Scale level B. His impairments included deficits in motor and sensory functioning, loss of voluntary bladder and bowel control, and orthostatic hypotension. His motor examination showed grade 3 hip flexion and knee extension, but absent strength in ankle dorsiflexion or plantar flexion, knee flexion, hip extension, and hip abduction (Table 20–6). ROM was normal throughout except straight leg raising (SLR) was possible to only 30° bilaterally owing to posterior thigh pain. His sensory examination to pinprick showed that he lost

normal sensation below the medical femoral condyles and had decreased sensation in the L-4 and L-5 dermatomes, absent sensation at S-1, but preservation of pinprick at S4-5, perianally. There were no problems with spasticity since cauda equina injuries result in lower motoneuron deficits with flaccid paralysis.

Functionally, he required assistance to move his legs while rolling in bed, coming to sit from supine, or during a transfer with a sliding board. His sitting tolerance was limited by orthostatic hypotension, and he could only sit up with the wheelchair back reclined 45°. From such a position, he could not propel his wheelchair. His FIM scores were complete independence (7) in communication and social cognition. In self-care, he was completely independent (7) for eating and grooming but needed moderate assistance (3) for bathing, set-up assistance (5) for upper body dressing, maximal assistance (2) for lower body dressing, and total assistance (1) for toileting and bladder and bowel management. For mobility and locomotion, he needed maximal assistance (2) for all transfers and total assistance (1) for locomotion, using a wheelchair. He was unable to ascend stairs.

His disabilities on admission included lack of independence in bed mobility, transfers, and indoor and community mobility. With his level of injury, long-term goals of independence in bed mobility and transfers were realistic as were goals of independent ambulation at home and in the community using AFOs and crutches. Short-term goals included tolerance to the upright position, improved hamstring ROM to allow long-sitting, improved upper extremity strength and endurance to allow independent transfers and wheelchair propulsion, and lower extremity strengthening of the weakened muscle groups.

His therapy initially included sessions on the tilt table, passive ROM exercises for the lower extremities, and instruction in turning and getting to a sitting position in bed. He progressed to work on upper extremity strengthening, sliding board transfers, and sitting balance, while also working on lower extremity strengthening. After 2 weeks, he had only rare episodes of symptomatic orthostatic hypotension. A lighter weight

TABLE 20–6. **CHANGES IN LOWER EXTREMITY GRADES OF STRENGTH OVER TIME**

	Left					Right				
	10/88	3/89	12/89	12/90	1/92	10/88	3/89	12/89	12/90	1/92
Hip flexion	3	4	4	4	5	3	4	4	4	5
Knee extension	3	4+	5	5	5	3	4+	5	5	5
Ankle dorsiflexion	0	1	2	2	2	0	0	0	0	0
Long toe extension	0	1	3	3	3	0	0	0	0	0
Ankle plantar flexion	0	1	2	3	3	0	0	0	0	2
Knee flexion	0	2	4	4	4	0	2	3	3	4
Hip abduction	0	2	3	4	4	0	0	3−	3−	4
Hip extension	0	1	3	4	4	0	1	2	3−	3+

wheelchair was substituted for the recliner wheelchair. His SLR improved to 45°, and he was noted to have developed trace muscle function in the knee flexors. He became independent in sliding board transfers and in bed mobility. He progressed to activities on the mat, including moving from prone to prone-on-elbows to quadruped positions. Bilateral AFOs were obtained with ankles fixed in a neutral position. He was able to pull himself to stand in the parallel bars but could not stand independently owing to his weak quadriceps and his ankle position. His AFOs were adjusted to place the ankles in about 5° of plantar flexion.

One month after admission to rehabilitation, Adam's strength had increased in his right leg for hip flexion and knee extension by half a grade, but no other changes were noted. Hamstring ROM continued to be limited owing to complaints of pain with stretching. Upper body strength improved, so that Adam could lift his trunk to do independent pressure relief and could transfer himself without a sliding board to level heights. He could propel his wheelchair independently to and from therapy sessions and was able to stand in the parallel bars with one-hand support.

Unfortunately, despite the hip flexion precaution that had been diligently followed, he developed acute pain in his lower back, radiating to the left anterior thigh, and was found to have developed a lateral subluxation of L-3 on L-4. A spica cast was applied, parents were trained to care for him, and he was discharged for 6 weeks with a home program for upper extremity strengthening. When his fusion was more stable, the cast was removed and replaced with the TLSO, and he returned to the inpatient rehabilitation program.

Upon readmission, Adam was found to have maintained upper body strength and to have lost little lower extremity strength, but SLR was still only 40°. He was also noted to have trace movements in left ankle inversion and toe flexion. He resumed his strengthening, ROM, and gait training programs. During the next month, SLR improved to 70°, knee flexion strength increased to grade 2, and he developed independent standing balance. His AFOs were returned to the neutral position, and he progressed to independent ambulation with a wheeled walker. He developed left patellar tendonitis, which responded well to ice massage and temporary discontinuation of resisted quadriceps exercises.

Five weeks after readmission, or 3.5 months after SCI, Adam began gait training with forearm crutches using a four point gait pattern. He was discharged to home the following week, in March 1989. Lower extremity strength at discharge is shown in Table 20-6, and he was reclassified as having L-3 paraplegia, ASIA Impairment Scale level C. SLR was 85° bilaterally and all other passive ROM was normal. He was independent with wheelchair mobility indoors and outdoors

but could not do wheelies to handle curb cuts owing to the presence of the TLSO and the restriction on hip flexion beyond 90°. He could ambulate for 150 feet using the AFOs and a wheeled walker.

Adam's FIM scores had improved to complete independence (7) in all areas of self-care except bathing; to modified independence (6) for bathing and bladder and bowel management; to complete independence (7) in transfers to bed, chair, wheelchair, and toilet; and to modified independence (6) for transfers to the bathtub chair and for locomotion using a wheelchair or ambulating with the walker and AFOs. He needed moderate assistance (4) to ascend stairs.

He returned home and began an outpatient physical therapy program twice weekly to continue working on gait training and lower extremity strengthening. A school physical therapist consulted with the physical education teacher to develop an adapted program focusing on weight training and use of a stationary bicycle. The school therapist remained available on a consultative basis for questions regarding the wheelchair, assistive devices, and the AFOs. Adam was essentially independent in his mobility throughout school. His orthopaedic surgeon allowed him to discontinue using his TLSO in May 1989, and all restrictions on movement were also lifted.

In August 1989, he was reevaluated in the SCI clinic. Questioning revealed that Adam had discontinued his participation in the outpatient physical therapy program the month before but was continuing to work on stretching and strengthening at home. His ROM was unchanged from his ROM at time of discharge. Increases in strength of one grade were noted in the left knee flexors, ankle dorsiflexors and plantar flexors, and in the extensors and abductors of both hips. He was ambulating independently with the forearm crutches and AFOs, using a bilateral reciprocal gait pattern or a swing-through pattern when in a hurry. His home ROM and strengthening programs were updated, but no further need for ongoing physical therapy was noted.

At reevaluation in December 1989, 14 months after SCI, Adam was found to have continued to improve in strength (see Table 20-6) and was reclassified with L-3 paraplegia, ASIA Impairment Scale level D. He used his forearm crutches only at school, and ambulated independently using his AFOs at home. He could ascend and descend stairs without using his crutches, but he used the rail. He used his wheelchair only after bathing to get from bathroom to bedroom without donning his AFOs. His left AFO was changed to one with a hinged ankle to allow free dorsiflexion but no plantar flexion past neutral to allow motion and the possibility of strengthening these muscle groups while walking. Continued home ROM and strengthening exercises were recommended.

Reevaluation 1 year later, in December 1990, revealed an essentially stable picture, although Adam did need new AFOs due to wear and tear. He had developed skin breakdown on the lateral border of his left foot and on his right shin from rubbing against the AFO and the Velcro closure. He no longer used his forearm crutches. ROM was well maintained. He was provided with new AFOs and counseled regarding care of insensate skin. Because he was working out in a gym several times a week, exercises were recommended to strengthen hip girdle and knee flexor muscles.

At last assessment, in January 1992, Adam had shown some improvement in right lower extremity strength of the targeted muscle groups. He also demonstrated new plantar flexion at the right ankle. Bilateral hinged AFOS were prescribed. Adam was a senior in high school and worked after school in a gas station. He had returned to an outdoor lifestyle, hiking, fishing, and hunting on a regular basis. He planned to enroll in a community college to study forestry. He was advised of state vocational rehabilitation services available to him and was referred to an adult rehabilitation facility for long-term monitoring of renal function and prescription of orthoses.

▌ SUMMARY

Physical therapy for the child with SCI can, at first glance, appear straightforward. Preserving ROM and promoting strength and endurance are the cornerstones for the functional achievement predicted by the level of injury. Yet predicting realistic long-term goals and attaining them require respect for the broader and more complex picture. The physical therapist must consider the cause of the injury (progressive vs stable), the completeness of the injury (preserved motor function, sensory function), and the potential for, or presence of, secondary complications (scoliosis, skin breakdown, contractures). The therapist must also be sensitive to the child's age, the child's adaptation to the disability, and the child's ability to meet age-appropriate expectations in the home, school, and community. Thus, it becomes imperative to provide the child and the family with a team approach, incorporating multiple disciplines and settings, to maximize the child's potential for functional independence.

Families and their children with SCI may be interested in joining the National Spinal Cord Injury Association (NSCIA) and their state chapters. NSCIA has literature regarding many practical aspects of life with SCI and publishes a quarterly newsletter. The address of NSCIA is 600 West Cummings Park, Suite 2000, Woburn, MA 01801. Schools and families may also be interested in having manuals as references for information on SCI. Two such books are currently available from Shriners Hospital (*Spinal Cord Injury, Self-Care Manual.* San Francisco: Shriners Hospital for Crippled Children, 1989) and the Paralyzed Veterans of America (*Yes, You Can!* Paralyzed Veterans of America, 1989. c/o Office Service, A01; 18th Street NW; Washington, DC 20006).

References

American Spinal Injury Association. International Standards for Neurological and Functional Classification of Spinal Cord Injury. Chicago: American Spinal Injury Association, 1992.

Bohn, D, Armstrong, D, Becker, L, & Humphreys, R. Cervical spine injuries in children. Journal of Trauma, *30*:463–469, 1990.

Bracken, MB, Shepard, MJ, Collins, WF, Holford, TR, Young, W, Baskin, DS, Eisenberg, HM, Flamm, E, Leo-Summers, L, Maroon, J. Marshall, LF, Perot, PL, Piepmeier, J, Sonntag, VKH, Wagner, FC, Wilberger, JE, & Winn, HR. A randomized, controlled trial of methylprednisolone or naloxone in the treatment of acute spinal-cord injury. New England Journal of Medicine, *322*:1405–1411, 1990.

Centers for Disease Control. Acute traumatic spinal cord injury surveillance—United States, 1987. MHWR. Morbidity and Mortality Weekly Report, *37*:285–286, 1987.

Committee on Sports Medicine. American Academy of Pediatrics. Atlantoaxial instability in Down syndrome. Pediatrics, *74*:152–153, 1984.

Crozier, KS, Graziani, V, Ditunno, JF, & Herbison, GJ. Spinal cord injury: Prognosis for ambulation based on sensory examination of inpatients who are initially motor complete. Archives of Physical Medicine and Rehabilitation, *72*:119–121, 1991.

Davidoff, GN, Roth, EJ, Haughton, JS, & Ardner, M.S. Cognitive dysfunction in spinal cord injury patients: Sensitivity of the Functional Independence Measure subscales versus neuropsychologic assessment. Archives of Physical Medicine and Rehabilitation, *71*:326–329, 1990.

DeVivo, MJ, Richards, JS, Stover, SL, & Go, BK. Spinal cord injury: Rehabilitation adds life to years. Western Journal of Medicine, *154*:602–606, 1991.

Ditunno, JF. New spinal cord injury standards, 1992. Paraplegia, *30*:90–91, 1992a.

Ditunno, JF. Functional assessment measures in CNS trauma. Journal of Neurotrauma, *9*:S301–S305, 1992b.

Ditunno, JF, Sipski, ML, Posuniak, EA, Chen, YT, Staas, WE, & Herbson, GJ. Wrist extensor recovery in traumatic quadriplegia. Archives of Physical Medicine and Rehabilitation, *68*:287–290, 1987.

Drory, Y, Ohry, A, Brooks, ME, Dolphia, D, & Kellerman, JJ. Arm crank ergometry in chronic spinal cord injured patients. Archives of Physical Medicine and Rehabilitation, *71*:389–392, 1990.

El Ghahit, AZ, & Hanson, RW. Educational and training levels and employment of the spinal cord injured patient. Archives of Physical Medicine and Rehabilitation, *60*:405–406, 1979.

Faden, AI. Recent pharmacological advances in experimental spinal injury: Theoretical and methodological considerations. Trends in Neurosciences, *6*:375–377, 1983.

Flett, PJ. The rehabilitation of children with spinal cord injury. Journal of Paediatric and Child Health, *28*:141–146, 1992.

Fordyce, WE. Behavioral methods in medical rehabilitation. Neuroscience and Biobehavioral Reviews, *5*:391–396, 1981.

Frankel, HL, Hancock, DO, Hyslop, G, Melzak, J, Michaelis, L,

Ungar, G, Vernon, J, & Walsh, JJ. The value of postural reduction in the initial management of closed injuries of the spine with paraplegia and tetraplegia. Paraplegia, 7:179–192, 1969.

Garber, SL, & Dyerly, LR. Wheelchair cushions for persons with spinal cord injury: An update. American Journal of Occupational Therapy, 45:550–554, 1991.

Graham, P, Weingarden, S, & Murphy, P. School reintegration. A rehabilitation goal for spinal cord injured adolescents. Rehabilitation Nursing, 16:122–127, 1991.

Granger, CV, Hamilton, BB, & Kayton, R. Guide for the use of the Functional Independence Measure for Children (WeeFIM) of the Uniform Data Set for Medical Rehabilitation. Buffalo, NY: State University of New York, Research Foundation, 1988.

Guttmann, L. Spinal Cord Injuries. Oxford: Blackwell, 1976.

Haley, SM, Faas, RM, Coster, WJ, Webster, H, & Gans, BM. Pediatric Evaluation of Disability Inventory. Boston: New England Medical Center, 1989.

Hamilton, BB, Granger, CV, Sherwin, FS, Zielezny, M, & Tashman, JS. A uniform national data system for medical rehabilitation. In Fuhrer, MJ (Ed.), Rehabilitation Outcomes: Analysis and Measurement. Baltimore: Paul H Brookes, 1987, pp. 137–147.

Haseltine, FP, Cole, SS, & Gray, DB (Eds.). Reproductive Issues for Persons with Physical Disabilities. Baltimore: Paul H Brookes, 1990.

Hirokawa, S, Grimm, M, Le, T, Solomonow, M, Baratta, RV, Shoji, H, & D'Ambrosia, RD. Energy consumption in paraplegic ambulation using the reciprocating gait orthosis and electric stimulation of the thigh muscles. Archives of Physical Medicine and Rehabilitation, 71:687–694, 1990.

Hobson, DA, & Tooms, RE. Seated lumbar/pelvic alignment. A comparison between spinal cord injured and noninjured groups. Spine, 17:293–298, 1992.

Jaeger, RJ, Yarkony, GM, & Roth, EJ. Rehabilitation technology for standing and walking after spinal cord injury. American Journal of Physical Medicine and Rehabilitation, 68:128–133, 1989.

Janssen, L, & Hansebout, RR. Pathogenesis of spinal cord injury and newer treatments: A review. Spine, 14:23–32, 1989.

Johnston, MV, & Keith, RA. Cost benefits of medical rehabilitation: Review and critique. Archives of Physical Medicine and Rehabilitation, 64:147–154, 1983.

Kewalramani, LS, Krauss, JF, & Sterling, HM. Acute spinal-cord lesions in a pediatric population: Epidemiological and clinical features. Paraplegia, 18:206–219, 1980.

Kliot, M, & Lustgarten, JH. Strategies to promote regeneration and recovery in the injured spinal cord. Neurosurgery Clinics of North America, 1:751–759, 1990.

LaHaye, PA, & Batzdorf, U. Posttraumatic syringomyelia. Western Journal of Medicine, 148:657–663, 1988.

Levine, SP, Kett, RL, Gross, MD, Wilson, BA. Cederna, PS, & Juni, JE. Blood flow in the gluteus maximus of seated individuals during electrical muscle stimulation. Archives of Physical Medicine and Rehabilitation, 71:682–686, 1990.

Massagli, TL, & Jaffe, KM. Pediatric spinal cord injury: Treatment and outcome. Pediatrician, 17:244–254, 1990.

McDonald, CM, Jaffe, KM, & Shurtleff, DB. Assessment of muscle strength in children with meningomyelocele: Accuracy and stability of measurements over time. Archives of Physical Medicine and Rehabilitation, 67:855–861, 1986.

Molnar, GE, & Kaminer, RD. History and examination. In Molnar, GE (Ed.), Pediatric Rehabilitation (2nd ed.). Baltimore: Williams & Wilkins, 1992, pp. 1–18.

Murphy, KP, Opitz, JL, Cabanela, ME, & Ebersold, MJ. Cervical fractures and spinal cord injury. Outcome of surgical and nonsurgical management. Mayo Clinic Proceedings, 65:949–959, 1990.

Nash, MS, Bilsker, S, Marcillo, AE, Isaac, SM, Bothelho, LA, Klose, KJ, Green, BA, Rountree, MT, & Shea, JD. Reversal of adaptive left ventricular atrophy following electrically-stimulated exercise training in human tetraplegics. Paraplegia, 29:590–599, 1991.

Pang, D, & Wilberger, JE. Spinal cord injury without radiographic abnormalities in children. Journal of Neurosurgery, 57:114–129, 1982.

Parziale, JR. Standard v light weight wheelchair propulsion in spinal cord injured patients. American Journal of Physical Medicine and Rehabilitation, 70:76–80, 1991.

Phillips, CA. Medical criteria for active physical therapy: Physician guidelines for patient participation in a program of functional electrical stimulation. American Journal of Physical Medicine, 66:269–286, 1987.

Pollack, SF, Axen, K, Spielholz, N, Levin, N, Haas, F, & Ragnarsson, KT. Aerobic training effects of electrically induced lower extremity exercises in spinal cord injured people. Archives of Physical Medicine and Rehabilitation, 70:214–219, 1989.

Priebe, MM, & Waring, WP. The interobserver reliability of the revised American Spinal Injury Association standards for neurological classification of spinal injury patients. American Journal of Physical Medicine and Rehabilitation, 70:268–270, 1991.

Ragnarsson, KT, Pollack, S, O'Daniel, W, Edgar, R, Petrofsky, J, & Nash, MS. Clinical evaluation of computerized functional electrical stimulation after spinal cord injury: A multicenter pilot study. Archives of Physical Medicine and Rehabilitation, 69:672–677, 1988.

Richards, JS, Hendricks, C, & Roberts, M. Prevention of spinal cord injury: An elementary education approach. Journal of Pediatric Psychology, 16:595–609, 1991.

Rothstein, JL, Levy, E, Fecher, R, Gordon, SK, & Banman, WA. Drug use and abuse in an urban veteran spinal cord injured population. Journal of the American Paraplegia Society, 15:217–219, 1992.

Seeger, BR, Law, D, Creswell, JE, Stern, LM, & Potter, MB. Functional electrical stimulation for upper limb strengthening in traumatic quadriplegia. Archives of Physical Medicine and Rehabilitation, 70:663–667, 1989.

Sipski, ML, Harris, M, & Alexander, C. Follow-up survey of use of home computerized bicycle ergometry. Journal of the American Paraplegia Society, 14:94–95, 1991.

Stotts, KM. Health maintenance: Paraplegia athletes and non-athletes. Archives of Physical Medicine and Rehabilitation, 67:109–114, 1986.

Stover, SL, & Fine, PR (Eds.). Spinal Cord Injury: The Facts and Figures. Birmingham, AL: University of Alabama Press, 1986.

Subbarao, JV. Walking after spinal cord injury: Goal or wish? Western Journal of Medicine, 154:612–614, 1991.

Sugarman, B. Medical complications of spinal cord injury. Quarterly Journal of Medicine, 54:3–18, 1985.

Tessler, A. Intraspinal transplants. Annals of Neurology, 29:115–123, 1991.

Waring, WP, & Karunas, RS. Acute spinal cord injuries and the incidence of clinically occurring thromboembolic disease. Paraplegia, 29:8–16, 1991.

Wilberger, JE. Spinal Cord Injuries in Children. New York: Futura, 1986.

Wu, L, Marino, R, Herbison, GJ, & Ditunno, JF. Recovery of zero grade muscles in the zone of partial preservation in motor complete quadriplegia. Archives of Physical Medicine and Rehabilitation, 73:40–43, 1992.

Yarkony, GM, Roth, EJ, Cybulski, G, & Jaeger, RJ. Neuromuscular stimulation in spinal cord injury: I. Restoration of functional movement of the extremities. Archives of Physical Medicine and Rehabilitation, 73:78–86, 1992.

Chapter 21

Brain Tumors, Traumatic Head Injuries, and Near-Drowning

WENDY E. PHILLIPS, PT, PCS, MA, MS

Physical therapists who work with children in acute care hospitals, rehabilitation centers, and community settings such as school systems are likely to treat patients with central nervous system (CNS) dysfunction. Three of the diagnoses that these physical therapists may treat include brain tumors, head trauma, and near-drowning.

BRAIN TUMORS

The reported incidence of brain tumors in children 15 years of age and younger in the general population has been estimated to be 2.5 to 3.5 per 100,000 (Lannering et al., 1990). Although this incidence in the general pediatric population is relatively low, physical therapists working in diagnostic and treatment centers, particularly in acute care hospitals, can expect to be involved in the treatment of these children.

Types of Pediatric Brain Tumors

Pediatric brain tumors are described as being either focal or diffuse. Diffuse tumors extend to a wider area of brain tissue than focal tumors, are associated with a short and rapidly declining clini-

cal course, and have a wide constellation of presenting signs and symptoms.

Tumors that are less than 2.5 cm. in diameter are considered focal (Shiminsky-Maher et al., 1991). Focal tumors, unlike diffuse tumors, are not associated with edema. Focal tumors are slow growing and have a long clinical history with symptoms evolving over a relatively long period of time. Clinical symptoms are more discrete and depend on the exact location of the tumor. Pediatric brain tumors may also be generally classified according to their location and include tumors occurring in the posterior fossa, the brain stem, or the midline region.

POSTERIOR FOSSA TUMORS

Three of the most common cerebellar tumors that occur in childhood are cerebellar astrocytomas, medulloblastomas, and ependymomas. Astrocytomas are tumors that are derived from astrocytic neuroglial cells and may arise from the vermis or the lateral lobes of the cerebellum. These tumors are usually well circumscribed and may be cystic. Ten year survival rates range from 29 to 96% depending on tumor subtype (Menkes & Till, 1990).

Medulloblastomas arise from primitive neurons in the fetal granular layer of the cerebellum and infiltrate the floor or lateral wall of the fourth ventricle and extend into its cavity. Metastasis frequently occurs by way of the cerebrospinal fluid to the subarachnoid space of the spinal canal. Like astrocytomas, the prognosis for medulloblastomas is variable, depending on the tumor subtype.

Ependymomas occur most frequently in the roof and floor of the fourth ventricle and occlude the ventricular cavity, protruding into the cisterna magna or extending through the foramen magnum to overlap the cervical spinal cord (Fokes & Earle, 1969). These tumors are slowly growing and may be asymptomatic. Evidence of malignancy is found in approximately 5% of cases, mostly in infants (Menkes & Till, 1990).

Clinical symptoms of posterior fossa tumors are related to increased intracranial pressure and involvement of cerebellar structures. Headaches that are nonlocalized or frontal are an early presenting symptom. Vomiting is the most common sign of cerebellar tumors and may be related to increased intracranial pressure or to direct pressure on the medullary vagal nuclei. Motor signs of cerebellar involvement include ataxia as a result of involvement of the cerebellar vermis. Cerebellar involvement may also contribute to an ataxic quality of speech that is sometimes present in children with cerebellar tumors.

Dysmetria, dysdiadochokinesia, intention tremor, and hypotonia may also be associated with cerebellar tumors. Hemiplegia and oculomotor signs may be clinical manifestations of cerebellar astrocytoma. When tumors extend into the brain stem, unilateral hearing loss and facial weakness may be found (Epstein & Wisoff, 1987). When the tumor extends rostrally or caudally from the medulla, quadriparesis or neck pain, torticollis, or both may be present (Epstein & Wisoff, 1987, 1988).

BRAIN STEM TUMORS

Brain stem tumors most frequently arise from the pons and on radiographic examination appear as a symmetric enlargement of the brain stem (Menkes & Till, 1990). Because of their location and close association with the centers that regulate vital functions, the prognosis for children with such tumors is usually poor.

Impairments associated with brain stem tumors include cranial nerve palsies, pyramidal tract signs, and cerebellar signs that occur without evidence of increased intracranial pressure (Bray et al., 1958; Stroink, 1986). If the tumor has progressed to include the spinal cord, quadriparesis or hemiparesis may be present (Shiminsky-Maher et al., 1991). Neck pain or torticollis may also be present (Epstein & Wisoff, 1987, 1988).

Vomiting and gait disturbances may occur, and pyramidal tract signs, eye squinting, and other signs of cranial nerve involvement may be present. Other clinical signs and symptoms that are less frequently noted as presenting problems include headache and dysarthria. In the case of brain stem tumors, vomiting occurs as a result of direct encroachment of the tumor on the vomiting center of the brain stem.

Gait deviations may be related to coordination problems or spasticity. Progression of the tumor to include cerebellar or spinal cord involvement or impingement on corticospinal tract fibers is likely to be related to impairments that will ultimately affect functional activities such as gait. Impairment of other functional skills, such as swallowing, may occur related to the involvement of the cranial nerve nuclei tracts.

MIDLINE TUMORS

The grouping together of a number of pathologically diverse tumors under the rubric of "midline tumors" has been proposed by Menkes and Till (1990). Craniopharyngiomas, optic nerve gliomas, and pineal tumors are considered here as examples of tumors that occur in midline brain regions.

Craniopharyngiomas are found either in the suprasellar region or in the infrasellar and suprasellar regions. The tumor is slowly growing, and symptoms may not be evident for several years. As this tumor grows forward, it may compress the optic chiasm. As it progresses downward, pressure is placed on the pituitary gland while upward compression affects the third ventricle.

Optic nerve gliomas arise from the optic nerve within or outside the orbit. Their progression is characterized by a spread through the photic foramen to the cranium. The tumor may also invade the third ventricle and hypothalamus and may compress the pituitary gland (Martin & Cushing, 1923).

Pineal tumors progress toward the tectal plate and result in compression of the cerebral aqueduct with resultant hydrocephalus. The tumor may also expand to compress the hypothalamus (Menkes & Till, 1990).

Clinical signs and symptoms of midline tumors, like other brain tumors, are determined by the tumor's size and location and its relationship to adjacent brain structures. In the case of craniopharyngiomas, progression of the tumor is related to symptoms of increasing intracranial pressure, visual complaints, and endocrine disturbances (Epstein & McCleary, 1986; Menkes & Till, 1990). Unilateral or bilateral optic atrophy may be present, resulting in visual impairments including unilateral or bilateral temporal field cuts (Menkes & Till, 1990). Changes in endocrine function are related to tumor involvement with the pituitary gland or the hypothalamus. Diabetes insipidus is a reported but less frequently occurring complication. Behavioral changes or personality changes and visual or olfactory hallucinations may also occur. If the tumor produces pressure effects on the temporal lobe, seizures may be present.

In the case of optic nerve gliomas, visual disturbances are the predominant clinical symptom. Poor vision or a perceived rapid deterioration of vision may be the presenting symptom. Nystagmus or an inability to focus on objects may occur. Optic nerve gliomas occur frequently in conjunction with neurofibromatosis, so that symptoms associated with neurofibromatosis are present in concert with the visual disturbances.

Symptoms of pineal tumors are often related to increased intracranial pressure. Headache is the predominant symptom, and the inability to direct eye movements outward bilaterally is sometimes present. If the tumor progresses to the third ventricle and causes pressure on adjacent structures, including the hypothalamus, diabetes insipidus may occur (Kageyama, 1987).

CEREBRAL HEMISPHERE TUMORS

Cerebral hemisphere tumors make up approximately 40% of pediatric brain tumors (Gjerris, 1978). The concomitants of increased intracranial pressure are frequent initial symptoms of cerebral hemisphere tumors, with headache being typical. When headaches are associated with increased intracranial pressure, they are often transitory, occurring in the morning or during the night.

Vomiting is another common sign of increased intracranial pressure. It may occur in conjunction with nausea and is not usually projectile. It often occurs in the morning and is not related to the child's eating pattern.

Seizures, particularly the complex partial variety, are also a common clinical sign of cerebral hemisphere tumors. Children who experience seizures often have no other neurologic deficits (Blume et al., 1982). Hemiparesis and sensory symptoms are rare.

Diagnostic Procedures

Magnetic resonance imaging (MRI) is a frequently used diagnostic tool in the evaluation of pediatric CNS problems. In fact, MRI has been suggested to be superior to other diagnostic tools

for this purpose (Gusnard & Zimmerman, 1990). For example, bone artifacts often noted on computed tomography (CT) of the posterior fossa are not a problem with MRI. MRI may also differentiate between benign structures such as a collection of cerebrospinal fluid and malignant masses such as cystic tumors. Additionally, MRI is very sensitive in the detection of blood and is particularly useful in the evaluation of hemorrhage.

CT is most successful in the assessment of areas of calcification, the evaluation of a foreign body in a sensitive location, and the identification of skull and bony abnormalities. CT may also be the evaluative tool of choice at times when a screening must be performed quickly. CT is less costly than MRI, and financial restraints may influence the selection of CT versus MRI diagnostic testing.

Treatment

Medical treatment of pediatric brain tumors includes surgery, radiation therapy, chemotherapy, or a combination of these therapies. The treatment selected depends on the type, location, and characteristics of the tumor.

SURGERY

Surgical excision of a brain tumor may be performed as a primary treatment or may be performed in conjunction with other treatments such as radiation therapy or chemotherapy. In cases in which full surgical excision of the tumor is not possible, radiation therapy is administered after surgery in an attempt to eradicate residual tumor cells. Surgical excision is the treatment of choice for cerebellar astrocytomas (Ingraham & Matson, 1954), ependymomas (Marsh & Laws, 1987), craniopharyngiomas (Till, 1982), certain pineal tumors (Lapras, 1987), and tumors of the cerebral hemispheres (Menkes & Till, 1990). When hydrocephalus is present secondary to the obstruction of cerebrospinal fluid by, for example, a posterior fossa tumor, surgical intervention may include the placement of a shunt.

RADIATION THERAPY

Radiation therapy is frequently administered as an adjunct to surgical intervention and is often begun a few weeks after surgery (Reilly, 1987). A radiation beam is directed at the tumor as a predetermined dose of energy is administered, and this process is repeated on a regular schedule for several days or weeks. The effect of the administration of the radiation is to slow or halt the proliferation of tumor cells. The effects of radiation are enhanced when this therapy is used in conjunction with certain chemotherapeutic agents. Hyperthermia, when combined with radiation treatment, is also considered to be an effective adjunctive treatment (Bernstein & Laperriere, 1990).

Although the goal of the administration of radiation is to kill tumor cells, adjacent cells and physiologic structures are often affected, and such damage results in various immediate and long-term side effects. Acute radiation encephalopathy occurs when vascular damage caused by the radiation results in increased vessel wall permeability. A loss of cortical neurons and fibrillary gliosis extending into the gray matter characterize this process (Menkes & Till, 1990).

Side effects noted in the patient who is undergoing radiation therapy include lethargy, nausea, and vomiting. Neurologic signs that existed before surgical intervention may reappear. Corticosteroids are often administered to treat edema and related symptoms. The frequent (i.e., daily) administration of less intense radiation has been suggested as an alternative that may prevent severe edema-related symptoms (Menkes & Till, 1990).

Radiation therapy is used in the treatment of various types of brain tumors, including medulloblastoma (Berry, 1981), brain stem gliomas (Stroink, 1987), optic nerve gliomas (Tenny et al., 1982), and certain tumors of the cerebral hemispheres (Menkes & Till, 1990).

Brachytherapy, in which irradiation is administered by an intracavitary route, has been proposed as a treatment for pediatric brain tumors (Bernstein & Laperriere, 1990). In this approach, a low-grade, radioactive colloid is permanently implanted within the skull.

The suggested advantages of brachytherapy over conventional radiation therapy include a more favorable distribution of the radiation with a rapid decrease in the dose outside the tumor volume and the ability to use a lower dose rate that allows greater recovery of normal versus tumor cells in the brain. Brachytherapy has been used as an experimental treatment for adults with brain tumors (Bernstein & Laperriere, 1990). Although not currently in pediatric use, brachytherapy may be a treatment modality more commonly used in the future.

CHEMOTHERAPY

The aim of chemotherapy is to kill significant numbers of tumor cells in each of the successive administrations of the chemotherapy. The erad-

ication of clonogenic cells that are capable of unlimited proliferation is a particular goal of chemotherapy. Antineoplastic drugs are frequently administered together to act against the tumor cells at different biochemical sites.

Antineoplastic drugs that affect tumor cells also affect other rapidly growing, normal tissues, such as bone marrow, gastrointestinal epithelium, and hair follicles. The toxic effect of antineoplastic drugs on normal tissues causes the frequently experienced side effects of chemotherapy, including hair loss, nausea and vomiting, and immune system depression.

Pediatric brain tumors treated with chemotherapy include pineal tumors (Stein & Fetall, 1985), neuroblastomas (Graham-Pole et al., 1991), brain stem gliomas (Menkes & Till, 1990), and medulloblastoma (Packer & Findlay, 1988; Packer et al., 1991). The chemotherapy regimen for patients whose treatment with antineoplastic agents is considered experimental is likely to vary from center to center.

Cognitive Considerations

Although medical interventions such as surgery, radiation therapy, and chemotherapy are often effective in the treatment of pediatric brain tumors, adjacent brain tissues and structures may be negatively affected. The side effects of commonly administered interventions have been related to toxicity to normal brain tissue (Castel & Caille, 1989). These effects have been classified as "acute," occurring within 1 to 6 weeks after treatment; "early delayed," occurring 3 weeks to 3 months after treatment; and "late delayed," occurring several months to years after treatment (Castel & Caille, 1989). Toxic treatment effects together with direct tumor effects have been associated with changes in neurologic status, including cognitive abilities (Cohen et al., 1983).

MEMORY FUNCTIONING

Memory is evaluated particularly with respect to a child's ability to learn new material. Although a child may retain and remember material learned before treatment of a brain tumor, learning new information may be problematic. Difficulties in the area of memory skills pose obvious problems for the child who will be returning to school. Less obvious are the influences of memory deficits on rehabilitative treatment.

The child who demonstrates difficulty learning new material may not progress as quickly as would be expected in learning an exercise program or in achieving independence in functional skills. For example, a child who demonstrates sufficient strength and coordination skills to perform a home exercise program may not be able to achieve the goal of independence in performing the program because of an inability to remember the component parts from one treatment session to the next.

Memory deficits may also be demonstrated by unsafe performance of functional skills. The omission of safety-related behaviors when performing transfers, for example, may limit the functional independence of a child whose balance and coordination skills when considered alone are sufficient for the performance of the task.

The limiting effect of memory deficits may be particularly frustrating for parents. A change in memory skills may increase the child's level of dependence. Such an apparent developmental regression may be perceived by a parent as the child's unwillingness to "try hard" or as a behavioral problem that is within the child's control. The results of an evaluation of a child's memory skills and capacity for new learning will be helpful in the development of an appropriate rehabilitation program and establishment of realizable functional goals. Working jointly with the child's family and the pediatric psychologist, the pediatric physical therapist may help determine the effect of memory and learning deficits on the child's functional abilities and the related need for assistance, environmental modification, or both.

EXECUTIVE SKILLS

The ability to formulate and switch conceptual sets, the ability to use feedback to initiate behavioral change, and the ability to exercise judgment in social and community settings are included under the rubric of "executive skills." Deficits in executive functioning are often associated with frontal lobe injury. They may be expressed as impulsive behavior resulting in failure to observe safety precautions or in an inability to recognize that behaviors are socially appropriate in particular settings.

The inability to change conceptual sets may be demonstrated in perseveration on a task or the inability to change activities without becoming disorganized. Difficulty switching conceptual sets may also influence the ability to perform reciprocal movements, alternating patterns of movement, or tasks with reciprocal or alternating components.

Arousal level and attentional ability may be impaired by frontal lobe lesions or lesions affecting the brain stem. A child's ability to follow commands or to benefit from feedback while learning motor and

functional skills may be affected by level of arousal. A child who is able to maintain a level of arousal at which incoming environmental stimuli are neither overstimulating nor insufficient to elicit the child's attention is likely to benefit more from training or instruction than the child who is hypoaroused or hyperaroused.

When possible, a determination of the time of day at which arousal level is not optimal or an alteration of therapeutic goals within a given treatment session in response to current arousal status may increase the effectiveness of intervention. Medications such as antiseizure or pain agents may also affect arousal. The time of least effect of the medication on arousal level will depend on the length of the half-life of that particular drug's activity.

VISUOSPATIAL SKILLS

Visuospatial and perceptual deficits may influence motor performance and functional mobility skills. Such deficits are frequently associated with lesions in the temporal or occipital lobes of the brain. A figure-ground deficit, or the inability to distinguish a given form from the background, may be related to difficulty with functional mobility skills. For example, problems with foot placement or the placement of an assistive device on a complex surface such as a step or ramp may be related to visuospatial skills. Visuospatial deficits may also limit the level of functional independence achieved. For example, a child who is unable to put on an orthosis because of visuospatial deficits may ultimately be dependent in functional mobility even though he or she is able to ambulate on flat surfaces independently after the orthosis is on. A child with visuospatial deficits related to memory skills may demonstrate difficulty developing a cognitive map of his or her environment and consequently may have difficulty functioning or moving from place to place in the home, school, or community.

LANGUAGE

Temporal lobe lesions may result in deficits in expressive or receptive language skills that will affect communication between therapist and patient and therefore will affect rehabilitative treatment. Language deficits are addressed in depth by speech and language pathologists.

Receptive language deficits impair a child's ability to comprehend the instructions that are given for the performance of a task or activity. Determination of the extent of a child's receptive language impairment and the best means of communication (e.g., gestures instead of speech for giving a direction) will increase the efficiency of communication and decrease both the therapist's and the child's level of frustration.

Expressive language disorders impair a child's ability to communicate information to others. A child with an expressive disorder may fully comprehend verbally communicated information and successfully formulate a cognitive response. A breakdown occurs, however, between the formulation of the response and the execution or verbal expression of what was intended. In this case, a child may not be able to express a related idea or concern. In this situation, as in the case of the child with a receptive disorder, knowledge of the child's most efficient mode of communication may lessen frustration related to the inability to express an intended response.

Conceptual Framework

Campbell (1992) has described a theoretical framework for the measurement of motor performance in children with cerebral palsy that may be generalized to the population of children with other diagnoses and disabilities including children with the diagnosis of pediatric brain tumor. This framework incorporates the terminology of the World Health Organization as used in documents that address individuals with disabilities. An extension of this model developed by the National Center for Medical Rehabilitation Research is presented in Chapter 7.

According to this framework, motor dysfunction may be considered in three different dimensions: an organ/systems or impairment dimension, a functional limitations dimension, and a disability dimension. Consistent with the described framework, rehabilitation of the child with the diagnosis of brain tumor may also be considered from these three perspectives.

IMPAIRMENT

Traditional medical treatments of brain tumors including radiation therapy, chemotherapy, and surgery address intervention at the impairment level. For example, medical intervention such as surgery that decreases pressure effects of a posterior fossa tumor on the cerebellum and adjacent brain structures acts at the organ level. This intervention directly affects the brain, an organ of the CNS.

Of particular interest to the pediatric physical therapist are ataxia and hypotonia or related weakness, which may be considered manifestations of the brain tumor pathology at the organ systems level.

Preserving range of motion (ROM) and flexibility are frequently goals in the treatment of a child with a diagnosis of brain tumor. Loss of functional active or passive ROM may be a risk for the child who is unable to continue with normal levels of activity either because of direct effects of the tumor or related to the side effects of medical treatment. A child with a diagnosis of brain stem glioma may demonstrate limited volitional movement in the lower extremities related to spasticity and, without ROM exercises, may develop hypoextensibility or contractures. On the other hand, a child who does not demonstrate motor dysfunction directly related to the tumor's effect may experience limited mobility related to the general or specific side effects of medical treatment. A child whose activity level is limited by nausea and vomiting or fatigue may also be at risk for loss of flexibility and ROM.

Specific side effects of chemotherapy have also been related to limited ROM or flexibility. Vincristine, an antineoplastic agent used in the treatment of medulloblastoma and other tumors, has been associated with peripheral neuropathy, especially when levels approach toxicity (Kosmidis et al., 1991). In this situation, ROM exercise and splinting are necessary to preserve ROM.

Muscle weakness that results from generally decreased activity may be present in children who are undergoing chemotherapy or radiation therapy or less frequently administered treatments such as bone marrow transplants. After extended periods of bed rest or sedentary behavior, muscle atrophy may be expected. In the case of a child with a peripheral neuropathy related to vincristine chemotherapy, atrophy is also likely to result.

Children whose tumors cause alterations in postural tone will also experience weakness. In the case of a child who presents with spasticity in agonist muscle groups, weakness can be expected in the antagonist groups. The child whose tumor caused hypotonia may also experience weakness related to less frequent functional use of muscle groups, especially antigravity muscles.

Increasing strength, therefore, is an appropriate treatment goal for children who experience weakness related to inactivity or whose weakness is limited to specific muscle groups. Careful consideration of the factors related to the side effects of medical treatment that may affect the rehabilitation of patients with the diagnosis of brain tumor is indicated.

The physical therapy selected for the child who is receiving medical treatment for a brain tumor is influenced by the associated side effects. For example, the child who is fatigued after radiation therapy or who is nauseated after chemotherapy may be scheduled for physical therapy before radiation therapy or chemotherapy. Because chemotherapy frequently affects blood parameters that are associated with clotting and tolerance of activity, blood cell counts should be considered when an exercise program is developed or modified.

For example, according to the hematology/oncology protocol at Egleston Children's Hospital, which was adapted from the work of Dietz (1980), no exercise is recommended for patients whose hematocrit is less than 25%, hemoglobin levels are less than 8 mg/dL, platelet counts are less than 20,000/mm^3 or white blood cell counts are less than 500/mm^3. Active exercise is recommended for patients whose hematocrit is greater than 25%, hemoglobin levels are 8 to 10 mg/dL, platelet counts are 20,000 to 50,000/mm^3 and white blood cell counts are greater than 500/mm^3. Resistive exercise is recommended only for patients whose hematocrit is greater than 25%, hemoglobin levels are greater than 10 mg/dL, platelet counts are greater than 50,000/mm^3, and white blood cell counts are greater than 500/mm^3.

Deficits in balance and coordination abilities may be anticipated in children whose tumors are located in the posterior fossa and affect the cerebellum (Menkes & Till, 1990). Coordination deficits may also be demonstrated in children who experience alterations of postural tone or weakness. In such cases, treatment approaches that focus on the improvement of strength, balance, and coordination are useful.

Changes in the child's cognitive status will also be an important consideration in the development of an exercise program that focuses on the improvement of balance and coordination skills, as well as other aspects of rehabilitation. Short-term memory deficits may make it difficult for a child to become independent in performing an exercise program. A lack of mastery of this task may be frustrating for both the child and family. Variable levels of arousal either within a given treatment session or from treatment to treatment will affect a child's ability to attend to instructions and to stay on task. A treatment plan for a given session may then need to be accordingly adjusted.

FUNCTIONAL LIMITATIONS

Functional limitation is defined as a potentially remediable inability to perform a task as a result of an impairment. Treatment is used to help the child regain the transfer and mobility skills needed for independent or assisted functioning in his or her

immediate environment. In the case of the child with a diagnosis of brain tumor, the amount of function that will be regained depends on whether the limitation is related to the lesion itself, to pressure effects, or to the effects of medical treatment such as surgery or radiation therapy.

For example, if a child's hemiparesis is related to direct pressure effects of a tumor or associated edema, surgical excision of the tumor, or treatment that shrinks or obliterates it, then it is likely to be followed by recovery of function. If the hemiparesis is related to an exacerbation of symptoms that has been noted to occur with radiation therapy (Menkes & Till, 1990), then a recovery of some function may also be expected. Alternately, if the hemiparesis is related to infiltration of the tumor into healthy tissue, function is less likely to be regained. Similarly, if healthy tissues have been surgically excised or damaged by radiation therapy, recovery is less likely to occur. When complete neurologic recovery does not occur, orthoses and adaptive equipment may be used to facilitate independent functioning in the child's environment. Recurrence of the tumor at a future time will also, of course, have an effect on the outcome of treatment.

In the functional limitations domain, increased independence in mobility skills, including bed mobility, transfer training, and gait, wheelchair, or other mobility training, are emphasized in treatment. Once again, the child's cognitive status must be considered. Difficulty learning new tasks and material or short-term memory problems or both may influence the method selected for instruction in transfer and mobility training.

A child's short-term memory deficits or variable levels of arousal may necessitate frequent repetition of instructions and additional cueing while learning a task. These factors will also influence safety. For example, a child may be physically capable of performing a transfer but may not be able to attend to the task sufficiently to observe the necessary safety precautions, such as positioning a wheelchair or locking the brakes.

DISABILITY

In the disability domain, a child's ability to function and be integrated into the community at large is a concern. Treatment is directed at assisting the child in the achievement of the highest possible levels of independent functioning in his or her home, school, and residential community. Treatment may be focused on the determination of the adaptive equipment, orthoses, and environmental modifications necessary for function in the community.

The role of the school physical therapist in intervention with a child who has undergone treatment and rehabilitation for a brain tumor provides an illustration of treatment focused at preventing disability. Goals of treatment may include determination of the mode of mobility and required assistive devices to promote efficient functioning in the classroom and school building. An evaluation of the child's general endurance in relation to the demands of daily activity and the formulation of recommendations for modifications in the child's schedule will also be included.

Intervention that focuses on helping the child become reintegrated into the community through the implementation of provisions in federal legislation such as the Americans With Disabilities Act (PL 101-336) may also be considered as an illustration of intervention to prevent disability. For example, working on improving the child's mobility in the community by securing public transportation mandated by federal legislation influences the child's ability to fully participate in the life of the community.

For children who experience tumor regrowth or for whom further treatment is not possible, physical therapists work with hospice organizations or home health care agencies. In such cases, the therapist collaborates with family members to help them cope with a progressively debilitating process in the child.

CASE HISTORY: BOB

Bob is a 13-year-old student and football player who initially experienced grand mal and petit mal seizures 5 months before admission to a pediatric hospital. At that time, a CT scan was performed and was determined to be negative. He was administered carbamazepine (Tegretol) for seizure control. Three months later his seizures returned and an MRI was performed. The MRI revealed a right temporal lobe mass.

Bob underwent radical resection (defined as removal of the tumor with less than 1.5 mL of tumor volume remaining) of the tumor, which was identified as a low-grade astrocytoma. Bob also underwent an anterior temporal lobectomy, an anterior amygdalectomy, and an anterior hippocampal resection as treatment for his seizures. A hemiplegia involving the left upper and lower extremities was noted in the recovery room.

The hemiplegia was believed to be related either to edema (in which case recovery of function was expected to occur) or to a cerebral infarct. The presence of left homonymous hemianopia suggested an infarct.

Bob began physical therapy within a few days of his surgery. He was noted to be initially alert and appropriate in his verbal responses but was intermittently agitated. He demonstrated difficulty with visual tracking into the left visual field and complained of headache and nausea. His left upper extremity was flaccid. In his left lower extremity, movements of knee flexion and extension and of hip abduction and adduction were available volitionally but were poorly controlled. He demonstrated difficulty with sitting balance and often fell toward the left side. He was able to transfer from bed to and from the commode with moderate assistance by three adults.

Initially, treatment focused on stretching to conserve ankle passive ROM, sitting balance activities, and transfer training. Bob also performed active ROM exercises and coordination exercises, particularly for the left lower extremity. As his balance improved, Bob began working on weight-shifting activities while standing in the parallel bars and also performed pregait foot placement exercises.

Bob was transferred to the rehabilitation unit of the hospital. His goals at this point included 1) standing with contact guarding for 1 minute; 2) transferring from sitting to standing with minimal assistance; and 3) ambulating 6 feet in the parallel bars with moderate assistance. Treatment included work on moving from sitting to standing and functional mobility activities such as rolling, moving from side-lying to sitting and from sitting to standing, and transfers.

As control improved, Bob began working on activities in the developmental progression (i.e., balance in quadruped and half kneel) and continued transfer and mobility training activities. His physical therapist noted a need for frequent reminders to Bob to move slowly and safely during transfers and transitional movements.

Bob's ambulation mode progressed to use of a quad cane with minimal assistance for up to 300 feet. His endurance was noted to be decreased. He continued to experience difficulty with left ankle dorsiflexion in gait, and a program including electrical stimulation for muscle re-education was implemented. Bob continued to work on balance activities including knee walking and balancing on one foot. His balance skills were addressed functionally as he ascended and descended stairs during gait training. At this time, Bob became increasingly aware of his functional deficits and his interactive style changed from outgoing and "happy-go-lucky" to more sad and withdrawn. He also expressed concern about increased dependence on his family and not being available to "help out" when needed.

Bob continued to demonstrate difficulty with left knee control and with transitions from sitting to standing. Treatment included continued work on getting up and down from the floor, as well as weight-shifting activities in standing. In addition to these activities,

Bob's physical therapist initiated a program of exercises for strengthening of his right extremities on the universal gym.

His gait training program progressed to include more work on stairs and ambulation outdoors in the hospital garden. He also began walking on a treadmill with assistance. Although Bob's balance in gait activities had improved significantly, his therapist continued to be concerned about his ability to handle extensive ambulation at home and decided to prescribe a wheelchair to be available at the time of discharge.

Bob returned to school the week after he was discharged from the rehabilitation program and was referred for outpatient physical therapy in his home community. Follow-up evaluation for his brain tumor included MRI at 6-month intervals for the first year after discharge.

Comments

When this case history is considered from the perspective of Campbell's (1992) framework, Bob's initial medical treatment (surgery) and his initial physical therapy may be considered to be focused at the organ systems impairment level. Removal of the tumor and adjacent tissue helped to restore function in the temporal lobe by halting the interference of the seizure activity. Initial physical therapy, including stretching exercises for the heelcords, balance and coordination activities, and active ROM exercises for strengthening, also addressed rehabilitation at the organ systems level. Rehabilitation of impairment continued to be addressed throughout Bob's hospital stay.

In the functional limitations domain, treatment was focused on regaining bed mobility and transfer skills. Gait training that helped Bob function in his immediate environment on the rehabilitation unit also addressed functional limitations. The use of electrical stimulation for muscle re-education addressed coordination and strength impairments, as well as initial functional gait and mobility training.

To limit disability in daily life, treatment was focused on mobility training outdoors in the garden and evaluation of Bob's safety in mobility skills. To address these needs, Bob's physical therapist determined that he would be likely to benefit from the use of a wheelchair for mobility over long distances outdoors but could use a quad cane inside. An evaluation of Bob's ability to function within his school could have also been considered.

The physical therapist's decision to include universal weight training in Bob's exercise program promoted the achievement of important physical performance goals while providing the opportunity for engaging in typical life experiences. Even though Bob had not regained sufficient skills to resume athletic activities at his school, he could be included in exercise training on the universal gym with his peers.

Bob's progress can be demonstrated by changes in his performance on the Functional Independence Measure for Children, WeeFIM (Braun & Granger, 1991), a pediatric functional assessment tool. At the time of admission to the rehabilitation unit, Bob required moderate assistance for self-care activities, transfers, and wheelchair mobility. He required maximal assistance for ambulation but was independent in the areas of communication and social cognition skills (Fig. 21–1). At the time of discharge, he was independent, or required assistive devices for self-care activities and transfers, and required supervision for ambulation. Improvements are reflected in an increase in his total score from 78 to 113 points (Fig. 21–1).

At the time of an outpatient follow-up visit, further improvements were noted and he was independent in all areas except for tub and shower transfers and ambulation, for which he required assistive devices. His total score increased further to 123 points (Fig. 21–2).

Treatment of the child with the diagnosis of brain tumor must take into consideration the characteristics of the treatment as well as the medical interventions administered in an attempt to ameliorate the problem. By addressing treatment for impairments, functional limitations, and disability, the pediatric physical therapist must formulate a treatment plan to address all aspects of a child's functioning that may be affected by the tumor.

▌TRAUMATIC HEAD INJURIES

Mechanics of Closed Head Injuries

Although both open and penetrating head injuries may be related to deficits for which the pediatric physical therapist provides rehabilitation, only closed head injuries are considered in this chapter.

Brain injury that results from closed head injury may be related to both primary and secondary mechanical factors. Primary injuries are related to the forces that occur at the time of the initial impact. Secondary injury results from the forces that occur in reaction to the impact forces.

PRIMARY INJURIES

Primary injuries, or those injuries related to the forces that occur at the time of initial impact, may be grouped with respect to the role played by acceleration factors.

Acceleration-dependent injuries are related to the effects that occur when a force is applied to a moveable head. They may be translational or rota-

UNIFORM DATA SYSTEM FOR MEDICAL REHABILITATION
WeeFIM INPATIENT CODING SHEET
Page 2 of 2

1. Facility Code ☐☐☐

2. Patient Code ☐☐☐☐☐☐☐☐

Admission Assessment

22. Admit From
1-Home 2-Board and Care 3-Transitional Living
4-Intermediate Care 5-Skilled Nursing Facility
6-Acute unit of own facility 7-Acute unit another facility
8-Chronic Hospital 9-Rehabilitation Facility 10-Other
12-Alternate Level of Care Unit ☐☐

23. Prehospital Living Setting
Use codes listed for item 22. ☐☐

24. Prehospital Living With
(Complete only if item 23 is coded 1-Home.)
1-Two Parents 2-One Parent 3-Foster care
4-Shelter 5-Relatives 6-Other ☐

25. Prehospital Educational Category
1-Not Student 2-Pre-School 3-Regular School ☐

26. Prehospital Educational Setting
1-Not student 2-Regular Class 3-Special Class
4-Home based 5-Day Care ☐

Discharge Assessment

27. Discharge to
1-Home 2-Board and Care 3-Transitional Living
4-Intermediate Care 5-Skilled Nursing Facility
6-Acute unit of own facility 7-Acute unit in another facility
8-Chronic Hospital 9-Rehabilitation Facility 10-Other
11-Died 12-Alternate Level of Care Unit ☐☐

28. Discharge Living With
(Complete only if item 27 is coded 1-Home.)
1-Two Parents 2-One Parent 3-Foster care
4-Shelter 5-Relatives 6-Other ☐

39. Functional Independence Measure (FIM)

(For Items 29-38 See Follow-Up Coding Sheet)

	ADMISSION	DISCHARGE
Self-Care		
A. Eating	6	7
B. Grooming	3	7
C. Bathing	3	6
D. Dressing-Upper Body	4	6
E. Dressing-Lower Body	2	6
F. Toileting	2	6
Sphincter Control		
G. Bladder Management	7	7
H. Bowel Management	7	7
Transfers		
I. Chair, Wheelchair	3	6
J. Toilet	2	6
K. Tub, Shower	2	4
Locomotion		
L. Walk/Wheelchair/Crawl	1 (⊗ Walk / ○ Wheelchair / ○ Crawl)	5 (⊗ / ⊗ / ○)
M. Stairs	1	5
Motor Subtotal Score	☐	☐
Communication		
N. Comprehension	7 (⊗ Auditory / ○ Visual / ○ Both)	7
O. Expression	7 (⊗ Vocal / ⊗ Nonvocal / ○ Both)	7
Social Cognition		
P. Social Interaction	7	7
Q. Problem Solving	7	7
R. Memory	7	7
Cognitive Subtotal Score	☐	☐
Total Motor and Cognitive Score	78	113

FIM Levels

NO HELPER
7 Complete Independence (Timely, Safely)
6 Modified Independence (Device)

HELPER
Modified Dependence
5 Supervision
4 Minimal Assistance (Subject = 75 % +)
3 Moderate Assistance (Subject = 50 % +)
Complete Dependence
2 Maximal Assistance (Subject = 25 % +)
1 Total Assistance (Subject = 0 % +)

(NOTE: Leave no blanks; enter 1 if not testable due to risk)

(Complete Both Pages)

COPY FREELY - DO NOT CHANGE

IPCS2-930625

FIGURE 21–1. Admission and discharge WeeFIM performance for Bob. (From Braun, SL, & Granger, CV. A practical approach to functional assessment in pediatrics. Occupational Therapy Practice, 2:46–51, 1991.)

UNIFORM DATA SYSTEM FOR MEDICAL REHABILITATION
WeeFIM OUTPATIENT OR FOLLOW-UP CODING SHEET

Page 2 of 2

9. Assessment Date   MONTH DAY YEAR

1. Facility Code

2. Patient Code

Assessment Information

34. Information Source
1-Patient 2-Family 3-Other

35. Method
1-In person 2-Telephone
3-Mailed questionnaire

36. Health Maintenance
1-Own care
2-Unpaid person or family   Primary
3-Paid attendant or aide
4-Paid, skilled professional   Secondary

37. Therapy
1-None
2-Outpatient therapy
3-Home-based paid professional therapy
4-Both 2 and 3
5-Inpatient Hospital
6-Long-term Care Facility
7-Other

39. Functional Independence Measure (FIM)

OUTPATIENT OR FOLLOW-UP

		Score
Self-Care		
A.	Eating	7
B.	Grooming	7
C.	Bathing	7
D.	Dressing-Upper Body	7
E.	Dressing-Lower Body	7
F.	Toileting	7
Sphincter Control		
G.	Bladder Management	7
H.	Bowel Management	7
Transfers		
I.	Chair, Wheelchair	7
J.	Toilet	7
K.	Tub, Shower	6
Locomotion		
L.	Walk/Wheelchair	6 ⊗ Walk / ○ Wheelchair / ○ Crawl
M.	Stairs	6

FIM Levels

NO HELPER	
7	Complete Independence (Timely, Safely)
6	Modified Independence (Device)
HELPER	
Modified Dependence	
5	Supervision
4	Minimal Assistance (Subject = 75 % +)
3	Moderate Assistance (Subject = 50 % +)
Complete Dependence	
2	Maximal Assistance (Subject = 25 % +)
1	Total Assistance (Subject = 0 % +)

Motor Subtotal Score

		Score
Communication		
N.	Comprehension	7 ⊗ Auditory / ○ Visual / ○ Both
O.	Expression	7 ⊗ Vocal / ○ Nonvocal / ○ Both
Social Cognition		
P.	Social Interaction	7
Q.	Problem Solving	7
R.	Memory	7

(NOTE: Leave no blanks; enter 1 if not testable due to risk)

Cognitive Subtotal Score

Complete Both Pages

Total Motor and Cognitive Score   113

FIGURE 21-2. Outpatient follow-up WeeFIM score for Bob. (From Braun, SL, & Granger, CV. A practical approach to functional assessment in pediatrics. Occupational Therapy Practice, 2:46–51, 1991.)

tional. In the case of translational injuries, a vector related to the force applied to the head passes approximately through the head's center of mass. In rotational injuries, the resultant force vector does not pass through the center of mass and angular acceleration results. For most closed head injuries, the resultant force is not purely translation or rotational but a combination of the two.

In the case of a *translational injury,* the response to a force applied to the side of the skull is lateral movement of both the skull and the brain. As the skull contacts an immovable object such as the door frame of an automobile, it rapidly decelerates. The brain, however, continues to move laterally until it is stopped by the lateral aspect of the skull. The injury that results from the initial impact of the brain on the skull is translational and is also termed a *coup* lesion. The lesion that occurs as the brain reacts secondarily to the initial force against the skull (moving in the opposite direction against the skull on the opposite side) is termed *contrecoup.* Contrecoup injuries may also cause significant brain damage.

Rotational injury occurs when the brain remains stationary while the skull rotates. The resultant forces are angular. Rotational injuries have been related to shearing trauma, which may be manifested as brain surface contusions and lacerations (Pang, 1985). Diffuse axonal injuries have also been related to shearing trauma.

Nonacceleration-dependent injuries are not related to acceleration factors. Brain injury that results from skull depression into brain tissue is one example. Vibration coinciding with the application of an initial force to the skull has also been hypothesized as a cause of nonacceleration-related injury (Marcal & Nickell, 1973).

SECONDARY INJURIES

Secondary injuries, or those that occur related to processes evoked in response to the initial trauma, account for a significant amount of the overall damage that occurs in closed brain injury. Perhaps one of the most frequently occurring causes of secondary injuries is *cerebral edema.* Unchecked cerebral edema and the resultant increase in intracranial pressure can lead to brain herniation, multiple cerebral infarctions, permanent brain stem necrosis, and irreversible coma (Pang, 1985). After a traumatic brain injury, cerebral edema is frequently a result of increased capillary permeability. Fluid leaks slowly, leading to clinically significant effects 4 to 6 hours after injury with peak effects at 24 to 36 hours after injury (Pang, 1985).

Epidural hematomas result when the middle meningeal artery, vein, or venous sinus bleeds into the epidural space between the dura and the skull. This usually follows a skull fracture or bending of the skull into the brain. As the skull recoils, a space that may fill with blood results. The rate of blood collection and the resultant increase in intracranial pressure determines the prognosis. The prognosis for rapidly accumulating hematomas is grave. The location of the hematoma has also been related to outcome. Temporal or posterior fossa hematomas are more likely to cause brain shift and brain stem compression than a hematoma in the frontoparietal area (Pang, 1985).

Acute subdural hematomas are related to extensive cortical injury and lacerated cortical vessels. Edema in the underlying brain tissue develops rapidly. Acute cerebral hematomas must be removed expediently. Their ultimate effect on recovery depends on both the time between development and evacuation of the hemorrhage and on the extent of damage to underlying brain tissue.

Increased intracranial pressure frequently occurs after brain injury as a result of edema and hematoma. Further damage to cerebral tissue from brain stem herniation may result. Initial increases in intracranial pressure are accommodated by expulsion of cerebrospinal fluid from the cavity into the subarachnoid space and ventricles and by expulsion of cerebral venous blood into the jugular veins or scalp (Lofgren & Awetnow, 1973). At the point that compensatory mechanisms are no longer effective, a rise in intracranial pressure occurs. When the magnitude of and increase in intracranial blood and fluid volume is compared with the resultant increase in intracranial pressure, the relation between the two increases exponentially (Pang, 1985). For these reasons, intracranial pressure is closely monitored in patients with brain injury.

Various evaluative procedures are used to monitor the effects of both primary and secondary trauma. Some of the methods used in the evaluation of pediatric brain tumors are also used to assess children with head injuries.

Evaluation Procedures

Brain imaging methods are useful in the evaluation of children with head injury. When the goal of assessment is determination of the extent of secondary injuries related to the circulatory system, such as hematoma, CT is likely to be used. When the goal of assessment is determination of the extent of a patient's injuries after the acute phase of the injury, MRI may be selected. The expense of MRI when compared with CT may also be a consideration in the selection of an evaluative measure. For example, the cost of MRI may not be reimbursable by some state or federally funded or private insurance companies.

Monitoring of intracranial pressure is frequently used, especially for assessment of the acute injury. When intracranial pressure is elevated to a level associated with risk for further brain damage, pressure caused by edema or hemorrhage may be surgically released.

BEHAVIORAL SCALES

Level of coma is frequently monitored using a criterion-based behavioral scale. Two frequently used measures are the Glasgow Coma Scale (Teasdale & Jennett, 1974) and the Rancho Los Amigos Scale (Hagen et al., 1979). Both of these scales assess a child's ability to respond to various stimuli ranging from a painful stimulus to a complex verbal command. A child's orientation to time and place is also considered. An increase in summary score of the Glasgow Coma Scale on successive administrations is an indicator of improvement. The administration of the Rancho Los Amigos Scale (Hagen et al., 1979) results in classification of a child into one of eight cognitive levels. Progression to a numerically higher level is an indicator of progress.

The Children's Orientation and Amnesia Test (COAT) (Ewing-Cobb et al., 1989) is also used to evaluate level of coma in children. Test items, particularly those that assess the appropriateness of verbal responses to orientation questions, are based on facts commonly known by children.

After an injury, a child may demonstrate behavior that falls at any point on the continuum described by the Glasgow Coma Scale (Teasdale & Jennett, 1974) or the Rancho Los Amigos Levels of Cognitive Recovery (Hagen et al., 1979). The pediatric physical therapist needs to be aware of a child's status relative to level of coma or cognitive status to plan appropriate treatment. A child who is generally unresponsive, or who responds only to pain or localized stimuli, may be exposed to sensory inputs designed to elicit arousal. Such stimuli include intermittent music or audiotaped voices or tactile or olfactory stimuli. An aspect of intervention at this level includes education for the family on the provision of appropriate levels of sensory stimulation.

When the child becomes agitated and confused, reducing the general amount of environmental stimulation is appropriate. Decreasing auditory and visual activity in the child's room or treatment area may help the child to focus on commands related to treatment. Keeping verbal communications simple with respect to sentence structure and the number of persons speaking is also recommended.

When the child has emerged from coma and is able to tolerate environmental stimulation in general, other cognitive deficits may become evident. The aspects of cognition described in the section on brain tumors are also likely to be evaluated in children with head injuries. Deficiencies in the areas of memory, executive functioning, and visuospatial skills may be present and should be taken into consideration in treatment planning.

Medical Interventions

Medical intervention for children with traumatic brain injury may include surgery, the use of pharmacologic agents, and the use of mechanical ventilation. Surgical interventions include evacuation of subdural or intracerebral hematomas. These procedures are used to decrease intracranial pressure and reduce pressure-related secondary brain injuries.

Pharmacologic agents are also frequently used to decrease cerebral edema and pressure-related secondary injuries. Drugs that are frequently used in the management of edema include mannitol and corticosteroids. Pharmacologic agents may also be used to induce paralysis in cases in which body movements would interfere with the administration of medical interventions.

Hyperventilation, or mechanically assisted ventilation at a rate greater than usual, may temporarily reduce intracranial pressure. Once hyperventilation is discontinued, intracranial pressure increases again. Hyperventilation is, therefore, a temporary measure used until other interventions such as surgery are available, or until pharmacologic agents take effect.

Rehabilitation

As medical technology improves survival rates, pediatric physical therapists can expect to be increasingly involved with the rehabilitation of patients with traumatic brain injury. An important consideration in treatment planning for this population is the developmental nature of the injury (Fletcher et al., 1987; Hale et al., 1990). Because children who have experienced a head injury may have not completed ontologic motor development, rehabilitation must take into consideration both recovery from the neurologic insult and what would have been normal developmental progression.

Similar to the child with a pediatric brain tumor undergoing rehabilitation, physical therapy intervention for the child with a traumatic brain injury may be described using Campbell's (1992) framework as a point of reference.

IMPAIRMENT

Interventions to maintain or improve joint flexibility and prevent musculoskeletal deformity are focused at the organ systems or impairment level. ROM, strengthening, and stretching exercises may be selected to address specific problems, such as weakness, or to remediate coordination or balance problems that are related to CNS injury.

When spasticity is present and contributes to the loss of functional ROM, serial casting may be an important component of treatment. Casting may also prevent loss of functional ROM when initiated in the intensive care unit and continued on the rehabilitation unit. Consideration must be given to the child's cognitive status if serial casting is selected. If the child is unresponsive or unable to communicate, particular care must be taken to ensure the maintenance of skin integrity because the child will not be able to reliably report pain or discomfort. If the child is agitated, responses to handling and other sensory stimuli associated with serial casting must be considered. For example, the noise associated with use of a cast saw may be overwhelming.

Positioning may also be considered as an intervention to prevent or reduce impairment. Positioning may be used to prevent contractures and deformities or to decrease the influence of abnormal postures. Positioning may also be used to increase the tolerance of the physiologic system to changes in body orientation with respect to gravity. For example, the physical therapist may develop a progressive program to increase tolerance for sitting in a wheelchair. For the patient who has spent an extended period of time in a gravity-eliminated position, a tilt-table may allow the circulatory system to gradually adapt to vertical body alignment.

Exercises and activities that focus on deficiencies in the areas of balance, coordination, and alignment address problems at the postural control level. When a child's cognitive status is considered, strategies selected to address postural control may also be part of cognitive remediation. For example, repetitive coordination exercises that involve alternating patterns of movement may remediate prob-

lems in the area of executive functioning, such as the ability to switch conceptual sets.

An activity involving maneuvering through an obstacle course addresses motor planning and balance skills and can also be useful in remediating short-term memory problems and difficulty learning and remembering new repertoires. The child who performs the obstacle course must remember instructions and negotiate the course in a predetermined order.

FUNCTIONAL LIMITATIONS

At this level, treatment focuses on improving mobility skills within the context of the immediate environment. Transfer training and bed and wheelchair mobility training are components of treatment. Treatment may also include evaluation for assistive devices and orthoses. Because children whose brain injuries are the result of a traumatic event may have other associated complications, such as fractures, the management of related mobility limitations must also be considered. For example, the child who demonstrates a hemiplegia related to brain injury but also has a fractured femur and humerus will be considerably more limited in mobility skills than the child who experiences either just a neurologic or an orthopaedic injury. Modalities such as electrical stimulation may be used to decrease strength impairment in a given muscle group to support mobility skills. For example, electrical stimulation of the quadriceps muscles may increase strength and stability for transfers.

A child's cognitive status will affect intervention in this domain. A child who demonstrates perseveration may have difficulty with reciprocal tasks (i.e., repetitive transfer training) or may become upset when asked to change from one activity to another. Short-term memory deficits may make it necessary for a child to have supervision even though the child's strength, balance, and endurance when considered alone are sufficient for the performance of a motor activity. Educating parents regarding the impact of a child's neurologic, orthopaedic, and cognitive status on his or her ability to function with respect to mobility skills is an important component of the treatment.

DISABILITY

In the area of disability, physical therapy is used to assist the child and family in making adaptations to facilitate functioning in the child's typical environment and roles. Evaluation for orthoses and mobility devices is appropriate, and the pediatric physical therapist may also make recommendations regarding environmental modifications within the child's home or school to promote independence. Educating and supporting parents as they adapt to changes in their child's physical and cognitive abilities as well as facilitating the child's transition to school and community living are appropriate goals to prevent disability and facilitate coping with inevitable societal barriers to full integration in society.

MEASURING CHANGE

During rehabilitation, assessment of change in both component motor skills and in level of functional independence is important. When a measure of change in the ability to perform motor developmental milestones as well as an evaluation of the components of gross motor skills is needed, a standardized tool such as the Peabody Developmental Motor Scales (Folio & Fewell, 1984) may be selected for preschoolers. The Bruininks-Oseretsky Test of Motor Proficiency (Bruininks, 1978) also purports to measure various aspects of gross motor performance in school-age children. Newly developed, functional measures such as the Pediatric Evaluation of Disability Inventory (Haley et al., 1992) and the WeeFIM (Braun & Granger, 1991) are criterion-referenced indicators of a change in functional skills such as mobility and self-care. The use of standardized measures to monitor motoric and functional change will also be useful to document progress as required by third-party payers.

CASE HISTORY: ELIZABETH

Elizabeth is a 10-year-old girl who experienced a traumatic brain injury. She was a passenger in an automobile who was thrown from the vehicle in an accident. She experienced a hemorrhage in the right thalamic area, a left tension pneumothorax, and a fracture of the right symphysis pubis. She was reportedly in a coma for 4 weeks at another facility where she required a tracheostomy for respiratory management. Reports indicated a left hemiplegia and elbow, ankle, and knee contractures as subsequent complications.

At the time of transfer to a pediatric rehabilitation facility, Elizabeth responded to one- and two-step commands and was described to be at a Rancho Los Amigos Scale Level III. As a result of tracheostomy closure, Elizabeth whispered as a primary mode of communication. Achilles tendon contractures were measured at 15° of plantar flexion on the right and 30° on the left. She was able to sit at the edge of the mat with moderate assistance and had difficulty in righting her head.

At this time, treatment included work on sitting balance and facilitation of head righting. The headrest on the wheelchair was removed intermittently to encourage independence in this skill. Elizabeth was also placed on a tilt-table to increase tolerance of a vertical position and to mechanically assist the stretching of her heelcords. A program of serial casting for the ankles was initiated with cast changes performed every 2 to 3 days. Elizabeth also began a program of strengthening and coordination exercises.

As rehabilitation continued, Elizabeth's treatment included mat and bed mobility exercises and stretching exercises for the hips and knees. When her head control improved, the wheelchair headrest was removed permanently. Serial casting for the right ankle resulted in increased ROM. Because of knee pain on the left that was not alleviated by positioning changes, casting for the left ankle was temporarily discontinued. Elizabeth continued standing on the tilt table for heelcord stretching.

By approximately 6 weeks after her injury, Elizabeth was able to transfer from supine to sitting with moderate assistance and to perform a standing pivot transfer with maximal assistance. Her strength was estimated to be in the fair range by manual muscle testing when the effects of postural tone were considered. Within 2 weeks, serial casting for the right ankle resumed. The casts were then bivalved to allow intermittent removal. Elizabeth began training in wheelchair mobility. Left lower extremity spasms limited her ability to control the wheelchair to negotiate around obstacles. Spasms also limited her ability to bear weight on her left leg during transfers. She became concerned about the appearance of her ankle contracture.

By 3½ months after her injury, Elizabeth was able to transfer from the wheelchair to the mat independently. She continued to experience difficulty in propelling her wheelchair, which her physical therapist believed to be related to coordination problems, particularly with her left arm. Elizabeth's physical therapist prescribed a one-arm drive wheelchair for continued mobility training. Elizabeth was then able to negotiate flat surfaces and a ramp.

The serial casting program continued in conjunction with standing on the tilt table. Elizabeth began ambulation with moderate assistance from her physical therapist and began riding an exercise bicycle as a coordination and strengthening exercise.

By 4½ months after her injury, Elizabeth was able to ambulate with her cane on a flat surface and climb stairs with standby assistance. At the time of discharge from the rehabilitation unit, Elizabeth walked with a cane but preferred the hand of an assistant for balance.

Before discharge, Elizabeth was evaluated by a neuropsychologist who reported deficiencies in several cognitive areas, including short-term memory, learning new material, and visuospatial skills. Elizabeth was discharged to an outpatient program for cognitive rehabilitation. She received outpatient physical and occupational therapy at a local hospital. At the time of a follow-up evaluation 4 months after discharge, she was ambulating using an ankle-foot orthosis; however, her function continued to be limited by ankle spasticity.

Comments

In the area of impairment reduction, Elizabeth's treatment included therapeutic interventions aimed at increasing muscle and soft tissue strength and flexibility. ROM and stretching exercises together with serial casting addressed limited flexibility related to muscle shortening after a period of abnormal ankle posturing. Management of Elizabeth's respiratory problems with a tracheostomy also addressed impairment at the organ systems level.

Serial casting for ankle impairment contributed to reduction of functional limitations. For example, placement of a cast that positioned the ankle more neutrally decreased the interference of extensor posturing when Elizabeth propelled her wheelchair. Serial casting and the resultant increase in ankle ROM allowed a more efficient gait pattern during ambulation with a cane.

Other mobility training such as bed mobility activities and transfer training were also focused on reducing functional limitations. Elizabeth's deficits in the areas of short-term memory and the ability to learn new material influenced her performance in these areas during treatment. For example, Elizabeth had difficulty remembering her physical therapist's instructions when learning to use the one-arm drive wheelchair. The influence of memory and learning defects may be expected to influence performance in other functional areas, such as activities of daily living skills.

To reduce disability, intervention was focused on achieving the greatest possible level of independence in mobility skills outdoors and in her community. At the time of discharge, Elizabeth was able to ambulate with a straight cane and standby assistance, allowing her to successfully negotiate her home and new school environments.

Elizabeth's progress in limiting disability may also be seen in her performance on the WeeFIM (Fig. 21–3). Initially, she required complete assistance for all self-care and mobility activities. She demonstrated less difficulty with communication and social cognition skills. At the time of discharge from the rehabilitation unit, Elizabeth was independent with an assistive device for self-care and mobility activities. She required supervision for ambulation on stairs and for tasks requiring memory. During the inpatient stay, Elizabeth's total WeeFIM score increased from 28 to 115 points (Fig. 21–3).

At the time of her follow-up rehabilitation clinic appointment, she required an assistive device for bathing

and for ambulation skills. Otherwise, Elizabeth was able to function independently at home and school. Her total WeeFIM score at her follow-up visit increased an additional 9 points compared with her score at discharge, for a total score of 124 points (Fig. 21–4).

NEAR-DROWNING

Near-drowning has been defined as an episode in which someone survives a period of underwater submersion (Fisher, 1993). Survivors may experience cardiac, CNS, or respiratory system complications and may require rehabilitation.

The brain and the heart are the organs most susceptible to injury related to a period of asphyxia and near-drowning injuries. Respiratory distress syndrome may occur related to pulmonary complications. Changes in fluid flux between the plasma and the alveoli alter surfactant properties and can lead to atelectasis and respiratory distress. Ischemia affecting cardiac muscle may lead to cardiac arrest.

Even when resuscitation is successful, the period of anoxia that has occurred may cause irreversible hypoxic-ischemic brain injury, including brain death (Cohn, 1980). Cerebral edema and herniation are complications associated with hypoxic-ischemic injury. When near-drowning occurs in cold water (less than 20°C), the diving reflex provides some protection from hypoxic-ischemic brain injury. The diving reflex causes bradycardia and peripheral vasoconstriction, with preferential shunting of blood to the heart and brain, reducing the magnitude of anoxic encephalopathy.

The factors that predict functional recovery in children who have experienced a near-drowning episode include the length of the period of submersion and the length of time before resuscitation is begun. More specifically, the length and severity of ischemia is an important factor (Beyda, 1991). In general, neuronal cells are not able to tolerate periods of complete ischemia lasting longer than 5 minutes without sustaining permanent injury; irreversible neuronal injury has been demonstrated to increase significantly after 10 minutes (Safar, 1988). The magnitude of the neuronal injury that occurs is also related to both the level of blood flow during the complete ischemic interval and the total duration of the ischemia. Although the return of blood flow that occurs after cardiopulmonary resuscitation was originally believed to have a restorative function, it is now believed to contribute significantly to morbidity and mortality (Beyda, 1991). Because cardiopulmonary resuscitation may not provide adequately oxygenated blood flow to the brain, significant ischemic injury may occur during

UNIFORM DATA SYSTEM FOR MEDICAL REHABILITATION

WeeFIM INPATIENT CODING SHEET

Page 2 of 2

1. Facility Code

2. Patient Code

Admission Assessment

22. Admit From
1-Home 2-Board and Care 3-Transitional Living
4-Intermediate Care 5-Skilled Nursing Facility
6-Acute unit of own facility 7-Acute unit another facility
8-Chronic Hospital 9-Rehabilitation Facility 10-Other
12-Alternate Level of Care Unit

23. Prehospital Living Setting
Use codes listed for item 22.

24. Prehospital Living With
(Complete only if item 23 is coded 1-Home.)
1-Two Parents 2-One Parent 3-Foster care
4-Shelter 5-Relatives 6-Other

25. Prehospital Educational Category
1-Not Student 2-Pre-School 3-Regular School

26. Prehospital Educational Setting
1-Not student 2-Regular Class 3-Special Class
4-Home based 5-Day Care

Discharge Assessment

27. Discharge to
1-Home 2-Board and Care 3-Transitional Living
4-Intermediate Care 5-Skilled Nursing Facility
6-Acute unit of own facility 7-Acute unit in another facility
8-Chronic Hospital 9-Rehabilitation Facility 10-Other
11-Died 12-Alternate Level of Care Unit

28. Discharge Living With
(Complete only if item 27 is coded 1-Home.)
1-Two Parents 2-One Parent 3-Foster care
4-Shelter 5-Relatives 6-Other

(For Items 29-38 See Follow-Up Coding Sheet)

39. Functional Independence Measure (FIM)

		ADMISSION	DISCHARGE
Self-Care			
A.	Eating	1	7
B.	Grooming	1	7
C.	Bathing	1	7
D.	Dressing-Upper Body	1	6
E.	Dressing-Lower Body	1	6
F.	Toileting	1	7
Sphincter Control			
G.	Bladder Management	1	5
H.	Bowel Management	1	7
Transfers			
I.	Chair, Wheelchair	1	6
J.	Toilet	1	7
K.	Tub, Shower	1	6
Locomotion		Walk / Wheelchair / Crawl	
L.	Walk/Wheelchair/Crawl	1	6
M.	Stairs		5

Motor Subtotal Score

FIM Levels

NO HELPER

7 — Complete Independence (Timely, Safely)

6 — Modified Independence (Device)

HELPER

Modified Dependence

5 — Supervision

4 — Minimal Assistance (Subject = 75 % +)

3 — Moderate Assistance (Subject = 50 % +)

Complete Dependence

2 — Maximal Assistance (Subject = 25 % +)

1 — Total Assistance (Subject = 0 % +)

		ADMISSION	DISCHARGE
Communication			
N.	Comprehension	3 (Auditory/Visual/Both)	7
O.	Expression	3 (Vocal/Nonvocal/Both)	7
Social Cognition			
P.	Social Interaction	3	7
Q.	Problem Solving	3	7
R.	Memory	3	5

(NOTE: Leave no blanks; enter 1 if not testable due to risk)

Cognitive Subtotal Score

Complete Both Pages

Total Motor and Cognitive Score — 28 — 115

COPY FREELY   DO NOT CHANGE

IPC02-800025

FIGURE 21-3. Admission and discharge WeeFIM performance for Elizabeth. (From Braun, SL, & Granger, CV. A practical approach to functional assessment in pediatrics. Occupational Therapy Practice, 2:46-51, 1991.)

UNIFORM DATA SYSTEM FOR MEDICAL REHABILITATION
WeeFIM OUTPATIENT OR FOLLOW-UP CODING SHEET

Page 2 of 2

9.Assessment Date

| MONTH | DAY | YEAR |

1. **Facility Code**

2. **Patient Code**

Assessment Information

34. Information Source
1-Patient 2-Family 3-Other

35. Method
1-In person 2-Telephone
3-Mailed questionnaire

36. Health Maintenance
1-Own care
2-Unpaid person or family
3-Paid attendant or aide
4-Paid, skilled professional

Primary

Secondary

37. Therapy
1-None
2-Outpatient therapy
3-Home-based paid professional therapy
4-Both 2 and 3
5-Inpatient Hospital
6-Long-term Care Facility
7-Other

---

39. Functional Independence Measure (FIM)

OUTPATIENT OR FOLLOW-UP

Self-Care
A.   Eating — 7
B.   Grooming — 7
C.   Bathing — 7
D.   Dressing-Upper Body — 7
E.   Dressing-Lower Body — 7
F.   Toileting — 7

Sphincter Control
G.   Bladder Management — 7
H.   Bowel Management — 7

Transfers
I.   Chair, Wheelchair — 7
J.   Toilet — 7
K.   Tub, Shower — 7

Locomotion
L.   Walk/Wheelchair — 6 ⊗ Walk ◯ Wheelchair ◯ Crawl
M.   Stairs — 6

Motor Subtotal Score —

Communication
N.   Comprehension — 7 ⊗ Auditory ◯ Visual ◯ Both
O.   Expression — 7 ⊗ Vocal ◯ Nonvocal ◯ Both

Social Cognition
P.   Social Interaction — 7
Q.   Problem Solving — 7
R.   Memory — 7

Cognitive Subtotal Score —

Total Motor and Cognitive Score — 124

FIM Levels	
NO HELPER	
7	Complete Independence (Timely, Safely)
6	Modified Independence (Device)
HELPER	
Modified Dependence	
5	Supervision
4	Minimal Assistance (Subject = 75 % +)
3	Moderate Assistance (Subject = 50 % +)
Complete Dependence	
2	Maximal Assistance (Subject = 25 % +)
1	Total Assistance (Subject = 0 % +)

(NOTE: Leave no blanks; enter 1 if not testable due to risk)

(**Complete Both Pages**)

FIGURE 21–4. Outpatient follow-up WeeFIM score for Elizabeth. (From Braun, SL, & Granger, CV. A practical approach to functional assessment in pediatrics. Occupational Therapy Practice, *2*:46–51, 1991.)

this emergency intervention. Coma, spasticity, and abnormal posturing are manifestations of CNS injury that may be present after near-drowning.

Impairment

Medical interventions that support respiration and attempt to prevent further injury and complications are focused at the organ systems level. Traditional and high-frequency mechanical ventilation, for example, treat acquired respiratory distress syndrome and may indirectly prevent further CNS complications. Extracorporeal membrane oxygenation is another intervention for the respiratory system in which blood is oxygenated mechanically outside the body, allowing the lungs to "rest." Mechanical ventilation and extracorporeal membrane oxygenation are frequently used in conjunction with pharmacologic paralysis of the musculoskeletal system, placing the child at risk for contractures, muscle weakness, and atrophy. (See Chapter 29 for further discussion of extracorporeal membrane oxygenation.)

Physical therapy for spasticity, rigidity, and abnormal posturing includes passive ROM and therapeutic exercise, which at least temporarily reduces spasticity. Positioning that prevents skin breakdown, contracture, and deformities is also directed at impairment of organ systems. For children who have received extracorporeal membrane oxygenation and been paralyzed pharmacologically, strengthening exercises and activities that improve endurance will be a component of treatment. If a child remains in coma indefinitely without regaining functional abilities, ongoing long-term treatment may be considered to be predominantly focused in the domain of reducing impairment.

Functional Limitations and Disability

Treatment of functional limitations and prevention of disability are accomplished in ways similar to that for children with head injuries and brain tumors. For children who remain in coma, with severe CNS injury, treatment may include intervention within the context of an extended-care facility or other residential setting. For children with severe spasticity and abnormal posturing, positioning and adaptive equipment prescription and fabrication constitute a significant component of treatment.

CASE HISTORY: JOHNNY

Johnny is a 23-month-old infant who was found unconscious in a swimming pool after submersion for an undetermined length of time. No respirations or pulse were noted at the time the emergency medical technicians arrived. Cardiopulmonary resuscitation was performed for 40 minutes, after which Johnny was intubated and mechanically ventilated. He was described as being in a coma, with occasional flailing of his extremities; sedative medication was administered along with mechanical hyperventilation.

Three days after the near-drowning incident Johnny was extubated. Four days after the near-drowning he was noted to be awake but unresponsive to verbal or visual stimuli. By day 5 he was resedated after being noted to be stiff and spastic with agitation.

Johnny was assessed by a physical therapist 5 days after the incident. He had Achilles tendon hypoextensibility on the right and demonstrated spontaneous, nonpurposeful movements. When placed in a supported sitting position, he was able to maintain an erect trunk for 4 to 5 seconds at a time. When he was placed in supported sitting, increased spasticity was noted in his right leg.

Treatment included the facilitation of head righting in supported sitting and passive ROM for the extremities. Johnny's mother was instructed in stretching his ankle muscles. Postural tone was noted to be increasing in a flexor pattern with plantar flexion in the ankles. Inhibitive cast boots were fabricated for both ankles to try to decrease spasticity. At this time treatment consisted of positioning in side-lying and prone over a ball, which had the effect of decreasing spasticity. Johnny also began standing next to a support in his inhibitive casts.

Johnny's casts were bivalved to allow intermittent applications. His treatment at this time consisted of passive ROM exercises, kneeling activities, and standing at a support. Decreased spasticity was noted in his hip adductors and plantar flexors. The facilitation of active hip extension in kneeling and standing while supported by a ball were the areas of emphasis in treatment.

Johnny's mother was instructed in assisting Johnny with sitting balance. At this time, Johnny was able to maintain his head erect for only 1 second at a time. Flexor positioning in the upper extremities interfered with righting and protective reactions in sitting. Because Johnny had not made significant progress in sitting balance and mobility skills, a custom-fitted wheelchair was ordered.

By 5 weeks after his injury, Johnny was not able to bring his hands to midline or to reach. His treatment continued to emphasize sitting balance and head-righting activities. Johnny became agitated at times, making it impossible to complete some treatment sessions.

Johnny was positioned in a supine stander to encourage active hip extension activity, which occurred for a few seconds at a time. When placed in a sitting position on a bench, Johnny could right his head for 2 to 3 seconds at a time.

Two months after his injury, Johnny became ill with respiratory syncytial virus pneumonia. Because the virus is highly contagious, he was moved to an isolation room. Treatment was limited by the layout of the isolation room and by increased agitation but continued to be focused on sitting balance and head righting. Johnny's therapist began working with Johnny on his upper extremity weight bearing in side-sitting and side-lying propped on his forearms. The therapist also began working on transitional movement from side-lying to quadruped.

By approximately 3 months after his injury, athetoid movements were noted in conjunction with difficulty in head and trunk control. Drooling also began. A week later, Johnny was observed to initiate movements, attempting to roll from supine to his side, toward a toy. He required assistance to complete this movement because of fluctuating tone. Johnny's mother was instructed in assisting him with movement transitions and supported standing activities.

Johnny's mother began to voice concerns about the extent of Johnny's disability and related changes in the life of the family. She expressed interest in his transfer to another long-term rehabilitation center after discharge. Nevertheless, Johnny was discharged home because admission to a long-term rehabilitation center could not be arranged. At the time of discharge, 3½ months after the near-drowning, Johnny was able to right his head for 10 seconds at a time and to roll from supine to prone on elbows with minimal assistance. In supported sitting he usually focused on a toy and attempted to manipulate it with greater control on the right than the left. Johnny received outpatient physical, occupational, and speech therapy at a local hospital.

By the time Johnny returned for a follow-up clinic visit 5 months after the near-drowning accident his head control had improved and he was able to right his head in the supported sitting position. Anterior-posterior righting reactions were also beginning to emerge in supported sitting. Johnny was able to roll from prone to supine and return independently. He was able to reach from the prone-on-elbows position.

Two-and-one-half years after the accident, Johnny was ambulating independently with a hemiplegic gait pattern that was ataxic. Ataxia increased as walking speed increased. Although Johnny regained functional mobility skills such as ambulation, he never regained verbal or expressive language skills.

Comments

Johnny's treatment during his hospitalization was focused primarily at impairment reduction through ROM and stretching exercises, serial casting, and exercises and activities that focused on balance improvement. Treatment in which rolling was facilitated as a mobility skill addressed functional limitations. The selection and fitting of a wheelchair was an intervention directed at limiting disability by supporting Johnny's integration into his home and community environments.

References

Bernstein, M, & Laperriere, NJ. A critical appraisal of brachytherapy for pediatric brain tumors. Pediatric Neurosurgery, 91:213–222, 1990.

Berry, MA. Radiation treatment for medulloblastoma: A 21-year review. Journal of Neurosurgery, 55:43–50, 1981.

Beyda, DH. Pathophysiology of near-drowning and treatment of the child with a submersion incident. Critical Care Nursing Clinics of North America, 3:273–280, 1991.

Blume, WT, Girvin, JP, & Kauffman, JCE. Childhood brain tumors presenting as chronic uncontrolled focal seizure disorders. Annals of Neurology, 12:538–549, 1982.

Braun, SL, & Granger, CV. A practical approach to functional assessment in pediatrics. Occupational Therapy Practice, 2:46–51, 1991.

Bray, PF, Carter, S, & Taveras, JM. Brainstem tumors in children. Neurology, 8:1–9, 1958.

Bruininks, RH. Bruininks-Oseretsky Test of Motor Proficiency. Circle Pines, MN: American Guidance Service, 1978.

Campbell, SK. Measurement of motor performance in cerebral palsy. In Forrsberg, H, & Hirschfeld, H (Eds.), Movement Disorders in Children. Basel: Karger, 1992, pp. 264–271.

Castel, JC, & Caille, JM. Imaging of irradiated brain tumors: Value of magnetic resonance imaging. Journal of Neuroradiology, 16:81–132, 1989.

Cohen, AM, Parker, JA, Donahoe, K, Jansons, D, & Kolodny, GM. Three years' experience with all-digital nuclear medicine department. Seminars in Nuclear Medicine, 20:225–233, 1983.

Cohn, AW, Edmonds, JF, & Barker, GA. Near-drowning in cold fresh water: Current treatment regimen. Canadian Anaesthetists Society Journal, 25:259–265, 1980.

Dietz, JH. Adaptive rehabilitation in cancer: A program to improve quality of survival. Postgraduate Medicine, 68:145–153, 1980.

Epstein, F, & McCleary, EL. Intrinsic brain stem tumors of childhood: Surgical indications. Journal of Neurosurgery, 64:11–24, 1986.

Epstein, F, & Wisoff, JH. Intra-axial tumors of the cervicomedullary junction. Journal of Neurosurgery, 67:483–487, 1987.

Epstein, F, & Wisoff, JH. Intrinsic brain stem functions tumors in childhood: Surgical indications. Journal of Neuro-oncology, 6:309–317, 1988.

Ewing-Cobb, L, Lewin, HS, Fletcher, JM, Miner, ME, & Eisenberg, HM. Post-traumatic amnesia in children: Assessment and outcome. Paper presented at the meeting of the International Neuropsychological Society. Vancouver, BC, 1989.

Fisher, DH. Near-drowning. Pediatric Review, 14:148–151, 1993.

Fletcher, JM, Miner, ME, & Ewing-Cobb, L. Age and recovery from head injury in children: Developmental issues. In Levin, HS, Greyman, J, & Eisenberg, HM (Eds.), Neurobehavioral Recovery from Head Injury. New York: Oxford University Press, 1987.

Fokes, EC, & Earle, KM. Ependymomas: Clinical and pathological aspects. Journal of Neurosurgery, 30:585–593, 1969.

Folio, MR, & Fewell, RR. Peabody Developmental Motor Scales and Activity Cards. Allen, TX: DLM Teaching Resources, 1984.

Gjerris, F. Clinical aspects and long-term prognosis in supratentorial tumors in infancy and childhood. Acta Neurologica Scandinavica, 57:445–456, 1978.

Graham-Pole, J, et al. High-dose chemoradiotherapy supported by marrow infusions for advanced neuroblastoma: A pediatric oncology group study. Journal of Clinical Oncology, 9:152–158, 1991.

Gusnard, DA, & Zimmerman, RA. Computed tomography versus magnetic resonance imaging. Clinical Pediatrics, 29:136–157, 1990.

Hagen, C, Makmus, D, Durham, P, & Bowman, K. Levels of cognitive functioning. In Rehabilitation of the Head-Injured Adult. Comprehensive Physical Management. Downey, CA: Professional Staff Association of Rancho Los Amigos Hospital, 1979, pp. 87–90.

Haley, SM, Cioffi, MI, Lewin, JE, & Baryza, MJ. Motor dysfunction in children and adolescents after traumatic brain injury. Journal of Head Trauma Rehabilitation, 5:77–90, 1990.

Haley, SM, Coster, WJ, Ludlow, LH, Halliwanges, JT, & Andrellos, PJ. Pediatric Evaluation of Disability Inventory (PEDI), version 1.0. Boston: New England Medical Center, 1992.

Ingraham, FD, & Matson, DD. Neurosurgery in Infancy and Childhood. Springfield, IL: Charles C Thomas, 1954.

Kageyama, N. Intracranial germinal tumors. Progress in Experimental Tumor Research, 30:255–264, 1987.

Kosmidis, HV, Bouhoutsou, DO, Varroutsi, MC, Papadatos, J, Stefanidis, CG, Vlachos, P, Scardoutsou, A, & Kostakis, A. Vincristine overdose experience with three patients. Pediatric Hematology and Oncology, 8:171–178, 1991.

Lannering, B, Marky, I, & Nordborg, C. Brain tumors in childhood and adolescence in West Sweden, 1970–1984: Epidemiology and survival. Cancer, 66:604–609, 1990.

Lapras, C. Direct surgery for pineal tumors: Occipital-transtentorial approach. Progress in Experimental Tumor Research, 30:268–275, 1987.

Lofgren, J, & Awetnow, NN. Cranial and spinal components of the cerebrospinal fluid pressure–volume curve. Acta Neurologica Scandinavica, 49:575–585, 1973.

Marcal, PV, & Nickell, RE. Assessment of coma and impaired consciousness: A practical scale. Lancet, 2:81–84, 1973.

Marsh, WR, & Laws, ER. Intracranial ependymomas. Progress in Experimental Tumor Research, 30:175–186, 1987.

Martin, P, & Cushing, H. Primary gliomas of chiasm and optic nerves in their intracranial portion. Archives of Ophthalmology, 52:209–229, 1923.

Menkes, JH, & Till, K. Tumors of the nervous system. In Menkes, JH (Ed.), Textbook of Child Neurology. Philadelphia: Lea & Febiger, 1990, pp 526–582.

Packer, RJ, & Findlay, K. Medulloblastoma: Presentation, diagnosis and management. Oncology, 2:35–45, 1988.

Packer, RJ, Sutton, LN, Goldwein, JW, Perilango, G, Borin, G, Ryan, J, Cohen, BH, D'Agio, G, Kramer, ED, & Zimmerman, RA. Improved survival with the use of adjuvant chemotherapy in the treatment of medulloblastoma. Journal of Neurosurgery, 74:4340–4343, 1991.

Pang, D. Pathophysiologic correlates of neurobehavioral syndromes followed closed head injury. In Ylviasaker, M (Ed.), Head Injury Rehabilitation. Austin, TX: Pro-Ed, 1985, pp 3–70.

Safar, P. Resuscitation from clinical death: Pathophysiologic limits and therapeutic potentials. Critical Care Medicine, 16:923–941, 1988.

Shiminsky-Maher, T, Abbott, R, Ursoff, JH, & Epstein, FJ. Current trends in the management of brain stem tumors in childhood. Journal of Neuroscience Nursing, 23:356–362, 1991.

Stein, BM, & Fetall, MR. Therapeutic modalities for pineal region tumors. Clinical Neurosurgery, 32:445–455, 1985.

Stroink, AR. Diagnosis and management of pediatric brain stem gliomas. Journal of Neurosurgery, 19:745–754, 1986.

Stroink, AR. Transependymal benign dorsally exophytic brain stem gliomas in childhood: Diagnosis and treatment recommendations. Journal of Neurosurgery, 20:439–459, 1987.

Teasdale, G, & Jennett, B. Assessment of coma and impaired consciousness: A practical scale. Lancet, 2:81–84, 1974.

Tenny, RT, Laws, ER, Younge, BR, & Rush, JA. The neurosurgical management of optic glioma. Journal of Neurosurgery, 57:452–460, 1982.

Till, K. Craniopharyngiomas. Childs Brain, 9:179–191, 1982.

Chapter 22

Myelodysplasia

KATHLEEN A. HINDERER, PT, MS, MPT
STEVEN R. HINDERER, PT, MD, MS
DAVID B. SHURTLEFF, MD

Children and adolescents with myelodysplasia represent one of the most exciting and challenging groups with which pediatric physical therapists can work. The multiple body systems affected by this malformation make the management of these clients much more complex than the congenital spinal cord defect alone might suggest. The physical therapist plays a key role in monitoring these individuals to prevent primary and secondary impairments and disabilities. The objectives of this chapter are to familiarize the physical therapist with the numerous manifestations of this myelodysplasia, describe its impact on body systems and functional skills, provide developmental expectations and prognosis based on the level of involvement, out-

line the roles of the various disciplines involved in team management, discuss methods of assessment, and highlight treatment strategies for specific problems.

GENERAL OVERVIEW

Types of Myelodysplasia

In *Dorland's Medical Dictionary*, myelodysplasia is described as "defective development of any part (especially the lower segments) of the spinal cord." The various types of myelodysplasia are illustrated in Figure 22–1. *Spina bifida* is a commonly used

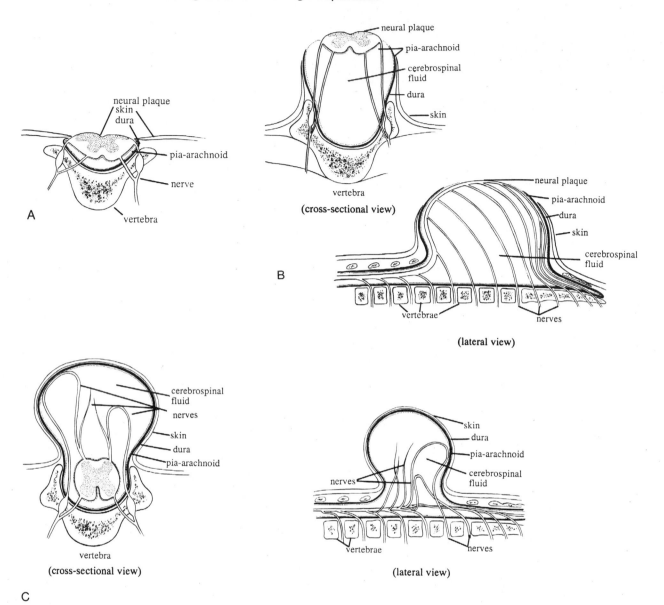

FIGURE 22–1. Types of myelodysplasia. *A,* An illustration of a *myelocele* with no cystic subarachnoid space anterior to the spinal cord as is observed with myelomeningocele. *B,* A *myelomeningocele* may barely protrude from the back or may be a large sessile lesion as pictured here. There is a covering membrane with nerves imbedded in the dome of the sac. These spinal nerves occasionally return to their appropriate neural foramina to exit from the spinal canal. *C,* This type of lesion may be incompletely covered or have a full-thickness skin covering as shown here. When such a lesion is completely skin covered and is associated with *no* paralysis, it is classified as a *meningocele.* Meningoceles have only a few or no nerves attached to the dome of the sac. (Adapted from Shurtleff, DB [Ed.], Myelodysplasias and Exstrophies: Significance, Prevention, and Treatment. Orlando, FL: Grune & Stratton, 1986, pp. 44 and 45.)

term referring to various forms of myelodysplasia. Spina bifida is classified into *aperta* (visible or open) lesions and *occulta* (hidden or not visible) lesions (Lemire et al., 1975; Lichtenstein, 1940). The degree of motor and sensory loss from these

lesions can range from no apparent loss to severe impairment. Regardless of initial level of neurologic impairment, individuals with *any* of these lesions are at risk for further loss of function over time. Paralysis may occur later in life as a complication of abnormal tissue growth (dysplasia) causing pressure on nerves (e.g., lipomatous or dermoid tissue). Lack of proper growth of associated connective tissues around the malformed spinal cord can also cause ischemia and progressive neurologic impairment by tethering of the cord.

Spina bifida aperta is commonly thought of as *myelomeningocele*, which is an open spinal cord defect that usually protrudes dorsally. Myelomeningoceles are not skin covered and are usually associated with spinal nerve paralysis (see Fig. 22–1*A* and *B*). Meninges and nerves can also protrude anteriorly or laterally, so that they are not visible externally but are still associated with nerve paralysis. Some individuals with myelomeningocele do not have associated paralysis. This has been particularly true since the introduction of planned prelabor caesarean delivery of fetuses with spina bifida aperta detected in utero to prevent trauma or infection of the neural sac from vaginal delivery (Luthy et al., 1991).

Meningoceles are also classified as spina bifida aperta. They are skin covered and are initially associated with no paralysis (see Fig. 22–1*C*). Meningoceles contain only membranes or nonfunctional nerves that end in the sac wall (Lemire et al., 1975). Other skin-covered lesions, however, can be associated with paralysis.

The next most common form of myelodysplasia is a *lipoma* of the spinal cord. Lipomas are classified as spina bifida occulta, but most are visible. They may be large or small and present as distinct, subcutaneous masses of fat, frequently associated with abnormal pigmentation of the skin, hirsutism, skin appendages, and dimples above the gluteal cleft. A lipomatous or fibrous tract descends ventrally from the subcutaneous lipoma to varying extents into the subdural space adjacent to the spinal cord. Lipomas of the spinal cord are therefore classified based on the location of the tract. They can be 1) lipomyelomeningoceles with paralysis, 2) lipomeningoceles with no paralysis, 3) lipomas of the filum terminale usually with no paralysis, 4) lipomas of the cauda equina or conus medullaris either with or without paralysis, and 5) myelolipomas that are lipomas within the dural sheath associated with paralysis. Some lipomas involving the spinal cord are not associated with an extension to subcutaneous fat. Lipomas of the spinal cord may or may not be associated with bifid vertebrae (true spina bifida).

Diastematomyelia is a fibrous, cartilaginous, or bony band or spicule separating the spinal cord into hemicords, each surrounded by a dural sac. It can occur as an isolated defect along with vertebral anomalies or in conjunction with either myelo-

meningocele or lipomyelomeningocele. Depending on the associated involvement of the spinal cord and meninges, diastematomyelia may be associated with paralysis initially or progressive weakness can develop later in occulta lesions as a result of cord tethering.

The least common of the myelodysplasias are separate or septated cysts. These *myelocystoceles* are separate from the central canal of the spinal cord and from the subarachnoid space. They occur in the low lumbar and sacral area and are skin covered. They may or may not be associated with nerve impairment or lipomas of the spinal cord. When a myelocystocele is associated with a primitive gut and an open abdomen, it is classified as an *exstrophy of the cloaca*. When the bony elements of the sacrum are missing or abnormal, such myelocystic lesions are termed *sacral agenesis*.

Pathoembryology

Embryologically, myelodysplastic lesions can be related to two different processes of nervous system formation: abnormal neurulation or canalization. *Neurulation* is the folding of ectoderm (primitive skin and associated structures) on each side of the notochord (primitive spinal cord) to form a tube that extends from the hindbrain to the second sacral vertebra. Meningoceles can therefore occur both over the skull and along the spinal column. Encephaloceles (containing brain if along the midline of the skull) and myelomeningoceles, which can occur along the spinal canal from the C-1 to S-2 vertebrae, result from a failure of complete entubulation with associated abnormal mesodermal (primitive connective tissue, muscle, and nervous tissue) development. Abnormal mesodermal development produces epidermal sinus tracts, lipomas, and diastematomyelia, as well as unfused posterior vertebral laminae (i.e., true spina bifida) (Lemire et al., 1975). Neurulation occurs early in development, before the 28th day of gestation.

The spinal cord distal to the S-2 vertebra develops by *canalization*. Groups of cells in the dorsal, central midline of the mesoderm, distal to the S-2 vertebra, become nerve cells. These cells clump together into masses, which develop cystic structures that join to form many canals. The canals ultimately fuse into one tubular structure that joins with the distal end of the spinal cord, which was developing from the neurulation process described previously. Failure of proper canalization, with subsequent retrogressive development of this region, embryologically explains the occurrence of skin-covered meningoceles, lipomas of the spinal cord, and myelocystoceles, all of which most frequently develop caudal to the L-3 vertebra (Lemire et al., 1975).

The much better formed, essentially normal, central nervous system (CNS) observed in lesions associated with abnormal canalization and the frequency of CNS malformations (e.g., Arnold-Chiari type II, mental retardation, cranial nerve palsies, and hydrocephalus) associated with neurulation can be explained by the way that neurulation takes place. The neural crests first fuse at approximately the C-1 vertebra, and closure of the neural tube progresses simultaneously in cephalad and caudal directions. The same embryologic neurulation processes are simultaneously forming the CNS from the tectal plate to the midlumbar area. It is therefore logical that an influence sufficient to interfere with neurulation along the spinal canal would also interfere with development of the cephalad end, producing CNS malformations above the spinal cord level, which are commonly exhibited in this population (Lemire et al., 1975). Because canalization occurs by different embryologic processes at a different time period than neurulation, any factor interfering with canalization will not necessarily impact neurulation so that the CNS forms normally above the midlumbar area.

Etiology

The cause of canalization disorders is unknown. This discussion therefore focuses on disorders of neurulation and, in particular, on myelomeningocele. These causes may also apply to other neural tube defects that can result from defective neurulation (i.e., anencephaly, encephalocele, meningocele, lipomyelomeningocele; all with or without diastematomyelia). For brevity, we refer to all these lesions throughout this chapter as MM for *myelo-meningocele* and its associated malformations (Shurtleff et al., 1986a).

GENETICS

MM is often associated with genetic abnormalities, including chromosomal aberrations as well as other classic "syndromes." Each child born with MM, therefore, warrants a careful physical examination by a pediatrician because the "syndrome" is usually more important than the spinal lesion for defining prognosis. The recurrence risk for siblings in the United States is 2 to 3% (Shurtleff et al., 1986a).

The occurrence of MM varies among races and regions of the world. African blacks have the lowest incidence of 1 in 10,000. Celts (Eastern Irish, Western Scots, and all Welsh) have a birth incidence recorded as high as 1 in 80 in the recent past. The Spanish also have a high birth incidence; however, these patients have unusually good leg function and minimal CNS abnormalities considering their thoracic and high lumbar level lesions. Sikhs living in Vancouver, British Columbia, have another form of MM, with a higher frequency in birth incidence than many other genetically related groups. One can conclude from these data that either there are many different genetic causes for MM or that there are many different genetically determined responses to one or more teratogens (Shurtleff et al., 1986a).

TERATOGENS

Teratogens can cause MM. Excess maternal alcohol intake can produce a classic fetal alcohol syndrome with MM. Ingestion of valproic acid (an anticonvulsant medication) during pregnancy is also associated with an increased birth incidence of MM. Many other possible teratogens have been studied, but inadequate descriptions of the pathology of the lesions and the relative infrequency of their occurrence have resulted in inconclusive observations. The rachitic lesion illustrated by Jacobson and Berlin (1972) suggests that the MM they observed among progeny of street-drug abusers is a specific entity that is likely due to nutritional deprivation, teratogen(s), or a combination of these influences. More studies combining detailed family histories, pathologic anatomy, and detailed physical examinations need to be conducted to determine the relative contribution of teratogens to MM formation (Shurtleff et al., 1986a).

NUTRITIONAL DEFICIENCIES

Folic acid deficiency has been identified as a cause of MM in some populations. A significant decrease in the incidence of MM births and abortions was observed for MM diagnosed prenatally in the United Kingdom during a placebo-controlled trial of prenatal folic acid administration (CIBA, 1994; MRC Vitamin Study Research Group, 1991). With the introduction of more foods containing folic acid in the Celtic regions of the United Kingdom, particularly during winter and early spring when potatoes are scarce (potatoes are high in folic acid and a staple of the diet in this region), there has been a decrease in the birth incidence of MM predating the research on folic acid supplementation (Elwood & Elwood, 1980). The decrease in birth incidence in the United Kingdom reflects a current worldwide trend. Conflicting reports raise the question whether the European and United Kingdom studies regarding the benefit of supplementation of folic acid can be applied to the culturally and genetically more diverse population of the United States where there are known racial and regional differences in the birth incidence of MM (Birth Defects & Genetic Diseases Branch of Birth Defects & Developmental Disabilities Office, 1991; Mills et al., 1989; Milunsky et al., 1989; Seller & Nevin, 1984).

Incidence and Prevalence

Superimposed on a general worldwide decrease in the birth incidence of MM are a number of influences to cause both a reduction in birth incidence and increased prevalence. Better nutrition mentioned earlier for the Celtic region of the United Kingdom and Ireland applies to many areas of the industrialized world. Wider availability of maternal serum α-fetoprotein screening and more highly refined resolution of diagnostic ultrasonography for fetal examination have given parents an option to terminate pregnancies because their fetus had MM (Main & Mennuti, 1986; Nyberg et al., 1988). Conversely, prenatal diagnosis has allowed other parents to select prelabor caesarean section, avoiding trauma to the neural sac from vaginal delivery. The outcome of prelabor caesarean delivery has been children with less paralysis and with minimal risk for CNS infection, both of which were previously a cause for increased morbidity and early death (Luthy et al., 1991). Improved medical care has allowed for increased survival and, secondarily, an increased prevalence. Incidence at birth in the United States has been reported to range from 0.4 to 0.9 per 1000 births, depending on the reporting source (Shurtleff et al., 1986a).

Diagnostic Techniques

The past decade has altered the management of MM from a postnatal crisis of horrendous magnitude to a prenatal option of either pregnancy termination or improved pregnancy outcome by prelabor caesarean section birth. This advance has been made possible by widespread use of maternal serum α-fetoprotein screening and improved resolution of ultrasonography (Main & Mennuti, 1986). Unfortunately, this type of screening will not detect skin-covered neural defects such as meningoceles or canalization defects distal to the S-2 vertebra.

Technical improvements are being made rapidly in ultrasonography so that minor variations in the frontal bones of the fetus and encapsulation of the midbrain by the cerebellum can be interpreted as the "lemon" and "banana" signs (Nyberg et al., 1988). These ultrasonographic signs are more accurate in defining the cranial malformations associated with MM than in detecting abnormalities of the spine. As discussed in the section on pathoembryology, these ultrasonographic signs are pertinent to neural tube defects cephalad to the S-2 vertebra (i.e., neurulation defects) but not to canalization defects, which are usually not associated with cranial malformations responsible for the Arnold-Chiari type II malformation (Shurtleff, 1986e), the cause of the "lemon" and "banana" signs. Some spinal dysraphic states and dorsal lumbosacral masses consistent with canalization defects such as myelocystocele or lipomyelomeningocele can be identified with ultrasonography. Other anomalies consistent with syndromes or organ malformations that are incompatible with survival beyond intrauterine life (e.g., anencephaly) can also be detected.

A third modality for prenatal diagnosis, amniotic fluid analysis, is critical in the evaluation of a fetus with a neural tube defect. Up to 10% of fetuses with a neural tube defect, detected in the first half of the second trimester or before, have an associated chromosome error, usually trisomy 13 or 18 (Luthy et al., 1991). Chromosome analysis of amniotic cells is therefore essential to the parental decision-making process regarding abortion of the pregnancy. From the same amniotic fluid specimen obtained for chromosome analysis, the acetylcholinesterase level can be determined. This test is more accurate than determination of the amniotic fluid level of α-fetoprotein used previously because the former is positive only in a fetus with an open neural tube defect (Main & Mennuti, 1986). The presence of a dorsal spine lesion and a negative result of an acetylcholinesterase test suggest a skin-covered meningocele or other skin-covered MM, which is an indication for normal vaginal delivery. An MM lesion containing nerves protruding dorsal to the plane of the back, in the presence of fetal knee or ankle function observed on ultrasonography, warrants prelabor caesarean section, sterile delivery, and closure of the open back lesion to preserve nerve function (Luthy et al., 1991).

IMPAIRMENTS

The discussions of pathoembryology and diagnosis describe the potential involvement of the brain and brain stem in addition to the spinal cord in individuals with MM. The multifocal involvement of the CNS results in several possible complex problems, making the care of these individuals more challenging and substantially different from children with traumatic spinal cord injuries. The broad spectrum of problems encountered with MM requires a multidisciplinary team approach in a comprehensive care outpatient clinic setting. In this section the variety of impairments that can occur with MM are described. In addition, general assessment and management issues related to each impairment are discussed. *Impairment*, for the purpose of this discussion, is defined as an abnormality of body system functions, whereas *functional limitation* is the inability to perform functional tasks as a consequence of impairments. Functional limitations and disabilities encountered at specific age levels, along with age-specific assessment and management issues, are discussed in subsequent sections of this chapter.

Musculoskeletal Deformities

Spinal and lower limb deformities and joint contractures occur frequently in children with MM. Orthopaedic deformities and joint contractures negatively affect positioning, body image, weight bearing (both in sitting and standing), activities of daily living (ADL), energy expenditure, and mobility from infancy through adulthood. Several factors contribute to abnormal posture, limb deformity, and joint contractures, including muscle imbalance secondary to neurologic dysfunction, progressive neurologic dysfunction, intrauterine positioning, coexisting congenital malformations, arthrogryposis, habitually assumed postures after birth, reduced or absent active joint motion, and deformities after fractures (Mayfield, 1991; Shurtleff, 1986d). The upper limbs can also be involved as a result of spasticity or poor postural habits. The upper limb region most likely to have restricted motion is the shoulder girdle due to overuse of the arms for weight bearing and poor postural habits.

Postural stability is essential to effectively perform functional tasks. Symmetric alignment is important to minimize joint stress and deforming forces and to permit muscles to function at their optimal length. Uncorrected postural deficits can result in joint contractures and deformities, stretch weakness, and musculoskeletal pain. Deficits that may appear insignificant during childhood often become magnified once an individual has adult body proportions, resulting in functional limitations and discomfort (e.g., low back pain resulting from an increased lumbar lordosis and hip flexion contractures). Consequently, limb, neck, and trunk range of motion (ROM), muscle extensibility, and joint alignment should be monitored throughout the life span so that appropriate interventions can be implemented as indicated.

Typical postural problems include forward head, rounded shoulders, kyphosis, scoliosis, excessive lordosis, anterior pelvic tilt, rotational deformities

of the hip or tibia (in-toeing, out-toeing, or windswept positions), flexed hips and knees, and pronated feet. It is important to observe posture and postural control after a given position has been maintained for a period of time to determine the effects of fatigue. Static and dynamic balance should be observed in sitting, four-point positioning, kneeling, half-kneeling, and standing, as well as during transitions between these positions. Symmetry and weight distribution should also be noted. In addition, typical sleeping and sitting positions should be identified to determine if habitual positioning is contributing to postural or joint deformities. Photographs or videotapes of sitting and standing postures are often useful to document current status and to provide a visual baseline for future reference.

Postural deviations and contractures that are typical for individual lesion levels are summarized below. Individuals with high-level lesions (thoracic to L-2) often have knee flexion, abduction, and external rotation contractures, knee flexion contractures, and ankle plantar flexion contractures. The lumbar spine is typically lordotic. Individuals with mid- to low-lumbar (L-3–L-5) lesion levels often have hip and knee flexion contractures, an increased lumbar lordosis, genu and calcaneal valgus malalignment, and a pronated position of the foot when bearing weight. They often walk with a pronounced crouched gait and bear weight primarily on their calcaneus. Individuals with sacral level lesions often have mild hip and knee flexion contractures and an increased lumbar lordosis, and the ankle and foot position can either be in varus or valgus, combined with a pronated or supinated forefoot. They may walk with a mild crouch gait and may bear weight primarily on their calcaneus unless plantar flexor muscles are at least grade 3/5.

Scoliosis occurring with MM can be congenital or acquired; the congenital form is usually related to underlying vertebral anomalies and the curve is often inflexible, whereas the acquired type is usually caused by muscle imbalance and the curve is flexible until skeletal maturity is reached (Mayfield, 1991), at which point little further progression is usually observed (Shurtleff, 1986d). Scoliosis is more frequently observed in higher lesion level groups and becomes more prevalent and increasingly severe with age in all groups (Mayfield, 1991).

Orthotic treatment, usually with a bivalved Silastic thoracolumbosacral body orthosis, is helpful in maintaining improved trunk position for functional activities but does not prevent progression of acquired spinal deformity (Mayfield, 1991). For children with progressive spinal deformities, orthotic management is continued until the child reaches a sufficient age to allow surgical fusion of the spine to prevent further progression of these deformities. Long spinal fusions before the skeletal age of 10 result in greater loss of trunk height because of ablation of the growth plates of vertebral bodies included in the fusion mass (Mayfield, 1991). Additionally, surgery at too young a skeletal age is associated with an increased frequency of instrumentation failure as a result of fragile bones and skin breakdown over the bulky spinal instrumentation (Mayfield, 1991). The ideal minimum age for spinal fusion is 10 to 11 years old in girls and 12 to 13 years old in boys (Mayfield, 1991). In general, children with spina bifida reach puberty and their growth spurt earlier than their able-bodied peers, so that only minimal truncal shortening occurs as a consequence of long spinal fusion when it is performed at the appropriate age.

Other spinal deformities that can occur in conjunction with, or separate from, scoliosis are kyphosis and lordosis deformities (Fig. 22–2). Kyphosis can occur in the lumbar spine with reversal of the lumbar lordosis, or the kyphosis can be more diffusely distributed over the entire spine. Hyperlordosis of the lumbar spine is another commonly observed deformity. Like scoliosis, both kyphosis and lordosis are more commonly observed in children with higher spinal lesions and the curves tend to progress with age (Mayfield, 1991). Severe kyphosis and scoliosis can limit chest wall expansion with consequent restriction of lung ventilation and frequent respiratory infections. This restrictive lung disease can limit exercise tolerance and can be life threatening in extreme cases (Mayfield, 1991).

Hip joints also are prone to deformity in children with MM. Children with high lumbar lesions (L-1, L-2) have unopposed flexion and adduction forces that gradually push the femoral head superiorly and posteriorly. The resulting contractures and secondary bony deformities of the proximal femur and acetabulum can lead to subluxation or dislocation (Fig. 22–3).

In children with hip subluxation or dislocation, long-term follow-up studies have indicated that reduction of the hips is not a prerequisite for ambulation. Mayfield (1991) states that a level pelvis and a good ROM are more important for function than hip reduction. Furthermore, he states that the presence of the femoral head in the acetabulum does not necessarily improve ROM at the hip or the ability to ambulate. Additionally, unlike in children with cerebral palsy, it does not appear to impact the amount of orthotic support, hip pain, or gait deviation (Ryan et al., 1991). The indications for hip surgery in children with MM continue to be controversial; however, a basic principle practiced at many centers is to operate only on children with a lesion level at or below L-3, when quadriceps muscle function is present, because these children are more likely to be functional ambulators into adulthood (Mayfield, 1991; Shurtleff, 1986d). An asymmetric pelvis caused by unilateral subluxation or dislocation, which interferes with sitting or

FIGURE 22–2. Spinal deformities. *A,* Collapsing type of lordoscoliosis. *B,* Kyphotic spinal deformity.

A   B

FIGURE 22–3. Lower limb deformities. *A*, Hip dislocation. *B*, Hip dysplasia and subluxation. *C*, Genu varus. *D*, Genu valgus. *E*, Equinovarus. *F*, Calcaneal valgus.

standing posture and contributes to scoliosis, is another potential indication for surgical relocation of the hip, *regardless* of lesion level or ambulatory potential.

Shurtleff (1986d) evaluated the frequency of all types of hip contractures in large numbers of children with various spinal lesion level groups. He noted that contractures measured in infancy tended to decrease in severity until approximately age 3 to 4 years, then increased to much higher values by adolescence. The initial decrease in severity of hip contractures can potentially be explained as a normal physiologic phenomenon resulting from intrauterine positioning. The increase in severity of contractures by adolescence, however, is of special concern to physical therapists. Mild contractures of minimal functional significance in young children can increase dramatically during later childhood and adolescence, necessitating persistent treatment and follow-up by the therapist to prevent significant functional loss. Consequently, physical therapists should be proactive in preventing the progression of contractures. Thoracic and high lumbar (L-1, L-2) groups of children have a higher incidence and greater severity of contractures owing to unopposed iliopsoas function, regardless of whether they were participating in a standing program or not (Liptak et al., 1992). Shurtleff (1986d) reports progressively declining frequency and severity of contractures in groups of children with lesions at L-3, L-4-5, and sacral levels, respectively. An unexpected finding from Shurtleff's study was that only a certain percentage of children in each lesion level group had hip contractures, subluxation, or both. These relative percentages were not altered by surgical procedures on the hip and stayed constant across age groups. No clear reasons were discerned why certain individuals were susceptible to contractures while others with similar neurologic function were not.

The knee joints frequently have contractures or deformities in children with MM. These include both flexion and extension contractures; the former more commonly occur in children who primarily use a wheelchair for mobility (Liptak et al., 1992), while the latter often occur after periods of immobility from fractures, decubitus ulcers, or surgical procedures. Varus and valgus deformities (see Fig. 22-3) are also observed. As described earlier for the hip joints, Shurtleff (1986d) studied the frequency of knee contractures and deformities in children with different lesion levels. An initial decrease from the contractures measured in infants was also noted at the knees, with the lowest prevalence occurring at age 4 to 5 years for patients with L-3 or higher lesions, and at age 2 to 3 years for

children with lesions below L-3. The frequency and severity of contractures increased in all groups from early childhood into adolescence. Knee joint contractures occurred in 65 to 70% of the thoracic and high lumbar groups by age 6 to 8, 20 to 25% of the L-4-5 group by age 9 to 12, and sporadically among the children with sacral level lesions. Valgus and varus deformities were most frequently observed in the L-3 and above groups, with a slight increase during adolescence.

Deformities of the ankles and feet can occur in both ambulatory and nonambulatory children and are most common in children with lesion levels at L-5 and above (Shurtleff, 1986d). Partial innervation and consequent muscle imbalance determine the type of deformity that occurs. Even with surgical correction these deformities will recur unless the deforming forces are removed. Progressive ankle and foot deformities can also be observed in conjunction with the development of spasticity and motor strength loss associated with tethering of the spinal cord. Children with "skip" lesions (see section on motor paralysis) are particularly prone to progressive foot deformities (Shurtleff, 1986d).

A variety of foot and ankle deformities can occur (see Fig. 22-3), including ankle equinovarus (clubfeet), forefoot varus or valgus, forefoot supination or pronation, calcaneal varus or valgus, pes cavus and planus, and claw-toe deformities. The most frequent contracture observed is of the ankle plantar flexor muscles. The frequency of foot deformities varies from 20 to 50% between lesion level groups (Shurtleff, 1986d). Although some deformities are more frequently associated with certain neurosegmental levels (e.g., clubfeet in thoracic and high lumbar lesions, claw-toes in sacral lesions), all types of ankle and foot deformities are observed in children at every lesion level. The presence of ankle and foot deformities can greatly impact sitting and standing posture, balance, mobility, and shoe fit, regardless of lesion level. Weight-bearing forces often result in ankle and foot deformities. Even partial weight bearing on wheelchair footrests in poor alignment over time can result in deformities and even in decubiti. Consequently, achieving a plantigrade position of the feet is a priority, regardless of ambulatory status. Orthoses and assistive devices should be adjusted properly to maintain neutral subtalar alignment and a plantigrade foot position.

Torsional deformities are common. Excessive foot progression angles and windswept positions of the lower limbs are often present (Fig. 22-4) as a result of hip anteversion, hip retroversion, or tibial torsion. These torsional deformities negatively impact sitting and standing balance, weight distribu

A

B

C

FIGURE 22-4. Torsional deformities. *A.* Femoral neck ante-version. *B.* External tibial torsion. *C,* Internal tibial torsion.

tion, and walking. The reader is referred to the article by Cusick and Stuberg (1992) for factors that contribute to torsional deformities in individuals with developmental disabilities, assessment procedures, normative values, and management suggestions.

Joint alignment and evidence of abnormal joint stress are often most apparent during dynamic activities, such as walking or wheelchair propulsion. Joint stresses are often magnified when walking on uneven surfaces, stairs, or curbs. Observing wear patterns on shoes and orthoses can provide additional clues to abnormal stress and malalignment. If joint deformities are supple, they may respond to stretching, combined with orthoses or positioning splints to maintain alignment. Fixed deformities may respond to serial casting (e.g., foot deformities) but will often require surgical intervention (e.g., scoliosis, unilateral hip dislocation, or tibial torsion). Habitual positions that produce deforming forces should be avoided, including the "frog-leg" position in prone or supine, W-sitting, ring sitting, heel sitting, or cross-legged sitting. If muscle imbalance is severe and the deforming forces are not effectively counteracted by stretching, strengthening, or positioning, muscle transfers may be indicated (e.g., partial transfer of the anterior tibialis muscle to the calcaneus to achieve a plantigrade foot position by balancing the unopposed dorsiflexion force in a child with L-5 motor function).

There are several reasons for maintaining joint ROM. Limited ROM can interfere with ADL, bed mobility, and transfers. Bed mobility is more efficient and self-care is easier for individuals who have maintained their flexibility (Hinderer & Hinderer, 1988). Restricted ROM, combined with muscle weakness, can result in poor postural habits and gait deviations. Adequate ROM needs to be maintained to perform ADL, such as bathing and toileting. Restricted joint motion can result in overlengthening of weak muscles, not permitting them to function in the optimal range of the length-tension curve. Limited ROM may result in discomfort, especially when lying down (e.g., tight hip flexors pulling on the lumbar spine). Severe contractures also can negatively impact body image. Contractures that may seem insignificant during childhood may become functionally limiting once the individual has adult-sized body proportions (e.g., knee extension contractures can interfere with the ability to maneuver in a wheelchair). In extreme cases, difficulty in managing paralyzed limbs due to joint contractures can put individuals at risk for skin breakdown and possibly amputations because of the increased incidence of injury (Hinderer et al., 1988). The impact of limited ROM on func-

tional performance should be considered before deciding whether treatment is indicated.

ROM and positioning of paralytic limbs should be done carefully, without excessive force, to avoid fractures (Schneider, 1985). Caution should also be exercised when adducting the hips to avoid hip dislocation. The prone hip extension test (Staheli, 1977) for measuring hip extension is the method of choice in this population because of interference of spinal and pelvic deformities and lower limb spasticity with the traditional Thomas test method (Bartlett et al., 1985). Ankle ROM should always be measured with the ankle joint in subtalar neutral so measurements are comparable.

There are several ways to minimize musculoskeletal trauma and reduce the incidence of acquired orthopaedic deformities. Improving traction of the hands by providing biking gloves for community wheelchair mobility reduces the grip forces required for wheelchair propulsion. Wheelchair seat positions influence propulsion effectiveness and the amount of stress on upper limb joints and muscles (Masse et al., 1992). For ambulators, shoes with nonskid soles improve foot traction. Symmetrical neutral joint alignment should be maintained in both sitting and standing via appropriate orthotics or seating devices. It is important to avoid shifting weight to one leg when standing and to avoid crossing the legs when sitting. Extreme ROM should be avoided, especially when bearing weight. Crutch and walker handgrips should be angled to avoid hyperextension of the wrists, and weight should be distributed across a broad, cushioned area. Orthoses should provide total contact to minimize the risk of development of pressure areas. Excessive pressure on tendons and the palms of the hand should be avoided to reduce the risk of developing carpal tunnel syndrome. Overhead reaching and work activities should be minimized by adapting the home, school, and work environments. In addition, long-distance mobility options need to be provided to reduce joint stresses. When sitting, weight bearing should be symmetric, pelvic tilt should be neutral with a slight lumbar lordosis, the hips and knees at 90°, and the feet flat on the floor. Good lumbar support should be provided. Inclining the seat backward 15° minimizes stress on the lumbar spine and helps keep the pelvis seated back in the chair (Chaffin & Andersson, 1991). Tilting the desk or table top upward improves the position of the upper trunk, head, and shoulders.

Osteoporosis

Decreased bone mineral density, thought to be secondary to hypotonic or flaccid musculature combined with decreased loading of long bones from altered mobility, is frequently observed in children with MM and often results in osteoporotic fractures. Stuberg (1992) suggests that standing programs are beneficial for children with developmental disabilities. He reports that the use of a standing program for 60 minutes, 4 or 5 times per week, appears to increase bone mineral density and enhances acetabular development in children with cerebral palsy. These issues need to be studied further in the MM population, however. Bone responses in children with flaccid paralysis may be quite different. Rosenstein and associates (1987) examined this issue in the MM population and reported that bone mineral density was 38 to 44% higher in household or community ambulators, compared with nonfunctional ambulators (exercise-only ambulators or nonambulators). Because the effects of lesion level were not controlled in this study, the potential contribution of muscle activity versus weight-bearing status to the differences in bone mineral density cannot be determined. In addition, neither study addressed the issue of reduction of the incidence of osteoporotic fractures.

Studying the frequency of fractures is a more direct and clinically significant method of examining the benefits of standing programs. Shurtleff (1986d) raised the question "Are fractures less common among those patients in standing or ambulatory programs than among similarly paralyzed sedentary peers?" Asher and Olson (1983) showed no correlation between fractures and the use of wheelchairs. DeSouza and Carroll (1976) reported no fractures in 7 nonambulators and 38 fractures in 16 ambulators. Their data imply that exposure to forces that can produce fractures (i.e., upright mobility) is the important risk factor for fractures, rather than the level of flaccid paralysis, as would be expected. Liptak and associates (1992) found no difference in the frequency of fractures between a group of children who were wheelchair users and a comparable group of children who ambulated with orthoses. Clinically, the use of standing frames, parapodiums, or hip-knee-ankle-foot orthoses (HKAFOs) in children with high lumbar and thoracic lesions does not appear warranted for the purpose of fracture prevention. For children with lower lumbar and sacral lesion levels, for whom upright positioning and mobility is an important functional skill, undue restriction of physical activity for fear of a fracture is not indicated. The fact that passive weight bearing does not decrease the risk of fractures in these children makes sense if one considers that bone density is more likely maintained by torque generated from volitional muscle activity. Active muscle contraction generates forces through the long bones that are several fold greater than the forces from passive weight bearing.

Motor Paralysis

The inherently obvious manifestation of MM is the paraplegia resulting from the spinal cord malformation. Upper limb weakness can also occur in this population, *regardless* of lesion level, and is often a sign of progressive neurologic dysfunction. Knowledge of the motor lesion level is useful for predicting associated abnormalities and for prognostication of functional outcome. A detailed discussion regarding developmental and functional expectations for each motor lesion level is provided later in the section on determinants of outcome and prognosis. Strategies for assessing strength and planning intervention programs to enhance motor function are provided in the section on specific evaluation and management strategies.

The motor level is defined as the lowest intact, functional neuromuscular segment. For example, an L-4 level indicates that the fourth lumbar nerve and the myotome it innervates are functioning, whereas segments below L-4 are not intact. Table 22-1 provides the International Myelodysplasia Study Group (IMSG) criteria for assigning motor levels from manual muscle strength test results (IMSG, 1993). The IMSG criteria have been shown to best reflect the innervation patterns of individuals with MM as opposed to other spinal segment classification systems. MM spinal lesions can be asymmetric when motor or sensory function of the right and left sides of the body are compared. Consequently, motor function should be classified individually for the right and left sides.

Neuromuscular involvement of individuals with MM may present in one of three ways: 1) lesions resembling complete cord transection, 2) incomplete lesions, and 3) skip lesions (Shurtleff, 1986d). Lesions resembling complete cord transection present as normal function down to a particular level, below which there is flaccid paralysis, loss of sensation, and absent reflexes. Incomplete lesions have a mixed presentation of spasticity and volitional control. Skip lesions are also observed, where more caudal segments are functioning despite the presence of one or more nonfunctional segments interposed between the intact more cephalad spinal segments. Individual "skip" motor lesions present either with isolated function of muscles noted below the last functional level of the lesion or with inadequate strength of muscle groups that have innervation higher than the lowest functioning group (Patient Data Management System, 1994). Conse-

TABLE 22–1. INTERNATIONAL MYELODYSPLASIA STUDY GROUP CRITERIA FOR ASSIGNING MOTOR LEVELS

Motor Level	Criteria for Assigning Motor Levels
T-10 or above T-11	Determined by sensory level and/or palpation of abdominal muscles.
T-12	Some pelvic control is present in sitting or supine (this may come from the abdominals or paraspinal muscles). Hip hiking from the quadratus lumborum may also be present.
L-1	Weak iliopsoas muscle function is present (grade 2).
L-1–2	Exceeds criteria for L-1 but does not meet L-2 criteria.*
L-2	Iliopsoas, sartorius, and the hip adductors all must be grade 3 or better.
L-3	Meets or exceeds the criteria for L-2 plus the quadriceps are grade 3 or better.
L-3–4	Exceeds criteria for L-3 but does not meet L-4 criteria.
L-4	Meets or exceeds the criteria for L-3 and the medial hamstrings or the tibialis anterior is grade 3 or better. A weak peroneus tertius may also be seen.
L-4–5	Exceeds criteria for L-4 but does not meet L-5 criteria.
L-5	Meets or exceeds the criteria for L-4 and has lateral hamstring strength of grade 3 or better plus one of the following: gluteus medius grade 2 or better, peroneus tertius grade 4 or better, or tibialis posterior grade 3 or better.
L-5–S-1	Exceeds criteria for L-5 but does not meet S-1 criteria.
S-1	Meets or exceeds the criteria for L-5 plus at least two of the following: gastrocnemius/soleus grade 2 or better, gluteus medius grade 3 or better, or gluteus maximus grade 2 or better (can pucker the buttocks).
S-1–2	Exceeds criteria for S-1 but does not meet S-2 criteria.
S-2	Meets or exceeds the criteria for S-1, the gastrocnemius/soleus must be grade 3 or better, and gluteus medius and maximus are grade 4 or better.
S-2–3	All of the lower limb muscle groups are of normal strength (may be grade 4 in one or two groups). Also includes normal-appearing infants who are too young to be bowel and bladder trained (see "no loss").
"No loss"	Meets all of the criteria for S-2–3 and has no bowel or bladder dysfunction.

*When description states "meets criteria . . .," strength of muscles listed for preceding levels should be increasing respectively.

Adapted with permission from Patient Data Management System. Myelodysplasia Study Data Collection Criteria and Instructions, 1994. (Available from D.B. Shurtleff, MD, Professor, Dept. of Pediatrics, Univ. of Washington, Seattle, WA 98195.)

quently, it is important to evaluate muscles with lower innervation than the last functional level, to determine if a "skip" lesion exists. The presence of

spasticity and reflexes should also be carefully documented.

McDonald and associates (1991b) demonstrated that muscle strength grades for the gluteus medius and medial hamstring muscles correlate more highly with strength grades of the hip adductors, hip flexors, and knee extensors than lower limb anterior compartment muscles that have been previously described as being innervated by the L-4, L-5, and sacral nerve roots. These data potentially explain the clinical observation that individuals with MM often have functional strength in the gluteus medius and medial hamstrings, despite having weak or nonactive lower limb anterior compartment muscles. It was concluded from this study that it is more useful clinically to group individuals with MM by the strength of specific muscle groups, as outlined in Table 22–1, rather than by traditional neurosegmental levels.

The measurement of muscle strength is an essential component of the evaluation of individuals with MM, who are at risk for loss of function from CNS complications. Careful and reliable serial measurements of both upper and lower limb muscle strength can aid in early detection of decreased function. Muscle strength test results are used in this population to determine the level of motor function (see Table 22–1), to identify muscle imbalance, and to predict present and future functional capabilities in the course of planning orthopaedic, surgical, and therapeutic management.

Sensory Deficits

Sensory deficits are often not clear-cut in this population, because sensory levels often do not correlate with motor levels and there may be "skip" areas that lack sensation. Because "skip" areas can occur within a given dermatome, it is important to test all dermatomes and multiple sites within a given dermatome to have an accurate baseline evaluation. Deficits should be recorded on a dermatome chart with areas of absent and decreased sensation color coded for the various sensory modalities (e.g., light touch, pinprick, vibration, and thermal). Proprioception and kinesthetic sense should also be evaluated in both the upper and lower extremities.

Based on the results of a study conducted on 30 adults with MM, testing with both light touch and pinprick stimuli is not necessary in this population because there is little discriminating value for detecting insensate areas (Hinderer & Hinderer, 1990). In contrast, vibratory stimuli could be felt one dermatome below light touch and pinprick sensation. Based on these results, vibration sensation should be evaluated in addition to either light touch or pinprick sensation.

Loss of sensation can be another sign of CNS complications and consequently should be closely monitored on a regular basis. It is important for individuals with MM to be aware of their sensory deficits and to be taught techniques to compensate by substituting other sensory modalities (e.g., vision). The impact of decreased sensation on safety should be emphasized, especially when checking temperature (e.g., bath water or when sitting near a fireplace) and when barefoot. Skin inspection and pressure relief techniques should be taught early so they are incorporated into the daily routine. The importance of pressure relief cushions and sitting push-ups for pressure relief should be emphasized. Proper management of lower limbs and joint protection techniques should be taught when learning how to perform ADL, such as transfers.

The impact of sensory deficits on functional performance should be kept in mind when teaching functional tasks. Individuals with MM may rely heavily on vision to compensate for sensory deficits (Shaffer et al., 1986). They may lack kinesthetic acuity that permits subconscious completion of many repetitive motor tasks. Consequently, visual attention may not be available to be directed at other factors in the environment (Andersen & Plewis, 1977). Adding small amounts of weight to the ankles or a walker may enhance proprioceptive awareness and facilitate gait training. Use of patellar tendon–bearing orthoses (Fig. 22–5) instead of traditional ankle-foot orthoses (AFOs) may also facilitate foot placement for individuals with innervation through L-3 because the orthosis contacts the skin in an area of intact sensation.

Hydrocephalus

Hydrocephalus is excessive accumulation of cerebrospinal fluid (CSF) in the ventricles of the brain. Approximately 25% or more of children with MM are born with hydrocephalus. An additional 60% develop it after surgical closure of their back lesion (Reigel, 1993). If left untreated, the continued expansion of the ventricles can cause loss of cerebral cortex with additional cognitive and functional impairment. Cerebellar hypoplasia with caudal displacement of the hindbrain through the foramen magnum, known as the Arnold-Chiari type II malformation, is usually associated with hydrocephalus.

The hydrocephalus will occasionally arrest spontaneously; however, 80 to 90% of children with

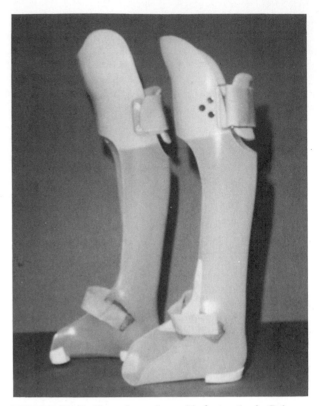

FIGURE 22–5. Ground-reaction ankle-foot orthosis. Polypropylene patellar tendon–bearing ground-reaction ankle-foot orthoses molded with the foot in a subtalar neutral position. Note the zero heel posts and posts under the first metatarsal heads.

hydrocephalus will require a CSF shunt (Shurtleff et al., 1986b). A ventriculoperitoneal catheter shunts excess CSF from the lateral ventricles of the brain to the peritoneal space, where the CSF is resorbed. Because a shunt is a foreign body, it can be a nidus for infection or can become obstructed, requiring neurosurgical intervention. Repeated or prolonged shunt dysfunction and infections often lead to additional functional and cognitive decline of the child. Shunt dysfunction is often gradual, with subtle symptoms. Therapists should be familiar with these symptoms to facilitate early detection and appropriate referral to a physician for further evaluation. Table 22–2 provides a list of early symptoms and signs of shunt obstruction. Of particular interest are the findings of Kilburn and associates (1985), which suggest that static or declining grip strength measurements are potentially an early indicator of neurologic dysfunction such as shunt malfunction or symptomatic Arnold-Chiari malformation. Hydrocephalus persists throughout life with consequent need of ongoing follow-up by a physician who is familiar with the medical complications associated with MM.

TABLE 22–2. **EARLY WARNING SIGNS AND SYMPTOMS OF SHUNT DYSFUNCTION**

Changes in speech
Fever and malaise
Recurring headache
Decreased activity level
Decreased school performance
Onset of or increased strabismus
Changes in appetite and weight
Incontinence begins or worsens
Onset or worsening of scoliosis
Onset of or increased spasticity
Personality change (irritability)
Decreased or static grip strength
Difficult to arouse in the morning
Decreased visuomotor coordination
Decreased visual acuity or diplopia
Decreased visuoperceptual coordination
Onset or increased frequency of seizures

Adapted with permission from Shurtleff, DB, Stuntz, JT, & Hayden, P. Hydrocephalus. In Shurtleff, DB (Ed.), Myelodysplasias and Exstrophies: Significance, Prevention, and Treatment. Orlando, FL: Grune & Stratton, 1986, p. 142.

Cognitive Dysfunction

Early closure of spinal lesions with antibiotic treatment to prevent meningitis and improved CSF shunt management have increased the expected cognitive function of children born with MM. The majority of children without hydrocephalus or with uncomplicated hydrocephalus (no infections or cerebral hemorrhage) will have intellect falling within the normal range on intelligence testing. The distribution of scores tends to be skewed toward the upper and lower ends of normal, however, with fewer children scoring in the middle of the curve and a greater proportion scoring at the lower end of the range (Shaffer et al., 1986). The intellectual performance of children who have had significant CNS infections is lower than those who have not had infection (Shurtleff et al., 1986b). Intelligence scores tend to be higher in lumbar and sacral lesion level groups than thoracic lesion level groups (Shaffer et al., 1986). Verbal subtest scores usually exceed performance subtest scores (Shaffer et al., 1986). The poorer scores on performance subtests, however, may not represent true differences in verbal versus nonverbal reasoning skills. Instead, these differences can potentially be explained by upper limb dyscoordination (discussed later) and by memory deficits (Shaffer et al., 1986). Dyscoordination and memory deficits are manifested as distractibility on subtests assessing acquired knowledge (e.g., arithmetic), integrated right-left hemisphere function (e.g., picture arrangement, block

design, and coding), speed of motor response (e.g., coding), and memory (e.g., digit span, coding, and arithmetic). Further controlled studies need to be conducted to determine the source or sources of discrepant verbal versus performance intelligence scores observed in individuals with MM.

The "cocktail party personality" is a cognitively associated behavioral disorder that occurs in some individuals with hydrocephalus, regardless of age or intelligence level (Hurley, 1993). These individuals are articulate and verbose, superficially appearing to have high verbal skills. Close examination of the content of their speech, however, shows frequent and inappropriate use of cliches and jargon. Individual words are often misused. Despite the initial appearance of being capable, these individuals are often quite impaired, and their performance in daily life is below what they superficially appear able to do (Hurley, 1993). It is important for the physical therapist to directly observe skills that these children report that they can perform and to confirm regular performance of the task at home with parents and care providers to determine if information provided by the client is accurate.

Upper Limb Dyscoordination

Upper limb dyscoordination is frequently observed in children with MM, especially those with hydrocephalus (Shaffer et al., 1986). The dyscoordination can potentially be explained by three possible causes: 1) cerebellar ataxia most likely related to the Arnold-Chiari type II malformation; 2) motor cortex or pyramidal tract damage secondary to hydrocephalus; or 3) motor learning deficits resulting from the use of upper limbs for balance and support rather than manipulation and exploration. These children perform poorly on timed fine motor skill tasks (Shaffer et al., 1986). Their movements can be described as halting and deliberate, rather than the expected smooth continuous motion of able-bodied children. It often appears that there is a heavy reliance on visual feedback instead of kinesthetic sense. Consequently, even with extensive training, these children often have difficulty integrating frequently used fine motor movements at a subconscious level (Shaffer et al., 1986). Practicing fine motor tasks has been found to be beneficial, however, and often carries over into functional tasks (Fay et al., 1986). These coordination deficits have been described by some authors as apparent motor apraxias or motor learning deficits (Brunt, 1980; Land, 1977). Given the frequent occurrence of upper limb dyscoordination in these children, true apraxias are likely less common than these studies indicate.

An additional factor that may contribute to upper limb dyscoordination is delayed development of hand dominance (Shaffer et al., 1986). A large number of children with MM have mixed hand dominance or are left handed, suggestive of possible left hemisphere damage (Shaffer et al., 1986). Brunt (1980) indicated that delayed hand dominance may contribute to deficits in bilateral upper limb function integration, resulting in further difficulty with fine motor tasks.

Visuoperceptual Deficits

Studies assessing visual perception have not clearly determined whether deficits in children with MM are common, as has been described in the literature (Miller & Sethi, 1971; Sand et al., 1973; Tew & Laurence, 1975). Tests that require good hand–eye coordination, such as the Frostig Developmental Test of Visual Perception, may artificially lower scores of children with MM as a result of the upper limb dyscoordination described earlier. When upper limb motor function has been removed as a factor in testing by using the Motor Free Visual Perception Test, children with MM have performed at age-appropriate levels (Shaffer et al., 1986). Consequently, results of visuoperceptual tests need to be interpreted carefully, in conjunction with other evaluations, before a diagnosis of a visual perception deficit is made.

Cranial Nerve Palsies

The Arnold-Chiari malformation, along with hydrocephalus or dysplasia of the brain stem, may result in cranial nerve deficits. Ocular muscle palsies can occur (Shurtleff, 1986e), such as involvement of cranial nerve VI (oculomotor) with consequent lateral rectus eye muscle weakness and esotropia on the involved side. Correction with patching of the eye, prescription lenses, or minor outpatient surgery is necessary to prevent amblyopia and for cosmesis (Reigel, 1993). Cranial nerves IX (glossopharyngeal) and X (vagus) can also be affected with pharyngeal and laryngeal dysfunction (croupy, hoarse cry) and swallowing difficulties (Shurtleff, 1986e). Apneic episodes and bradycardia may occur with a severely symptomatic Arnold-Chiari type II malformation and can potentially be life threatening. These severe symptoms usually appear within the first few weeks of life but can occur at any time (Reigel, 1993). The survival rate is only about 40% in these severe cases (Shurtleff, 1986c). Those infants who do survive, however, have been noted to have gradual improvement in cranial nerve function. Neurosurgical posterior fossa decompression and high cervical laminectomies do not seem to substantially improve the outcome (Griebel et al., 1991; Shurtleff, 1986c). In contrast, surgical decompression of the Arnold-Chiari malformation has been shown to be beneficial for the treatment of progressive upper and lower limb spasticity (Griebel et al., 1991).

Spasticity

The muscle tone of infants and children with MM can range from flaccid to normal to spastic. Stack and Baber (1967) found that some upper motoneuron signs were present in approximately two-thirds of children with MM whom they examined; however, only about 9% had true spastic paraparesis. The remainder of this group had predominantly a lower motoneuron presentation with scattered upper motoneuron signs (e.g., flexor withdrawal reflex). In the group of children without upper motoneuron signs, most had totally flaccid paralysis below the segmental level of their spinal lesion, but a small percentage had normal tone.

Spasticity and abnormal reflexes can affect function and positioning in individuals with MM; however, the greater area of concern is with regard to progression of neurologic dysfunction. The emergence of upper motoneuron signs in a child where none were detected previously, or an increase in spasticity or abnormal reflexes over prior levels, is presumed to be related to an underlying pathologic process (see next section on progressive neurologic dysfunction), *requiring urgent attention* until proven otherwise. The physical therapist should notify the child's physician of such changes so that appropriate evaluation can be pursued. Early detection and treatment of these processes can prevent or limit permanent neurologic loss.

Progressive Neurologic Dysfunction

In addition to progression of spasticity, decline in motor or sensory function, pain, and change in bladder or anal sphincter function can also be observed in many individuals with MM. Several causes have been identified, including hydrocephalus, syringomyelia, syringobulbia, and tethered cord syndrome. Because of the risk of progressive loss of function, it is *essential* that the previous parameters be closely monitored in individuals with MM throughout their life span.

Spinal cord tethering at the site of initial spinal defect repair is a relatively common cause for this phenomenon. Cord tethering occurs from scarring of the neural placode or spinal cord to the overlying dura or skin with resultant traction on neural structures. The tethered cord syndrome may also result from a number of congenital anomalies, including thickening of the filum terminale, diastematomyelia, and intraspinal lipomas or dermoid cysts (Rekate, 1991). An acquired cause of progressive spinal cord dysfunction that has been reported is severe herniation of intervertebral disks into the spinal canal, causing compression of the cord (Shurtleff & Dunne, 1986). As described above in the section on hydrocephalus, shunt malfunction or latent reactivation of hydrocephalus can also produce signs and symptoms of progressive neurologic loss. Additionally, syringes occurring either in the brain stem (syringobulbia) or anywhere within the spinal cord (syringomyelia) can lead to progressive neurologic dysfunction.

Seizures

Seizures have been reported to occur in 10 to 30% of children and adolescents with MM (Shurtleff & Dunne, 1986). The etiologies of seizure activity include associated brain malformation, CSF shunt malfunction or infection, and residual brain damage from shunt infection or malfunction. Anticonvulsant medications, which are necessary for prophylaxis against seizures, unfortunately can also accentuate any cognitive deficits or dyscoordination already present (Gadow, 1986; Reynolds, 1983). Untreated seizures, however, can lead to permanent cognitive or neurologic functional loss, or even death.

Neurogenic Bowel

Fewer than 5% of children with MM develop voluntary control of their urinary or anal sphincter (Reigel, 1993). Abnormal or absent function of spinal segments S-2 through S-4, which provide the innervation to these organs, is the primary reason for the incontinence. The anal sphincter can be flaccid, hypotonic, or spastic, causing different manifestations of dysfunction during defecation. Anorectal sensation is also often impaired, preventing the individual from receiving sensory input of an imminent bowel movement so that he or she can take appropriate action. In addition to incontinence, constipation and impaction can also occur. Fortunately, conscientious attention to individually designed bowel programs can have effective results, minimizing problems of incontinence and constipation (King et al., 1994; Reigel, 1993; Wicks & Shurtleff, 1986a, 1986b). King and associates (1994) report that instituting bowel training before age 7 years correlates with improved outcomes by means of better compliance. When stool incontinence is interfering with a child's school and social activities, the physical therapist may want to become involved to help address the problem. Incontinence often impacts feelings of self image and competence, which in turn can affect performance in other activities pertinent to the therapist's treatment program.

Neurogenic Bladder

Just as the nerves to control defecation are impaired, so are the nerves that produce bladder control. A variety of different types of dysfunctions can occur depending on the relative tonicity of the detrusor muscle in the bladder wall and the outlet sphincters of the bladder. Bladder management strategies are directed toward the point or points of dysfunction. The goal is infection-free social continence with preservation of renal function. Retrograde flow of urine from the bladder up the ureters to the kidneys, called vesicoureteral reflux, can occur without symptoms or signs being evident until the later stages of irreversible renal failure. Inadequate emptying of the bladder with residual urine retention within the bladder provides an optimal culture media for bacteria to grow, causing recurrent urinary tract infections and possible generalized sepsis. Adequate bladder management is therefore an essential component of health maintenance and normal longevity of people with MM, in addition to being an important social issue.

For most individuals, effective bladder management is achieved with clean intermittent catheterization on a regularly timed schedule for voiding. A small catheter is inserted into the bladder through the urethra until urine begins to flow. After the bladder is empty or urine stops flowing, the catheter is withdrawn, cleansed with soap and water, and stored for future use. It has been shown that the clean method of catheterization, as opposed to sterile technique, is sufficient for prevention of urinary tract infections (Reigel, 1993). The risk of injury to the urethra or bladder from clean intermittent catheterization is sufficiently low to allow young children to be taught to catheterize themselves. Mastery of the technique is usually achieved by the age of 6 to 8 years depending on the severity of the involvement (Shurtleff & Mayo, 1986). Supplementation of clean intermittent catheterization with oral medication for spastic detrusor muscle function (e.g., oxybutynin [Ditropan] or propantheline [Pro-Banthine]), spastic sphincter function (phenoxybenzamine), or hypotonic sphincter function (ephedrine) is required in some children to achieve treatment goals. It is recommended that individuals with MM have regular follow-up with a urologist every 6 months until the age of 2 and yearly thereafter, throughout the life span (Kimura et al., 1986). The physical therapist needs to be aware of the method used for urine drainage as it relates to wheelchair positioning, transfer techniques, and orthoses so that assistive devices do not interfere with effective performance of urine drainage techniques. It is important to allow adequate time for clients with MM to attend to bowel and bladder needs before and after evaluation and therapy sessions so that they are comfortable and continent during physical activities. Discomfort from a distended bladder or rectum may impair performance. Clients are often not assertive in requesting necessary time for personal care, and therapists should encourage them to do so to avoid embarrassing accidents.

Skin Breakdown

Decubitus ulcers and other types of skin breakdown occur in 85 to 95% of all children by the time they reach young adulthood (Shurtleff, 1986a). Okamoto and associates (1983) performed an extensive study of skin breakdown on 524 patients with MM who were 1 to 20 years old. Perineal decubiti and breakdown over the apex of the spinal kyphotic curve (gibbus) occurred in 82% of children with thoracic level lesions, 62% of those with high lumbar level lesions, and 50 to 53% of those with lower level lesions. Lower limb skin breakdown was approximately equivalent in all lesion level groups (30–46%). Although the sites and causes of skin breakdown varied among lesion level groups, the overall frequency was the same. The prevalence of skin breakdown at any one time was 20 to 25% for the population sampled. Several etiologies for skin breakdown were ascertained. In 42% of the children, tissue ischemia from excessive pressure was the cause. In 23% a cast or orthotic device produced the breakdown. In another 23% urine and stool soiling produced skin maceration. Friction and shear accounted for another 10%; burns accounted for 1%; and 1% of causes were not recorded or were unknown.

Other authors have described additional causes of skin breakdown (Shurtleff, 1986a). These include excessive weight bearing over bony prominences of the pelvis as a result of spinal deformity, obesity, lower limb autonomic dysfunction with vascular insufficiency or venous stasis, and tenuous tissue postoperatively over bony prominences.

Age is an important factor in the etiology of skin breakdown. Shurtleff (1986a) showed that young children who are not toilet trained have the greatest problem with breakdown from skin soiling (ammonia burns). Young active children with MM have the greatest frequency of friction burns on knees and feet from scooting along rugs, hot water scalds, and pressure ulcers from orthoses or casts. Older children, adolescents, and young adults develop skin breakdown over lower limb bony prominences (even if they did not have ulcers when they were younger) from the increased pressure of a larger body habitus, asymmetric weight bearing resulting from deformities, abrasions of the buttocks or lower limbs due to poor transfer skills, improperly fitted orthoses, and lower limb vascular problems. Strategies for prevention taught by the physical therapist therefore need to be directed to the likely causes of skin breakdown for the age of the individual.

Obesity

Obesity is a common and difficult multifactorial problem occurring in children with MM. For children who are ambulatory, a greater expenditure of energy is required to participate in physical play activities, so that it is likely that less time will be spent engaged in physical play and more sedentary activities (e.g., watching television) are often adopted. Children with mobility limitations, whether they are ambulatory or wheelchair mobile, may not be well accepted by able-bodied peers when they attempt to participate in physically challenging play, or they may feel conspicuous because of having difficulty keeping up. The likelihood of participation under these circumstances is diminished. As obesity develops, this further complicates participation and negatively impacts self-image, creating an undesirable cycle perpetuating weight gain. Additionally, children with MM probably are at a disadvantage physiologically. Studies evaluating the caloric intake required for children with MM (Shurtleff, 1986b) have shown that the intake should be lower than for able-bodied obese peers. This is likely not just a function of the decreased activity level of children with MM. Decreased muscle mass of large lower limb muscle groups diminishes the ability to burn calories (i.e., the basal metabolic rate of children with MM is probably lower than normal). This is consistent with the observation that children with high lumbar and thoracic lesions have greater problems with obesity. Weight control is therefore not just a function of decreased caloric intake for children with MM. The challenge of the physical therapist is to find age-appropriate physical activities for their clients that are fun and at which they can succeed, so that physical activity is positively reinforced and a life-long pattern of engaging in such activities is developed.

The usual mechanism to screen for obesity in the general population is height-weight ratios; however, arm span–weight ratios are more appropriate for monitoring individuals with MM. Shurtleff (1986b) notes that height-weight ratios are not useful in children with MM because of their short stature, decreased linear length secondary to spine or lower limb deformities, and decreased growth of paretic limbs. He recommends monitoring individuals with MM by measuring serial subscapular skin-fold thickness, linear length measured along the axis of long bones to take into consideration hip and knee joint contractures, arm span measured with a spanner, and weight measured on a platform scale (subtracting the weight of the wheelchair or adaptive aids). Results should be recorded on National Center for Health Statistics percentile charts (Hamill et al., 1979). Arm span measurements should be adjusted using correction factors to avoid underestimating body fat content; 0.9 arm span for children with no leg muscle mass (thoracic and high-lumbar levels), 0.95 arm span for those with partial loss of muscle mass (mid- and low-lumbar lesions), and 1.0 arm span for children with minimal or no muscle mass loss.

DETERMINANTS OF OUTCOME AND PROGNOSIS

The motor function present is the most important factor for predicting outcome and prognosis. Common characteristics of each lesion level are described in this section. Motor function is classified according to the IMSG criteria (see Table 22–1), which differ from the traditional classification system used for individuals with spinal cord injuries, as discussed earlier in the section on motor paralysis. The functional motor level does not always correspond to the anatomic lesion level because of individual variations in nerve root innervation of muscles. The information presented here is intended to serve as general guidelines for expectations at a given level of motor function. Many factors besides muscle strength influence an individual's functional potential and result in variations of performance within a given lesion level group. These factors include age, body proportions, weight, sensation, orthopaedic deformities, joint contractures, spasticity, upper limb function, and cognition. The relative contribution of these factors is highly individual, and a thorough evaluation and follow-up of each child is necessary to maximize potential capabilities.

Thoracic Level

Individuals with thoracic level muscle function have innervation of neck, upper limb, shoulder girdle, and trunk musculature, but no volitional lower limb movements are present. Neck, upper limb, and shoulder girdle muscle groups are innervated by the C-1 to T-4 spinal nerves; back extensors by the C-2 to L-4 spinal nerves; intercostals by the thoracic nerves; and abdominals by T-5 to L-1. Consequently, individuals with motor function at or above T-10 have strong upper limbs and upper thoracic and neck motions but their lower trunk musculature is weak. They have difficulty with unsupported sitting balance and may have decreased respiratory function. Sliding boards may be required to perform wheelchair transfers because of the combination of poor trunk control and upper limb dyscoordination.

Individuals with motor function at T-12 have strong trunk musculature and good sitting balance and may have weak hip hiking by means of the quadratus lumborum (innervated by T-12 to L-3). Ambulation may be attempted for exercise at this level using a parapodium. A wheelchair, however, is required for functional household and community mobility.

Children with thoracic level lesions also tend to have greater involvement of other areas of the central nervous system, with corresponding cognitive deficits. Consequently, even though many of these people achieve independence with basic self-care skills and mobility by late childhood, they often require a supervised living situation throughout life. They are rarely competitively employed but often participate in sheltered workshop settings or perform volunteer work (Hinderer et al., 1988).

High Lumbar (L-1–L-2) Level

Individuals with high lumbar motor function have weak hip movements. The iliopsoas muscle is supplied by nerve roots L-1 through L-4, with its primary innervation at L-2 and L-3. The sartorius muscle is supplied by L-2 and L-3 and the adductors by L-2 through L-4. With L-1 motor function, weak hip flexion may be present, and with L-2 motor function the hip flexors, adductors, and rotators are grade 3 or better. According to Schafer and Dias (1983), unopposed hip flexion and adduction contractures are often present at the L-2 motor level and this muscle imbalance often results in dislocated hips. Short-distance household ambulation is possible with high lumbar innervation (L-1 and L-2) when body proportions are small, using knee-ankle-foot orthoses (KAFOs) or reciprocating gait orthoses (RGOs) and upper limb support. These children generally use a wheelchair for community distances. By the second decade of life, a wheelchair is typically the sole means of mobility commensurate with increased energy requirements and enlarged body proportions (Hinderer et al., 1988; Shurtleff, 1986d).

The prognosis of children with high lumbar lesions for function and independent living as adults is similar to the thoracic group described earlier (Hinderer et al., 1988). More individuals in this group, however, achieve independent living status (approximately 50%) but they are still rarely able to maintain competitive employment as adults.

L-3 Level

Individuals with L-3 muscle function have strong hip flexion and adduction, weak hip rotation, and at least antigravity knee extension. The quadriceps muscle group is innervated by nerve roots L-2 through L-4. Children with grade 3 quadriceps strength usually require KAFOs and forearm crutches to ambulate for household and short community distances and a wheelchair for long community distances. By adulthood, most individuals with L-3 level lesions are primarily wheelchair mobile (Hinderer et al., 1988; Shurtleff & Lamers, 1978; Stillwell & Menelaus, 1983).

Approximately 60% of individuals with lesions at this level achieve independent living status as adults (Hinderer et al., 1988). Despite their higher level of independence, only a small percentage (about 20%) actively participate in full-time competitive employment (Hinderer et al., 1988).

L-4 Level

At the L-4 motor level, antigravity knee flexion and grade 4 ankle dorsiflexion with inversion may be present. The medial hamstrings are innervated by nerve roots L-4 through S-2, and the anterior tibialis is innervated primarily by L-4 and L-5, with some innervation from S-1. An individual is considered to have L-4 motor function if the medial hamstrings or anterior tibialis is at least grade 3. Calcaneal foot deformities are common at this motor level as a result of the unopposed action of the tibialis anterior muscle (Schafer & Dias, 1983). Knee extension is usually strong, and these individuals are generally functional ambulators with AFOs and forearm crutches. When first learning to walk, however, KAFOs, a walker, or both may be required. A wheelchair is often needed for long distances.

In the adult follow-up study that we conducted, only 20% of individuals with L-4 motor function continued to ambulate as adults (Hinderer et al., 1988). Many individuals stopped ambulation after their adolescent growth spurt. Others were unable to maintain ambulation because of ankle and knee valgus joint deformities and elbow and wrist pain resulting from years of weight bearing in poor alignment. To increase the likelihood of maintaining biped ambulation for individuals with L-4 motor function throughout adulthood, upright posture should be emphasized when ambulating to minimize the weight-bearing stress on upper limb joints. Orthoses must be aligned properly and posted to support the ankle in a subtalar neutral position. If the ankle joint is malaligned, the knee joint position is adversely affected. It is essential to maintain the knee and ankle in neutral alignment when weight bearing. A flexed and valgus position should not be permitted. Often a patellar tendon–bearing, ground-reaction force orthotic design is optimal to protect the knee and increase the knee extension moment. The proximal medial trim line can be extended higher to provide additional medial knee support, if needed, to reduce a genu valgus deformity (see Fig. 22–5). Knee musculature should be strengthened to assist in maintaining the knee in neutral alignment when weight bearing. Every effort shold be made to progress ambulation to using AFOs and forearm crutches to allow short-distance ambulation to easily be combined with long-distance wheelchair mobility. Crutches can be transported on the wheelchair, and AFOs are optimal because, unlike KAFOs, they do not interfere with dressing or toileting and do not cause skin breakdown when sitting. The prognosis for independent living and employment is similar to that for the group with L-3 lesions.

L-5 Level

According to the IMSG criteria, classification of an L-5 motor level is based on the presence of lateral hamstring muscles with at least grade 3 strength, and either grade 2 gluteus minimus and medius muscles (L4–S1), grade 3 posterior tibialis muscles (L-5–S-1), or grade 4 peroneus tertius muscles (L-4–S-1). Therefore, an individual with an L-5 motor level has at least antigravity knee flexion and weak hip extension using the hamstrings and may have weak hip abduction as well as weak plantar flexion with inversion, strong dorsiflexion with eversion, or both. Weak toe movements may also be present. Hindfoot valgus deformities or calcaneal foot deformities are common as a result of muscle imbalance. Individuals with motor function through L-5 are able to ambulate without orthoses, yet require them to correct foot alignment and substitute for lack of push-off. A gluteal lurch is typically evident unless upper limb support is used. Bilateral upper limb support is usually recommended for community distances to decrease energy expenditure, decrease gluteal lurch and trunk sway, maintain symmetric alignment, protect lower limb joints, and improve safety. The need for upper limb support often becomes more apparent with increased height following growth spurts. Traversing uneven terrain is often difficult. A wheelchair may be required when there is a rapid change in body proportions (e.g., pregnancy) or for long distances on rough terrain. A bike is also useful for long community distances.

Approximately 80% of individuals with lesions at L-5 and below achieve independent living status as adults (Hinderer et al., 1988). About 30% are employed full time (20% part time), well below the average employment rate of the general adult population.

S-1 Level

With muscle function present through S-1, at least two of the following additional muscle actions are present: gastrocnemius/soleus (grade 2), gluteus medius (grade 3), or gluteus maximus (grade 2). Individuals with S-1 motor function have improved hip stability and can walk without orthoses or upper limb support. A weak push-off is evident when running or climbing stairs. A mild to moderate gluteal lurch is often present. Gait deviations and functional limitations are often more pronounced after the adolescent growth spurt. The toe musculature is generally strong. Foot deformities are less common at this level, but foot orthoses or AFOs may be required to improve lower limb alignment and permit muscle groups to function at a more optimal length. Medial and lateral stability at the ankle appears to be required for adequate

function of the plantar flexor muscles during push-off (Lehmann et al., 1986).

S-2, S-2–3, and "No Loss" Levels

Motor function is classified at the S-2 level if the plantar flexor muscles are at least grade 3 and the gluteals grade 4. The only obvious gait abnormality present at this level is generally a decreased push-off and stride length when walking rapidly or running as a result of the decreased strength of the plantar flexor muscles. If all lower limb muscle groups have grade 5 strength except for one or two groups with grade 4 strength, the motor level is classified as S-2–3, according to the IMSG criteria. The term "no loss" is used if the bowel and bladder function normally and lower limb strength is judged to be normal through manual muscle testing. Substantial strength deficits (e.g., 50 to 60%), however, may be undetected by traditional manual muscle testing (Agre et al., 1987; Aitkens et al., 1989; Beasley, 1956, 1961; Bohannon, 1986; Griffin et al., 1986; Miller et al., 1988). Functional deficits may therefore be present even for individuals classified as having "no loss." Foot orthoses are often beneficial to maintain the ankle in the subtalar neutral position and optimize ankle muscle function by maintaining optimal muscle length.

ASSESSMENT AND MANAGEMENT OF MUSCULOSKELETAL ISSUES, MOBILITY, AND FUNCTIONAL SKILLS

There are three primary reasons for evaluating the individual with MM: 1) to define an individual's current status so that appropriate program planning can occur, 2) to identify the potential for developing secondary impairments so that preventative measures can be implemented, and 3) to monitor changes in status that could indicate progressive neurologic dysfunction. Because of the complexity of problems associated with MM, numerous dimensions of disability must be assessed by various disciplines. The physical therapist provides essential information to other team members for program planning and to monitor status. Careful documentation is important for communication among team members and for serial comparisons over time. General assessment and management strategies will be discussed in this section. Considerations that are specific to certain age categories are discussed in the section on age-specific assessment and physical therapy.

Assessment Strategies

The dimensions typically assessed by physical therapists include ROM, muscle extensibility, joint alignment or orthopaedic deformities, muscle tone, muscle strength and endurance, sensation, posture, motor development, ADL, mobility skills, equipment needs, and environmental accessibility. It is important to use standardized protocols, when available, which have good reliability and validity to permit comparison within and between individuals (Hinderer & Hinderer, 1993b). If more than one measurement method exists (e.g., hip extension ROM), the specific method employed should be documented and used consistently. Comprehensive assessments should be conducted at regular intervals throughout the life span on all individuals with MM. In addition, it is recommended that therapists remain blind to previous results of the more subjective measures (e.g., manual muscle testing scores or gait deviations) until the assessment is complete to avoid potential biases. Videotapes and photographs are often a useful adjunct to clinical assessment of gait, joint deformities, and posture. These visual records provide an excellent baseline for comparison purposes if deterioration in status is suspected. It is beneficial to conduct assessment of activities that are influenced by environmental or endurance factors (e.g., wheelchair mobility, gait, or ADL) in more natural settings.

The IMSG recommends a comprehensive, multidisciplinary evaluation for *all* individuals with MM, *regardless* of functional level, because they *all* are at risk for progressive neurologic dysfunction, as discussed earlier. The following assessment intervals are recommended: newborn preoperatively, newborn postoperatively, 6 months, 12 months, 18 months, 24 months, and annually thereafter, continuing through adulthood (Shurtleff, 1986c). Annual examinations are suggested to occur around an individual's birth date so that they are not forgotten. ROM, muscle extensibility, strength, endurance, coordination, and functional parameters should be monitored more closely during periods of rapid growth, when individuals with MM are at increased risk for loss of function. Preintervention and postintervention measurements should be obtained for individuals undergoing surgery or other therapeutic procedures. More frequent assessment of specific goal attainment is indicated for individuals receiving ongoing therapeutic intervention. Mobility and independence with ADL should be re-evaluated when body proportions or environmental demands change to determine if the individual has the strength, endurance, coordination, and adaptive equipment required to function effectively.

Shurtleff (1986c, 1991) advocates using the Patient Data Management System (PDMS) standardized protocol and recording format to serially monitor individuals with MM. The PDMS is composed of a comprehensive, interdisciplinary recording format, which consists of the dimensions typically assessed by each discipline. In addition, intervention data (e.g., surgery, medications, and therapy) are also documented. Scoring and recording criteria can be obtained by contacting the IMSG (IMSG, 1993). The PDMS computerized recording format is beneficial for monitoring this population because serial test results from birth to present can be efficiently scanned for each parameter to detect improvements or deterioration in status. In addition, an individual client's status can be directly compared with that of other individuals with similar characteristics by using the interactive database. The standardized format facilitates communication between and within disciplines and treatment centers and promotes clinical research. Duplication of effort by the various health care professionals involved in the management of individuals with MM is minimized because each discipline is assigned specific PDMS areas to assess, yet all disciplines share the information in the combined database. The PDMS format has also been applied to several other pediatric populations, including those with cerebral palsy, cystic fibrosis, hemophilia, and traumatic brain injury (Shurtleff, 1991).

Individuals with MM should be evaluated on at least a yearly basis by multiple disciplines at a comprehensive care center. It is important, however, for comprehensive care centers and local school and treatment settings to coordinate their assessments, goals, and treatment programs to avoid duplication of effort and to ensure appropriate prioritization of treatment goals. The use of the PDMS facilitates communication. The School Needs Identification and Action Forms (Rowley-Kelly & Kunkle, 1993) also provide a useful format for identifying impairments, academic and functional limitations, and the remedial action recommended. The areas assessed by the school needs forms include health-related services required, physical management instructions, accessibility, safety and fire drills, preparation for school entry, educational rights and related services, academic difficulties, psychological assessment, perceptuomotor deficits, visuoperceptual deficits, self-help skills, social acceptance, social and emotional issues, parent and school relationships, transitional services, and other needs.

Management Strategies

Once primary and secondary impairments and disabilities are identified through a comprehensive evaluation, the functional significance needs to be determined to appropriately plan management strategies. Treatment of an impairment is indicated if it currently interferes with function or if the deficit can progress to a point where it may negatively impact future function. Treatment is also indicated if the efficiency, effectiveness, or safety of performance can be improved. Strength, endurance, and efficiency of performing tasks should be emphasized. Weight-bearing joints need to be protected to prevent early onset of osteoarthritis and to prolong mobility. In addition, the most efficient and effective means of mobility for a given environment should be determined. Goal setting for intervention must consider the impact of the multiple impairments discussed earlier on functional performance expectations. The cognitive, social, and behavioral issues discussed in the impairments section should also be considered.

Fay and associates (1986) recommend three specific treatment approaches for developmental delays in this population. The first is developmental programming in which children are encouraged by parents, teachers, and therapists with a "high dose" of normal developmental activities in "at risk" areas. The philosophy behind this approach is that supplemental early emphasis and practice in potential problem areas will minimize later deficits. These early intervention programs are often initiated for children with MM before measurable delays are identified. The second approach, remediation, is implemented once problem areas are clearly identified. This approach consists of repetition of a set of graded tasks in the domain of concern. Improved performance through practice theoretically carries over into functional activities. The third approach is teaching compensatory skills. Compensation is often implemented when the other two approaches have not produced sufficient results or when the child is older or more severely inpaired. This treatment approach involves identifying functional impairments and developing strategies to help the child become as independent as possible or providing adaptive equipment to compensate for underlying problems and minimize disability in daily life.

Specific Assessment and Management Strategies

Specific assessment and management strategies as they pertain to strength, mobility, gait, and equipment issues are highlighted in this section because of the magnitude of the impact of these factors on function in this population, regardless of age or lesion level. Suggestions for impairment-specific parameters (e.g., ROM, orthopaedic deformi-

ties, and sensation) were discussed in the section on impairments. Developmental issues are discussed in the section on age-specific assessment and physical therapy.

STRENGTH

Upper limb, neck, and trunk musculature should be screened for weakness. If evidence of weakness exists, then a more specific assessment of strength should be conducted. For individuals with thoracic or high lumbar level involvement, it is important to palpate trunk musculature to determine which portions of muscle groups are functioning. Dynamometer values of grip and pinch strength should also be obtained. Kilburn and associates (1985) suggest that grip strength measurements can be a sensitive measure of progressive neurologic dysfunction. A standardized protocol for obtaining grip strength measurements and normative values for children has been provided by Level (1984).

Specific testing of isolated motions of lower limb muscles is essential to determine if individual muscles are functioning. Standardized test protocols should be used (e.g., Daniels & Worthingham, 1986; Janda, 1983; Kendall et al., 1993). It is essential to detect changes in strength in this population as soon as possible, since loss of strength can be a sign of progressive neurologic dysfunction. As a result, we recommend using quantitative strength measurements in conjunction with traditional manual muscle testing techniques. It is also important to distinguish between reflexive and voluntary movements. Reflexive movements should be documented, but they should not be considered when determining motor lesion levels.

Manual muscle testing is the most common method used to assess strength in this population because of its adaptability in a typical clinic setting. Manual muscle testing is the method of choice for *screening* muscle strength to determine the presence of volitional activity in specific muscles and to determine whether an individual muscle's function varies throughout the ROM. There are several limitations to relying only on manual muscle testing scores for *serially monitoring* strength, as discussed in Chapter 4.

Manual muscle testing has limited inter-rater and test-retest reliability (Hinderer & Hinderer, 1993a). Manual muscle test scores must change more than one full grade to be confident that a true change in strength has occurred. In addition, manual muscle testing has poor concurrent validity compared with more quantitative measures. Several studies have demonstrated that deficits in strength exceeding 50% are *not* detected by manual muscle testing (Agre et al., 1987; Aitkens et al., 1989; Beasley, 1956, 1961; Bohannon, 1986; Griffin et al., 1986; Miller et al., 1988). Agre and colleagues (1987) examined this issue in 33 adolescents with MM. Individuals who had been classified as having "no motor deficits" by means of manual muscle testing actually had strength deficits compared with normative data. These deficits were 40% for the hip extensor and 60% for the knee extensor muscles. The lack of concurrent validity of manual muscle testing compared with quantitative measurements demonstrates that the sensitivity of manual muscle testing in detecting weakness is very limited and is inadequate for detecting early strength loss in individuals with MM.

The *predictive validity* of manual muscle testing has been examined in two studies on children with MM. Murdoch (1980) examined the predictive validity of neonatal manual muscle testing assessments using a truncated three-point scale. The correlation between muscle power of the newborn and subsequent mobility of the child at age 3 to 8 years was "very poor." In contrast, McDonald and associates (1986) examined the predictive validity of manual muscle testing for individual muscle groups on 825 children with MM using the complete 0- to 5-point grading scale. Predictive validity of manual muscle testing generally increased from birth to age 5. The probability that a given manual muscle test score precisely predicted future scores varied with age and the particular muscle group tested. These probabilities ranged from 23 to 68% for newborns and from 54 to 87% in older children. The probability that a single test score predicted future strength within ± one manual muscle test grade, however, was considerably higher, ranging from 70 to 86% for newborns and from 87 to 97% for older children. These results indicate that manual muscle testing is useful for predicting future muscle function within one manual muscle test grade. Strength test results obtained in infancy using the complete manual muscle test scale, therefore, appear to provide useful information for prognosis and for planning the course of treatment.

The limited reliability and concurrent validity of manual muscle testing indicates that it is not the method of choice for monitoring changes in strength over time. In contrast, strength testing using hand-held instruments has been found to be a reliable and sensitive method for assessing strength in children and adolescents with MM. Intraclass inter-rater and test-retest correlation coefficients using this technique ranged from .73 to .99 (Effgen & Brown, 1992; Hinderer, 1988). Other authors report good to high levels of reliability when testing the strength of other populations of children and adolescents with hand-held instrumentation (Florence et al., 1988; Hinderer & Gutierrez, 1988, Hinderer & Hinderer, 1993a; Hosking et al., 1976;

Hyde et al., 1983; Mendell & Florence, 1990; Stuberg & Metcalf, 1988). Several portable, hand-held instruments are available for use in conjunction with manual muscle testing (Hinderer & Hinderer, 1993a). The advantages of these instruments over nonportable instruments are that they are easily applied in typical clinic settings and can be used with standard manual muscle testing techniques to obtain objective force readings from most muscle groups.

It is best to obtain three myometry trials and report the average score because the mean is more stable over time and between raters (Hack et al., 1981; Hinderer, 1988). Torque values should be reported (force × lever arm length) to permit comparison over time, regardless of changing body proportions, at least until skeletal maturity has been attained. Torque values also permit direct comparison of force production capabilities between individuals with different body proportions. Standardized testing techniques must be implemented when assessing strength with hand-held instruments to ensure the consistency of measurements. Many factors influence test results and must be controlled for when testing, including test positions, instructions and commands provided, use of reinforcement and feedback, application of resistance, the type of contraction, and the examiner's body mechanics. For more information regarding techniques used in testing with hand-held instruments, the reader is referred to the work of Hinderer and Hinderer (1993a).

There are several factors that should be considered when testing the muscle strength of children with MM, including age, developmental level, cognitive level, ability to follow directions, attention span, motivation, motor planning skills, sensation, and proprioception. The examiner must carefully watch for muscle substitutions. This is particularly challenging in the MM population because of altered angles of pull from orthopaedic deformities. It is often difficult for multijoint muscles such as the hamstrings to initiate motions. Any differences in function between end-range and mid-range positions should be noted. Special considerations when testing infants and young children are discussed in the section on age-specific assessment and physical therapy.

As discussed in the impairments section, several CNS complications can account for loss of muscle function in this population. There are many factors that can result in normal variations in strength, however, that should also be considered when interpreting test results. These factors include changes in body proportions, hormonal influences, motor learning, illness, injury, surgery, immobilization, physical or psychological fatigue, the prior state of activity, seasonal variations, temporal factors, motivation, cooperation, and comprehension. Discussion of the specific influences of these factors is beyond the scope of this chapter. For further information regarding the impact of these factors on force production, the reader is referred to the work of Hinderer and Hinderer (1993a). Because of the multiple factors that can influence force production, it is important to repeat the testing at more frequent intervals, if strength loss is suspected, to determine whether consistent test results are obtained. There are several variables that should be considered when interpreting muscle test results, including the reliability and standard error of measurement of the testing method used, the concurrent and predictive validity of test results, and factors that can account for fluctuations in strength (Hinderer & Hinderer, 1993a).

Static strength measurements should be correlated with functional measures to observe effects of fatigue and to determine the effect of reduced strength and limited endurance on function. Individuals with neurogenic muscle weakness may have a higher degree of variability in force production as a result of the lower threshold of fatigue and slower rate of recovery of weak musculature (Steindler, 1955). Local muscle endurance appears to be deficient in some neuromuscular diseases (Bar-or, 1986; Milner-Brown & Miller, 1989). Although this issue has not been specifically tested in the MM population, these results suggest that force production may be more variable in weak muscle groups of individuals with MM.

If function is present but weakness exists in muscle groups that are important for postural stability, ADL, mobility, or balance of muscle forces around joints, then strengthening exercises are indicated. The specific muscle groups to emphasize vary depending on the lesion level and functional requirements. In general, strong upper limb muscle groups are required for performing transfers, wheelchair propulsion, and when using assistive devices to walk. Increasing the strength of trunk musculature improves sitting balance and postural stability. Increasing the strength of key lower limb muscle groups that are critical for ambulation can improve gait and can possibly minimize the need for orthoses and assistive devices. For example, increasing the quadriceps and hamstrings strength in an individual with L-4 motor function may enable progression of ambulation from using KAFOs to using AFOs (see the case history at the end of this chapter).

Muscle groups should be strengthened within functional ROM. In addition to traditional strengthening exercises, many play activities promote strengthening (Embry et al., 1903). Muscle

re-education techniques such as functional electrical stimulation and biofeedback are useful to teach muscles to function in new parts of the ROM. Electrical stimulation has also been found to be beneficial to increase strength and enhance functional performance in this population (Karmel-Ross et al., 1992). Strengthening programs should be implemented during periods when an individual is at risk for loss of muscle strength and endurance (e.g., after recent surgery, immobilization, illness, or bed rest) and during periods of rapid growth when individuals often lose function as a result of changes in body proportions.

Endurance activities are also important for weight control and to enhance aerobic capacity. Individuals with MM must have adequate endurance to meet the challenges of community mobility. Low-impact aerobic activities to minimize joint stress are preferable. In general, jumping activities should be avoided because joint stress is increased as a result of the inadequate deceleration provided by weak lower limb muscles. Indications for endurance training and instruction in energy conservation techniques include decreased aerobic capacity, a high energy cost of mobility, and limited endurance.

MOBILITY

Ineffective mobility is a hallmark of MM. Effective mobility is defined as any efficient and effective means of moving about in space that enables the individual to easily traverse and explore the environment, grow and develop, and independently pursue an education, vocation, or avocation (Shurtleff, 1986d). Mobility options provided should meet these criteria for all environments encountered by the individual so that lifestyle is not limited by endurance and difficulty traversing uneven terrain.

Changes in body proportions can significantly impact mobility. Mobility options, orthoses, and assistive device requirements that are ideal at one time may not be effective once body proportions, environmental demands, or both change. Consequently, the appropriateness of adaptive equipment and mobility options needs to be re-evaluated throughout the life span. Emphasis of this point to clients by their health care providers helps to prevent the feeling of failure if alternate mobility options are required in the future. Too often, individuals with MM grow up being praised for walking instead of using a wheelchair or for walking without assistive devices, depending on their lesion level. This emphasis gives the impression that normal biped ambulation is the only socially acceptable form of mobility. Several of the adults in our follow-up study reported that it was difficult to accept the use of a wheelchair or other assistive devices as they grew up because they felt like they were a failure or that they would disappoint their parents and health care providers (Hinderer & Hinderer, 1988). It is important to emphasize that wheelchairs and other assistive devices are aids for effective mobility and that their use does not represent a failure of biped ambulation.

Bed mobility, floor mobility, wheelchair mobility, ambulation, and transfers should be assessed and compared with the requirements for independent function. Criteria for assessing mobility parameters are endurance, efficiency, effectiveness, safety, degree of independence, and accessibility. Objective information regarding these parameters is often helpful to convince clients and their parents that alternative methods of mobility should be considered. Efficiency can be estimated by measuring the time required to complete a task. Energy expenditure can be estimated by measuring heart rate. Regression equations have been determined for this population to equate heart rate with the energy expenditure required for a given task (Williams et al., 1983). The regression equations for energy expenditure and efficiency of this population are

Energy cost (ml O_2/kg min) = 0.073 (HR) + 6.119
Energy efficiency (ml O_2/kg meter) =
$$0.006 \text{ (HR)} - 0.313.$$

Criteria for determining the most practical and effective mode of mobility for household and community distances are provided in Table 22–3. Standardized tests that are useful for evaluating mobility in this population are discussed in Chapters 1 and 2. In addition, the Timed Test of Patient Mobility (Jebsen et al., 1970) is beneficial for assessing the efficiency of mobility because the time required to perform bed mobility, transfers, wheelchair mobility, and gait mobility tasks is documented. Normative data are available for comparison purposes. We suggest augmenting the efficiency time score of the Timed Test of Patient Mobility with a rating scale for the level of independence, safety, practicality, and assistive devices required for each task (Hinderer & Hinderer, 1988). Other assessments that are specific to function in wheelchairs include the Functional Task Performance Wheelchair Assessment of positioning, reaching, and driving tasks (Deitz et al., 1991) and the Seated Postural Control Measure for sitting posture and functional movements (Fife et al., 1991).

GAIT

Thorough evaluation and documentation of gait status are essential to monitor functional motor

TABLE 22–3. FEASIBILITY OF WHEELCHAIR AND BIPED AMBULATION: CRITERIA FOR EVALUATION

Household Distances

ENDURANCE
Adequate to go between rooms in house?
Adequate to get to yard and car?

EFFICIENCY
Record heart rate and calculate energy expenditure.
Record normal and fast household walking speeds.
Is fast pace adequate for emergency situations?
Is normal pace practical for everyday activities?

EFFECTIVENESS
Independent with all transfers?
Able to carry, reach, lift, and climb?
Able to perform activities of daily living?
Able to go forward, backward, sideways, and turn?

SAFETY
Has good stability and balance?
Observes joint and skin protection?
Able to maneuver around obstacles?
Safe on smooth surfaces and rugs?
Safe when turning?

ACCESSIBILITY
Maneuvers in and out of house independently?
Necessary household rooms accessible?
Emergency exit routes accessible?

Community Distances

ENDURANCE
Sufficient at a functional speed for average community distances? (e.g., going to school, store, medical appointments, and social activities)
Adequate for play and recreational activities? (e.g., playground, park, beach, theater, sports arenas, sports participation)
Adequate for long-distance community distances? (e.g., shopping mall, zoo, concert, sporting events, hiking)

EFFICIENCY
Record heart rate and calculate energy expenditure.
Record normal and fast walking paces.
Adequate speed to cross intersections?
Is typical pace practical for community distances?

EFFECTIVENESS
Independent with all transfers?
Able to maneuver in all directions?
Able to climb and step over obstacles?
Able to carry packages and groceries?
Able to reach and lift items from shelves?

SAFETY
Has good stability and balance?
Observes joint and skin protection?
Safe on wet or slippery surfaces?
Able to maneuver around obstacles?
Able to maneuver in congested areas?
Safe on uneven terrain, curbs, inclines, and steps?

ACCESSIBILITY
Maneuvers in and out of car and bus independently?
Necessary community buildings accessible?

status and to watch for signs of progressive neurologic dysfunction. Clients or their parents typically notice changes in gait patterns and walking endurance before they notice increased muscle weakness. Careful gait observation is also needed to determine the most appropriate orthoses and assistive devices.

Examination of orthoses and assistive devices for wear patterns helps to determine if they are being used on a regular basis or just to perform in the clinic setting. Gait should be evaluated in a natural environment on a variety of walking surfaces. Clients should be observed walking for typical household and community distances to determine the effects of fatigue.

All too often decisions regarding gait problems and the need for orthoses and assistive devices are made by observing short-distance ambulation on a smooth clinic floor. Performance in the home or community environment may be vastly different than in a clinic situation, especially when walking around a number of obstacles, in congested areas, when traversing uneven terrain, or with inclement weather. The impact of these factors must be considered when making recommendations.

Requirements for orthoses and ambulatory aids should be documented. Gait deviations should be closely observed and recorded. If possible, gait deviations and efficiency parameters should be observed both with and without orthoses and assistive devices. Typical gait parameters evaluated include arm swing, trunk position and sway, pelvic tilt and rotations, compensated or uncompensated Trendelenburg position, excessive hip flexion and rotation, excessive knee flexion or hyperextension, toe clearance, foot position, push-off effectiveness, and foot progression angle.

Observational gait analysis is the technique used most commonly to assess gait in clinical settings (Krebs et al., 1985). Video analysis augments clinical observations by allowing the evaluator to observe gait multiple times at slow speeds and by providing a permanent record that is invaluable for comparison purposes if deterioration of functional status is suspected. The inter-rater reliability of observational analysis through videotapes, however, has been reported to be low to moderate (Eastlack et al., 1991; Krebs et al., 1985). Footprint analysis is a low-cost method of obtaining objective information regarding velocity, cadence, foot progression angle, base of support, toe clearance, stride length, and step length (Shores, 1980). More sophisticated methods of objective gait analysis are described in Chapter 3.

Criteria for the effectiveness, efficiency, and safety of household and community ambulation are provided in Table 22–3. Efficiency and practicality of ambulation can be estimated by monitoring heart rate, normal and fast walking velocity, and maximum walking distance. Other time-distance variables (e.g., step and stride length, cadence, and cycle time) provide useful information regarding symmetry, stability, and function. These variables can be used for comparison purposes if they are normalized (adjusted) for stature (Rose et al., 1991).

Time-distance variables provide information about gait symmetry by comparing right-left differences in step lengths and stance to swing phase ratios. Examining cadence and the percentage of time spent in the stance phase versus the swing phase provides information regarding the stability of gait. For instance, a high cadence or an imbalance in the stance versus swing phase duration may indicate instability. Parameters such as walking velocity and cadence provide information regarding the functional practicality of gait. If the velocity is too low or step rate is too high, the individual may not be able to meet environmental demands.

It is essential to normalize time-distance variables for stature to compare these parameters serially over time for a given individual or to compare between individuals of different stature (e.g., comparing with normative data). These parameters are normalized by dividing by leg length. An alternate but less precise method of normalizing time-distance parameters is to divide by height because overall height is closely correlated to individual limb lengths. If these parameters are not normalized for stature, conclusions regarding differences in function may be confounded by changes in body proportions over time.

Indications for lower limb orthoses are provided in Table 22–4. Specifications and their effect on gait are outlined in Table 22–5. Indications for gait training include when a child is first learning to walk, when there is potential for progression to a new type of orthosis or upper limb aid, for progression to a more efficient gait pattern (e.g., from a 4-point to a 2-point alternate gait), when there is potential for improving gait (e.g., crouched gait pattern, excessive foot progression angle), to improve safety and confidence with advanced walking activities (e.g., walking on inclines, rough terrain, steps, learning to fall safely and stand up independently from floor, carrying and lifting objects), and to improve the efficiency and safety of gait, transfers, and management of aids.

Strength of the quadriceps muscles has been suggested by some authors to be the best predictor of ambulatory potential in children with MM (Schopler & Menelaus, 1987; Williams et al., 1983), while others indicate that iliopsoas muscle strength is better (McDonald et al., 1991b). McDonald and associates (1991b) examined the relationship between the patterns of strength and mobility in 291 children with MM who had received at least three serial standardized strength assessments after age 5 and who were classified for their mobility status as community ambulators, partial (household) ambulators, and nonambulators. Iliopsoas muscle

TABLE 22–4. INDICATORS FOR LOWER LIMB ORTHOSES

Foot Orthoses, UCBL, or Supramalleolar Orthoses

ADVANTAGES

Permits full active dorsiflexion and plantar flexion.
Maintains the subtalar joint in neutral alignment.
Provides medial and lateral ankle stability.

MOTOR FUNCTION

S-1 to "No loss"
Must have adequate toe clearance and sufficient gastrocnemius/soleus strength to provide adequate push-off and decelerate forward movement of tibia.

INDICATIONS

Unequal weight distribution, resulting in skin breakdown, foot deformities, or abnormal shoe wear.
Medial and lateral ankle instability, resulting in balance problems, especially difficulty traversing uneven terrain.
Poor alignment of the subtalar joint, forefoot, or rearfoot.

Ankle-Foot Orthoses (standard AFOs and ground-reaction force AFOs)

ADVANTAGES

In general, the ground-reaction force (Fig. 22–5) is advantageous for this population. The proximal trim line can be extended medially to control genu valgus. The ground-reaction force AFO also facilitates push-off and knee extension during the stance phase and improves static standing balance. The ground-reaction force AFO has a patellar tendon–bearing design. This design distributes pressure across a broad area, preventing skin breakdown and lower leg deformities, which are common when traditional AFO anterior straps have been worn for an extended period of time. If traditional AFOs are used in this population, the anterior straps must be well padded.

MOTOR FUNCTION

L-4 to S-1
Weak or absent ankle musculature
Knee extensors at least grade 4

INDICATIONS

Medial and lateral instability of knee or ankle
Insufficient knee extension moment
(ground-reaction force AFO)
Lack of or ineffective push-off
Inadequate toe clearance
Crouched gait pattern

Knee-Ankle-Foot Orthoses

ADVANTAGES

If unable to maintain upright posture due to joint contractures or muscle weakness, or if the knee joints are unstable, KAFOs are indicated.
If the knee joint is primarily required for medial and lateral stability so the knee joint is unlocked, or if there is potential to progress to ambulation with the knee joints unlocked, it is best to incorporate the ground-reaction force AFO component into the KAFO design to provide the advantages listed earlier in the AFO section.

MOTOR FUNCTION

L-3 to L-4
Weak knee musculature
Absent ankle musculature

INDICATIONS

Medial and lateral instability of knee
Weak quadriceps (grade 4– or less)

Reciprocating Gait Orthoses or Hip-Knee-Ankle-Foot Orthoses

ADVANTAGES

The reciprocating gait orthosis (RGO) cable system facilitates hip extension during stance phase and hip flexion during swing phase by coupling flexion of one hip with extension of the opposite hip.
Release of both cables permits hip flexion when sitting.
The RGO reduces the energy required for ambulation compared with walking with traditional KAFOs.

MOTOR FUNCTION

L-1 to L-3 (some centers also advocate for thoracic level)
Weak hip flexion is required to effectively operate the cables.

INDICATIONS

Unable to maintain an upright posture with the hip joints extended
RGO is indicated to facilitate hip extension and swing phase.

Thoracic-Hip-Knee-Ankle-Foot Orthoses, Parapodiums, or Verlos

ADVANTAGES

Upright positioning for high-level lesions
Generally for exercise walking only

MOTOR FUNCTION

Thoracic to L-2 (Walking is usually nonfunctional for these high-level lesions because of the high energy expenditure required and the slow, cumbersome walking pace.)

INDICATIONS

Limited distance mobility
Upright positioning
"Exercise" walking

TABLE 22–5. **LOWER LIMB ORTHOTIC SPECIFICATIONS, OBJECTIVES, AND EVALUATION CRITERIA**

Orthotic Specifications

SHOE HEEL HEIGHT

A low heel (¼ to ½ inch) may improve balance by shifting the center of gravity forward in a person with a calcaneal weight-bearing position.

A low heel (¼ to ½ inch) may decrease knee hyperextension by shifting the center of gravity forward.

A high heel shifts the center of gravity too far forward and causes balance problems in a person with weak plantar flexors.

A high heel may result in increased hip and knee flexion, combined with an increased lordosis or swayback posture.

ANKLE ANGLE

Ideally molded or set in 5° *plantar flexion* with a rigid anterior and posterior stop to reduce energy requirements and to increase the knee extension moment (Lehmann et al., 1985), as long as toe clearance is adequate and the knee does not hyperextend. If foot clearance is a problem, then set angle more acutely, no higher than neutral, at the minimum angle required to clear the foot during swing phase. Plastic orthoses must enclose the malleoli to effectively resist dorsiflexion and provide a rigid anterior stop (Lehmann et al., 1983).

Do not set ankle angle more acutely than a neutral angle unless trying to control a knee hyperextension problem, because the energy expenditure will increase.

KEEL

Generally, keel should be rigid to the distal aspect of the metatarsal heads (to decrease energy expenditure by providing a longer lever). The plastic should extend to the end of the toes to maintain proper toe alignment, but it must be pulled thin distal to the metatarsal heads to provide a flexible toe break. If a flexible toe break is not provided, the knee extension moment may be excessive, resulting in knee hyperextension. The alternative is to trim the plastic at the metatarsal heads, but the toes are not adequately supported in this latter case.

Extending a rigid keel out to the end of the toes may be indicated to increase the extension moment at the knee. Do not extend the rigid lever arm to the end of the toes if it results in knee hyperextension or difficulty with balance (especially on stairs).

PLANTAR ASPECT

Posting may be required to accommodate the hindfoot and rearfoot position so that the subtalar joint is maintained in a neutral position, yet a plantigrade position is achieved (Weber & Agro, 1990).

Posting helps distribute the weight across the plantar aspect and prevents varus or valgus.

STRAPS

All straps should be well padded.

An instep strap angled at 45° helps hold the heel in place and prevents pistoning and friction.

KAFOs should have a three-point pressure distribution. A suprapatellar and infrapatellar strap combined distributes the pressure best. A spider knee cap pad can also be used but results in greater shear forces through the knee joint.

An infrapatellar strap often deforms the lower leg when worn for a prolonged period of time because the pressure is not well distributed. The patellar tendon–bearing orthotic trim line is preferred in this population because the pressure is better distributed.

Orthotic Fabrication Objectives

INCREASE MEDIAL AND LATERAL STABILITY

Mold in subtalar neutral position (Knutson & Clark, 1991; Weber & Agro, 1990).

Proximal trim line should be sufficiently proximal and anterior to provide adequate leverage to control the ankle and to distribute pressure evenly.

Increase base of support and equalize weight-bearing forces by means of external posting.

Valgus or pronated foot:

Post medially under first metatarsal head and medial aspect of calcaneus.

Flare posting medially to increase the base of support and to prevent deviation into valgus.

Varus or supinated foot:

Post medially under first metatarsal head to accommodate supinated position of forefoot and equalize pressure distribution.

Zero posting under calcaneus (with lateral flare if needed) to prevent deviation into supination at heel strike.

Orthoses must sit level in shoes, and the shoes should be fastened securely so they do not slide on orthoses.

DECREASE ENERGY EXPENDITURE

Ankle angle ideally molded or set at 5° plantar flexion with rigid anterior stop (see ankle angle, earlier)

Distal trim line at metatarsal heads to provide a long rigid lever arm

PROVIDE ADEQUATE TOE CLEARANCE AND SIMULATE PUSH-OFF

Plantar flexion stop, ideally set at 5° of plantar flexion if able to adequately clear toe without increasing knee flexion during swing phase (see ankle angle, earlier).

Generally a rigid dorsiflexion stop required, unless client has sufficient plantar flexor strength to control forward movement of tibia during stance phase.

INCREASE KNEE EXTENSION MOMENT

Ground-reaction force, patellar tendon–bearing orthosis

Solid ankle, cushioned heel or wedge heel anteriorly to move ground-reaction force forward at heel strike

Rigid dorsiflexion stop set in 5° plantar flexion (see ankle angle, earlier)

Keel rigid to distal aspect of metatarsal heads to provide a long rigid lever and yet still permit a flexible toe break (see keel, earlier). An even greater extension moment can be provided by extending the rigid lever to the end of the toes. This is usually contraindicated, however, because it results in difficulties with balance (especially on stairs).

PREVENT KNEE HYPEREXTENSION

(By increasing knee flexion moment)

Flare heel posteriorly to move ground-reaction force behind knee joint axis at heel strike to produce a flexion moment.

Ankle set at neutral angle with rigid dorsiflexion and plantar flexion stop (if this does not adequately prevent knee hyperextension, the angle may need to be set more acutely, into dorsiflexion). The more acute the angle, however, the greater the energy expenditure (Lehmann et al., 1985).

Table continued on following page

TABLE 22-5. LOWER LIMB ORTHOTIC SPECIFICATIONS, OBJECTIVES, AND EVALUATION CRITERIA *Continued*

A low heel (¼ to ½ inch) may decrease knee hyperextension by shifting the center of gravity forward.
Keel rigid to the distal aspect of the metatarsal heads to provide a long rigid lever to decrease energy expenditure. Plastic must be pulled thin beyond this point, however, to provide a flexible toe break (*do not* extend the rigid keel to the end of the toes, since this will increase the knee extension moment at push-off).
KAFOs with knee extension stops, if knee hyperextension cannot be adequately controlled with previously described modifications.

IMPROVE PRESSURE DISTRIBUTION
Total contact orthoses
All straps should be well padded.
Bony prominences should be padded (e.g., malleoli, prominent naviculi, patellar tendon region).
Posting to equalize pressure distribution on foot and minimize pressure on malleoli and naviculi.
Patellar tendon–bearing orthosis distributes pressure better than a proximal strap.
KAFOs: the combination of a suprapatellar and infrapatellar strap distributes pressure most effectively.

IMPROVE BALANCE
Adding a low heel (¼ to ½ inch) may improve balance by shifting the center of gravity forward in a person with a calcaneal weight-bearing position.
A high heel shifts the center of gravity too far forward and causes balance problems, particularly in a person with weak or absent plantar flexors.

Orthotic Evaluation Criteria
Check for pressure areas.
Heel must seat well in orthosis.
Check for rigid keel and flexible toe break.
Check knee alignment and congruency of knee joint axis.
All straps and bony prominences should be well padded.
Check medial and lateral alignment and make sure the orthosis is posted properly with subtalar joint in neutral.
Check angle at ankle (anterior/posterior and medial/lateral).
Check anterior and posterior stops to make sure they adequately control motion, facilitate push-off, and permit toe clearance during swing phase.
Insert orthosis in shoe to check alignment. If molded properly, the orthosis should be able to balance and stand without support on a flat surface.

---

strength was found to be the best predictor of ambulation. The quadriceps, anterior tibialis, and gluteal muscles also were determined to have significant importance for ambulation in these children. Grade 0 to 3 iliopsoas strength was always associated with partial or complete reliance on a wheelchair. Patients with grade 4 to 5 iliopsoas and quadriceps muscle strength were almost all community ambulators, and none of this group were completely wheelchair dependent. Children with grade 4 to 5 gluteal and anterior tibialis muscle strength were all classified as community ambulators and did not require the use of an assistive device or orthoses.

Key muscle groups for community ambulation, listed in order of importance, are the iliopsoas, gluteus medius and maximus, quadriceps, anterior tibialis, and hamstring muscles (McDonald et al., 1991b). Specific strength of these muscles accounted for 86% of the variance in mobility status. Gluteus medius muscle strength was found to be the best predictor of requirements for aids or orthoses. In individuals with gluteus medius strength grade 2 to 3, 72.2% required aids, orthoses, or both. If activity in this muscle was absent or trace, 95.7% required aids, orthoses, or both. In contrast, if gluteus medius strength was grade 4 to 5, only 11.2% required aids, orthoses, or both.

Agre and associates (1987) reported that maximum walking velocity was correlated with hip and knee extensor muscle strength. They compared the energy expenditure and efficiency of ambulation in children with MM versus able-bodied peers and found that children with MM exhibited 218% lower energy efficiency and a 41% lower ambulation velocity. They also reported that mobility in a wheelchair was considerably more efficient than walking, approximating normal gait in terms of energy requirements. In addition, individuals classified as having "no loss" by means of manual muscle testing had a decreased walking velocity and increased energy expenditure compared with able-bodied peers.

EQUIPMENT

A wide variety of adaptive equipment is often required for individuals with MM. Equipment needs vary considerably with level of lesion and age. Therapists must be aware of the available options and be able to select the most appropriate type of equipment for a given situation. In addition, it is important to educate parents and clients regarding the fit and appropriateness of adaptive equipment so that they can be knowledgeable consumers. It is beyond the scope of this chapter to discuss specific equipment items. The reader is referred to the work of Baker and Rogosky-Grassi (1993), Knutson and Clark (1991), and Pomatto (1991) for further information regarding adaptive equipment and orthoses for this population. In the following section the focus is on factors to consider when evaluating the appropriateness and fit of adaptive equipment. Indications for lower limb orthotics are provided in Table 22–4. Design specifications and objectives for orthoses are included in Table 22–5.

Orthoses should be closely evaluated to determine their fit, condition, and appropriateness. Skin tolerance should be monitored on a daily basis. All straps should be well padded, and there should be total contact of the orthosis with the limb, so that pressure is distributed broadly. The heel should be seated well in the orthosis. Joint alignment and congruency of orthotic and anatomic joint axes should be observed. The subtalar joint should be in a neutral position with appropriate posting, if required, so that the plantar surface of the orthosis is flat on the floor (Knutson & Clark, 1991; Weber & Agro, 1990). The anterior and posterior angles at the ankle should be set to optimize push-off yet provide adequate toe clearance (Lehmann et al., 1985).

Assessments of adaptive equipment and orthotics should be conducted on at least a yearly basis. Assessments should occur more often during periods of rapid growth; when environmental demands change (e.g., changing school or work settings); when there are changes in lifestyle, goals, or vocation; or when there is a change in status that may affect motor control or mobility. The reader is referred to Table 22–5 for considerations when evaluating the components and fit of orthoses in this population.

Orthoses decrease energy expenditure, if set at the proper angle, by substituting for weak muscles and simulating the normal path of the center of mass. Energy requirements are lowest and the gait pattern is more normal if the ankle joint is set at 5° of plantar flexion (Lehmann et al., 1985). Plastic orthoses must enclose the malleoli to effectively resist dorsiflexion and provide a good substitute for the gastrocnemius and soleus muscles during the latter part of stance (Lehmann et al., 1985). In addition, provision of medial and lateral stability at the ankle appears to be indicated for adequate function of the plantar flexors during push-off (Lehmann et al., 1986).

AGE-SPECIFIC ASSESSMENT AND PHYSICAL THERAPY

In addition to the dimensions of disability discussed earlier, there are issues that are of particular importance for specific age groups. Intervention should be provided to keep pace with the normal timing of development (Bleck & Nagel, 1982; Shurtleff, 1966). Throughout the life span, it is important to keep in mind the overall picture of the needs of the client and family. The medical problems and the number of health care professionals involved in the care of individuals with MM can be overwhelming. Many members of other disciplines in addition to the physical therapist may also be making requests of the family's time. Each professional needs to prioritize his or her goals, relative to those of other disciplines, and coordinate planning so that the demands placed on the client and the family are realistic. It is best to work as a team with the family and other disciplines to integrate appropriate intervention programs into the client's daily routine. In addition, if conflicting information is provided to parents, they often become confused and may lack appropriate information to set realistic goals for their children and adolescents (e.g., goals for mobility, self-care, employment, and independent living). Consequently, multidisciplinary team collaboration with the family is important to establish appropriate goals and expectations.

The following section focuses on special considerations throughout the life span. Four age groups are discussed: infancy, preschool age, school age, and adolescence. Disabilities that are typically present, as well as the causes and impact of functional limitations on expected life roles, are discussed for each of the four age groups. Assessment of impairments, functional limitations, and disabilities, along with recommendations for ongoing monitoring, typical physical therapy goals, intervention, and strategies to prevent secondary impairments and functional limitations, are also discussed. In addition, typical secondary disabilities and functional limitations encountered during adolescence and their impact on the transition to adulthood are discussed in the section on adolescence and transition to adulthood. The information presented in this latter section has important implications for preventative management during childhood and adolescence to minimize the incidence of acquired impairments and functional limitations that often surface later in life.

It is important to keep in mind that the interaction of a multitude of impairments may impact on an individual's functional performance, yet only a few key impairments are discussed later for each age group. The reader is referred to the previous section on impairments for a more thorough discussion of other factors. Similarly, only key assessment and intervention strategies that are specific to a given age category are discussed in each section.

Infancy

TYPICAL DISABILITIES: CAUSES AND IMPLICATIONS

The multiple impairments and overwhelming medical needs of a newborn with MM may interfere with parent–infant interaction. Parents are often afraid to handle their infant with MM, and the opportunities for handling and interacting with their child may be further limited by medical complications. Parents and extended family members may be cautious in handling the infant, resulting in decreased stimulation. Naturally occurring opportunities for early environmental stimulation, observation and exploration, and social interaction also may be limited as a result of somatosensory and motor deficits, hypotonia, and visual deficits. Family and infant interaction may be further impeded by the additional duties required of patients (e.g., bowel and bladder management), frequent medical visits, and hospitalizations for complications.

The achievement of fine motor and gross motor developmental milestones is usually delayed during infancy because of multiple impairments, including joint contractures and deformities, motor and sensory deficits, hypotonia, upper limb dyscoordination, CNS dysfunction, visual and perceptual disorders, and cognitive deficits. The lack of normal infant movements, combined with impaired sensation, results in decreased kinesthetic awareness and inhibits perceptuomotor development. Independence with early ADL, such as holding a bottle or finger feeding, is also negatively affected by impairments resulting from MM, especially swallowing disorders, upper limb dyscoordination, and visuoperceptual deficits.

ASSESSMENT OF IMPAIRMENTS

As discussed in Chapter 4, therapists must be aware of normal physiologic flexion of the hips and knees when assessing newborns. Limitations of up to 35° are present in normal newborns. These contractures may be more pronounced at birth in the infant with MM after prolonged intrauterine positioning of the relatively inactive fetus. Physiologic flexion spontaneously reduces in able-bodied infants from the effects of gravity and spontaneous lower limb movements. Physiologic flexion of infants with MM typically does not spontaneously reduce, because of decreased or absent spontaneous

lower limb activity secondary to muscle weakness. Consequently, contractures may develop even in children with sacral level function if they lack full strength of the gluteal muscles.

Two primary orthopaedic concerns during this period are to identify and manage dislocated hips and foot deformities. Early orthopaedic management of these deformities results in improved potential for standing balance and more timely achievement of motor milestones such as sitting and walking (Mayfield, 1991; Menelaus, 1976). Achieving a plantigrade foot position is important, regardless of ambulatory prognosis. Plantigrade alignment is optimal for shoe fit, positioning and weight distribution in sitting, and stability when bearing weight for standing pivot transfers or ambulation.

When assessing muscle tone in infants, the Movement Assessment of Infants (Chandler et al., 1980) is a useful tool. Hypotonia is typical in infants with MM, even if sacral level function is present (Wolf & McLaughlin, 1992). Poor head control, delayed neck and trunk righting, automatic reactions, and low trunk and lower limb muscle tone are typical. A mixture of hypotonia, hypertonia, and spastic movements may be present in the limbs. It is important to distinguish between voluntary and reflexive movements when assessing muscle function.

One of the key physical therapy considerations in managing the newborn with MM is to establish a reliable baseline of muscle function before and after back closure. This baseline is important for predicting future function and for monitoring status. In addition, it is important to identify muscle imbalance around joints and existing joint contractures that are unlikely to reduce spontaneously.

In the newborn, muscle function is assessed before and after surgical closure of the back to determine the extent of motor paralysis. Side-lying is usually the position of choice for testing the newborn, to avoid injury to the exposed neural tissue (Schneider, 1985). The state of alertness must be considered and documented when testing newborns or infants. Repeated evaluations may need to be conducted at different times of the day to observe the infant's muscle activity in various behavioral states. Optimal performance cannot be elicited if the infant is in a sleepy state. Muscle activity is best observed when the infant is alert, hungry, or crying. If the infant is drowsy, several techniques can be used to arouse the infant, including assessing limb ROM, rocking vertically to stimulate the vestibular system, and providing tactile and auditory stimulation (Hinderer & Hinderer, 1993a; Schneider, 1985). Ideally, the infant's spontaneous activity should be observed in supine, prone, and side-lying positions before the examiner starts handling the infant. Handling the infant may suppress spontaneous activity. Movement can often be elicited through sounds, visual tracking, reaching for toys, tickling, placing limbs in antigravity positions to elicit holding responses, and moving limbs to end-range positions to see if the infant will move out of the position (Hinderer & Hinderer, 1993a). For older infants, muscle activity can be observed, palpated, and resisted in developmental positions.

Therapists often do not record specific strength grades for infants and young children. Instead, either a dichotomous scale (present or absent) or a 3-point ordinal scale (apparently normal, weak, or absent) is often advocated (Murdoch, 1980; Pact et al., 1984; Schneider, 1985). This 3-point scale, however, lacks sensitivity and predictive validity (Murdoch, 1980). In contrast, specific manual muscle test strength scores (grades 0 to 5) have been found to provide useful information for infants and young children with MM and are predictive of later function (McDonald et al., 1986). Consequently, when strength is assessed manually, we recommend using the full manual muscle testing scale, regardless of age. The estimated quality of the examination should also be recorded, indicating the examiner's degree of confidence in the results, based on the child's level of cooperation. Neck and trunk musculature should be graded as "normal for age" if the child is able to perform developmentally appropriate activities (Kendall et al., 1993).

Testing sensation in infants and young children presents special challenges. Complete testing of multiple sensory modalities is not possible until the child has acquired sufficient cognitive and language abilities to accurately respond to testing (Schneider, 1985). Parents can often provide useful information to help focus on probable insensate areas. It is best to test the child in a quiet state. Testing with a pin or other sharp object should begin at the lowest level of sacral innervation and progress to more proximally innervated dermatomes until a noxious response is noted (e.g., crying or facial grimace).

ONGOING MONITORING

During the first year of life, it is important to monitor joint alignment, muscle imbalance, and the development of contractures. Typical lower limb contractures that often develop are hip and knee flexion contractures, combined with external rotation at the hips. Children with weak or absent hip musculature often lie in a "frog-legged" position with the hips flexed and externally rotated and the knees flexed. Consequently, these muscle groups are typically in a shortened position. It is important to closely monitor ROM and muscle extensibility during periods of rapid growth. Soft

tissue growth typically lags behind skeletal changes, resulting in decreased extensibility. Stretching exercises should be initiated early on, if indicated, when contractures are relatively flexible and respond well to treatment. If orthoses or night-positioning splints are used to correct orthopaedic deformities, the fit of these devices should be monitored to prevent skin breakdown.

Because therapists often see infants more frequently than other health care professionals do, they should watch for early signs of neurologic complications and report suspected changes in status to the primary care physician. Changes in muscle tone and muscle function are observed with progressive neurologic dysfunction. Baseline measurements, therefore, are essential, and these parameters should be closely monitored. Therapists should also watch for behavioral changes, decreases in performance, and other subtle signs of shunt malfunction (see Table 22–2) or seizure disorders. Motor development must also be observed to determine if an infant is keeping pace with normal developmental expectations.

TYPICAL PHYSICAL THERAPY GOALS AND STRATEGIES

During the newborn period, physical therapists must be sensitive to the feelings and needs of parents and other extended family members who are learning to cope with the overwhelming problems of a child with MM. Parents go through a period of tremendous adjustment. They are required to meet the demands of a normal infant, plus deal with the extensive medical and surgical needs of their newborn, and adjust to the long-term implications of their child's multiple impairments. Not all instructions may be assimilated at any one time given the large amount of information to which parents are asked to attend. Often instructions need to be reviewed and reinforced during subsequent visits. Written instructions should be provided to augment verbal explanations.

If ROM is limited, parents should be instructed in positioning techniques. It is optimal to maintain ROM by means of positioning because little additional time is required of the family. If contractures do not resolve with positioning, or if contractures are not supple, parents should also be instructed in stretching exercises and soft tissue mobilization techniques. It is usually most efficient to perform stretching exercises and soft tissue mobilization techniques in conjunction with diaper changes.

For infants who exhibit hypotonia, parents should be instructed in handling techniques to facilitate head and trunk control. Techniques advocated for children with hypotonic cerebral palsy (e.g., Finnie, 1975) are often beneficial. Parents should be encouraged to provide sitting opportunities for the infant to facilitate the development of head and trunk control. Additional head and trunk support is often required in high chairs, strollers, and car seats. If motor development is significantly delayed and requires therapeutic intervention, a combination of neurodevelopmental treatment and proprioceptive neuromuscular facilitation techniques is beneficial. Therapeutic interventions and adaptive equipment should be planned to ideally keep pace with the normal timing of development, so that the child is provided with normal developmental experiences. During the later half of the first year, preparatory activities for mobility are indicated. Emphasis should be placed on balance, trunk control, and facilitating an upright posture as the child progresses through the developmental sequence.

PREVENTION OF SECONDARY IMPAIRMENTS AND FUNCTIONAL LIMITATIONS

Parents should be instructed in proper positioning, ROM, and handling techniques with the lower limbs in neutral alignment to prevent the development of contractures. If the hips are dislocated or subluxed, parents should be instructed in proper positioning, double diapering, and the use of a night-positioning orthosis, if indicated (Rowley-Kelly & Kunkle, 1993; Schafer & Dias, 1983). If surgery is indicated to relocate hip dislocations (see previous section on orthopaedic deformities), it is generally performed after 6 months of age. Foot deformities are generally treated through serial casting or positioning splints.

Parents should also be instructed to inspect insensate skin areas during diaper changes and dressing for signs of pressure or injury. Parents need to understand the importance of skin inspection and that insensate areas should be inspected on a daily basis throughout life.

Toddler and Preschool Years

TYPICAL DISABILITIES: CAUSES AND IMPLICATIONS

The achievement of fine motor and gross motor developmental milestones continues to be delayed. Mobility is typically impaired in this population owing to orthopaedic, motor, and sensory deficits. As the child nears the end of the first year of life, it is important to provide opportunities for environmental exploration. If the child does not have an efficient, effective mode of independent mobility

by the end of the first year, provision of a mobility device is indicated.

Environmental exploration is essential for the development of initiative and independence. Limited early mobility may result in a lack of curiosity and initiative and may negatively affect other aspects of development (Becker, 1975; Burlingham, 1953; Butler et al., 1984; Oakland & Sherman, 1969; Shurtleff, 1986d; White et al., 1979). If a toddler does not have an effective means of independently exploring and interacting with the environment, he or she may learn to be passively dependent. The negative influence of limited early mobility on personality and behavior development can persist throughout life. Passive-dependent behavior is a commonly observed personality trait of adolescents and adults with MM.

Limited mobility also negatively affects socialization, especially interaction with other children. If a stroller is used as the primary mode of community mobility beyond the normal age of weaning a child from a stroller, other children will view the child with MM as a "baby." Play opportunities are also limited if a child does not have an effective means of mobility.

Independence with ADL is often impaired in this population because of fine and gross motor impairments, upper limb dyscoordination, and CNS dysfunction. Children who are not independent with ADL may miss out on normal childhood experiences (e.g., play time) while waiting for others to assist them with basic skills. Their self-esteem may also be negatively affected if other children tease them regarding their dependency.

It is important that parents, child care personnel, and preschool teachers be aware of other motor deficits that are often exhibited in this population, such as poor eye-hand coordination. The potential impact of these deficits on functional performance in handwriting and the acquisition of ADL skills such as feeding and dressing should be realized, so that reasonable goals can be established and the use of appropriate adaptive equipment implemented.

ASSESSMENT OF IMPAIRMENTS AND FUNCTIONAL LIMITATIONS

By the end of the first year, ROM is expected to be within normal limits. If limited ROM persists, it is important to distinguish between fixed and supple contractures. Muscle extensibility should also be determined. Orthopaedic deformities should be evaluated to determine if they are fixed or flexible.

To assess strength, functional muscle testing techniques are advocated for young children 2 to 5 years old because they may not cooperate with traditional test procedures (Hinderer & Hinderer,

1993a; Pact et al., 1984). Functional activities that are helpful in determining the strength of key lower limb muscle groups include gait observations, heel- and toe-walking, climbing up and down a step, one-legged stand, toe touching, squat to stand, bridging, bicycling in supine, the Landau position, prone kicking, the wheelbarrow position, sit-ups, pull to sit, and sitting and standing push-ups. It is often possible for young children to cooperate with isolated muscle actions by having them push against a puppet to show how strong they are. To elicit the cooperation of older preschoolers (3- to 4 year olds), it is often helpful to name the muscle and describe its "job" (the muscle action). The children think that the muscle names are humorous, maintaining their attention. Asking children to have the muscle do its "job" makes strength testing more understandable (Hinderer & Hinderer, 1993a). We have found it possible to obtain objective, reliable measures of strength from children as young as 4 years of age using hand-held myometry techniques (Hinderer & Hinderer, 1993a). The degree of confidence regarding whether the child's optimal performance was elicited should be recorded.

Once the child is 2 years of age, light touch and position sense can usually be assessed by eliciting tickling responses or having the child respond to the touch of a puppet. Other sensory modalities can ordinarily be accurately tested once the child is 5 to 7 years old. The accuracy of responses often needs to be double checked because of short attention span and response perseveration. Two sensory testing techniques help to minimize perseveration of responses. The first is to randomly alternate between testing light touch and pinprick and have the child identify the type of sensation. The second is to have the child point to the spot that was touched and correctly state when no area was touched.

Fine and gross motor development should be assessed using appropriate standardized tests such as those discussed in Chapters 1 and 2. Evaluation of ADL should focus on what the individual actually does on a daily basis, in addition to what he or she is capable of doing. If independence with ADL is limited, appropriate adaptations and interventions should be implemented to foster independence. The Functional Activities Assessment (Okamoto et al., 1984; Sousa et al., 1976, 1983) is useful for this population (Fig. 22–6). Items may be scored by direct observation or by parent report. Assistive devices required to perform a given task are also documented. The "Can" and "Does" scoring format permits the examiner to record what the child can do versus what the child actually does on a regular basis. In addition, if the child is directly observed performing the task, the degree of inde-

pendence and the time to complete the task are recorded.

ONGOING MONITORING

Joint alignment, muscle imbalance, contractures, posture, and signs of progressive neurologic dysfunction should continue to be monitored. Contractures that seem insignificant during childhood may become functionally limiting once the individual has adult-sized body proportions. For example, knee extension contractures can interfere with the ability to maneuver in a wheelchair.

TYPICAL PHYSICAL THERAPY GOALS AND STRATEGIES

Joint alignment, contractures, muscle strength, and postural alignment should continue to be treated, as necessary. Proper positioning in sleeping and sitting should continue. If stretching or strengthening exercises are indicated, it is often helpful to involve other family members in the exercise program so that the child does not feel singled out. For ambulatory candidates with weak hip and knee musculature, strengthening activities may be beneficial if the child is cooperative. In addition to traditional posture exercises (Kendall et al., 1993), many play activities promote strengthening and the development of good posture (Embrey et al., 1983). The use of therapy ball techniques to strengthen postural muscles is also beneficial. Muscle re-education techniques, such as functional electrical stimulation and biofeedback, are useful to teach muscles to function in new ROM after stretching exercises. Electrical stimulation has also been found to be beneficial in increasing strength and enhancing functional performance in this population (Karmel-Ross et al., 1992).

During the preschool years, the focus is on improving the independence, efficiency, and effectiveness of ADL and mobility. Development of independence with dressing and feeding should be encouraged. Appropriate guidance should be provided, so that parents have age-appropriate expectations. It is important for young children to actively participate in skin inspection, bowel and bladder management, donning and doffing orthoses, wheelchair management, and other ADL tasks. Teaching these skills early on and actively involving the child facilitates independence and incorporation of these activities into the daily routine. As a result, these extra responsibilities required of the child with MM become as natural as other ADL, such as brushing teeth. Waiting to introduce tasks until the child is older is often met with resistance, especially when the child observes that siblings do not have the same requirements.

By kindergarten age, children without disabilities are able to dress and toilet themselves (with the exception of some fasteners), eat independently, and be mobile (Fay et al., 1986). These skills need to be emphasized at an early age in the MM populations so that independence is achieved by the time the child begins school. A wide range of age of achievement of independence with ADL is evident in this population when examining the normative data provided on the Functional Activities Assessment (see Fig. 22–6). This wide variability in age of achieving skills within a given motor level suggests that a significant percentage of children are delayed in ADL skill acquisition because of attitudes and expectations. Fay and associates (1986) suggest that these delays may be partially caused by low parental expectations and protective attitudes, perceptions that it is faster for the parent to perform the

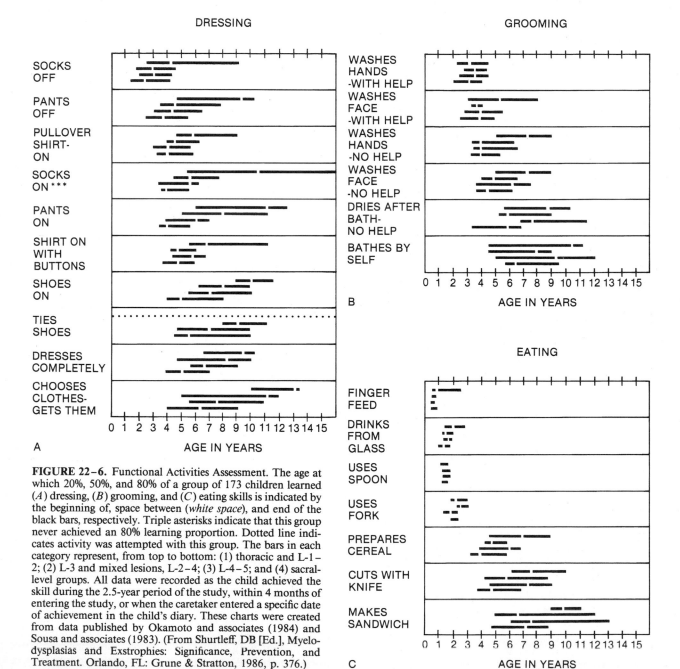

FIGURE 22–6. Functional Activities Assessment. The age at which 20%, 50%, and 80% of a group of 173 children learned (*A*) dressing, (*B*) grooming, and (*C*) eating skills is indicated by the beginning of, space between (*white space*), and end of the black bars, respectively. Triple asterisks indicate that this group never achieved an 80% learning proportion. Dotted line indicates activity was attempted with this group. The bars in each category represent, from top to bottom: (1) thoracic and L-1–2; (2) L-3 and mixed lesions, L-2–4; (3) L-4–5; and (4) sacral-level groups. All data were recorded as the child achieved the skill during the 2.5-year period of the study, within 4 months of entering the study, or when the caretaker entered a specific date of achievement in the child's diary. These charts were created from data published by Okamoto and associates (1984) and Sousa and associates (1983). (From Shurtleff, DB [Ed.], Myelodysplasias and Exstrophies: Significance, Prevention, and Treatment. Orlando, FL: Grune & Stratton, 1986, p. 376.)

task, and parental difficulty accepting the reality of the child's functional impairments. Showing parents the ADL normative data for children with MM and promoting positive parental expectations of independence are beneficial. It is important for parents to positively reinforce the child's attempts to be independent so he or she is motivated to achieve.

Skin inspection and pressure relief techniques should be taught early so that they are incorporated into the daily routine. Proper management of lower limbs and joint protection techniques should be taught to avoid injury of insensate areas when learning how to perform ADL, such as transfers. The impact of sensory deficits on functional performance should be kept in mind during gait training and when teaching other functional tasks.

Provision of an effective means of independent mobility is *essential* for young children. Consequently, if a child does not begin maneuvering effectively within the environment by 1 year of age, alternative means of mobility need to be considered to achieve independent home and short-distance community mobility (Butler et al., 1984; Shurtleff, 1986d). Mobility options should be explored and implemented as frequently as is needed so that the child is able to actively participate in normal childhood activities. Various mobility options are available, from manual devices such as a castor cart to electric wheelchairs. Electric wheelchair use has been found to be feasible and beneficial for children as young as 24 months of age (Butler et al., 1984). If a wheelchair is indicated, it is important to present this option to the parents in a positive way. The use of a wheelchair does not preclude walking. In fact, children who use wheelchairs at an early age generally are more interested in mobility, independence, and environmental exploration. Consequently, they tend to be more independent in all forms of mobility later in life. Ryan and associates (1991) recommend introducing a wheelchair as early as 18 months to enable children to keep up with their peers, boost self-confidence, facilitate independence, and increase activity levels.

Preparatory activities for mobility are indicated for 1 to 2 year olds. Emphasis should be placed on balance, trunk control, and facilitating an upright posture. For ambulatory candidates, once the child begins to pull to stand, the need for orthoses to improve weight-bearing alignment should be considered. It is important to anticipate future ambulatory needs when recommending orthoses to maximize their utility.

For children with high-level lesions (thoracic to L-2), preparatory activities for wheelchair mobility should be emphasized (e.g., sitting balance, arm strengthening, transfer training, wheelchair propulsion, and electrical switch operation if indicated). The focus of wheelchair training for toddlers and preschoolers with high-level lesions should include mobility, environmental exploration, safety, and transfer skills. Household distance ambulation using a parapodium, HKAFO, KAFO, or RGO may be attempted, but energy expenditure is very high. Consequently, wheelchairs are generally used for community mobility of children with thoracic to L-2 motor function, particularly once body proportions increase.

Biped ambulation is feasible for toddlers and preschoolers with L-3 and below motor function. It is essential to maintain adequate ROM and to emphasize an upright posture so that weight-bearing forces are properly distributed and muscles can function at their optimal length. Therapeutic activities that promote trunk control and balance are beneficial. Children with lumbar level lesions will require upper limb support for walking. In general, a reverse-facing walker is best when learning to walk, so that the child is upright and upper limb weight bearing is minimized. Reverse-facing walkers have been found to promote better postural alignment than anterior-facing walkers (Logan et al., 1990). Once an upright gait is established, the child can be advanced to forearm crutches.

If children with sacral level motor function require upper limb support to begin walking, a reverse-facing walker is also usually best to minimize upper limb weight bearing. Alternatively, forearm crutches can be used if the child is able to walk upright while manipulating the crutches. Children with L-5 and S-1 level lesions often abandon their upper limb aids when they are young and their center of mass is low to the ground. Upper limb aids may still be indicated for endurance and to decrease trunk sway when walking long distances, for balance when walking on rough terrain, or to minimize the stress on weight-bearing lower limb joints. The need for upper limb aids should be re-evaluated when the child is older and body proportions and environmental demands have changed.

The use of positive reinforcement is often recommended for this population to enhance cooperation with assessment procedures and treatment programs. In general, food is not an appropriate form of reinforcement because obesity is often a concern. Verbal reinforcement is preferred at this age.

PREVENTION OF SECONDARY IMPAIRMENTS AND FUNCTIONAL LIMITATIONS

Individuals are at risk for joint contractures when there is muscle imbalance around joints, when a substantial portion of the day is spent sitting, when there is a prolonged period of immobilization or bed rest, after recent surgery, and during periods of rapid growth when soft tissue growth may lag behind skeletal changes. It is important to closely monitor individuals with MM during these periods so that treatment can be initiated early on, if needed, when contractures are still flexible and respond well to treatment. Early detection and treatment of contractures is important to prevent fixed deformities and stretch weakness of overlengthened muscles.

Habitual postural positions that contribute to deforming forces should be discouraged. Positions that should be avoided include the "frog-leg" position in prone or supine, W-sitting, ring sitting, heel sitting, and cross-legged sitting. The importance of skin inspection of insensate areas, use of pressure relief cushions, and sitting push-ups for pressure relief should be emphasized at an early age so that these preventative measures become routine.

It is essential to emphasize an upright posture when a child is learning to walk. If children are permitted to walk in a crouched position, hip and knee flexion contractures develop, muscles are required to function at a mechanical disadvantage, and weight-bearing joint stress is increased (especially for upper limb joints). Once a crouched gait pattern has become established, it is difficult to teach a more upright posture because of the joint contractures and stretch weakness of excessively lengthened muscles that have developed over time. Therapists must closely observe joint alignment and posture when a child is upright. Postural deviations that look insignificant when a child is young are often magnified once body proportions increase. The importance of an upright posture should be emphasized to clients, parents, and other care providers.

School Age

TYPICAL DISABILITIES: CAUSES AND IMPLICATIONS

Independence with ADL often continues to be impaired in this age group. Children who are not independent with ADL may miss out on normal childhood experiences (e.g., play time or recess) while waiting for parents or teachers to assist them with basic skills. Their self-esteem may continue to be negatively affected if other children tease them regarding their dependency.

Mobility limitations are magnified once a child begins school because of the increased community mobility distances and skills required. Advanced mobility skills are needed because of environmental barriers such as curbs, ramps, uneven terrain,

and steps. Ineffective or inefficient community mobility can further reinforce dependent behaviors if other children carry his or her school books and lunch tray or push the wheelchair.

The negative effects of limited mobility and physical limitations on socialization become more apparent at this age. Play and recreational opportunities are restricted if a child does not have an effective method of mobility. Often children with MM are excluded from recess or physical education class. Consequently, they miss out on opportunities for social interaction. Even if they are included in these activities, often their involvement is peripheral (e.g., score keeper during physical education class). Mobility limitations, dependency with ADL, difficulties with toileting, and the difficulty of managing adaptive equipment often interfere with other aspects of peer interaction, such as going over to friends' houses to play or spending the night with friends.

Finally, it is important that parents and teachers be aware of perceptuomotor, visuoperceptual, and sensory deficits. The potential impact of these deficits on writing speed, legibility, and accuracy, the efficiency and effectiveness of performing ADL skills, problem solving, and cognitive abilities should be realized so that reasonable goals can be established and the use of appropriate adaptive equipment can be implemented. Multiple hospitalizations or medical complications can also negatively impact school performance.

ASSESSMENT OF IMPAIRMENTS AND FUNCTIONAL LIMITATIONS

As with younger children, joint alignment, strength, muscle imbalance, contractures, muscle extensibility, and posture should continue to be monitored. Other parameters that should be assessed include sensation, coordination, fine motor skills, ADL, mobility, gait, body awareness, and functional skills.

Reliable, sensitive, objective measures of strength can be obtained in school-aged children (Hinderer & Hinderer, 1993a). We recommend that objective methods of strength assessment, such as hand-held myometry, be used to serially monitor strength of individuals with MM who are old enough to cooperate (typically age 4 or older). Stationary isokinetic or strain gauge devices can also provide objective measures of strength, but these devices are not available in the typical clinic or school setting.

Independence with ADL should be assessed. In addition to the basic ADL skills evaluated in the Functional Activities Assessment, the school-aged child's ability to carry items and assist with basic household chores should be evaluated. The adequacy of clearance, duration, frequency, and reliability of performance of wheelchair push-ups are also assessed by the physical therapist. Bowel and bladder function and the degree of continence are usually evaluated by a nurse. It is important that the physical therapist understand the functional impairments and degree of independence with bowel and bladder function, however, because positioning, adaptive equipment, and mobility issues can often restrict independence with bowel and bladder management programs.

The home, school, and community environments should be accessible so that individuals with MM can participate fully in all activities. The Americans with Disabilities Act of 1990 mandates access to all buildings, programs, and services used by the general public in the United States. Even partial exclusion from a school program can have lasting negative effects on a student's social and emotional development (Baker & Rogosky-Grassi, 1993). Providing accessibility to the entirety of school, home, and community activities lets individuals with MM know that they have the same opportunities and rights of access as everyone else. Limited access broadcasts a message of exclusion and estrangement. Both physical and social barriers to participation need to be addressed. For a more thorough discussion of evaluating environmental accessibility in the school setting, see the work of Baker and Rogosky-Grassi (1993). Community accessibility should also be evaluated. Ideally, the client should have access to the community school, church, grocery and drug stores, post office, bank, cleaners, stores and shopping malls, library, restaurants, theaters, sports arenas, hospital, physician's office, work environment, and public transportation. Streets, sidewalks, crosswalks, and parking lots should also be accessible.

ONGOING MONITORING

Joint alignment, muscle imbalance, contractures, posture, and signs of progressive neurologic dysfunction should continue to be monitored. As school-aged children mature, they should become more responsible for daily inspection of insensate skin areas when they are bathing and dressing. Appropriate performance of pressure relief strategies also should be monitored. Areas of skin breakdown should be noted so that appropriate adjustments in equipment and preventative behaviors can be implemented or reviewed.

School-aged children should be observed closely during periods of rapid growth because they are at risk for loss of function as a result of cord tethering. Parents and teachers should be made aware of signs of progressive CNS complications so that they know when to refer the child to a primary care physician.

TYPICAL PHYSICAL THERAPY GOALS AND STRATEGIES

The stretching and strengthening strategies discussed for the two previous age groups also apply to the school-aged child. Improving the flexibility of low back extensor, hip flexor, hamstrings, and shoulder girdle musculature should be emphasized. When possible, stretching and strengthening exercises should also be incorporated into the physical education program. It is important that children with MM participate in physical education classes and sport activities in a meaningful way.

Proper positioning while sleeping and sitting should continue. In the classroom, seating should provide stability and symmetric alignment. Feet should be flat on the floor or on wheelchair footrests. The seat and desk height should be adjusted to fit the child's body proportions. The desk top should be tilted up to improve neck and upper trunk alignment. Appropriate cushioning should be provided. The child's chair should be positioned in the room so that the teacher and blackboard can easily be viewed while maintaining neutral alignment, without having to turn in the chair.

If a child has not achieved independence with a given ADL task by the age at which 50% of the normative group achieved independence on the Functional Activities Assessment, the child's performance should be assessed to determine if adaptive equipment is required or if further interventions are indicated. Goals for ADL performance should include efficiency in addition to independence. If the child is not as efficient as the primary caretaker, the caretaker will most likely perform the task. The target goal, therefore, is for the child to be able to perform the task as efficiently as the primary caretaker. Showing parents the ADL normative data for children with MM and promoting positive parental expectations of independence are beneficial (see Fig. 22–6). It is important for parents to positively reinforce the child's attempts to be independent so he or she is motivated to achieve. Pressure relief techniques should be incorporated into the daily routine. Joint protection measures also should be implemented early on to prevent the development of future degenerative changes.

Once children with MM begin school, it is important that they have an independent, efficient, and effective means of mobility for home and community distances. Alternative means of mobility may need to be considered for long distances to ensure that children with MM are able to keep up with their peers and still have energy left to attend to classroom activities. Various mobility options should be evaluated according to the criteria outlined in Table 22–3 to determine the most effective means of mobility for a given environment. Community level wheelchair and ambulation skills should be taught, emphasizing efficiency and safety. Community, home, and school environments should be assessed to determine if there are architectural barriers that interfere with daily activities. It is essential for normal social development to permit accessibility to all of the school, home, and community activities, including recess, physical education, and field trips (Baker & Rogosky-Grassi, 1993).

A functional environment should be created at home and school by removing obstacles and adapting the environment to facilitate efficient and independent function. Adaptive equipment and effective mobility devices should be provided to maximize function. Community mobility skills may need to be practiced to facilitate independent function. Endurance training may also be indicated to ensure that the individual has sufficient endurance and efficiency to function effectively in all activities.

Recreation and physical fitness are important for physical, psychological, and social reasons. Psychosocial benefits of participation in recreational activities include enhancing confidence and self-esteem, increasing socialization, improving group participation skills, provision of a means of exercising in a more normal way, and increasing interest and motivation in maintaining flexibility, strengthening, and endurance. In contrast, perceived physical restrictions result in a sedentary lifestyle, potentially predisposing these individuals to problems with obesity and degenerative diseases. It is important to stimulate a life-long interest in fitness and recreation. In addition, community resources, feasibility of transportation, and the family's lifestyle must be taken into account.

Recreation activities must be carefully selected to ensure that they are beneficial and feasible yet enjoyable so they will be continued on a regular basis. Ideally, recreation activities should incorporate forms of aerobic exercise, along with socialization. It is important for individuals with MM to be involved in regular aerobic exercise to maintain their physical fitness and effectively control their weight. Recreational and physical fitness goals include maintaining and improving flexibility, strength, endurance, aerobic capacity and cardiovascular fitness, coordination, and controlling weight. Low-impact aerobics are preferred to minimize stress on joints. Aerobic exercise videotapes have been developed for individuals with disabilities. Swimming is

an ideal sport for this population, because they are often able to be competitive with their able-bodied peers and there is minimal stress on joints. Other low-impact activities include cycling, rowing, cross-country skiing, roller and ice skating, and aerobic dance.

Verbal reinforcement or implementation of a token economy system to earn special privileges is preferred at this age to enhance cooperation with assessment procedures and treatment programs. As was mentioned earlier, food is not an appropriate form of reinforcement.

PREVENTION OF SECONDARY IMPAIRMENTS AND FUNCTIONAL LIMITATIONS

As discussed earlier, it is important to monitor the development of joint contractures. Postural deficits, if uncorrected over time, can result in joint contractures and deformities, stretch weakness, and musculoskeletal pain. Deficits that may appear insignificant during childhood often become magnified once an individual has adult body proportions, resulting in functional limitations and discomfort (e.g., low back pain resulting from an increased lumbar lordosis and hip flexion contractures).

Joint protection is also important, even at this early age. Joint trauma from excessive stress is cumulative over the life span. Children do not typically complain of pain, and children with MM may not be able to reliably detect pain in insensate areas. Consequently, sources of excess joint stress need to be identified by carefully observing children while they perform ADL and transfers, walk, and propel their wheelchair.

Children and their parents should be involved as much as possible in the decision-making and management of their disability. The rationale for assistive devices and therapeutic interventions should be explained so that they are in agreement with treatment plans and become knowledgeable regarding acquisition of medical care and services, rather than being passive recipients.

Adolescence and Transition into Adulthood

TYPICAL DISABILITIES: CAUSES AND IMPLICATIONS

Adolescence often brings expanded domains of travel for individuals with MM. School buildings become larger, with more environmental barriers for people with physical disabilities. To keep up with peers, community mobility must include mobility skills to travel long distances quickly and efficiently between classrooms, out to athletic fields as a participant or spectator, around shopping malls, and into crowded movie theaters, dances, and night clubs. Independent adult living also requires mobility and balance skills that permit completion of advanced ADL tasks such as cooking, cleaning, clothes washing, shopping, yardwork, house and equipment maintenance, driving, riding on public transportation, and going to work. Children who have gotten by with slow, inefficient ambulation skills using cumbersome adaptive equipment or have had basic wheelchair mobility on level surfaces but suddenly cannot handle ramps, hills, curbs, and uneven ground are "left in the dust." Nearly all of the adults in a study of 30 individuals with MM (Hinderer et al, 1988) required referral to a physical therapist to address advanced mobility or equipment issues. It has been the observation of the authors that many adolescents and young adults do not have sufficient mobility skills to succeed independently in the community and must play "catch-up " to achieve their functional potential. The price paid for this delayed development of functional community mobility and lack of independence is social incompetence, dependence for advanced living skills, and unemployability, all of which must subsequently be addressed once mobility skills are improved.

Changes in functional mobility skills often occur concurrently with the rapid changes of adolescence. Individuals who have previously been ambulatory often become more reliant on a wheelchair. Dudgeon and associates (1991) reported that adolescents with MM often exhibit changes in ambulation that are not explained by progressive complications. They suggest that these changes reflect adaptation of mobility to new environmental and social demands that require different speed, accessibility, and energy demands than those encountered in childhood. If orthotic stabilization of the hip, knee, or both is required, it is unlikely that adolescents with MM will maintain community ambulation; instead, most become nonambulators (Dudgeon et al., 1991). Wheelchair transfer skills are also observed to decline in some individuals. The study of 30 adults with MM (Hinderer et al., 1988) showed that 43% had declined in their mobility status from previous examinations performed during adolescence. Several potential factors can play a role in this decreased function.

Changes in body proportions and body composition occur throughout the growing years, but the rate of these changes is accelerated dramatically during adolescence (Hinderer & Hinderer, 1993a). Increases in limb length affect the torque generated by muscles as a result of increased muscle length and resistance force moment arms. In addition,

increases in height raise the location of the center of mass higher off the ground, making upright balance more difficult and energy expenditure greater to perform mobility tasks. Changes in body composition also alter the biomechanics of movement and affect performance. The relative percentage of force-generating muscle to fat and bone tissue changes the ratio of force-producing tissue to the load of the limbs. The development of obesity often occurs during adolescence and can further accentuate these changes. Additionally, it is known that during the adolescent growth spurt, the rate of skeletal growth exceeds the increase in muscle mass; the latter catches up after skeletal growth slows in late adolescence. Decreased flexibility of the trunk and two-joint limb muscles is often observed as part of this process. Normal adolescents frequently become clumsy during this period of adjustment while learning how to coordinate their longer limb lengths and increased muscle mass. Adolescents with MM already have a mechanical disadvantage and are consequently more susceptible to dyscoordination and decreased flexibility. It is likely that these developmental changes contribute to the decline in mobility that often occurs in adolescents with MM.

Progression of the neurologic deficit is another potential cause for decline in mobility function, and adolescents are particularly at risk during rapid periods of growth. Forty percent of the participants in our adult follow-up study (Hinderer et al., 1988) had lower limb strength loss compared with previous strength examinations as adolescents. Twenty-seven percent had a reduction in lower limb sensory perception. The greatest motor and sensory losses occurred in the groups with lesions at L-5 and below—the individuals with the most function to lose. Additionally, 10% of study participants demonstrated upper limb strength loss. Progressive neurologic loss, therefore, appears to be an important factor in the changes in mobility status of many individuals during adolescence.

Immobilization for treatment of secondary complications of MM can also contribute to decreased mobility skills. The development of decubiti, fractures, and orthopaedic surgeries such as spinal fusions often require extended periods of immobilization with consequent disuse weakness, decreased endurance, and contracture development, all of which can contribute to decreased performance of mobility and transfer tasks.

Prolonged periods of bed rest are often necessary to heal decubitus ulcers to avoid bearing weight on pressure areas. Adolescents often have an increased incidence of decubiti compared with younger children. This is due to their increased body mass causing greater pressure over bony prominences around the buttocks and because of the development of adult sweat patterns in these areas. Fifty-six percent of the adults evaluated in our study (Hinderer et al., 1988) had a history of skin breakdown since their last evaluation as adolescents; nearly 17% had breakdown present at the time of the evaluation. An alarming number of these people had little insight into the causes or methods for preventing skin breakdown despite their previous care in a large multidisciplinary pediatric clinic. Even more disturbing was the fact that three individuals (10%) had sustained lower limb amputations since adolescence (two bilateral, one unilateral) as a result of nonhealing ulcers that had progressed to osteomyelitis. Clearly, functional mobility is impacted by decubitus ulcers and especially by limb loss.

Musculoskeletal problems can also impact the mobility of adolescents. Progression of spinal deformities often occurs during the growth spurt or in conjunction with one of the neurologic complications previously discussed. Sitting and standing balance can be affected by these spinal changes, leading to decreased mobility and transfer skills. Spinal orthoses prescribed to maintain optimal postural alignment also limit trunk ROM and hip flexion, interfering with wheelchair transfers and moving from sitting to standing. Surgical fusion of the spine to correct deformity and prevent its further progression can lead to immobilization with its consequent effects on mobility described earlier. Lower limb fractures secondary to osteoporosis can also necessitate immobilization with increased risk of functional loss.

Adolescents often begin to develop wear and tear changes of weight-bearing joints as a result of the excessive loading of these joints necessitated by their neurologic deficit. Joint pain, ligamentous instability, or tendinitis can further limit mobility capabilities. Fifty percent of the adult study participants (Hinderer et al., 1988) complained of joint pain and 100% had joint or spinal deformities noted at the time of their examination.

Several other issues become important for the physical therapist to be cognizant of during adolescence. Independence with self-care and other daily activities is essential for normal socialization and for preparing individuals to lead normal adult lives. Bowel and bladder continence and independent management of bowel and bladder emptying are essential for social acceptance by peers and are even more critical at this stage because of the impact on dating, sexuality, higher education, employment, and independent living. Design and fit of wheelchair equipment, mobility aids, and orthoses affect independence with these tasks. Cosmesis is also a consideration with regard to equipment selection because body image and appearance become increasingly important issues during adolescence. Improper design or fit of equipment can significantly limit normal development in these areas.

ASSESSMENT OF IMPAIRMENTS AND FUNCTIONAL LIMITATION

Based on the discussion of disabilities and their causes, several impairments should be assessed by the physical therapist. Emphasis of specific impairments should be based on the known or suspected concurrent medical problems.

Joint ROM and muscle extensibility of two-joint muscles (especially hip and knee flexors) and trunk muscles should be assessed. Neck and low back motions are often restricted, particularly in adolescents and adults because of muscle imbalance and poor postural habits. Joint swelling, ligamentous instability, crepitus, and pain with or without joint motion should be documented. If these conditions are progressive or severe enough to interfere with function, the client should be referred to a physician for further evaluation and treatment. The distribution of degenerative joint changes should be noted with regard to performance of mobility tasks and obesity to determine the contribution of abnormal joint stresses to joint pain and dysfunction.

Muscle strength should continue to be monitored for all major upper and lower limb muscle groups. When progressive neurologic dysfunction is suspected, coordination testing and serial grip strength measurements can also be helpful. Posture and trunk balance in sitting and standing (for ambulators) should be assessed. Real or apparent leg length discrepancy may be present in individuals with foot and ankle deformities, lower limb contractures, unilateral or bilateral hip dislocation, or pelvic obliquity related to spinal curves.

Thorough assessment of bed mobility, floor mobility, wheelchair mobility and transfers, and appropriateness and fit of wheelchair equipment is essential for wheelchair users. Endurance and effectiveness of mobility should be assessed to determine if the individual's current mode of mobility is practical for community level function. Table 22–3 provides further detail regarding important areas to assess. When orthoses are needed to maintain proper alignment or to facilitate efficient ambulation, the appropriateness and fit of the orthoses must be assessed by the physical therapist. Tables 22–4 and 22–5 provide further information regarding lower limb orthoses used in this population.

ONGOING MONITORING

Given the multitude of potential problems that can occur during adolescence and adulthood, comprehensive evaluations should continue on at least a yearly basis, and potentially more frequently when problems are suspected or known to be present. Without regular re-evaluation, these individuals often "fall through the cracks" and endure permanent loss of function that was avoidable. An unfortunate example was one of the adult study participants with a diagnosis of lipomeningocele and a neurosegmental classification of "no loss" as an adolescent. His lesion level was reclassified at an L-5 level at the time of our study. His loss of neurologic function was caused by a recurrent lipoma on his spine that went undetected and was not surgically removed until permanent neurologic loss had occurred. This individual thought that because his original lesion was removed as an infant with preservation of his spinal cord function, he had no risk of future problems and therefore did not seek medical care until neurologic loss was irreversible. Early detection of progressive muscle strength loss, scoliosis, progression of spasticity, or contractures by the physical therapist with timely referral to a physician familiar with the potential complications associated with MM and aggressive physical therapy (see section on prevention of secondary impairments and functional limitations) to reverse lost function can avoid this scenario. This patient's story underscores the need for all individuals with MM to be followed *throughout* life, even if there are seemingly no current problems or their lesion has been classified as "no loss" after surgical closure.

TYPICAL PHYSICAL THERAPY GOALS AND STRATEGIES

Functional goals for adolescents and adults are based on a number of factors that have been discussed in preceding sections of this chapter. The section on determinants of outcome and prognosis provides guidelines for outcome expectations based on neurologic system function. In general, the goal for all but the most severely involved clients is to achieve independent basic and community mobility skills. The physical therapist must, therefore, be aware of all environments, distances, and barriers the individual is required to negotiate to adequately prepare the client for all eventualities. Instruction in advanced community skills, along with endurance training, is often indicated. Physical and occupational therapists often need to be involved with driver's education programs and with the provision of adaptive equipment required for driving.

Goodwyn (1990) expanded the Functional Activities Assessment format to include adolescent skills required for independent living. The items were selected from existing adult-oriented skill achievement tests, and normative data were studied in this population. The Kohlman Evaluation of Living Skills (McGourty, 1988) is also a useful screening tool for determining independence with adult living skills such as self-care, safety, health maintenance, money management, transportation, telephone use, and work and leisure activities. For adolescents and adults, the ability to lift and carry items such as a hot dish, grocery bags, a laundry basket, and heavy household items is also important to evaluate. It is particularly important to observe safety issues and the use of proper body mechanics for advanced living skills. In addition, the maximum carrying distance should be determined and contrasted to functional demands. If independence and effectiveness with ADL are limited, appropriate adaptations and interventions should be made to foster independence. Environmental adaptations or assistive devices required to perform functional tasks should be determined and specifically selected for application to social, educational, vocational, and work capacity requirements of the adolescent and adult. Vocational counseling and planning should begin early during the high school years. A social worker may need to be involved with the family to assist with the transition toward independent living because a mutually dependent relationship is often fostered by the intense lifelong involvement of parents and siblings in assisting the individual with MM. Recreation therapy may be used to assist with shopping for and purchasing personal items, use of public transportation, and developing appropriate adult leisure activities. Occupational therapy may be useful to address advanced living skills such as cooking, cleaning, laundry, money management, and driver's training for appropriate candidates. Depending on the practice setting, however, it may be necessary for the physical therapist to manage these areas. The expectation for individuals with MM who have intelligence in the normal range and sufficient motor function to care for themselves is the ability to thrive as an independent adult in our society.

PREVENTION OF SECONDARY IMPAIRMENTS AND FUNCTIONAL LIMITATIONS

The physical therapist plays an important role in anticipating the potential for functional loss when one of the medical complications of MM previously described increases the risk of secondary impairments. For example, when an adolescent undergoes a surgical procedure that requires extended bed rest, then maintenance of muscle extensibility, joint ROM, and strength at the bedside followed by resumption of physical mobility tasks as soon as possible postoperatively can prevent long-term or permanent decline in mobility skills. Unfortunately, care providers are often not aware of these issues and intervention is not instituted until it is too late to recover lost function. The physical therapist must serve as an advocate for the client under these circumstances.

Another mechanism for preventing secondary impairments is education of clients and their parents regarding the fit, specifications, condition, and maintenance of their adaptive equipment. They should know how to monitor skin tolerance and the fit of adaptive equipment. They should also understand the rationale for equipment and design features that are recommended. Knowledgeable consumers can detect and report potential problems before they result in complications such as decubiti. They need to be aware of the potential consequences of poorly fitted equipment so that they can advocate for the provision of quality equipment. The majority of adults in our follow-up study had improperly fitted equipment or lacked equipment that was essential for optimal function. These adults were also unaware of proper equipment maintenance techniques (Hinderer et al., 1988). As a result, many adults were functioning well below their capabilities and had skin breakdown, back pain, or joint pain as a result of poorly fitted orthoses or improper wheelchair design and seating.

Summary

There are few populations who challenge the skill and knowledge domains of the physical therapist as extensively as individuals with MM. The previous discussion has highlighted the multitude and complexity of problems encountered by children and adolescents with MM. Each lesion level group has general functional expectations that help direct physical therapy goals from an early age. While MM is a congenital onset problem requiring intervention by the physical therapist during infancy and childhood, most of the impairments and functional deficits described in this chapter occur throughout the life span. Individuals with MM should be followed on a regular basis, even as adults, in multidisciplinary specialty clinics by care providers familiar with this population. Because the physical therapist has extended contact with these individuals from infancy through adolescence, the therapist plays an important role in screening and triaging for potential problems, in addition to more traditional physical therapy roles. The challenges and rewards of working with this population are therefore extraordinary. The following case history illustrates the principles of assessment and management discussed in this chapter.

CASE HISTORY: SALLY

BACKGROUND INFORMATION

Sally is a 6-year-old girl with L-4 level paraplegia resulting from a myelomeningocele. She was referred for physical therapy assessment. She was born at term by vaginal delivery (7.2 lb, 48 cm) and was transferred immediately to a tertiary-care medical center where back closure was done on day 1 and a ventriculoperitoneal shunt for hydrocephalus placed on day 7. A subsequent infection necessitated removal and replacement of the shunt. Sally remained in the hospital for about 2 months. She has a neurogenic bladder with recurring urinary tract infections. Sally's mother performs intermittent bladder catheterization every 4 hours and assists with her daily bowel movement by performing manual extraction. Academics have been difficult for Sally, and she performs fine motor activities slowly. She is social, happy, and self-confident, however, and makes friends easily.

At 7 months Sally rolled prone to supine but could not sit independently. At 15 months she commando crawled and was able to get into quadruped. She pulled to stand and had a modified quadruped crawl with little lower limb reciprocation at 2 years of age. She did not have an effective method of mobility until 3½ years old when she was able to walk with AFOs and a wheeled anterior-facing walker. By 4 years of age, her gait with AFOs and the walker was crouched with little reciprocation and a wheelchair was her primary method of mobility. Her walking improved by switching to use of long-leg braces (knees locked) at age 4½ years, and she began to walk with forearm crutches and KAFOs at age 5 years.

PHYSICAL EXAMINATION

Range of motion was within functional limits except for bilateral 15° hip flexion contractures and 20° knee flexion contractures. Her forefeet and hindfeet had a varus inclination when examined in a non–weight-bearing position with her subtalar joint positioned in neutral. This resulted in a valgus, everted position of her feet when bearing weight.

Motor level was L-4 with weak quadriceps muscle strength (grade 4−), particularly in the shortened part of the range (from 40° to 20° of active knee extension), and grade 3+ hamstring muscle strength. Weakness in the terminal knee extension range had not been noted previously but was consistent with her history of knee flexion contractures and crouched gait. No volitional activity was present in the gluteal muscles or distal to the knee. Minimal spasticity was present in the hip adductor and hamstring muscles.

Sensory level was intact through L-3 but absent below this level.

Sally propelled independently in a lightweight wheelchair on level surfaces and on gradual inclines. She was independent for all transfers except to and from the floor because she was unable to independently operate the knee locks on her KAFOs. She walked with locked KAFOs and forearm crutches using a 4-point gait pattern and was independent on level surfaces and gradual inclines. She had difficulty traversing uneven terrain and more severe inclines. When she attempted to walk without upper limb support, she had a severe gluteal lurch with lateral trunk sway and lost her balance after a few steps. She was a short-distance community ambulator (primarily walked at home and school and used a wheelchair for long distances). When bearing weight without orthoses or with the knees of her KAFOs unlocked, her hips and knees were severely flexed and her feet were dorsiflexed, everted, and pronated.

Her KAFOs were set in 5° of dorsiflexion and were aligned in valgus at the subtalar joint. The KAFO knee joint axis was not congruent with her anatomic knee joint axis. Only a narrow, infrapatellar anterior knee strap was present, and there was no padding on any of the KAFO straps. She was unable to independently manipulate the knee locks because of her knee flexion contractures. She had pressure marks from the infrapatellar straps and decubiti on her heels.

Physical Therapy Concerns and Recommendations

At the time of her initial assessment, Sally's orthoses did not fit properly and were causing pressure sores. Her parents requested that she progress to AFOs, if possible, so that she could be more independent with transfers. Her hip and knee flexion contractures prevented her from achieving the stable upright stance required for efficient ambulation with AFOs. Her weakness in terminal knee extension, in conjunction with the contractures, presented further difficulties for maintaining upright posture and ambulating with AFOs. Because this weakness had not been noted previously, and she exhibited mild lower limb spasticity, it was important to serially monitor her strength and muscle tone over the next several months to determine if she was experiencing progressive neurologic loss.

Despite the problems, in Sally's favor were the volitional quadriceps and hamstring muscle function present, a supportive family, and her personality with a willingness to try new and difficult tasks. Hip and knee flexion contracture reduction and healing of the heel decubitus ulcers were initial steps that had to be completed before AFOs could be fabricated. The unavailability of physical therapy at school provided an additional challenge. Her father worked full time and her mother had 4 other siblings to care for in addition to

Sally so frequent outpatient physical therapy sessions were not a practical alternative. Discontinuance of the improperly fitting KAFOs and good wound care healed the decubitus ulcers. In the meantime, an aggressive program of stretching and strengthening was implemented.

An initial physical therapy session consisting of soft tissue mobilization followed by passive stretching resulted in 10° reductions in the hip and knee contractures. Sally's mother was instructed by the therapist in techniques for stretching the hip and knee flexors, which Sally performed daily. Strengthening exercises for the quadriceps and hamstring muscles were also implemented, including short arc quads, straight-leg raises, knee flexion, and squat to stand exercises. Sally was seen biweekly by the therapist for re-evaluation and progression of her program. After 2 weeks of therapy, she continued to have difficulty with terminal knee extension and initiation of knee flexion. A home program of functional electrical stimulation was implemented to enhance volitional contractions of the quadriceps and hamstring muscles and to assist with muscle re-education (Karmel-Ross et al., 1992). Strengthening exercises augmented with functional electrical stimulation resulted in significant increases in strength.

After 2 months of treatment, Sally had only 5° hip flexion contractures and her knees could fully extend. Quadriceps and hamstring muscle strength were grades 4 and 4−, respectively. Her decubiti were fully healed and she was anxious to resume bipedal ambulation. The child could stand and walk short distances with her knees and hips extended when she used a reverse-facing walker and concentrated on walking with an upright posture. She fatigued and was distracted easily, however, and still required support at the knees for community distances. The long-term goal remained progression to independent ambulation using AFOs and forearm crutches. Ground-reaction force AFOs (see Fig. 22–5) would most likely be the optimal design for advancing her to ambulation with AFOs, for the reasons outlined in Table 22–4. KAFOs were still currently indicated, however, to maintain an upright posture for community distances. If she regressed to a crouch gait pattern, contractures and stretch weakness could recur. After consultation with the orthotist, new KAFOs were fabricated that incorporated a ground-reaction force AFO component, along with removable metal knee joints, uprights, and thigh cuff sections. These orthoses enabled Sally to practice upright walking using a posture-control walker at home, with the knee joints either locked or unlocked. In therapy sessions, and under her mother's supervision, the thigh and knee components could be removed so that she could practice walking with the ground-reaction force AFOs.

Orthotic specifications included those listed in Table 22–5 for increasing medial and lateral stability, enhancing the knee extension moment, decreasing energy expenditure, providing adequate toe clearance, simulated push-off, distributing pressure evenly, and improving balance. The orthotist molded the feet in subtalar neutral, and the footplates of the AFOs were posted to accommodate forefoot and hindfoot varus and forefoot supination. The posting provided a wider base of plantigrade support to improve balance and prevented her feet from rolling over into pronation when weight bearing, thus maintaining good biomechanical alignment of the ankles and knees. The ankles were set in 5° of plantar flexion, providing an extensor moment at the knees to encourage more upright stance and gait.

Strengthening exercises and functional electrical stimulation were continued. Gait training began at home and in therapy sessions, initially using a posture-control walker and then progressing to forearm crutches. Gait training emphasized an upright posture and terminal knee extension with the KAFO knee joints unlocked and removed. Functional electrical stimulation was used in conjunction with gait training for muscle re-education (Kieklak & DeVahl, 1986; Packman & Ewaski, 1983). Videotaping of her gait pattern was used throughout the treatment process to provide visual feedback. Sally quickly progressed to ambulation with forearm crutches with the knee joints unlocked. Strength continued to increase; after 3 months of strengthening and gait training, quadriceps and hamstring muscle strength were grades 4+ and 4, respectively, and she was able to walk with ground-reaction force AFOs and forearm crutches for short community distances using a 4-point gait pattern. She continued to use a wheelchair for long distances. Progression to a more efficient 2-point gait was then emphasized. She mastered the 2-point gait pattern following another month of gait training. Strengthening exercises and stretching have continued prophylactically 3 times a week. Her mother understood that it was essential to avoid regression to a crouched gait pattern and continued to monitor her ROM and posture closely, especially during periods of rapid growth. Sally continues to ambulate independently for short community distances with ground-reaction force AFOs and forearm crutches and uses a wheelchair for longer distances. She also has mastered wheelchair-to-floor transfers. It will be important to continue to teach her advanced wheelchair skills, including ramps and curbs, so that she is independent with the chair in the community because she, like many individuals with L-4 level function, will most likely continue to use the chair for long-distance community mobility as an adolescent and adult.

References

Agre, JC, Findley, TW, McNally, MC, Habeck, R, Leon, AS, Stradel, L, Birkebak, R, & Schmalz, R. Physical activity capacity in children with myelomeningocele. Archives of Physical Medicine and Rehabilitation, 68:372–377, 1987.

Aitkins, S, Lord, J, Bernauer, E, Fowler, W, Lieberman, J, & Berck, P. Relationship of manual muscle testing to objective strength measurements. Muscle and Nerve, 12:173–177, 1989.

Andersen, EM, & Plewis, I. Impairment of motor skill in children with spina bifida cystica and hydrocephalus: An exploratory study. British Journal of Psychology, 68:61–70, 1977.

Asher, M, & Olson, J. Factors affecting the ambulatory status of patients with spina bifida cystica. Journal of Bone and Joint Surgery (American), 65:350–356, 1983.

Baker, SB, & Rogosky-Grassi, MA. Access to the school. In Rowley-Kelly, FL, & Reigel, DH (Eds.), Teaching the Student with Spina Bifida. Baltimore, MD: Paul H. Brookes Publishing, 1993, pp. 31–70.

Bar-or, O. Pathophysiological factors which limit the exercise capacity of the sick child. Medicine and Science in Sports and Exercise, 18:276–282, 1986.

Bartlett, MD, Wolf, LS, Shurtleff, DB, & Staheli, LT. Hip flexion contractures: A comparison of measurement methods. Archives of Physical Medicine and Rehabilitation, 66:620–625, 1985.

Beasley, WC. Influence of method on estimates of normal knee extensor force among normal and postpolio children. Physical Therapy Review, 36:21–41, 1956.

Beasley, WC. Quantitative muscle testing: Principles and applications to research and clinical services. Archives of Physical Medicine and Rehabilitation, 42:398–425, 1961.

Becker, RD. Recent developments in child psychiatry: I. The restrictive emotional and cognitive environment reconsidered: A redefinition of the concept of therapeutic restraint. Israeli Journal of Psychiatry and Related Sciences, 12:239–258, 1975.

Birth Defects and Genetic Diseases Branch of Birth Defects and Developmental Disabilities Office, National Center for Environmental Disease and Injury. Use of folic acid prevention of spina bifida and other neural tube defects, 1983–1991. Morbidity and Mortality Weekly Report, 40:1–4, 1991.

Bleck, EE, & Nagel, DA. Physically Handicapped Children—A Medical Atlas for Teachers. Orlando, FL: Grune & Stratton, 1982.

Bohannon, RW. Manual muscle test scores and dynamometer test scores of knee extension strength. Archives of Physical Medicine and Rehabilitation, 67:390–392, 1986.

Brunt, D. Characteristics of upper limb movements in a sample of meningomyelocele children. Perceptual Motor Skills, 51:431–437, 1980.

Burlingham, D. Notes on problems of motor restraint during illness. In Lowenstein, RM (Ed.), Drives, Affects, Behavior. New York: International Universities Press, 1953, pp. 169–175.

Butler, C, Okamoto, GA, & McKay, TM. Motorized wheelchair driving by disabled children. Archives of Physical Medicine and Rehabilitation, 65:95–97, 1984.

Chaffin, DB, & Andersson, GBJ. Occupational Biomechanics (2nd ed.). New York: John Wiley & Sons, 1991.

Chandler, LS, Andrews, MS, & Swanson, MW. Movement Assessment of Infants: A Manual. Rolling Bay, WA: Authors, 1980.

CIBA. CIBA Symposium No. 191: Neural Tube Defects. London: CIBA Foundation, 1994.

Cusick, BD, & Stuberg, WA. Assessment of lower extremity alignment in the transverse plane: Implications for management of children with neuromotor dysfunction. Physical Therapy, 72:3–15, 1992.

Daniels, L, & Worthingham, C. Muscle Testing Techniques of Manual Examination (5th ed.). Philadelphia: WB Saunders, 1986.

Deitz, JC, Jaffe, KM, Wolf, LS, Massagli, TL, & Anson, DK. Pediatric power wheelchairs: Evaluation of function in the home and school environments. Assistive Technology, *3*:24–31, 1991.

DeSouza, L, & Carroll, N. Ambulation of the braced myelomeningocele patient. Journal of Bone and Joint Surgery (American), *58*:1112–1118, 1976.

Dudgeon, BJ, Jaffe, KM, & Shurtleff, DB. Variations in mid-lumbar myelomeningocele: Implications for ambulation. Pediatric Physical Therapy, *3*:57–62, 1991.

Eastlack, ME, Arvidson, J, Snyder-Mackler, L, Danoff, JV, & McGarvey, CL. Interrater reliability of videotaped observational gait-analysis assessments. Physical Therapy, *71*:465–472, 1991.

Effgen, SK, & Brown, DA. Long-term stability of hand-held dynamometric measurements in children who have myelomeningocele. Physical Therapy, *72*:458–465, 1992.

Elwood, JM, & Elwood, JH. Epidemiology of Anencephalus and Spina Bifida. Cambridge: Oxford University Press, 1980.

Embrey, D, Endicott, J, Glenn, T, & Jaeger, DL. Developing better postural tone in grade school children. Clinical Management in Physical Therapy, 3:6–10, 1983.

Fay, G, Shurtleff, DB, Shurtleff, H, & Wolf, L. Approaches to facilitate independent self-care and academic success. In Shurtleff, DB (Ed.), Myelodysplasias and Exstrophies: Significance, Prevention, and Treatment. Orlando, FL: Grune & Stratton, 1986, pp. 373–398.

Fife, SE, Roxborough, LA, Armstrong, RW, Harris, SR, Gregson, JL, & Field, D. Development of a clinical measure of postural control for assessment of adaptive seating in children with neuromotor disabilities. Physical Therapy, *71*:981–993, 1991.

Finnie, NR. Handling the Young Cerebral Palsied Child at Home (2nd ed.). New York: EP Dutton, 1975.

Florence, JM, Pandya, S, King, W, Schierbecker, J, Robison, JD, Signore, LC, Mandel, S, & Arfken, C. Strength assessment: Comparison of methods in children with Duchenne muscular dystrophy (Abstract). Physical Therapy, *68*:866, 1988.

Gadow, K. Children on Medication. San Diego, CA: College Hill Press, 1986.

Goodwyn, MA. Biomedical psychological factors predicting success with activities of daily living and academic pursuits. Unpublished doctoral dissertation. Seattle: University of Washington, 1990.

Griebel, ML, Oakes, WJ, & Worley, G. The Chiari malformation associated with myelomeningocele. In Rekate, HL (Ed.), Comprehensive Management of Spina Bifida. Boca Raton, FL: CRC Press, 1991, pp. 67–92.

Griffin, JW, McClure, MH, & Bertorini, TE. Sequential isokinetic and manual muscle testing in patients with neuromuscular disease: Pilot study. Physical Therapy, *66*:32–35, 1986.

Hack, SN, Norton, BJ, & Zahalak, GI. A quantitative muscle tester for clinical use (Abstract). Physical Therapy, *61*:673, 1981.

Hamill, PV, Drizd, TA, Johnson, CL, Reed, RB, Roche, AF, & Moore, WM. Physical growth: National Center for Health Statistics percentiles. American Journal of Clinical Nutrition, *32*:607–629, 1979.

Hinderer, KA. Reliability of the myometer in muscle testing children and adolescents with myelodysplasia. Unpublished master's thesis. Seattle: University of Washington, 1988.

Hinderer, KA, & Gutierrez, T. Myometry measurements of children using isometric and eccentric methods of muscle testing (Abstract). Physical Therapy, *68*:817, 1988.

Hinderer, KA, & Hinderer, SR. Mobility and transfer efficiency of adults with myelodysplasia (Abstract). Archives of Physical Medicine and Rehabilitation, 69:712, 1988.

Hinderer, KA, & Hinderer, SR. Muscle strength development

and assessment in children and adolescents. In Harms-Ringdahl, K (Ed.), International Perspectives in Physical Therapy, Vol. 8, Muscle Strength. London: Churchill Livingstone, 1993a, pp. 93–140.

Hinderer, SR, & Hinderer, KA. Sensory examination of individuals with myelodysplasia (Abstract). Archives of Physical Medicine and Rehabilitation, *71*:769–770, 1990.

Hinderer, SR, & Hinderer, KA. Quantitative methods of evaluation. In DeLisa, JA (Ed.), Rehabilitation Medicine: Principles and Practices (2nd ed.). Philadelphia: JB Lippincott, 1993b, pp. 96–121.

Hinderer, SR, Hinderer, KA, Dunne, K, & Shurtleff, DB. Medical and functional status of adults with spina bifida (Abstract). Developmental Medicine and Child Neurology, *30*(suppl 57):28, 1988.

Hosking, GP, Bhat, US, Dubowitz, V, & Edwards, RHT. Measurements of muscle strength and performance in children with normal and diseased muscle. Archives of Disease in Childhood, *51*:957–963, 1976.

Hurley, AD. Conducting psychological assessments. In Rowley-Kelly, FL, & Reigel, DH (Eds.), Teaching the Student with Spina Bifida. Baltimore, MD: Paul H. Brookes Publishing, 1993, pp. 107–124.

Hyde, S, Goddard, C, & Scott, O: The myometer: The development of a clinical tool. Physiotherapy, *69*:424–427, 1983.

International Myelodysplasia Study Group Database Coordination, David B. Shurtleff, MD, Department of Pediatrics, University of Washington, Seattle, WA 98195, 1993.

Jacobson, CB, & Berlin, CM. Possible reproductive determent in LSD users. Journal of the American Medical Association, *222*:1367–1373, 1972.

Janda, V. Muscle Function Testing. Boston, MA: Butterworths, 1983.

Jebsen, RH, Trieschman, RB, Mikulic, MA, Hartley, RB, McMillan, JA, & Snook, ME. Measurement of time in a standardized test of patient mobility. Archives of Physical Medicine and Rehabilitation, *51*:170–175, 1970.

Karmel-Ross, K, Cooperman, DR, & Van Doren, CL. The effect of electrical stimulation on quadriceps femoris muscle torque in children with spina bifida. Physical Therapy, *72*: 723–731, 1992.

Kendall, FP, McCreary, EK, & Provance, PG. Muscles: Testing and Function (3rd ed.). Baltimore: Williams & Wilkins, 1993.

Kieklak, H, & DeVahl, J. Respond II: Protocol for Pediatric Applications, Medtronics, Inc., Minneapolis, MN, 1986.

Kilburn, J, Saffer, A, Barnes, L, Kling, T, & Venes, J. The vigorimeter as an early predictor of central neurologic malformation in myelodysplastic children. Paper presented at the meeting of the American Academy for Cerebral Palsy and Developmental Medicine, Seattle, 1985.

Kimura, DK, Mayo, M, & Shurtleff, DB. Urinary tract management. In Shurtleff, DB (Ed.), Myelodysplasias and Exstrophies: Significance, Prevention, and Treatment. Orlando, FL: Grune & Stratton, 1986, pp. 243–266.

King, JC, Currie, DM, & Wright, E. Bowel training in spina bifida: Importance of education, patient compliance, age, and anal reflexes. Archives of Physical Medicine and Rehabilitation, *75*:243–247, 1994.

Knutson, LM, & Clark, DE. Orthotic devices for ambulation in children with cerebral palsy and myelomeningocele. Physical Therapy, *71*:947–960, 1991.

Krebs, DE, Edelstein, JE, & Fishman, S. Reliability of observational kinematic gait analysis. Physical Therapy, *65*:1027–1033, 1985.

Land, LC. Study of the sensory integration of children with myelomeningocele. In McLaurin, RL (Ed.), Myelomeningocele. Orlando, FL: Grune & Stratton, 1977, pp. 113–140.

Lehmann, JF, Condon, SM, de Lateur, BJ, & Price, R. Gait abnormalities in peroneal nerve paralysis and their corrections by orthoses: A biomechanical study. Archives of Physical Medicine and Rehabilitation, 67:380–386, 1986.

Lehmann, JF, Condon, SM, de Lateur, BJ, & Smith, C. Ankle-foot orthoses: Effect on gait abnormalities in tibial nerve paralysis. Archives of Physical Medicine and Rehabilitation, 66:212–218, 1985.

Lehmann, JF, Esselman, PC, Ko, MJ, de Lateur, BJ, & Dralle, AJ. Plastic ankle-foot orthoses: Evaluation of function. Archives of Physical Medicine and Rehabilitation, 64:402–404, 1983.

Lemire, RJ, Loeser, JD, Leech, RW, & Alvord, ED (Eds.). Normal and Abnormal Development of the Human Nervous System. Hagerstown, MD: Harper & Row, 1975.

Level, MB: Spherical grip strength of children. Unpublished master's thesis. Seattle: University of Washington, 1984.

Lichtenstein, BW. Spinal dysraphism; spina bifida and myelodysplasia. Archives of Neurology and Psychiatry, 44:792–810, 1940.

Liptak, GS, Shurtleff, DB, Bloss, JW, Baitus-Hebert, E, & Manitta, P. Mobility aids for children with high-level myelomeningocele: Parapodium versus wheelchair. Developmental Medicine and Child Neurology, 34:787–796, 1992.

Logan, L, Byers-Hinkley, K, & Ciccone, CD. Anterior versus posterior walkers: A gait analysis study. Developmental Medicine and Child Neurology, 32:1044–1048, 1990.

Luthy, DA, Wardinsky, T, Shurtleff, DB, Hollenbach, KA, Hickok, DE, Nyberg, DA, & Benedetti, TJ. Cesarean section before the onset of labor and subsequent motor function in infants with myelomeningocele diagnosed antenatally. New England Journal of Medicine, 324:662–666, 1991.

Main, DM, & Mennuti, MT. Neural tube defects: Issues in prenatal diagnosis and counseling. Journal of the American College of Obstetrics and Gynecology, 67:1–16, 1986.

Masse, LC, Lamontagne, M, & O'Riain, MD. Biomedical analysis of wheelchair propulsion for various seating positions. Journal of Rehabilitation Research and Development, 29:12–28, 1992.

Mayfield, JK. Comprehensive orthopedic management in myelomeningocele. In Rekate, HL (Ed.), Comprehensive Management of Spina Bifida. Boca Raton, FL: CRC Press, 1991, pp. 113–164.

McDonald, CM, Jaffe, KM, Mosca, VS, & Shurtleff, DB. Ambulatory outcome of children with myelomeningocele: Effect of lower-extremity muscle strength. Developmental Medicine and Child Neurology, 33:482–490, 1991a.

McDonald, CM, Jaffe, K, & Shurtleff, DB. Assessment of muscle strength in children with meningomyelocele: Accuracy and stability of measurements over time. Archives of Physical Medicine and Rehabilitation, 67:855–861, 1986.

McDonald, CM, Jaffe, KM, Shurtleff, DB, & Menelaus, MB. Modifications to the traditional description of neurosegmental innervation in myelomeningocele. Developmental Medicine and Child Neurology, 33:473–481, 1991b.

McGourty, LK. Kohlman Evaluation of Living Skills (KELS). In Hemphill, BJ (Ed.), Mental Health Assessment in Occupational Therapy. Thorofare, NJ: Black Publishers, 1988, pp. 131–146.

Mendell, JR, & Florence, J. Manual muscle testing. Muscle and Nerve, 13(suppl):16–20, 1990.

Menelaus, MB. Orthopedic management of children with myelomeningocele: A plea for realistic goals. Developmental Medicine and Child Neurology, 18(suppl 37):3–11, 1976.

Miller, E, & Sethi, L. The effect of hydrocephalus on perception. Developmental Medicine and Child Neurology, 13(suppl 25):77–81, 1971.

Miller, LC, Michael AF, Baxter, TL, & Kim, Y. Quantitative muscle testing in childhood dermatomyositis. Archives of Physical Medicine and Rehabilitation, 69:610–613, 1988.

Mills, JL, Rhoads, GG, Simpson, JL, Cunningham, GC, Conley, MR, Lassman, MR, Walden, ME, Depp, R, & Hoffman, HJ. The absence of a relation between the periconceptual use of vitamins and neural tube defects. New England Journal of Medicine, 321:430–435, 1989.

Milner-Brown, HS, & Miller, RG. Increased muscular fatigue in patients with neurogenic muscle weakness: Quantification and pathophysiology. Archives of Physical Medicine and Rehabilitation, 70:361–366, 1989.

Milunsky, A, Jick, H, Jick, SS, Bruell, CL, MacLaughlin, DS, Rothman, KJ, & Willett, W. Multivitamin/folic acid supplementation in early pregnancy reduces the prevalence of neural tube defects. Journal of the American Medical Association, 262:2847–2852, 1989.

MRC Vitamin Study Research Group. Prevention of neural tube defects: Results of the Medical Research Council vitamin study. Lancet, 338:131–137, 1991.

Murdoch, A. How valuable is muscle charting? A study of the relationship between neonatal assessment of muscle power and later mobility in children with spina bifida defects. Physiotherapy, 66:221–223, 1980.

Nyberg, DA, Mack, LA, Hirsch, J, & Mahoney, BS. Abnormalities of fetal cranial contour in sonographic detection of spina bifida: Evaluation of the "lemon" sign. Radiology, 167:387–392, 1988.

Oakland, JA, & Sherman, WE. An examination of Erickson's theory from the perspective of a study of congenitally paraplegic children. In Proceedings of 46th Annual Meeting of American Orthopsychiatric Association, New York, 1969.

Okamoto, GA, Lamers, JV, & Shurtleff, DB. Skin breakdown in patients with myelomeningocele. Archives of Physical Medicine and Rehabilitation, 64:20–23, 1983.

Okamoto, GA, Sousa, J, Telzrow, RW, Holm, RA, McCartin, R, & Shurtleff, DB. Toileting skills in children with myelomeningocele: Rates of learning. Archives of Physical Medicine and Rehabilitation, 65(4):182–185, 1984.

Packman, RA, & Ewaski, B. Respond II: Gait Training Protocol. Minneapolis, MN: Medtronics, 1983.

Pact, V, Sirotkin-Roses, M, & Beatus, J. The Muscle Testing Handbook. Boston: Little, Brown & Co., 1984.

Patient Data Management System. Myelodysplasia Study Data Collection Criteria and Instructions, 1994. (Available from D.B. Shurtleff, MD, Professor, Department of Pediatrics, University of Washington, Seattle, WA 98195.)

Pomatto, RC. The use of orthotics in the treatment of myelomeningocele. In Rekate, HL (Ed.), Comprehensive Management of Spina Bifida. Boca Raton, FL: CRC Press, 1991, pp. 165–183.

Reigel, DH. Spina bifida from infancy through the school years. In Rowley-Kelly, FL, & Reigel, DH (Eds.), Teaching the Students with Spina Bifida. Baltimore, MD: Paul H. Brookes Publishing, 1993, pp. 3–30.

Rekate, HL. Neurosurgical management of the newborn with spina bifida. In Rekate, HL (Ed.), Comprehensive Management of Spina Bifida. Boca Raton, FL: CRC Press, 1991, pp. 1–28.

Reynolds, EH. Mental effects of antiepileptic medication: A review. Epilepsia, 24(suppl 2):S85–S95, 1983.

Rose, SA, Ounpuu, S, & DeLuca, PA. Strategies for the assessment of pediatric gait in the clinical setting. Physical Therapy, 71:961–980, 1991.

Rosenstein, BD, Greene, WB, Herrington, RT, & Blum, AS. Bone density in myelomeningocele: The effects of ambulatory status and other factors. Developmental Medicine and Child Neurology, 29:486–494, 1987.

Rowley-Kelly, FL, & Kunkle, PM. Developing a school outreach program. In Rowley-Kelly, FL, & Reigel, DH (Eds.),

Teaching the Student with Spina Bifida. Baltimore, MD: Paul H. Brookes Publishing, 1993, pp. 395–436.

Ryan, KD, Pioski, C, & Emans, JB. Myelodysplasia—the musculoskeletal problem: Habilitation from infancy to adulthood. Physical Therapy, 71:935–946, 1991.

Sand, PL, Taylor, N, Rawlings, M, & Chitnis, S. Performance of children with spina bifida manifesta on the Frostig Developmental Test of Visual Perception. Perceptual Motor Skills, 37:539–546, 1973.

Schafer, MF, & Dias, LS. Myelomeningocele: Orthopaedic Treatment. Baltimore, MD: Williams & Wilkins, 1983.

Schneider, JW. Congenital spinal cord injury. In Umphred, DA (Ed.), Neurological Rehabilitation, Vol. 3. St. Louis: CV Mosby, 1985, pp. 289–313.

Schopler, SA, & Menelaus, MB. Significance of strength of the quadriceps muscles in children with myelomeningocele. Journal of Pediatric Orthopaedics, 7:507–512, 1987.

Seller, MJ, & Nevin, NC. Periconceptual vitamin supplementation and the prevention of neural tube defects in south-east England and northern Ireland. Journal of Medical Genetics, 21:325–330, 1984.

Shaffer, J, Wolfe, L, Friedrich, W, Shurtleff, H, Shurtleff, D, & Fay, G. Developmental expectations: Intelligence and fine motor skills. In Shurtleff, DB (Ed.), Myelodysplasias and Exstrophies: Significance, Prevention, and Treatment. Orlando, FL: Grune & Stratton, 1986, pp. 359–372.

Shores, M. Footprint analysis in gait documentation. Physical Therapy, 60:1163–1167, 1980.

Shurtleff, DB. Timing of learning in the myelomeningocele patient. Journal of the American Physical Therapy Association, 46(2):136–148, 1966.

Shurtleff, DB. Decubitus formation and skin breakdown. In Shurtleff, DB (Ed.), Myelodysplasias and Exstrophies: Significance, Prevention, and Treatment. Orlando, FL: Grune & Stratton, 1986a, pp. 299–312.

Shurtleff, DB. Dietary management. In Shurtleff, DB (Ed.), Myelodysplasias and Exstrophies: Significance, Prevention, and Treatment. Orlando, FL: Grune & Stratton, 1986b, pp. 285–298.

Shurtleff, DB. Health care delivery. In Shurtleff, DB (Ed.), Myelodysplasias and Exstrophies: Significance, Prevention, and Treatment. Orlando, FL: Grune & Stratton, 1986c, pp. 449–514.

Shurtleff, DB. Mobility. In Shurtleff, DB (Ed.), Myelodysplasias and Exstrophies: Significance, Prevention, and Treatment. Orlando, FL: Grune & Stratton, 1986d, pp. 313–356.

Shurtleff, DB. Selection process for the care of congenitally malformed infants. In Shurtleff, DB (Ed.), Myelodysplasias and Exstrophies: Significance, Prevention, and Treatment. Orlando, FL: Grune & Stratton, 1986e, pp. 89–116.

Shurtleff, DB. Computer data bases for pediatric disability: Clinical and research applications. In Jaffe, KM (Ed.), Physical Medicine and Rehabilitation Clinics of North America: Pediatric Rehabilitation. Philadelphia: WB Saunders, 1991, pp. 665–688.

Shurtleff, DB, & Dunne, K. Adults and adolescents with myelomeningocele. In Shurtleff, DB (Ed.), Myelodysplasias and Exstrophies: Significance, Prevention, and Treatment. Orlando, FL: Grune & Stratton, 1986, pp. 433–448.

Shurtleff, DB, & Lamers, J. Clinical considerations in the treatment of myelodysplasia. In Crandal, DB, & Brazier, MAB (Eds.), Prevention of Neural Tube Defects: The Role of Alpha-fetoprotein. New York: Academic Press, 1978, pp. 103–122.

Shurtleff, DB, Lemire, RJ, & Warkany, J: Embryology, etiology and epidemiology. In Shurtleff, DB (Ed.), Myelodysplasias and Exstrophies: Significance, Prevention, and Treatment. Orlando, FL: Grune & Stratton, 1986a, pp. 39–64.

Shurtleff, DB, & Mayo, M. Toilet training: The Seattle experience and conclusions. In Shurtleff, DB (Ed.), Myelodysplasias and Exstrophies: Significance, Prevention, and Treatment. Orlando, FL: Grune & Stratton, 1986, pp. 267–284.

Shurtleff, DB, Stuntz, JT, & Hayden, PW. Hydrocephalus. In Shurtleff, DB (Ed.), Myelodysplasias and Exstrophies: Significance, Prevention, and Treatment. Orlando, FL: Grune & Stratton, 1986b, pp. 139–180.

Sousa, JC, Gordon, LH, & Shurtleff, DB. Assessing the development of daily living skills in patients with spina bifida. Developmental Medicine and Child Neurology, 18(suppl 37):134–142, 1976.

Sousa, JC, Telzrow, RW, Holm, RA, McCartin, R, & Shurtleff, DB. Developmental guidelines for children with myelodysplasia. Journal of the American Physical Therapy Association, 63:21–29, 1983.

Stack, GD, & Baber, GC. The neurological involvement of the lower limbs in myelomeningocele. Developmental Medicine and Child Neurology, 9:732, 1967.

Staheli, LT. Prone hip extension test: Method of measuring hip flexion deformity. Clinical Orthopedics, 123:12–15, 1977.

Steindler, A: Kinesiology of the Human Body Under Normal and Pathological Conditions. Springfield, IL: Charles C Thomas, 1955.

Stillwell, A, & Menelaus, MB. Walking ability in mature patients with spina bifida. Journal of Pediatric Orthopedics, 3:184–190, 1983.

Stuberg, WA. Considerations related to weight-bearing program in children with developmental disabilities. Physical Therapy, 72:35–40, 1992.

Stuberg, WA, & Metcalf, WK. Reliability of quantitative muscle testing in healthy children and in children with Duchenne muscular dystrophy using a hand-held dynamometer. Physical Therapy, 68:977–982, 1988.

Tew, B, & Laurence, KM. The effects of hydrocephalus on intelligence, visual perception, and school attainments. Developmental Medicine and Child Neurology, 17(suppl 35):129–134, 1975.

Weber, D, & Agro, M. Clinical Aspects of Lower Extremity Orthotics. Winnipeg, Manitoba: Canadian Cataloguing in Publication Data/Canadian Association of Prosthetists and Orthotists, 1990.

White, BL, Kaban, BT, & Attanucci, JS. The Origins of Human Competence. Lexington, MA: Lexington Books, 1979.

Wicks, K, & Shurtleff, DB. An introduction to toilet training. In Shurtleff, DB (Ed.), Myelodysplasias and Exstrophies: Significance, Prevention, and Treatment. Orlando, FL: Grune & Stratton, 1986a, pp. 203–219.

Wicks, K, & Shurtleff, DB. Stool management. In Shurtleff, DB (Ed.), Myelodysplasias and Exstrophies: Significance, Prevention, and Treatment. Orlando, FL: Grune & Stratton, 1986b, pp. 221–242.

Williams, LV, Anderson, AD, Campbell, J, Thomas, L, Feinell, E, & Walker, JM. Energy cost of walking and of wheelchair propulsion by children with myelodysplasia: Comparison with normal children. Developmental Medicine and Child Neurology, 25:617–624, 1983.

Wolf, LS, & McLaughlin, JF. Early motor development in infants with myelomeningocele. Pediatric Physical Therapy, 4:12–17, 1992.

Chapter 23

Assistive Technology

SHIRLEY J. CARLSON, PT, PCS, MS
CAROLE RAMSEY, OTR/L

Physical therapists have long been involved in the practice of providing individuals with physical impairments with devices or pieces of equipment that are designed to help achieve or improve independent function. Attempts to increase carryover of therapy goals in the home and classroom settings often included homemade "adaptive equipment" for positioning, mobility, and communication. The application of technologic advances to health care, rehabilitation, and special education settings began slowly several decades ago and has rapidly accelerated. Assistive, or rehabilitation, technology now encompasses a vast range of materials, designs, and applications. It is used to promote the development and acquisition of skills that a client lacks as a result of disease or injury. It can also provide compromises or adaptations in motor function when the attainment of certain skills is unrealistic or impossible. Also referred to as "enabling technology," assistive technology can often generate new opportunities and open new doors for individuals with physical impairments.

In the past 20 years there has been a virtual explosion in the number and type of assistive devices. The creation of several federally funded rehabilitation engineering centers in 1972 focused efforts on research and development of new products, as well as on the delivery of services to the consumer (Hedman, 1990). This process began to bring together professionals from many fields, such as biomedical and rehabilitation engineering, physical therapy, occupational therapy, speech and, language pathology, and special education. As these professionals became aware of their shared clients, problems, and methods, they gradually came to work together toward common goals, as evidenced by the increase in number and sophistication of seating, augmentative communication, and technology teams and clinics across North America. Federal legislation such as Public Laws 94-142 and 99-457 and the Americans with Disabilities Act (see Chapters 31 and 33) ensures the rights of people with disabilities to inclusion in natural education and work environments. These laws have helped to focus attention on, and create a growing market for, new technologies and products. Consumer demands for increased durability and performance have induced manufacturers to borrow technologies created by the aerospace, medical, and information industries. The recent Technology-Related Assistance for Individuals with Disabilities Act (1988, PL 100-407) has given individual states the impetus to develop their own statewide service delivery plans (Hedman, 1990). The field of assistive technology has rapidly moved toward the status of a new professional specialty.

The purpose of this chapter is to discuss four major elements of assistive technology frequently employed in pediatric physical therapy, focusing on the role physical therapists play in selecting and obtaining appropriate pieces of equipment for their clients. The four elements include postural support systems (adaptive seating), wheeled mobility, augmentative and alternative communication (AAC), and environmental control units (ECUs). Emphasis is on application of these devices to individuals with severe physical impairments.

PRESCRIBING ASSISTIVE TECHNOLOGY: THE TEAM CONCEPT

In spite of the diversity of technologic devices, most still require modification or customization in design, implementation, or attachment (Hedman,

1990). The complexity and expense of most of the devices required by individuals with severe physical impairments demand a thorough and careful process of selection and construction. Many professionals and lay people may need to be involved, each contributing a particular area of knowledge and expertise. All individuals who will be interacting with the client and the equipment on a regular basis need to be considered part of the team and may contribute important information.

The configuration of the team (Fig. 23–1) varies depending on the types of assistive technology needed as well as on the setting in which the evaluation and prescription are being conducted. The core of the team is shared by the consumer, or user, of the equipment and the professionals who prescribe and obtain the devices. The recent focus on family-centered intervention stresses the need to involve the client and primary caregivers in the goal-setting and decision-making process to ensure

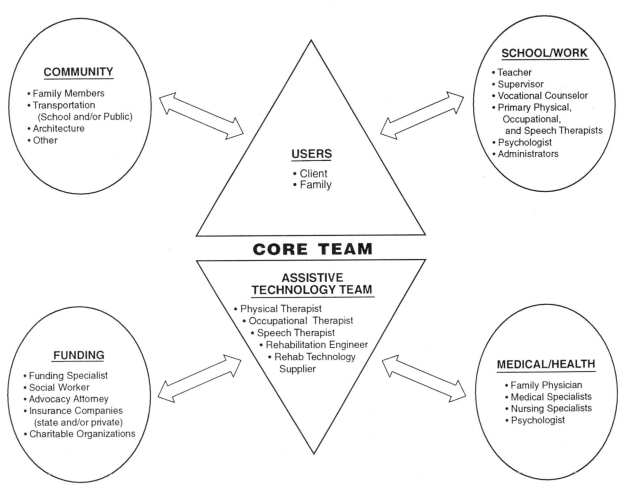

FIGURE 23–1. Core team interactions important in selecting and procuring assistive technology. Members and roles of each component may fluctuate depending on specific client problems and settings.

realistic and meaningful solutions (Foster & Phillips, 1992; see also Chapter 30). The professional component of the core should include experts with thorough training and experience in the areas being examined (mobility, seating, AAC, and ECUs) and usually includes some or all of the following: physical therapist, occupational therapist, speech and language pathologist, rehabilitation engineer, and rehabilitation technology supplier.

Surrounding this core are several groups who share important roles and information. In the client's school or work setting, classroom teachers and aides, administrative personnel, psychologists, vocational counselors, and work supervisors may all need to be consulted. The client may have primary physical, occupational, and speech and language therapists in these settings with whom the development of goals and strategies needs to be coordinated. Within the medical setting, the client's family physician, as well as other medical specialists and nurses, may need to be involved. Problems requiring collaboration with medical personnel may include management of deformity and contracture, pressure ulcerations, incontinence, self-injury and safety, and visual and other sensory deficits. The issue of funding establishes a third group of contributors, including third-party payers, state-sponsored medical equipment programs, civic organizations, and other outside funding agencies. Many clinics and centers now employ a funding specialist whose role is to identify and obtain funding for prescribed technology. A social worker, who may or may not be part of the core team, and, in contested cases, an advocacy attorney, may also assist with this function. A final group within the team includes other community and family members who engage in day-to-day interactions or who provide special support services such as transportation or revision of architectural barriers.

As mentioned, the makeup of the team and the setting in which it functions can vary. For example, in many hospitals and rehabilitation centers with comprehensive technology service delivery programs, physicians (especially physiatrists and orthopaedic surgeons) may be an integral part of the core team. In residential centers and schools, one or more of the client's primary therapists, along with an equipment vendor, may function as the core team.

A successful team will recognize that each of these members, even a minor player, has important information and perspective. Equally important is the message that communication must be bidirectional. The core team must impart information regarding proper use, training, maintenance, respon-

sibility, and safety relative to the prescribed devices to appropriate individuals.

Through a survey of 227 adults with various disabilities, Phillips and Zhao (1993) studied factors that predict abandonment of assistive technology devices. Nearly 30% of all devices were completely abandoned, with mobility devices abandoned most often. Devices were most frequently abandoned in the first year or after the fifth year. Four factors were significantly related to abandonment. The first was lack of consideration of the user's opinion during the selection process. Ease of procurement was a second factor, with easily obtained items purchased directly from a vendor (without team consultation) the most likely to be abandoned. A third factor was poor device performance, which reflected the user's perception of the device's ability to enhance his or her own performance in an easy, reliable, and comfortable manner. The fourth factor was the change in users' needs and priorities over time, including functional changes as well as changes in lifestyle and activities.

The evolving role of the rehabilitation technology supplier, previously known as an equipment vendor or durable medical equipment dealer, deserves special mention. The National Association for Medical Equipment Suppliers is a trade association for durable medical equipment suppliers. The rehabilitation section of this organization has defined Standards of Practice and Protocol for rehabilitation technology suppliers in an attempt to increase recognition as a profession rather than as a commercial industry. In addition, the rehabilitation section of NAMES is developing a National Registry of Rehabilitation Technology Suppliers that will adopt these Standards of Practice and Protocol as its standards of practice. Criteria established by the National Registry's board of directors include a minimum standard of experience, continuing education, and statements of recommendation from referral sources. Qualified rehabilitation technology suppliers will be registered as "members" of the National Registry. A testing and certification process is expected to follow in the future (NAMES Rehab Section, 1992). The significance of these actions is to fill a gap that has often existed in the past between the therapists, who knew the outcomes they were trying to achieve, and the equipment provider, who sold a given line of wheelchairs. The rehabilitation technology supplier will have an intimate product knowledge of sophisticated technology, and enough understanding of clinical applications and issues, to be able to work with therapists and rehabilitation engineers to solve difficult problems. In this manner a certain level of involvement, quality, and ongoing service can be ensured by the rehabilitation technology team.

LEVELS OF INTERVENTION

Several chapters in this book refer to the use of assistive technology to achieve the goals of physical therapy for children with particular disorders. The benefits of assistive technology can be grouped and discussed according to the National Center for Medical Rehabilitation Research (NCMRR) model of the disabling process presented in Chapter 7. At the first level of the model, no claims were found in the literature that the types of assistive technology discussed in this chapter can alter the underlying pathophysiology of the clients' conditions, such as muscle disease or central nervous system damage.

Correctly prescribed and used, assistive technology, especially therapeutic positioning (adaptive seating), may address the dimension of impairment, particularly by helping to prevent secondary impairments such as skin breakdown, cardiopulmonary compromise due to scoliosis or slouched posture, and contractures or deformity due to inadequately supported body segments. Other potential benefits at this level are the reduction of tone or excessive muscle activity and a decrease in pathologic movements.

Assistive technology devices are essentially functional devices, and the most common reason for their use is to provide alternatives to functional limitations imposed by the client's disorder, thereby preventing or minimizing disability in activities of daily life. The inability to sit unsupported, the inability to walk or move from one place to another, the inability to use the hands well as the result of a weak, unstable trunk, or the inability to produce speech are often primary reasons for prescribing a seating system, a power wheelchair, or an electronic communication device.

Assistive devices intervene in the disability dimension of the NCMRR model by improving the ability to perform socially appropriate activities. A power wheelchair may allow independent access to school or work. An AAC system may facilitate interactions with peers or promote social skills. An ECU system may make the difference between less restricted living in a supervised apartment or living in a nursing home or intermediate care facility. On the other hand, if careful thought is not given to the selection of appropriate devices, we may potentially add to the disability by limiting transportation options or increasing the client's reliance on others during repairs or maintenance.

Regarding societal impact, we need to consider whether the use of technology can decrease medical or care costs, such as hospitalizations for decubitus healing or the need for live-in personal attendants. Social policies and attitudes may have an impact on the success of clients in obtaining and using their assistive devices productively. Technology also has the potential to alter those attitudes and policies as clients' appearance and visibility improve and their capabilities become recognized.

Documentation of these benefits is often based empirically on clinical experience and observation. The literature is replete with descriptions of creative solutions for individual client problems. More difficult to find are carefully controlled studies of the effectiveness of assistive technology intervention on any of these dimensions of the disabling process. In this chapter we examine some of the literature within the framework of the NCMRR model.

LIFE-SPAN TECHNOLOGY

Assistive technology can be applied across the life span, and, indeed, the individual's needs change with growth and development. Intervention at each stage must be carefully planned to achieve maximum benefits. For example, positioning the infant is essential to promote social interaction and development of early concepts such as cause-and-effect and object permanence. Switch-activated toys and power-driven mobility toys can help the preschooler learn how to self-initiate movement and control the organization of his or her environment. The school-aged child needs the postural support and comfort to enable learning and to help reinforce functional goals of therapy. He or she needs a reliable way to indicate needs and make choices. The adolescent needs to keep up with peers and be accepted socially. He or she should be included in decision making regarding choice of mobility, seating, or communication options whenever possible. The young adult needs to be able to get to and from a job or day setting and rely as little as possible on others to achieve basic functions, such as position changes, communicating, eating, and toileting. This group tends to spend many more hours at a time in one position, and hygiene and skin care become especially important.

THE SELECTION PROCESS

An environment is a person's surroundings or a setting in which he or she spends a great deal of time. Children function in a series of environments throughout the day. Selection of assistive technologies must consider all of those environments in which they are to be used. Additionally, the wheelchair itself, with its adaptive seating and communication systems, becomes a primary microenvironment for many severely impaired clients (Bergen, 1992). The ultimate responsibility of the assistive technology team must be to solve the client's identified problem without creating new problems, in an affordable manner with obtainable and durable equipment that can and will be serviced as needed and will meet the client's needs for the foreseeable future until a new device is appropriate (Hedman, 1990).

Once a referral has been made to an assistive technology team, there are several steps to be followed in the prescription of devices (American Board of Physical Therapy Specialties, 1987; Attermeier, 1987; Bergen et al, 1990; Mann & Lane, 1991):

Step 1. *Identify the problem.* Interviews, questionnaires, and occasionally site visits are used to seek information and identify the client's overall needs and specific problems. There are three components to this process (Mann & Lane, 1991). *Client information* includes diagnosis, age, and developmental levels and the problems and needs to be addressed. Current equipment and its shortcomings should be identified. Recent assessments of performance and skills are included. *Environment information* identifies the context in which the problems occur, that is, where and when potential devices will be used and for what tasks. Other individuals who will be involved with the training and the use and care of the equipment are also identified. *Product information* includes the functional specifications of devices with potential for solving the identified problems.

Step 2. *Establish realistic goals.* The therapist, in concert with the client and family, prioritizes the needs identified in step 1. The desired functional gains must be considered as well as resource constraints, such as funding and availability of devices (American Board of Physical Therapy Specialities, 1987).

Step 3. *Perform the physical assessment.* Each type of assistive technology requires particular measurements, such as body dimensions (e.g., hip and shoulder width, trunk height, thigh and leg length), range of motion (ROM), functional strength and endurance, postural control, functional skills, and communication skills. Simulation with trial devices is especially helpful at this point. Referral to other specialists may be indicated for remediation or treatment of certain problems, such as surgery to correct severe deformity.

Step 4. *Plan the intervention.* The team formulates a global concept of the assistive technology package while considering the relationship among the various components. The key to this step is to match the products and their features to the client's problems and capabilities. What types of equipment are needed to meet the client's needs, and can the various pieces be interfaced with each other? The length of time the devices will be required and their ability to "grow" or be modified in the future are considered. The rehabilitation technology supplier is instrumental in identifying appropriate equipment choices at this point, and a rehabilitation engineer is invaluable in creating unique solutions to difficult problems. This step also identifies who will be responsible for each task and a time line for completion. The amount and type of training required by the client, the family, school personnel, and others who interact with the child on a regular basis and those responsible for providing that training are identified.

Step 5. *Select components and interfaces.* A list of equipment items is generated, and the correct size, style, and model (when appropriate) of each component are specified. For equipment with component pieces, mounting hardware such as brackets, extension arms, and locking pins must be carefully selected to provide correct alignment, as well as strong and durable interfaces between components. This will ensure safety, easy detachment when taking apart a system for cleaning or transportation, and adjustability and growth of the system.

Step 6. *Secure funding.* The equipment justification and itemized price list are submitted to the funding agency at this point; however, it is wise to be well aware of the client's funding options throughout the selection process (see step 2). Customarily, equipment and devices that are considered to be "medically necessary" (wheelchairs, walkers, braces) will be approved before devices that might be considered "recreational," such as ECUs, computer equipment, switches, and, sometimes, communication devices. The team must be prepared to justify a more expensive choice if indicated by the client's needs, when a less costly alternative exists. Although new legislation is gradually providing and mandating financial support for assistive devices, implementation and interpretation of the laws may vary considerably from state to state. Possible sources for funding and reimbursement include federal, state, and local agencies (Medicaid, Medicare, Department of Veterans Affairs, Social Security Administration, Easter Seals, United Cerebral Palsy, Muscular Dystrophy Association, and special education and developmental disability agencies); private insurance plans; personal savings; trust funds; personal loans; and private corporate, civic, and religious groups. Strategies for obtaining funding include 1) determining the eligibility guidelines of the particular agency; 2) determining the agency's definition of need and using appropriate language and terminology that reflects that definition; 3) learning to negotiate with the agency, preferably establishing an ongoing dialogue between the funding advocate on the team and the agency contact; 4) keeping accurate records of all correspondence and telephone conversations with dates and times noted; 5) if a claim is denied, exploring the reasons why (e.g., sometimes a person must be ineligible for one type of assistance to receive another); and 6) appealing the decision through the correct procedures for that agency or approaching other funding sources (Funding Strategies, 1993).

Step 7. *Assemble or construct the assistive technology package.* Commercial equipment is ordered and customized pieces, such as molded seats and backs, are fabricated. The timing of the latter may need to be delayed until the former are received to ensure the least amount of error due to growth and structural or functional changes. Fittings with the client are performed frequently, and the team should be prepared for the need for revisions to the original plan.

Step 8. *Deliver the system.* This step includes the final fittings (or programming of electronic devices), testing, and adjustments. The primary users (the client and family or caregivers) should be instructed in proper use of all parts. Warranty, safety, and maintenance information must be shared with the client and family.

Step 9. *Provide training.* In many cases, extended training will be required for devices such as power wheelchairs, electronic speech devices, and ECUs; and this may occur in a different setting such as the home or school. Therefore, the team may need to train family members or the child's primary therapists or teachers both in the use of the device and in the best way to train the child.

Step 10. *Schedule follow-up.* For the child who is physically challenged, the previous process is usually only one of many repetitions of a cycle. Mechanical and electronic equipment wears out and breaks down, making repairs and fine-tuning necessary. The child's problems and needs change with age, development of new skills, and change of environments. As technologies continue to improve or be introduced, new solutions become available.

POSTURAL SUPPORT SYSTEMS

The purpose of the adaptive seating system is to provide external postural support for the child with functional limitations in sitting as a result of impairments in musculoskeletal alignment, postural control, muscle tone, or strength. The goal is to enable the child to compensate for functional limitations and thereby prevent or minimize disability. Letts (1991) stated that to achieve stable sitting, biomechanical forces and moments in all planes must be balanced. In a 1987 review of the literature, MacNeela found a consensus among authors for achieving an upright "midline orientation of the entire body with a near vertical alignment of the trunk and head." The "90-90-90 rule" (referring to degrees of flexion at the hips, knees, and ankles) was upheld as the golden standard until recently, when therapists recognized that to preserve the trunk stability necessary for head and upper extremity control, pelvic and lower extremity alignment may need to be altered to accommodate contracture or deformity (Bergen, 1992). Kangas (1991) has gone further in seriously challenging the idea of static positioning, stating that it is unnatural and impedes function. In this section, studies that have examined the effectiveness of postural support systems are reviewed using the NCMRR model as outlined earlier. Considerations in the prescription of postural support systems are then discussed.

Efficacy Studies

Major concerns in the seating management of individuals with cerebral palsy (CP) or head injuries are normalization of muscle tone and improvement of upper body postural control to enhance functional skills of the head and hands. Much of the research on therapeutic seating for this group has examined the effects of variables such as hip flexion angles (or seat-to-back angles) and orientation of the trunk and head (or angle-in-space). The former is achieved by wedging the seat or reclining the back; the latter is achieved by tilting the entire system. There has been considerable interest in the anteriorly tipped (or forward-inclined) seat, in which the front edge of the seat is rotated downward, thus increasing the seat-to-back angle while maintaining a near-vertical back. Most clients with myelodysplasia or spinal cord injuries tolerate and function well in a typical upright position, however, sitting pressures and the prevention of skin ulcerations are of concern. Various types of sitting surfaces and adjustments to postural alignment have been studied in the attempt to reduce pressure and decrease the incidence of decubiti. In children with muscular dystrophy, prevention of spinal collapse, preservation of upper extremity function, and comfort are major goals of positioning.

IMPAIRMENT

Neuromuscular Function and Pathologic Movement Patterns. A long-standing principle of therapeutic seating is that increased muscle tone, here defined as muscle activity at rest, can be reduced by altering seating angles. Nwaobi and colleagues (1983) tested the hypothesis that hip flexion of greater than 90° decreases extensor tone by examining the effect of various seat and back angle relationships on the electromyographic (EMG) activity of the lumbar paraspinal muscles in 11 children with spastic CP. EMG activity was least when the seat and back angles were oriented at 0°/90° (horizontal seat and vertical back). EMG activity was greatest at an orientation of 0°/75° (back inclined forward on a horizontal seat, thus increasing hip flexion). Activity at 15°/90° (hip flexion greater than 90° but with a vertical back) was higher than at 0°/90°. In two additional comparisons, 0°/90° with 15°/105° (hip flexion constant at 90°) and 0°/105° with 15°/120° (hip flexion less than 90°), the lumbar EMG activity was greater in each of the more reclined positions. The authors concluded that orientation of the body in space played a more important role than hip flexion in the reduction of extensor tone. However, the authors also cited a previously unpublished study (Nwaobi & Cusick, 1980) in which hip adductor activity was decreased in the 15°/90° (flexed) position compared with the other positions studied.

Nwaobi (1986) then studied the effect of orientation in space on myoelectric activity while keeping hip flexion constant at 90° in 12 subjects with CP. The two orientations compared were sitting in an upright, vertical position and sitting in a position of 30° posterior tilt. Myoelectric activity in the lumbar paraspinal, hip adductor, and ankle plantar flexor muscles was measured. The mean integrated EMG activity was significantly lower in the vertical position and higher in the tilted position for the paraspinal and hip adductor muscle groups. The difference in integrated EMG activity for the ankle plantar flexors was not significant.

Pile and colleagues (1988) measured EMG activ-

ity from bilateral back extensors and medial hamstrings in 8 subjects with spastic quadriplegia. All subjects had fixed deformities, had no reliable method of communication, and were classified in the most severe category of seating needs. Two seat-back angles were examined in each of four orientation-in-space angles, yielding eight different positions. The seat-back angles were the open position of 96° and the closed position of 84°. The orientation angles were the vertical plane and three angles of posterior tilt in 12° increments to a maximum of 36°. The subjects had very individualized responses to the changes in position on EMG activity. When analyzed by subject, the data showed significant effects of position on EMG activity, but the direction of these effects was variable between subjects and even between muscles. In addition, the effect of changing the orientation was different for the two seat-back angles, suggesting an interaction effect between these two variables.

Bablich and co-workers (1986) measured EMG activity in the midthoracic, lumbar paraspinal, and hamstring muscles of 12 children with CP for two conditions: sitting on level seats and sitting on anteriorly tipped seats. They found a decrease in the midthoracic activity and an increase in the lumbar activity when the subjects sat on the anteriorly tipped seat.

Myhr and von Wendt (1991) attempted to evaluate the effects of position on muscle activity using a more clinical approach. They photographed and videotaped 23 subjects with various types and severity of CP sitting in either their own seating system and chair or on an anteriorly tipped chair with an abduction orthosis and a cutout table for upper extremity weight bearing. They counted the frequency of typical pathologic movements, described as spastic or tonic reflex patterns, over a 5-minute period. To reduce subjective interpretation of this measure, the authors identified and defined a single pattern for each subject. Pathologic movements were significantly reduced in the experimental sitting position when compared with the subjects' original positions.

Physiological Functions. Nwaobi and Smith (1986) studied pulmonary function in sitting in 8 children with spastic CP. Each child was tested in a nonadapted wheelchair with standard sling seat and back and in an adapted seating system consisting of modular plastic inserts with lateral trunk and thigh supports incorporated into a frame with independent adjustments of orientation in space, hip flexion angle, foot support height, and headrest height.

When positioned in the adapted system, the children demonstrated significant improvement in the three pulmonary functions measured: vital capacity, forced expiratory volume in 1 second calculated as a percentage of vital capacity, and expiratory time. The differences were attributed to changes in the shape, structure, and capacity of the thorax and abdomen and to improved control of the respiratory muscles in the supported, upright position.

Noble-Jamieson and co-workers (1986) studied the effect of position changes and bracing on pulmonary function in two groups of children with muscle weakness as a result of neuromuscular disease. The first group of 20 children was ambulatory and without scoliosis. They showed a slight decrease (6%) in forced vital capacity (FVC) when supine compared with sitting, but it was not significantly different from a similar decrease seen in children without disease. In a second group of nonambulatory children with scoliosis, however, the decrease in FVC while supine compared with sitting was significant (mean reduction of 12%). The children in the second group were also tested while sitting with their spinal brace (lightweight polypropylene body jacket) on and off. FVC showed a mean reduction of 22% with the brace on compared with the brace off. Subjects with more severe scoliosis showed a greater decrease in FVC. The greater the reduction in Cobb's angle achieved with the brace on, the greater was the decrease in FVC.

Skeletal Deformity, Contracture, and Passive ROM. The only studies found that pertained to these types of impairments examined the management of scoliosis in patients with Duchenne's muscular dystrophy. Carlson and Payette (1985) used a combination of molded seating systems with soft spinal corsets and found a reduction of curves on radiography. Seeger and associates (1984b), however, found no significant difference in spinal curves when modular seats, custom-molded seats, unmodified wheelchair seats, and spinal jackets were used in boys aged 14 to 16 with Duchenne's muscular dystrophy.

The principle that postural support systems can maintain or increase ROM or prevent and control contracture and deformity, particularly for clients with increased postural tone, has not been studied. In theory, maintaining normalized skeletal alignment of the trunk and lower extremities should help to prevent structural changes such as scoliosis and hip dislocation, particularly for the young child without contractures. It can be argued, however, that for those with severely increased tone, strong deforming muscle forces cannot be overcome through seating.

Postural Stability and Control. In the study by Bablich and colleagues (1986), postural stability of the subjects was measured with a tracking system that monitored a point on the body (the top of the head) in three-dimensional space while the subjects were seated on flat or anteriorly tipped seats. The anteriorly tipped seat resulted in a more upright and stable posture by increasing trunk extension and decreasing deviation from the midline in the subjects with CP.

Myhr and von Wendt (1991) also included clinical measures of head and postural control in their study of sitting in children with CP. The mean duration of head control during a 5-minute test period was significantly increased in the anterior sitting position compared with the subjects' usual positions. Postural control of the head, trunk, and feet (ability to keep feet on the footrests) was scored on a 4-point sitting assessment scale developed by the authors. Median scores for all three measures improved in the anterior position. The validity of the scale is questionable, however, because head and trunk control were scored based on whether external support was needed. For many subjects, such external support was an integral part of their original seating system. In at least some cases, the subjects would have received the lowest possible score because the support was present as part of the chair rather than because the subject required it.

Miedaner (1990) also used a 4-point scale to rate active control of trunk extension while sitting on a bench in 15 children between 2 and 6 years of age. The subjects had various types of motor impairment, including hypotonia, hypertonia, and developmental delay. The Modified Schober Measurement (distance between defined marks on the spine) was then used to measure trunk extension when the subjects sat on the floor, a level bench, a bench tipped anteriorly 20°, a bench tipped anteriorly 30°, and a commercial TherAdapt Posture Chair (TherAdapt Products, Bensonville, IL). The latter is an anteriorly tipped seat with an anterior leg support to provide weight bearing through the knees and shins rather than the feet. The subjects' back extension in the TherAdapt Chair was significantly greater compared with all other positions except level bench sitting.

Reid and colleagues (1991) used an instrumented system to track changes in position of the C-7 spinous process during quiet sitting in children with and without neurologic impairment. The tracking system yielded a calculated measurement termed *the radius of stability.* A smaller radius was interpreted to indicate reduced postural sway and thus increased postural stability. In the control group, postural sway when sitting on a horizontal flat seat decreased with age. Children with CP (aged 5 to 6 years) and children with head injury (aged 13 to 15 years) showed no statistically significant difference in the amount of postural sway when compared with children of the same age in the control group, although they showed more variability.

The children with neurologic impairment were then tested in a 10° anteriorly tilted sitting position. Group data revealed no differences in postural sway between the horizontal and the anterior sitting positions. Inspection of individual data revealed that half of the children with CP (described as having spasticity with tight hamstrings) had a decrease in sway and a more upright posture (vertical measurement of C-7 height) on the anterior seat. The other half of the children with CP (described as having low trunk tone and tight hamstrings) had an increase in sway on the anterior seat but also a more upright posture. Reid and colleagues surmised that because both groups had a more upright posture, reduced postural sway may not necessarily indicate improved postural control.

McClenaghan and co-authors (1992) used a video digitizing system to measure segmental displacements of the head, shoulder, hip, knee, and ankle and an instrumented seating surface to measure seat reaction forces. Two measures of the reaction forces were used as indicators of postural stability: 1) the trial variability of the path of the center of pressure and 2) the mean location of the center of pressure. The subjects included 20 children, aged 4 to 15 years, of whom 10 were non-impaired and 10 had mild to moderate spastic cerebral palsy. The three experimental sitting conditions studied were with the seat surface in a horizontal position (0°), tipped 5° anteriorly, and tipped 5° posteriorly. Data were collected in each position for 2 minutes during both quiet sitting and active sitting (while performing an upper extremity task).

During quiet sitting, the children with CP exhibited greater displacements of the head, shoulder, and hip than did the children without impairment; during active sitting, only the difference in shoulder displacement was significant. The change in seat orientation did not significantly affect displacements for either group during active sitting, but during quiet sitting on the anterior seat the group with CP had increased displacement of the head. The children with CP showed greater variability in the center of pressure than the children in the control group for all conditions, and variability was greater during active sitting compared with quiet sitting for both groups. Altering the seat angle did not significantly change the variability for either group. The location of the center of pressure was

farther forward in the children with CP, particularly during active sitting on the anterior seat. In summary, significant differences were found between children with and without motor impairment, as well as between quiet and active sitting for both groups; however, seat inclination did not affect most dependent measures of postural stability.

Pressure and Prevention of Decubiti. Several factors contribute to the development of pressure sores (Crenshaw & Vistnes, 1989), including skin temperature, moisture, shear, and compression. Pressure has perhaps been the most studied variable, since it has a clear relationship to the development of decubiti and is relatively easy to measure and manipulate during wheelchair seating. The risk of a pressure sore is directly related to the length of time soft tissue is compressed and inversely related to the area being compressed. Serious pressure sores are a common impairment in children with spinal cord injury and myelodysplasia in which immobility and insensate tissue compound the problem of prolonged sitting. Clients who are immobilized by severe CP or other neuromuscular impairment also need special considerations for pressure relief in sitting. Skeletal asymmetries such as pelvic obliquity, hip dislocation, and scoliosis predispose children who sit in wheelchairs to pressure problems.

Researchers have developed a number of devices to measure pressures over the entire sitting surface, allowing the mapping of pressure patterns. These are used to study differences in pressure distribution between subjects with and without motor impairment, as well as the effect that altering the seating surface has on reducing seat interface pressure and preventing decubiti. Drummond and co-workers (1982) found that normal adult subjects displayed an even distribution of pressure from side to side and a biphasic pattern of pressure concentration with a posterior concentration on the ischial tuberosities and a second, but lesser, concentration on the anterior thighs. The center of pressure was generally centrally located just in front of the perineum. Pate (1988) found a similar biphasic pattern in adolescent boys without impairment; however, he sampled sitting pressures over a 3-hour period and found that pressure tended to be skewed slightly to one side or the other. Drummond and colleagues (1982) also studied 15 patients with "unbalanced sitting" due to pelvic obliquity or scoliosis. They found a pronounced shift of pressure laterally and often posteriorly, thereby severely loading one of the ischial tuberosities.

Gilsdorf and colleagues (1990) found that, for subjects without impairment, returning to upright after a short period of reclining in a wheelchair resulted in higher pressures and shear forces than in the original upright position. Leaning forward off the backrest returned the forces to initial values. They also found that as the footrests were elevated, pressure under the ischial tuberosities was increased.

Shields and Cook (1988) studied pressures under the ischial tuberosities in adults without impairment in various sitting configurations. They found no difference in pressure between upright sitting and 10° of recline; however, there was a significant reduction of pressure in both positions when a lumbar support was added. They recommended using the lumbar support with the reclined position for patients with spinal cord injury based on the observation that these individuals slide or rotate off the lumbar support when positioned upright because of tight hamstrings or weak trunk musculature.

Reger and colleagues (1986) used magnetic resonance imaging to evaluate soft tissue contours of the buttocks during loading in one subject with paraplegia and one normal subject. For the subject with paraplegia, less sitting pressure was required before soft tissue became compressed by a bony prominence. There was also increased stiffness and lateral shifting of the gluteal muscle mass of the subject with paraplegia. The authors recommended matching the shape and material of the seating support to the tissue contours to preserve soft tissue padding.

Sprigle and co-workers (1990a) developed a system to measure body contours and custom-contoured a foam cushion to match those measurements. They reported that foam cushions that were contoured to match the shape of the buttocks, as opposed to flat foam, improved the load transfer from buttocks to cushion. The total contact surface area of the contoured foam was greater than for the flat foam. Foam stiffness was also important in determining the seat contours, with a stiffer foam having less deflection under the load. In a related study, the same authors examined the sitting pressures of 11 clients with spinal cord injury when seated on flat compared with contoured foam cushions of different stiffness (Sprigle et al., 1990b). They found that pressures were lower on the contoured cushions than on the flat cushions and were lower on the more compliant foam than on the stiffer foam. The buttocks were encompassed more on the contoured and softer cushion with less tissue distortion. Sprigle and co-workers cautioned against using too soft a foam that would deform too much and "bottom out" quickly.

Several studies have compared sitting pressures, skin temperature, and relative humidity in subjects seated on a number of commercially available cushions (Fisher et al., 1978; Garber, 1985; Garber & Dyerly, 1991; Garber et al., 1978; Palmieri et al., 1980; Seymour & Lacefield, 1985; Stewart et al., 1980). In general, the findings indicate that no one type of cushion is universally effective for all clients and that a variety of cushion options are needed to meet a variety of needs. In addition, the subjects in most of these pressure studies were adults with spinal cord injury and the unique needs of children, particularly those with severe pelvic and spinal deformity, as in myelodysplasia and CP, have not been studied.

FUNCTIONAL LIMITATIONS

Upper Extremity Control and Hand Function. Several authors have investigated the effect of varying seating configurations on upper body control and function. Seeger and associates (1984a) found that increased hip flexion angle in three 10° increments past 90° did not improve hand function on a joystick-controlled targeting task in 9 subjects with marked extensor spasticity. Nwaobi and colleagues (1986) also varied hip angle to measure its effect on upper extremity performance time in triggering a touch-activated switch with a shoulder horizontal adduction movement. They positioned 10 subjects with CP upright and then altered the hip flexion angle for 50°, 70°, 90°, and 110° of flexion. Movement time was fastest at the 90° position and slowest at the 50° position. Contrary to Seeger's results, when the faster time in the 90° position was compared with that in the 110° position there was a statistically significant difference.

In another study, Nwaobi (1987) seated his subjects with CP in a positioning device that maintained the hips at 90° of flexion but varied the orientation in space from vertical to 15° and 30° of posterior tilt and 5° of anterior tilt. Performance on the same shoulder adduction task was best in the vertical position and worst in the anterior position.

Myhr and von Wendt (1991) and McClenaghan and co-workers (1992) both included upper extremity performance measures in their previously described studies. Myhr and von Wendt reported higher mean scores on the 4-point scales for arm and hand function in the anteriorly tipped position. McClenaghan and co-workers measured performance on six different upper extremity tasks and found that seat inclination angle (level, tipped 5° anteriorly or 5° posteriorly) did not affect performance for subjects either with or without CP, except for a linear tapping task that decreased significantly in the posterior position and a thumb press task that was better in the anterior position.

In a single-subject study, McCormack (1990)

found that allowing an 8-year-old boy with spastic athetoid CP to sit in his typical position of posterior pelvic rotation (sacral sitting) did not affect his typing speed and accuracy when compared with sitting in a more therapeutic alignment with neutral pelvic rotation.

Oral-Motor, Speech, and Communication Functions. Hulme and co-workers (1987) positioned 11 children with multiple handicaps between the ages of 1 and 4 years in individually selected therapeutic seating devices and then assessed their eating and drinking skills. Data were collected every 6 weeks, with three baseline measurements taken before receiving the seating device and four measurements taken after. Significant improvements were seen in oral-motor skills associated with eating and drinking as assessed using a clinical rating scale and direct observation; however, no significant improvements were seen in self-feeding or independent drinking.

In another study, Hulme and colleagues (1988) explored the relationship between adaptive seating and vocalizations in 8 children between 1.5 and 2.8 years of age with spasticity or hypotonia. Samples of spontaneous vocalizations were taken monthly, from 3 months before to 6 months after delivery of the seating system. Increased frequency of speech sounds was found in 7 children, and increased types of sounds were found in 6 after receipt of the system. The authors did not indicate that they controlled for maturation over the 9-month period.

Bay (1991) did a single-subject study of a 37-year-old woman with spastic athetoid CP to determine the effect of therapeutic positioning in a wheelchair on her ability to activate her electronic communication device with a head-mounted light sensor. Eight observations were made during a baseline period. She was seated in her manual wheelchair, which had no foot support, no lateral trunk support, and a seat height greater than her lower leg length. During the intervention period, an additional eight observations were made while she was seated in her power wheelchair with lateral trunk supports and properly adjusted foot support. There was an increased rate (hits per minute) in head-controlled typing but decreased accuracy (correct hits as percentage of total hits) during the intervention period.

Mobility. Several researchers have examined the effect of seating position on efficiency of manual wheelchair propulsion in adults (Brubaker et al., 1984; Hughes et al., 1992; Van der Woude et al., 1989). Altering seat height, seat inclination, or anterior-posterior orientation for individual subjects affected upper extremity patterns of joint motion and wheeling efficiency. Wheeling performance can

be optimized by adjusting seating configurations in relation to the propulsion mechanism (hand-rims or lever), based on the functional characteristics of each user. The effect that standard wheelchair configurations and the addition of seating systems has on the ability of young children with disabilities to learn self-wheeling has not been considered in the literature.

DISABILITY

The assumption is often made that individuals who experience an increase in functional skills also decrease their level of disability and improve their ability to fill societal roles. Little research has been done to test this assumption, however, and anecdotal descriptions are much more plentiful in the literature.

Hulme and co-workers (1983) used a survey to retrospectively evaluate families' perceptions of clients' motor and social interaction behaviors after receipt of adaptive seating equipment. The clients were 41 individuals who were nonambulatory and developmentally disabled. They ranged in age from 1 to 67 years, and most received some sort of motor or sensory training program (individually determined) in conjunction with the equipment. The seating devices included wheelchairs, travel chairs, and strollers, with custom adaptations as needed. Improvements were seen in most of the motor and social behaviors surveyed. Improvements in motor behaviors included increased ability to sit upright without leaning, more time spent in sitting and less time lying down, increased ability to grasp an object, and improved ability to eat with a spoon. Social behavior changes included an increased number of community places visited, more time during the day spent with someone else, and less time spent in the bedroom. Although there was no change in frequency of leaving the home, caregivers reported an improvement in ease of taking the clients out of the home. The authors recommended further research to separate the effects related to the equipment and the effects related to the training programs.

McEwen (1992) studied the effects of assistive positioning on social-communicative interactions between 10 students, 6 to 12 years of age, with profound multiple disabilities, and their classroom staff. The subjects were divided into a higher-functioning group and a lower functioning group. Positions included a wheelchair, a sidelyer, and a freestyle position on a mat on the floor. The interactions measured included adult-initiated interactions, student initiated interactions, and maintenance of communication during a structured interaction. Adults initiated interactions more often when the students were in the wheelchair, whereas there was no difference in student initiations between the positions. For the lower-functioning group, the average duration of interaction during the structured session was higher in the free-style position than in either of the other two positions. For the higher-functioning group, there was no difference in duration of interaction between positions.

SUMMARY

When the above studies are summarized, the gaps in information and the number of questions that remain to be answered regarding best options in seating become evident. There is supporting evidence in the literature that therapeutic seating systems that provide external postural support may improve pulmonary function in subjects with CP, reduce scoliosis when combined with a soft orthosis in subjects with muscular dystrophy, possibly have some effects on upper extremity function in subjects with CP, and potentially improve oral-motor skills, vocalizations, and social interaction behaviors in subjects with multiple disabilities. More specifically, an upright orientation appears to correlate with decreased myoelectric activity of extensor muscles at rest in cerebral palsy, improve pulmonary function in subjects with muscle weakness compared with supine positioning, improve an upper extremity (shoulder adduction) task in subjects with CP, and increase the number of adult-initiated interactions with subjects that have profound involvement compared with floor-lying positions. Hip flexion greater than 90° did not reduce myoelectric activity in extensors, nor did it improve upper extremity function. From Fife and colleagues' (1988) study, it appears that, in clients with the most severe involvement, effects of orientation in space and seat-to-back angles are more variable and individualized than for clients with mild-to-moderate involvement reported in other studies. This must be considered when assessing clients with severe impairments and supports the need for postural support system simulation. The purpose in providing a postural support system for these clients usually is focused more on improving comfort and alignment than function.

The effects of anteriorly tipping the seat are more controversial. Although anteriorly tipped seats appear to increase back extension and improve spinal alignment, it is unclear whether they improve stability or upper extremity function. Clinically, anteriorly tipped seats are usually used to encourage more "active sitting," with the goal of improving pelvic and spinal alignment in the presence of tight lower extremity musculature. The more vertical orientation of the pelvis that is possible with an anteriorly tipped seat may place the lumbar extensors at a better biomechanical advantage and reduce the need for the thoracic extensors to be excessively active to compensate for upper body flexion. As an active sitting position, the effects of long-term seating on performance and fatigue need to be studied.

There is evidence that use of contoured cushions improves pressure distribution in subjects with spinal cord injury. Lumbar rolls tend to decrease pressure under the ischial tuberosities. The results with commercially available pressure relief cushions are variable, but of interest is the number of manufacturers of these cushions that are adding blocks and foam pieces to provide custom-contouring of their products.

Much work remains to be done in defining the features and components of postural support systems that reduce impairment, improve function, and increase social access for individuals with severe physical impairments. Identifying the specific disorders and severity of involvement and consistently reporting this information in all research reports are also necessary. Objective clinical tools for identifying functional levels and measuring change as a result of intervention with a postural support system, such as the Level of Sitting Scale (Fife et al., 1991) and seat interface pressure monitors, need to be developed and refined in terms of validity, reliability, and ease of clinical use.

The societal impact of use of adaptive seating, as well as of assistive technology clinics and programs, has yet to be studied in detail. Potentially, these can reduce costs of hospitalizations due to decubiti and corrective surgery. It is likely that the establishment of comprehensive regional centers is the most cost-effective way to deliver advanced technology to the greatest number of people. One interesting paradox that should be examined is that in spite of receiving expensive assistive technology and vocational training that theoretically increases clients' employability, persons with disability frequently end up unemployed because they lose Medicaid or other social funding and employers are unwilling to assume the high cost of their insurance.

Principal Concepts in the Prescription of Postural Support Systems

STANDARDIZATION OF TERMINOLOGY

Assistive seating technology has been evolving rapidly in many different regions of North America, creating a confusion of locally adopted language and terminology. The Rehabilitation Engineering Society of North America (RESNA) has published a list of standardized seating terminology that will be helpful in improving communication among research and service centers, clients, and funding sources (Medhat & Hobson, 1992).

MATCHING THE INTERVENTION TO THE CLIENT'S LEVEL OF NEED

Classification schemes have been developed by many authors and are based on different dimensions of the NCMRR model. Two methods of classification are compared in Table 23–1. Trefler (1984) described three classifications of seating clients based on the level of impairment of neuromotor control and deformity, whereas Tredwell (1988; Tredwell & Roxborough, 1991) used functional criteria to describe three similar categories.

Fife and colleagues (1991) described a Level of Sitting Scale that included seven levels of functional sitting ability. They intend it to be a clinical index of the need for adaptive seating and part of a tool for evaluating effectiveness of seating programs for groups of children. Reliability tests for scoring the scale are underway.

The levels of intervention achieved with postural support systems have also been classified in many ways, but most investigators agree on three basic categories based on the amount of support the systems provide (Bergen et al., 1990). The first level of intervention is the *planar system* and consists of a flat seat and back. Good postural stability and sitting balance, with a minimum of deformity, are required, and this type of system is most appropriate for clients at the first level of the classification schemes. The seat and back consist of a solid base (plywood or plastic), covered by foam, and upholstered with vinyl or knit fabric. Flat trunk or pelvic supports may be added laterally. Many commercial variations are available, or they can be easily constructed in the clinic.

The second level of intervention is the *contoured system*, which provides external postural control by increasing the points of contact, especially laterally. The seat and back surfaces are rounded by shaping layers of firm foam to correspond to the curves of the body. Contours also help distribute pressures more evenly. Contouring can range from simple to aggressive. Although contoured systems are most typically used for clients at the second classification level, simple contouring can improve comfort and stability for many clients at the first level and aggressive contouring may provide enough support for some clients at the third level. Many varieties are fabricated in the clinic of a solid base with varying densities and configurations of foam, or there are a number of standardized modules commercially available.

The third level of intervention is the *custom-molded system*. It provides an intimate fit by closely conforming to the shape of the client's body, thereby giving the most postural support. When carefully molded it also provides the greatest amount of pressure relief. The time and expense involved in the fabrication of these systems is considerable, and the molding process requires a great deal of skill. Production of the mold usually involves either a vacuum consolidation method or a chemical reaction of liquid foams injected into a special bag. Several varieties of custom-molded systems are available, including those that can be completed on site and those that are sent to a central fabrication center.

ASSESSMENT AND SIMULATION

Physical assessment of the client for evaluation and prescription of postural support systems is a pivotal role of the physical therapist on the technology team. The physical therapist applies knowledge of anatomy, kinesiology, biomechanics, and principles of neuromuscular control of posture and function when assessing the child. Early strategies for seating intervention used by therapists often fo-

TABLE 23–1. TWO METHODS OF CLASSIFICATION OF SITTING NEEDS

Trefler (1984)	Tredwell (1988)
Group I	Hand-Free Sitter
Good head control	Sits for long periods
Good to fair trunk control	without using hands for
Good to fair fine motor skills	support
Symmetric posture readily attainable	
Joint ROM within normal limits	
Group II	Hand-Dependent Sitter
Good to fair head control	Needs one or both hands
Fair to poor trunk control	to maintain sitting
Fair to poor fine motor skills	Needs some form of trunk
Up to and including moderate deformities	or pelvic support to be able to use hands for ADL
Group III	Propped Sitter
Fair to poor head control	Unable to sit without
Poor trunk control	major modification for
Poor fine motor skills	pelvis and trunk
Deformities at the severe end of the scale, with limitation in ROM due to contractures	Often requires head support
	Severe structural and functional deformity

cused on controlling tone and reflexes according to Bobath-based principles. MacNeela (1987) and Letts (1991) stressed the critical need to thoroughly understand and apply the principles of biomechanics to seating intervention as well.

Bergen has provided the most current and complete discussion of the assessment process (Bergen, 1992; Bergen et al., 1990). The client should be assessed both supine and sitting. A simulator chair works especially well for measuring linear dimensions, determining seating angles, and determining the amount of contouring needed, particularly for the more severely involved client who requires a very individualized solution. Two seating simulators that are commercially available are shown in Figures 23–2 and 23–3; however, many centers have made their own using modular components.

The assessment of posture in a wheelchair begins with the pelvis and its relationship to its adjacent segments. The orientation and range of mobility of the pelvis in all three planes will in turn determine the alignment and support needed at the trunk, head, and extremities. The measurements taken with the client supine and sitting are summarized in Figures 23–4 through 23–7. The effect of hip flexion and knee extension ROM on the vertical orientation of the pelvis is among the most critical factors in selecting seating angles and components. If there are minimal contractures of the hamstrings, hip extensors, and hip flexors, the pelvis should

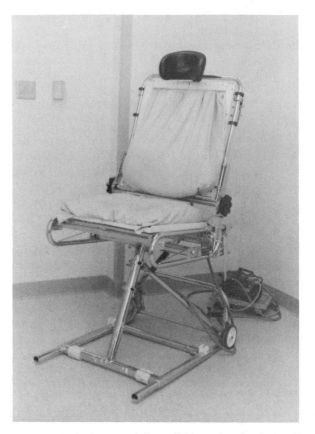

FIGURE 23–3. Commercially available seating simulator with adjustable angles. Shown with Contour-U (PinDot Products, Chicago, IL) vacuum-molding units for custom-contoured seat and back inserts.

retain a considerable amount of mobility and vertical orientation of the pelvis with a well-aligned trunk above will be possible. If any or all of these muscles are tight, the pelvis may be locked in either an anterior or posterior tilt and the client will require a much more individualized solution.

FIGURE 23–2. Commercially available seating simulator with multiadjustable components and angles. Shown mounted on a power mobility base that also allows assessment of driving ability and appropriate controls and switches.

FIGURE 23–4. The examiner must monitor the lumbar curve as the hips are flexed and the knees extended. (Redrawn with permission from Bergen AF, Presperin, J, & Tallman, T. Positioning for Function: Wheelchairs and Other Assistive Technologies. Valhalla, NY: Valhalla Rehabilitation Publications, 1990.)

FIGURE 23-5. Hip (C) and knee (D_{sup}) angles, thigh/hip length (A_{sup}), and calf length (B) are measured first in supine. (Redrawn with permission from Bergen, AF, Presparin, J, & Tallman, T. Positioning for Function: Wheelchairs and Other Assistive Technologies. Valhalla, NY: Valhalla Rehabilitation Publications, 1990.

Identification of the severity and type of deformities during assessment and simulation will influence the type of system and components chosen. A flexible deformity—one that can be manually corrected and maintained with a reasonable amount of

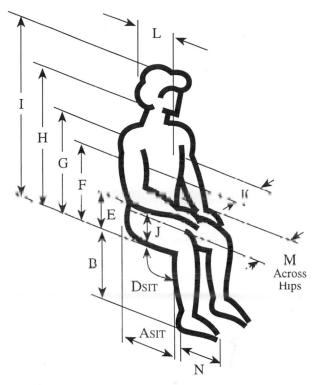

FIGURE 23-7. The following measurements are added to those taken with the client supine: A_{sit} (R & L), behind hips to popliteal fossa; B (R & L), popliteal fossa to heel; D_{sit}, knee flexion angle; E, sitting surface to pelvic crest; F, sitting surface to axilla; G, sitting surface to shoulder; H, sitting surface to occiput; I, sitting surface to crown of head; J, sitting surface to hanging elbow; K, width across trunk; L, depth of trunk; M, width across hips; N, heel to toe. (Redrawn with permission from Bergen, AF, Presparin, J, & Tallman, T. Positioning for Function: Wheelchairs and Other Assistive Technologies. Valhalla, NY: Valhalla Rehabilitation Publications, 1990.)

FIGURE 23-6. Measurements in sitting must be taken with the client sitting on a surface with a thin top. This will allow the knees to flex as needed. (Redrawn with permission from Bergen, AF, Presparin, J, & Tallman, T. Positioning for Function: Wheelchairs and Other Assistive Technologies. Valhalla, NY: Valhalla Rehabilitation Publications, 1990.

force—can often be maintained in optimal alignment with the appropriate and balanced use of support components. Postural support systems, however, are not intended to stretch tight musculature or correct bony deformity. Stretching invariably results in sacrifice of the optimum posture because the child will attempt to move and avoid the uncomfortable forces. Fixed deformities—those that are not correctable without an undue amount of force—and severe muscle contractures must be accommodated in the postural support system, and reduction must be addressed through other interventions. Letts (1991) strongly advocates surgical intervention to achieve a balance of sitting forces in much the same way that a goal of surgery is to improve symmetry of gait for individuals who are ambulatory.

Although the primary focus of the assessment is the pelvis, the primary goal of intervention is to provide a stabilized trunk for upright posture and for function (Bergen et al., 1990). With many individuals, the trunk alignment is achieved by first establishing the optimum pelvic positioning. For clients with severe scoliosis and pelvic obliquity, however, neutral alignment of the pelvis is not always possible and does not result in acceptable trunk and head alignment. In such cases, it is better to start with a relatively vertical head and level shoulders and allow the pelvis to be tilted and rotated.

In clients prone to pressure problems, evaluation of sitting pressures should also be included in the assessment process. Many rehabilitation technology centers use instrumented pressure-monitoring chairs as client evaluation tools as well as for research. There are a few simpler devices, such as the Texas Interface Pressure Evaluator (T-KAT, Inc., Stafford, TX), available to the clinician to measure pressure while seated on various cushions (Stefans & Creitz, 1986). Shortcomings of such devices are that accuracy of the monitor decreases with an increasingly contoured cushion and the monitor itself can interfere with the cushion's ability to conform to the bony prominence. In addition, pressure in deep tissues, especially near bone, can be higher than a reading of seat interface pressures might indicate (Crenshaw & Vistnes, 1989). Some companies and centers that manufacture custom-molded cushions are taking advantage of computer-aided design technology. A computer makes a graphic image of the seating surface contours. This is stored on disk and sent to the company where the contoured cushion is fabricated from the image, allowing a precise fit. Variable-tilt and variable-recline features of manual and power wheelchairs can provide another source of pressure relief throughout a long day of sitting for some clients.

CONSIDERATIONS IN SELECTING POSTURAL SUPPORT SYSTEMS

The scope of this chapter precludes a thorough discussion of all options and features of postural support systems. Many excellent resources exist describing these in more detail and provide problem-solving lists and charts (Bergen et al., 1990; Letts, 1991; Trefler, 1984; Trefler et al., 1993). In this section attention is focused on some of the most salient points in the decision-making process.

Seats. In most cases, the seat is the most critical element of the postural support system. The use of true planar seats is becoming rare since most clinicians are finding that a small amount of lateral contouring for even the highest-level sitter adds comfort and stability (Bergen, 1992; Bergen et al., 1990). The benefit of adding contours to help re-

FIGURE 23–8. An antithrust seat can help to hold the pelvis back on the seat. (Redrawn with permission from Bergen AF, Presparin, J, & Tallman, T. Positioning for Function: Wheelchairs and Other Assistive Technologies. Valhalla, NY: Valhalla Rehabilitation Publications, 1990.)

lieve pressure problems is evidenced by the number of commercially available pressure cushions, such as Jay and ROHO, that are adding foam blocks and wedges to allow customization of cushion shape. Antithrust seats (Fig. 23–8) have a block of high-density foam placed just anterior to the ischial tuberosities that keeps the pelvis from sliding forward and equalizes pressure distribution along the thighs (Siekman & Flanagan, 1983). Antithrust seats can be added to planar as well as contoured systems.

Seat placement within the wheelchair frame is another important consideration. A thick cushion or inappropriate mounting hardware can place the seat too high, causing loss of independent transfers or wheeling, or can change the center of gravity to an unsafe position. Forward or backward placement, especially in very small children, can affect the knee angle required for foot placement on the footrests and can change the ease of wheeling by affecting access to the wheel rims or loading or unloading the front casters.

Backs. A back support with a gently curved surface can improve lateral trunk stability and comfort. Simple contouring for a prominent rib hump can be achieved by cutting a hole in the plywood or plastic to allow the overlying foam some give. More aggressive contouring can be achieved using blocks of high-density foam to form the shape (Bergen et al., 1990). A custom-molded back should be used for clients with severe fixed spinal deformity.

Sagittal plane alignment of the spine has traditionally been adjusted using lumbar rolls. Margolis (1992; Margolis et al., 1988) pointed out that control of sagittal curves begins with the pelvis and sacrum rather than the lumbar spine. The use of a "bi-angular back" in which the portion behind the pelvis was oriented vertically and the portion above the pelvis was angled back a few degrees to encourage lumbar extension was advocated. Others have added sacral discs or pads to the back surface.

Pelvic Stabilization. Pelvic stabilization has traditionally been achieved with a seatbelt placed at a 45° angle at the junction of back and seat. For highly functional individuals, placement of the belt across the anterior thighs, just in front of the hips, allows more natural active trunk and pelvic mobility (Bergen et al., 1990).

Margolis and colleagues (1985, 1988) introduced the subASIS bar as a form of rigid pelvic stabilization. Maintaining the pelvis in a vertical orientation is essential or the client will slide under the bar. A less rigid variation of the subASIS bar is the Semi-Rigid Pelvic Stabilizer (SRPS) shown in Figures 23-9 and 23-10 (Carlson, 1987; Carlson & Grey, 1988). Constructed of high-density foam mounted on a reinforcing strip of thermoplastic splinting material, it incorporates wedges that fit under the anterior superior iliac spine while providing relief across the lower abdomen. Like the subASIS bar, the SRPS provides direct control of the pelvis for stabilization, yet the angle of placement can be varied as with a seatbelt, making it an option for clients with a mild fixed posterior pelvic tilt. The flexibility of the SRPS may result in fewer pressure problems than the subASIS bar, and it works especially well for clients who demonstrate a strong asymmetric thrusting pattern. Another form of pelvic stabilization is anterior knee blocks (Fig. 23-11), which direct a force up the length of the femurs to counter sliding of the pelvis (Bergen et al., 1990; Carlson, 1988).

Angles. From the studies reviewed in this chapter, there apparently is not a consensus as to the effects of seat and spatial angles on alignment and function in sitting. Factors that need to be considered in determining angles include severity and nature of postural tone abnormalities, contractures, and deformities; level of motor control for sitting; and design and purpose of the mobility base. Although the concept of upright (90 90 90) sitting is theoretically sound, it is neither a natural functional sitting position (Kangas, 1991) nor a logistically possible option for many clients. Slight wedging of the seat or posterior tilt may improve head

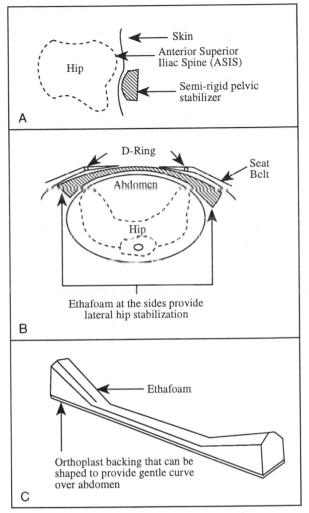

FIGURE 23-9. Placement of the semi-rigid pelvic stabilizer from a side view (*A*) and from a top view (*B*). *C*, detail of the stabilizer shape. (Redrawn with permission from Carlson, SJ. The semi-rigid pelvic stabilizer for seating control. Assistive Devices Information Network Newsletter [University of Iowa, Iowa City, IA], *1*[1]:2–3, 1987.)

alignment or keep very young children from sliding. Opening the hip angle may be necessary when hip extension contractures are present. By allowing the knees to flex, thus bringing the feet back under the seat, the amount of rotatory force on the pelvis may be significantly reduced in the presence of tight hamstrings.

The anteriorly tipped seat has exciting potential for clients with hyperextensible lower extremity musculature but fair to good upper body control who "sacral sit" on a flat surface. Good pelvic stabilization must be achieved to prevent sliding. Unfortunately, the client often lacks enough knee ex-

FIGURE 23–10. Completed, upholstered semi-rigid pelvic stabilizer with webbing belt and Velcro adjustments attached.

tension to keep the heels from interfering with caster movement in wheelchair seating. Figure 23–12 shows one solution for a young man with severe spastic athetoid CP in which one legrest arrangement was used for functional tasks in the stationary chair and the other, while not an ideal position, was used for wheeling.

Upholstery. Vinyl upholstery is easy to clean and durable and protects the cushions from urine and

FIGURE 23–11. Knee blocks used to stabilize pelvis and prevent sliding on an anteriorly tipped seat. (From Carlson, SJ. Knee gate for control of forward sliding in wheelchair. Assistive Devices Information Network Newsletter [University of Iowa, Iowa City, IA], 2[3]:2–3, 1988.)

food spills. On the other hand, a knit fabric breathes better to decrease temperature and moisture and is less slippery to decrease shear in decubitus-prone clients. Contoured cushions are easier to cover with a knit fabric, but a fabric that is pulled too tightly will interfere with deep contours. Vacuum methods allow use of thick vinyl upholstery on even aggressively contoured cushions. Color selection is now much more fun than it used to be and allows clients to express their own tastes, preferences, and even school spirit!

Leg Supports. Leg supports are usually a component of the mobility base but are discussed here because of their direct influence on the entire seating system. Elevating legrests should never be ordered unless that option is specifically required because they are offset forward of the seat more than fixed legrests. This contributes to forward sliding on the seat or to poor positioning of the lower legs and feet for weight bearing. Leg and foot positioning can be especially difficult with small, pediatric chairs because they frequently interfere with caster action. Footplates that extend backward are helpful when clients have tight hamstrings. Foot straps hold the feet in the desired location to assist with lower body stability and weight bearing. For clients with deformity or limited joint movement, forcing the foot into neutral alignment on the footrest may impose undesirable stresses at the knees or hips (Bergen et al., 1990). Other clients exhibit natural postural adjustments and placement of the feet during weight shifting and active movement, and their feet should be left free.

Lateral and Medial Supports. Lateral trunk supports (or scoliosis pads) range from simple, flat, padded blocks to elaborately contoured, wraparound supports. Swivel or swing-away mounting hardware is usually needed for wraparound supports. Square or rectangular blocks used as lateral thigh or pelvic pads are usually not very effective, and a contoured seat should be considered. Medial thigh supports (abductor wedges or pommels) are

FIGURE 23–12. Anteriorly tipped seat mounted in a manual wheelchair. *A*, An anterior knee and shin support was used to decrease stretch on the hamstrings and improve pelvic and trunk alignment; this support is used for stationary sitting only, since the feet interfere with caster motion. *B*, An alternate foot position on the footrests allowed wheeling but contributed to sliding and slouching.

intended to maintain hip alignment in neutral or slight abduction and must not be used to stretch tight adductors or prevent sliding of the pelvis. Removable or swingaway supports facilitate transfers and urinal or catheter use (Bergen et al., 1990).

Anterior Supports. The purpose of an anterior trunk support is to keep the spine erect over the pelvis. Butterfly-shaped straps are often more effective than single horizontal belts or even H- or Y-straps because they apply more direct control at the sternum and shoulders. The lower end of the straps should be attached to the back or the seat behind the pelvis to improve the line of pull of the device. Rigid shoulder retractor pads provide even more anterior shoulder control, but the client's tolerance to these must be monitored.

Headrest. Good head positioning can be one of the most difficult tasks in seating a client. In an otherwise totally immobile client, the head is the one part that is likely to move. Poor head positioning can make an otherwise effective postural support system look awful. On the other hand, our own recent observations of barium swallow studies suggest that some clients with the most severe physical and mental impairments may need to adopt a forward-hanging head position to cope with increased oral secretions or reflux. Correcting these clients' heads to a position that "looks good" may increase their risk of aspiration or choking.

Support under the occiput is generally deemed better than a flat contact on the back of the head. Neck rings, two-step (with an occipital ledge), and contoured head supports increase the options. Halos encircle the forehead and should always be used with caution, particularly during vehicular transport, because of the potential for neck injury. Collars with soft anterior chin support are being used more often for the client who has constant neck flexion regardless of seating angles.

Upper Extremity Supports. Cutout trays are the most typical form of upper extremity support and can be designed for a multitude of special purposes. Posterior elbow blocks and scapular pads are used to reduce the tendency to retract the arms; however, if these are needed, it may be necessary to reassess whether the seating angles are appropriate. Clients with severe dystonia often like wrist or arm cuffs for restraint of one or both arms.

WHEELED MOBILITY

The purpose of the mobility base is dependent on the child's level of function. For some, the primary purpose will be independent mobility and the therapist must then determine how this independence will be achieved. For others, the purpose of the base is to provide a means of dependent transportation, and this must be accomplished in a comfortable and efficient manner. In either case, the base serves the additional role of supporting the seating system. Selection of a mobility base requires consideration of the client's lifestyle, the seating system it will support, and the environments in which it will function. Assessment for a new mobility base should ideally be done at the same time as assessment and simulation for the postural support system, since much of the same information and data regarding the client and the environment needs to be gathered.

Research on Mobility

A physiologic *impairment* common among people with movement dysfunction is excessive energy expenditure during locomotion. Fisher and Gullickson (1978) stated that persons with disability decrease their walking speed so that energy expenditure approaches a normal range and that assistive devices that increase effort will be abandoned. Ten-year-old children with CP walked at nearly half the velocity of age-matched children without disability and consumed more oxygen per kilogram of body weight per minute doing so (Campbell & Ball, 1978). DeSouza and Carroll (1976) reported that 50% of children with myelomeningocele who were ambulatory with braces stopped walking between the ages of 10 and 20 years.

Williams and colleagues (1983) studied oxygen consumption in 15 children with myelomeningocele during ambulation and wheelchair propulsion. Eight children used crutches, 1 used a walker, and 6 used no assistive device. The authors reported that ambulation was 218% less energy efficient than for children without disability; energy expenditure was significantly lower during wheelchair propulsion than during walking; and wheelchair propulsion was as fast and as energy efficient as normal walking.

Agre and colleagues (1987) also measured oxygen consumption during crutch walking and wheelchair propulsion in 33 children with myelomeningocele. Children with a higher lesion (L-2 or above) expended energy at an amount equal to their maximal aerobic capacity when walking at the slowest speed measured (26.6 m/min). Children with lower lesions (L3–4) used 85% of their maximal aerobic capacity. Wheelchair propulsion at a speed of 53 m/min required 42% less energy than crutch walking at the same speed. When the children with myelomeningocele propelled the wheelchair at the usual walking speed of children without disability (66 m/min), oxygen consumption was only 9% greater than for the nondisabled children during walking.

Future studies of wheelchair ergometrics in children with other disabilities would be useful as well. For example, it is likely that energy expenditure is also excessive during wheeling a manual wheelchair in children with CP who have upper extremity involvement. Power wheelchair driving will most likely allow a reduction of energy expenditure to near normal levels during locomotion.

One concern about the amount of energy expenditure during locomotion is that it leads to *functional limitation*, such as fatigue, and to *disability*, such as poor academic performance. Franks and associates (1991) studied the effect of walking with an assistive device and using a wheelchair on school performance in 3 children with myelomeningocele. The subjects propelled their wheelchair at school for 5 days, then walked with crutches or walker for 5 days, and then used the wheelchair again for 5 days. Performance measures were taken at the end of each school day and included reading fluency, visuomotor accuracy, and manual dexterity. Visuomotor accuracy was significantly decreased for all three subjects during the ambulation phase compared with the wheelchair phase. Manual dexterity during the ambulation phase decreased for one subject, did not change for one subject, and increased for one subject. Reading fluency did not change for any of the subjects. The authors concluded that excessive energy expenditure associated with walking with assistive devices can have potentially negative effects on academic performance and that physical therapists need to consider these effects when selecting mobility devices.

Brubaker (1986, 1988b) has proposed that there are several factors that affect performance and mobility in users of manual wheelchairs. Some of the human factors are physiologic capacities, such as strength and endurance, and are dependent on the user's diagnosis, age, sex, lifestyle, and build. Another factor is the position of the individual within the wheelchair, particularly in relation to the handrims or other propulsion method, which determines the mechanical advantage of the user to act on the chair. Wheelchair factors that affect mobility are rolling resistance, control, maneuverability, stability, and dynamic behavior. These are dependent on the quality and construction of the wheelchair, such as weight, rigidity of the frame, wheel alignment, mass distribution, and suspension.

The developmental consequences of impaired movement is another area of functional limitation and disability that has been documented (Campos,

1988; Rosenbloom, 1975). The nondisabled infant's experience with independent forward progression has a profound impact on perceptual, cognitive, emotional, and social processes. For the immobile child, early provision of artificial forms of locomotion has the potential to minimize the deficits in spatial cognitive, affective, and social functions (Campos, 1988). Prone scooters, caster carts, and walkers are alternatives for young children with functional upper extremities. For the child with severe upper extremity involvement, however, power mobility offers the best choice.

Several researchers have studied the benefits of providing power wheelchairs to young children (Butler, 1986; Butler et al., 1983; Butler et al., 1984; Paulsson & Christoffersen, 1984; Schiaffino & Laux, 1986; Verburg et al., 1984). Traditionally, prescription of power wheelchairs has been put off until children reached their teens when all attempts at effective ambulation have been exhausted. Power wheelchairs were considered too expensive and too difficult for young children to learn to drive, and walking was too important a goal to "give up." Studies indicate that children as young as 24 months can successfully learn independent power mobility within a few weeks (Butler, 1986; Butler et al., 1983). Benefits attributed to the use of power mobility include increases in self-initiated behaviors including change in location, rate of interaction with objects, and frequency of communication (Butler, 1986). Other benefits reported are increased peer interaction, increased interest in other forms of locomotion, including walking, increased family integration such as inclusion in outings, and decreased perception of helplessness by family members (Butler et al., 1983; Paulsson & Christoffersen, 1984; Schiaffino & Laux, 1986; Verburg et al., 1984).

Performance characteristics of various power bases is another important area of study. Deitz and colleagues (1991) studied the performance of children without disability on functional tasks while using four different power wheelchairs representing different design classes, including a standard chair, a modular (all-terrain) base, a three-wheeled scooter, and a unique pediatric base with a power elevating seat (Turbo). Functional positioning tasks required the subjects to position themselves at a standard table, at a classroom desk, and at the blackboard. Access to the environment tasks had the children opening a door, retrieving books from shelves, retrieving a book from the floor, turning on a water faucet, and turning on a light switch. Wheelchair maneuvering skills included U-turns, making left and right turns on a pathway, and speed and accuracy in straight driving. No chair

was superior in all the tasks, although certain designs were advantageous for some tasks. The scooter and Turbo allowed positioning at the table and desk, respectively, whereas the other two bases did not. The Turbo offered the widest range of reaching; however, maneuverability was least for the Turbo and greatest for the conventional chair.

Jones (1988) evaluated performance characteristics of 15 power devices from six manufacturers driven by an unimpaired adult. He tested straight driving speed, speed on a graded run with a 90° turn, a curb jump of varying thicknesses, and load pulling. The chairs included two conventional chairs, three "all-terrain" bases, seven three-wheelers, and one children's all-terrain model. His results showed that each chair had advantages and disadvantages, and performance characteristics must be matched with the client's intended use, lifestyle, and comfort during the selection process.

An interdisciplinary U.S. Wheelchair Standards Committee, administered through RESNA and approved by the American National Standards Institute, has completed a document on wheelchair standards. The standards represent a comprehensive approach to testing and disclosing information about wheelchairs (Bryant, 1991). Manufacturers, suppliers, and consumers can use this information to improve their products, select chairs with the best performance for the cost, and identify chairs that meet specific performance needs.

Selection of a Mobility Base

The goal in selecting a mobility base is to provide an appropriate means of getting from one location to another efficiently. It is inappropriate to require someone to rely on his or her everyday mobility for exercise. As the previously mentioned research indicates, prohibiting the use of a manual wheelchair for a child with marginal ambulation or that of a power wheelchair for a child with marginal manual wheelchair skills places their functional and academic performance at risk owing to excessive energy expenditure. A creative and structured fitness program is a more appropriate way of addressing strength and cardiovascular endurance goals (Franks et al., 1991; Leonard, 1992).

Jones (1990) and Brubaker (1988a) agreed that positioning needs take precedence over the issuance of a mobility device. At the same time, the design of the postural support system should maximize potential for independent function in the wheelchair whenever possible. This, in turn, may influence chair modifications and the type of interface hardware ordered. For example, if a 5-inch, modular composite foam cushion is deemed necessary for pressure relief, yet the client has short extremities as in myelodysplasia, both independent transfers and independent wheeling will be more difficult. A possible solution is to order a chair with a lower seat height and request it without upholstery so that drop brackets can be used to lower the cushion between the seat rails.

Some seating simulators have been mounted on a power base and can be used to assess driving skills and control-box placement once the desired seating position has been obtained. Several manufacturers now have evaluation power chairs with a remote, attendant-held control that can override the user's control. Ideally, for whichever class of wheelchair the client is being assessed, he or she should be offered test drives in a variety of bases with as appropriately simulated postural support as possible.

There are four major considerations in selecting a mobility base: class, style, size, and model (or brand). Four general classes of mobility bases include transporter chairs, standard manual wheelchairs, one-arm drive manual wheelchairs, and power bases. These are discussed in further detail below. Ideally, choice of class should be based primarily on the potential level of independent mobility. In reality, other factors often come into play, including methods of transportation, availability of training or supervision, and even availability of funding.

The second consideration is choice of style of the base. Within each class, there are several styles with different features and performance characteristics. Factors that influence this choice are the level and type of postural support system required, the level of independence in other skills such as transfers and activities of daily living, the specific environments in which the chair will be used, the method of transportation, and the needs of caregivers.

Selection of size is another important step and may influence both the style and class chosen. This is based on client size and expected growth rate, growth capabilities of the chair itself, and the size and style of the postural support system. More and more styles of mobility bases are becoming available in a variety of sizes.

The final consideration is the model or brand of chair. Often the finer details of construction are important at this stage, such as the proportions of the chair, angles, orientations, adjustability of parts such as footrests and armrests, and swingaway, detachment, or folding mechanisms. Other important influencing factors are performance characteristics, styling, comfort, rate of breakdown, availability of parts, and service record. Regional preferences for various models and manufacturers are evident across North America.

TRANSPORTER CHAIRS

Transporter chairs (Fig. 23–13) are generally intended for individuals who will not need to access the wheels for independent mobility, including the most severely impaired and very young children. In other cases, this type of chair may be used as a back-up method of transportation for a child who ambulates or uses a power wheelchair. Transporter chairs often come with firm seats and backs and have a wide variety of positioning components as options. Alternatively, contoured or custom-molded postural support systems can be fabricated and mounted on the frames. Some of these chairs can be used as vehicular transport seats and comply with federal safety standards. Others are designed for very young children and look and perform like a stroller.

When choosing a dependent mobility base, the primary caregiver must be considered a user as well. Attention should be given to his or her comfort and ease of use, including push handle height, rolling resistance, maneuverability, and ease of disassembly and transport. Parents of young children who are receiving their first mobility base and seating system may be very sensitive to the need for a wheelchair. Stroller bases that look least like a wheelchair are popular and are often much less threatening.

Manual tilt and recline features are incorporated into many transporter chairs. A fixed angle of tilt or recline can be useful when designing the postural support system for some clients. For others, the ability to vary the amount of tilt or recline throughout the day is critical for prevention of pressure sores, fatigue, and discomfort.

MANUAL WHEELCHAIRS

The standard manual wheelchair has two large wheels, usually in back, for independent propulsion, and two small swiveling casters in front. Manual wheelchairs are often chosen as dependent mobility, or transporter, bases as well, because of their ability to accept custom-designed postural support systems, their ease of use, and their tilt and recline options (Fig. 23–14). For independent wheelers, the 1980s was the "new age" of manual wheelchairs when lightweight chairs and chairs designed for recreational use and athletic competition became widely available. Lightweight and durable metals and fabrics, alternate wheel placement, improved frame proportions and designs, adjustability, and

FIGURE 23-15. Transporter chairs. *A,* Stroller base. *B,* Travel chair. *C,* Manual wheelchair-style base with smaller rear wheels, stroller handles, and tilt mechanism to 45°.

FIGURE 23–14. Standard lightweight manual wheelchair with manual tilt mechanism, shown with a contoured seating system.

adaptability to custom seating have all helped to streamline the manual wheelchair to improve efficiency and control, ease of transfers, portability, and appearance (Brubaker, 1988a). Lightweight chairs with the large wheels in front are much easier for young children to propel for short distances indoors. For the very active person, ultra-lightweight, high-performance chairs incorporate rigid frames and high-quality bearings for the best chair responses (Bergen et al., 1990). The serious athlete can find specialized designs dedicated to specific performance needs and which sometimes barely resemble the traditional concept of a wheelchair.

ONE-ARM DRIVE MANUAL WHEELCHAIRS

One-arm drive wheelchairs (Fig. 23–15) are designed for individuals with significant asymmetry of upper extremity strength and function that prevents bimanual propulsion. The classic style is the double-handrim propulsion method, with a linkage system to the other wheel. Another style uses a pumping action with a lever and ratchet system. The lever systems are generally easier and more efficient for both wheeling and steering, although they create more problems in dependent wheeling by caregivers (Bergen et al., 1990). A one-arm drive

FIGURE 23–15. One-arm drive manual wheelchairs. *A*, Double handrim model. *B*, Pump handle model with a lever and ratchet mechanism.

chair should generally not be recommended for clients with tonal disorders such as CP if existing asymmetry is exacerbated while operating the wheelchair.

POWER MOBILITY

Hays (1988) described four functional categories of children for whom power mobility is indicated. The first group includes children who will never ambulate and who experience no independent mobility without the use of a power device. The second group includes children with insufficient mobility, that is, they ambulate or use a manual wheelchair but with unacceptable speed or endurance. The third group consists of children who have lost independent mobility through disease, brain injury, or spinal cord trauma. For this group, the developmental implications of independent mobility may be less important but the acceptance of assisted mobility is a more significant issue. The fourth group includes children who require assisted mobility temporarily, either because they gain new ambulation skills through surgery or maturation or they recover lost function.

In the past decade, advances in technology have brought independent power mobility to a greater number of individuals with severe disabilities than ever before. Today a variety of power bases and options are available (Fig. 23–16), including the standard model, modular or all-terrain base, add-on power units, and three-wheeled scooters (Field, 1992). Power chairs may be ordered with seats that tilt-in-space, backs that recline, units that recline and tilt, legrests that elevate, and headrests that adjust, all with the touch of a switch. Manufacturers have responded to an increased demand for pediatric-sized power wheelchairs by producing wheelchairs that are now lighter in weight, correctly proportioned for children, and have growth capabilities (Kemper, 1991). Major advances in electronics have produced a greater variety of controls that are easier to access, more durable, and relatively easy to adjust.

The style of power base chosen will depend in part on the client's upper body control. The three-wheeled scooters are steered using a tiller that requires a significant amount of upper extremity active range of motion and sitting balance. The control functions are usually mounted on the tiller and require a grip-type action of the thumb or fingers. Jones described a range of scooters from "light duty mall crawlers to heavy duty barnyard rut jumpers" (Jones, 1990). Scooters are often easier to transport in the trunk of a car and are popular because they look least like a wheelchair.

The standard and modular bases offer the greatest range of seating and control options. The standard chair is usually belt driven; the modular base has direct drive motors to improve power as well as control in turning. The entire seating unit can be removed from the pedestal mount of the modular base.

Power recline and power tilt wheelchairs offer an excellent alternative to individuals who need position changes throughout a long day of sitting to perform different functions or because of pain, fatigue, or pressure concerns associated with sitting too long (Fields, 1992; Jones & Kanyer, 1992). The act of reclining, however, causes shearing of tissues due to the disproportionate movement between the client and the postural support system. On returning to the upright position, most clients will have shifted position in the system, and the more complex the seating system, the more significant the effects. Power recliners are now available in low-shear and zero-shear models to help address these problems. Power tilt models work well for the client with severe hypertonia or contractures who cannot tolerate having the seat-to-back angle opened up or who, once having done so, cannot return to an upright position without significant sliding.

Controls for power wheelchairs are available in two basic types: proportional and microswitch. The former has a proportional relationship between movement of the joystick and speed of the chair or sharpness of turning, whereas the latter has an on/off relationship to chair movement. The proportional control is the standard joystick found on most power wheelchairs (Fig. 23–16A). It is customarily mounted on either armrest and will move in a 360° arc. The movement of the joystick controls the speed as well as the direction of the wheelchair. An alternative to the standard joystick is a remote proportional joystick (Fig. 23–17) that is smaller and more compact. This feature allows a great deal of flexibility for joystick placement, provided sturdy mounting hardware is used. Proportional joysticks are also available in short-throw models that require less movement and force for activation and in heavy-duty models that will withstand a great deal of force. Head control units are also available for some wheelchairs (Field, 1992).

A microswitch control consists of four separate switches, with each switch controlling one direction—forward, reverse, left, and right. All four switches might be in one control box (resembling a standard proportional control) or assembled into a smaller, more compact, remote control. Microswitches are also available in heavy-duty and short-throw models, as are the proportional controls. Microswitches are somewhat more flexible in

FIGURE 23–16. Power wheelchairs. *A,* Conventional, belt-drive model (pediatric-sized), shown with standard armrest-mounted proportional control. *B,* All-terrain, direct-drive model. *C,* Three-wheeled power chair or "scooter."

assessment purposes. For example, they may be separated and set up in arrays to evaluate head control or each of the four switches may be positioned at different body sites. The wafer board and arm-slot control are examples of microswitch technology. Microswitch-driven chairs tend to be less precise and smooth while turning and changing directions because each direction is controlled by a separate switch (Field, 1992). Figures 23–18 and 23–19 illustrate some popular wheelchair controls.

With the recognition that age is no longer the determining factor in successful use of power mobility has come the need to define appropriate selection criteria. Schiaffino and Laux (1986) reported that children needed a cognitive level of at least 2 years of age, although these children would take longer to train than children with cognitive skills at the 3-year level or above. Barnes (1991) described a "motoric language" needed to learn to drive a powered chair that includes relational vo-

FIGURE 23–17. Smaller remote joystick, center-mounted with adjustable mounting system.

cabulary (in, on, under), substantive vocabulary (nouns), directionality (forward, backward, right, left), perceptual concepts (visual and auditory feedback with switch activation), spatial concepts (depth perception, location of self in an environment, and problem solving to avoid obstacles), and serial or sequential concepts (first, second; before, after). Given the results of the research discussed earlier, it is possible that many of these concepts could actually be taught through training in a power device. Power toys that are available at local toy stores make an excellent inexpensive alternative for power training of young children when the devices can be suitably adapted for seating and control.

Galka and Lombard (1992) described functional criteria for safe driving including the ability to turn the chair on and off, follow a straight course, turn both left and right, back the chair up, maneuver around objects and persons, and stop quickly. The "marginal driver" is one of any age who may show borderline cognitive or physical skills or whose visuoperceptual problems significantly interfere with driving ability. With supervision, these children may do well driving in a very specific setting, such as their school, but are not successful in novel or unpredictable community settings. The value of a power chair in increasing self-esteem and promoting independence in specific skills must be carefully weighed against the expense and amount of training and supervision required.

Besides the client criteria, there are several practical considerations that are unique to selection of a power device (Galka & Lombard, 1992):

FIGURE 23–18. Examples of power wheelchair controls. *From left to right:* arm slot control, pneumatic switch and hardware, heavy-duty joystick.

FIGURE 23-19. Examples of power wheelchair controls. *From left to right*: proportional joystick, wafer switch, chin control mounted on collar.

1. Where and how will the power chair be used? Is there sufficient space at home as well as school? If not, will the device be kept and maintained at school? Are buildings accessible? Since power chairs are generally too heavy to lift, do ramps need to be built?

2. What care and maintenance will the power wheelchair require? Routine cleaning of seats and cushions, checking tires for proper air pressure, and battery care are necessary. The wheelchair will need to be stored in a warm, dry place with an electrical outlet for charging the batteries. Sealed lead acid and gel batteries are more expensive and require less maintenance but have less storage capacity and usable life. Unsealed lead acid batteries are least expensive, with the greatest storage capacity, but fluid levels must be maintained and there is potential for spillage of the acid (Jones, 1990).

3. How will the device be transported? Is the school bus equipped with a crash-tested tie-down system for the style of chair being considered? Some school districts refuse to transport certain types of power wheelchairs. The family may need a van for transporting the chair, and a ramp or a lift may be required for loading and unloading. If the chair needs to be broken down into manageable pieces to fit into the family car, who will do this?

4. Is a back-up manual wheelchair available for times when the power chair is in the shop?

5. How expensive will the power wheelchair be? What funding options are available? How much funding are third-party payers willing to approve for a power device?

6. Will the power mobility device provide proper support, or will specialized seating be required? What types of postural support systems can be interfaced with the base?

7. How much supervision will be needed? If a client is found to be a marginally safe driver, who will provide supervision in what environments?

The evaluation process is also more complicated than for other types of wheelchairs. First, a variety of power bases should be available for trial and preferably with capabilities to adjust speed, acceleration, deceleration, turning speed, sensitivity, and tremor-dampening of the joystick. Children will generally perform better in a pediatric-sized wheelchair rather than an adult-sized wheelchair, so that option should be available. Because proper support is critical to performance in a power wheelchair, the therapist needs access to a variety of seating components (seats, backs, thoracic supports, headrests, foot supports), straps, and perhaps a laptray to provide stability to the client that will, in turn, enhance best functional movement patterns for operating the controls. A variety of controls and mounting options should also be available for trial as needed. Evaluation may need to take place over a period of several days to weeks, especially for the young and inexperienced drivers who require much practice with the different options before a final decision is made.

A standard proportional control mounted on the armrest should be the first option the therapist evaluates if a child is found to have reasonable upper extremity control since this is the simplest and least expensive. If a more midline position of the joystick is desired, placement of the control bracket on the inside of the wheelchair armrest is relatively easy.

Site options for the control increase with the use of a remote joystick and the proper hardware. Some possibilities include center mounting of the joystick either close to the user to compensate for decreased ROM or strength, mounting the joystick at arm's length on top of a laptray to provide support and increased stability for an individual with dyskinetic movements or fluctuating muscle tone, or mounting the joystick for chin or foot operation. An integrated control is another option for a client with limited functional movements and site options because it permits operation of not only the wheelchair but also of other equipment such as a communication aid, ECU or computer equipment (Guerette et al., 1992).

Transportation Safety

Safety in transportation of clients in wheeled mobility devices is an important issue. More and more testing is being done of various wheelchairs and restraint systems (Shaw, 1987). Wheelchairs in vans or buses should never be in a side-facing position. There should be two sets of restraints, one for the chair and one for the occupant, and, ideally, only tie-downs that meet federal safety standards should be used. Letts (1991) provides a list of restraint options for children with special needs such as premature infants, children with poor head and trunk control, children dependent on ventilators, and children in hip spica casts. Concern for transportation safety must also extend to the components of postural support systems, especially to stress tolerances of straps, buckles, D-rings, and mounting hardware (Arnold, 1988).

AUGMENTATIVE AND ALTERNATIVE COMMUNICATION

Children with severe neuromotor impairments often have difficulty communicating effectively with others; that is, they are unable to convey information in a way that it is readily and clearly understood by others. Communication is not limited to spoken or verbal output but also includes use of body language, gestures, facial expressions and written output. When the ability to communicate and interact is not functional, some form of augmentative or alternative communication (AAC) should be explored. Augmentative communication is the use of aids or techniques to supplement a child's existing vocal or verbal communication. Alternative communication refers to the communication method used by a person without vocal ability (Reichle et al., 1991).

Speech impairments in children may occur as a result of congenital or acquired dysarthria, developmental apraxia, developmental aphasia, congenital anomalies, mental retardation, autism, or deafness (Coker, 1985). The following classifications of dysarthria, apraxia, and aphasia were given by Munson and colleagues (1987). Dysarthria is defined as the neuromotor impairment of speech production and may affect to varying degrees any or all systems composing the speech mechanism. Apraxia (dyspraxia) is defined as a problem in motor planning without the presence of neuromotor impairment. Apraxia may affect not only gross and fine motor development but also speech development. In children, it is often called developmental apraxia of speech or developmental verbal apraxia to differentiate it from acquired apraxia in adults. Aphasia is a disorder in understanding or expressing spoken or written language secondary to injury or disease of the brain.

As with other facets of assistive technology, identifying AAC systems is best accomplished through the interdisciplinary team process. The speech and language pathologist along with the child and family members should assume the lead roles on the team. Other participants may include the physical therapist, occupational therapist, educator, social worker, psychologist, rehabilitation engineer, and physician.

Before an evaluation for AAC, a child who is nonambulatory should have acquired a proper mobility base and be well positioned. Proper postural support will minimize the effects of abnormal muscle tone and pathologic movement patterns that interfere with controlled movement and function. Stowers and colleagues (1987) described a motor screening process and detailed motor assessment guidelines for therapists on the AAC team. Information to be gathered included the child's ability to maintain postural and head control, the variety and quality of available movements, the ability to isolate one joint movement from another, the effect of voluntary movement on associated movements throughout the body, reflexes and involuntary movements, and contractures and deformities.

York and Wiemann (1991) also offered comprehensive guidelines for evaluation of children with motor impairments for AAC devices. Although communication often takes place in a seated position, they suggested assessing children in other positions as well, including weight bearing on knees or feet and lying with the body elongated. A change in body position may affect the ability to produce a controlled movement for activating a switch used with a communication device. Within the classroom setting, the physical therapist plays an important role in preparation of the child for communication activity and in helping the speech and language pathologist and teacher in selection of positions and access modes.

According to Attermeier (1987), early intervention therapists are in a unique position to influence development of effective communication skills in infants and young children. She suggested that therapy sessions include developing head control along with the ability to separate head and neck movements from eye movements, providing opportunities to make choices, developing a method of indication, and encouraging family members to talk to and read to their youngsters.

A number of techniques and devices for augmenting communication are available and may or may not employ electronics. Supplementation techniques are often referred to as "unaided" or "aided" communication (Mann & Lane, 1991; Stowers et al., 1987). Unaided techniques such as eye gaze, signing, or gesturing do not require external devices or equipment but rely on the user's ability to physically respond in some consistent manner. Aided techniques include the use of an external device, which may or may not be electronic. A communication sheet (Fig. 23–20) or notebook (with pictures, symbols, or words) is an example of a nonelectronic aided device.

Electronic communication aids offer a much greater range of capabilities and options for the user. One simple example is a tape recorder equipped with a loop tape message that repeats each time the switch is activated. This device is often a good starting place when assessing young children for augmentative communication because it is relatively inexpensive and can be readily adapted with a number of different switches for assessment purposes. Other electronic devices are far more sophisticated and feature different input methods, voice output options, storage capability for vocabulary and phrases, possibility of printouts, and capability to run a computer through the communication device (Fig. 23–21).

FIGURE 23–20. Communication board mounted inside a Plexiglas-covered laptray with a built-in language board frame. This is an example of direct selection using a nonelectronic device.

Selection capability is an important feature of each electronic device and includes three choices: direct, scanning, and encoding. Direct selection is preferred over scanning to operate a communication device, whenever possible, because it is faster. The most logical method for direct selection is pointing with a finger; however, other methods of pointing or indicating may need to be explored such as using a fisted hand, hand or finger splint (one finger is splinted in extension), hand-held

FIGURE 23–21. This electronic communication device may be directly operated with an optical headpointer. Many other selection techniques are also possible, including row and column scanning, two-switch scanning, and joystick use.

FIGURE 23–22. Devices for pointing or indicating that may be used with communication aids or environmental control units. *From left to right*: chin pointer, thermoplastic hand splint with stylus, headstick

T-bar, or stylus. When hand use is not feasible, eye gaze or various head control methods (headstick, chinstick, mouthstick, or lightbeam) should be considered before other body parts are used (Fig. 23–22).

With scanning, the device runs through a sequence of choices (usually rows, then columns), repeating the sequence until the user makes a selection. The scanning rate is usually adjustable, which allows beginners ample time to become familiar with the new equipment and to build confidence and accuracy before increasing the speed. In most cases the selection is made by using a special switch or switches mounted specifically to allow the user independent access. Examples include a pressure switch mounted on a laptray and operated with the hand, a leaf switch positioned near the child's temporal region and operated with lateral head movements, and a chin switch mounted on a collar (Fig. 23–23) and operated by flexion and extension movements of the head.

Encoding is the third access option and uses symbols (such as the dots and dashes used in Morse code) to represent words. This mode requires less motor control than the other options, but cognitive demands are higher since the user must be able to remember where messages are stored and how to sequence stored messages and, in some cases, how to program the device independently if a knowledgeable assistant is not available (Mann & Lane, 1991). Encoding may be used with either direct or scanning modes.

A comprehensive team evaluation should ensure that the end product for the child is a functional "communication system" rather than just a "communication device." This generally means combining the advantages of electronic and nonelectronic aids (Munson et al., 1987). Once a communication system has been identified and obtained for a child, the team needs to mount the equipment appropri-

ately, train the child and other users, and schedule regular follow-up appointments.

ENVIRONMENTAL CONTROL UNITS

An ECU is a device or system of devices that allows an individual with motor impairment to operate electrical appliances or equipment in a variety of ways and places. This technology is available to all of us in the form of energy- and time-saving devices such as electronic garage door openers and remote controls for television and

FIGURE 23–23. A lever switch can be mounted on a chin switch bracket to access a communication device.

audio equipment. The purpose of an ECU is to apply technology to facilitate the user's control over the environment, to promote independence, and to improve the quality of life (Prentke Romich, 1982).

Benefits of ECU use include increased personal satisfaction, increased participation in life activities, possible return to work, and possible reduction in cost for personal care attendants (Dickey & Shealy, 1987). Symington and colleagues (1986) demonstrated that the use of ECUs in one residential facility to operate televisions, radios, lights, tape recorders, and stereos reduced the amount of nursing care required by about 2 hours per day per participant. Both residents and nursing staff reported reduced frustration following introduction of ECUs. Efthimiou and co-workers (1981) found that persons with spinal cord injuries who used ECUs participated more often in telephone use, were more inclined to travel, and spent more time in educational pursuits than nonusers. In a study of elderly nursing home residents with mobility and fine motor impairments, Mann (1992) found that radio use increased threefold (compared with the control group) once the participants were equipped with and trained in the use of remote devices to turn radios on and off.

An ECU generally includes three parts: the main control unit (central processing unit), the switch (transducer), and any devices (peripherals) to be controlled or activated (Prentke Romich, 1982). Most units provide the user with some type of feedback (tactile, visual, or auditory) that immediately indicates which function has been selected before the function is activated. Feedback can be an essential feature to the user with memory impairments and is helpful in initial assessment and training sessions with systems capable of multiple functions.

Two basic types of ECUs include direct and remote. In a direct system, the devices to be controlled are plugged directly into the main control unit. In a remote system, the control unit acts as a transmitter, sending radio waves, ultrasonic signals, or infrared light beams to remote receivers. The receivers, in turn, are connected to the devices to be activated. The remote system has the advantages of operating a number of devices or appliances from one location such as a wheelchair or bed and the absence of wires running from the unit to the device (Vanderheiden & Borden, 1988).

Capabilities among systems vary greatly from simply turning on and off one device to operating whole house configurations and integrated computer work stations. Common functions include operation of a small electrical appliance, stereo, television, videocassette recorder, light fixture, door lock, intercom or call signal, electric bed, and telephone and computer equipment. ECUs can be activated through a wide variety of switches and controls (described later in this chapter), through voice activation, or through the user's power wheelchair controller, electronic communication aid, or computer.

Control of the environment for a preschooler might include operating a blender with a head-activated leaf switch to prepare treats at school or by activating a pressure switch with the hand to operate a battery toy during free time (Fig. 23–24). An older child may use a headstick to operate the television's remote control to select a channel, control the volume, and turn off the set when done, thereby giving the child a sense of responsibility and independence from caregivers. Adapted phone equipment that can be programmed to store several numbers, automatically dial a number, and answer calls with the touch of a switch can allow a teenager access to important, age-appropriate socialization.

In most cases each part of an ECU (main control unit, switch/control, peripherals) is evaluated and ordered separately. When selecting a system, Haataja and Saarnia (1990) recommended that the team evaluate 1) the user's level of impairment and residual functions; 2) the user's motivation for acquiring and using a device; 3) the specific appliances or equipment the user wants to control; and 4) the environment in which the control will operate.

Dickey and Shealy (1987) recommended that the therapist perform a comprehensive physical assessment of the client, including muscle strength, ROM, endurance, gross and fine motor control, sensation, and perceptual status. This information will assist in determining the best control sites (e.g., hand, chin, elbow) and possible methods of input (e.g., rocker switch, sip and puff, eye gaze). Information about the client's cognitive skills such as learning style, long and short-term memory, and processing skills is also important. The technology team must consider whether the client's abilities are likely to change over time, such as improvement of skills as a result of therapy or loss of function due to a progressive condition. If either option is likely, the ECU selected should be readily and affordably adaptable to ensure continued benefit to the user. Thorough team assessment will provide clients with accurate information that will allow them to select an ECU and an appropriate controller that satisfies their needs, complements their abilities, and increases their independence.

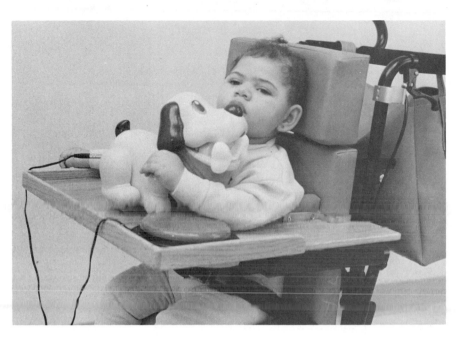

FIGURE 23-24. A large pressure switch can be used to activate a battery-operated toy placed on a laptray.

SWITCHES, CONTROLS, AND ACCESS SITES

Principles that guide the assessment and selection process for assistive technology, as well as the needed switches and controls to operate the equipment, tend to be very similar whether looking at power mobility, communication, or environmental control. Generally the switch site is selected first and then the switch or control is chosen.

As part of the interdisciplinary team, the physical therapist evaluates neuromotor status to provide information about the child's functional movement patterns. When sites are evaluated for switch access, these functional movements need to be voluntary, reliable, and, in some cases, sustainable. The movements should not contribute to fatigue or pain nor elicit pathologic reflexes or increase postural tone (TASH, 1992). Individual therapy goals (such as improvement in active ROM or strength in certain joints or muscle groups) should not be incorporated into assessment or treatment sessions for switch technology. It is more important to determine efficient and highly motivating methods of access for children requiring technology. Secondary therapeutic benefits may or may not occur over time.

Sensory information is important, including visual and auditory processing and how the client reacts to tactile, kinesthetic, and proprioceptive input. Young children often learn to operate switches that provide a variety of sensory cues (clicks, beeps, light displays) more quickly than switches that do not. Level of cognitive functioning is important, as are attention span, memory, ability to follow directions, ability to sequence, and problem-solving skills. Psychosocial factors include the motivation and willingness of the client and family to accept and use assistive devices. It is not uncommon to see children use sophisticated electronic communication aids in their school environment but use only eye gaze and facial and body gestures at home because family members may not perceive the need for assistive technology in the same way professionals do. If funding is difficult to obtain, devices may not be readily available for children in environments outside their school settings.

A variety of switches and controls are available from manufacturers who specialize in technologic aids for people with disabilities. They vary in size, shape, cost, performance capabilities, and ways in which they are activated (Fig. 23-25). Switches may be single (perform an on/off function), dual (perform on/off and a select function), or multiple (perform on/off and several functions). Examples of multiple switch configurations are joysticks, wafer boards, slot controls, and key boards (Mann & Lane, 1991) (see Figs. 23-18 and 23-19).

Methods for activating switches include air pressure, light reception, magnetic fields, sound waves, and physical contact (Mann & Lane, 1991). Switches vary in sensitivity (force required for acti-

FIGURE 23–25. A variety of switches that can be used to activate communication or ECU devices. *Clockwise from far left*: membrane switch, lever switch, cylindrical switch, Jelly Bean pressure switch, eye blink switch, large pressure pad, lever or leaf switch, dual rocker switch, and Big Red large pressure switch.

vation) as well as in movement excursion, durability, and size (TASH, 1992). If a client is capable of any purposeful, controlled movement of any body part, an appropriate switch can be identified. The use of hands to access switches is the logical and preferred mode for most children; however, switches that require physical contact such as touch or pressure may be activated by other body parts (e.g., head, chin, tongue), eyebrow movements, or lower extremity movements. "Extensions" to body parts may be needed, such as head or chin pointers, mouth sticks, light beams, splints, or styluses (see Fig. 23–22). Clients with high-level spinal cord injuries often use the pneumatic breath control switches to operate devices, whereas heavy-duty contact switches are most appropriate and functional for clients with fluctuating muscle tone. Technologic aids are also available (and continually evolving) that can be operated by voice or other sound input, light activation, and even eye movements.

An "integrated control" may be considered for certain clients if the optimum input device is the same for activating several aids such as a power wheelchair, communication device, computer equipment, and ECU. For example, a power wheelchair joystick can be designed as an integrated control. There are several disadvantages to integrated controls, including higher cost for more complicated electronics, ability to operate only one device at a time, and loss of all functions if repairs are needed (Guerette et al., 1992).

Mounting of devices and switches also needs to be considered by the rehabilitation technology team. Equipment must be secure and stable while being used but also easily moveable or removable as needed.

CASE HISTORY: SCOTT

Scott was born in 1963 with spastic athetoid CP (Fig. 23–26). Scott is dependent on others for all personal care including feeding, dressing, grooming, hygiene, toileting, transfers, and mobility, unless he is in his power wheelchair. Functional arm and hand usage is limited, with purposeful movement dominated by reflexive patterns and fluctuating tone. His speech is dysarthric, but his ability to communicate is excellent. Scott agreed to be featured in this chapter to provide a consumer's viewpoint of assistive technology. His words and thoughts (in italics) reflect many of the points made in this chapter regarding the need for team consultation, communication, respect for the client's opinion, customization of equipment and devices, and the revisions to equipment required over a lifetime.

Before passage of Public Law 94-142 in 1975, few local school districts were able or inclined to provide educational services for children with severe physical disabilities. Scott's early education (from preschool in 1967 to junior high in 1975) was at a residential program at the University of Iowa. After he returned to his home school district, he continued to receive assistive technology services at the same facility, which was converted to a regional evaluation and consultation center.

In addition to classes, his early years were filled with individual therapy sessions, including speech, occupational, and physical therapy. A variety of assistive devices (called adaptive equipment at the time) were used over the years in Scott's therapeutic management, including Pope night splints; short-leg braces; long-leg braces with pelvic band; stand-up boxes; bilateral upper arm restraints; pelvic restraints; chest restraints;

FIGURE 23–26. Scott, sitting in his custom-molded seating system, mounted in his power wheelchair with swing-away chin control joystick. He is using his custom headstick to activate a Light Talker. His communication sheet, scaled in the frame on his laptray, is also visible.

wooden armchairs; footboards with footstraps; cutout tables; various bowls, spoons, cups, and straws for feeding; communication boards; headsticks; electric typewriters with keyshield; and last, but not least, wheelchairs.

"Manual wheelchairs . . . at first these required little or no adapting. As I got older, we tried one fancy chair I remember well. The back was in sections and could adjust to different positions. I remember about five people in the P.T. room working all day to adapt it to fit me." Wheelchairs were generally not adapted in the 1960s, and children relied on seat belts and pelvic or chest restraints; in some cases, their long-leg braces locked in flexion at the hips and knees kept them safely in their chairs.

Records indicate that Scott was evaluated for his first seating system in 1973 and was provided with *"a wedged seat with 15° angle, a wedge between thighs, and a high back."* His long-leg braces were discontinued because the seating inserts were believed to provide adequate postural support for sitting. Over the next 20 years, Scott's seating systems changed from simple linear wood and foam inserts, to wood and foam with contouring, to orthotic molded inserts, to his currently used, custom molded Comfort (Pindot Products, Chicago, IL) seat and back cushions. Changes in his seating requirements closely paralleled changes in his musculoskeletal status over the years, which included slowly progressing kyphoscoliosis, hip flexion and adduction contractures, and knee flexion contractures.

Scott began using a headstick between 3 and 4 years of age for pointing and to manipulate objects in his environment. He soon developed proficiency with his head stick and eventually switched to a custom-made chin pointer style that he has had for over 15 years. *"I'm careful picking equipment out. I want the least amount of equipment on me as possible. This is so no more extra attention, looks, or glares come my way. However, I wear my headstick because it's my life. People see it before they see my face. But I think of it as a part of me. Once people get to know me, the headstick becomes less noticeable and everyone's happy."*

While Scott was learning headstick skills, he was introduced to picture and word boards for communication. The combination of headstick skill plus his ability to spell and write to communicate progressed over the years, as did his selection and use of technology. *"Language boards/Touch Talkers . . . This has been a very 'lucky' area for me. I've had a word board ever since age 3. As I grew, so did my boards. My first try at a voice (electronic device with voice output) was a bomb! Other people were telling ME what I wanted! Finally, I took a stand and said 'No' to that device, and most people took that as my not wanting a 'voice.' That wasn't so, it was just too much work with a poor voice. I was saying, 'let's wait.' My word board did fine back then. But as my life got busier, I had a greater need to communicate. I knew that was when I needed a voice output. The 1989 Touch Talker had a pretty good voice to it and so I fell in love with it. Now, with the Liberator (a highly sophisticated AAC device from Prentke Romich Co. [Shreve, OH] with voice or print output, ability to operate computers and ECUs, and perform math and calculator functions), I'm in heaven."*

"Power wheelchairs . . . I still remember my first electric chair. I had a big say in the driving method. Everyone was thinking 'headstick,' and I said, 'No, try my

chin!' I was shocked at how well I could drive power chairs once the right method was found. Now better controls are coming out so who knows what will be next." Scott received his first power wheelchair in 1981 and his second chair in 1988. "My power wheelchair. It is my legs, my little home. I have everything in my backpack, it holds as much as a small house." Following fabrication and assembly of seating components, a custom swingaway mounting arm to hold the chin control was designed and fabricated by a rehabilitation engineer who worked closely with Scott to meet his needs. With this custom device, Scott is able to move the chin control into position for driving or swing it out of the way with his arm to access his communication equipment independently. Most importantly, the mounting hardware is sturdy, is durable, and does not slip out of alignment. The capability to customize cannot be over-emphasized when providing technology for individuals with severe physical disabilities. One-of-a-kind designs and devices often provide the best solutions to technology puzzles. "My chin control arm. It has no wires or batteries, it works off my power. Being homemade, it's made to last. My headstick is another good example."

In the early years, much of Scott's therapeutic management and adaptive equipment reflected an attempt to intervene at the impairment level, such as by preventing contractures and increasing weight bearing with braces and standing boxes. Functional limitations were also addressed by providing alternatives to speech and walking, such as headsticks, communication boards, and wheelchairs. As Scott became older, it was evident that many of his impairments (scoliosis and contractures) needed to be accommodated, rather than corrected, to maximize function. Now, as a young adult, Scott's priorities lie with minimizing his disabilities and increasing acceptance of his role in society.

Technology has made a definite impact on Scott's life over the years. "In general, special devices have changed my life in a good way. I'm doing more and more for myself. However, rapid changes in equipment design makes knowing what to buy very hard." Scott lives in a group home in Iowa City, Iowa, with four other young men with physical disabilities. He works 6 hours a day in an adult program entering data on an IBM computer. Future plans include working toward getting his own apartment with one or two hired personal care attendants and perhaps taking classes at the university or community college.

References

Agre, JC, Findley, TW, McNally, MC, Habeck, R, Leon, AS, & Stradel, L. Physical activity capacity in children with myelomeningocele. Archives of Physical Medicine and Rehabilitation, 68:372–377, 1987.

American Board of Physical Therapy Specialities, Pediatric Specialty Council. Physical Therapy Advanced Clinical Competencies: Pediatrics, 1987. (Available from American Physical Therapy Association, 1111 North Fairfax Street, Alexandria, VA, 22314.)

Arnold, RL. Safe transportation for persons with disabilities. Assistive Devices Information Network Newsletter (University of Iowa, Iowa City, IA), 2(1):1–2, 1988.

Attermeier, SM. Augmentative communication: An interdisciplinary challenge. Physical and Occupational Therapy in Pediatrics, 7(2):3–11, 1987.

Bablich, K, Sochaniwskyj, A, & Koheil, R. Positional and electromyographic investigation of sitting posture of children with cerebral palsy (Abstract). Developmental Medicine and Child Neurology, 28(suppl. 53):25, 1986.

Barnes, KH. Training young children for powered mobility. Developmental Disabilities Special Interest Section Newsletter (American Occupational Therapy Association), 14(2):1–2, 1991.

Bay, JL. Positioning for head control to access an augmentative communication machine. American Journal of Occupational Therapy, 45:544–549, 1991.

Bergen, AF. Seating and positioning principles for the neurologically involved client. Presented at the American Physical Therapy Association Combined Sections Meeting, San Francisco, February 1992.

Bergen, AF, Presperin, J, & Tallman, T. Positioning for Function: Wheelchairs and Other Assistive Technologies. Valhalla, NY: Valhalla Rehabilitation Publications, 1990.

Brubaker, CE. Wheelchair prescription: An analysis of factors that affect mobility and performance. Journal of Rehabilitation Research and Development, 23(4):19–26, 1986.

Brubaker, CE. Impact of changes in manual wheelchair design. Presented at the Fourth International Seating Symposium, Vancouver, BC, February 1988a.

Brubaker, CE. Manual mobility. Presented at the Fourth International Seating Symposium, Vancouver, BC, February 1988b.

Brubaker, CE, McClay, IS, & McLaurin, CA. Effect of seat position on wheelchair propulsion efficiency. In Proceedings of the 2nd International Congress on Rehabilitation Engineering. Washington, DC: RESNA Press, 1984, pp. 12–14.

Bryant, L. Wheelchair standards ready to roll. TeamRehab Report, May/June, 1991, pp. 44–45.

Butler, C. Effects of powered mobility on self-initiated behaviors of very young children with locomotor disability. Developmental Medicine and Child Neurology, 28:325–332, 1986.

Butler, C, Okamoto, GA, & McKay, TM. Powered mobility for very young disabled children. Developmental Medicine and Child Neurology, 25:472–474, 1983.

Butler, C. Okamoto, GA, & McKay, TM. Motorized wheelchair driving by disabled children. Archives of Physical Medicine and Rehabilitation, 65:95–97, 1984.

Campbell, J, & Ball, J. Energetics of walking in cerebral palsy. Orthopedic Clinics of North America, 9:374–377, 1978.

Campos, JJ. Locomotor experience and psychological development. Presented at the Fourth International Seating Symposium, Vancouver, BC, February 1988.

Carlson, JM, & Payette, M. Seating and spine support for boys with Duchenne muscular dystrophy. In Proceedings of the 8th Annual RESNA Conference. Washington, DC: RESNA Press, 1985, pp. 36–38.

Carlson, SJ. The semi-rigid pelvic stabilizer for seating control. Assistive Devices Information Network Newsletter (University of Iowa, Iowa City, IA), 1(1):2–3, 1987.

Carlson, SJ. Knee gate for control of forward sliding in wheelchair. Assistive Devices Information Network Newsletter (University of Iowa, Iowa City, IA), 2(3):2–3, 1988.

Carlson, SJ, & Grey, TL. The semi-rigid pelvic stabilizer for seating control. Presented at the Fourth International Seating Symposium, Vancouver, BC, February 1988.

Cohen, C. Augmentative communication: A perspective for pediatricians. Pediatric Annals, *14*:3, 1985.

Crenshaw, RP, & Vistnes, LM. A decade of pressure sore research: 1977–1987. Journal of Rehabilitation Research and Development, *26*:63–74, 1989.

DeSouza, LJ, & Carroll, N. Ambulation of the braced myelomeningocele patient. Journal of Bone and Joint Surgery (American), *58*:1112–1118, 1976.

Dickey, R, & Shealy, SH. Using technology to control the environment. American Journal of Occupational Therapy, *41*:717–721, 1987.

Deitz, J, Jaffe, KM, Wolf, LS, Massagli, TL, & Anson, D. Pediatric power wheelchairs: Evaluation of function in the home and school environments. Assistive Technology, *3*:24–31, 1991.

Drummond, DS, Narechania, RG, Rosenthal, AN, Breed, AL, Lange, TA, & Drummond, DK. A study of pressure distributions measured during balanced and unbalanced sitting. Journal of Bone and Joint Surgery (American), *64*:1034–1039, 1982.

Efthimiou, MA, Gordon, WA, Sell, GH, & Stratford, C. Electronic assistive devices: Their impact on the quality of life of high-level quadriplegic persons. Archives of Physical Medicine and Rehabilitation, *62*:131–134, 1981.

Field, D. Advanced power mobility systems. Presented at the Eighth International Seating Symposium, Vancouver, BC, February 1992.

Fields, CD. Finding comfort in recliners: Looking at power. TeamRehab Report, January/February 1992, pp. 34–37.

Fife, SE, Roxborough, LA, Armstrong, RW, Harris, SR, Gregson, JL, & Field, D. Development of a clinical measure of postural control for assessment of adaptive seating in children with neuromotor disabilities. Physical Therapy, *71*:981–993, 1991.

Fife, SE, Roxborough, LA, Cooper, D, & Steinke, T. Tonic electromyographic activity in seated subjects with spastic quadriplegia: A pilot study. Presented at the Fourth International Seating Symposium, Vancouver, BC, February 1988.

Fisher, SV, & Gullickson, G. Energy cost of ambulation in health and disability: A literature review. Archives of Physical Medicine and Rehabilitation, *59*:124–133, 1978.

Fisher, SV, Szymke, TE, Apte, SY, & Kosiak, M. Wheelchair cushion effect on skin temperature. Archives of Physical Medicine and Rehabilitation, *59*:68–71, 1978.

Foster, MA, & Phillips, W. Family systems theory as a framework for problem solving in pediatric physical therapy. Pediatric Physical Therapy, *4*:70–73, 1992.

Franks, CA, Palisano, RJ, & Darbee, JC. The effect of walking with an assistive device and using a wheelchair on school performance in students with myelomeningocele. Physical Therapy, *71*:570–579, 1991.

Funding Strategies. Iowa Program for Assistive Technology, 1993. (Brochure available from Iowa University Affiliated Program, Unversity Hospital School, The University of Iowa, Iowa City, IA, 52242.)

Galka, G, & Lombard, T. So . . . You're considering power mobility. Unpublished booklet, 1992. (Available from Occupational Therapy Department, Division of Developmental Disabilities, University Hospital School, University of Iowa, Iowa City, IA 52242.)

Garber, SL. Wheelchair cushions for spinal-cord injured individuals. American Journal of Occupational Therapy, *39*:722–725, 1985.

Garber, SL, & Dyerly, LR. Wheelchair cushions for persons with spinal cord injury: An update. American Journal of Occupational Therapy, *45*:550–554, 1991.

Garber, SL, Krouskop, TA, & Carter, RE. A system for clinically evaluating wheelchair pressure-relief cushions. American Journal of Occupational Therapy, *32*:565–570, 1978.

Glisson, F, Patterson, R, Fisher, S, & Appel, H. Sitting forces

and wheelchair mechanics. Journal of Rehabilitation Research and Development, *27*:239–246, 1990.

Guerette, P, Caves, K, & Goss, K. One switch does it all. TeamRehab Report, *3*(2):26–29, 1992.

Haataja, S, & Saarnia, I. An evaluation procedure for environmental control system. In Proceedings of the 13th annual conference on rehabilitation technology. Washington, DC: RESNA Press, 1990, pp. 25–26.

Hays, RM. Childhood motor impairments: Clinical overview and scope of the problem. Presented at the Fourth International Seating Symposium, Vancouver, BC, February 1988.

Hedman, G. Overview of rehabilitation technology. Physical and Occupational Therapy in Pediatrics, *10*(2):1–10, 1990.

Hughes, CJ, Weimar, WH, Sheth, PN, & Brubaker, CE. Biomechanics of wheelchair propulsion as a function of seat position and user-to-chair interface. Archives of Physical Medicine and Rehabilitation, *73*:263–269, 1992.

Hulme, JB, Bain, B, & Hardin, MA. The influence of adaptive seating devices on vocalization (Abstract). Developmental Medicine and Child Neurology, *30*(suppl 57):35, 1988.

Hulme, JB, Poor, R, Schulein, M, & Pezzino, J. Perceived behavioral changes observed with adaptive seating devices and training programs for multihandicapped, developmentally disabled individuals. Physical Therapy, *63*:204–208, 1983.

Hulme, JB, Shaver, J, Acher, S, Mullette, L, & Eggert, C. Effects of adaptive seating devices on the eating and drinking of children with multiple handicaps. American Journal of Occupational Therapy, *41*:81–88, 1987.

Jones, CK. A sampler of available powered mobility bases: Hard facts and a little opinion. Presented at the Fourth International Seating Symposium, Vancouver, BC, February 1988.

Jones, CK. In search of power for the pediatric client. Physical and Occupational Therapy in Pediatrics, *10*(2):47–68, 1990.

Jones, CK, & Kanyer, B. Review of tilt systems. Presented at the Eighth International Seating Symposium, Vancouver, BC, February 1992.

Kangas, KM. Seating, positioning and physical access. Developmental Disabilities Special Interest Section Newsletter (American Occupational Therapy Association), *14*(2):4, 1991.

Kemper, K. Case study: Power to the preschooler. TeamRehab Report, *2*(4):42–47, 1991.

Leonard, RB. A question of power. TeamRehab Report, May 1992, pp. 22–23.

Letts, RM (Ed.). Principles of Seating the Disabled. Boca Raton, FL: CRC Press, 1991.

MacNeela, JC. An overview of therapeutic positioning for multiply-handicapped persons, including augmentative communication users. Physical and Occupational Therapy in Pediatrics, *7*(2):39–60, 1987.

Mann, WC. Use of environmental control devices by elderly nursing home patients. Assistive Technology, *4*(2):60–65, 1992.

Mann, WC, & Lane, JP. Assistive Technology for Persons with Disabilities: The Role of Occupational Therapy. Rockville, MD: American Occupational Therapy Association, 1991.

Margolis, S. Lumbar support issues. Presented at the Eighth International Seating Symposium, Vancouver, BC, February 1992.

Margolis, SA, Jones, RM, & Brown, BE. The subASIS bar: An effective approach to pelvic stabilization in seated positioning. In Proceedings of the 8th annual RESNA conference. Washington, DC: RESNA Press, 1985, pp. 45–47.

Margolis, SA, Wengert, ME, & Kolar, KA. The subASIS bar: No component is an island: A five year perspective. Presented at the Fourth International Seating Symposium, Vancouver, BC, February 1988.

McClenaghan, BA, Thombs, L, & Milner, M. Effects of seat-surface inclination on postural stability and function of the upper extremities of children with cerebral palsy. Developmental Medicine and Child Neurology, *34*:40–48, 1992.

McCormack, DJ. The effects of keyguard use and pelvic positioning on typing speed and accuracy in a boy with cerebral palsy. American Journal of Occupational Therapy, 44:312–315, 1990.

McEwen, IR. Assistive positioning as a control parameter of social-communicative interactions between students with profound multiple disabilities and classroom staff. Physical Therapy, 72:634–647, 1992.

Medhat, MA, & Hobson, DA. Standardization of Terminology and Descriptive Methods for Specialized Seating: A Reference Manual. Washington, DC: RESNA Press, 1992.

Miedaner, JA. The effects of sitting positions on trunk extension for children with motor impairment. Pediatric Physical Therapy, 2:11–14, 1990.

Munson, JH, Nordquist, CL, & Thuma-Rew, SL. Communication Systems for Persons with Severe Neuromotor Impairment: An Iowa Interdisciplinary Approach. Iowa City, IA: University of Iowa, 1987.

Myhr, U, & von Wendt, L. Improvement of functional sitting position for children with cerebral palsy. Developmental Medicine and Child Neurology, 33:246–256, 1991.

NAMES Rehab Section. Quarterly Report. Spring, 1992.

Noble-Jamieson, CM, Heckmatt, JZ, Dubowitz, V, & Silverman, M. Effects of posture and spinal bracing on respiratory function in neuromuscular disease. Archives of Disease in Childhood, 61:178–181, 1986.

Nwaobi, OM. Effects of body orientation in space on tonic muscle activity of patients with cerebral palsy. Developmental Medicine and Child Neurology, 28:41–44, 1986.

Nwaobi, OM. Seating orientations and upper extremity function in children with cerebral palsy. Physical Therapy, 67:1209–1212, 1987.

Nwaobi, OM, Brubaker, CE, Cusick, B, & Sussman, MD. Electromyographic investigation of extensor activity in cerebral-palsied children in different seating positions. Developmental Medicine and Child Neurology, 25:175–183, 1983.

Nwaobi, OM, & Cusick, B. The effect of hip flexion angle on the electrical activity of the hip adductors in cerebral palsied children. Unpublished report, 1980.

Nwaobi, OM, Hobson, DA, & Trefler, E. Hip angle and upper-extremity movement time of children with cerebral palsy. Developmental Medicine and Child Neurology, 28(suppl 53):24, 1986.

Nwaobi, OM, & Smith, PD. Effect of adaptive seating on pulmonary function of children with cerebral palsy. Developmental Medicine and Child Neurology, 28:351–354, 1986.

Palmieri, VR, Haelen, GT, & Cochran, GV. Comparison of sitting pressures on wheelchair cushions as measured by air cell transducers and miniature electronic transducers. Bulletin of Prosthetic Research, 17(1):5–8, 1980.

Pate, G. Patterns of pressure during normal sitting. Presented at the Fourth International Seating Symposium, Vancouver, BC, February 1988.

Paulsson, K, & Christoffersen, M. Psychological aspects of technical aids: How does independent mobility affect the psychosocial and intellectual development of children with physical disabilities? In Proceedings of the 2nd International Conference on Rehabilitation Engineering. Washington, DC: RESNA Press, 1984.

Phillips, B, & Zhao, H. Predictors of assistive technology abandonment. Assistive Technology, 5:36–45, 1993.

Prentke Romich Company. Environmental Control Systems. Shreve, OH, 1982.

Reger, SI, Chung, KC, & Paling, M. Weightbearing tissue contour and deformation by magnetic resonance imaging. In Proceedings of the 9th Annual Conference on Rehabilitation Technology. Washington, DC: RESNA Press, 1986, pp. 387–389.

Reichle, J, York, J, & Sigafoos, J. Implementing Augmentative and Alternative Communication: Strategies for Learners with Severe Disabilities. Baltimore: Paul H Brookes, 1991.

Reid, DT, Sochaniwskyj, A, & Milner, M. An investigation of postural sway in sitting of normal children and children with neurological disorders. Physical and Occupational Therapy in Pediatrics, 11(1):19–35, 1991.

Rosenbloom, L. The consequences of impaired movement: A hypothesis and review. In Holt, KS (Ed.), Movement and Child Development. Philadelphia: JB Lippincott, 1975.

Schiaffino, S, & Laux, J. Prerequisite skills for the psychosocial impact of powered wheelchair mobility on young children with severe handicaps. Developmental Disabilities Special Interest Section Newsletter (American Occupational Therapy Association), 9(2):1, 3, 8, 1986.

Seeger, BR, Caudrey, DJ, & O'Mara, NA. Hand function in cerebral palsy: The effect of hip-flexion angle. Developmental Medicine and Child Neurology, 26:601–606, 1984a.

Seeger, BR, Sutherland, AD, & Clark, MS. Orthotic management of scoliosis in Duchenne muscular dystrophy. Archives of Physical Medicine and Rehabilitation, 65:83–86, 1984b.

Seymour, RJ, & Lacefield, WE. Wheelchair cushion effect on pressure and skin temperature. Archives of Physical Medicine and Rehabilitation, 66:103–108, 1985.

Shaw, G. Vehicular transport safety for the child with disabilities. American Journal of Occupational Therapy, 41:35–42, 1987.

Shields, RK, & Cook, TM. Effect of seat angle and lumbar support on seated buttock pressure. Physical Therapy, 68:1682–1686, 1988.

Siekman, AR, & Flanagan, K. The anti-thrust seat: A wheelchair insert for individuals with abnormal reflex patterns or other specialized problems. In Proceedings of the 8th Annual Conference on Rehabilitation Engineering. Washington, DC: RESNA Press, 1983, pp. 203–205.

Sprigle, S, Chung, KC, & Brubaker, CE. Factors affecting seat contour characteristics. Journal of Rehabilitation Research and Development, 27:127–134, 1990a.

Sprigle, S, Chung, KC, & Brubaker, CE. Reduction of sitting pressures, with custom contoured cushions. Journal of Rehabilitation Research and Development, 27:135–140, 1990b.

Stefans, V, & Creitz, L. Effect of wheelchair cushion design on interface pressures in pelvic obliquity. Developmental Medicine and Child Neurology, 28(suppl 53):26, 1986.

Stewart, SFC, Palmieri, V, & Cochran, GVB. Wheelchair cushion effect on skin temperature, heat flux, and relative humidity. Archives of Physical Medicine and Rehabilitation, 61:229–233, 1980.

Stowers, S, Altheide, MR, & Shea, V. Motor assessment for unaided and aided augmentative communication. Physical and Occupational Therapy in Pediatrics, 7(2):61–77, 1987.

Symington, DC, Lywood, DW, Lawson, JS, & Maclean, J. Environmental control systems in chronic care hospitals and nursing homes. Archives of Physical Medicine and Rehabilitation, 67:322–325, 1986.

TASH, Inc. Making your World Accessible. Markham, Ontario, Canada, 1991–1992.

Tredwell, SJ. The basic approach to seating. Presented at the Fourth International Seating Symposium, Vancouver, BC, February 1988.

Tredwell, S, & Roxborough, L. Cerebral palsy seating. In Letts, RM (Ed.), Principles of Seating the Disabled. Boca Raton, FL: CRC Press, 1991.

Trefler, E (Ed.). Seating for Children with Cerebral Palsy. Memphis: University of Tennessee, 1984.

Trefler, E, Hobson, DA, Taylor, SJ, Monahan, LC, & Shaw, CG. Seating and Mobility for Persons with Physical Disabilities. Tucson, AZ: Therapy Skill Builders, 1993.

Vanderheiden, G, & Borden, P. Environmental controls using technology to control technology. In The Source, April 1988, pp. 16–17. (Available from Trace R & D Center, University of Wisconsin, Madison, WI.).

van der Woude, LHV, Veeger, DJ, Rozendal, RH, & Sargeant, TJ. Seat height in handrim wheelchair propulsion. Journal of Rehabilitation Research and Development, *26*:31–50, 1989.

Verburg, G, Snell, E, Pilkington, M, & Milner, M. Effects of powered mobility on young handicapped children and their families. In Proceedings of the 2nd International Conference on Rehabilitation Engineering. Washington, DC: RESNA Press, 1984.

Williams, LO, Anderson, AD, Campbell, J, Thomas, L, Feiwell, E, & Walker, JM. Energy cost of walking and of wheelchair propulsion by children with myelodysplasia: Comparison with normal children. Developmental Medicine and Child Neurology, *25*:617–624, 1983.

York, J, & Weimann, G. Accommodating severe physical disabilities. In Reichle, J, York, J, & Sigafoos, J (Eds.), Implementing Augmentative and Alternative Communication. Baltimore: Paul H Brookes, 1991.

Section Four

Management of Cardiopulmonary Conditions

SUZANN K. CAMPBELL, PT, PhD, FAPTA
Section Editor

Chapter 24

Children with Ventilator Dependence

M. KATHLEEN KELLY, PT, MS

INCIDENCE

One of the ironies of the recent advances in medicine and technology is that a new category of patients has been created—those who are dependent on technology for their very survival. The U.S. Government Office of Technology Assessment (OTA) (1987) defines the technology-dependent child as "one who needs both a medical device to compensate for the loss of a vital body function, and substantial and ongoing nursing care to avert death or further disability." This technology may range from apnea monitors and intravenous medications to dialysis and mechanical ventilators. The number of infants and children who are mechanically ventilated has increased steadily because the early neonatal course of infants with respiratory compromise is now optimized by the use of aggressive respiratory management and because of significant improvements in the technical aspects of ventilation that have reduced the incidence of barotrauma and oxygen toxicity (Leonard et al., 1989).

Although the number of children who depend on technology is small in comparison to the rates of other disabilities, their medical expenses are quite costly because many require prolonged hospitalizations in an intensive-care environment well beyond the acute stages of their disease. According to a 1987 technical memorandum from OTA, the number of children who are dependent to some degree on mechanical ventilation is estimated to be between 680 and 2000 per year. As a result of advances in health care, experts predict that this number will increase in the years to come (Mallory & Stillwell, 1991; OTA Memorandum, 1987; Raulin & Shannon, 1986). Geographic differences in the number of children who are ventilator dependent exist largely as a result of differing parental attitudes and differing medical practices (Mallory & Stillwell, 1991; OTA Memorandum, 1987).

Because home ventilator programs were first developed in response to the polio epidemic of the 1940s and 1950s, the child who is ventilator dependent represents the prototype of a technology-dependent child (Gillis et al., 1989). Because the needs of these children are able to be met with increasingly sophisticated equipment, the scope of home health care has continued to widen and is no longer restricted to the treatment of minor illnesses. In recent years there has been a rapid growth in high-tech pediatric home care and increasing support for managing children with chronic illnesses at home (Andrews & Nielson, 1988; Lantos & Korman, 1992; Quint et al., 1990). Changes in health care financing also reflect a greater acceptance of home care as an alternative to hospitalization.

Since 1981, U.S. legislative efforts in the area of financial assistance have made it more feasible for families to care for children at home. The Omnibus Reconciliation Act of 1981 (OBRA) resulted in an expansion of Medicaid benefits by financing medical and nonmedical support services and allowing the purchase of equipment to be used in the home. It also expanded Medicaid eligibility by considering only the child's income and essentially disregarding parental income when calculating the allotment of funds. Originally, these waivers were individually approved through the Health Care Financing Administration (HCFA), but in 1982 the Medicaid Home and Community Based waiver program (also known as the Katie Beckett waiver) was developed, which allowed each state to establish its own program under the waiver (Burr et al., 1983). This legislative change removed the necessity for individual states to file with HCFA. For example, this model waiver program has saved the state of Maryland $79,000 and $83,000 for the home care of ventilator-dependent and oxygen-dependent children, respectively, and it has essentially expanded Medicaid eligibility criteria to include middle and upper income families whose private insurance has reached its maximum (Fields et al., 1991).

Provided the home is safe and nurturing, children with chronic illnesses or disabilities have a better chance of optimal development when cared for in the home. The cost of home care, although usually less expensive than that of hospital care, is still high because many of the children are expected to survive well beyond early childhood (Billeaud et al., 1992; Burr et al., 1983; Fields et al., 1991; OTA Memorandum, 1987). Although home care has been shown to be more cost-effective than institutional care, the burden on the family continues to be great since the family is often expected to bear some portion of the financial cost. In addition, there are enormous psychological, social, and personal resources necessary to keep a child who is dependent on technology at home. The decision to send the child home needs to take more than economic considerations into account. The high degree of medical and technologic expertise required by parents or caregivers can be a tremendous drain on a family, and it "strains the traditional conceptions of parental responsibilities" (Mallory & Stillwell, 1991). Successfully caring for a child who is ventilator dependent at home requires cooperative efforts on the part of the family and community (Fields et al., 1991; Goldberg & Monahan, 1989).

The population of infants and children who are dependent on a ventilator is quite diverse since there are many diseases that may result in prolonged dependence on assisted ventilation. Although the degree of care and support varies from child to child, all of these children require care that is expensive and that demands sophisticated equipment and round-the-clock vigilance and monitoring.

PATHOPHYSIOLOGY OF CHRONIC RESPIRATORY FAILURE

Adequate respiratory function requires effective pulmonary exchange of oxygen and carbon dioxide. Respiration requires an organ of gas exchange, the lungs, and a "pump" mechanism consisting of the rib cage, respiratory muscles, and the central control centers (Watchko et al., 1991). Under normal conditions, the pump mechanism can adapt to satisfy the changing metabolic needs that may occur during exercise, hyperthermia, or other demands (Bureau & Begin, 1983). However, when these systems are unable to deliver oxygen and remove carbon dioxide from the pulmonary circulation, respiratory failure ensues and gas exchange is impaired (Pagtakhan & Chernick, 1983).

Chronic respiratory failure is not a specific disease entity but a pathophysiologic state defined by treatment with mechanical ventilation for more than 28 days, usually as a result of abnormal gas exchange caused by either primary lung failure or failure of the respiratory pump (Roussos, 1985). Primary lung failure is typically associated with acute respiratory disease such as bronchopulmonary dysplasia (BPD). In this case, primary lung or airway disease compromises pulmonary gas exchange. On the other hand, failure of the respiratory pump mechanism may be caused by inadequate control of respiration from either the brain stem, spinal cord, or peripheral nervous system or by inadequate force generation or respiratory muscle efficiency as the result of primary muscle disease, chest wall defects, or muscle fatigue.

A number of conditions may predispose children to chronic respiratory failure, but the most common pathophysiologic process is respiratory distress leading to respiratory failure (Table 24–1). Some of the more common diagnoses requiring long-term ventilation in the pediatric population include BPD, neuromuscular disease, traumatic or congenital spinal cord injuries, congenital anomalies such as congenital heart disease and various airway abnormalities, and central hypoventilation syndrome (Ondine's curse). The pathophysiologic mechanisms that can lead to respiratory failure can be broadly categorized into four major groups: central nervous system disease; muscle disease and musculoskeletal abnormalities; intrinsic pulmo-

TABLE 24-1. **CRITERIA OF RESPIRATORY FAILURE**

Clinical signs
RESPIRATORY
Tachypnea
Altered depth and pattern of respiration (deep, shallow, apnea, irregular)
Chest wall retractions
Nasal flaring
Cyanosis
Decreased or absent breath sounds
Expiratory grunting
Wheezing or prolonged expiration
GENERAL
Fatigue
Excessive sweating
CARDIAC
Tachycardia
Hypertension
Bradycardia
Hypotension
Cardiac arrest
CEREBRAL
Restlessness
Irritability
Headache
Mental confusion
Papilledema
Seizures
Coma
LABORATORY FINDINGS
Hypoxemia (acute or chronic)
Hypercapnia (acute or chronic)
Acidosis (metabolic or respiratory)

From Pagtakhan, RD, & Chernick, V. Intensive care for respiratory disorders. In Kendig, EL, & Chernick, V (Eds.), Disorders of the Respiratory Tract in Children. Philadelphia: WB Saunders, 1983, p. 148.

nary disease; and airway abnormalities (Table 24-2).

Central nervous system disease is characterized by disorders affecting the central respiratory centers (i.e., the brain stem or cervical spinal cord) (Fig. 24-1). Congenital central hypoventilation syndrome (CCHS) is a rare primary brain stem disorder that presents very shortly after birth or early in infancy. The mechanism of central dysfunction is not known but is postulated to be an abnormal integration of chemoreceptor input (Woo et al., 1992). Patients with CCHS have chronic respiratory failure in the absence of primary pulmonary or neuromuscular disease. This disorder is generally diagnosed in the neonatal period when the infant experiences apneic episodes during sleep or while awake. CCHS may be associated with other systemic or oncologic conditions such as Hirschsprung's disease or neuroblastoma (Woo et al., 1992).

Although the incidence of CCHS is low, this group of patients faces a lifelong dependence on mechanical ventilation. The severity of CCHS varies, as does the degree of dependence on a mechanical ventilator. Because these children have absent or negligible ventilatory sensitivity to hypercapnia and variable sensitivity to hypoxemia during sleep, they are dependent on a ventilator during the night or during sleep (Weese-Mayer et al., 1992; Woo et al., 1992). Artificial ventilation in these patients is done almost exclusively with positive-pressure ventilators or diaphragmatic pacemakers. For children who require 24-hour-a-day ventila-

TABLE 24-2. **COMMON PATHOPHYSIOLOGIC MECHANISMS LEADING TO CHRONIC RESPIRATORY FAILURE**

Central Nervous System	Intrinsic Muscle Disease	Intrinsic Pulmonary Disease	Congenital Airway Abnormalities
Congenital hypoventilation syndrome	Congenital abnormalities of thoracic rib cage	Congenital heart disease	Tracheoesophageal fistula
Viral encephalitis	Congenital myopathies	Respiratory distress syndrome or bronchopulmonary dysplasia	Subglottic stenosis
Brain tumors	Duchenne's muscular dystrophy		Laryngomalacia
Arnold Chiari malformation	Phrenic nerve trauma	Tumors	Choanal atresia
Traumatic spinal cord injuries	Diaphragmatic dysfunction	Aspiration syndromes	Various syndromes
Anterior horn cell disease	Myasthenia gravis	Pneumothorax	
Apnea of prematurity	Botulism		
Intracranial hemorrhage			
Hypoxic encephalopathy			

Data from Mallory, GB, & Stillwell, PC. The ventilator-dependent child: issues in diagnosis and management. Archives of Physical Medicine and Rehabilitation, 72:43-55, 1991; Goldsmith, JP, & Karotkin, EH. Introduction to assisted ventilation. In Goldsmith, JP, & Karotkin, EH (Eds.), Assisted Ventilation of the Neonate (2nd ed.). Philadelphia: WB Saunders, 1988; and Pagtakhan, RD, & Chernick, V. Intensive care for respiratory disorders. In Kendig, EL, & Chernick, V (Eds.), Disorders of the Respiratory Tract (4th ed.). Philadelphia: WB Saunders, 1983.

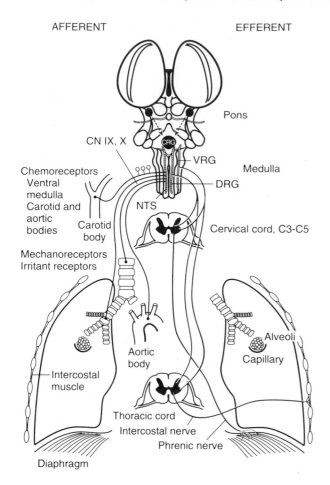

AFFERENT   EFFERENT

Pons

CN IX, X

VRG

Chemoreceptors
Ventral
medulla

Medulla

DRG

Carotid and
aortic
bodies

NTS

Carotid
body

Cervical cord, C3-C5

Mechanoreceptors
Irritant receptors

Aortic
body

Alveoli

Capillary

Intercostal
muscle

Thoracic cord

Intercostal nerve

Phrenic nerve

Diaphragm

FIGURE 24–1. Schema outlining the various contributions to the neural control of respiration. NTS, nucleus tractus solitarius; VRG, ventral respiratory group; DRG, dorsal respiratory group. (From Brazy, JE, Kinney, HC, & Oakes, WJ. Central nervous system structural lesions causing apnea at birth. Journal of Pediatrics, *111*:163–175, 1987.)

tion, these options seem to be the most reasonable and the least invasive.

Children with CCHS usually have otherwise unremarkable medical histories. The most vulnerable period is before the diagnosis is made when the infant may experience hypoxic episodes resulting in permanent neurologic damage. With early diagnosis and aggressive management of respiratory failure, the adverse sequelae of hypoxia should be minimized and most of these children can enjoy a relatively "normal" and productive life.

Acquired disorders of the brain stem that affect respiration typically result from either infectious disease processes, brain stem tumors, or complications of Arnold-Chiari malformations. In these instances chronic respiratory failure may be transient or long term. Spinal cord injury or disease can also result in chronic respiratory failure, leading to dependence on mechanical ventilation. The rate of recovery of breathing and motor function after the

injury separates those infants and children with satisfactory outcomes from those with poor outcomes (i.e., complete dependence on mechanical ventilation). The level of spinal cord injury dictates the degree of respiratory compromise. Typically, with injuries involving the upper cervical or cervicothoracic area, respiration is compromised because of phrenic and intercostal nerve root damage affecting the function of the diaphragmatic and accessory muscles of respiration. Patients with cervical-level injuries usually require mechanical ventilation either throughout the entire day or only at night. The prognosis for dependence on mechanical ventilation depends on the level of the lesion, the extent of nerve damage, and the nature of the lesion (MacKinnon et al., 1993).

Anterior horn cell disease represents another group of disorders affecting the spinal cord. Spinal muscular atrophy is one of the most common anterior horn cell diseases seen in children since the polio era (Mallory & Stillwell, 1991). There are different types of spinal muscular atrophy, the most common being type I (Werdnig-Hoffman disease). Werdnig-Hoffman disease is an hereditary and progressive disease that typically leads to respiratory failure within a few months after birth. The infant with Werdnig-Hoffman disease typically presents with generalized hypotonia and paralysis of the limb and trunk musculature with facial sparing. The presence of bulbar weakness results in difficulty with swallowing and sucking, putting these infants at great risk of aspiration, which complicates their already compromised respiratory status. If respiratory involvement is present and noted in the early postnatal period, it is usually severe, leading to respirator dependence very early in the child's life (Chapter 13).

Intrinsic muscle disease is another common cause of chronic respiratory failure in children. Those with congenital myopathies typically manifest symptoms of respiratory failure early in the course of the disease, whereas those with muscular dystrophies typically do not present with respiratory compromise until late childhood or early adolescence. In either case, mechanical ventilation may be warranted to compensate for the significantly reduced respiratory muscle function (Bureau & Begin, 1983).

Congenital anomalies of the thorax may also predispose the infant to respiratory failure. Thoracic abnormalities are associated with a variety of syndromes (e.g., asphyxiating thoracic dystrophy and dwarfism) as well as scoliosis. In all cases, the rib cage abnormalities result in pulmonary hypoplasia and significantly decreased lung volumes. Treatment of these various impairments will vary; however, in some cases the child may require mechanical ventilation.

Respiratory failure associated with preterm birth probably represents the most common category of pediatric patients who are dependent on a ventilator. The unique properties of the developing respiratory system, such as narrow, compliant airways, increased thoracic compliance (with a subsequent decrease in pump efficiency), respiratory muscle fatigue, and a vulnerability to respiratory infections, all place the infant and child at risk for acute and chronic lung disease and subsequent respiratory failure. Preterm birth may lead to respiratory failure for a number of reasons, the most common of which are perinatal asphyxia, lung immaturity, respiratory distress syndrome (RDS), pneumonia, pneumothorax, and congenital malformations (Haney & Allingham, 1992). Although the advent of mechanical ventilation has decreased the mortality and morbidity rates of neonates with RDS, res-

piratory failure continues to be a major cause of neonatal mortality. RDS accounts for 30% of all neonatal deaths and 50 to 70% of preterm infant deaths. The anatomic and physiologic immaturity of the infant's airways and the high pressures necessary to maintain alveolar distention and adequate gas exchange are believed to be responsible for iatrogenic damage to lung tissue. These conditions often lead to the diagnosis of BPD, which is the most common example of intrinsic lung disease. A subset of infants with BPD go on to develop chronic respiratory failure. In these cases, the cause of the respiratory failure is lung failure and eventually "pump" failure as the disease progresses.

BPD, first described by Northway in 1967, is a relatively common iatrogenic sequela to RDS in infants born prematurely. It is a gradually emerging chronic lung disease that is superimposed on an acute lung injury. It is thought that structural changes in the lung parenchyma occur as a result of both increased ventilatory pressures over a period of time and prolonged exposure to high levels of oxygen tension. Only after the acute disease has subsided, can BPD be accurately distinguished from complications of other acute lung injury (Northway, 1979). The definition of BPD varies, although the single criterion that is universally agreed on is oxygen dependence greater than 30% beyond 28 to 30 days.

BPD is characterized by tachypnea, dyspnea, hypoxemia, hypercarbia, and characteristic radiologic findings (Northway, 1979). The manifestations of chronic BPD are variable since the disease severity can range from mild, resembling RDS, to severe, requiring supplemental oxygen for extended periods of time. Ten to 30% of infants requiring mechanical ventilation go on to develop BPD, the incidence being inversely related to gestational age and birth weight. In low birth weight infants weighing less than 1500 g, the incidence increases to 30 to 40%; in those with birth weights less than 1000 g, the incidence can be as high as 70% (Bozynski et al., 1987). In the first year of life, the mortality rate can be as high as 40%, usually as a result of respiratory failure, sepsis, or intractable cor pulmonale (Bancalari & Sosenko, 1990). Once an infant survives beyond the first year, the majority will demonstrate ongoing clinical improvement.

The morbidity associated with BPD does not necessarily result from the primary disease but is more likely associated with problems that may occur during the acute phase of lung disease. Linear and anthropometric growth are often adversely affected by BPD (Bregman & Farrell, 1992; Kurzner et al., 1988; Meisels et al., 1986). Early in their postnatal course, premature infants are vulnerable to undernutrition as a result of body composition and the lack of acquisition of nutrients during the last trimester of gestation. It is during the third trimester that an accumulation of fatty acids and fat-soluble vitamins takes place. Because a small percentage of the preterm infant's birth weight is fat, marginal reserves of these specific nutrients, supply very little caloric reserve and decrease the antioxidant functions that play a role in lung repair and protection from lung injury. Postnatally, inadequate nutrition in the very low birth weight infant may also affect lung growth and development, increasing the infant's susceptibility to hyperoxia and barotrauma.

Although optimal nutrition is an important goal in the care of infants with respiratory distress, it is often difficult to achieve because of the increased energy expenditure, increased work of breathing, and limited fluid intake (Bregman & Farrell, 1992; Kurzner et al., 1988). Weinstein and Oh (1981) have reported a 25% increase in resting oxygen consumption of preterm infants with BPD compared with normal infants. In addition, the caloric requirements of the infants with BPD are 25% to 50% greater than those of normal infants. Kao and colleagues (1988) found that oxygen consumption did not decrease when pulmonary mechanics were improved and work of breathing decreased, suggesting that other factors such as inflammation, repair processes of the lung, and pulmonary tension might account for the increased metabolic rate, hence, the increased oxygen consumption (Weinstein & Oh, 1981). These children may also experience a failure to thrive because of an intolerance for feeding secondary to oral motor sensitivity, a poor suck, or decreased physical stamina to sustain the demands of feeding (Bregman & Farrell, 1992; Yu et al., 1983).

A common neurologic sequel to preterm birth is intraventricular or subdural hemorrhage resulting from large pressure swings acting on the delicate vasculature. Intraventricular hemorrhage is commonly associated with respiratory distress, prolonged mechanical ventilation, and BPD (Dykes et al., 1988). The additive effects of these associated problems place infants with respiratory distress at risk for developmental delays and neuromotor impairments. Because lung tissue continues to grow postnatally, most infants will recover from BPD and eventually function independent of assisted ventilation and supplemental oxygen if conditions for growth are optimized (Farrell & Fost, 1989). However, a relatively small proportion of the infants who develop BPD go on to require prolonged ventilation. Many of these children get past the

acute medical crises and do not require the intensive-care environment; but for those who are not as fortunate, their young lives are filled with uncertainty, insecurity, and an abnormal environment in which to grow and develop. A higher incidence of developmental delays has been reported in infants who are maintained on mechanical ventilators for prolonged periods of time (Bozynski et al., 1987).

The treatment of BPD, as well as of other forms of chronic lung disease, includes nutritional support, respiratory support, and pharmacologic management, in addition to addressing the child's psychosocial and developmental needs. Commonly used pharmacologic approaches include bronchodilators and diuretics to improve airway conductance, decrease edema, and increase gas exchange; sedatives for persistent agitation; and high-dose corticosteroids to decrease inflammation of the respiratory tract. All of these have adverse side effects that may alter the child's developmental and medical course. The respiratory management may range from supplemental oxygen given by nasal cannula to a tracheostomy with mechanical ventilatory support and oxygen. Nevertheless, these infants and children require ongoing monitoring of their physiologic status to ensure physiologic stability.

Although there have been no major breakthroughs in the prevention of BPD, the long-term outcomes have improved and the disease severity is reduced as a result of medical and pharmacologic improvements (Bancalari & Sosenko, 1990). Two of the most recent additions to the armamentarium for treatment of neonatal respiratory distress are the use of high-frequency ventilators (high-frequency jet ventilator or high-frequency oscillatory ventilator) and surfactant replacement in the early neonatal period. High-frequency ventilation achieves adequate ventilation at lower intrapulmonary pressures, thereby reducing the degree of barotrauma to the airways and reducing the risks of pulmonary air leaks. The collaborative trials comparing high frequency jet ventilation to conventional forms of mechanical ventilation have thus far failed to *consistently* demonstrate a significant decrease in the incidence of BPD. However, in light of various design problems, the results appear to be encouraging (Truog & Jackson, 1992).

The introduction of surfactant to treat RDS was a major breakthrough in neonatal medicine. To date, clinical trials have not demonstrated a *significant* reduction in the incidence of BPD, however, the results appear to be promising in demonstrating a reduced severity of the complications associated with respiratory distress syndrome (Speer et al., 1992). Thus far, it appears that the best prevention of BPD is the ability to avoid prematurity, barotrauma, overuse of the ventilator, and the release of free oxygen radicals (possibly with the use of antioxidants) associated with the inflammatory process. The prevention of BPD is quite difficult, since it is often a result of the aggressive medical management for acute survival of a preterm infant in the neonatal period.

▌MECHANICAL VENTILATION

Regardless of the pathophysiologic mechanism involved in respiratory disease, respiratory failure can be classified into two types (Pagtakhan & Chernick, 1983). Type I failure is characterized by hypoxemia with a normal or low arterial PCO_2, the primary cause being a ventilation-perfusion mismatch. The hallmark of type II respiratory failure is alveolar hypoventilation in which arterial carbon dioxide levels are elevated in conjunction with hypoxemia. Chronic alveolar hypoventilation may be associated with airway or parenchymal disease or can be found in children with central nervous system dysfunction or peripheral abnormalities who have normal lung tissue (American Thoracic Society, 1990). Mechanical ventilation is usually indicated once an individual progresses from type I to type II failure. Even in the absence of type II failure, mechanical ventilation is usually needed in any case in which the patient demonstrates the potential for hypoventilation and subsequent hypoxemia (Pagtakhan & Chernick, 1983) (Table 24–3).

Mechanical ventilation is designed to either assist or substitute for a person's respiratory efforts (i.e., moving air into and out of the lungs) (Pagtakhan & Chernick, 1983). This is achieved by a periodic transfer of gas between the ventilator and the thorax and lungs (Tremolieres, 1991). Mechanical ventilators have played and continue to play a very important role in critical care medicine for both adults and children. Since the beginning of the modern era of mechanical ventilation in the 1950s, ventilators have undergone significant technologic advances (Goldsmith & Karotkin, 1988; Perel & Stock, 1992).

Over the past 35 years, 300 to 400 different types of ventilators have been on the market at one time or another (Perel & Stock, 1992; Tremolieres, 1991). Contemporary knowledge of respiratory physiology and a more detailed understanding of the pathophysiologic mechanisms underlying diseases of the respiratory system continue to drive research and development in this area. It is beyond the scope and intent of this chapter, as well as of physical therapy practice, to detail the information

that exists on mechanical ventilation. Broadly speaking, however, ventilators can be classified according to the mode of artificial lung inflation (Table 24–4), the type of ventilation (Table 24–5), or the cycling mechanism (Table 24–6).

The type of mechanical ventilation and the various parameters chosen depend on a number of considerations, including an understanding of the pathophysiology that precipitated ventilatory failure; the available equipment; knowledge of the current literature; and previous experience (Perel &

TABLE 24–3. SELECTION CRITERIA FOR MECHANICAL VENTILATION

Parameter*	Findings
Clinical†	
Respiratory	Apnea; decreased breath sounds; rigorous chest wall movement; weakening ventilatory effort
Cardiac	Asystole; peripheral collapse; severe bradycardia or tachycardia
Cerebral	Coma; lack of response to physical stimuli; uncontrolled restlessness; anxious facial expression
General	Limpness; loss of ability to cry
Laboratory‡	
$PaCO_2$	Newborn: > 60–65 mm Hg Older child: > 55–60 mm Hg Rapidly rising > 5 mm Hg
PaO_2	Newborn: < 40–50 mm Hg Older child: < 50–60 mm Hg

*Clinical and laboratory data may indicate need for mechanical ventilation.

†More than one episode of apnea with bradycardia or an episode of cardiac arrest is adequate indication for initiating mechanical ventilation even in the absence of blood gas data.

‡Laboratory values less extreme than those indicated must be supplemented by clinical evidence of severity to warrant initiating mechanical ventilation.

From Pagtakhan, RD, & Chernick, V. Intensive care for respiratory disorders. In Kendig, EL, & Chernick, V (Eds.), Disorders of the Respiratory Tract in Children. Philadelphia: WB Saunders, 1984, p. 160.

TABLE 24–4. MODES OF ARTIFICIAL LUNG INFLATION

Positive-Pressure Ventilation: inflates the lung by increasing airway pressures above atmospheric pressure; the peak inflation pressure generated depends on lung–thorax compliance, airway resistance of the patient, delivered tidal volume and inspiratory flow rate, and baseline level of continuous positive airway pressure from the ventilator.

Negative-Pressure Ventilation: a subatmospheric pressure gradient is created around the body while the nose and mouth are exposed to ambient air (atmospheric); as a result of the pressure differential, air enters the lungs.

In types of ventilation there is a positive transpulmonary pressure; that is, airway pressure is greater than pleural pressure.

TABLE 24–5. **COMMON CLASSIFICATION OF POSITIVE-PRESSURE VENTILATION**

Type of Ventilation	Description
Controlled mechanical ventilation (CMV)	Delivers a preselected ventilatory rate, tidal volume, and inspiratory flow rate independent of spontaneous effort by the patient.
Continuous positive-pressure ventilation (CPPV)	Similar to CMV except the airway pressure never returns to 0.
Assisted mechanical ventilation	Also known as "patient triggered" positive-pressure ventilation; the ventilator will not deliver a breath unless the patient initiates a spontaneous breathing effort.
Assist control ventilation	Combines assisted mechanical ventilation and CMV, whereby the ventilator may be triggered by the patient's spontaneous efforts or by a timing device, whichever comes first. There is a minimal preselected rate determined so CMV acts as a backup in the event of apnea or an attempt to breathe at a rate lower than that preselected.
Intermittent mandatory ventilation (IMV)	Allows the patient to breathe spontaneously with a mechanical inflation provided at preset intervals; the ventilatory rate cannot be influenced by the patient. In addition to the spontaneous breaths from the patient, IMV should be titrated to only deliver the support needed to maintain normal alveolar ventilation and $PaCO_2$.
Synchronized intermittent mandatory ventilation (SIMV)	Similar to IMV, however, at regular intervals the mandatory breath is synchronized to begin with the next spontaneous inhalation. (This technique was introduced to avoid the phenomenon of "breath stacking.")
Mandatory minute ventilation	Patient is guaranteed a preselected minute volume either through spontaneous ventilation or as a positive-pressure breath from the ventilator. (If the desired minute volume is achieved by the patient's spontaneous breaths, then no mandatory breaths are delivered by the ventilator.)
Continuous positive airway pressure ventilation (CPAP)	Positive-pressure modes are used in conjunction with spontaneous breaths; can be used individually or with mechanical ventilation.
Expiratory positive-pressure ventilation	Similar to CPAP except that the airway pressure is 0 or negative during inhalation but increases at the end of exhalation to a predetermined positive pressure.

From Perel, A, & Stock, MC (Eds.), Handbook of Mechanical Ventilatory Support. Baltimore: Williams & Wilkins, 1992, pp. 7–30. Copyright © 1992, the Williams & Wilkins Co., Baltimore.

Stock, 1992). Because there are many combinations of ventilatory attributes that can obtain the same desirable results, practices are far from uniform, tend to vary widely (Froese, 1991), and often cannot be supported by scientific research (Rasanen & Downs, 1990). Although mechanical ventilation can support gas exchange in the presence of severe disease processes, it is not without significant sequelae or serious associated risks (Table 24–7). In most instances, prolonged dependence on mechanical ventilation necessitates tracheal intubation with a tracheostomy. The presence of a tracheostomy tube contributes a certain degree of risk and morbidity, however, the advantages over prolonged endotracheal intubation typically outweigh the risks (Bartlett, 1984). There are numerous complications that can occur with mechanical ventilation, and it is essential that individuals who work with children on ventilators have a knowledge of normal and pathologic respiratory physiology, as well as an intimate knowledge and understanding

of how the machine interfaces with the patient's physiology (Kirby et al., 1990; Perel & Stock, 1992).

Advances in their design, efficiency, and portability have all contributed to an increasing use of mechanical ventilators outside the acute care environment. In the past 5 to 10 years there has been a shift in the emphasis on home care, and it is feasible for children who are ventilator dependent to be cared for outside the hospital. Positive-pressure ventilators are the most frequently used mode of ventilation for pediatric patients. These ventilators offer features that allow for easy portability, and they are equipped with reliable low- and high-pressure alarms (Mallory & Stillwell, 1991). The cycling mode chosen varies depending on the patient's age and diagnosis. Negative-pressure ventilators are not as commonly used as positive-pressure ventilators, especially in those children who require continuous mechanical ventilation, because they are not meant for 24-hour-a-day support.

TABLE 24–6. CYCLING MECHANISMS ON POSITIVE-PRESSURE VENTILATORS

Time: may be divided into inspiratory and expiratory phases; expressed as an inspiration-expiration ratio in seconds
Time-cycled ventilation: mechanical ventilation terminates after a preselected inspiratory time (T_1) elapses.
Volume: a measure of the tidal volume delivered to the patient; expressed in milliliters for tidal volume and liters for minute volume
Volume-cycled ventilation: mechanical inhalation terminates after a preselected volume (V_T) has been ejected from the ventilator irrespective of changes in pulmonary mechanics.
Pressure: a measure of the impedance to gas flow rate encountered in the ventilator breathing circuit and patient's airways and lungs, expressed in centimeters of water, millimeters of mercury, or kilopascals (kPa) (1 mm Hg = 1.36 cm H_2O)
Pressure-cycled ventilation: mechanical ventilation terminates when a preselected peak inspiratory pressure is achieved within the breathing circuit tubing.
Flow rate: a measure of the rate at which the volume is delivered to the patient; expressed in liters per second or minute
Flow-cycled ventilation: mechanical ventilation is terminated when the inspiratory flow rate delivered by the ventilator decreases to a critical value, independent of inspiratory time or tidal volume.

From Perel, A, & Stock, MC (Eds.), Handbook of Mechanical Ventilatory Support. Baltimore: Williams & Wilkins, 1992, pp. 7–30. Copyright © 1992, the Williams & Wilkins Co., Baltimore.

A number of complex decisions are made before choosing the appropriate method of ventilation, as well as the plan regarding long-term management. If home care is an option for a child, the decision to send the child home is not made solely on the basis of medical stability. Rather, family and social support as well as financial resources are as important as the medical and technical management required. The American Thoracic Society (1990) has adopted an official statement regarding the home management of pediatric patients who are ventilator dependent. For detailed information on the specifics of planning and implementing effective home care for these children, the reader is referred to the American Thoracic Society, as well as to several other resources (Jackson, 1986; Mallory & Stillwell, 1991; Schreiner et al., 1987).

▌WEANING

During the acute stages of respiratory failure, the goals of mechanical ventilation are to support gas exchange and give the respiratory muscles a rest. In most cases, immediately after a patient is put on a ventilator the goal of weaning should be considered. The primary goal of assessing weaning capa-

bility is to determine at what point the patient is capable of maintaining adequate alveolar ventilation while breathing spontaneously. This requires the ventilatory pump to support the work required for breathing (Hodgkin et al., 1984). Various determinants of physiologic and medical stability such as pulmonary function, gas exchange, neuromuscular function, respiratory muscle strength, and ventilatory pattern are used to determine weaning capabilities. Knisely and co-workers (1988) found an association between prolonged ventilatory dependence in infants and diaphragmatic muscle atrophy. These investigators suggested that these changes could certainly affect the weaning process because the diaphragm would be predisposed to fatigue. For those children who are able to be weaned, it is primarily done by trial and error where the time off the ventilator is variable, dependent on when hypercapnia and hypoxia develop (Gozal et al., 1993).

TABLE 24–7. COMPLICATIONS ASSOCIATED WITH MECHANICAL VENTILATION

Respiratory
Tracheal lesions (erosion, edema, stenosis, granuloma, obstruction, perforation)
Accidental endotracheal tube displacement or actual extubation
Air leaks (pneumothorax, pneumomediastinum, interstitial emphysema)
Infection (tracheitis, pneumonitis)
Trapping of gas (hyperinflation)
Excessive secretions (atelectasis)
Oxygen hazards (depression of ventilation, bronchopulmonary dysplasia)
Pulmonary hemorrhage
Circulatory
Impairment of venous return (decreased cardiac output and systemic hypotension)
Oxygen hazard (retrolental fibroplasia, cerebral vasoconstriction)
Septicemia
Intracranial hemorrhage
Hyperventilation (decreased cerebral blood flow)
Metabolic
Increased work of breathing ("fighting the ventilator")
Alkalosis (potassium depletion, excessive bicarbonate therapy)
Renal and Fluid Balance
Antidiuresis
Excess water in inspired gas
Equipment Malfunction
Power source failure
Improper humidification (overheating of inspired gas, inspiratory line condensation)
Improper tubing connections (kinked line, disconnection)
Ventilation malfunction (leaks, valve dysfunction)

Adapted from Pagtakhan, RD, & Chernick, V. Intensive care for respiratory disorders. In Kendig, EL, & Chernick, V (Eds.), Disorders of the Respiratory Tract in Children. Philadelphia: WB Saunders, 1983, p 162.

Weaning from the ventilator is an individualized process and can be a very arduous task both physiologically and psychologically (Hodgkin et al., 1984). During that time, the child's schedule of activities may need to be altered. It is imperative that the physical therapist communicate with the medial team as to the amount of physical exertion that can be tolerated. At all costs both muscular and respiratory fatigue must be avoided.

Regardless of the cause for requiring chronic mechanical ventilation, once a child is diagnosed with chronic respiratory failure and the decision is made to begin artificial ventilation, prevention and treatment of the associated complications need to be a primary goal of medical and rehabilitative management. These children require early and aggressive developmental intervention. Although the degree and intensity may vary, the intervention approach should maximize the child's developmental and functional potential. After the acute medical condition of any of these patient groups is stabilized, considerable efforts should be aimed at promoting growth and development. In many centers, specialized units exist that exclusively serve the medical and developmental needs of infants and children who are ventilator dependent (Mallory & Stillwell, 1991; Schreiner et al., 1991). These units often attempt to provide individualized care and management while trying to maintain as normal an environment as possible. The need for multidisciplinary involvement is of utmost importance throughout infancy and early childhood to address the varied developmental needs of these children.

DISABILITIES ASSOCIATED WITH MECHANICAL VENTILATOR DEPENDENCE

In addition to a new category of patients being "created," chronic dependence on assisted ventilation has also created a new category of developmental disabilities. As elucidated previously, there is a wide range of pathophysiologic mechanisms that underlie dependence on mechanical ventilation. Hence, this "medical" diagnosis represents a very diverse and heterogeneous group of children with varying impairments and developmental capabilities. Despite these differences, however, these children are all medically fragile and vulnerable. It has been known for a number of years that the medically fragile infant and child is at risk for physical as well as mental and social disabilities. Although the predictive value of any one risk factor is not well established, it appears that long-term outcome depends on a number of risk factors and their

interactions (Resnick et al., 1988; Schaaf & Davis, 1992), including the predisposing medical problem such as respiratory failure (Gillis et al., 1989).

In addition to the risks associated with prolonged intubation and mechanical ventilation, the additive effects of secondary problems such as recurrent hypoxic episodes, recurrent infections, poor weight gain and physical growth, and extended hospitalization can result in any number of impairments. For example, because of the often prolonged periods of immobility or restricted activity early in the course of their disease, these children may demonstrate such problems as sensory defensiveness, generalized weakness, and soft tissue or muscular tightness. Likewise, if the child has had some type of hypoxic or ischemic episode, there may be neurologic damage that limits normal motor skill acquisition. Infant development research suggests that the development of mobility allows the child to progress through other areas of cognitive and perceptual development such as the acquisition of object permanence (Bai & Bertenthal, 1992). Thus, it appears that these impairments could result in functional limitations in other areas of development. These children often present with global developmental delays, despite having no history of neurologic insults.

The relationship between multiple risk factors is seen in Figure 24–2. Schaaf & Davis (1992) suggest that environmental factors become increasingly more important to the child's eventual outcome, a concept that is receiving much attention in the literature on the outcome of children with disabilities (Escalona, 1982; Hunt et al., 1988; Schafer et al., 1987; Slater et al., 1987). Even in the presence of an otherwise unremarkable medical history, the child on a ventilator is at risk for functional limitations related to communication, mobility, and cardiorespiratory endurance.

The context for motor learning is quite limiting for the child who is hospitalized for prolonged periods or who is constrained by life-saving equipment. The lack of practice and of variable practice opportunities makes skill acquisition difficult. Larin states that physical practice remains essential to motor learning (see Chapter 6 for further details on motor learning concepts).

Certainly, in terms of secondary prevention of the potential for "mild motor dysfunction" or global motor delays, physical therapists have the opportunity to encourage variable practice of motor skills from infancy onward. Recognition of the need for variable practice of motor skills in differing contexts needs to extend well into the school-aged years since different motor competencies are expected of these children as they attempt

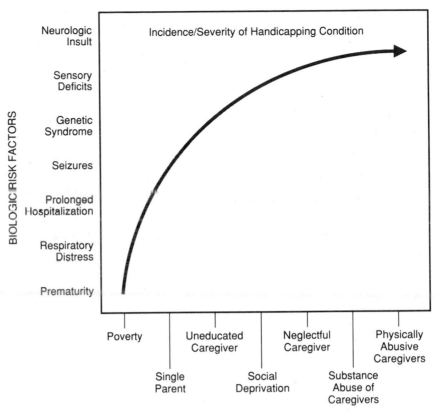

FIGURE 24-2. Relationship between multiple risk factors. This example illustrates how various biologic risk factors in combination with multiple environmental risks can magnify the incidence of disabilities associated with the given pathophysiologic process. (From Schaaf, RC, & Davis, WS. Promoting health and wellness in the pediatric disabled and "at risk" population. In Rothman, J, & Levine, R (Eds.), Prevention Practice: Strategies for Physical Therapy and Occupational Therapy. Philadelphia. WB Saunders 1992, p 273.)

to keep up with their peers and be independent in school and community activities.

Few studies have specifically examined the developmental outcome of children who are ventilator dependent. Current developmental assessments, although useful to some degree with this population, are inadequate and fail to take into account the effects of medical and physiologic instability; long-term hospitalization; decreased mobility; and separation from "normal" social, emotional, and physical life experiences.

One group that has probably been studied most extensively is infants and children with BPD. Bozynski and colleagues (1987) assessed the relationship between mechanical ventilation and developmental outcome and found prolonged ventilator dependence to be the best predictor of poor developmental progress during the first 18 months. This finding is disputed by Bregman and Farrell (1992), who have asserted that length of mechanical ventilation does not necessarily correlate with developmental outcome. In general, a paucity of literature exists on the long-term outcomes of chronically ventilated infants with BPD, as well as on the out-

comes of other diagnostic groups requiring prolonged mechanical ventilation.

Regardless of the reason for being dependent on assisted ventilation, appreciation of the fact that the child is at a disadvantage in terms of developmental risks is a compelling reason to begin early intervention as soon as the infant or child is medically stable. The vulnerability of young children can be affected by both biological and environmental circumstances, which may result in developmental delays with minor or major consequences (Brooks-Gunn et al., 1992). However, if these children have been spared the associated problems (most commonly the frequent hypoxic episodes), then there is a good chance that they can grow and develop normally. For example, children with CCHS have a favorable prognosis and the capacity for normal or near normal intelligence if they are diagnosed early and managed aggressively (Weese-Mayer et al., 1992). Similarly, infants with BPD who have not had major neurologic insults also have an excellent chance of being weaned from oxygen dependence and the ventilator, as well as functioning independently in their school years (Mallory & Stillwell,

1991). Because of the risks for abnormal neurodevelopmental sequelae in this population and in other children who are ventilator dependent, physical therapists are often involved with providing developmental intervention early in the course of an infant's hospitalization. Delays in the initiation of rehabilitation or habilitation can place the child at risk for developing secondary impairments and functional limitations that could otherwise be prevented.

ASSESSMENT AND PROBLEM DEFINITION

The physical therapy assessment of the infant or child who is mechanically ventilated needs to encompass a wide range of skills and observations. In addition to an understanding of motor skill development, one needs to have a knowledge of developmental cardiorespiratory physiology and of the implications of a compromise to those systems. The complexity of the technical environment makes this a challenging population. First, the physical therapist needs to be comfortable with the equipment, both the ventilator and its attachments, as well as the physiologic monitoring devices (Table 24–8). Although the infant or child may be medically stable, the presence of an artificial airway creates a critical situation because of the potential for its being dislodged or occluded. Because the infant or young child may not yet communicate well, it is up to the therapist to interpret any signs of impending or actual distress. The essence of our intervention is to ensure that no harm be done in the delivery of services and to optimize the child's developmental potential.

Before any assessment or treatment session, the therapist should confer with the child's primary nurse or caregiver to determine the child's most recent medical status, in addition to their baseline physiologic parameters. Depending on the nature and severity of the predisposing condition, the cardiorespiratory parameters may vary from what is considered to be normal for the child's age (Table 24–9). It is always prudent to establish the "safe" physiologic parameters within which to work. Typically, heart rate, respiratory rate, and oxygen saturation are monitored while the child is on the ventilator. In the home or outpatient setting, one may choose to monitor these parameters periodically, however, there is no substitute for the keen visual observation of signs of distress.

Physical Therapy Assessment

The physical therapy assessment essentially consists of three parts: respiratory, neuromuscular and neurodevelopmental, and functional assessments. A respiratory evaluation is essential even if the physical therapist is not involved with postural drainage, percussion, and vibration. At a minimum, the therapist should be comfortable observing the patient for signs of respiratory distress, skin color changes indicative of hypoxia, changes in respiratory rate, breathing pattern, symmetry of chest expansion, posture, and general comfort (DeCesare & Graybill, 1990). (In neonates, visual inspection of hypoxia is not effective since neonates generally do not appear cyanotic until the Pao_2 is dangerously low, below 40 mm Hg [Null et al., 1990].) Signs of respiratory distress such as retractions, nasal flaring, expiratory grunting, and stridor may not be evident when a child is on a mechanical ventilator (Crane, 1990). For more information specific to the assessment of the cardiorespiratory system, the reader is referred elsewhere (DeCesare & Graybill, 1989; Gould, 1991; Waring, 1983).

The neuromuscular assessment should provide

TABLE 24–8. **COMMONLY ENCOUNTERED NONINVASIVE MONITORING DEVICES**

Equipment	Physiologic Parameters Monitored
Cardiorespiratory monitors	Heart rate and respiratory rate
Pulse oximeter*	Transcutaneous arterial oxygen saturation to monitor hypoxemia
Ventilator alarms	Various modes chosen for the individual case as well as airway pressures, gas concentrations, and expiratory tidal volumes
Trancutaneous PO_2 and PCO_2	Partial pressure of oxygen and carbon dioxide in the arterial blood
Oxygen analyzers on the ventilator	Oxygen supply in the ventilator circuit
Sphygmomanometer	Blood pressure

These are some noninvasive devices that one may use to monitor response to activity and general status. Before any evaluation or treatment session the therapist should be familiar with *all* of the equipment used for the child.

*Pulse oximeters are not useful for discriminating hyperoxia since the blood is fully saturated at PaO_2 of 150 mm Hg.

TABLE 24–9. **APPROXIMATE NORMAL PHYSIOLOGIC VALUES**

Parameter	Newborn	Older Infant & Child
Respiratory rate	40–60	20–30 (≤6 years)
		15–20 (>6 years)
Heart rate	120–200	100–180 (≤3 years)
		70–150 (>3 years)
PO_2 (mm Hg)	60–90	80–100
PCO_2 (mm Hg)	30–35	30–35 (≤2 years)
		20–24 (>2 years)
Blood pressure (mm Hg)		
Systolic	60–90	75–130 (≤3 years)
		90–140 (>3 years)
Diastolic	30–60	45–90 (≤3 years)
		50–80 (>3 years)
Arterial oxygen saturation (%)	87–89 (low)	95–100
	94–95 (high)	
	90–95 (preterm infant)	

These values represent "normal" physiologic values; in the case of infants and children with varying pathophysiologic processes, the "normal" values may be different.

Data from Comer, DM. Pulse oximetry: Implications for practice. Journal of Obstetrics, Gynecology and Neonatal Nursing, 21:35–41, 1992; and Pagtakhan, RD, & Chernick, V. Intensive care for respiratory disorders. In Kendig, EL, & Chernick, V (Eds.), Disorders of the Respiratory Tract in Children (4th ed.). Philadelphia: WB Saunders, 1983, pp. 145–168.

information about the infant or child's general musculoskeletal status, strength, sensation, posture, and general movement competencies. The evaluation procedures vary depending on the age and cognitive level of the child, and the areas of emphasis may be different depending on the diagnosis. The neurodevelopmental assessment is an important contribution for these children. Because they are at great risk for global developmental delays that may or may not have a pathophysiologic component, ongoing assessment of how the child is progressing is vital. It cannot be emphasized enough that a multidisciplinary team approach is necessary. The physical therapy assessment alone does not begin to represent the wide range of competencies that need to be monitored. Ideally, all aspects of the child's development will be evaluated periodically by members of the health care team.

The type of developmental assessments used vary with the age of the child (Chapter 1). The use of any standardized assessment requires that the therapist be familiar with the purpose of the test, its limitations, and its relevance to the outcome measures of interest. Specifically, the user needs to understand the generalizability of the test results because many assessments are normed on children without disabilities. Supplementing any standardized assessment should be the therapist's individualized assessment of the infant or child's developmental competencies.

The child needs to be functional within the context of his or her environment; therefore, an evaluation of the child's functional level is as important as the respiratory and neuromotor assessments that the physical therapist would typically perform. The functional assessment should include age-appropriate basic and instrumental activities of daily living; general mobility skills; communication skills; and an evaluation of the child's role within the family and within the relevant environment. At the very least, the functional assessment provides an indication of how well the child is integrated into the family and community lifestyle.

The importance of the disablement framework (see Chapter 7) relative to the assessment of motor function is nicely elucidated by Haley and colleagues (1993). These authors stress the significance of assessing motor skills during spontaneous activity and of obtaining parental impressions of function. Their emphasis on functional considerations is translated into the recommendation that the environment and social context be an essential part of any evaluation to determine the nature of the child's functional limitations, disabilities, and handicaps. The child on assisted ventilation exemplifies this concept because it would be impossible to isolate the effects of the restrictive environment in an assessment of the child's sensorimotor development.

Haley and colleagues (1993) caution that standardized and criterion-referenced testing of neuromotor behaviors and movement analyses do not always give information at all levels of the disablement spectrum. They recommend sampling motor outcomes across the entire disablement framework and suggest the use of judgment based assessments, which can provide additional information that is a useful adjunct to that obtained from standardized or criterion-based assessments. Judgment-based assessments do not require observation of the *actual* performance of the motor task; however, the respondent is asked to make a judgment about the ability of the child to perform a task based on prior observations and a knowledge of how the child would typically perform. This allows one to distinguish between what the child is capable of and how the child actually performs during day-to-day functional tasks. Parent or caregiver participation should be encouraged in the actual assessment, as well in the formulation of therapy goals (see Chapter 30).

TREATMENT CONSIDERATIONS

No one intervention approach is unanimously embraced by physical therapists for any diagnostic group. Similarly, in the case of children with ventilator dependence, physical therapy varies widely because of differing philosophies of management and the wide range of problem areas that might be identified. Thus, the intent of this section is not to prescribe specific treatment ideas but to present a conceptual framework from which one can organize an appropriate treatment plan and to emphasize considerations unique to this group of children.

The vast majority of healthy infants and children are capable of using a variable repertoire of motor skills to explore and learn. This normal acquisition of skills presumes a normal interaction of the cardiopulmonary and musculoskeletal systems, as well as the presence of the necessary cognitive requirements. Inactivity in children is never normal, and they usually require minimal encouragement to be active and spontaneous. In the case of a child with chronic respiratory insufficiency, however, a compromised physiologic system alone may limit the seemingly endless exploration and practice in which children typically engage. In children with a chronic illness a reduced capacity for activity or exercise can be a direct or indirect result of their pathophysiologic process (Bar-Or, 1986). Regardless of the cause, a vicious cycle of inactivity→ reluctance to move and explore→decreased endurance and "fitness"→inactivity ensues. Another consideration is that these children may associate movement with negative experiences such as fatigue, hypoxia, and pain, therefore limiting their "motivation" to be as active as their peers. It is not always easy to distinguish among the various factors that lead to a paucity of movement, especially in the absence of neurologic deficits.

A major goal of the physical therapist in the management of children who are dependent on ventilators should be secondary prevention, that is, to prevent deprivation of sensory and motor experiences and all of the various sequelae that result from that deprivation. Regardless of the child's diagnosis, treatment should be aimed at providing a variety of opportunities for movement challenges and for exploration, as well as to increase their capacity for exercise. Depending on whether the child has a specific motor impairment, these goals may be accomplished with or without the use of assistive devices. For example, in the case of a child with BPD who also had an intraventricular hemorrhage, assistive devices may be needed for ambulation because of lower extremity weakness and spasticity. Alternatively, the child with CCHS with no neurologic injuries leading to motor impairments may be completely independent in all motor skills. In the context of functional limitations, exercise intolerance is certainly a problem in this group of children. Physical therapists should use developmental intervention as a means of improving the child's tolerance for exercise. Any activity in which these infants or children engage should be viewed as "exercise" and seen as a means of improving their tolerance for movement. A paucity of literature exists on the role developmental intervention plays in improving cardiopulmonary status and exercise tolerance, *in addition* to achieving developmental goals.

The beneficial effects of exercise have been well documented in certain populations such as those individuals with cystic fibrosis and asthma (Darbee & Cerny, 1990); however, less information exists that objectively documents the effects of any type of structured exercise program on either short- or long-term outcomes of children who are dependent on ventilators. Bader and colleagues (1987) examined the long-term pulmonary sequelae and exercise tolerance of 10 children with BPD at a mean of 10 years of age. All children in the study had required either mechanical ventilation or oxygen therapy for at least 30 days. Half of the group had exercise-induced bronchospasms. No significant differences were found in maximal oxygen consumption, suggesting that their aerobic fitness was comparable to the "normal" group.

Despite similarities in cardiovascular function, the BPD group demonstrated pulmonary limitations to exercise evidenced by a decrease in arterial oxygen saturation and an increased $Paco_2$. Although some of the children were mechanically ventilated for a very short time during their acute disease course, it would be erroneous to extrapolate the findings to the population of children who remain chronically dependent on mechanical ventilation. Certainly there is a need for more long-term studies to determine the effectiveness of exercise programs in this group.

Simply stated, the "normal" response to exercise is an increase in heart rate, followed by a return to baseline. Ventilation also increases linearly with the metabolic rate until approximately 60% of the oxygen consumption at which time it increases more rapidly. (See Chapter 5 for a summary of the cardiorespiratory and musculoskeletal components of exercise and fitness.) These relationships, as well as the other physiologic processes that support adequate ventilation and perfusion during exercise, are altered in conditions of lung disease. Whereas exercise is normally cardiac limited, in those with chronic lung disease, exercise may be ventilatory limited as a result of deficient exercise capacity, gas exchange, or poor pulmonary mechanics (Darbee & Cerny, 1990). Each child's specific pathophysiologic process determines the response to exercise and the capacity for improvement. Regardless of the diagnosis there is usually no reason not to encourage some type of physical activity in children who are dependent on a ventilator.

Although one of the ultimate goals of physical therapy is to facilitate age-appropriate motor skill acquisition and function, therapists need to recognize the potential for physiologic jeopardy when implementing intervention with these infants and children. The amount and type of motor activities must be individualized and graded to the child's level of tolerance so that the risks associated with the physiologically immature or unstable systems are not magnified. Decisions regarding the mode, intensity, and frequency of activity should be made in conjunction with the other members of the child's medical team and modified as the disease process changes.

ROLE OF THE INTERDISCIPLINARY TEAM

The lives of infants and children who are ventilator dependent are complex, and these children require a variety of services to meet their needs. It is known that children at risk benefit most from effective interaction and collaboration of many members of a health care team. The most effective outcomes occur when the focus of the team is on the integration of the child into the family and then, at the right time, into the community (Raulin & Shannon, 1986; Schaaf & Davis, 1992).

Although physical therapists play an important role in direct treatment, consultation, parent teaching, and discharge planning, they represent only one aspect of the care that these children require. For these children to progress optimally they must be managed by a multidisciplinary team rather than by fragmented individual services. Typically, a multidisciplinary team might consist of physicians, nurses, therapists, nutritionists, and other professionals who address the psychosocial aspects of the child, family, and community (Table 24–10). Ideally the "team" is involved with the child at all stages of the child's care and development, certainly well beyond the acute care hospitalization. It is essential that the goals be re-evaluated throughout the child's various stages of life and, if necessary, various stages of the disease.

As health care professionals, physical therapists need to shift their focus from traditional medical models to child- and family-centered intervention. Treatment goals should be directed toward "maintenance, restoration and development of a sense of well being, social productivity, and self actualization" (Schaaf & Davis, 1992). The physical therapist has an obligation to "treat" the family in addition to treating the child. This includes ongoing parental and family teaching, communication of future needs and expectations, and a commitment to respecting the limitations each family may have.

TABLE 24–10. INTERDISCIPLINARY TEAM OF CAREGIVERS FOR VENTILATOR-DEPENDENT CHILDREN

Physicians
Pediatric pulmonologists or critical care specialist
Pediatric physiatrist or developmental specialist
General pediatrician
Pediatric neurologist
Nurses
Special care unit nurse
Discharge planning nurse
Pediatric pulmonary nurse
Home nursing agency
Therapists
Physical therapist
Occupational therapist
Speech therapist
Respiratory therapist
Durable medical equipment company representative
Other Professionals
Nutritionist
Social worker
Psychologist/family therapist
Child life therapist
Third party payer representative

Adapted from Mallory, GB, & Stillwell, PC. The ventilator-dependent child: Issues in diagnosis and management. Archives of Physical Medicine and Rehabilitation, 72:43–55, 1991.

By nature of the predisposing medical condition, a child dependent on mechanical ventilation for prolonged periods of time is already "identified" as being at some degree of risk at least from a medical perspective. It is hoped that the caregivers, both medical and personal, appreciate the fact that the child is at a developmental risk and that the family unit is also at risk for problems secondary to the intense demands placed on the family when caring for a child with chronic medical needs.

As the degree and complexity of impairment and disabilities increase, the general quality of life decreases, especially if financial, psychosocial, and emotional supports dwindle. Keeping this in mind, one of the most important roles of the interdisciplinary team is to work closely with family members as the child is being considered for discharge. Parents should expect the health care professionals to give them as much information as needed to make an informed decision about their abilities to care for their child at home. The risks and the benefits of home care need to be thoroughly explained.

The dilemma of whether a child can be cared for at home on a ventilator not only involves the decision of the parents and medical staff but also must take into account the complexities of health care financing, insurance, and community resources. It is imperative that the family or designated caregivers be involved in, and capable of learning, all aspects of the child care (American Thoracic Society, 1990; Frates et al, 1985; Mallory, 1991). This includes not only managing the ventilator and other monitoring equipment, but also being able to provide emergency medical procedures if the child experiences distress. The critical nature of this type of family teaching goes beyond our normal expectations of the family unit, and therefore caregivers need extensive support from the interdisciplinary team members. Parents who decide *not* to have their child cared for at home on a ventilator, or those who do not have a choice, will also need ongoing support as they continue to be parents from a distance and without the luxury of the home environment.

Communication and collaboration among team members are essential to the child and family's well-being and to an understanding of the disability. Short- and long-term goals developed by the interdisciplinary team should be formulated in conjunction with the family, keeping in mind the ultimate goal of maximizing function from a physical, cognitive, social-emotional, and family dynamics perspective. It is not uncommon for parents to be naive to the disease process and the implications for future function. As a protective mechanism, many parents are often overprotective of a "sick" child and actually contribute to sustaining the child's fear of movement challenges or lack of activity. Especially in relation to functional mobility and fitness, the physical therapist has an important role to play in educating the family toward maximizing the child's *abilities* rather than imposing limitations because of the child's *disabilities*. In the case of the child who is at home, this role may extend to community therapists and school personnel as well.

Family-centered intervention is mandated by law, representing a departure from the traditional child-focused programs (Kolobe, 1992). For reasons other than legal ones, however, the involvement of the parents and family in the life of the child with a disability is essential for optimal child development and family dynamics. Probably no situation better demonstrates the need for inclusion of the family in the child's entire care plan more than in the case of the child who is dependent on mechanical ventilation.

The parents and extended family of these children have a crucial role to play in shaping the child's environment to be the most conducive to learning and optimal development. More importantly, from a practical point of view, the child's life depends on the parents' knowledge about the intensive care needed to maintain the child's fragile life. Although most would agree that having a child who is dependent on a ventilator remain at home is physically, financially, developmentally, and emotionally beneficial, the impact of having a child with chronic medical needs and disabilities causes varying degrees of stress on families and on their coping strategies (American Thoracic Society, 1990; Bach et al., 1992; Fields et al., 1991; Frates et al., 1985).

Quint and associates (1990) found that the coping skills of the primary caregivers decreased as the length of home ventilation increased beyond 2 years. The implications of poor coping strategies are numerous, especially since the primary caregiver is often a parent who has other family members to care for. Although the sample studied was small, this finding supports the concept that caring for a ventilator-dependent child can possibly contribute to family dysfunction. The parents of a child who is dependent on mechanical ventilation also have the added burden of needing highly qualified child care resources, making leisure time or needed respite care difficult to arrange. The family's coping skills and lifestyle needs should always be at the forefront of any parent–professional relationship and a major consideration of any rehabilitation program that might be recommended. It is essential that the child's therapy program be integrated into the family's daily routine and not be the sole focus of the family's daily schedule (Kolobe, 1992).

CASE HISTORY: LISA

This case history illustrates a very representative course of a child with chronic respiratory failure (Figs. 24–3 through 24–9).

Medical and Surgical History

Lisa is a 19 month old girl who was born prematurely at 28 weeks' gestation. Her birth weight was 1 lb 10 oz. Her medical course was complicated by intrauterine growth retardation, RDS leading to BPD, grade II intraventricular hemorrhage, retinopathy of prematurity, gastroesophageal reflux, anemia, moderate tracheomalacia, and multiple infections. She continues to have difficulties gaining weight and is below the 50th percentile for height and weight (adjusted age).

She had a tracheostomy placed when she was 4 months old, and gastrostomy and jejunostomy tubes were placed when she was 6 months old.

Hospital Course

Lisa was hospitalized for the first 15 months of life, and she has been mechanically ventilated since birth. She began receiving physical, occupational, and speech therapy when she was deemed to be medically stable at 9 months of age. Up until that time, physical therapy had been involved on a consulting basis for a positioning program that nursing staff had carried out. For the

FIGURE 24–4. With some encouragement, Lisa is able to briefly lift her head and prop on her forearms. She was only able to hold this position for about 10 seconds before collapsing. Note that she is off of the ventilator, which she is able to tolerate for brief periods.

first 5 to 6 weeks after beginning her therapies, Lisa's therapy sessions were often canceled secondary to her agitation with handling; she often required sedatives for prolonged periods of agitation that would result in arterial oxygen desaturations. She was also followed by professionals in social work, child development, neu-

FIGURE 24–3. Note Lisa's difficulty with antigravity head and upper trunk control. She has difficulty achieving and maintaining weight bearing through her arms.

FIGURE 24–5. Note the inability to sustain lower extremity weight bearing even when given the support of the walker.

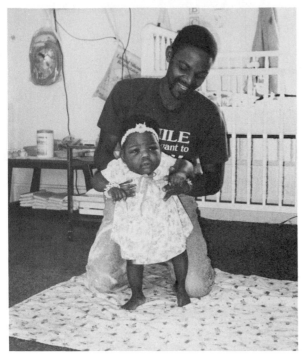

FIGURE 24–6. With support, there is brief weight acceptance through the right lower extremity. Note the degree of trunk support required in this position.

FIGURE 24–8. The pulse oximeter is attached to Lisa's great toe, during her therapy sessions. This monitoring device is a useful adjunct to observation of her clinical signs, especially during the weaning period.

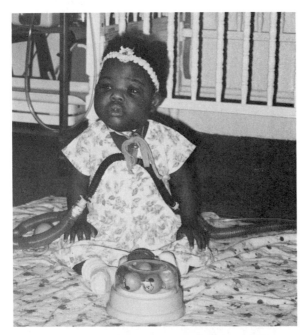

FIGURE 24–7. Lisa achieved independent sitting at 18 months of age. She was not, however, able to move out of the sitting position. This photograph illustrates her lack of exploratory behaviors since she demonstrated no interest in the toy placed in front of her. Note her wide base of support and hip external rotation for stability.

rology, pulmonology, ophthalamology, infectious diseases, and critical care medicine, in addition to her general pediatrician.

Lisa's parents were involved with her medical care throughout her entire hospital stay. They consistently demonstrated a good knowledge of her respiratory care, including trouble shooting with the ventilator, tracheal suctioning, and recognizing Lisa's signs of distress.

At the age of 13 months, Lisa was diagnosed with cerebral palsy because of her extremely delayed motor skills and signs of hypertonia (primarily brisk reflexes, increased resistance to passive movement, and dystonic movement patterns). At 14 months of age, discharge plans were begun. Her social worker began working with the insurance company and the state to file for approval in the state's model waiver program. This program approved 24 hours of nursing care for the first week and then between 12 and 18 hours following that time. Extensive training sessions were held with the parents who were able to demonstrate significant competence in Lisa's care. They also had numerous sessions with all of the different therapists to learn Lisa's home program. The plan was for Lisa to be discharged as soon as the nursing coverage could begin.

Once discharge was definite, Lisa was switched to a ventilator that was specifically intended for home use, and both the parents and home nursing agency repre-

FIGURE 24-9. The surroundings of a child with a disability may need to become a high-tech environment for survival. Missing from this photograph is a feeding pump.

sentatives were trained with that specific ventilator. In addition to the various ventilator alarms, the monitoring devices for home use included a cardiorespiratory monitor and a pulse oximeter.

Physical Therapy Involvement

The initial physical therapy evaluation was very limited secondary to her medical instability. Treatment sessions focused primarily on increasing tolerance to handling, gentle passive range of motion, continuation of Lisa's positioning program and ongoing parent teaching about how to recognize her signs of distress. Because of the practices at the hospital, physical therapists were not involved in chest physical therapy.

At 12 months chronologic age (9 months adjusted age), the Peabody Developmental Motor Scales were administered and Lisa's gross motor age equivalent was 2 months. The occupational therapist reported a Bayley Scales of Infant Development mental age equivalent of 2.3 months. At 15 months of age, before discharge from the hospital, these significant delays continued. The Peabody Scales were administered before discharge. Lisa had demonstrated improvements in socialization skills and increased tolerance for activity and handling and was beginning to demonstrate increased spontaneous movement; however her Peabody score did not reflect these qualitative changes. She passed 7 of 10 items in the 2- to 3-month category. The failed items required lower extremity weight acceptance and mobility. In the 4- to 5-month items, she passed only 2 of 10 skills.

The physical therapist had identified the following as Lisa's major strengths and weaknesses at discharge (12 months adjusted age; 15 months chronological age):

Weaknesses

- Paucity of active movements and exploratory behaviors for adjusted age
- Limited endurance for active movement
- Lack of protective responses in supported sitting
- Lack of active trunk mobility
- Increased resistance to passive movement, more predominant in the lower extremities
- Interference of the asymmetric tonic neck reflex with activities requiring eye–hand coordination
- Decreased strength of antigravity postural muscle groups and the extremities (evidenced by inability to sustain body weight in weight-bearing positions)
- Lack of weight acceptance through lower extremities

Strengths

- Improved antigravity head control in supported sitting
- Briefly able to use arms to prop in sitting
- Tolerance to the prone position improved with attempts at lifting head against gravity
- Increased spontaneous movements and attempts at transitions

At discharge, recommendations were made that addressed all of the above areas. Because she was so inactive, the importance of increasing her activity level was emphasized as a means of improving Lisa's "fitness" level. The parents were involved in coming up with activities that accomplished the various goals established and suited their schedules.

Lisa is enrolled in an early intervention program for home-bound children. She receives physical therapy once a week, occupational therapy twice a month, and speech therapy twice a month. She is also followed in a multidisciplinary pulmonary follow-up clinic every 3 to 4 months. At those visits, she is evaluated by physical, occupational, and speech therapists.

Her respiratory status is stable at 19 months. She has evidence of tracheomalacia, a sequela of prolonged intubation. This may complicate or prevent extubation until she has significant airway growth. Because she is capable of spontaneous breaths, she is using the synchronized intermittent mandatory ventilation mode and most recently is on room air (no supplemental oxygen from the ventilator). She is currently beginning to be weaned from the ventilator. The parents have taken an active role in this process and keep detailed logs of her responses to being off the ventilator for short periods of time. They are able to recognize her signs of fatigue and distress and monitor her using the pulse oximeter and cardiorespiratory monitors during periods of activity. When Lisa becomes stressed or exhibits signs of respiratory fatigue, her respiratory rate increases and she tends to desaturate below her usual 94 to 96%.

Disablement Framework

The case history outlined here can be summarized using the disablement framework to illustrate some of the major areas of concern for this child. This example illustrates the varying nature of disablement in a ventilator-dependent child. Given the very same medical history and pathophysiologic processes, another child could present with very different impairments, functional limitations, and disabilities.

The following processes are not inclusive of *all* areas relevant to this child's development, rather those that have an impact on her motor skill development.

Pathophysiology

- Immature lung development
- RDS leading to pathophysiologic changes in the lung parenchyma consistent with BPD
- Intraventricular hemorrhage
- Gastroesophageal reflux (hypotonic lower esophageal sphincter)

Impairments

- Decreased lung compliance
- Increased work of breathing
- Weakness
- Decreased muscular and cardiorespiratory endurance

- Poor postural control
- Delayed physical development (height and weight for age)
- Increased resistance to passive movement
- Poor oral motor coordination
- Oral motor hypersensitivity

Functional Limitations

- Motor skill delays, fine and gross motor
- Decreased repertoire of movement skills
- Poor protective extension skills in sitting
- Lack of environmental exploration
- Lack of transitional skills
- Lack of adequate nutritional intake from oral feedings
- Intellectual delays
- Speech and communication delays

Disabilities

- No attempts at any self-care activities
- Lack of age-appropriate play skills
- Limited home and community mobility

(One would assume that since she has demonstrated abnormal movement patterns, in addition to her significant motor delays, that the scope of her disabilities will increase as she gets older.)

SUMMARY

It is ironic that the very technology that has prolonged the survival of infants and children with chronic respiratory failure has also contributed to their morbidity. Because of improved medical and technologic management, a large number of children who are mechanically ventilated are likely to survive and eventually be discharged from the intensive-care environment. More than likely, the rate of medical and technologic progress will continue to exceed the strides made in the rehabilitation and prevention of disabilities and the policies that support an uncomplicated transition into the home and community.

Although physical therapists can do little to prevent chronic respiratory failure and ventilator dependence, they have an important role to play in fostering the child's development. Uncertainty regarding the prognosis for weaning from the ventilator or a child's prognosis for a productive and independent life may persist for an extended period of time. For the family there is the additional stress relating to the child's fragile medical status and the constant possibility of sudden death if the mechanical equipment should fail. When children go home on mechanical ventilation, normal family routines are replaced with highly structured schedules with no room for spontaneity. It is essential that health care professionals present the parents with a realistic picture of the benefits, cost, and burden of caring for a child at home and help them to realize that advanced technologic capacity does not necessarily ensure or equate to a benefit for the patient or the family (Mallory & Stillwell, 1991).

From early on in the neonatal intensive care unit through school age, physical therapists are in a unique position to be involved with these children and families. Some aspects of care may be specific medically related interventions, such as percussion and postural drainage; however, the majority of time is spent addressing various aspects of the child's development. In dealing with any population at risk for disability, one of the major roles of physical therapists is to integrate treatment goals into everyday activities and help the caregivers or parents appreciate the relevance of their involvement. The ecologic validity of the treatment goals increases if those goals are made a part of functionally relevant tasks.

The care of this group of children will continue to be a challenge to physical therapists and other health care professionals because they possess a wide range of impairments, functional limitations, and disabilities. One should not expect uniformity in the assessment and treatment of these children. This should not be discouraging, but should force physical therapists to organize clinical judgments according to the "disabling" dimension that most clearly affects the child's ultimate functional outcome.

References

American Thoracic Society. Home mechanical ventilation of pediatric patients. American Review of Respiratory Disease, 141:258–259, 1990.

Andrews, MM, & Nielson, DW. Technology-dependent children in the home. Pediatric Nursing, 14:111–151, 1988.

Bach JR, Intinola, P, Alba, AS, & Holland, IE. The ventilator-assisted individual: Cost analysis of institutionalization vs rehabilitation and in-home management. Chest, 101:26–30, 1990.

Bader, D, Ramos, AD, Lew, CD, Platzker, ACG, Stabile, MW, & Keens, TG. Childhood sequelae of infant lung disease: Exercise and pulmonary function abnormalities after bronchopulmonary dysplasia. Journal of Pediatrics, 110:693:699, 1987.

Bai, DL, & Bertenthal, BI. Locomotor status and the development of spatial search skills. Child Development, 63:215–226, 1992.

Bancalari, E. Neonatal chronic lung disease. In Fanaroff, AA, & Martin, RJ (Eds.), Neonatal-Perinatal Medicine: Diseases of the Fetus and Infant. St. Louis: CV Mosby, 1992, pp 861–874.

Bancalari, E, & Sosenko, I. Pathogenesis and prevention of neonatal chronic lung disease: Recent developments. Pediatric Pulmonology, 8:109–116, 1990.

Bar-Or, O. Pathophysiological factors which limit the exercise capacity of the sick child. Medicine and Science in Sports and Exercise, 18:276–282, 1986.

Billeaud, C, Piedboeuf, B, & Chessex P. Energy expenditure and severity of respiratory disease in very low birth weight infants receiving long-term ventilatory support. Journal of Pediatrics, 120:461–464, 1992.

Bozynski, MEA, Nelson, MN, Matalon, TAS, O'Donnell, KJ, Naughton, PM, Vasan, U, Meier, WA, & Ploughman, L. Prolonged mechanical ventilation and intracranial hemorrhage: Impact on developmental progress through 18 months in infants weighing 1,200 grams or less at birth. Pediatrics, 79:670–676, 1987.

Brazy, JE, Kinney, HC, & Oakes, WJ. Central nervous system structural lesions causing apnea at birth. Journal of Pediatrics, 111:163–175, 1987.

Bregman, J, & Farrell, EE. Neurodevelopmental outcome in infants with bronchopulmonary dysplasia. Clinics in Perinatology, 19:673–694, 1992.

Brooks-Gunn, J, Gross, RT, Kraemer, HC, Spiker, D, & Shapiro, S. Enhancing the cognitive outcomes of low birth weight, premature infants: For whom is the intervention most effective? Pediatrics, 89:1209–1215, 1992.

Bureau, MA, & Begin, R. Chest wall diseases and dysfunction in children. In Kendig, EL, & Chernick, V (Eds.), Disorders of the Respiratory Tract in Children. Philadelphia: WB Saunders, 1983, pp. 601–616.

Burr, BH, Guyer, B, Todres, ID, Abrahams, B, & Chiodo, T. Home care for children on respirators. New England Journal of Medicine, 21:1319–1323, 1983.

Comer, DM. Pulse oximetry: Implications for practice. Journal of Obstetric, Gynecologic, and Neonatal Nursing, 21:35–41, 1992.

Crane, LD. Physical therapy for the neonate with respiratory disease. In Irwin, S, & Tecklin, JS (Eds.), Cardiopulmonary Physical Therapy. St. Louis: CV Mosby, 1990, pp. 389–416.

Darbee, J, & Cerny, F. Exercise testing and exercise conditioning for children with lung dysfunction. In Irwin, S, & Tecklin, JS (Eds.), Cardiopulmonary Physical Therapy. St. Louis: CV Mosby, 1990, pp. 461–476.

DeCesare, JA, & Graybill, CA. Physical therapy for the child with respiratory dysfunction. In Irwin, S, & Tecklin, JS (Eds.), Cardiopulmonary Physical Therapy. St. Louis: CV Mosby, 1990, pp. 417–460.

Dykes, FD, Ahmann, PA, & Brann, AW. Central nervous system morbidity. In Goldsmith, JP, & Karotkin, EH (Eds.), Assisted Ventilation of the Neonate (2nd ed). Philadelphia: WB Saunders, 1988.

Escalona, SK. Babies at double hazard: Early development of infants at biologic and social risk. Pediatrics, 70:670–676, 1982.

Fallat, RJ, & Osborn, JJ. Patient monitoring techniques. In Burton, GG, & Hodgkin, JE (Eds.), Respiratory Care: A Guide to Clinical Practice. Philadelphia: JB Lippincott, 1984, pp. 940–950.

Farrell, PM, & Fost, NC. Long-term mechanical ventilation in pediatric respiratory failure: Medical and ethical considerations. American Review of Respiratory Disease, 140:S36–S40, 1989.

Fields, AI, Rosenblatt, A, Pollack, MM, & Kaufman, J. Home care cost-effectiveness for respiratory technology–dependent children. American Journal of Diseases in Children, 145:729–733, 1991.

Frates, RC, Splaingard, ML, Smith, EO, & Harrison, GM. Outcome of home mechanical ventilation in children. Journal of Pediatrics, 106:850–856, 1985.

Froese, AB. Mechanical ventilation. In Chernick, V, & Mellins, RB (Eds.), Basic Mechanisms of Pediatric Respiratory Disease: Cellular and Integrative. Philadelphia: BC Decker, pp. 418–431, 1991.

Ganong, WF. Review of Medical Physiology. Norwalk: Appleton & Lange, 1993, p. 605.

Gillis, J, Tibballs, J, McEniery, J, Heavens, J, Hutchins, P, Kilham, HA, & Henning, R. Ventilator-dependent children. Medical Journal of Australia, 150:10–14, 1989.

Goldberg, AI, & Monahan, CA. Home health care for children assisted by mechanical ventilation: The physician's perspective. Journal of Pediatrics, 114:378–383, 1989.

Goldsmith, JP, & Karotkin, EH. Assisted Ventilation of the Neonate (2nd ed.). Philadelphia: WB Saunders, 1988.

Gould, A. Cardiopulmonary evaluation of the infant, toddler, child, and adolescent. Pediatric Physical Therapy, 3:9–13, 1991.

Gozal, D, Shoseyev, D, & Keens, TG. Inspiratory pressures with CO_2 stimulation and weaning from mechanical ventilation in children. American Review of Respiratory Diseases, 147:256–261, 1993.

Haley, SM, Baryza, MJ, & Blanchard, Y. Functional and naturalistic frameworks in assessing physical and motor disablement. In Wilhelm, IJ (Ed.), Physical Therapy Assessment in Early Infancy. New York: Churchill Livingstone, 1993, pp. 225–256.

Haney, C, & Allingham, TM. Nursing care of the neonate receiving high-frequency jet ventilation. Journal of Obstetric, Gynecologic, and Neonatal Nursing, 21:87–195, 1992.

Hodgkin, JE, Gray, LS, & Burton, GG. Techniques of ventilatory weaning. In Burton, GG, & Hodgkin, JE (Eds.), Respiratory care: A Guide to Clinical Practice. Philadelphia: JB Lippincott, 1984, pp. 648–655.

Hunt, J, Cooper, B, & Tooley, W. Very low birthweight infants at 8 and 11 years of age: Role of neonatal illness and family status. Pediatrics, 82:596–603, 1988.

Jackson, DF. Nursing care plan: Home management of children with BPD. Pediatric Nursing, 12:342–348, 1986.

Kao, LC, Durand, DJ, & Nickerson, BG. Improving pulmonary function does not decrease oxygen consumption in infants with bronchopulmonary dysplasia. Journal of Pediatrics, 112:616–621, 1988.

Kirby, RR, Banner, MJ, & Downs, JB (Eds.). Clinical Applications of Ventilatory Support. New York: Churchill Livingstone, 1990, pp. 173–198.

Knisely, AS, Leal, SM, & Singer, DB. Abnormalities of diaphragmatic muscle in neonates with ventilated lungs. Journal of Pediatrics, 113:1074–1077, 1988.

Kolobe, THA. Working with families of children with disabilities. Pediatric Physical Therapy, 4:57–62, 1992.

Kurzner, SI, Garg, M, Bautista, DB, Sargent, CW, Bowman, M, & Keen, TG. Growth failure in bronchopulmonary dysplasia: Elevated metabolic rates and pulmonary mechanics. Journal of Pediatrics, 112:73–80, 1988.

Lantos, JD, & Kohrman, AF. Ethical aspects of pediatric home care. Pediatrics, 89:920–924, 1992.

Leonard, BJ, Brus, JD, & Choi, T. Medicaid model waiver program. Public Health Reports, 104:465–472, 1989.

MacKinnon, JA, Perlman, M, Kirpalani, H, Rehan, V, Sauve, R, & Kovacs, L. Spinal cord injury at birth: Diagnostic and prognostic data in twenty-two patients. Journal of Pediatrics, 122:431–437, 1993.

Mallory, GB, & Stillwell, PC. The ventilator-dependent child: Issues in diagnosis and management. Archives of Physical Medicine and Rehabilitation, 72:43–55, 1991.

Meisels, SJ, Plunkett, JW, Roloff, DW, Pasick, PL, & Steifel, GS. Growth and development of preterm infants with respiratory distress syndrome and bronchopulmonary dysplasia. Pediatrics, 77:345–352, 1986.

Northway, WH. Observations on bronchopulmonary dysplasia. Journal of Pediatrics, 95:815–817, 1979.

Null, D, Berman, LS, & Clark, R. Neonatal and pediatric ventilatory support. In Kirby, RR, Banner, MJ, & Downs, JB (Eds.), Clinical Applications of Ventilatory Support. New York: Churchill Livingstone, 1990, pp. 199–238.

Office of Technology Assessment: Technology-Dependent Children: Home vs Hospital Care. A Technical Memorandum. Washington, DC: U.S. Government Printing Office, 1987.

Pagtakhan, RD, & Chernick, V. Intensive care for respiratory disorders. In Kendig, EL, & Chernick, V (Eds.), Disorders of the Respiratory Tract in Children (4th ed.). Philadelphia: WB Saunders, 1983, pp. 145–168.

Perel, A, & Stock, MC. Introduction to ventilatory support. In Perel, A, & Stock, MC (Eds.), Handbook of Mechanical Ventilatory Support. Baltimore: Williams & Wilkins, 1992, pp. 3–6.

Quint, RD, Chesterman, E, Crain, LS, Winkleby, M, & Boyce, WT. Home care for ventilator-dependent children: Psychosocial impact on the family. American Journal of Diseases in Children, 144:1238–1241, 1990.

Rasanen, J, & Downs, JB. Modes of mechanical ventilatory support. In Kirby, RR, Banner, MJ, & Downs, JB (Eds.), Clinical Applications of Ventilatory Support. New York: Churchill Livingstone, 1990, pp. 173–198.

Raulin, AM, & Shannon, KA. PNPs: Case managers for technology-dependent children. Pediatric Nursing, 12:338–340, 1986.

Resnick, MB, Armstrong, S, & Carter, RL. Developmental intervention program for high-risk premature infants: Effects on development and parent-infant interaction. Developmental & Behavioral Pediatrics, 9:73–78, 1988.

Roussos, C. Ventilatory failure and respiratory muscles. Lung Biology in Health and Diesease, 29:1253–1279, 1985.

Schaaf, RC, & Davis, WS. Promoting health and wellness in the pediatric disabled and "at risk" population. In Rothman, J, & Levine, R (Eds.), Prevention Practice: Strategies for Physical Therapy and Occupational Therapy. Philadelphia: WB Saunders, 1992, pp. 270–283.

Schafer, DS, Spalding, JB, & Bell, AP. Potential predictors of child progress as measured by the Early Intervention Developmental Profile. Journal of the Division for Early Childhood, 11(2):106–117, 1987.

Schreiner, MS, Donar, ME, & Kettrick, RG. Pediatric home ventilation. Pediatric Clinics of North America, 34:47–60, 1987.

Silvestri, JM, Weese-Mayer, DE, & Nelson, MN. Neuropsychologic abnormalities in children with congenital central hypoventilation syndrome. Journal of Pediatrics, 120:388–393, 1992.

Sinkin, RA, Cox, C, & Phelps, DL. Predicting risk for bronchopulmonary dysplasia: Selection criteria for clinical trials. Pediatrics, 86:728–736, 1990.

Slater, MA, Naqvi, M, Andrew, L, & Haynes, K. Neurodevelopment of monitored vs nonmonitored very low birth weight infants: The importance of family influences. Developmental and Behavioral Pediatrics, 8:278–285, 1987.

Speer, CP, Robertson, B, Curstedt, T, Halliday, HL, Compagnone, D, Gefeller, O, Harms, K, Herting, E, McClure, G, Reid, M, Tubman, R, Herin, P, Noack, G, Kok, J, Koppe, J, van Sonderen, L, Laufkotter, E, Kohler, W, Boenisch, H, Albrecht, K, Hanssler, L, Haim, M, Oetomo, SB, Okken, A, Altfeld, PC, Groneck, P, Kachel, W, Relier, JP, & Walti, H. Randomized European multicenter trial of surfactant replacement therapy for severe neonatal respiratory distress syndrome: Single versus multiple doses of Curosurf. Pediatrics, 89:13–20, 1992.

Tremolieres, F. Description of a ventilator. In Lemaire, F (Ed.),

Mechanical Ventilation. New York: Springer-Verlag, 1991, pp. 3–18.

Truog, WE, & Jackson, JC. Alternative modes of ventilation in the prevention and treatment of bronchopulmonary dysplasia. Clinics in Perinatology, 19:621–647, 1992.

Waring, WW. The history and physical examination. In Kendig, EL, & Chernick, V (Eds.), Disorders of the Respiratory Tract in Children. Philadelphia: WB Saunders, 1983, pp. 57–78.

Watchko, JF, Mayock, DE, Standaert, TA, & Woodrum, DE. The ventilatory pump: Neonatal and developmental issues. Advances in Pediatrics, 38:109–134, 1991.

Weese-Mayer, DE, Silvestri, JM, Menzies, LJ, Morrow-Kenny, AS, Hunt, CE, & Hauptman, SA. Congenital central hypoventilation syndrome: Diagnosis, management, and long-term outcome in thirty-two children. Journal of Pediatrics, 120:381–387, 1992.

Weinstein, MR, & Oh, W. Oxygen consumption in infants with BPD. Journal of Pediatrics, 99:958–961, 1981.

Woo, MS, Woo, MA, Gozal, D, Jansen, MT, Keens, TG, & Harper, RM. Heart rate variability in congenital central hypoventilation syndrome. Pediatric Research, 31:291–296, 1992.

Yu, VYH, Orgill, AA, Lim, SB, Bajuk, B, & Astbury, J. Growth and development of very low birthweight infants recovering from bronchopulmonary dysplasia. Archives of Disease in Childhood, 58:791–794, 1983.

Resources

Parents and professionals might be interested in the International Ventilators Users Network (IVUN), 5100 Oakland Ave, #206, St. Louis, MO 63110-1406. The IVUN is a worldwide network of ventilator users and health professionals. This group is a strong advocate for home care and long-term ventilation and provides numerous resources for professionals, patients, and families of ventilator-dependent children.

Ventilators: Alternatives for Long-Term and Home Use (A manual for people who are considering the long-term use of a ventilator at home) by E.A. Oppenheimer, M.D., and A.S. Baldwin-Meyers, R.N.C., M.S.N.

This manual provides information on many aspects of mechanical ventilation, such as the various types of ventilators, phrenic nerve pacers, and issues related to chronic mechanical ventilation. It also has an extensive bibliography and a list of organizations and equipment companies. It can be obtained by writing to Dr. E.A. Oppenheimer, Pulmonary Medicine, 4950 Sunset Blvd., Los Angeles, CA 90027-5822.

Chapter 25

Cystic Fibrosis

JO A. ASHWELL, BScPT
JENNIFER L. AGNEW-COUGHLIN, BScPT, BHK
STEPHANIE BOYD, BScPT
DINA BROOKS, BScPT, MSc

Cystic fibrosis (CF) was first defined as a clinical entity just over 50 years ago when Andersen published a paper describing the clinical course of a number of children who had died of pulmonary and digestive problems. She labeled the disorder "cystic fibrosis of the pancreas" (Andersen, 1938). This disease was thereafter classified as a disorder of exocrine gland function, influencing the respiratory system, pancreas, reproductive organs, and sweat glands. At times the first presenting sign has been the subjective report "my child tastes salty to kiss"; the "sweat test" has confirmed the diagnosis. Subsequent study and interest led to clearer understanding of the disease and a coordinated approach to treating the associated impairments. Over time the disorder that had so intrigued Andersen has come to be known as cystic fibrosis, and research has continued, yielding a vast knowledge base about this chronic illness. In 1989, a major scientific breakthrough occurred with discovery of the precise locus on chromosome 7 of the gene responsible for CF (Riordan et al., 1989). Investigations and research have followed to define the pathologic basis of the physical manifestations of CF.

Although at present the time-honored definition of this disease as the most commonly inherited life-shortening illness in the white population remains appropriate, our present growing understanding of CF may prove to temper its impact. More research needs to be done before treatment may allow people with CF to lead lives free of the complications currently implicit in this diagnosis. Current management of the manifestations of CF has however promoted improved quality of life and a better prognosis for life expectancy for people with CF (MacLusky & Levison, 1990).

Classified as a hereditary disease, CF has long been understood to be inherited in an autosomal recessive pattern (MacLusky & Levison, 1990). Two copies of the gene responsible for CF are inherited by an affected individual. Both parents of a child diagnosed with CF are, therefore, known to be carriers of at least one copy of a mutation at the gene locus responsible for CF. Those persons with one copy of the CF gene are called heterozygote carriers and are not diagnostically positive for CF.

CF is diagnosed in 1 in 2000 children born to white parents, and statistical analysis of this incidence yields a best estimate of the rate of heterozygote carriers as about 5% of the population in areas of the world where significant white populations have settled (MacLusky et al., 1987). The incidence of CF in African, African-American, and Asian peoples is considerably lower than that in whites — approximately 1 in 17,000 births in the African-American population and an estimated 1 in 90,000 births in Asian societies (MacLusky et al., 1987). Recent research and new possibilities for carrier screening are producing more precise statistical estimates of the actual incidence of individuals who are heterozygote CF carriers, suggesting that previous rates were underestimated (Witt et al., 1992). Prenatal diagnosis of CF is now sometimes possible, as is screening for carrier status, which is discussed in detail later in this chapter.

The identification in 1989 of the site of the gene responsible for CF by an international team of researchers, led by Drs. Tsui, Collins, and Riordan, was an extraordinary achievement in molecular genetics (Kerem et al., 1989). Subsequent research advances in numerous laboratories worldwide have yielded an unprecedented quantity of data on the genetic and pathologic components of CF. According to Collins (1992), the Michigan-based genetic researcher who collaborated on the CF gene discovery, more than 200 separate mutations have now been identified at the CF gene locus. There are 12 prominent or more common mutations of the gene, with mutation deltaF508 occurring the most often. These 12 mutations are responsible for 85 to 90% of documented cases of CF.

The basic molecular defect in CF has now been revealed. The CF gene product, called the cystic fibrosis transmembrane regulator (CFTR), is under extensive study with the hope that a cure for CF may result from a clear understanding of the functional defect accounted for by this protein. CFTR is an operative factor in transepithelial transport and plays a key role in chloride channel functioning. With our present level of understanding, CFTR seems to be most abundantly expressed in the apical membrane surface of epithelial cells of the respiratory, gastrointestinal, reproductive, and sweat glands (Collins, 1992). Historically, these systems have received much scrutiny as the organ systems most affected by CF, with impairments of the respiratory system representing the major cause of morbidity and mortality in this disease. Abnormal expression of the CFTR protein in airway epithelial cells is likely the primary cause of the respiratory manifestations of CF (Crystal, 1992).

The nature of the disease, its multisystemic involvement, and the variety of needs of affected individuals and their families dictate that professional intervention in the management of CF is generally concentrated in regional CF clinics. Comprehensive treatment programs for CF were only established about 30 years ago (Doershuk et al., 1964) but are now the primary mode of delivery of associated health care needs. CF centers can offer their clients the services of respirologists, gastroenterologists, physical therapists, dietitians, psychological and genetic counselors, social workers, and specialty care nursing personnel. These multidisciplinary teams are dedicated to the delivery of the most effective and palatable treatments available in promoting the optimal level of well-being for their patients with CF. The team can offer crucial support to affected families. Worldwide, CF centers are also dedicated to the collaborative process, as clinical expertise and the knowledge base expand to suggest new possibilities in the treatment of this disease and new hopes for an ultimate cure.

PATHOPHYSIOLOGY

The primary pathologic feature of CF is obstruction of mucus-secreting exocrine glands by hyperviscous secretions (MacLusky et al., 1987). Blockage of exocrine gland products prevents their delivery to target tissues and organs and creates clinical abnormalities in these body systems. The most predominantly impaired organs are the lungs and pancreas, with significant involvement of the reproductive system, sinuses, and sweat glands. An elevated level of sodium chloride in the sweat has been the principal diagnostic indicator for CF for almost 40 years (Gibson & Cooke, 1959).

The pulmonary impairments of CF are characterized by accumulation of hyperviscous secretions leading to progressive airway obstruction, secondary infection by opportunistic bacteria, inflammation, and subsequent bronchiectasis and irreversible airway damage. Airways may be further obstructed by bronchoconstriction. Impaired respiratory muscle function under conditions of malnutrition and weakness or deconditioning also impacts on the progression of the functional limitations of the respiratory system in patients with CF, as does the mechanical disadvantage that results from chronic lung hyperinflation.

The obstruction of the small airways in CF and subsequent air trapping and atelectasis result in ventilation and perfusion mismatching, which leads to hypoxemia. Long-standing hypoxemia may result in pulmonary artery hypertension and cor pulmonale or right ventricular failure. Large airway bronchiectasis combined with small airway obstruction reduces vital capacity and tidal volume and results in decreased volumes of air flow at the alveolar level and a progressively increasing arterial carbon dioxide tension ($Paco_2$), which may lead to hypercapnic respiratory failure (Yankaskas, 1992). Respiratory failure accounts for 95% of the mortality in CF (Orenstein, 1989).

Viscous secretions begin to obstruct the pancreatic duct in utero, and periductal inflammation and fibrosis cause the loss of the pancreatic exocrine function. The resulting maldigestion of fats and protein leaves the pancreatic-insufficient patient with clinical steatorrhea (Durie et al., 1984); the stools are described as bulky, frequent, and "greasy" and, perhaps most noticeably, as having a strongly offensive odor. In infancy, patients with CF can display evidence of protein–calorie malnutrition with a protruding abdomen, muscle wasting, and initial diagnosis of failure to thrive despite the reports from parents of these children's hearty appetites (MacLusky & Levison, 1990). Compensating for loss of pancreatic function remains a critical feature of management throughout these children's lives.

Another pathologic finding in CF can be the first seen, presenting clinically in the 10 to 15% of diagnosed cases who demonstrate meconium ileus as neonates (Park & Grand, 1981). Abnormal secretions resulting in an increase in viscosity have been found in analysis of in vitro tissue (Cheng et al., 1988). In combination with abnormal pancreatic function and the hyperviscous secretions of the intestinal glands, the viscosity of the meconium is altered and causes an obstruction at the distal ileum, thus preventing passage of meconium in the first neonatal days (MacLusky & Levison, 1990). Distal intestinal obstruction is seen in older patients, associated with abnormal intestinal secretions and increased adherence of mucus in the intestines (Durie, 1988).

Abnormal secretions may cause hepatobiliary involvement, recurrent pancreatitis, and, for about 7% of patients with CF, diabetes mellitus (MacLusky & Levison, 1990). Obstruction of the vas deferens causes infertility in 98% of males with CF (Taussig et al., 1972). The fertility rate in females with CF is estimated as 20 to 30% of normal (Matson & Capen, 1982).

In the upper respiratory tract, sinusitis may cause persistent headache while nasal polyps occur in 7 to 26% of CF patients and often necessitate surgical resection. There is a 50 to 80% recurrence rate of nasal polyps once polypectomy is performed (MacLusky et al., 1987). Hypertrophic pulmonary osteoarthropathy is often associated with advanced severity of pulmonary disease and is most noticeable in the clinical finding of "clubbing," which is rounded hypertrophic changes in the terminal phalanges of the fingers and toes (MacLusky & Levison, 1990).

ETIOLOGY

The etiology of CF is traced to the abnormal gene product, the CFTR protein. The exact properties of CFTR and its impairment of function in CF have been the subject of intense scientific scrutiny, escalating in intensity since the CF gene discovery. To understand the molecular pathology of CF the precise mechanism of action of CFTR needed to be clarified. Attempts were made to replicate CFTR with coordinated investigations of the structure of its DNA engineering. If correction of the basic defect in CF by transferring normally functioning genes into the CFTR gene locus can be accomplished, a cure for the impairments in CF may be possible in the near future. Research has identified a gene transfer using retrovirus mediation in vitro that corrects the cystic fibrosis defect in animal tissue (Drumm et al., 1990). An application of the corrected gene for patients with CF through methods of gene transfer into the epithelial cells is one goal of current research (Crystal, 1991). Clinical trials to investigate the feasibility of gene transfer using a mediated human adenovirus are under way. With the emerging knowledge of the chloride channel regulatory abilities of CFTR, new therapeutics aimed at normalizing the defective electrolyte transport of the airway epithelium of patients with CF look promising (Boucher, 1992).

DIAGNOSIS AND MEDICAL MANAGEMENT

Early diagnosis, including prenatal determination of the presence of CF gene mutation, has enabled researchers to follow the expression and progression of the disease from birth in many patients. Impairment of the respiratory system does not manifest immediately, and at birth the lungs appear normal on radiologic examination. In the most distal small airways, however, dilatation and hypertrophy of mucus-secreting goblet cells begins early in life and subsequent impaired mucociliary clearance can cause obstructive mucus plugs and associated air trapping and atelectasis. Signs of hyperinflation may be present on radiography. The presentation of infants with failure to thrive and nutritional losses through steatorrhea accounts for up to 85% of the cases of CF diagnosed in infancy. A history of respiratory illness such as repeated respiratory tract infections, recurrent bronchiolitis, or even pneumonia is often reported, but in 80% of newly diagnosed cases there is no known family history of CF (MacLusky & Levison, 1990).

A quantitative pilocarpine iontophoresis sweat test, an analysis of chloride levels in the sweat, is the accepted test to confirm the diagnosis of CF. Because of the quantity of sweat required to provide an accurate analysis and the difficulty in inducing adequate amounts when testing infants in the first few months of life, positive diagnosis may be delayed until a valid test can be performed. Values above 60 mEq/l of sweat chloride are considered positive for CF (MacLusky & Levison, 1990).

Screening tests for prospective parents who are known carriers (with prior offspring with CF or with CF themselves) are now possible and raise a number of ethical issues when CF is suggested neonatally. Genetic counseling is therefore available at CF centers. Analysis of the blood of known heterozygote parents and tissue from the fetus obtained through amniocentesis or chorionic villi sampling can determine the presence of the CF gene mutation common to the family history. With identity of the same pattern of inherited genetic material in the fetus as in an affected sibling there is a 98% probability the fetus is also affected (Dean et al., 1987). Mass carrier screening in prenatal populations of up to 4000 women has been undertaken in both the United States and England to investigate the value and feasibility of population screening for CF heterozygotes. In California, where 6 to 12 of the most common mutations were sought, this type of screening identified over 90 female heterozygotes. Screening of their partners revealed 5 male heterozygotes and therefore five high-risk pregnancies (Witt et al., 1992). Among adults with CF and parents of affected children, attitudes and debate about prenatal diagnosis and heterozygote screening reflect a variety of concerns. Although up to 74% of questioned adults with CF in one study reported supporting carrier testing of their siblings (Lemke et al., 1992) and 93% supported screening for carriers in the general population, only a minority saw prenatal diagnosis as an absolute indication for termination of pregnancy (Conway & Allenby, 1992). The future of carrier screening and any possible effects prenatal diagnosis may have on the incidence rate of CF remain to be seen.

Medical management of pulmonary disability in CF generally focuses on attempts to limit the effects of impairments in the disease, namely, the airway obstruction due to chronic bronchorrhea (the abnormal mucus secretions) and the progressive inflammation that is secondary to chronic bacterial colonization (MacLusky et al., 1987). Nutritional management is also vitally important because the majority of patients with CF will have some pancreatic insufficiency and therefore require enzyme supplementation to compensate for losses of enzymes crucial to fat and protein digestion. Patients are followed periodically, and quantitative sputum cultures are regularly performed. (Clinics vary as to frequency of assessment; generally, appointments are made every 3 months.) Radiologic assessment and pulmonary function testing, nutritional status, and any pattern of weight loss combined with subjective reports of treatment compliance assist the CF clinical team to gauge the ever-changing therapeutic needs of their patients with CF and to initiate treatment regimens with the aim of preventing or slowing development of the functional limitations of CF.

Throughout their lives, most people with CF battle the tendency toward malnutrition that comes from protein and calorie deficits. Special attention to a properly balanced, high-calorie diet with supplementary pancreatic enzymes requires acceptance and compliance in patients of all ages with CF but may aid in slowing the rate of deterioration of lung function. During acute episodes of respiratory exacerbations, the anorexia that accompanies the frequent racking cough, increase in mucus production, and increased work of breathing poses a challenge to provide adequate nutritional intake. Levels of resting energy expenditure are reportedly higher in patients with CF with more progressive pulmonary disease (Fried et al., 1991; Spicher et al., 1991), and this has implications for the degree of caloric input necessary for patients with advanced pulmonary dysfunction. Caloric supplementation may be necessary in the form of feedings given nasogastrically or intravenously. Nutritional management for patients with intractable weight loss can be provided by nocturnal feedings through indwelling gastrostomy or jejunostomy tubes (MacLusky & Levison, 1990).

Most of the morbidity seen in CF is associated with deteriorating pulmonary status; medical intervention is, therefore, focused on attempts to influence the rate of progression of the pathogenesis of pulmonary dysfunction in CF. Antibiotic therapy appears to have significantly influenced the effects of the chronic endobronchial colonization that typifies CF and has been a mainstay of treatment regimens for 30 years (MacLusky & Levison, 1990). Sputum cultures show colonization by a number of organisms in a common pattern that changes with severity of disease and age of the patient. *Staphylococcus aureus, Pseudomonas aeruginosa, P. cepacia, Haemophilus influenzae,* and *Klebsiella* are the organisms most commonly seen.

Combinations of colonizing organisms are very common, particularly when disease severity and age of the patient advances. Prophylactic antibiotics are advocated by some but remain controversial. Inhaled antibiotics, such as the aminoglycosides tobramycin and gentamicin, which have shown some effect on *Pseudomonas* species, have not shown universal therapeutic value (MacLusky et al., 1989). Ceftazidime and aminoglycosides are used intravenously to target *Pseudomonas* infections in the hospitalized patient, but eradication of this organism is rare. *P. aeruginosa* is now the most common pathogen in CF, with reported clinic rates as high as 70% of patients affected (Corey et al., 1984a). Pharmacologic therapies are needed to inhibit the adherence of the initiating bacteria in *P. aeruginosa* colonization since this pathogen has demonstrated an extraordinary affinity for the airways of patients with CF (Prince, 1992). Several of the virulent products of *P. aeruginosa* cause airway inflammation and progressive epithelial destruction and therefore contribute significantly to the severity of the pulmonary impairment in CF (MacLusky & Levison, 1990). Anti-inflammatory corticosteroids may slow the progressive pulmonary deterioration (Auerbach et al., 1985) but are associated with numerous side effects when used on a long-term basis and require careful consideration before use.

Although 25 to 50% of patients with CF have evidence of increased airway hyperactivity, the mechanism for bronchoconstriction in CF appears to differ from that of asthma (MacLusky & Levison, 1990). When assessed by methacholine challenge, higher doses are necessary to produce a response and the bronchodilation achieved through salbutamol (Ventolin) therapy is both slower and less dramatic than in patients with asthma (Skorecki et al., 1976). Evaluation by exercise challenge, using a bicycle ergometer or treadmill and using the change in peak expiratory flow rate as a measure of lung function, indicates that a majority of children with CF demonstrate bronchial hyperreactivity with the increased respiratory effort of exercise (Day & Mearns, 1973). Inhaled sympathomimetic agents do demonstrate the effect of bronchodilation in many patients and may also improve mucociliary function and therefore serve to complement airway clearance techniques (Ormerod et al., 1980) (Fig. 25–1). When used immediately before exercise or pulmonary physical therapy, bronchodilators may help to prevent induced bronchospasm and are therefore often prescribed as an important adjunct to physical therapy (MacLusky & Levison,

FIGURE 25–1. Receiving inhalation therapy in hospital.

1990). Anticholinergics, such as ipratropium bromide (Atrovent), have also been shown to be effective bronchodilators in patients with CF (Wiebicke et al., 1990).

PHYSICAL THERAPY

Providing effective pulmonary hygiene by promoting improved clearance of mucus-obstructed airways benefits the pulmonary environment, allowing for improvements in gas exchange and limiting the tissue damage associated with infection. Physical therapy techniques to promote airway clearance include postural drainage and manual or mechanical percussion of segmental lobes, vibratory facilitation of ciliary function, directed breathing techniques such as the forced expiration technique and autogenic drainage, and use of positive expiratory pressures (PEP) through valve-equipped facial masks, as well as exercise prescription, assisted coughing, and postural realignment exercises.

Much more research is needed to scientifically support the efficacy of the use of pulmonary physical therapy modalities in CF. A comparative study of the current literature that we undertook demonstrated a need for more adequate controls, randomized design and sampling larger sample sizes, and use of valid outcome measures. The studies reviewed were evaluated and classified according to the level of evidence supported by the research design as proposed by Sackett (1986). Our analysis suggested support for exercise, "conventional" physical therapy (postural drainage, percussion, and vibration), and PEP mask therapies in treatment of children with CF in chronic stages of the disease when pulmonary function test (PFT) results were used as an outcome measure. In acute exacerbations of respiratory status, both PEP mask therapy and conventional physical therapy showed some evidence of improving pulmonary function scores. A moderate cycling program used to replace two of the three daily conventional physical therapy sessions produced equivalent improvement in PFT results. More critical analysis is needed before the effectiveness of autogenic drainage is known, but new studies may clarify its significance as an airway clearance technique.

In this chapter considerations for choosing appropriate treatment modalities for patients with CF are outlined. An increasing number of people with CF are reaching the third and even fourth decades of life (Orenstein, 1989), and surgical advances in lung transplantation offer hope of prolonging life for some people with chronic pulmonary disabilities. Physical therapists are serving an expanded role in treatment programs for people with cystic fibrosis. It is of crucial importance that clinical decisions be directed by careful consideration of the available scientific evidence and that therapists continue to seek out the means to scientifically evaluate empiric experiences of using various physical therapy modalities in the management of CF.

LUNG TRANSPLANTATION

Organ transplantation is now a treatment option in many different terminal illnesses, including CF. In the past decade advances in surgical technique and postoperative care with improved immunosuppressive therapies have given some patients with CF a new lease on life. (See Chapter 27 for a more detailed discussion of the involvement of physical therapy in postsurgical care.)

Heart-lung transplantation for selected patients with CF experiencing respiratory failure has been performed in England with varying measures of success since 1984. Seventy-nine patients with CF received heart-lung transplants between 1984 and 1991 at one British hospital; the actuarial survival for the group was 69% at 1 year and 54% at 2 years after surgery (Khaghani et al., 1991). Improvement in postoperative lung function was maintained by the patients who survived, and the mean forced expiratory volume in 1 second (FEV_1) of this group was 75% (of the predicted value for normal subjects) at 1 year (Khaghani et al., 1991).

In North America, both heart-lung and double-lung transplants have been performed on patients with CF with end-stage pulmonary disease. The Toronto Lung Transplant Group were pioneers in this field and performed the world's first successful double-lung transplant in 1987 (Pizer, 1991). In 1992, the St. Louis International Lung Transplant Registry reported that 170 lung transplants had been performed on patients with CF, including 29 pediatric cases (Trulock, 1992). The actuarial 1-year and 2-year survival rates for the entire group were 64% and 59%, respectively (Trulock, 1992). Complications arising from postoperative infections or development of obliterative bronchiolitis accounted for most of the mortality in the transplanted group (Egan, 1992). It has been postulated that the development of obliterative bronchiolitis may be evidence of chronic rejection since there has been some success in arresting its development with immunosuppressive augmentation (Paradowski, 1992). The problem with malabsorption that patients with CF have dictates difficulties with the therapeutic regimen for adequate immunosuppression after transplantation. High doses of immunosuppressive drugs, such as cyclosporine, must be taken. One major complication of large doses of cyclosporine is the development of nephrotoxicity (observed in 10% of one transplant center's patients), necessitating careful postoperative monitoring (Paradowski, 1992).

Criteria for acceptance on a waiting list for lung transplantation include severe pulmonary disease with marked hypoxemia, no significant dysfunction or disease of other vital organs, a history of compliance with medical treatment, and an acceptable psychosocial profile (Patterson & Cooper, 1988). There were 702 persons registered on the February 1992 U.S. lung transplant waiting list, and the average wait for transplant was recorded as 236 days (Trulock, 1992). A referral for transplant (and acceptance onto the waiting list) must be made early enough to allow for a substantial wait for a suitable donor. The results of PFTs and blood gas measurements are correlated with mortality in patients with CF; 2-year mortality rates are greater than 50% in patients with an FEV_1 of less than 30% of predicted value, and an arterial oxygen pressure (Pao_2) of less than 55 mm Hg or a $Paco_2$ of more than 50 mm Hg (Kerem et al., 1992). Careful consideration of these parameters is therefore essential in assessment of suitability for transplantation. The long wait for donor organs also creates a need for the development of a preoperative program of conditioning for these patients. Participation in a pre-operative rehabilitation program is a component of the lung transplantation program in many centers. These conditioning programs are designed to optimize the patient's functional ability and exercise tolerance as well as helping to maintain emotional well-being during the long wait for a transplant (Craven et al., 1990). Physical therapists play a primary role in development and implementation of these exercise programs, which are described later in this chapter.

Double-lung transplantation is now performed by bilateral anterolateral thoracotomies using bilateral submammary incisions as first described in 1990 (Pasque et al., 1990). The lungs are transplanted as sequential single-lung grafts. The lung with the worst pulmonary function is replaced first while oxygenation and ventilation are maintained by the native lung. Replacement of the second lung can then proceed with the newly implanted lung supporting the patient (Winton, 1992). Use of this technique has reduced to 30 to 35% the number of patients requiring anticoagulation and cardiopulmonary bypass during surgery (Winton, 1992). This surgical innovation has also reduced the degree of complication from perioperative bleeding, which can be a significant problem for patients with CF because of the presence of inflammatory adhesions within the pleural space (Winton, 1992).

Single-lung transplants are not performed on patients with CF because the remaining native lung continues to be ventilated after transplantation and its overexpansion will compress the transplanted lung (MacLusky & Levison, 1990). Contamination of the native lung could also spread infection to the transplanted lung (Egan, 1992).

IMPAIRMENTS

Assessment and Prognosis

The primary physiologic abnormalities in CF include 1) a dysfunctional chloride channel in trans-epithelial electrolyte transport creating abnormal increases in the concentrations of sodium and chloride in serous gland secretions; 2) blocked exocrine gland function due to obstruction by hyperviscous secretions; and 3) an extraordinary susceptibility to chronic endobronchial colonization by specific groups of bacteria, apparently compounded by impaired or deficient ciliary clearance. Although patients with CF show marked differences in levels of clinical impairment, all patients with CF have these three abnormalities (MacLusky & Levison, 1990).

The degree of functional limitation that these impairments impose varies greatly among people with CF. Proper measurement of these limitations is crucial to determining the proper interventions. Assessment techniques to quantify the impairments seen in CF measure the functioning of the respiratory and gastrointestinal systems and the limitations in exercise tolerance. Quality of life questionnaires and school attendance records provide information on the patient's perceived level of disability.

A number of clinical scoring systems have been proposed in an attempt to standardize assessment of CF. The most frequently used is the Shwachman score (Shwachman & Kulczycki, 1958). Points are awarded under four categories: 1) chest radiography, 2) growth and nutrition, 3) pulmonary (physical findings and cough), and 4) case history, which includes subjective reports of activity tolerance. Findings that reflect no impairment or limitation ("normal" findings) are awarded 25 points; therefore a "perfect" Shwachman score is 100. The lower the score, the worse the clinical condition of the patient. A patient scoring 40 points may present with an increased anterior-posterior diameter on chest radiography with atelectatic patches and noticeable hyperinflation, subnormal weight and height, poor muscle strength, marked reduction of fat on skinfold testing, chronic productive cough, rapid respiration and pulse, moderate to severe overexpansion of the lungs, rattles and wheezes on auscultation, breathlessness on exertion, listlessness or lethargy, poor school attendance, limited exercise tolerance, postural abnormalities of protracted shoulders and extended neck, clubbing of the phalanges, and poor appetite or anorexia (Shwachman & Kulczycki, 1958) (Fig. 25–2). This scoring system has good interobserver reliability and correlates well with PFT scoring systems (Lewiston & Moss, 1987), permitting use in clinical comparisons of disease morbidity.

Assessing Pulmonary Impairment

PFT scores provide incremental knowledge of the extent of bronchial obstruction and a means of tracing the degree of restriction of lung function. PFTs include measurement of static and dynamic lung volumes and air flow. Evidence of reactive airway disease can be quantified. Spirometry can be used to record acute deterioration of pulmonary function and to monitor recovery. Vital capacity (VC), total lung capacity (TLC), inspiratory reserve volume (IRV), and expiratory reserve volume (ERV) are directly measured by spirometry. Spirometry can measure air flow rates during different

FIGURE 25–2. An example of postural changes in one individual: elevation of the shoulders and an increased anterior-posterior diameter of the chest. Also note intercostal indrawing.

phases of expiration, yielding an indication of the amount of bronchial obstruction. The measure of FEV_1 chronicles the early portion of expiration, whereas FEV_3 reflects the terminal stages of a maximal expiratory effort. FEV_1 is frequently reported as a ratio to forced vital capacity (FVC). In a healthy individual, FEV_1/FVC is 0.70 to 0.80, indicating that 70 to 80% of the FVC is expired in the first second of a forced exhalation (Miller, A, 1987). Changes in this ratio can reflect an obstructed expiratory air flow.

Analysis of spirometric flow–volume curves enables the early detection of abnormalities in the smaller airways (Orenstein, 1989). Convexity of the curve in relation to the volume axis is one of the most sensitive indicators of early obstruction of the peripheral airways (Mellins, 1969). $FEF_{25-75\%}$ is the measurement of flow between 25 and 75% of vital capacity and reflects air flow at high lung vol-

umes. Miller (1987) suggests that $FEF_{25-75\%}$ is more sensitive than FEV_1 or FEV_1/FVC in detecting changes in small airway obstruction and provides an important indication of early pulmonary disease in individuals with CF because initial abnormalities involve the small airways (Mellins et al., 1968). Timed volumes at high lung volumes (e.g., FEV_1) may remain within normal limits because the contribution of the small airways to overall resistance is low (Kattan, 1987). FEV_1 is therefore not a sensitive test in early lung disease but indicates obstruction of the central bronchi and becomes markedly abnormal as disease progresses (MacLusky & Levison, 1990).

With more severe pulmonary dysfunction, air trapping results in increases in residual volume (RV) and functional reserve capacity (FRC) (both are measured by a more complicated PFT than spirometry) and an increase in RV/TLC. Restrictive disease can be reflected in decreases in TLC and VC (Altose, 1979). The presence of both restrictive and obstructive components of pulmonary dysfunction may compensate for each other in some measurements (Miller, WF, et al., 1987). For example, restrictive disease (in the absence of an obstructive component) results in a normal RV/TLC and obstructive disease (in the absence of a restrictive component) results in an increase in this ratio. When both components coexist, RV/TLC "may not reflect the anatomic changes" (Miller, WF, et al., 1987).

Spirometry is the simplest type of PFT performed in hospital or clinic. Spirometric measurements are all generated by "effort-dependent" means, however, and cannot be used as a test for young children. Children younger than age 6 cannot perform the necessary forced expirations in a reliable way. Modifications to the classic methods of measuring ventilatory parameters in infants and young children are described in the literature (Buist et al., 1980; Doershuk et al., 1970; England, 1988; Sammut & Morgan, 1987; Taussig, 1977; and Tepper et al., 1988).

In older children and adults, many other factors, such as sputum retention, poor nutrition, and fatigue, can influence the individual's performance on spirometric PFTs. Notably, many children with CF show performance scores on repeat tests that have a significantly greater range of variability than that of scores of normal test subjects (Cooper et al., 1990). Interpretation of the pulmonary function of an individual with CF therefore also must include other PFTs, such as the closed-circuit helium dilution method, the open-circuit nitrogen washout technique, or a method colloquially known as the "body box"—total-body plethysmography. Ruppel (1991) provides detailed descriptions of these tests. In the plethysmograph, the volume of air is a constant; the test measures the changes in air pressure within the sealed chamber as the patient breathes through a mouthpiece. These measures yield an accurate calculation of the patient's lung volumes, the FRC and RV (Altose, 1979). Some claustrophobia may be experienced by subjects undergoing testing in the "body box," and plethysmography may not be appropriate for all young children.

The National Institute of Health's comparative review of 307 cases of CF reported that PFT scores showed a common pattern: progressive declines in flow rates and VC and an increase in the RV/TLC ratio, correlating with clinically gauged worsening of disease (di Sant'Agnese & Davis, 1979). As pulmonary disease becomes progressively more severe, deteriorating PFT scores can be used to help predict life expectancy. In one study patients with poor arterial gases and an FEV_1 of less than 30% of predicted value had 2-year mortality rates of greater than 50% (Kerem et al., 1992). Individuals with CF demonstrate a characteristic decline in midexpiratory flow rate ($FEF_{25-75\%}$); noting the rate of this decline becomes an important prognostic indicator (Gurwitz et al., 1979). Steadily worsening PFT scores reliably correlate with declining clinical condition and are used as an indicator in assessment for lung transplantation (Khaghani et al., 1991).

Progressive hypoxemia is one of the earliest signs of increasing pulmonary disease and can occur before any other detectable abnormality in lung function (Lamarre et al., 1972). Mucous plugging and bronchiolitis in the patient's airways cause ventilation-perfusion abnormalities, and the subsequent hypoxemia worsens as severity of the obstruction increases (MacLusky & Levison, 1990). Further declines in arterial oxygenation can occur during sleep so blood gases may have to be monitored throughout the night to assess the need for nocturnal supplementation of oxygen (Muller et al., 1980). Increased oxygen demands during exercise can be a contributing factor to hypoxemia in the patient with CF. Although arterial blood gas measures are considered the "gold standard" in blood gas analysis (Zadai, 1992), they are not commonly used in patients with CF because of their invasive nature. Other noninvasive techniques such as pulse oximetry are preferred. Pulse oximetry to gauge the level of oxygen saturation in the blood as the patient performs exercise contributes to assessment of the suitability of supplemental oxygen during exercise.

Other changes in blood gas readings forewarn of serious disability. Hypercapnia in CF indicates advanced pulmonary disease and carries a poor prognosis. In a study of survival patterns of patients with CF who demonstrated hypercapnia, it was found that morbidity usually occurred within 1 year of the development of chronic hypercapnia (Wagener et al., 1980).

Chest radiographs can provide detailed evidence of the progressive nature of pulmonary disease in CF. In the initial stages of pulmonary involvement, the chest radiograph may reveal signs of hyperinflation and peribronchial thickening. As the disease progresses, bronchiectasis can become apparent, particularly in the upper lobes, and pulmonary infiltrates appear as nodular shadows on radiographs. With severe pulmonary disease the hyperexpanded lungs can precipitate flattening of the diaphragm, thoracic kyphosis, and bowing of the sternum, all detectable on radiograph (MacLusky & Levison, 1990) (Fig. 25–3). Confirmation of the development of a pneumothorax can also be provided by examining the chest radiographs. When pulmonary disease is advanced, pulmonary artery hypertrophy may be noticed on radiography as a sign of the pulmonary hypertension associated with cor pulmonale (MacLusky & Levison, 1990).

Cultures from sputum of a patient with CF identify the variety of bacteria that has infected the lower respiratory tract (Gilljam et al., 1986). Sensitivity studies can then be performed to identify effective antibiotic therapies (Orenstein, 1989). CF centers perform regular sputum bacteriology tests to ensure adequate antibiotic coverage for their patients and to help monitor the state of bacterial colonization (MacLusky et al., 1987).

Physical examination of the patient also renders valuable information. Chest assessment includes inspection, palpation, percussion, and auscultation. Inspection can reveal postural abnormalities, modifications of breathing pattern (Fig. 25–4), or signs of respiratory distress. Evidence of a chronic productive cough may be apparent. Evaluation of the comparative dimensions of the chest in the anterior-posterior and transverse planes may reveal the barrel chest deformity common to obstructive lung diseases (Humberstone, 1990). Palpation and accurate interpretation of the findings of tactile fremitus will reveal atelectasis, pneumothorax, or large airway secretions (Humberstone, 1990). Evaluation of the resonance pattern of the chest, as demonstrated by audible changes on percussion, can provide an indication of abnormally dense areas of the lungs (Humberstone, 1990).

Age of the patient may highly influence the reliability and clinical usefulness of different components of the physical examination. In an infant, measurement of chest wall expansion may be diffi-

FIGURE 25-3. Two chest radiographs of same individual showing marked deterioration over course of 8 years. *A,* On diagnosis there is evidence of bronchial wall thickening and slight prominence of pulmonary arteries. *B,* At the preterminal stage there is diffuse bilateral bronchiectasis and fibrosis, with severe hyperinflation and bilateral areas of consolidation.

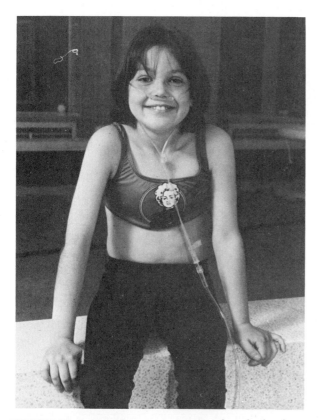

FIGURE 25-4. Use of accessory muscles of respiration is apparent on physical inspection.

cult and percussion may not be appropriate (Crane, 1990).

Careful auscultation of the chest can contribute information on the quality of air flow and evidence of obstruction in different areas of the lungs. Reduced ventilation is suggested by decreased breath sounds or presence of inspiratory crackles (also called rales). If crackles are heard throughout the ventilatory cycle, it suggests impaired secretion clearance. Diffuse airway obstruction may present as polyphonic wheezing (Humberstone, 1990).

The examiner needs to be aware that chronically hyperinflated lungs tend to mask or make it difficult to hear adventitious sounds on auscultation (Humberstone, 1990). It is also important to note that use of a stethoscope, described as the "most frequently used tool in medicine" (Loudon, 1987), is not consistent or reliable among health care providers (Pasterkamp et al., 1987). Validity and reliability of auscultation may be affected by a disparity in nomenclature, the quality of the stethoscope used, and a lack of correlation between pathologic findings and lung sounds (Aweida & Kelsey, 1989). When various health care workers were compared, significant differences were noted in the terminology used to describe tape-recorded adventitious sounds (Pasterkamp et al., 1987). Despite auscultation's limitations in interobserver reliability, it continues to serve as a valuable element of clinical assessment. Familiarization with the usual pattern of a patient's lung sounds can be a critical component of assessment because an alteration of the typical pattern may signal a pulmonary change that might otherwise have gone undetected.

The long-term prognosis of CF patients with significant pulmonary disease worsens when there is also evidence of protein–calorie malnutrition (Park & Grand, 1981). Patients who are pancreatic-insufficient need oral supplementary enzymes to enable them to absorb adequate nutrients from their diet and prevent the devastating effects of malnutrition. Identifying the need for enzyme supplementation is, therefore, a critical component in the treatment of CF. Pancreatic function may be determined by a number of testing methods, including fecal fat assessment, pancreatic substrate assays, and direct collection of pancreatic secretions by duodenal intubation (MacLusky & Levison, 1990). Individuals with CF who have significant preservation of pancreatic function and therefore can maintain normal fat absorption have less pulmonary dysfunction and a better prognosis than those individuals who have pancreatic insufficiency (Corey et al., 1984b).

A number of clinicians and researchers have examined various prognostic indicators in CF. Sustaining adequate nutritional requirements to ensure the maintenance of appropriate growth percentiles is one such indicator (Corey et al., 1984b). Other factors that are associated with a preferred prognosis include single organ involvement at diagnosis, absent or single organism sputum colonization, and a normal chest radiograph 1 year after diagnosis. Multiple organ involvement, abnormal chest radiographs at diagnosis, colonization of multiple organisms in the sputum, a falloff from typical growth curves, and recurrent hemoptysis are all factors associated with a poor prognosis. There also appears to be a gender bias in severity of disease expression, with male patients possessing a better prognosis than their female counterparts (MacLusky et al., 1987).

PHYSICAL THERAPY: ASSESSMENT AND TREATMENT

Infancy

A diagnosis of CF for their child can mean many things to parents. At the most basic level, it means they have a child with "special needs," and those needs can be seen to influence the family dynamics (Lloyd-Still & Lloyd-Still, 1983). At the time of diagnosis, education needs to be provided for the family and this seems best achieved by regional CF centers, because a number of different specialty services can be provided in one place. A physical therapist at a CF center is part of a cohesive team of interested investigators and caregivers. Educating the patients and their families while assessing and treating the myriad of complications in this disease is the ongoing goal of a CF center's staff.

PREVENTING DISABILITY: PARENTAL EDUCATION

At the time of diagnosis the child's family members are forced to familiarize themselves with CF and both the psychological and practical demands implicit with this diagnosis. Treatment often needs to be implemented immediately, and the family needs help in making the necessary adjustments and provisions to ensure compliance with any suggested therapeutic regimen. Physical therapists ascertain which essential elements of the child's care must be addressed by them and then provide instruction for the family in the proper administration of the physical therapy modalities that appear appropriate. The therapist needs to demonstrate sensitivity and equanimity while interacting with these children and their families, remembering that this is a very stressful time for those involved and that what the family may "hear" can differ from what is actually said to them (Maxwell, 1991).

What families seem to need most is information that acknowledges the seriousness of the disease while still emphasizing the likelihood of a happy and fulfilling family life. Developing the types of strategies that permit some flexibility in treatment regimens promotes a better integration of the child's treatment needs into the family's routines (Maxwell, 1991). Parents may have many concerns and a host of questions and can be especially confused by all the uncertainty that typifies the disease. Since the progression of CF is so variable in each case, an ongoing assessment of the child's status is the only way to ensure meeting the child's individual requirements. This means that the family members must have continued association with the CF center and need to appreciate their role as functioning members of the caregiving team.

Children with a chronic condition have been shown to have increased risk of psychosocial dysfunction, particularly when parental anxiety is overwhelming (Cappelli et al., 1989; Green & Solnit, 1964). Since excessive parental overprotection is strongly linked to the existence of psychosocial maladjustment in children, the parents of a child with CF need to be alerted to the dangers of unnecessarily shielding their child from aspects of normal life. In infancy, this may take the form of overdressing the child to guard against drafts or neglecting to allow the child to participate in normal exploratory play. Physical therapists need to reassure parents that infants with CF have the same requirements as other infants with respect to physical and emotional development. Excellent reference materials are available in most CF centers. Teaching manuals, designed to supplement the information imparted by the CF center staff, are often distributed to families and can be made available to other interested caregivers such as child-care workers or school teachers. Orenstein's book (1989) *Cystic Fibrosis: A Guide for Patient and Family* is highly recommended.

MANAGEMENT OF IMPAIRMENT

In the neonate, the most frequently seen symptoms of CF are meconium ileus, malabsorption of nutrients, and failure to thrive, all of which are associated with the gastrointestinal tract (Rosenstein, 1984). Overt pulmonary involvement is not apparent in the neonatal period, since the lungs are morphologically normal at birth (Hardy et al., 1989; MacLusky & Levison, 1990). Within a few months, however, some infants with CF will develop signs of impaired respiratory function, presenting with symptoms suggesting bronchiolitis. Pronounced wheeze, an indication of hyperactive airways, is sometimes apparent, and chest radiographs can reveal evidence of hyperinflation (Phillips & David, 1987). Obstruction of air flow in these infants may be related to airway inflammation, mucosal edema, copious mucus secretions, and increased airway tone (Tepper, 1992). The bronchioles are considered the main site of air flow obstruction in infancy (Taussig et al., 1984).

Measurements to assess possible limitation of pulmonary function cannot be taken in the conventional way (e.g., spirometry) in this population; therefore, researchers have had to modify standard methods to accommodate testing in this age group. Infants with CF demonstrate low values of pulmonary compliance (Phelan et al., 1969), decreased lung compliance, and a less homogeneous distribution of ventilation when compared with normal controls (Tepper et al., 1988). Tepper and colleagues (1987) found these changes present in both symptomatic and asymptomatic infants. Abnormalities in flow–volume curves (Godfrey et al., 1983) and low values of maximal expiratory flow (Hiatt et al., 1988) indicate that the limitations to air flow in infancy are associated with bronchoconstriction (Hardy et al., 1989). Infants with CF have indeed displayed altered bronchial tone after the administration of a bronchodilator, as revealed by the fact that air flow rates showed significant in-

creases not seen in a control group (Hiatt et al., 1988). Methacholine challenge testing also revealed heightened airway responsiveness (Ackerman et al., 1991).

These research studies have yielded valuable insight into the early pulmonary manifestations of CF in infancy. The formal PFTs used in these studies, however, are not feasible or practical for the infant population of most clinics or CF centers. Assessment of pulmonary involvement in infancy is usually limited to physical examination findings, history of respiratory symptoms, and chest radiographs. Carefully observing for signs of respiratory distress, such as nasal flaring, expiratory grunting, retractions of the chest wall, tachypnea, pallor, or cyanosis, produces an indication of respiratory status. Auscultation of an infant or young child is less than ideal owing to the deceptively easy transmission of sounds from the close structures underlying the thin chest wall (Crane, 1990), but careful auscultation is necessary to ascertain if there is any evidence of wheezing. Changes visible on radiography are the most reliable indication of early pulmonary involvement, because it has been demonstrated that air flow obstruction may precede the presence of overt respiratory symptoms and because lack of cooperation in this population diminishes the reliability of the physical examination. Historical accounts of respiratory illness must also be carefully considered.

It has been suggested that the rate of deterioration of pulmonary function in individuals with CF might be slowed by early initiation of treatment (Taussig et al., 1984). Since research has shown changes in respiratory patterns and mechanics in asymptomatic infants newly diagnosed with CF (Tepper et al., 1988), these findings suggest that early therapeutic intervention might actually delay the onset of overt symptoms of respiratory impairment (Eid et al., 1991). The value of initiating pulmonary treatment before development of symptoms remains controversial, however, and there is little documentation supporting the prophylactic benefit following from commencement of physical therapy before the onset of significant pulmonary disease.

A study was conducted to evaluate the combined effect of a bronchodilator and chest physical therapy on infants newly diagnosed with CF, addressing the controversy surrounding treatment for asymptomatic children (Hardy et al., 1989). Baseline, preintervention measurements of the mechanics and energetics of breathing were obtained for all subjects. Twenty minutes after the inhalation of a bronchodilator, chest physical therapy was given to the subjects, consisting of 20 minutes of chest percussions and vibrations applied in five different postural drainage positions. Immediately after the physical therapy session, repeat pulmonary function measurements were taken. A majority of the infants (10 of 13) demonstrated decreases from baseline values in pulmonary resistance, with subsequent decreases in the work of breathing, after the administration of the bronchodilator and chest physical therapy (Hardy et al., 1989). The researchers postulated that the bronchodilator relieved subclinical bronchospasm and aided the reduction of mucosal edema, and that chest physical therapy, assisting the immature mucociliary system, was effective in mobilizing secretions, thereby improving the patency of the airways (Hardy et al., 1989). The possibility of initiating effective therapeutic procedures before pulmonary dysfunction has caused significant disability is intriguing. When serial PFTs are possible, objective measures of the progression of impairment and the effects of specific treatments may provide future evidence of the efficacy of early intervention (Hardy et al., 1989).

Prevention of obstructive mucus plugging is the initial goal of pulmonary physical therapy in this population. The primary modalities used for promotion of clearance of secretions for infants with CF are postural drainage, percussion, and vibrations. The physiologic rationale and precise methodology of these modalities are well described in most comprehensive texts on physical therapy (e.g., Frownfelter, 1987; Irwin & Tecklin, 1990; Mackenzie, 1989), but important modifications to the proper use of these modalities for infants will be discussed.

In obstructive airway diseases such as CF, the effectiveness of the antireflux mechanism at the esophagogastric junction is reduced (Orenstein & Orenstein, 1988). The increases in intra-abdominal pressure that can be associated with coughing also promote gastroesophageal reflux (Scott et al., 1985). Thirty-five percent of newly diagnosed infants with CF had symptomatic gastroesophageal reflux in one study (Vinocur et al., 1985), and 24-hour esophageal monitoring revealed abnormalities in 10 successive infants newly diagnosed with CF in another (Dab & Malfroot, 1988). Since gastroesophageal reflux can result in aspiration of gastric contents, head-down positions for postural drainage may have to be modified. Timing the physical therapy around feeding schedules may also be necessary to reduce the risk of gastroesophageal reflux. Postural drainage positions are easily achieved by arranging the infant in the required manner on the caregiver's lap. Holding the small child in this way also seems to offer the child an extra measure of

security. Adapting hand position (by "tenting" of the middle finger) suits the application of percussion on a tiny chest wall. The applied force of percussion should vary with size and condition of the infant, and conscientious monitoring of the infant's response to treatment should guide the amount of vigor used in percussion. Timing of manual vibrations to coincide with the expirations of an infant is difficult owing to the infant's rapid respiratory rate, and this technique may be very difficult to teach to parents.

Education for the family in the application of prescribed physical therapy modalities should be ongoing. Periodically asking the parent or caregiver to demonstrate treatment positions and manual technique allows the therapist to identify possible problems with proper application. In some CF centers the physical therapist is also responsible for ordering, demonstrating, and arranging for the maintenance of the equipment necessary for the aerosol delivery of medications. Instruction in the care and use of these nebulizers is vitally important to ensure correct delivery of prescribed medications.

Compliance with any suggested therapeutic regimen requires commitment on the part of the caregiver. The demands of caring for a child with CF can seem extreme when considering the extra attention to nutritional issues, medications, and physical therapy that this diagnosis entails. Signs of excessive stress or evidence that the family is having difficulty in coping with the caregiving requirements may become obvious. Referral to a social worker might help identify the family in crisis. Social workers can then aid the family in developing strategies to enable adjustment to the various challenges that lie ahead of them as they nurture their child with CF.

Preschool- and School-Aged Period

PREVENTION OF DISABILITY

Approximately 75% of children with CF are now diagnosed before their third birthday (Lloyd-Still & Lloyd-Still, 1983). When there is a positive family history of CF, parents are familiar with the disease, but in many cases there is no prior knowledge of the disorder and the diagnosis can be startling. Initial shock may be followed by disbelief, anger, or grief (Lloyd-Still & Lloyd-Still, 1983). The age of the child when diagnosed affects parental reaction to some extent. The longer the prediagnostic stage (the older the child), the greater the likelihood of the parents experiencing extreme shock at time of diagnosis (Burton, 1975). Sensitivity for the anguish experienced by the family must be shown.

The clinical status of children with CF is highly variable. Some toddlers may have already experienced pulmonary complications and been hospitalized repeatedly, while others exhibit little or no detrimental impact on their respiratory status. The effects of protein–calorie deficits due to malabsorption may be manifest in stunted development such as small stature or a lower than average weight-for-height ratio; therefore, a difference in appearance from their healthy siblings or friends may already be perceptible.

Young children need to develop the ability to function socially outside the family circle. Demands of school and new friendships dictate a lessening of parental attachments and a capacity for some measure of independence (Lloyd-Still & Lloyd-Still, 1983). This type of autonomy may be difficult to achieve for the child with CF. If parents perceive that their child is fragile with exceptionally vulnerable health, they may become overprotective. McCollum and Gibson (1970) examined issues of family adaptation to CF and found that 47% of parents in the study admitted granting less independence to their child with CF than to their healthy children. Cappelli and colleagues (1989) found a strong correlation between parental overprotection and psychological maladjustment in the child; the attempt to shield her or him from harm can negatively affect a child's ability to adapt to social pressures. Behavior problems such as restlessness, excessive daydreaming, and inattentiveness are found more often in children with medical conditions such as CF than in their healthy peers (McCollum and Gibson, 1970). Encouraging the child with CF to participate in a variety of social and physical activities could prove beneficial to both their physical and emotional health. The physical therapist should stress the importance of incorporating an active lifestyle into the family dynamic.

ASSESSMENT OF FUNCTIONAL LIMITATIONS

Evaluation of impairment and functional limitations in the young child includes history, physical examination, chest radiographs, blood gases, oximetry, and sputum bacteriology. The pulmonary function of children who are able to execute the necessary voluntary maneuver (usually by age 6) can now be assessed by spirometry. A history of poor exercise tolerance; peribronchial thickening and noticeable hyperinflation on a chest radiograph; hypoxemia; quantitative sputum cultures that reveal endobronchial bacterial colonization;

presence of persistent, productive cough; symptoms of chronic bronchitis; and decreases in flow rates measured by spirometry are symptomatic of obstructive lung disease in CF.

Assessment by the physical therapist should include thorough history taking, physical examination including postural assessment, and, when applicable, some type of exercise tolerance testing. Young children with CF may have a chronic cough, hypoxemia, and decreased compliance of the lungs (Tepper et al., 1988), leading to restrictions in maximal oxygen consumption and an increase in work of breathing and an increase in resting energy expenditure (Shepherd et al., 1988). These factors will all compromise exercise tolerance.

Exercise testing is an objective method in which the physical therapist can assess and quantitate the subject's pulmonary deterioration as well as determine the subject's response to physical therapy. Individuals with CF will often not be aware of the extent of their physical limitations owing to the slow progression of their disease (Cerny & Darbee, 1990). An exercise test will often detect mild pulmonary dysfunction, which may go undetected with investigations at rest, and will also help reveal how the individual copes with work despite their disability (Godfrey, 1974).

When choosing an exercise test protocol, the purpose for the test and the age and disease severity of the subject should be carefully considered. To assess functional limitations, the exercise test should be progressive and stress the subject's cardiorespiratory system to a symptom-limited maximum. It should also be reproducible and capable of providing meaningful results (Singh, 1992).

Cycle ergometers are often used for testing exercise capacity in children with pulmonary disease (Cerny et al., 1982; Godfrey & Mearns, 1971; Marcotte et al., 1986; Nixon et al., 1992). An accurate prediction of oxygen consumption can be obtained since the mechanical efficiency for pedaling a cycle is independent of body weight and therefore is almost identical for all individuals (Cerny & Darbee, 1990). Although the treadmill test generally yields higher oxygen consumption values, the cycle ergometer has the advantages of being relatively inexpensive, portable, and safe. Because cycling is also a familiar exercise for many people, it is less likely to cause apprehension. As with the treadmill test, cycle ergometry is reproducible (Fox & Mathews, 1981). In addition, the subject is relatively stationary and therefore vital signs are easily monitored. Most ergometers have adjustable seat heights suitable for children, and it is important to also be able to adjust handlebars and pedal crank length.

Several progressive exercise protocols are used on

the cycle ergometer to determine maximum oxygen consumption or individual peak work capacity (see Chapter 5). Cerny and colleagues (1982) examined subjects with CF matched to a normal control sample to monitor cardiopulmonary response to incrementally increased workloads with cycle ergometry. Workloads were increased every 2 minutes until the subject could not continue. The study demonstrated that normal subjects needed an increased workload of 0.32 W/kg on average to effect an increase in heart rate of 10 beats per minute. Subjects with CF required workload increases ranging from 0.13 to 0.35 W/kg, depending on the severity of their disease, to demonstrate the same change in heart rate. Cerny and colleagues concluded that the limiting factor in exercise tolerance was severity of pulmonary involvement and not cardiovascular limitation (Cerny et al., 1982).

If the child is too small to successfully use a cycle ergometer, a treadmill can be used because only the ability to walk is required (Fig. 25–5). The child should be monitored closely to maintain a sense of confidence during the test. The elevation and speed are adjusted according to the size and skill of the subject and should be selected to allow even the subject with severe dysfunction to exercise at two to three levels of difficulty (Cerny & Darbee, 1990).

For individuals with severe lung disease, field walking tests such as 6- or 12-minute walks (Butland et al., 1982) or the shuttle walking test (Scott, et al., 1990) may be preferred. Walking tests are simple, are inexpensive, and can be performed by individuals of all ages and abilities with little risk of injury (Porcari et al., 1989). Because they are highly reproducible, walking tests correspond closely to the demands of everyday activity (Guyatt et al., 1985).

Subjects performing an exercise test need to be closely monitored and special notice given to signs of increased work of breathing, disproportionate to what is expected (Cerny & Darbee, 1990). Subjective measures of the perceived level of respiratory labor with a dyspnea scale such as Borg's Scale of Ratings of Perceived Exertion (Borg, 1982) can be taken before, during, and after the exercise test.

Maximal work capacity is limited by ventilation in individuals with pulmonary disease (Cerny & Darbee, 1990). Deficiencies in gas exchange and poor pulmonary mechanics compound the effects of decreased exercise capacity (Cerny et al., 1982; Dantzker et al., 1982; Henke & Orenstein, 1984). That limitation in exercise is due to pulmonary restrictions is further evidenced by the failure to reach predicted peak heart rates in exercise test subjects with CF, suggesting that exercise capacity

FIGURE 25–5. Treadmill testing with a young patient on oxygen.

is not limited by cardiovascular factors (Canny & Levison, 1987).

A complete physical examination should assist in revealing the individual's level of fitness, thus aiding the physical therapist in choosing the most appropriate exercise testing protocol. Individual exercise programs can then be designed to improve exercise capacity and fitness level.

The goals of physical therapy for the young child should encompass the improvement of exercise tolerance with continued attention to secretion clearance techniques. Correction and maintenance of proper postural alignment are also stressed. Goals of treatment should be explained to the child as fully as possible with the aim of eliciting his or her cooperation and, conceivably, compliance with the proposed treatment plan. Parental support for implementation of the physical therapy recommendations is also vitally important.

MANAGEMENT OF PULMONARY IMPAIRMENT

The chronic hypersecretions of the mucus glands of the tracheobronchial tree characteristic of CF (Lloyd-Still, 1983) result in obstructive lung disease. Incompetent mucus clearance, inflammatory infiltrate, and mucopurulent plugging obstruct air flow and contribute to the debilitation of pulmonary function (Lloyd-Still, 1983). The small peripheral airways are the site of most of the early pulmonary changes in CF. Patchy atelectasis and ventilation-perfusion abnormalities lead to increases in functional dead space and discernible hypoxemia (MacLusky & Levison, 1990). People with CF demonstrate a wide variance in the severity of illness, since the disease progresses in individuals at different rates, but some amount of chronic air flow obstruction is often already present in childhood.

Postural drainage, percussion, and vibration ("conventional" physical therapy) remain the primary modalities for secretion mobilization. Once children have grown too large to be positioned in the caregiver's lap for postural drainage, equipment such as a drainage board will have to be introduced. Mechanical percussors may be used to ease the work involved with manual percussion and to provide the child with an aid for self-treatment (Fig. 25–6). Children with a chronic illness should be encouraged to assume a degree of responsibility for their own treatment. Feeling some level of control over one's own health fosters self-esteem and helps to subdue anxiety (Kellerman et al., 1980). Children with CF may find it difficult to sustain the performance of manual percussion, even on easily accessible lung segments, and mechanical percussors can therefore help to alleviate this problem.

Although conventional physical therapy has long been used in the treatment of CF, it has been criticized as being too time-consuming and difficult to perform independently. Compliance with a daily physical therapy regimen is reported as lower than with all other aspects of treatment (Passero et al., 1981). Proof of efficacy might promote compliance, but research studies to examine the effectiveness of conventional physical therapy are difficult to evaluate owing to use of a wide variety of outcome measures, including different PFTs, volume of secretions produced, and participants' subjective impressions, to name a few (Starr, 1992). It is also problematic to compare studies done in different stages of the disease or with differences in study populations. Identifying the independent variable is sometimes troublesome because of the diverse combinations of techniques used; for example, percussion is rarely performed independently of postural drainage and coughing, making it difficult to definitively state which aspect of the treatment investigated has proven effective.

In a study by Lorin and Denning (1971), the short-term effect of conventional physical therapy for patients with CF, compared with cough alone, was production of more sputum. Other studies support the effectiveness of conventional physical therapy in increasing amounts of sputum expector-

FIGURE 25–6. Self-administered postural drainage and percussion using a mechanical percussor.

ated by subjects when excess secretion production is already a feature of the patient's condition (Bateman et al., 1979; Mazzacco et al., 1985). The amount of sputum produced may be quantified by volume or weight, but caution must be used when interpreting the findings from this type of measurement. Because many individuals may swallow a portion of their sputum, the output can underestimate the true volume produced. The amount of saliva that contaminates the product is difficult to determine, and this has resulted in the measurement of the dry weight of sputum in some studies. Measurement of dry weight is not practical in most clinical settings. In addition, the amount of sputum produced does not indicate where it originated.

Alternative methods for mobilizing secretions and stimulating cough have been suggested, usually involving directed breathing techniques. These include huffing, PEP, autogenic drainage, and the forced expiration technique (FET), now known as the active cycle of breathing. A limited number of studies have been conducted to compare the efficacy of these treatment modalities in CF. A comprehensive discussion of the feasibility, rationale, and precautions resulting from studies examining the use of conventional physical therapy, FET, huffing, and isolated coughing has been presented by Starr (1992).

The rationale for use of huffing, a type of forced expiration with a similar mechanism to coughing, was suggested by a study that bronchoscopically demonstrated that maintenance of an open glottis throughout the maneuver stabilized the collapsible airway walls of subjects with chronic air flow obstruction (Hietpas et al., 1979). The glottis normally closes in the compression phase of a cough, translating high compressive pressures on the tracheobronchial tree that may cause bronchiolar collapse (Starr, 1992). Uncontrolled coughing is often nonproductive and exhausting. To perform huffing, the subject is asked to take a deep inspiration and then, without allowing the glottis to close, to render a strong contraction of the abdominal muscles to aid in forceful expiration. Maintaining an open glottis can be compared to vocalizing "ha" (Starr, 1992). Huffing is an uncomplicated breathing technique that can be easily taught to young children. Although its precise value is not well known, performing huffs can introduce the child to the concept of controlled or directed breathing techniques.

Descriptions of the FET vary. Generally, it employs forceful expirations combined with an open glottis as in huffing, interspersed with controlled breathing at mid to low lung volumes. A 3-year

study was conducted by Reisman and associates (1988) to compare the treatment effects of FETs in isolation (without postural drainage) versus conventional physical therapy in subjects with mild to moderate pulmonary involvement. The study assessed the rates of deterioration in PFT scores, exercise challenge tests, and Shwachman clinical scores for all study subjects. The subjects who performed only FETs had significantly greater rates of decline in measures of FEV_1, mid-expiratory flow rates ($FEF_{25-75\%}$), and Shwachman score than the group performing conventional physical therapy.

Other studies support the use of FET when used as an adjunct to postural drainage for secretion clearance (Pryor et al., 1979; Sutton et al., 1983; Sutton et al., 1985; Van Hengstrum et al., 1988). These studies describe FETs differently than Reisman and associates did, use dissimilar outcome measures (sputum yield and clearance of radioaerosol particles), and combine the maneuver with postural drainage, so the results are not easily compared with those of Reisman and associates. The consensus seems to be that FET has some benefit in mobilizing secretions from the peripheral airways but should be used in conjunction with postural drainage or conventional physical therapy.

Use of PEP (Fig. 25-7) as a means of secretion mobilization for individuals with CF has been proposed. Introduced for use in this population in the 1980s in Denmark, PEP has been shown to be as effective as conventional physical therapy in both chronic (baseline) stages of CF (Oberwaldner et al., 1986; Steen et al., 1991; Tyrrell et al., 1986; Van Asperen et al., 1987) and during an acute exacerbation of pulmonary complications (Oberwaldner et al., 1991). The transmural pressure generated by maintaining resistant pressure throughout the expiration phase is thought to allow air flow to reach some obstructed alveoli through use of collateral airway channels. Airways are "splinted open" through the maintenance of PEP, thereby facilitating movement of peripheral secretions toward central airways (Lannefors, 1992). The reader is urged to refer to the studies mentioned earlier to gain a better understanding of PEP as an airway clearance modality for CF.

Exercise has also been shown to be a useful therapeutic modality for secretion clearance, as evidenced by improved expiratory flow rates in subjects with stable CF with mild pulmonary disease (Zach et al., 1981). A 30-month study of the effects of discontinuing other airway clearance modalities in favor of participation in aerobic exercise activities demonstrated no significant declines in clinical status (Shwachman score), radiographic results, or PFT outcomes (Andreasson et al., 1987). In an

FIGURE 25–7. Use of a PEP mask.

acute exacerbation, exercise proved as effective as conventional physical therapy for the study subjects when pulmonary function was reviewed (Cerny, 1989). The group assigned to "exercise" continued to receive one bronchial hygiene treatment session by a physical therapist daily, whereas the CPT group received three of these sessions per day. Cerny concluded that hospitalized patients could substitute exercise for part of the standard in-hospital care (Cerny, 1989).

Salt and fluid requirements need special attention in the individual with CF who is participating in exercise, especially in hot weather. The higher sodium and chloride concentrations in the perspiration of people with CF impose an elevated demand for salt and fluid replacement while exercising, which may not always be apparent to the individual (Orenstein et al., 1983).

Benefits of an exercise program extend beyond increases in peak oxygen consumption, increased maximal work capacity, improved mucus expectoration, and improved expiratory flow rates (Heijerman et al., 1991; Orenstein et al., 1981; Zach et al., 1981). Participation in a prescribed exercise program has also been shown to improve self-concept (Folkins, 1972) and may provide increased social interaction.

Fitness level has implications as a prognostic indicator. An improved survival rate is found in individuals with CF who demonstrate higher levels of aerobic fitness. Although this may simply reflect less severe illness, the ability to maintain aerobic fitness appears to have value in improving longevity (Nixon et al., 1992). Further research is necessary to determine what precise role prescriptive exercise programs play in improving survival.

Young children with CF should be encouraged to use those treatment modalities that best suit their requirements for adequate secretion clearance and prevention of deterioration of clinical status. Attitudes toward compliance with treatment can greatly influence the effectiveness of any therapeutic regimen, and the challenge for the physical therapist is to design a treatment strategy for these children that is useful both for efficacy and practicality. Children who learn to adopt their physical therapy treatments as an aspect of daily living, as opposed to a burden or punishment, will be more likely to comply with treatment plans.

Adolescence

Adolescence is a time of rapid transformation in many areas of development. Sexual maturation comes about as a result of the major changes in circulating hormones occurring around the time of maturity of the skeletal system, normally when the child is about 11 or 12. These hormonal secretions cause a "growth spurt" in the adolescent (Green, 1983). "Delay of maturity" occurs when there has been slowed or prolonged skeletal maturation. This is often the cause of delayed puberty in adolescents with CF (di Sant'Agnese & Davis, 1979; Mitchell-Heggs et al., 1976). Arrested sexual development, combined with a smaller than average physical build, can intensify feelings of isolation from healthy peers (McCollum & Gibson, 1970). A need for increasing independence can conflict with the demands of daily medical care, making compliance with the routine seem arduous. The adolescent with CF who looks and feels disparate from the perceived "norm" may rebel against the continuation of time-consuming treatments that reinforce his or her sense of being dissimilar or abnormal (Boyle et al., 1976).

Compliance with the "conventional" physical therapy routine of daily postural drainage and percussion sessions is poor in the adolescent population (McCollum & Gibson, 1970; Passero et al., 1981). Alternate methods of treatment such as the use of PEP or a program of regular exercise have already been discussed. Another treatment modality that has garnered attention of late is the technique known as autogenic drainage.

A self-generated airway clearance technique that requires no equipment or special environment to execute, autogenic drainage relies on the user's ability to control both inspiratory and expiratory air flow to generate maximum air flow within the different generations of bronchi (Chevaillier, 1984). Three separate phases of the technique are believed to "unstick" mucus in the peripheral airways, "collect" the mucus in the middle airways, and "evacuate" it from the central airways according to the volume level of the controlled breaths (McIlwaine et al., 1992). Mobilization of airway secretions by autogenic drainage does not rely on the gravity assistance needed for postural drainage and can be performed in a sitting position.

Autogenic drainage was originally developed for treating asthma by Chevaillier, a Belgian physical therapist, but was then adopted for use with the CF population in many European CF centers. North American CF centers have been slower to incorporate autogenic drainage as a treatment modality. This may be due to the scarcity of research studies validating its long-term efficacy. Studies have been published that promote the effectiveness of autogenic drainage with secretion clearance in patients with asthma (Dab & Alexander, 1977) and as a comparison treatment method to conventional physical therapy and PEP with patients with CF (McIlwaine et al., 1988). A 2 year comparison trial of autogenic drainage and conventional physical therapy has also been reported and showed no significant differences between treatment groups when clinical status and PFT scores were used as outcome measures (Davidson et al., 1992).

Autogenic drainage requires concentration and the ability to use proprioceptive and sensory cues to localize the secretions in the various levels of bronchi. When instructing an individual in autogenic drainage, the therapist must use a hands on ap-

proach, with a minimum of environmental distractions. A one-on-one teaching process is recommended. This type of concentrated self-directed activity is usually not achievable by children younger than age 12. The mechanism for collateral ventilation through the channels of Lambert and pores of Kahn is not fully developed in young children (DeCesare and Graybill, 1990), and this provides another limitation to the use of autogenic drainage before adolescence.

Maintenance of proper posture is important for individuals with CF to provide efficient breathing mechanics. The changes in the length-tension relationships of the respiratory musculature that may occur with increases in FRC create a mechanical disadvantage and contribute to increased work of breathing and muscle fatigue (Cerny & Darbee, 1990). Several postural changes are found in CF to varying degrees, associated with chronically hyperinflated lungs, including increased anterior-posterior diameter of the chest, shoulder elevation, and forward protraction and abdominal flexion (Rose & Jay, 1986). The incidence of thoracic kyphosis in CF is approximately 15% (Denton et al., 1981), which predisposes affected individuals to chronic back pain. Estimates of the rate of back pain among people with CF are as high as 80% (Rose & Jay, 1986).

The physical therapist must assess postural abnormalities and determine which changes may be reversible or amenable to treatment. Exercises to promote improved posture include a strengthening program for the supporting muscles of the back and spine, stretching of contracted musculature, and training the subject to develop a keener sense of his or her postural alignment. Projecting a good appearance is usually very important to teenagers, and informing the teenager with CF of the benefits of a good postural maintenance program may provide the incentive necessary to ensure compliance with recommendations for exercises.

Secondary effects of strength training with weights may be an improvement in self-confidence in the adolescent since it has been shown to be beneficial in promoting weight gain (Strauss et al., 1987). As pulmonary impairment worsens, nutritional status is a consideration that requires a great deal of focus. Individuals who are malnourished have reduced exercise capacity; therefore, the ability to maintain adequate weight gain is essential to the goal of improving exercise tolerance (Canny & Levison, 1987). The dietitian serving the population with CF contributes considerable expertise in identifying situations in which intervention is necessary and may be a valuable ally to reinforce the message that exercise can promote weight gain when appropriately managed. A liaison with the dietitian can ensure coordination of dietary and physical therapy recommendations.

Transition to Adulthood

When CF was first described in 1938, fewer than half of its victims survived their first year (Davis, 1983), but CF is no longer a purely pediatric disease. With contemporary methods of management, almost 80% of patients should reach adulthood (MacLusky & Levison, 1990), and it is currently estimated that the life expectancy of children born with CF in 1990 is 40 years (Elborn et al., 1992). Although many of the issues physical therapists are concerned with in the pediatric patient are similar for adults, some special differences should be considered.

The psychosocial issues in adulthood are distinct because the normal progression of psychological maturation brings new concerns with each developmental stage (Davis, 1983). Greater clinical awareness, early treatment, and more effective management of CF have all contributed to the improvement of prognosis (Pinkerton, 1985). Choices regarding education, employment, marriage, and family will have to be made. These choices are more complex than usual for the adult with CF who has to consider not only present health status but also attempt to predict future health status.

Physically demanding occupations may not be appropriate for the adult with CF with pulmonary limitations; therefore, a careful consideration of the physical demands of any task must be undertaken. Jobs involving constant exposure to dust, chemical fumes, or smoke should be avoided (Davis, 1983; Orenstein, 1989). Many adults with CF will be socially and vocationally fully functioning members of society, however, and their physical therapy plan must accommodate their busy lifestyles. Physical therapists need to help the adult incorporate strategies for fitting treatment into work schedules. Methods that are more convenient and promote independence, such as the PEP mask and autogenic drainage, may be more agreeable to the adult at work or school.

Because many adults with CF witness mortality among their peers, deterioration of their own health may have heightened significance for them. The adult who as an adolescent chose to be noncompliant with a physical therapy regimen may decide to initiate one again. Generally, individuals with CF have a strong positive outlook and are able to fully enjoy many of the normal pleasures of adulthood despite having to contend with unusual diffi-

culties (Orenstein, 1989). Patients' attitudes and outlook on life can have a tremendous influence on the medical progression of CF, so significantly so that they are included in prognostic scores (Davis, 1983).

Because of the progressive nature of CF, many adults will have more symptoms and functional limitations than they had as children (Orenstein, 1989). Minor hemoptysis occurs in up to 60% of adults with CF (di Sant'Agnese & Davis, 1979), and, in most cases, the cause is an increase in bronchial infection that has irritated a blood vessel (Orenstein, 1989). Massive hemoptysis, which is also strongly related to advancing age (Davis, 1983), is defined as a rupture of a bronchial blood vessel into the airways producing greater than 300 ml of blood in 24 hours (Cohen, 1992). It is reported to occur in 5 to 7 % of adults with CF (Porter et al., 1983) and warrants hospitalization and possible blood transfusion (Lloyd-Still, 1983).

Pneumothorax, which is one of the most common respiratory complications in adulthood, occurs in approximately 19% of individuals older than 13 years of age (MacLusky & Levison, 1990). A common cause of pneumothorax is the spontaneous rupture of apical bullae, which develop due to increased air trapping and microabscess formation in the diseased lung (MacLusky & Levison, 1990).

Episodes of hypertrophic pulmonary osteoarthropathy also increase in prevalence with advancing age (Davis, 1983). Digital clubbing can become more noticeable in people whose pulmonary disease is severe (Orenstein, 1989).

In general, cardiac status is related to severity of pulmonary involvement: the more severe the pulmonary adaptation to hypoxemia, the worse the pulmonary hypertension and right-sided heart strain. With comparable degrees of pulmonary disease, adults, especially those with mild lung disease, have more severe echocardiographic abnormalities than children. This may reflect the accumulative effects of episodes of mild hypoxemia and nocturnal oxygen desaturation that occur in even minimally affected individuals (Davis, 1983).

Because the incidence of respiratory complications increases with age, physical therapists need to continually adapt the individual's treatment program according to these changes. For the individual experiencing hemoptysis, physical therapy may have to be altered, although there are conflicting opinions in the literature as to the extent of the modification necessary. MacLusky and Levison (1990) report that conventional physical therapy is usually discontinued until there is no longer blood in the sputum. Lloyd-Still (1983) is also in favor of temporarily discontinuing conventional physical therapy. Orenstein (1989), however, believes that if the cause of minor hemoptysis is an increase in bronchial infection irritating a blood vessel, treatment should be the same as for other types of increased infection. He believes that bleeding within the lungs can worsen infection by providing a more hospitable environment for bacteria. He does caution that if a particular treatment position aggravates the bleeding, then that position should be avoided.

Other reports in the literature on hemoptysis include the opinion that chest physical therapy should not be withheld for all individuals who produce blood in their sputum (Mackenzie, 1989). The use of postural drainage, percussion, and shaking along with huffing or FETs may be less likely to increase the amount of bleeding than the frequent uncontrolled coughing that may occur with abandonment of the manual techniques (Starr, 1992). DeCesare and Graybill (1990) conclude that decisions should be based on individual situations and stress the importance of modified but continued physical therapy. In summary, it would seem logical that if a particular technique, such as percussion, makes the individual's situation worse, it should be discontinued. Other modalities, such as breathing techniques, may be introduced at this time.

Chest physical therapy is contraindicated in the presence of an untreated, progressing, or tension pneumothorax (DeCesare & Graybill, 1990); however, treatment can continue with a small, stable pneumothorax (DeCesare & Graybill, 1990; Mackenzie, 1989) and with a pneumothorax that has resolved through treatment with a thoracotomy and insertion of a chest tube for vacuum drainage of air (DeCesare & Graybill, 1990). Percussion must not be performed directly over the chest tube site owing to the danger of displacement, but percussion may be safely performed elsewhere on the thorax as tolerated. The PEP mask would not be the treatment of choice, since theoretically it could make the pneumothorax worse as a result of increased pressures generated in the airways.

Treatment of joint pain associated with hypertrophic pulmonary osteoarthropathy is usually symptomatic, using standard anti-inflammatory agents (Phillips & David, 1986). Physical therapists have a role in helping to relieve pain while maintaining joint range of motion. A home treatment program consisting of stretching, muscle strengthening, and range of motion exercises for the specific joints involved can be easily added to the individual's existing exercise program.

When pulmonary disease becomes so disabling that the individual is having difficulty performing activities of daily living, physical therapy goals should encompass these needs. The patient may have to be instructed in energy conservation techniques such as diaphragmatic pursed-lip breathing and assuming positions that relieve breathlessness. These positions should promote comfort and relaxation and should encourage mobility of the thorax and support of the spinal column. They should also include hip flexion to relax the abdominal area and aid in increasing intra-abdominal pressure for coughing (DeCesare & Graybill, 1990). Examples of energy conservation positions are shown in Figure 25–8. Retraining of the respiratory pattern using pursed-lip breathing in conjunction with diaphragmatic excursion has shown temporary benefits in increased tidal volume, decreased respiratory rate, reduction in $Paco_2$ levels and improved Pao_2 levels, as well as subjective benefits reported by patients (Ciesla, 1989). It may be that pursed-lip breathing improves confidence and decreases anxiety by providing some temporary control over oxygenation (Ciesla, 1989).

Oxygen needs with exercise may have to be assessed at this time. Continuation of an active lifestyle should be promoted for all individuals with CF to optimize physical condition and maintain an optimistic outlook. If the individual is considering lung transplantation as an option, then physical therapists need to involve the individual in a formalized exercise program.

Suitability for lung transplantation is determined by a multidisciplinary team of health care professionals. After meeting criteria for evaluation, the patient is usually admitted to a hospital to undergo a detailed assessment process. This includes an extensive review of pulmonary, cardiac, and immune functions and also a thorough psychological assessment of the patient and family. The physical therapist's role is to determine the candidate's exercise capacity.

The Toronto Lung Transplant Program at the Toronto Hospital has a well-established rehabilitation program. Exercise capacity is determined by using the 6-minute walk test and ear oximetry, or the Modified Bruce Protocol on the treadmill, which Craven and colleagues (1990) describe as follows. The 6-minute walk test is conducted with the individual walking a level measured distance of 75 meters. The subject is instructed to walk as quickly and comfortably as possible throughout the 6-minute test. If the patient becomes short of breath or too exhausted to continue, he or she is allowed to rest but then must continue the test as soon as symptoms subside. The number of laps (distance) and the rest periods the subject takes are

FIGURE 25–8. *A* and *B*, Positioning for energy conservation, promoting relaxation, and ease of breathing.

recorded, and pulse and respiratory rates are measured before and after the test. If there is concern regarding potential desaturation during the test, monitoring can be done throughout with a portable pulse oximeter.

The ear oximetry test is performed on the treadmill with the subject walking at 1 mph with a 4% gradient for a period of 5 minutes or to his or her tolerated limit. If the subject finds the speed or gradient too difficult, the test is stopped and repeated at a slower speed on the level. During the exercise test oxygen is titrated to ensure an arterial oxygen saturation of greater than 85% with exercise. For subjects who find this test too easy, the Modified Bruce Protocol Treadmill Test can be used.

The modified test differs from the Bruce Treadmill Test in that it has two added stages at the beginning of the test: stage 0 and stage ½. These stages were incorporated to enable the testing of patients at lower intensity levels. During the treadmill test the patient is monitored by electrocardio-

graphic recording and ear oximetry. The results of this test help to determine if severity of disability warrants consideration for transplant. Individuals can also be monitored at regular intervals with this test to gauge potential deterioration in their functional status. Once accepted into the lung transplantation program, most centers require attendance at a formal rehabilitation program (Grossman, 1988) featuring aerobics, muscle strengthening, stretching, and light calisthenics.

Physical therapy goals for the adult with CF include optimizing functional ability, physical exercise tolerance, and emotional well-being. For the individual awaiting a lung transplant, improvement in overall function should enable him or her to handle the actual surgery and immediate postoperative period with less difficulty (Craven et al., 1990). Arnold and associates (1991) found that 13 patients with end-stage CF showed improvement in their functional exercise capacity by participation in pulmonary rehabilitation while awaiting double-lung transplantation. Pulmonary rehabilitation entailed treadmill walking and lower-extremity ergometry 3 to 5 times per week, initiated at the time of listing for double-lung transplant. Six-minute walks were performed biweekly to assess changes in functional exercise capacity, while workload on the treadmill and bicycle ergometer was recorded. Six-minute walk distances and treadmill and bicycle workloads all increased significantly. The conclusions from these data confirm the possibility of improving functional exercise capacity with patients with end-stage CF awaiting double-lung transplantation, despite severe limitations in pulmonary function, and imply a role for aerobic exercise to improve conditioning, exercise tolerance, and quality of life for all patients with CF.

The physical therapist's contact with those individuals in the terminal stages of their disease should not be discontinued. Goals at this stage must include the provision of comfort measures and be directed by the patient's wishes. Treatment sessions may have to decrease in duration and be offered with increased frequency throughout the day. Adaptations to postural drainage positions may have to be adopted so treatment can be tolerated. As the work of coughing becomes too tiring or painful, other modalities such as splinting and huffing can be reviewed. Relaxation and anxiety-reducing techniques, such as massage, may be the primary need of the dying patient. Simply listening to the concerns of these patients can be therapeutic. The value of a compassionate ear should not be underestimated. Physical therapists treating terminally ill patients should be careful to incorporate the families' needs, respecting the fact that this is an emotionally volatile time for all involved.

CASE HISTORY: SUZETTE

Suzette is a 17-year-old girl with CF. She was diagnosed with CF at age 5 months following an admission to hospital with failure to thrive. The diagnosis of CF was based on her presenting symptomatology of poor appetite, vomiting following feedings, bulky and foul-smelling stools, chronic cough, and a recurrent rectal prolapse and laboratory investigations that demonstrated right lower lobe pneumonia and partial atelectasis of the right middle lobe on a chest radiograph, presence of *Staphylococcus aureus* in nasopharyngeal aspirate, and elevated sweat chloride level. Suzette was discharged with prescriptions for enzyme supplements, multivitamins, cloxacillin, bronchodilators, and physical therapy consisting of postural drainage and manual percussions concentrating on the right middle and lower lobes.

Suzette was next admitted to hospital in 1977 with recurrent vomiting. During this admission, her sputum culture showed colonization by *Pseudomonas aeruginosa*. In 1980, she was again admitted to hospital for treatment of acute bronchitis. Her chest radiographs showed patchy atelectasis and peribronchial thickening of the right middle lobe and a partial collapse of the right lower lobe. After a 10-day course of treatment with intravenously administered antibiotics, Suzette was discharged on the same medications as previously mentioned except for the change of her oral antibiotic to cephalexin. She remained stable for the next few years.

In 1982, Suzette participated in a standardized series of exercise challenge tests administered in the school system based on the Canada Fitness Awards Test (Canadian Association for Health, Physical Education and Recreation, 1980) and scored in the top third percentile for her age category. The exercise assessment included an endurance run, speed sit-ups, flexed arm hang, standing broad jump, sit and reach, and flexibility assessments. Also in 1982, Suzette underwent her first PFT assessment. Her FVC was 1.05 liters, 72% of the predicted value of 1.45 liters; and her FEV_1 was 0.82 liter, 78% of predicted value. She was classified as having "mild obstruction."

In January 1983, Suzette was admitted to hospital with an exacerbation of respiratory symptoms. Immediately after discharge she was tested at school with the same series of exercise challenge tests as before and was awarded a gold medal for consistently excellent results. Two weeks later she was readmitted to hospital for acute bronchitis. At this time, because of her chronic chest radiographic findings of bronchiectasis of the right middle lobe and collapsed right lower lobe, the possibility of lobectomy was considered. A bronchoscopy revealed mild bronchiectasis and secretions in both right- and left-stem bronchi. After consulting with Suzette's parents and considering her clinical presentation with the maintenance of good fitness levels, the decision was made to defer performing a lobectomy. Suzette was not judged to have severe enough impairment to justify this course of action.

On a routine clinic appointment in August, 1983, Suzette and her parents reported that her recurrent vomiting was interfering with completion of physical therapy. She was also experiencing mild, streaky hemoptysis with severe coughing. On questioning, the family related that physical therapy was regularly given 30 minutes after meals to accommodate parental work schedules. The physical therapist aided the family in devising a schedule that allowed treatment sessions to be completed before meals. A recommendation was also made to modify treatment with the use of FETs if Suzette continued to experience vomiting. The family was instructed in this technique, and Suzette demonstrated good performance of FETs. It was suggested to the family that Suzette should also attempt to regularly perform controlled coughing, following the physical therapy sessions, with some huffing. The family was requested to keep a record of when episodes of hemoptysis occurred.

During the following year, a subjective record of continued frequent hemoptysis was reported, correlating with severe bouts of uncontrolled coughing. Between October and December of 1984, Suzette was admitted to hospital twice with hemoptysis. The bleeding typically persisted for 2 to 7 days and occurred about every 2 weeks.

Physical examination revealed no cyanosis, moderate clubbing, decreased breath sounds in the right lower lobe, and diffuse coarse inspiratory crepitations heard throughout both lower lobes posteriorly. The parents were again consulted and asked to consider a right middle lobe lobectomy because this was the presumed causative site of Suzette's recurrent hemoptysis. Her parents were resistant to this course and asked to defer the decision until the following spring with the hopes that the frequency of Suzette's hemoptysis would decrease. They vowed to continue with the treatment plan of attempting to control coughing with the previously learned breathing techniques combined with relaxed diaphragmatic pursed-lip breathing because they believed this was effective in reducing the incidence of blood in the sputum. When she was followed up in clinic in May 1985, she showed marked clinical improvement with no further episodes of hemoptysis. In view of this, along with the previous bronchoscopic evidence of involvement in more than one lobe, a lobectomy was not indicated.

Suzette next performed spirometric PFTs in August 1985, during a routine clinic appointment. Her FVC was 83% of predicted, FEV_1 was 79% of predicted, and $FEF_{25-75\%}$ was 60% of predicted. Obstruction was still considered to be mild. Suzette told the physical therapist on this occasion that she was "sad," and mentioned the recent separation of her parents as being the source of her mood.

In October 1985, Suzette presented at her clinic visit looking drawn and pale. She complained of frequent nocturnal wakings caused by a racking cough that was productive of a large amount of thick yellowish sputum. She reported that she had no appetite and had lost 2.5 kg (5.5 lb) since August. She admitted to reduced compliance with her postural drainage and percussion treatments as a result of severe epigastric pain when in a head-down position. Evidence of chronic colonic loading was subsequently found.

Suzette was admitted to hospital for 2 weeks, and received intravenous antibiotic therapy and physical therapy sessions 3 times a day, which were modified to tolerance. During a physical therapy session Suzette began to relate a number of fears surrounding her attendance at a new school. She had recently moved with her mother into a home with her mother's boyfriend, and Suzette had concerns about fitting in with her new classmates. She had to leave the classroom once a day for inhalation therapy and physical therapy, making her feel different from the other students. She was afraid they would ask her many questions about CF, and she did not feel comfortable answering these types of questions. All of the concerns were related to the social worker responsible for Suzette's case.

The social worker arranged for one of the nurses from the CF clinic to travel to the school and give a talk on CF to Suzette's class. This reassured Suzette greatly, and she started to look forward to returning to school. With the social worker's help, Suzette also began to confront some of her feelings about her parents' separation. Ongoing counseling was made available to the entire family.

Suzette remained clinically stable for the next year until she was again admitted to hospital in November of 1986 with a respiratory exacerbation. She was discharged after 10 days but reported never feeling "right" for the next few months and was readmitted to hospital in February 1987. Suzette's performance on spirometric PFTs revealed an FVC of 60%, an FEV_1 of 52%, and an $FEF_{25-75\%}$ of 23% of expected values at the time of admission. A decision was made to add an inhaled antibiotic (tobramycin) to Suzette's usual medications to be continued after discharge. During her next clinic visits, Suzette relayed a positive subjective response to the new medication and showed steady clinical improvement. In September 1987 the results of her PFTs demonstrated significant improvement over the test results in February: her FVC was 85%, FEV_1 was 85%, and $FEF_{25-75\%}$ was 72% of predicted values. Suzette continued on the inhaled tobramycin for the next year and remained clinically stable.

In July 1990, the clinic physical therapist discovered that Suzette was rebelling against compliance with her physical therapy regimen. Suzette did not feel that she wanted to do daily treatments since they interfered with the time she wanted to spend with her friends. Suzette's mother admitted to being frustrated with the "continual struggle" against compliance and sought alternatives to Suzette's treatment plan. The physical therapist suggested a cycle ergometer test to establish a baseline measure of Suzette's exercise tolerance. Suzette only completed 2 minutes on the ergometer before being overcome with a prolonged spell of coughing, necessitating discontinuation of the test. A discussion of the benefits of regular exercise followed. Suzette admitted to being fearful of exertion as a result of her embarrassment over the severe, productive coughing that usually ensued. An exercise program was proposed by the physical therapist that featured a walking program of very gradually increasing difficulty, and Suzette agreed to try the program for 2 months. Suzette then underwent a 6-minute walk test, and although she complained of some shortness of breath, completed 250 yards.

Over the next three clinic appointments, Suzette remained clinically stable and reported steady improvement with her exercise program but continued problems with maintaining a daily schedule of postural drainage and percussion. She admitted to noncompliance with the treatments.

In April 1992, Suzette came to clinic complaining of a prolonged malaise and her weight had dropped 2 kg (4.4 lb). She suffered from intermittent fevers and had a frequent cough, productive of large amounts of thick, green sputum that was occasionally tinged with blood. Chest radiography revealed new extensive infiltrates in her right middle lobe and a complete right lower lobe collapse. Results of her PFTs were FVC of 59%, FEV_1 of 52%, and $FEF_{25-75\%}$ of 31% of predicted values. She required an intravenous course of antibiotics and was hospitalized.

Suzette was admitted to hospital again in late summer and had a further admission in November 1992. Both admissions were for respiratory exacerbations. During these two admissions, Suzette was instructed in the use of a PEP mask. She quickly demonstrated the proper application of the mask and reported that she "liked" using it. The physical therapist proposed that she attempt to use the mask twice daily, in addition to one daily session of postural drainage and percussion, and Suzette agreed to try this regimen.

In February 1993, Suzette came to her clinic appointment in obvious distress. She complained of "almost continuous" shortness of breath, daily fevers, a severely decreased tolerance for exercise, and frequent episodes of hemoptysis. Chest radiography revealed a lobar consolidation. She reported feeling "very sick" for about 10 days but had not come in earlier because she was reluctant to submit to another hospitalization. Unfortunately, Suzette did need to be hospitalized. The social worker became involved as Suzette became very withdrawn during this admission and was found to be severely depressed. The frequency of Suzette's hospital admissions and declining clinical status over the past few years had exacted an emotional toll. With psychological counseling and emotional support from all members of the multidisciplinary team, Suzette gradually came to embody a more optimistic demeanor. On discharge, Suzette thanked various members of the team who had cared for her and vowed to "keep fighting." She envisaged a "new beginning" and resolved to comply with her entire therapeutic regimen, "even physical therapy." Just before discharge Suzette performed a 6-minute walk test and finished 480 yards. She maintained a broad smile throughout the distance.

CONCLUSION

The treatment of CF poses many challenges for physical therapists. The multisystemic involvement of the disorder means that physical therapists need to continually interact with a team of professionals to shape appropriate treatment plans. Collaboration with this type of multidisciplinary health care team is always stimulating and fosters a creative and fulfilling area of practice in physical therapy. New advances suggest exciting possibilities for the future care of people with CF, and physical therapists serving this population are required to continually adapt their approach to treatment in light of new research. The aspiration to discover a cure seems to be approaching fulfillment. Meanwhile, the challenge for all those involved is in finding effective means to slow (or prevent) the disabling effects of this disease.

References

Ackerman, V, Montgomery, G, Eigen, H, & Tepper, R. Assessment of airway responsiveness in infants with cystic fibrosis. American Review of Respiratory Disease, 144:344–346, 1991.

Altose, MD. The physiological basis of pulmonary function testing. Clinical Symposia, 31(2):1–39, 1979.

Andersen, DH. Cystic fibrosis of the pancreas and its relation to celiac disease: A clinical and pathologic study. American Journal of Diseases of Children, 56:344–395, 1938.

Andreasson, B, Jonson, B, Kornfalt, R, Nordmar, E, & Sandstrom, S. Long-term effects of physical exercise on working capacity and pulmonary function in cystic fibrosis. Acta Paediatrica Scandinavica, 76:70–75, 1987.

Arnold, CD, Westerman, JH, Downs, AM, & Egan, TM. Benefits of an aerobic exercise program in C.F. patients waiting for double lung transplant. Pediatric Pulmonology Supplement, 6:287, 1991.

Auerbach, HS, Williams, M, Kirkpatrick, JA, & Colten, HR. Alternate-day prednisone reduces morbidity and improves pulmonary function in cystic fibrosis. Lancet, 2:686–688, 1985.

Aweida, D, & Kelsey, CJ. Accuracy and reliability of physical therapists in auscultating tape-recorded breath sounds. Physiotherapy in Canada, 42(6):279–282, 1989.

Bateman, JRM, Newton, SP, Daunt, KM, Pavia, D, & Clarke, SW. Regional lung clearance of excessive bronchial secretions during chest physiotherapy in patients with stable chronic airway obstruction. Lancet, 7:294–297, 1979.

Borg, GAV. Psychophysical bases of perceived exertion. Medicine and Science in Sports and Exercise, 14:377–381, 1982.

Boucher, RC. The new pharmacology: Tools to arrest CF lung disease. Pediatric Pulmonology Supplement, 8:65–66, 1992.

Boyle, IR, di Sant'Agnese, PA, & Sack, S. Emotional adjustment of adolescents and young adults with cystic fibrosis. Journal of Pediatrics, 88:318–326, 1976.

Buist, AS, Adams, BE, Sexton, GJ, & Azzam, AH. Reference values for functional residual capacity and maximal expiratory flow in young children. American Review of Respiratory Disease, 122:938–900, 1980.

Burton, L. The Family Life of Sick Children: A Study of Families Coping with Chronic Childhood Disease. London: Routledge and Kegan Paul, 1975.

Butland, RJA, Pang, J, Gross, ER, Woodcock, AA, & Geddes, DM. Two, six and 12-minute walking test in respiratory disease. British Medical Journal, 284:1607–1608, 1982.

Canadian Association for Health, Physical Education and Recreation. Fitness Performance: Second Test Manual—Canadian Youths, Ages 6–17. Ottawa: CAHPER, 1980.

Canny, GJ, & Levison, H. Exercise response and rehabilitation in cystic fibrosis. Sports Medicine, 4:143–152, 1987.

Cappelli, M, McGrath, PJ, MacDonald, NE, Katsanis, J, & Lascelles, M. Parental care and overprotection of children with cystic fibrosis. British Journal of Medical Psychology, 62:281–289, 1989.

Cerny, FJ. Relative effects of bronchial drainage and exercise for in-hospital care of patients with cystic fibrosis. Physical Therapy, 69:633–639, 1989.

Cerny, FJ, & Darbee, J. Exercise testing and exercise conditioning for children with lung dysfunction. In Irwin, S, & Tecklin, JS (Eds.), Cardiopulmonary Physical Therapy. St. Louis: CV Mosby, 1990, pp. 461–475.

Cerny, FJ, Pullano, TP, & Cropp, GJA. Cardiorespiratory adaptations to exercise in cystic fibrosis. American Review of Respiratory Disease, 126:217–220, 1982.

Cheng, PW, Boucher, RC, & Yankaskas, JM. Glycoconjugates secreted by cultured human nasal epithelial cells. In Mastella, G, & Quinton, PM (Eds.), Cellular and Molecular Basis of Cystic Fibrosis. San Francisco: San Francisco Press, 1988.

Chevaillier, J. Autogenic drainage. In Lawson, D (Ed.), Cystic Fibrosis: Horizons. New York: John Wiley & Sons, 1984, p. 235.

Ciesla, N. Postural drainage, positioning and breathing exercises. In Mackenzie, CF (Ed.), Chest Physiotherapy in the Intensive Care Unit. Baltimore: Williams & Wilkins, 1989, pp. 93–133.

Cohen, AM. Hemoptysis: Role of angiography and embolization. Pediatric Pulmonology Supplement, 8:85–86, 1992.

Collins, FS. The C.F. gene: Perceptions, puzzles and promises. Pediatric Pulmonology Supplement, 8:63–64, 1992.

Conway, SP, & Allenby, K. Parental and patient attitudes in an adult CF clinic to prenatal screening programmes. Pediatric Pulmonology Supplement, 8:238, 1992.

Cooper, PJ, Robertson, CF, Hudson, IL, & Phelan, PD. Variability of pulmonary function tests in cystic fibrosis. Pediatric Pulmonology, 8:16–22, 1990.

Corey, M, Allison, L, Prober, C, & Levison, H. Sputum bacteriology in patients with cystic fibrosis in a Toronto hospital during 1970–1981. Journal of Infectious Diseases, 149:283, 1984a.

Corey, M, Gaskin, K, Durie, P, Levison, H, & Forstner, G. Improved prognosis in C.F. patients with normal fat absorption. Journal of Pediatric Gastroenterology and Nutrition, 3 (Suppl 1):99–105, 1984b.

Crane, L. Physical therapy for the neonate with respiratory disease. In Irwin, S, & Tecklin, JS (Eds.), Cardiopulmonary Physical Therapy. St. Louis: CV Mosby, 1990, pp. 389–416.

Craven, JL, Bright, J, & Dear, CL. Psychiatric, psychosocial, and rehabilitative aspects of lung transplantation. Clinics in Chest Medicine, 11:247–257, 1990.

Crystal, RG. New frontiers in therapy. Pediatric Pulmonology Supplement, 6:64, 1991.

Crystal, RG. In vivo gene transfer strategies for the respiratory manifestations of cystic fibrosis. Pediatric Pulmonology Supplement, 8:67, 1992.

Dab, I, & Alexander, F. Evaluation of the effectiveness of a particular drainage procedure called autogenic drainage. In Baran, D, & VanBogaert, E (Eds.), Cystic Fibrosis. Ghent, Belgium: European Press, 1977, pp. 185–187.

Dab, I, & Malfroot, A. Gastroesophageal reflux: A primary defect in cystic fibrosis. Scandinavian Journal of Gastroenterology Supplement, 143:125–131, 1988.

Dantzker, DR, Patten, GA, & Bower, JS. Gas exchange at rest and during exercise in adults with cystic fibrosis. American Review of Respiratory Disease, 125:400–405, 1982.

Davidson, AGF, McIlwaine, PM, Wong, LTK, & Pirie, GE. Long-term comparative trial of conventional percussion and drainage physiotherapy versus autogenic drainage in cystic fibrosis. Pediatric Pulmonology Supplement, 8:a298, 1992.

Davis, PB. Cystic fibrosis in adults. In Lloyd-Still, JD (Ed.), Textbook of Cystic Fibrosis. Stoneham, MA: Wright, 1983, pp. 351–370.

Day, G, & Mearns, M. Bronchial lability in cystic fibrosis. Archives of Disease in Childhood, 48:355–359, 1973.

Dean, M, O'Connell, P, Leppert, M, Park, M, Amos, JA, Phillips, DG, White, R, & Vande Woude, GF. Three additional DNA polymorphisms in the met gene and D7S8 locus: Use in prenatal diagnosis of cystic fibrosis. Journal of Pediatrics 111:490–495, 1987.

DeCesare, JA, & Graybill, CA. Physical therapy for the child with respiratory dysfunction. In Irwin, S, & Tecklin, JS (Eds.), Cardiopulmonary Physical Therapy. St. Louis: CV Mosby, 1990, pp 417–460.

Denton, JR, Tietjen, R, & Gaerlan, PF. Thoracic kyphosis in cystic fibrosis. Clinical Orthopaedics and Related Research, 155:71–74, 1981.

di Sant'Agnese, PA, & Davis, PB. Cystic fibrosis in adults: 75 cases and a review of 232 cases in the literature. American Journal of Medicine, 66:121–132, 1979.

Doershuk, CF, Downs, TD, Matthews, LW, & Lough, MD. A method for ventilatory measurements in subjects one month to five years of age: Normal results and observations in disease. Pediatric Research, 4:165–174, 1970.

Doershuk, CF, Matthews, LW, & Tucker, AS. A five-year clinical evaluation of a therapeutic program for patients with cystic fibrosis. Journal of Pediatrics, 65:1112–1113, 1964.

Drumm, ML, Pope, HA, Cliff, WH, Rommens, JM, Marvin, SA, Tsui, L-C, Collins, FS, Frizzell, RA, & Wilson, JM. Correction of the cystic fibrosis defect in vitro by retrovirus-mediated gene transfer. Cell, 62:1227–1233, 1990.

Durie, PR. Gastrointestinal motility disorders in cystic fibrosis. In Willa, JP (Ed.), Disorders of Gastrointestinal Motility in Childhood. New York: John Wiley & Sons, 1988, pp. 91–99.

Durie, PR, Gaskin, KJ, Corey, M, Kopelman, H, Weizman, Z, & Forstner, GG. Pancreatic function testing in cystic fibrosis. Journal of Pediatric Gastroenterology and Nutrition, 3:89–98, 1984.

Egan, TM. Overview of lung transplantation for cystic fibrosis. Pediatric Pulmonology Supplement, 8:204–205, 1992.

Eid, N, Buchheit, J, Neuling, M, & Phelps, H. Chest physiotherapy in review. Respiratory Care, 36:270–282, 1991.

Elborn, JS, Shale, DJ, & Britton, JR. Cystic fibrosis: Current survival and population estimates to the year 2000. Thorax, 45:783a, 1992.

England, SJ. Current techniques for assessing pulmonary function in the newborn and infant: Advantages and limitations. Pediatric Pulmonology, 4:48–53, 1988.

Folkins, C. The effects of physical training on mood. Journal of Clinical Psychology, 32:583–588, 1972.

Fox, EL, & Mathews, DK. The Physiological Basis of Physical Education and Athletics (3rd ed.). Philadelphia: Saunders College Publishing, 1981.

Fried, MD, Durie, PR, Tsui, L-C, Corey, M, Levison, H, & Pencharz, PB. The cystic fibrosis gene and resting energy expenditure. Journal of Pediatrics, 119:913–916, 1991.

Frownfelter, DL (Ed.): Chest Physical Therapy and Pulmonary Rehabilitation. Chicago: Year Book Medical Publishers, 1987.

Gibson, LE, & Cooke, RE. A test for the concentration of electrolytes in sweat in cystic fibrosis of the pancreas utilizing pilocarpine by iontophoresis. Pediatrics, *23*:545–549, 1959.

Gilljam, H, Malmborg, A, & Strandvik, B. Conformity of bacterial growth in sputum and contamination free endobronchial samples in patients with cystic fibrosis. Thorax, *41*:641–645, 1986.

Godfrey, S. Exercise Testing in Children. Philadelphia: WB Saunders, 1974.

Godfrey, S, Bar-Yishay, E, Arad-I, Landau, LI, & Taussig, LM. Flow-volume curves in infants with lung disease. Pediatrics, *72*:517–522, 1983.

Godfrey, S, & Mearns, M. Pulmonary function and response to exercise in cystic fibrosis. Archives of Disease in Childhood, *46*:144–151, 1971.

Green, M, & Solnit, AJ. Reactions to the threatened loss of a child: A vulnerable child syndrome. Pediatrics, *34*:58–66, 1964.

Green, OC. Endocrinological complications associated with cystic fibrosis. In Lloyd-Still, JD (Ed.), Textbook of Cystic Fibrosis. Stoneham, MA: Wright, 1983, pp. 329–349.

Grossman, RF. Lung transplantation. Medical Clinics of North America, *24*:4572–4579, 1988.

Gurwitz, D, Corey, M, Francis, PWJ, Crozier, D, & Levison, H. Perspectives in cystic fibrosis. Pediatric Clinics of North America, *26*(3):603–615, 1979.

Guyatt, GH, Sullivan, MJ, Thompson, PJ, Fallen, EL, Pugsley, SO, Taylor, DW, & Berman, LB. The 6-minute walk: A new measure of exercise capacity in patients with chronic heart failure. Canadian Medical Association Journal, *132*:919–923, 1985.

Hardy, KA, Wolfson, MR, Schidlow, DV, & Shaffer, TH. Mechanics and energetics of breathing in newly diagnosed infants with cystic fibrosis: Effect of combined bronchodilator and chest physical therapy. Pediatric Pulmonology, *6*:103–108, 1989.

Heijerman, HGM, Bakker, W, Sterk, P, & Dijkman, JH. Oxygen-assisted exercise training in adult cystic fibrosis patients with pulmonary limitation to exercise. International Journal of Rehabilitation Research, *14*:101–115, 1991.

Henke, KG, & Orenstein, DM. Oxygen saturation during exercise in cystic fibrosis. American Review of Respiratory Disease, *129*:708–711, 1984.

Hiatt, P, Eigen, H, Yu, P, & Tepper, RS. Bronchodilator response in infants and young children with cystic fibrosis. American Review of Respiratory Disease, *137*:119–122, 1988.

Hietpas, B, Roth, R, & Jensen, W. Huff coughing and airway patency. Respiratory Care, *24*:710, 1979.

Humberstone, N. Respiratory assessment and treatment. In Irwin, S, & Tecklin, JS (Eds.), Cardiopulmonary Physical Therapy. St. Louis: CV Mosby, 1990, pp. 283–322.

Irwin, S, & Tecklin, JS (Eds.), Cardiopulmonary Physical Therapy. St. Louis: CV Mosby, 1990.

Kattan, M. Pediatric pulmonary function testing. In Miller, A (Ed.), Pulmonary Function Tests: A Guide for the Student and House Officer. Philadelphia: WB Saunders, 1987, pp. 199–212.

Kellerman, J, Zeltzer, L, & Ellenberg, L. Psychological effects of illness in adolescence: Anxiety, self-esteem and perception of control. Journal of Pediatrics, *97*:126–131, 1980.

Kerem, E, Reisman, J, Corey, M, Canny, GJ, & Levison, H. Prediction of mortality in patients with cystic fibrosis. New England Journal of Medicine, *326*:1187–1191, 1992.

Kerem, B-S, Rommens, JR, Buchanan, JA, Markiewicz, D, Cox, TK, Chakravarti, A, Buchwald, M, & Tsui, L-C. Identification of the cystic fibrosis gene: Gene analysis. Science, *245*:1073–1080, 1989.

Khaghani, A. Heart-lung transplantation for cystic fibrosis. Pediatric Pulmonology Supplement, *6*:128–129, 1991.

Khaghani, A, Madden, B, Hodson, M, & Yacoub, M. Heart-lung transplantation for cystic fibrosis. Pediatric Pulmonology Supplement, *6*:128–129, 1991.

Lamarre, A, Reilly, BJ, & Bryan, AC. Early detection of pulmonary function abnormalities in cystic fibrosis. Pediatrics, *50*:291–298, 1972.

Lannefors, L. Different ways of using positive expiratory pressure to loosen and mobilize secretions. Pediatric Pulmonology Supplement, *8*:136–137, 1992.

Lemke, A, Lester, L, Lloyd-Still, J, & Powers, C. Attitudes toward genetic testing among adults with cystic fibrosis. Pediatric Pulmonology Supplement, *8*:238, 1992.

Lewiston, N, & Moss, R. Interobserver variance in clinical scoring for cystic fibrosis. Chest, *91*:878–882, 1987.

Lloyd-Still, DM, & Lloyd-Still, JD. The patient, the family and the community. In Lloyd-Still, JD (Ed.), Textbook of Cystic Fibrosis. Stoneham, MA: Wright, 1983, pp. 443–446.

Lloyd-Still, JD. Pulmonary manifestations. In Lloyd-Still, JD (Ed.): Textbook of Cystic Fibrosis. Stoneham, MA: Wright, 1983, pp. 165–198.

Lorin, MI, & Denning, CR. Evaluation of postural drainage by measurement of sputum volume and consistency. American Journal of Physical Medicine and Rehabilitation, *50*:215–219, 1971.

Loudon, RG. The lung exam. Clinics in Chest Medicine, *8*:265, 1987.

Mackenzie, CF. Undesirable effects, precautions, and contraindications of chest physiotherapy. In Mackenzie, CF (Ed.), Chest Physiotherapy in the Intensive Care Unit. Baltimore: Williams & Wilkins, 1989, pp. 321–344.

MacLusky, IB, Canny, GJ, & Levison, H. Cystic fibrosis: An update. Paediatric Reviews and Communications, *1*:343–384, 1987.

MacLusky, IB, Gold, R, Corey, M, & Levison, H. Long-term effects of inhaled tobramycin in patients with cystic fibrosis colonised with *Pseudomonas aeruginosa*. Pediatric Pulmonology, *7*:42–48, 1989.

MacLusky, IB, & Levison, H. Cystic fibrosis. In Chernick, V (Ed.), Kendig's Disorders of the Respiratory Tract in Children, Vol. 5. Philadelphia: WB Saunders, 1990, pp. 692–730.

Marcotte, JE, Grisdale, RK, Levison, H, Coates, AL, & Canny, GJ. Multiple factors limit exercise capacity in cystic fibrosis. Pediatric Pulmonology, *2*:274–281, 1986.

Matson, JA, & Capen, CV. Pregnancy in the cystic fibrosis patient. Journal of Reproductive Medicine, *26*:373, 1982.

Maxwell, B. Nursing aspects of C.F. care. Pediatric Pulmonology Supplement, *6*:85–86, 1991.

Mazzacco, MC, Owens, GR, Kiriloff, LH, & Rogers, RM. Chest percussion and postural drainage in patients with chronic bronchiectasis. Chest, *88*:360–363, 1985.

McCollum, AT, & Gibson, LE. Family adaptation to the child with cystic fibrosis. Journal of Pediatrics, *77*:571–578, 1970.

McIlwaine, PM, Davidson, AGF, Wong, LTK, & Pirie, GE. Autogenic drainage. Pediatric Pulmonology Supplement, *8*:134–135, 1990.

McIlwaine, PM, Davidson, AGF, Wong, LTK, Pirie, GE, & Nakielna, EM. Comparison of positive expiratory pressure and autogenic drainage with conventional percussion and drainage therapy in the treatment of cystic fibrosis. Pediatric Pulmonology, *4*(Suppl 2):132a, 1988.

Mellins, R. The site of airway obstruction in cystic fibrosis. Pediatrics, *44*:315–318, 1969.

Mellins, R, Levine, OR, Ingram, RH, Jr, & Fishman, AP. Obstructive disease of the airways in cystic fibrosis. Pediatrics, *41*:560–573, 1968.

Miller, A. Spirometry and maximum expiratory flow volume curves. In Miller, A (Ed.), Pulmonary Function Tests: A

Guide for the Student and House Officer. Philadelphia: WB Saunders, 1987, pp. 15–32.

Miller, WF, Scacci, R, & Gast, LR. Laboratory Evaluation of Pulmonary Function. Philadelphia: JB Lippincott, 1987, pp. 105–176.

Mitchell-Heggs, P, Mearns, M, & Batten, JC. Cystic fibrosis in adolescents and adults. Quarterly Journal of Medicine, 45: 479–504, 1976.

Muller, N, Frances, P, Gurwitz, D, Levison, H, & Bryan, AC. Mechanisms of hemoglobin desaturation during rapid-eye movement sleep in normal subjects and in patients with cystic fibrosis. American Review of Respiratory Disease, 119:338, 1980.

Nixon, PA, Orenstein, DM, Kelsey, SF, & Doershuk, CF. The prognostic value of exercise testing in patients with cystic fibrosis. New England Journal of Medicine, 327:1785–1788, 1992.

Oberwaldner, B, Evans, JC, & Zach, MS. Forced expirations against a variable resistance: A new chest physiotherapy method in cystic fibrosis. Pediatric Pulmonology, 2:358–367, 1986.

Oberwaldner, B, Theissl, B, Rucker, A, & Zach, MS. Chest physiotherapy in hospitalized patients with cystic fibrosis: A study of lung function effects and sputum production. European Respiratory Journal, 4:152–158, 1991.

Orenstein, DM. Cystic Fibrosis: A Guide for Patient and Family. New York: Raven Press, 1989.

Orenstein, DM, Franklin, BA, Doershuk, CF, Hellerstein, HK, Germann, KJ, Horowitz, JG, & Stern, RC. Exercise conditioning and cardiopulmonary fitness in cystic fibrosis. Chest, 80:292–298, 1981.

Orenstein, DM, Henke, KG, & Cerny, FJ. Exercise and cystic fibrosis. Physician and Sports Medicine, 2:57–63, 1983.

Orenstein, SR, & Orenstein, DM. Gastroesophageal reflux and respiratory disease in children. Journal of Pediatrics, 112: 847–858, 1988.

Ormerod, LP, Thompson, RA, & Anderson, CM. Reversibility of airways obstruction in cystic fibrosis. Thorax, 35:768–772, 1980.

Paradowski, LJ. The CF patient post lung transplant: The UNC experience. Pediatric Pulmonology Supplement, 8:210–212, 1992.

Park, RW, & Grand, RJ. Gastrointestinal manifestations of cystic fibrosis: A review. Gastroenterology, 81:1143–1161, 1981.

Pasque, MK, Cooper, JD, Kaiser, LR, Haydock, DA, Triantafilloy, A, & Trulock, EP. Improved technique for bilateral lung transplantation: Rationale and initial clinical experience. Annals of Thoracic Surgery, 49:785–791, 1990.

Passero, MA, Remor, B, & Solomon, J. Patient-reported compliance with cystic fibrosis therapy. Clinical Pediatrics, 20: 264–268, 1981.

Pasterkamp, H, Montgomery, M, & Wiebicke, W. Nomenclature used by health care professionals to describe breath sounds in asthma. Chest, 92:346–352, 1987.

Patterson, GA, & Cooper, JD. Status of lung transplantation. Surgical Clinics of North America, 68:545–558, 1988.

Phelan, PD, Gracey, M, Williams, HE, & Anderson, CM. Ventilatory function in infants with cystic fibrosis. Archives of Disease in Childhood, 44:393–400, 1969.

Phillips, BM, & David, TJ. Pathogenesis and management of arthropathy in cystic fibrosis. Journal of the Royal Society of Medicine, 79(Suppl 12):44–49, 1986.

Phillips, BM, & David, TJ. Management of the chest in cystic fibrosis. Journal of the Royal Society of Medicine, 80(Suppl 15):30–37, 1987.

Pinkerton, P, Trauer, T, Duncan, F, Hodson, M, & Batten, J.

Cystic fibrosis in adult life: A study of coping patterns. Lancet, 2:761–763, 1985.

Pizer, HF. Organ transplants: A patient's guide. Cambridge, MA: Harvard University Press, 1991.

Porcari, JP, Ebbeling, CB, Ward, A, Freedson, PS, & Rippe, JM. Walking for exercise testing and training. Sports Medicine, 8:189–200, 1989.

Porter, DK, Van Every, MJ, Anthracite, RF, & Mack, JW, Jr. Massive hemoptysis in cystic fibrosis. Archives of Internal Medicine, 143:287–290, 1983.

Prince, A. Pseudomonas aeruginosa gene products associated with epithelial colonization. Pediatric Pulmonology Supplement, 8:75–76, 1992.

Pryor, JA, Webber, BA, Hodson, ME, & Batten, JC. Evaluation of the forced expiration technique as an adjunct to postural drainage in treatment of cystic fibrosis. British Medical Journal, 2:417–418, 1979.

Reisman, JJ, Rivington-Law, B, Corey, M, Marcotte, J, Wannamaker, E, Harcourt, D, & Levison, H. Role of conventional physiotherapy in cystic fibrosis. Journal of Pediatrics, 113: 632–636, 1988.

Riordan, JR, Rommens, JM, Kerem, B-S, Alon, N, Rozmahel, R, Grzelczak, Z, Zielensky, J, Lok, S, Plavsic, N, Drumm, ML, Iannuzzi, MC, Collins, FS, & Tsui, L-C. Identification of the cystic fibrosis gene: Cloning and characterization of complementary DNA. Science, 245:1066–1073, 1989.

Rose, J, & Jay, S. A comprehensive exercise program for persons with cystic fibrosis. Journal of Pediatric Nursing, 1:323–334, 1986.

Rosenstein, B, & Langbaum, T. Diagnosis. In Taussig, LM (Ed.), Cystic Fibrosis. New York: Thieme-Stratton, 1984, pp. 85–115.

Ruppel, G. Manual of Pulmonary Function Testing. St. Louis: CV Mosby–Year Book, 1991.

Sackett, DL. Rules of evidence and clinical recommendations on the use of antithrombotic agents. Chest, Supplement, 89:25–35, 1986.

Sammut, P, & Morgan, WJ. Volume-independent assessment of forced expiratory flow in young children. American Review of Respiratory Disease, 135:A238, 1987.

Scott, RB, O'Loughlin, EV, & Gall, DG. Gastroesophageal reflux in patients with cystic fibrosis. Journal of Pediatrics, 106:223–227, 1985.

Scott, SM, Walters, DA, Singh, SJ, Morgan, MDL, & Hardman, AE. A progressive shuttle walking test of functional capacity in patients with chronic airflow limitation. Thorax, 45:781a, 1990.

Shepherd, R, Vasques-Velasquez, L, Prentice, A, Holt, TL, Coward, W, & Lucas, A. Increased energy expenditure in young children with cystic fibrosis. Lancet, 2:1300–1303, 1988.

Shwachman, H, & Kulczycki, LL. Long-term study of 105 patients with cystic fibrosis. American Journal of Diseases of Children, 96:6–15, 1958.

Singh, S. The use of field walking test for assessment of functional capacity in patients with chronic airways obstruction. Physiotherapy, 78:102–104, 1992.

Skorecki, K, Levison, H, & Crozier, DN. Bronchial lability in cystic fibrosis. Acta Paediatrica Scandinavica, 65:39–44, 1976.

Spicher, V, Roulet, M, & Schultz, Y. Assessment of total energy expenditure in free-living patients with cystic fibrosis. Journal of Pediatrics, 118:865–972, 1991.

Starr, JA. Manual techniques of chest physical therapy and airway clearance techniques. In Zadai, CC (Ed.), Pulmonary Management in Physical Therapy. New York: Churchill Livingstone, 1992, pp. 99–133.

Steen, HJ, Redmond, AOB, O'Neill, D, & Beattie, F. Evaluation of the PEP mask in cystic fibrosis. Acta Paediatrica Scandinavica, 80:51–56, 1991.

Strauss, GD, Osher, A, Wang, CI, Goodrich, E, Gold, F, Colman, W, Stabile, M, Dobrenchuk, A, & Keens, T. Variable weight training in cystic fibrosis. Chest, 92:273–276, 1987.

Sutton, PP, Lopez-Vidriero, MT, Pavia, D, Newman, SP, & Clay, MM. Assessment of percussion, vibratory-shaking and breathing exercises in chest physiotherapy. American Review of Respiratory Disease, 66:147–152, 1985.

Sutton, PP, Parker, RA, Webber, BA, Newman, SP, & Garland, N. Assessment of the forced expiration technique, postural drainage and directed coughing in chest physiotherapy. European Journal of Respiratory Disease, 64:62–68, 1983.

Taussig, LM. Maximal expiratory flows at functional residual capacity. A test of lung function for young children. American Review of Respiratory Disease, 116:1031–1038, 1977.

Taussig, LM, Landau, LI, & Marks, MI. Respiratory system. In Taussig, LM (Ed.), Cystic Fibrosis. New York: Thieme-Stratton, 1984, pp. 115–174.

Taussig, LM, Lobeck, CC, di Sant'Agnese, PA, Ackerman, DR, & Kattwinkel, J. Fertility in males with cystic fibrosis. New England Journal of Medicine, 287:587–589, 1972.

Tepper, RS. Assessment of pulmonary function in infants with cystic fibrosis. Pediatric Pulmonology Supplement, 8:165–166, 1992.

Tepper, RS, Hiatt, P, Eigen, H, Scott, P, Grosfeld, J, & Cohen, M. Infants with cystic fibrosis: Pulmonary function at diagnosis. Pediatric Pulmonology, 5:15–18, 1988.

Tepper, RS, Hiatt, PW, Eigen, H, & Smith, J. Total respiratory compliance in asymptomatic infants with cystic fibrosis. American Review of Respiratory Disease, 135:1075–1079, 1987.

Trulock, EP. Assessment of patients with CF for lung transplantation: Indications, contraindications and expectations. Pediatric Pulmonology Supplement, 8:206–207, 1992.

Tyrrell, JC, Hiller, EJ, & Martin, J. Face mask physiotherapy in cystic fibrosis. Archives of Disease in Childhood, 61:598–611, 1986.

Van Asperen, PP, Jackson, L, Hennessy, P, & Brown, J. Comparison of a positive expiratory pressure (PEP) mask with postural drainage in patients with cystic fibrosis. Australian Paediatric Journal, 23:283–284, 1987.

Van Hengstrum, M, Festen, J, & Beurskens, C. Conventional physiotherapy and forced expiration technique maneuvers have similar effects on tracheobronchial clearance. European Respiratory Journal, 1:758, 1988.

Vinocur, CD, Marmon, L, Schidlow, DV, & Weintraub, WH. Gastroesophageal reflux in the infant with cystic fibrosis. American Journal of Surgery, 149:182–186, 1985.

Wagener, JS, Taussig, LM, Burrows, B, Hernried, L, & Boat, T. Comparison of lung function survival patterns between cystic fibrosis and emphysema or chronic bronchitis patients. In Sturgess, JM (Ed.), Perspectives in Cystic Fibrosis. Mississauga, Can. Imperial Press, Ltd, 1980, pp. 236–243.

Wiebicke, W, Pownter, A, Montgomery, M, & Pagtakhan, R. The effect of dipratropium bromide on lung function in patients with cystic fibrosis. Pneumonologie, 44 (Suppl 1):277–278, 1990.

Winton, T. Double lung transplantation for cystic fibrosis: Operative technique and early post-operative care. Pediatric Pulmonology Supplement, 8:208–209, 1992.

Witt, DR, Blumberg, B, Schaefer, C, Fitzgerald, P, Fishbach, A, Holtzman, J, Kornfeld, S, Lee, R, Nemzer, L, Palmer, R, Sato, M, & Jenkins, L. Cystic fibrosis carrier screening in a prenatal population. Pediatric Pulmonology Supplement, 8:235, 1992.

Yankaskas, JR. Respiratory failure in CF: Pathophysiology and treatment, including the role of mechanical ventilation. Pediatric Pulmonology Supplement, 8:87–88, 1992.

Zach, MS, Purrer, B, & Oberwaldner, B. Effect of swimming on forced expiration and sputum clearance in cystic fibrosis. Lancet, 2:1201–1203, 1981.

Zadai, CC. Comprehensive physical therapy evaluation: Identifying potential pulmonary limitations. In Zadai, CC (Ed.), Pulmonary Management in Physical Therapy. New York: Churchill Livingstone, 1992, pp. 55–78.

Chapter 26

Asthma

CYNTHIA L. MAGEE, PT, MS

Bronchial asthma is a chronic disorder of the respiratory system manifested by intermittent, reversible episodes of dyspnea, wheezing, and coughing (Paul & Fafoglia, 1988). In susceptible individuals, the airways are hypersensitive to stimuli or triggers that result in shortness of breath, coughing episodes, or both. These stimuli are classified as extrinsic or intrinsic. Extrinsic or allergic stimuli include pollen, mold, animal dander, cigarette smoke, foods, drugs, and dust. Intrinsic or nonallergic stimuli include viral infections, inhalation of irritating substances, exercise, emotional stress, and environmental factors such as the weather or climate changes. An individual may be sensitive to either type of stimuli or to both types. A study of 298 children with asthma, aged 5 months to 14 years 11 months, revealed that the most common triggers included upper respiratory tract infections (virtually all children), exercise (60% of children), changes in the weather (63%), grass pollen (63%), animal danders (cats 55%, dogs 36%, and feathers 21%), and even strong odors (about 50%) (Mercer & Van Niekerk, 1991).

The prevalence of asthma is increased in the extended families of persons who demonstrate asthma or allergic rhinitis. Mercer and Van Niekerk (1991) reported that 76.8% of 298 children with asthma had allergic rhinitis, 17.1% had eczema, and 91% had a family history of allergy in first- or second-degree relatives.

Genetic research has located the gene responsible for asthma on the long arm of chromosome 11 (Cookson et al., 1989; Julier et al., 1990). An autosomal dominant pattern of inheritance with variable patterns of expression is demonstrated. Cookson and colleagues (1989) reported that 85% of those who carry the gene display some symptoms, 60% had wheezing, and 20% had been diagnosed with asthma. Although it is not possible to predict which individuals who carry the gene will be more severely affected, a child who has two parents with asthma has a greater chance of having severe symptoms.

The prevalence of reported asthma in children younger than the age of 17 is 8 to 10%, making asthma the most common lung disease in children (Evans et al., 1987). The prevalence ratio in childhood of boys to girls is 1.5 : 1. A study conducted in Great Britain (Burney et al., 1990) demonstrated an increasing prevalence of asthma in children 5 to 12 years of age over the period from 1973 to 1986. Although the prevalence of bronchitis decreased over this same time period (down 4.7% for boys and 5.8% for girls), the prevalence of asthma in creased by 6.9% for boys and 12.8% for girls. The increase in asthma, therefore, cannot be explained solely by a change in diagnosis.

In a survey conducted in the United States over the years 1976 to 1980 involving 7399 children aged 3 to 17 years there was an overall prevalence of asthma of 6.7% (Gergen et al., 1988). The prevalence was 7.8% for boys and 6.7% for girls. Rates were higher in blacks (9.4%) than in whites (6.2%) and higher in urban areas (7.1%) than in rural areas (5.7%). The prevalence also varied by area of the country: 5.4% northeast, 5.6% midwest, 6.3% south, and 7.1% west. The first attack occurred before age 3 in 66.1% of boys and 48.1% of girls. By age 10, 93.9% of the boys and 92.7% of the girls had experienced their first attack.

PATHOPHYSIOLOGY

The physical, neurogenic, chemical, or pharmacologic factors that are associated with asthma are specific to each individual (Bierman & Pearlman, 1983). They stimulate or trigger the immune system to release chemical mediators, which in turn cause constriction of the bronchial muscles, increased mucus production, and swelling of the mucus membranes. These effects result in increased resistance to air flow, increasing the work of breathing and decreasing pulmonary ventilation. Mucus accumulation may cause blockage of the airways, resulting in further air trapping, hyperinflation, and, eventually, atelectasis.

The pathophysiology of asthma is one of five types of hypersensitivity reactions mediated by the immune system (Male, 1986). Asthma is considered a type 1 or immediate-type hypersensitivity reaction. Subsequent to exposure to a bronchial challenge there is an immediate reaction of bronchoconstriction resulting mainly from the release of histamine and bradykinin. Accumulation of inflammatory cells may result in a secondary late reaction (6 to 8 hours later). Serum molecules and cells of the immune system migrate to the site of inflammation where they stimulate increased blood supply, increased capillary permeability, migration of cells out of the blood vessels into the tissues, and smooth muscle contraction.

Three main types of cells are associated with the immune system: lymphocytes, phagocytes, and accessory cells (Male, 1986). Lymphocytes react to foreign material by producing antibodies. The phagocytes, which include blood monocytes, neutrophils, and tissue macrophages, take up and break down pathogens, foreign material, and debris. The accessory cells, which include eosinophil and basophil granulocytes, mast cells, platelets, and antigen-presenting cells, play a role in inflammation. Eosinophil chemotactic factor and neutrophil chemotactic factor are derived from lymphocytes and attract eosinophils and neutrophils to the site of inflammation.

In sensitive individuals, mast cell responses are critical in production of an asthmatic reaction (Friedman & Kaliner, 1987). Mast cells are located immediately adjacent to small airways, in alveolar septa, and in connective tissue often adjacent to blood vessels and unmyelinated nerves. They are also located in smooth muscle, beneath the capsule of mucus glands, and in airway lumina. Mast cells are distributed in approximately equal proportions in the airway connective tissue and in the peripheral lung. Mast cells are also associated with nonallergic asthma. They can be activated by stimulation of sensory nerves in the airway mucosa, by neuropeptides, by opioids generated during temperature regulation, or by psychic stimuli.

When chemical mediators are released from the cells of the immune system, an immune response is set up (Male, 1986). Mast cells and basophils release histamine. Basophils, neutrophils, and macrophages release platelet-activating factor. Platelets release serotonin. Arachidonic acid is released from mast cells and produces prostaglandins and thromboxanes through the cyclo-oxygenase pathway and leukotrienes and slow reactive substance of anaphylaxis through the lipoxygenase pathway. These different mediators have specific adverse effects, which are summarized in Figure 26–1.

The release of chemical mediators of the allergic response depends on the relative intracellular concentrations of cyclic adenosine monophosphate (AMP) and cyclic guanosine monophosphate (GMP) (Crofton & Douglas, 1981). A higher concentration of cyclic AMP will inhibit the release of mediators, resulting in bronchodilation, decreased mucus production, and decreased histamine production. A higher concentration of cyclic GMP will enhance the release of mediators, resulting in bronchoconstriction, increased mucus production, and increased histamine production. Cyclic AMP can be increased by stimulation of the sympathetic nervous system through the β-adrenergic receptors. Cyclic GMP can be increased by stimulation of the sympathetic nervous system through the α-adrenergic receptors or by stimulation of the parasympathetic nervous system. Knowledge of the pathophysiology of immune system hypersensitivity

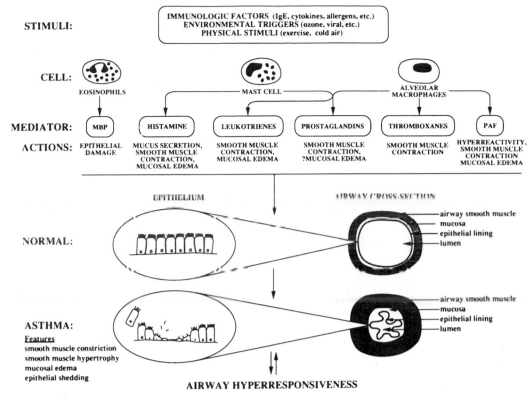

FIGURE 26-1. The stimuli, important cell types and their mediator products, the tissue response to these factors, and how they relate to the development of airway hyperresponsiveness and the pathogenesis of asthma. (Adapted from Hill, MR, & Kamada, AK. Pathogenesis of asthma: Implications for therapy. Drug Intell Clinical Pharmacy 25:993–1005, 1991; with permission from Hill, MR, Szefler, SJ, & Larsen, GL. Asthma pathogenesis and the implications for therapy in children. Pediatric Clinics of North America, 39:1211, 1992.)

reactions has been used to develop effective pharmacologic control of asthma and other conditions.

Mucociliary transport in patients with asthma has been investigated and found to be abnormal (Mezey et al., 1978; Kurashima et al., 1992). Six patients with ragweed hypersensitivity, aged 18 to 48 years, and 7 controls, aged 19 to 29 years, participated in one study (Mezey et al., 1978). Tracheal mucus velocity (TMV) was measured before and after antigen challenge. Forced expiratory volume during the first second of exhalation (FEV_1) was measured by spirometry and used to determine lung function. Mean baseline TMV was 54% of normal ($p < .01$) even though FEV_1 was normal or only slightly abnormal. After the antigen challenge when FEV_1 had reached maximal decrease ($p < .01$), the mean TMV had decreased to 72% of baseline ($p < .05$). TMV continued to decrease to 47%

of baseline ($p < .05$) even though FEV_1 had returned to baseline values.

PRIMARY IMPAIRMENT

Diagnosis

The diagnosis of asthma is made on the basis of history, physical examination, auscultation and palpation, and pulmonary function tests (PFTs). Wheezing and rhonchi will be detected and may even be present when the child demonstrates no breathing difficulty. During an acute asthma attack, the child may evidence an increased respiratory rate, expiratory grunting, intercostal muscle retractions and nasal flaring, an alteration in the inspiration–expiration ratio, and coughing. In severe cases, a bluish color of the lips and nails may be noted.

PULMONARY FUNCTION TESTS

PFTs are performed to determine the degree of respiratory impairment. Various PFT equipment is available to obtain specific PFT parameters. The Wright Peak Flow Meter (Armstrong Medical Industries, Northbrook IL) is the most commonly used device because of the relative ease of use, availability, and cost of the unit. Spirometry can be used to obtain several PFT measurements during one test. Plethysmography or the "body box" is the least used and is found in pulmonary clinics. Obtained test values are compared with predicted values based on age, sex, height, and air temperature. Many computer programs are available that provide actual values, predicted values, and percentage of predicted values. An unofficial interpretation of the results may also be given. The degree of impairment may be classified on four or five levels (normal to severe or very severe) based on results of percentage of predicted values. Different laboratories may use different values for determining degree of impairment (Miller, 1968). An example is given in Table 26–1.

Asthma is a disease of both the large and the small airways. The predominant site of flow limitation varies with the individual (McFadden et al., 1977). Various PFT parameters are sensitive to different areas of obstruction (Buckley & Souhrada, 1985; Ruppel, 1982). The airway obstruction in asthma typically results in difficulties during expiration. PFT measurements may reveal decreases in forced vital capacity (FVC), FEV_1, forced expiratory volume compared with forced vital capacity (FEV/FVC), and peak expiratory flow rate (PEFR) owing to airway obstruction in large or small airways; decreases in forced expiratory flow during 25 to 75% of forced vital capacity ($FEF_{25-75\%}$) owing to airway obstruction specifically in small airways; and increases in residual volume (RV) and func-

TABLE 26–1. DEGREE OF RESPIRATORY IMPAIRMENT

Normal: >85% of predicted value*
Mild: 70–85% of predicted value
Moderate: 55–70% of predicted value
Severe: <55% of predicted value

*Predicted value based on age, height, sex, and air temperature. Adapted from American Medical Association Committee on Rating of Mental and Physical Impairment. Guidelines to evaluation of permanent impairment: The respiratory system. Journal of the American Medical Association, *194*:919–932, 1965.

TABLE 26–2. RESULTS OF SPIROMETRY IN 14-YEAR-OLD BOY WITH ASTHMA*

Test	Actual	Predicted	% Predicted
FVC	2.57	2.51	102
FEV_1	2.17	2.16	100
PEFR	5.36	3.62	148
$FEF_{25-75\%}$	2.22	2.94	76
FEV_1/FVC	84	86	

*Results show normal values for FVC, FEV_1, and PEFR and mild impairment for $FEF_{25-75\%}$. This boy was free of symptoms at the time of testing.

tional residual capacity (FRC) due to air trapping. Decreases in $FEF_{25-75\%}$ are common in early stages of obstructive disease before other measurements are abnormal (Ruppel, 1982).

Even when the child is free of symptoms, some impairment may be noted (Crofton & Douglas, 1981). Table 26–2 shows the PFT results of a 14-year-old boy who was symptom-free at the time of the test. Values within the normal range are noted for FVC, FEV_1, and PEFR; however, impairment of a mild degree in $FEF_{25-75\%}$ was found.

The most commonly reported PFT measurements are PEFR and FEV_1. Many investigators, however, recommend using more than one PFT parameter to detect individual differences in the predominant site of airway obstruction (Buckley & Souhrada, 1975; Cropp, 1979; Kattan et al., 1978). In the PFT results in Table 26–2, if only PEFR or FEV_1 was used to determine airway obstruction, no impairment would have been reported. By including $FEF_{25-75\%}$ a mild degree of impairment would be reported and proper treatment could be initiated.

PRIMARY IMPAIRMENT IN INFANCY AND EARLY CHILDHOOD

During infancy and early childhood, asthma attacks are often triggered by viral infections, in particular by respiratory syncytial virus. A diagnosis of wheezy bronchitis or acute bronchiolitis rather than a diagnosis of asthma may be made (de Benedictis et al., 1990).

Although the majority of children with asthma experience their first episode before age 3, it is difficult to obtain objective measurements for diagnosis in toddlers. PFTs are not usually used with this age group. Asthma severity scales using parameters other than PFTs have been investigated. One study (Kerem et al., 1991) compared clinical signs (accessory muscle use, heart rate, respiratory rate, pulsus paradoxus, dyspnea, and wheezing) to spirometric values (FEV_1) and transcutaneous arterial oxygen saturation (tcSao$_2$) in 71 children, aged 5 to 17 years, during an acute asthmatic attack. Significant correlations were found between FEV$_1$ and accessory muscle use ($p < .001$), dyspnea ($p < .001$), and wheezing ($p < .001$). Significant correlations were also found between tcSao$_2$ and FEV$_1$ ($p < .001$) and accessory muscle use ($p < .001$); however, a low FEV$_1$ was not always associated with a low tcSao$_2$ or a high clinical score. Kerem and colleagues emphasize the need to use both subjective and objective measures in evaluating the severity of an asthma attack.

Another study (Bishop et al., 1992) investigated the ability of a clinical asthma severity scale, clinical judgment rating, and oxygen saturation level to predict the severity of an acute asthma attack for 60 children, aged 6 months to 17 years. The asthma severity scale score was obtained by pediatricians' ratings of accessory muscle use, wheeze, and heart rate, each on a 4-point scale. The clinical judgment rating was obtained by the pediatricians' clinical judgment of the severity of the asthma attack, also on a 4-point scale (mild, moderate, severe, or very severe). Severity of oxygen desaturation, obtained by pulse oximetry, was rated on a 3-point scale (mild, moderate, severe). The severity of the asthma attack was determined by admission, length of inpatient stay, frequency and duration of inhalation therapy, and parental assessment of subsequent days unwell. Wheezing and accessory muscle use were found to be the most valuable in predicting the severity of the asthma attack.

In a study by Wennergren and co-workers (1986), a clinical symptom grading system based on respiratory rate; rhonchi; wheezing; retractions, fatigue; anxiety, cyanosis, pallor, and cold sweat; and breath sounds and degree of consciousness was compared with transcutaneous oxygen pressure (tcPo$_2$) and transcutaneous carbon dioxide pressure (tcPco$_2$) in children younger than 2 years of age during an acute asthmatic attack. At very slight signs of obstruction, tcPo$_2$ was decreased and continued to decrease with severity of signs and symptoms. The tcPco$_2$ remained almost unchanged until moderate obstruction was evident.

These studies demonstrate that objective measurements can be obtained for children who are too young or in too much distress to adequately perform PFTs. The acute asthmatic attack can be monitored with standardized protocols for documentation of signs and symptoms.

Physicians seem to be hesitant to make the diagnosis of asthma. Wheezy bronchitis and acute bronchiolitis are considered temporary diseases, whereas asthma is a chronic and recurring condition. Unfortunately, if a diagnosis of asthma is not made, the child will receive inappropriate treatment and will not benefit from prophylactic treatment of asthma. Unnecessary or inappropriate medication may be prescribed, and the child may continue to have undiagnosed respiratory problems.

A retrospective study in an "asthma aware" medical practice examined the medical records of 52 children with diagnosed asthma aged 18 months to 11 years (Levy & Bell, 1984). Eight of these children were diagnosed in the hospital, and 44 were diagnosed by general practitioners. An average of 16 to 20 (range, 1–48) consultations for respiratory problems was required before the diagnosis of asthma was recorded. Thirty-five of the 52 children had their first consultation for respiratory problems before age 1, another 10 (total 45) between 1 and 2 years of age, another 6 (total 51) by age 4, and all 52 by age 5. In 31 patients, an objective diagnosis was made based on a change in PEFR of at least 20%. In 21 patients, a subjective diagnosis was made based on a history suggestive of asthma combined with a positive response to bronchodilators or asthma prophylaxis. Symptoms recorded during consultations included cough (96% of children), wheeze (75%), difficulty sleeping (31%), and difficulty breathing (25%). A preoccupation with infection as the primary cause of recurrent respiratory problems in the children was revealed by physicians' treatments. Before the diagnosis of asthma was made and recorded, 43% of prescriptions were for antibiotics, 38% were for cough suppressors, and 17% were for bronchodilators.

IMPAIRMENT IN CHILDHOOD

An increased prevalence of asthma during childhood has been reported in children who have a history during infancy of wheezy bronchitis, croup, respiratory syncytial virus infection, bronchopulmonary dysplasia, and viral bronchiolitis and in children with extremely low birth weight (500–999 g) (Crofton & Douglas, 1981; Gold et al., 1989; Li & O'Connell, 1987; McConnochie & Roghmann, 1984; Pullan & Hey, 1982; Rickards et al., 1987; Smyth et al., 1981). An increased prevalence of chronic or recurrent otitis media with effusion has been reported in children with upper respiratory tract allergy (Fireman, 1988). Otitis media with effusion has been related to an abnormal function of the eustachian tube and has been associated with allergy, infection, and enlarged adenoids. It may be an intrinsic trigger for asthma.

During childhood, PFT measures become an easy and effective diagnostic tool. Overt wheezing is the major presenting sign. Some children may only exhibit respiratory difficulty after exercise, at night, or in cold air (de Benedictis et al., 1990). Some children may have trouble keeping up with peers or with strenuous exercise. Routine PFT results may be normal; however, the history may indicate that an allergen or exercise challenge test should be performed. The prevalence of exercise-induced asthma (EIA) is 70 to 90% in individuals with documented asthma who have performed an exercise challenge test; however, a positive history of EIA is not always given (Schroeckenstein & Busse, 1988; Sly, 1986; Voy, 1986).

The exercise challenge test requires the child to run on a treadmill for 6 to 8 minutes at the slope and speed needed to attain a heart rate of 75 to 90% of the predicted maximum heart rate for the child's age. PFT measures are then taken at 5-minute intervals for 20 to 30 minutes after the run. The test is positive if PFT measures drop by more than 15% from pre-exercise baseline measures or if the child develops a cough or wheeze (Burr et al., 1974; Cropp, 1979; Taussig et al., 1980). If bronchospasm is elicited, the diagnosis is made if signs and symptoms are reversed by administration of bronchodilator medications (de Benedictis et al., 1990). Table 26–3 shows the results of an exercise challenge test for a 17-year-old girl who did not have positive results for EIA. In fact, the exercise resulted in some bronchodilation. Table 26–4 shows the positive test results of an exercise challenge test for a 14-year-old boy and the reversal of bronchoconstriction 15 minutes after the administration of bronchodilator medication by nebulizer. After the 6-minute exercise challenge, this boy demonstrated severe impairment in $FEF_{25-75\%}$, mild impairment in FEV_1, and within normal values for PEFR. His PFT measures, however, dropped by more than

15% from pre-exercise baseline values for each parameter. The time at which the lowest value is reached may vary among individuals and between parameters for one individual. Even though this boy had severe bronchoconstriction his oxygen saturation remained at or above 98%.

IMPAIRMENT IN ADOLESCENCE

By adolescence, symptoms often decrease. Even when free of symptoms, however, the adolescent may have significant impairment revealed by PFT measures. Continued decrease in severity and frequency of asthma attacks during adolescence results in the belief that children "outgrow" asthma. Research has not demonstrated this to be true. In a study of 286 subjects at age 28, first studied at age 7 and again at ages 10, 14, and 21, it was found that asthma severity at age 28 was similar to that at age 14 (Kelly et al., 1988). Asthma that had worsened during adolescence continued to worsen in early adulthood. In another study, 331 children with asthma and 77 controls were examined at ages 7, 14, and 21 (Martin et al., 1980). Although in some subjects there was amelioration of symptoms, they did continue to wheeze.

Medical Management

Episodes of asthma attacks are usually reversible and can be prevented or modified to some degree when the individual-specific triggers have been identified. The frequency, duration, and severity of attacks are highly variable even for the same individual.

Acute treatment is aimed at reversing the bron-

TABLE 26–3. **EXERCISE CHALLENGE TEST RESULTS***

Time (min)	PEFR	FEV₁	FEF₂₅₋₇₅%	RPE	Heart Rate	% O₂ Saturation
0	5.08/112%	2.36/84%	2.82/75%	7	105	94
1				14	165	94
3				15	177	94
5				14	175	94
6/0				14	175	94
3	5.42/119%	2.49†/89%	2.98/79%			94
5	5.42/119%	2.49/89%	2.98/79%			94
10	5.34/118%	2.62/93%	2.90†/77%			94
15	4.83†/106%	2.49/89%	3.19/85%			94
20	4.91/108%	2.49/89%	3.02/80%			94
		Change from Baseline				
	4.9% drop	5.5% rise	2.8% rise			

*Results of an exercise challenge test for a 17-year-old girl with asthma. Test consisted of a 6-minute run on a treadmill followed by 20 minutes of monitoring. Results are negative for exercise-induced asthma.
†Lowest value after exercise.

TABLE 26-4. **EXERCISE CHALLENGE TEST RESULTS***

Time (min)	PEFR	FEV$_1$	FEF$_{25-75\%}$	RPE	Heart Rate	% O$_2$ Saturation
0	6.01/166%	2.53/117%	2.42/82%	6	96	98
1	—	—	—	11	160	100
3	—	—	—	12	166	99
5	—	—	—	13	167	98
6/0	—	—	—	14	167	98
3	3.98/110%	1.69/78%	1.10/37%	—	—	100
5	3.98/110%	1.77/82%	1.02†/35%	—	—	99
10	3.39†/94%	1.60†/74%	1.03/35%	—	—	100
15	3.81/105%	1.65/76%	1.35/46%	—	—	100
20	4.83/133%	1.90/88%	1.49/51%	—	—	100
		Change from baseline				
	43.5% drop	36.8% drop	57.3% drop			
		15 minutes after nebulizer				
	5.42/150%	**2.66/125%**	**3.02/103%**			

*Results of an exercise challenge test for a 14-year-old boy with asthma. Test consisted of a 6-minute run on a treadmill followed by 20 minutes of monitoring. Results are positive for exercise-induced asthma. Reversal of bronchoconstriction 15 minutes after nebulizer treatment with albuterol is indicated in bold type.

†Lowest value after exercise.

choconstriction. Bronchodilator medications are administered by injection or inhalation (Bierman & Pearlman, 1983). If the asthma attack is severe and does not respond to bronchodilator medications, the diagnosis of status asthmaticus may be made and is considered a life-threatening medical emergency. Hospitalization will be required to administer medications intravenously, to monitor blood gases, and to administer oxygen.

The main goal of long-term management is to aid the child in living a life as similar as possible to his or her peers. The approach depends on the specific stimuli or triggers (Spector, 1989). Some allergens such as cigarette smoke, animal dander, or dust can be handled by environmental control. Desensitization ("allergy shots") may be used for triggers such as pollen or mold. Triggers such as emotional stress may be handled by relaxation exercises and education.

MEDICATIONS

Many individuals with asthma require daily medication. The primary medications in current use are xanthines (e.g., theophylline [Slo-phyllin, Quibron]), β-sympathomimetics (e.g., albuterol [Proventil, Ventolin] and metaproterenol [Alupent]), disodium cromoglycate (e.g., Cromolyn, Intal), and corticosteroids (e.g., prednisone, beclomethasone [Beclovent]) (Anderson, SD, 1981; Barnes, 1991, Paul & Fafoglia, 1988, Spector, 1989).

Theophyllines have been important in the treatment of asthma for more than 50 years, but their mode of action is not yet clearly known. It is unlikely that the role is bronchodilation but more likely that there is an anti-inflammatory or immunoregulatory effect. It has been proposed that xanthines inhibit the breakdown of cyclic AMP. Slow-release formulations allow once- or twice-daily dosing. Xanthines that reduce side effects such as diuresis, increased heart rate, and stimulation of the nervous system, are under investigation (Barnes, 1991).

Bronchodilators reverse the contraction of the smooth muscles. The most widely used and most effective are the β$_2$-agonists, which have been available for the past 20 years. They are equally effective on the large and small airways and may have an effect on other cells, such as mast cells, to prevent release of mediators. Recently, inhaled β$_2$-agonists with a longer duration of action have been introduced. Salmeteral and formoterol are available in European countries (Lofdahl & Chung, 1991). They have anti-inflammatory and bronchodilatory properties and protect against bronchoconstriction for over 12 hours. Formoterol inhibits the release of histamine and leukotrienes, and salmeterol inhibits the release of histamine, leukotrienes C$_4$ and D$_4$, prostaglandin D$_2$, and thromboxane B$_2$.

Disodium cromoglycate works by inhibiting the release of the immune system mediators. It also has anti-inflammatory properties and inhibits both immediate and late hypersensitivity reactions. Cromolyn has been shown to improve mucociliary transport in patients whose transport is abnormal and to offer partial protection from antigen-induced bronchospasm (Mezey et al., 1978). It is one of the safest medications but is inconvenient in that dosage is required 4 times a day. The administration of 20 mg of cromolyn 3 times per day over 3 years has been shown to decrease histamine sensitivity and overall asthma severity (Wantanabe, 1992). Newer cromolyn-like drugs are being studied (Spector, 1989). Ketotifen is administered orally and is long acting (12–24 hours). Nedocromil is administered by aerosol twice daily. Azelastine, which is used for rhinitis, has antiallergic properties (Spector, 1989; Spector et al., 1987). It inhibits release of histamine and other mediators, inhibits EIA and early and late allergen challenge reactions, and has demonstrated bronchodilatory properties.

Corticosteroids are highly effective antiasthmatic agents, especially when given by inhalation. They decrease inflammation and may decrease the amount of arachidonic acid available for conversion to prostaglandins or other substances. Budesonide is an experimental drug in the United States (King & Chang, 1987). It has a high topical-to-systemic ratio of anti-inflammatory effect and is 10 to 20 times more effective than beclomethasone. Research in the area of corticosteroids is directed toward inhaled agents with higher topical potency but without the systemic side effects; corticosteroids that are targeted for specific inflammatory cells, such as macrophages; and the use of liposomes to deliver corticosteroids to specific sites (Barnes, 1991). Another important goal of research is to develop nonsteroidal drugs that mimic the benefits of corticosteroids but without the side effects.

Other mechanisms to induce bronchodilation are under investigation (Barnes, 1991). Drugs that stimulate production of cyclic AMP have been investigated. Forskolin has been shown to increase cyclic AMP but has not proven effective as a bronchodilator. Drugs that inhibit the breakdown of cyclic AMP have been investigated. At this time, however, their use is limited by cardiovascular side effects, nausea, and vomiting. Anticholinergics, calcium antagonists, and potassium channel activators have demonstrated some potential for benefit, but selectivity and side effects continue to need research.

Researchers have recently placed an increased emphasis on asthma as an inflammatory disease. Inflammation is critically involved at an early stage, leading to airway hyperresponsiveness (Sykes & Cochetto, 1992). Drugs that reduce the inflammatory response are also being investigated. Leukotriene, platelet-activating factor, and thromboxane antagonists have been developed and are undergoing clinical trials (Manning et al., 1990; Rasmussen et al., 1992; Taylor, et al., 1991). Inhibitors of enzymes involved in mediator synthesis and inhibitors of neurogenic inflammation are fu-

ture possibilities. The use of immunomodulators such as methotrexate, cyclosporin-A, and gold is under investigation (Barnes, 1991; Spector, 1989).

Another problem area of asthma under investigation is decreased mucociliary clearance. Nineteen adults with asthma aged 28 to 75 years and 30 controls participated in a study to investigate the drug thromboxane A_2 synthetase inhibitor (OXY-046) (Kurashima et al., 1992). Before the treatment period, the mean velocity of mucociliary transport for the group with asthma was 25% of the mean for the control group. OXY-046 was administered orally twice daily for 4 weeks. Following the treatment period, the frequency of asthma attacks decreased. Mean sputum volume decreased by 28.3% ($p < .01$) at 2 weeks and by 44.5% ($p < .001$) at 4 weeks. The mean score for difficulty of sputum expectoration decreased by 64% ($p < .001$) at 2 weeks and by 60% ($p < .01$) at 4 weeks. Mean velocity of mucociliary transport improved by 119.7% ($p < .01$) from baseline, but remained significantly ($p < .01$) decreased from the control group. No significant changes were found in the velocity of mucociliary transport in the control subjects who received OXY-046.

In the study by Mezey and co-workers (1978), after administration of cromolyn sodium, mean TMV increased to 132% of baseline in patients with asthma. Following antigen challenge when FEV_1 had significantly ($p < .05$) decreased, mean TMV was 162% of baseline. After 1 hour, mean TMV continued to be increased to 134% of baseline. No change in TMV was reported in the control group.

At the present time, long-acting β_2-agonists and corticosteroids are the treatment of choice for asthma, but the future holds many possibilities for new drugs. Future research must consider disease severity, disease volatility, concurrent medications and comorbidity, age, and gender as factors in drug responsivity. The exciting field of genetic research should aid in the development of a drug that can specifically turn off the asthma gene.

▌SECONDARY CONDITIONS

Recurrent asthma attacks may result in secondary impairments, functional limitations, and disabilities beginning in early childhood and continuing throughout life. Restricted physical activity, school absences, school difficulties, changes in family lifestyle, and increased use of health care facilities are examples of some disabilities that may begin in early childhood. As the child approaches adolescence, self-esteem concerns become prominent. As adulthood is reached, concerns such as choice of vocation and living location become increasingly more important to consider.

Restrictions in Daily Life

Asthma is a condition that may alter or interfere with the daily life of the individual and his or her family. Asthma accounts for approximately 25% of school absentee days caused by chronic illness and accounts for 33% of doctor visits (Evans et al., 1987). It results in long-term limitation of daily activity for 23% of children with asthma. Bed rest for 1 or more days per year is required by 12% of children with asthma. In a study of 420 children with asthma, aged 7 to 16 years, 13% had school absences of more than 5 days due to asthmatic symptoms (Braback & Kalvesten, 1988). The results of a third study (Anderson, HR et al., 1983) of 284 children with asthma and 92 controls are presented in Table 26–5. Fortunately, little effect on social activities was reported. Belonging to clubs, swimming, and special lessons, such as music lessons, were reported as equally frequent among the children with asthma and the controls.

Townsend and associates (1991) investigated the impact of asthma on the lives of 100 children aged 7 to 18 years who were diagnosed with mild-to-moderate asthma and on the lives of their parents. The children and their parents were asked if each item on their respective questionnaires was a prob-

lem for them and then to rate those items on a 5-point scale (1 = does not bother you much; 5 = bothers you very, very much). The children's questionnaire consisted of 77 items, which included 29 items dealing with respiratory symptoms and fatigue, 21 items dealing with emotional function, and 16 items dealing with limitations in physical activities. A separate medication side effects category and a wishes category were included for each child. The children reported that respiratory symptoms such as wheezing, asthma attacks, shortness of breath, and feeling out of breath were the most bothersome. Emotional items such as fear, frustration, and anger were identified by more than 45%. Feeling frightened by an asthma attack was reported by 49%. In the limitations in physical activity category, running was reported by 85%. In the medication side effects category, 32% reported difficulty in falling asleep, and 22% reported not being able to sit still and feeling restless. Seventy-six percent reported at least one problem including inability to concentrate in school. The wishes focused mostly on being able to perform a current activity better or longer. Thirty-nine percent wished they could own a pet. For the parents, the questionnaire consisted of 69 items: 13 dealing with interference of the disease in day-to-day activities, and 56 dealing with the emotional impact on parents, which included basic health concerns as well as financial concerns. The emotional items scored higher than interference with daily life items. Major areas were concern about drug side effects and long-term effects, permanent lung damage, and feeling helpless during an attack.

The effect of asthma on the daily life of 150 adults, aged 18 to 70 years, was investigated by Juniper and colleagues (1992). A questionnaire consisting of 32 items assessed asthma symptoms, emotional problems caused by asthma, activities restricted by asthma, and troublesome environmental stimuli. The subjects were asked to rate each item on a 5-point scale (not very important to extremely important). Major asthma symptoms reported included shortness of breath, chest tightness, and wheezing. Emotional problems were not rated very highly. Major restrictions in physical activities included jogging and running. Major environmental triggers included cigarette smoke, dust, and air pollution. Exposure to and avoidance of environmental stimuli were classified as two different types of limitations. Choosing not to go to a party due to cigarette smoke was a different problem than choosing to go and then dealing with the consequent symptoms. Limitations were reported to be greater for younger than older adults and greater for women than for men.

TABLE 26–5. **EFFECTS OF ASTHMA ON DAILY LIFE**

Activity Affected by Asthma	Percent of Children Affected
School absence due to wheezing	58%
School absences of more than 30 days	12%
At least one day of bed rest required	34%
Wheezing severe enough to interfere with speaking	13%
Nocturnal wheezing interrupting sleep	40%
Activities around the house	29%
Mother's activities affected	42%
Activities affected a lot	7%
Special household arrangements required	13%
Special arrangements of child's bedroom	29%
Special allowances made for child	29%
Family pet removed	20%
Family choice of holiday activities	11%

Data compiled from a study of 284 children with asthma: Anderson, HR, Bailey, PA, & Cooper, JS. Morbidity and school absence caused by asthma and wheezing illness. Archives of Disease in Childhood, 58:919–933, 1983.

RESTRICTIONS IN PHYSICAL ACTIVITY

In 70 to 90% of individuals with diagnosed asthma, exercise has been identified as a trigger (Sly, 1986). The degree of bronchial spasm caused by exercise is variable among individuals and may vary on a daily basis depending on other triggers to which the child has been exposed. Asthma caused by exercise can be inhibited or modified by proper medication, proper warm-up and cool-down, or both.

Children with asthma may restrict their physical activity on their own. Teachers or parents may discourage the child from participation due to fear of an asthma attack. Regular physical education may be modified, and the child may avoid sports activities to prevent an asthma attack. In a study of 420 children with asthma, aged 7 to 16 years, 40% reported restricted physical activity of more than 10 days per year because of asthmatic symptoms; an additional 24% reported occasional restriction (Braback & Kalveston, 1988). This hypoactivity may lead to decreased cardiovascular fitness (Bar-Or, 1986). A pattern of hypoactivity, isolation from peers, and focus on disability may then become established.

The need for physical activity and the normal effects of conditioning and training on the cardiovascular and pulmonary systems are discussed in Chapter 5. The need for fitness in children with asthma is no less important than in children without asthma.

Cardiopulmonary responses other than PFT measures before, during, and after exercise and during bronchoconstriction have been studied in children with asthma. These responses as reported by various researchers are summarized in Table 26-6. In children with severe asthma, obstructive changes and disturbed pulmonary gas exchange have been reported even at rest when asymptomatic (Bevegard et al., 1976; Hedlin et al., 1986).

Repeated asthma attacks with increased production and accumulation of mucus combined with the abnormal mucociliary clearance associated with asthma may result in an altered breathing pattern, poor posture, and decreased cardiovascular fitness. Expiration may become an active rather than a passive process. Continued use of the accessory muscles of inspiration rather than the diaphragm may result in decreased thoracic mobility, hypoextensibility of pectoral muscles, elevated and adducted shoulders, winging scapulae, kyphosis, hypertrophied neck muscles, forward-head posture, and hypoextensibility of the hip and knee flexor muscles. Chronic lung hyperinflation may result in chest deformities (Bolton et al., 1956).

MEDICATION SIDE EFFECTS

Although the medications used in the management of asthma are necessary, the side effects of these medications also may have an impact on daily life (Brumback et al., 1984; Furukawa et al., 1984; Rachelefsky et al., 1986; Springer et al., 1985). Side effects of theophylline include nausea and heartburn, headaches, restlessness, insomnia, muscle spasms, anxiety, irritability, tremulousness, muscle incoordination, speech disturbances, heart

TABLE 26-6. **REPORTED CARDIOPULMONARY RESPONSES IN CHILDREN WITH ASTHMA AT REST, DURING EXERCISE, AFTER EXERCISE, AND DURING BRONCHOSPASM**

Response	Rest	During Exercise	After Exercise	During Bronchospasm
Cardiac output	N	N	N	I
Blood pressure	N	N		
Blood volume	N			
Heart volume	N			
Stroke volume	N			N/I
Total hemoglobin	N			
Alveolar-arterial O_2 gradient	N/I		N/I	I
PaO_2/$tcPO_2$	N	N/I/D	D	I/D
$PaCO_2$/$tcPCO_2$	N	N/I		N/I
Ventilation-perfusion	N/abn		abn	abn
Minute ventilation	N	I	I/N	
Physiologic dead space	N/I			I
Arterial blood lactate		I		

Reported results do not include pulmonary function test measurements.
N, normal; abn, abnormal; I, increased from normal; D, decreased from normal.
Data from Anderson (1972), Bevegard (1976), Chryssanthopoulos (1984), Freyschus (1984), Hedlin (1984, 1986), & Wennergren (1986).

palpitations, excessive perspiration, and frequent urination. Side effects of β-sympathomimetics include nervousness, headache, trembling, heart palpitations, dizziness or light-headedness, dryness or irritation of the mouth and throat, heartburn, and bad taste in the mouth. Side effects of oral corticosteroids in the typical doses used for treatment of asthma include increased appetite and weight gain, fluid retention, increased bruising, and mild elevation of blood pressure. In corticosteroid-dependent individuals, increased body fat composition, myopathy of type II (fast twitch) fibers, decreased proximal muscle strength, acne exacerbation, hirsutism, linear growth suppression, and osteoporosis have been reported (Hollister & Bowyer, 1987). A study by Picado and associates (1990) investigated respiratory and skeletal muscle strength and endurance time, examined biopsy specimens of deltoid muscles for type I and type II fibers, and assessed nutritional status of oral corticosteroid-dependent subjects and of controls. No difference was found in respiratory or skeletal muscle strength or endurance time. Atrophy of type II muscle fibers was found to be associated with decreased nutritional status rather than with corticosteroid use. Another study evaluating fitness in children with moderately severe to severe asthma found increased skinfold thickness (body fat) present more frequently than normal (Strunk et al., 1988). The investigators, however, did not believe it to be likely that corticosteroids played a primary role in this finding.

The side effects and dosage schedule of medication may call attention to the child. During the school day, the child may need to leave the classroom to receive medication. Theophylline has side effects that may interfere with school work. Increased attention, concentration, and memory ability were noted by psychological testing of children with asthma after 2 weeks off theophylline and on cromolyn (Furukawa et al., 1984). Parents reported decreased restlessness, distractibility, and irritability; increased manageability; and better sleeping during the time off theophylline. In a second study comparing theophylline and cromolyn therapy over 4 weeks, psychological tests revealed abnormal visuospatial planning in children with an intelligence quotient (IQ) of 87 to 105 compared with children with IQs of 111 to 134 when on theophylline (Springer et al., 1985).

Another study of children 6 to 12 years of age with mild asthma who had not been on any long-term oral medications for at least 6 months evaluated the effect of short-term (4 weeks) use of theophylline (Rachelefsky et al., 1986). Assessments were made by psychological tests, parent questionnaire and daily diary, and teacher checklist. Psychological tests were used to measure memory and learning, attention span, spatial visualization, and IQ. The parent questionnaire was designed to evaluate the child's behavior and consisted of 26 associated behaviors and 21 activity-attention behaviors. The daily diary was used to record medications and signs and symptoms. The teacher checklist was designed to characterize the child's ability to control activity and attention. Thirty-three associated behaviors and 20 activity-attention behaviors were rated comparing the child with other students. Significant ($p < .001$) negative effects were reported during theophylline use. Specific areas noted by teachers were "trouble finishing task," "seems to do things fast without thinking," "easily distracted from work," "gets into fights," and "gets angry easily."

Attention needs to be given to asthma-related behaviors used to get attention or to avoid demanding situations. Conditioned fear and anxiety may occur owing to repeated breathlessness and unpleasant treatments (Dahl et al., 1990). Vividly remembered incidents of intense fear and anger have been shown to significantly ($p < .05$) decrease FEV_1 (Tal & Micklich, 1976).

GROWTH AND DEVELOPMENT

Another effect of asthma that is particularly important for self-esteem in adolescence is delayed growth and development. Both sexual and skeletal maturation are frequently delayed. Bone age has been correlated to height rather than to age (Snyder et al., 1967). In infancy, no delay is evident, but a small consistent delay has been recorded in childhood (Hauspie et al., 1977). By adolescence, growth delay is marked. The adolescent growth spurt is delayed by approximately 1.3 years. The total length of the growth period is extended, however, and children with asthma eventually reach normal height and weight. The more severe the asthma, the greater the delay. This delay has not been found to be related to allergies or to short-term use of corticosteroids, and the explanation is still unknown (Shohat et al., 1987).

IMPACT ON SOCIETY

Asthma is thought to be a mild chronic disorder, but increases in morbidity and mortality have been reported over the past few decades (Evans et al., 1987). Between the years 1965 and 1983, a 200% increase in hospitalizations for asthma was reported. Hospitalizations were more frequent for males than for females and for nonwhites than for whites. An increase in deaths due to asthma for children older than 5 years of age was reported between 1979 (2598 deaths) and 1982 (3151 deaths). Death rates in 1982 were higher for 15- to 24-year-olds (0.4/100,000) than for 5- to 14-year-olds (0.2/100,000). Death rates were higher for blacks than for whites in both age groups: 0.7/100,000 black and 0.1/100,000 white for 5- to 14-year-olds and 1.1/100,000 black and 0.3/100,000 white for 15- to 24-year-olds. Death rates were also higher for children living below the poverty level (13.1/100,000) than for those living at or above the poverty level (10.3/100,000).

Asthma also has a major impact on the national economy. The cost related to asthma was estimated to be $6.2 billion in 1990. Hospitalizations were the largest single direct expense, accounting for $1.6 billion. Forty-three percent of the economic impact of asthma was associated with emergency department use, hospitalizations, and death (Weiss et al., 1992).

PHYSICAL THERAPY: ASSESSMENT AND TREATMENT

The goal of physical therapy is prevention of secondary difficulties resulting from recurrent asthma attacks. Education, relaxation, increasing or maintaining range of motion and muscle strength, improving thoracic mobility and posture, improving breathing pattern and bronchial hygiene, and improving exercise tolerance would be applicable to all ages, although different goals may be stressed at different points in the life cycle.

Infancy and Preschool-Aged Period

For the infant or preschool child, parent education and involvement are most important. The parent can learn to recognize signs of an impending asthma attack. Administering medication and calming the child can prevent the attack from progressing. The parent can be sure that the child drinks plenty of liquids to help thin any secretions. Research has demonstrated that postural drainage with percussion will help to clear the lungs when mucus accumulations occur (Huber et al., 1974). Twenty-one children with mild to moderate airway obstruction were divided into treatment and control groups. The treatment group received chest physical therapy with vibration and percussion. Thirty minutes after treatment, the treatment group demonstrated up to 40% increases in FEV_1. Many children also find percussion to be calming.

School-Aged and Adolescence Period

The older child can and should become more actively involved in independently managing his or her asthma. The child can receive education on identifying specific triggers, signs and symptoms of an impending attack, and proper medication technique. Exercises to improve or maintain range of motion, muscle strength, and posture can be taught. Relaxed diaphragmatic breathing and effective coughing techniques should be practiced often and in settings that cause difficulties. Relaxed diaphragmatic breathing may be performed to prevent or lessen the severity of an attack (Bolton et al., 1956). Deep inspirations, however, should be avoided since they have been shown to induce bronchoconstriction (Gayrard et al., 1975). Pursed lip exhalation helps to maintain the intra-airway pressure and prevent collapse of the airways (King, JT et al., 1984). Relaxed diaphragmatic breathing exercises and pursed lip exhalations can slow the respiratory rate and give the child a sense of control (King, JT et al., 1984). The forced expiration technique or "huffing" combined with relaxed diaphragmatic breathing does not increase airway obstruction and is effective in clearing airway secretions (Pryor & Webber, 1979).

EXERCISE-INDUCED ASTHMA

Because EIA is so common, any breathing difficulties associated with exercise should be evaluated by means of a standardized exercise challenge test conducted by qualified laboratory personnel. If a positive test is obtained, the child may be given medication to be used before exercising. In some children, however, medication does not totally prevent bronchoconstriction following exercise. Table 26–7 shows the results of an exercise challenge test performed 15 minutes following the proper administration of a bronchodilator inhaler for the 14-year-old previously presented in Table 26–4. Although the bronchodilator provided some protection against the exercise-induced bronchoconstriction, a positive test for EIA was still obtained with a moderate degree of respiratory impairment noted in $FEF_{25-75\%}$. For these children, enjoyable physical activities and sports activities may need to be specifically selected to encourage exercising for fitness. Frequency, duration, and intensity should then be gradually increased.

An interesting aspect of EIA is that the degree of bronchoconstriction experienced is affected by type, duration, and intensity of exercise; air temperature and humidity; and time since the previous

TABLE 26-7. **EXERCISE CHALLENGE TEST RESULTS***

Time (min)	PEFR	FEV$_1$	FEF$_{25-75\%}$	RPE	Heart Rate	% O$_2$ Saturation
0	3.52/97%	2.50/116%	2.08/71%	6	83	98
1	—	—	—	8	159	99
3	—	—	—	11	161	98
5	—	—	—	12	163	97
6/0	—	—	—	13	168	98
3	3.43†/95%	2.29/106%	1.86/63%	—	—	100
5	6.18/187%	2.25/104%	2.73/83%	—	—	98
10	5.44/150%	1.92†/89%	1.80†/61%	—	—	98
15	3.43/95%	2.34/108%	2.05/70%	—	—	98
20	3.94/109%	2.42/112%	1.98/67%	—	—	99
		Change from baseline				
	2.1% drop	23.3% drop	14.1% drop			

*Results of an exercise challenge test 15 minutes following proper inhalation of a bronchodilator for a 14 year old boy with asthma. Test consisted of a 6-minute run on a treadmill followed by 20 minutes of monitoring. Results indicate a positive exercised induced asthma response.
†Lowest value after exercise.

exercise (Sly, 1982). Short exercise periods (less than 2 minutes) are less likely to cause difficulty than prolonged exercise of 5 minutes or more. Exercise at a lower heart rate is also less problematic. For example, baseball would cause fewer difficulties than basketball. Swimming is less likely to cause difficulty than running. Exercising in cold, dry air will cause heat loss from the respiratory mucosa and result in more problems than exercising in warm, humid air (Ben-Dov et al., 1982; Strauss et al., 1978). Hyperventilation at rest under conditions that simulate the hyperpnea of exercise (same minute ventilation) has been shown to induce bronchoconstriction equivalent to that during exercise (Deal et al., 1979). The bronchoconstriction was increased when dry, cold air was breathed and inhibited when warm, humid air was breathed. It has been concluded, therefore, that the major stimulus for EIA may be heat loss caused by the hyperpnea of exercise rather than by the exercise itself.

Previous strenuous exercise can result in a refractory period during which there is a decreased bronchoconstriction response to exercise. This refractory period can last up to 2 hours and has been related to the intensity of the first exercise period (Edmunds et al., 1978). Exercising in warm, humid air, however, can inhibit EIA and also result in a refractory period to a second exercise period (Ben-Dov et al., 1982). A prolonged submaximal warm-up lasting 30 minutes and completed 21 minutes before a standard EIA test has also been shown to inhibit EIA (Reiff et al., 1989). Seven repeated 30-second short sprints with a 2½-minute rest between them completed 20 minutes before a standard exercise test have also been shown to inhibit EIA

(Schnall & Landau, 1980). Refractoriness, therefore, is not dependent on the degree of bronchoconstriction occurring during previous exercise.

CONDITIONING PROGRAMS AND PHYSICAL FITNESS

Conditioning programs can improve the response of the cardiovascular and respiratory systems to exercise. An increase in cardiac output results from an increase in cardiac stroke volume. A similar oxygen requirement can then be met by a lower heart rate. Ventilation improves with lower frequency and higher tidal volume. Improved oxygen utilization can result from an increase in the size and number of muscle mitochondria (Orenstein et al., 1985; Sharkey, 1979). An increase in fitness will result in an improved minute ventilation with a consequent decreased stimulus for EIA. Children with asthma have been shown to be able to attain normal maximum oxygen consumption (Vo$_2$max) levels (Bevegard et al., 1976; Chryssanthopoulos et al., 1984; Hedlin et al., 1986). Fit adults with asthma have been shown to be able to exercise significantly ($p < .001$) longer than unfit adults with asthma even though both groups were able to attain the same heart rate (Haas et al., 1985).

Children with asthma have participated safely in various exercise programs to improve their physical fitness when receiving preventative medication (Fitch et al., 1976; Henrickson & Nielson, 1983; Nickerson et al., 1983; Orenstein, 1985; Svenonius et al., 1983; Varray et al., 1991). Three types of programs will be described. In the first study (Henrickson & Nielson, 1983), 12 children with

EIA and generally poor physical fitness were divided into a training group of 28 and a control group of 14. The training group participated in a 6-week endurance training program consisting of 15 minutes of warm up, 15 minutes of ball games, 10 minutes of running, 20 minutes of gymnastic exercises, 20 minutes of circuit training, and 10 minutes of team games. The training sessions lasted 90 minutes and were scheduled twice per week. Following the 6-week program, the training group demonstrated a significantly increased aerobic capacity ($p < .05$) and a significantly decreased resting heart rate ($p < .05$). The second study (Fitch et al., 1976) examined the effects of a swimming program. Forty-six children participated in a 5-month program. The program began with three sessions per week and increased in intensity, duration, and frequency up to 5 1-hour sessions per week. At the conclusion of the program, improved posture and fitness, decreased fat folds measures, and enhanced swimming ability were reported, although no statistical analysis was reported. The third study (Nickerson et al., 1986) examined the effect of a running program. Fifteen children ran 4 days per week for 6 weeks. The daily distance was gradually increased over 2 weeks to 3.2 km. Fitness was assessed by measuring the distance run in 12 minutes. At the conclusion of the program, the average distance the children could run in 12 minutes was significantly increased above baseline measures ($p < .005$).

Varray and associates (1991) have emphasized the need to individualize physical fitness or aerobic training. Fourteen children with asthma, aged 9 to 13 years, were divided into a training group and a control group. The training group participated in two types of swimming training: aerobic training and high-intensity training, each conducted 2 times per week for 3 months. During the aerobic training the individual's ventilatory threshold (VTh, the point at which a nonlinear increase in ventilation occurs) was used to determine the training swimming speed (VTh velocity, the speed required to maintain the heart rate at VTh). During each session, the children swam 3 times for 10 minutes at their individual VTh velocity. The high-intensity training sessions were conducted during the second 3 months and consisted of two series of 6- to 25-meter laps at maximal speed with a 1-minute rest between laps at each session. After aerobic training, Vo_2max was significantly ($p < .001$) higher for the training group than for the controls. Mean VTh increased in the training group by 20% from baseline ($p < .001$). A significant ($p < .001$) increase in O_2 pulse max ($Vo_2/HRmax$) in the training group was also found, indicating improved cardiac adaptation and oxygen extraction. After high-intensity

training, Vo_2max did not change. VTh and O_2 pulse max decreased after the high-intensity training sessions and were not significantly different from baseline. The use of VTh to determine exercise intensity decreases the hyperventilation stimulus for EIA during training and individualizes the aerobic training protocol.

The effect on EIA itself of programs to improve fitness has been reported, but results are contradictory. On closer examination, it can be observed that the programs that reported a decrease in EIA (Henricksen & Nielsen, 1983; Svenonius et al., 1983) retested the children at the same heart rate, whereas the programs that reported no change in EIA (Fitch et al., 1976; Nickerson et al., 1983) altered the exercise stress level on retesting to compensate for the improved fitness and to ensure the same EIA stimulus. As previously mentioned, one of the benefits of improved fitness is a lower respiratory rate, which has been shown to then decrease the stimulus for EIA. This is an interesting and important observation demonstrating the value of improving and maintaining cardiovascular fitness in children with asthma.

Other areas of fitness have been evaluated by Strunk and associates (1988). Seventy-six children, aged 9 to 17 years, with moderately severe to severe asthma were evaluated for fitness by a timed 9-minute run, skin-fold thickness, number of sit-ups completed in 60 seconds, and flexibility determined by reaching toward the toes while sitting on the floor with outstretched legs. The primary area of difficulty was found to be endurance: 91% of the children scored at or below the 50th percentile, 74% at or below the 25th percentile, and 51% at or below the 10th percentile. An increase in skin-fold thickness was also present more frequently than normal: 21% at or below the 10th percentile. The results were not well explained by the severity of the disease.

Some children with EIA may reach Olympic levels of physical fitness. In the 1984 summer Olympics, 67 of 597 U.S. Olympic athletes had EIA. These athletes participated in 29 different events and won 41 medals (Voy, 1986).

The psychological adjustment to asthma has been found to be at least as important as the severity in determining fitness (Strunk et al., 1989). Ninety children, aged 9 to 17 years, with moderate to severe asthma, were tested by bicycle ergometry to determine cardiovascular fitness. Forty-eight percent were found to be more than 2 standard deviations below the mean with an additional 5% 1 to 2 standard deviations below the mean. Medical variables (recent exacerbation of disease, FEV_1, and specific airway conductance) and the psychological adjustment in terms of the child's relationship to family and peers, overall school adaptation, and the presence of psychiatric symptoms then were correlated with fitness separately and jointly. Medical variables as predictors of fitness resulted in an $R^2 = 0.08$ ($p < .19$). When psychological variables were added to the equation, the variance increased to 0.18 ($p < .003$). Psychological variables alone resulted in an R^2 of 0.12 ($p < .001$). Psychological variables were, therefore, more important in predicting fitness than medical factors.

EDUCATION

The proper use of medications must be discussed as part of an educational program. Many teenagers may underdose or overdose to "belong." With the present stress on drug education, some teenagers may be hesitant to take their medications for fear of being teased about "being on drugs." Other teenagers may have such a strong desire to participate in activities that they take extra doses, especially of metered-dose inhalers, at the slightest feeling of tightness. Still others may deny the symptoms and not take their medication when it is appropriate (Dahl et al., 1990).

The proper use of metered-dose inhalers has been taught to children as young as preschoolers. The majority of children, however, do not use a correct technique. An increased number of errors has been demonstrated by children younger than 6 years of age (Pedersen et al., 1986). Lee (1983) found that when time was taken to ensure that the child performed the maneuver correctly, use of proper technique was retained on retesting 6 months later.

Children with asthma and EIA do not always feel that they receive sufficient support from instructors at school. In a study of 420 children with asthma, aged 7 to 16 years, 29% of those who had occasional restrictions and 62% of those who had frequent restrictions stated that they had insufficient support from the instructor (Braback & Kalvesten, 1988). Physical education teachers may not have an adequate knowledge of asthma and, in particular, of EIA. The child who experiences EIA may be accused of being out of shape or lazy and pushed too much. Conversely, the instructor may not encourage the child to participate to his or her ability.

Another area in which physical therapists in the educational environment may be helpful is in teacher education. In many classrooms, a child may be exposed to a variety of triggers (classroom pets, plants, chalk dust, laboratory chemicals, and carpeting are a few examples. School performance may be affected by some of the asthma medications as previously mentioned (Brumback et al., 1984;

Furukawa et al., 1984; Rachelefsky, et al., 1986; Springer et al., 1985). School personnel should be instructed in the signs and symptoms of asthma and in relaxation and breathing exercises. They should know what to do to assist a child who is experiencing an asthma attack. Advanced notification of planned class experiences that might trigger attacks should be given to parents so that proper medications can be used if necessary. Occasionally, it may be necessary to alter the planned experience.

Behavioral management programs have proven helpful in increasing the child's participation in his or her own monitoring of asthma. Easily available specific programs include "Superstuff" (Superstuff [Item 0317], American Lung Association, New York), "Open Airways", (Open Airways/Respiro Abierto: Asthma Self Management Program, National Heart, Lung, and Blood Institute, Bethesda, MD), and "Asthma Care Training" (Asthma Care Training for Kids, Asthma and Allergy Foundation of America, Washington, DC) These programs are aimed at increasing self-management skills, helping families adjust to the demands that asthma imposes on family life, changing the use of health care services (e.g., decreased use of emergency departments), and improving school attendance and performance. Learning to discriminate early asthma symptoms is important for the proper use of relaxation and breathing exercises and of medication. A significant ($p < .05$) positive correlation has been found between subjectively experienced asthma and experienced panic in connection with asthma and school absenteeism (Dahl et al., 1990). Significant ($p < .05$) positive correlation has also been found between the perception of panic in asthmatic situations and the number of "as needed" doses of medication.

Education programs have been found to assist the child and family in developing coping skills. In one study, changes in compliance behavior and reductions in emergency department visits and days in the hospital were noted after education sessions (Lewis et al., 1984). The children demonstrated increased self-care and increased use of relaxation exercises. The parents demonstrated improved communication with their children and changes in smoking behavior and played a more active role during an attack. Another study (Dahl et al., 1990) examined the effect of behavioral intervention on children with severe asthma who were on oral β_2-agonists and used inhalers on an "as needed" basis. The behavioral intervention consisted of symptom discrimination, self-management techniques for breathlessness and to decrease the psychological dependence on spray medications, and modification of asthma-related behaviors (e.g., using asthma as a way to gain an advantage or to avoid a demanding situation). Relaxation and breathing exercises were taught to decrease anxiety and panic, to allow more appropriate use of the spray medication, and to aid in symptom discrimination. The intervention group demonstrated a significantly ($p < .05$) decreased use of "as needed" β_2-agonist sprays and significantly ($p < .05$) decreased number of school absences when compared with a control group.

Physical therapy can assist the child with asthma and his or her family in prevention of secondary impairments that can lead to functional limitations and disabilities. Maintenance of a good breathing pattern and bronchial hygiene for elimination of secretions will minimize poor posture and thoracic deformities. Improving or maintaining range of motion, muscle strength, and cardiovascular endurance will result in good physical fitness. Education will help the family learn to accept some lifestyle changes that will be necessary and to deal with the asthma attacks that do occur. Consultation with school personnel, scout leaders, camp counselors, and coaches will allow the child to participate in activities to his or her maximum ability.

Transition to Adulthood

During transition to adulthood, the individual-specific triggers may need to be considered when selecting future living and employment. When selecting a college roommate, for example, whether the person is a smoker may need to be considered. Reserve Officers' Training Corps and the military academies will not accept a candidate who has a history of asthma. The military services will not enlist a person with a history of asthma. Employment may be limited by allergens or asthma. Continued physical fitness should be stressed. Although it is believed that children outgrow asthma owing to a decrease in the number and severity of asthma attacks, adults who had asthma as children often demonstrate a positive bronchoconstriction response when sufficiently challenged (de Benedictis et al., 1990).

CASE HISTORY: TERRY

Terry was born in December 1974. He had signs and symptoms as an infant suggestive of allergies to cow's milk and eggs. These foods were avoided and Terry drank a soy formula. During his infancy and toddler years, he also experienced several episodes of croup. At the age of 19 months, he had a severe reaction to baby aspirin. Urticarial lesions appeared on his legs and arms, and the pediatrician was concerned about the reaction spreading to his lungs.

At the age of 2 years 6 months, Terry experienced his first asthma attack. It occurred after midnight and, therefore, he was seen in the emergency department of the local hospital. Wheezing, nasal flaring, expiratory grunting, intercostal retractions, and abdominal respirations were noted. Terry was treated and released. He was examined the following morning by his pediatrician and within 1 week had recovered. Of significance to his asthmatic attack is that he had been treated by the pediatrician 5 days earlier for upper respiratory tract infection, gastroenteritis, and otitis media.

At this time, Terry was referred to an allergist for evaluation. Skin prick allergen testing was positive for nearly every allergen tested. Very strong reactions to chicken, turkey, cow's milk, and eggs, as well as to mold, cat, and tobacco were found. A familial history of asthma was strong on the father's side and minimal on the mother's side. The allergist recommended placing Terry on theophylline, eliminating as many of the reactive foods as possible, and then gradually reintroducing them to obtain a more definite picture of the response to allergens. The parents were instructed in environmental control and to encourage liquids.

Terry experienced strong nervous system and gastrointestinal system side effects to the theophylline, and the medication was changed to metaproterenol (Alupent). Although the side effects decreased, they did not disappear.

During the 15 months (aged 2 years 6 months to 3 years 9 months) after Terry's first episodes of otitis media and asthma, he experienced four more episodes of otitis media and five episodes of respiratory congestion, wheezing, and bronchioasthmatic-type attacks that required examination and treatment by the pediatrician. A myringotomy with tubes was performed at age 2 years 11 months. Other mild asthma attacks were handled by medication at home. Terry's mother performed chest physical therapy as needed, along with calming, encouraging fluids, and administering medications.

At the age of 3 years 9 months, Terry was hospitalized for status asthmaticus. He was in significant respiratory distress with intercostal and substernal retractions, nasal flaring, expiratory stridor, and wheezing. Terry recovered quickly and was discharged after 4 days. While Terry was hospitalized, his parents were questioned about a family history of cystic fibrosis. After the hospitalization, the allergist recommended desensitization (allergy shots). Terry received an injection once per week for 6 weeks, and, interestingly, he would grind his teeth throughout that night.

After the myringotomy tubes fell out, Terry began to experience otitis media again. A second myringotomy with tubes and an adenoidectomy were performed when Terry was 4 years old.

During the next 2 years (aged 4 to 6), Terry was followed by a different allergist who recommended discontinuing the desensitization series and continuing with the daily medications and encouraging fluids. Subsequent wheezing episodes were milder and were handled with medications, fluids, and chest physical therapy. Between acute asthmatic attacks, signs and symptoms were negative and peak flow rates were greater than 100% of predicted values. Relaxed diaphragmatic breathing was practiced, and Terry would request chest physical therapy when he began to feel congestion. Terry was aware of the foods and situations that would cause difficulty and would try to avoid them if possible. If at a friend's house for lunch, for example, he would inform the friend's mother that he was allergic to milk and refuse to drink it even though often the mother was skeptical.

From age 6 to the present age of 19, Terry required treatment in the doctor's office for an acute asthma attack only once. Terry and his parents became aware of signs and symptoms that would indicate the beginning of an asthma attack. These were often associated with a cold. A home stethoscope was used to detect wheezing or decreased air flow. Using relaxation techniques, breathing exercises, and chest physical therapy, as well as medication, Terry was able to lessen or inhibit asthma attacks. Medication was not used daily but only as needed.

At age 13, Terry's mother learned that while playing with friends, Terry often had to stop to rest and catch his breath or to recover from coughing. He had not been interested in playing organized team sports but had enjoyed playing games with his friends just for fun. Unfortunately, the possibility of EIA had never been examined. After a consultation with the doctor, Terry was prescribed and instructed in the use of an albuterol (Ventolin) inhaler to use before physical education or other physical activity. A cromolyn (Intal) inhaler was also prescribed. At age 14, Terry participated in a research project on EIA. Until that time, the severity of his EIA had never been documented. The results in Tables 26–4 and 26–7 are for Terry. His physical education teachers were informed of his condition and worked with Terry in improving his physical fitness. At age 13,

TABLE 26–8. RESULTS OF STANDARDIZED PHYSICAL EDUCATION FITNESS TESTING FOR 13-YEAR-OLD BOY WITH ASTHMA

Test	Score	Percentile Rank
Sit-ups in 60 seconds	33	30th
Pull-ups	0	<20th
Long jump	5 feet 2 inches	25th
Shuttle run	10.2 seconds	60th
50-yard dash	7.8 seconds	30th
60-yard run	3 minutes 5 seconds	<5th*

*Major difficulty was found on prolonged running.
Data from Hunsicker, P. & Reiff, G. AAHPER Youth Fitness Test Manual (rev. ed.). Reston, VA: AAHPER Publications (American Alliance for Health, Physical Education, and Recreation), 1976, pp. 38–53.

Terry was tested in physical education class using the test from the American Alliance for Health, Physical Education, Recreation, and Dance (Reston, VA). Results are presented in Table 26–8. At the time of the testing, Terry had not yet started using the Ventolin inhaler before physical activity. It can be seen that Terry was at or below the 30th percentile in all tests but shuttle run and that his major difficulty was in the 600-yard run. Results from testing at age 17 are reported in Table 26–9. The high school physical education teachers were very strict in assessing quality of performance. The improvement in his physical fitness can be seen. The testing was completed during the fall when the pollen was high, and, therefore, Terry did not complete the 1-mile test as per physician recommendation.

This history exemplifies the need to question any child who seems to demonstrate the possibility of having EIA. Terry had reasoned that he had asthma; just as he could not eat turkey on Thanksgiving, he had difficulty with running. He had never known any different and so had never mentioned it.

Terry and his parents have learned to recognize signs and symptoms of an impending asthma attack and how to inhibit or minimize the attack, as well as allergens that need to be avoided. This awareness has resulted in

TABLE 26–9. RESULTS OF STANDARDIZED PHYSICAL EDUCATION FITNESS TESTING FOR 17-YEAR-OLD BOY WITH ASTHMA

Test	Score	Attainment Standard* (45th percentile)	Outstanding Achievement* (80th percentile)
Sit-ups	53	46	55
Sit and reach	20	17	20
Pull-ups	7	8	11

*Standards are from the Chrysler Fund – Amateur Athletic Union Physical Program, Poplars Building, Bloomington, IN 47405.

decreased visits to the doctor and decreased absences from school. Family life and vacations and teenage social life always take potential asthma attacks into account. Medication is carried by Terry for use as needed.

Unfortunately, not all asthma attacks could be prevented. Occasionally, a decision was made to try a potentially asthma-inducing situation after preventative medication. A hay ride resulted in bronchoconstriction. An overnight school camping experience resulted in a severe reaction to the mold and pollen. A Boy Scout back-pack hike and sleep out was cancelled at the last minute when asthma symptoms were noted; however, a 12-mile bike ride was accomplished without difficulties and a skiing trip was experienced with minimal problems. Terry participates in school dances and sporting activities with friends. He occasionally has problems in his school science laboratories when strong chemicals are used, but a second dose from his inhaler and relaxed breathing usually inhibit the bronchoconstriction.

Terry has always been short for his age, usually at or below the 5th percentile. Decreased height was not a problem that needed to be discussed, however, because he was one of the oldest students in his class because of the cutoff date for starting school and was within the 10th to 25th percentile for the class. At his present age of 19, Terry is continuing to grow. He is above the 25th percentile for his age for both height and weight, which is greater than was predicted at age 2.

Terry is now in college in a University Honors Program, majoring in biotechnology. He is already involved in research, which has heightened his interest in genetic research as a career. Perhaps he will be involved in work on a genetic cure for asthma.

CONCLUSION

Asthma is a common childhood condition that may produce functional limitations and interfere with daily life. Much is available to assist the child and family in dealing with asthma. Asthma is a life-long condition and, therefore, the main objective is to accept the condition and learn how to best avoid or minimize primary and secondary impairments that limit function and lead to disability. New developments in genetic research, however, hold promise for major advances in prevention and management of asthma.

REFERENCES

American Medical Association Committee on Rating of Mental and Physical Impairment. Guidelines to evaluation of permanent impairment: The respiratory system. Journal of the American Medical Association, 194:919–932, 1965.

Anderson, HR, Bailey, PA, Cooper, JS, Palmer, JC, & West, S. Morbidity and school absence caused by asthma and wheezing illness. Archives of Disease in Childhood, 58:777–784, 1983.

Anderson, SD. Drugs affecting the respiratory system with particular reference to asthma. Medicine and Science in Sports and Exercise, 13:259–265, 1981.

Anderson, SD, Silverman, M, & Walker, SR. Metabolic and ventilatory changes in asthmatic patients during and after exercise. Thorax, 27:718–725, 1972.

Bar-Or, O. Pathophysiological factors which limit the exercise capacity of the sick child. Medicine and Science in Sports and Exercise, 18:276–282, 1986.

Barnes, PJ. New therapeutic approaches. British Medical Bulletin, 48:231–247, 1991.

Ben-Dov, I, Bar-Yishay, E, & Godfrey, S. Refractory period after exercise-induced asthma unexplained by respiratory heat loss. American Review of Respiratory Disease, 125:530–534, 1982.

Bevegard, S, Eriksson, BO, Graff-Lonnevig, V, et al. Respiratory function, cardiovascular dimensions and work capacity in boys with bronchial asthma. Acta Paediatrica Scandinavica, 65:289–296, 1976.

Bierman, CW, & Pearlman, DS. Asthma. In Kendig, EL, & Chernick, L (Eds.), Disorders of the Respiratory Tract in Children (4th ed.). Philadelphia: WB Saunders, 1983, pp. 496–543.

Bishop, J, Carlin, J, & Nolan, T. Evaluation of the properties and reliability of a clinical severity scale for acute asthma in children. Journal of Clinical Epidemiology, 45:71–76, 1992.

Bolton, JH, Gandevia, B, & Ross, M. The rationale and results of breathing exercises in asthma. Medical Journal of Australia, 2:675–680, 1956.

Braback, L, & Kalvesten, L. Asthma in schoolchildren: Factors influencing morbidity in a Swedish survey. Acta Paediatrica Scandinavica, 77:826–830, 1988.

Brumback, RA, Wilson, H, & Station, RD. Behavior problems in children taking theophylline. Lancet, 1:958, 1984.

Buckley, JM, & Souhrada, JF. A comparison of pulmonary function tests in detecting exercise-induced bronchoconstriction. Pediatrics, 56(suppl):883–889, 1975.

Burney, PGJ, Chinn, S, & Rona, R. Has the prevalence of asthma increased in children? Evidence from the national study of health and growth 1973–86. British Medical Journal, 300:1306–1310, 1990.

Burr, ML, Eldridge, BA, & Borysiewicz, LK. Peak expiratory flow rates before and after exercise in schoolchildren. Archives of Disease in Childhood, 49:923–926, 1974.

Chryssanthopoulos, C, Maksud, MG, Gallen, WG, & Hause, LL. Cardiopulmonary responses of asthmatic children to strenuous exercise. Clinical Pediatrics, 23:384–388, 1984.

Cookson, WO, Sharp, PA, Faux, JA, & Hopkin, JM. Linkage between immunoglobulin E response underlying asthma and rhinitis and chromosome 11q. Lancet, 1:1292–1295, 1989.

Crofton, J, & Douglas, A (Eds.). Bronchial asthma. In Respiratory Diseases (3rd ed.). Boston: Blackwell Scientific Publications, 1981, pp. 478–515.

Cropp, GJA. The exercise bronchoprovocation test: Standardization of procedures and evaluation of response. Journal of Allergy and Clinical Immunology, 64:627–633, 1979.

Dahl, J, Gustafsson, D, & Melin, L. Effects of a behavioral treatment program on children with asthma. Journal of Asthma, 27:41–46, 1990.

de Benedictis, FM, Canny, GJ, & Levison, H. The progressive nature of childhood asthma. Lung, 168:278–285, 1990.

Deal, EC, McFadden, ER, Ingram, RH, & Jaeger, JJ. Hyperpnea and heat flux: Initial reaction sequence in exercise-induced asthma. Journal of Applied Physiology, 46:476–483, 1979.

Edmunds, AT, Tooley, M, & Godfrey, S. The refractory period

after exercise-induced asthma: Its duration and relation to the severity of exercise. American Review of Respiratory Diseases, *117*:247–254, 1978.

Evans, R, Mullally, DI, Wilson, RW, Gergen, PJ, Rosenberg, HM, Grauman, JS, Chevarley, FM, & Feinleib, M. National trends in the morbidity and mortality of asthma in the US: Prevalence, hospitalization and death from asthma over two decades: 1965–1984. Chest, *91*(suppl):65S–74S, 1987.

Fireman, P. Otitis media and its relationship to allergy. Pediatric Clinics of North America, *35*:1075–1090, 1988.

Fitch, KD, Morton, FR, & Blanksby, BA. Effects of swimming training on children with asthma. Archives of Disease in Childhood, *51*:190–194, 1976.

Freyschus, U, Hedlin, G, & Hedenstierna, G. Ventilation-perfusion relationships during exercise-induced asthma in children. American Review of Respiratory Disease, *130*:888–894, 1984.

Friedman, MM, & Kaliner, MA. Symposium on mast cells and asthma: Human mast cells and asthma. American Review of Respiratory Disease, *135*:1157–1164, 1987.

Furukawa, CT, Shapiro, GG, DuHamel, T, Weimer, L, Pierson, WE, & Bierman, CW. Learning and behaviour problems associated with theophylline therapy. Lancet, *1*:621, 1984.

Gayrard, P, Orehek, J, Grimaud, C, & Charpin, J. Bronchoconstrictor effect of a deep inspiration in patients with asthma. American Review of Respiratory Disease, *111*:433–439, 1975.

Gergen, PJ, Mullally, DI, & Evans, R. National survey of prevalence of asthma among children in the US, 1976 to 1980. Pediatrics, *81*:1–7, 1988.

Gold, DR, Trager, IB, Weiss, ST, Tosteson, TD, & Speizer, FE. Acute lower respiratory illness in childhood as a predictor of lung function and chronic respiratory symptoms. American Review of Respiratory Disease, *140*:877–884, 1989.

Haas, F, Pineda, H, Axen, K, Gaudino, D, & Haas, A. Effects of physical fitness on expiratory airflow in exercising asthmatic people. Medicine and Science in Sports and Exercise, *17*:585–592, 1985.

Hauspie, R, Susanne, C, & Alexander, F. Maturational delay and temporal growth retardation in asthmatic boys. Journal of Allergy and Clinical Immunology, *59*:200–206, 1977.

Hedlin, G, & Freyschuss, U. Cardiac output and blood pressure in asthmatic children before and during induced asthma. Acta Paediatrica Scandinavica, *73*:441–447, 1984.

Hedlin, G, Graff-Lonnevig, V, & Freyschuss, U. Working capacity and pulmonary gas exchange in children with exercise-induced asthma. Acta Paediatrica Scandinavica, *75*:947–954, 1986.

Henricksen, JM, & Nielson, TT. Effect of physical training on exercise-induced bronchoconstriction. Acta Paediatrica Scandinavica, *72*:31–36, 1983.

Hollister, JR, & Bowyer, SL. Adverse side effects of corticosteroids. Seminars in Respiratory Medicine, *8*:400–405, 1987.

Huber, AL, Eggleston, PA, & Morgan, J. Effect of physiotherapy on asthmatic children (Abstract). Journal of Allergy and Clinical Immunology, *53*:109, 1974.

Julier, C, Nakamura, Y, Lathrop, M, O'Connell, P, Leppert, M, Litt, M, Mohandas, T, Lalouel, JM, & White, R. A detailed map of the long arm of chromosome 11. Genomics, *7*:335–345, 1990.

Juniper, EF, Guyatt, GH, Epstein, RS, Ferrie, PJ, Jaeschke, R, & Hiller, TK. Evaluation of impairment of health related quality of life in asthma: Development of a questionnaire for use in clinical trials. Thorax, *47*:76–83, 1992.

Kattan, M, Keens, TG, Mellis, CM, & Levinson, H. The response to exercise in normal and asthmatic children. The Journal of Pediatrics, *92*:718–721, 1978.

Kelly, WJ, Hudson, I, Raven, J, Phelan, PD, Pain, MC, & Olinsky, A. Childhood asthma and adult lung function. American Review of Respiratory Disease, *138*:26–30, 1988.

Kerem, E, Canny, G, Tibshirani, R, Reisman, J, Bentur, L, Schuh, S, & Levison, H. Clinical-physiological correlations in acute asthma of childhood. Pediatrics, *87*:481–486, 1991.

King, JT, Bye, MB, & Demopoulos, JJ. Exercise programs for asthmatic children. Comprehensive Therapy, *10*:67–71, 1984.

King, TE, & Chang, S. Corticosteroid therapy in the management of asthma. Seminars in Respiratory Medicine, *8*:387–399, 1987.

Kurashima, K, Ogawa, H, Ohka, T, Fujimura, M, & Matsuda, T. Thromboxane A_2 synthetase inhibitor (OXY-046) improves abnormal mucociliary transport in asthmatic patients. Annals of Allergy, *68*:53–56, 1992.

Lee, HS. Proper aerosol inhalation technique for delivery of asthma medications. Clinical Pediatrics, *22*:440–443, 1983.

Levy, M, & Bell, L. General practice audit of asthma in childhood. British Medical Journal, *289*:1115–1116, 1984.

Lewis, CE. A randomized trial of ACT. Pediatrics, *74*:478–486, 1984.

Li, JT, & O'Connell, EJ. Viral infections and asthma. Annals of Allergy, *59*:321–328, 1987.

Lofdahl, CG, & Chung, KF. Long-acting β_2-adrenoreceptor agonists: A new perspective in the treatment of asthma. European Respiratory Journal, *4*:218–226, 1991.

Male, D. Immunology: An Illustrated Outline. St Louis: CV Mosby, 1986.

Manning, PJ, Watson, RM, Margolskee, DJ, Williams, VC, Schwartz, JI, & O'Byrne PM. Inhibition of exercise-induced bronchoconstriction by MK-571, a potent leukotriene D_4 receptor antagonist. New England Journal of Medicine, *323*:1736–1739, 1990.

Martin, AJ, McLennan, LA, Landau, LI, & Phelan, PD. The natural history of childhood asthma to adult life. British Medical Journal, *280*:1397–1400, 1980.

McConnochie, KM, & Roghmann, KJ. Bronchiolitis as a possible cause of wheezing in childhood: New evidence. Pediatrics, *74*:1–10, 1984.

McFadden, ER, Ingram, RH, Haynes, RL, & Wellman, JJ. Predominant site of flow limitation and mechanisms of post-exertional asthma. Journal of Applied Physiology, *42*:746–752, 1977.

Mercer, MJ, & Van Niekerk, CH. Clinical characteristics of childhood asthma. South African Medical Journal, *79*:77–79, 1991.

Mezey, RJ, Cohn, MA, Fernandez, RJ, Januszkiewicz, AJ, & Wanner, A. Mucociliary transport in allergic patients with antigen-induced bronchospasm. American Review of Respiratory Disease, *118*:677–684, 1978.

Miller, A. The role of the computer in pulmonary function tests. In Miller, A. (Ed.), Pulmonary Function Tests in Clinical and Occupational Lung Disease. Orlando, FL: Grune & Stratton, 1968, pp. 285–304.

Nickerson, BG, Bautista, DB, Namey, MA, Richards, W, & Keens, TG. Distance running improves fitness in asthmatic children without pulmonary complications or changes in exercise-induced bronchospasm. Pediatrics, *71*:147–152, 1983.

Orenstein, DM. Exercise tolerance and exercise conditioning in children with chronic lung disease. Journal of Pediatrics, *106*:556–560.

Orenstein, DM, Reed, ME, Grogan, FT, et al. Exercise conditioning in children with asthma. Journal of Pediatrics, *106*:556–560, 1985.

Paul, GH, & Fafoglia, BA. All About Asthma and How to Live with It. New York: Sterling Publishing, 1988.

Pederson, S, Frost, L, & Arnfred, T. Errors in inhalation technique and efficiency in inhaler use in asthmatic children. Allergy *41*:118–124, 1986.

Picado, C, Fiz, JA, Montserrat, JM, Grau, JM, Fernandez-Sola, J, Luengo, MT, Casademont, J, & Agusti-Vidal, A. Respiratory and skeletal muscle function in steroid-dependent bronchial asthma. American Review of Respiratory Disease, 141:14–20, 1990.

Pryor, JA, & Webber, BA. An evaluation of the forced expiration technique as an adjunct to postural drainage. Physiotherapy, 66:304–307, 1979.

Pullan, CR, & Hey, EN. Wheezing, asthma, and pulmonary function dysfunction ten years after infection with respiratory syncytial virus in infancy. British Medical Journal, 284:1665–1669, 1982.

Rachelefsky, GS, Wo, J, Adelson, J, Mickey, MR, Spector, SL, Katz, RM, Siegel, SC, & Rohr, AS. Behavior abnormalities and poor school performance due to oral theophylline use. Pediatrics, 78:1133–1138, 1986.

Rasmussen, JB, Eriksson, L-O, Margolskee, DJ, et al. Leukotriene D_4 receptor blockade inhibits the immediate and late bronchoconstrictor responses to inhaled antigen in patients with asthma. Journal of Allergy and Clinical Immunology, 90:193–201, 1992.

Reiff, DB, Choudry, NB, Pride, NB, & Ind, PW. The effect of submaximal warm-up exercise on exercise-induced asthma. American Review of Respiratory Disease, 139:479–484, 1989.

Rickards, AL, Ford, GW, Kitchen, WH, Doyle, LW, Lissenden, JV, & Keith, CG. Extremely low-birthweight infants: Neurological, psychological, growth, and health status beyond five years of age. Medical Journal of Australia, 147:476–481, 1987.

Ruppel, G. Manual of Pulmonary Function Testing. St. Louis: CV Mosby, 1982.

Schroeckenstein, DC, & Busse, W. Exercise and asthma: Not incompatible. Journal of Respiratory Diseases, 9:29–45, 1988.

Schnall, RP, & Landau, LI. Protective effects of repeated short sprints in exercise-induced asthma. Thorax, 35:828–832, 1980.

Sharkey, BJ. Physiology of Fitness. Champaign, IL: Human Kinetics Publishers, 1979.

Shohat, M, Shohat, T, Kadeem, R, Mimouni, M, & Danon, YL. Childhood asthma and growth outcome. Archives of Disease in Childhood, 62:63–65, 1987.

Sly, RM. History of exercise-induced asthma. Medicine and Science in Sports and Exercise, 18:314–317, 1986.

Sly, RM. Management of exercise-induced asthma. Drug Therapy, 12(March):95–100, 1982.

Smyth, JA, Tabachnik, FE, Duncan, JW, Reilly, BJ, & Levison, H. Pulmonary function and bronchial hyperreactivity in long-term survivors of bronchopulmonary dysplasia. Pediatrics, 68:336–340, 1981.

Snyder, RD, Collip, PJ, & Greene, JS: Growth and ultimate height of children with asthma. Clinical Pediatrics, 6:389–392, 1967.

Spector, SL. Outpatient treatment of asthma. Annals of Allergy, 63:591–597, 1989.

Spector, SL, Perhach, JL, Rohr, AS, Rachelefsky, GS, Katz, RM, & Siegel, SC. Pharmacodynamic evaluation of azelastine in subjects with asthma. Journal of Allergy and Clinical Immunology, 80:75–80, 1987.

Springer, C, Goldenberg, B, Ben Dov, I, & Godfrey, S. Clinical, physiologic, and psychologic comparison of treatment by cromolyn or theophylline in childhood asthma. Journal of Clinical Immunology, 76:64–69, 1985.

Strauss, RH, McFadden, ER, & Ingram, RH. Influence of heat and humidity on the airway obstruction induced by exercise in asthma. Journal of Clinical Investigation, 61:433–440, 1978.

Strunk, RC, Mrazek, DA, Fukuhara, JT, Masterson, J, Ludwick, SK, & LaBrecque, JF. Cardiovascular fitness in children with asthma correlates with psychological functioning of the child. Pediatrics, 84:460–464, 1989.

Strunk, RC, Rubin, D, Kelly, L, Sherman, B, & Fukuhara, J. Determination of fitness in children with asthma: Use of standardized tests for functional endurance, body fat composition, flexibility, and abdominal strength. American Journal of Disease in Childhood, 142:940–944, 1988.

Svenonius, E, Kautto, R, & Arborelius, M. Improvement after training of children with exercise-induced bronchospasm. Acta Paediatrica Scandinavica, 72:22–30, 1983.

Sykes, RS, & Cochetto, DM. Antiasthma drugs: Key issues in clinical trial methodology. Journal of Asthma, 29:79–90, 1992.

Tal, A, & Miklich, DR. Emotionally induced decreases in pulmonary flow rates in asthmatic children. Psychosomatic Medicine, 38:190–199, 1976.

Taylor, IK, O'Shaughnessey, KM, Fuller, RW, & Dollery, CT. Effect of cysteinyl-leukotriene antagonist ICI204.219 on allergen-induced bronchoconstriction and airway hyperreactivity in atopic subjects. Lancet, 337:690–694, 1991.

Taussig, LM, Chernick, V, Wood, R, et al. Standardization of lung testing in children. Journal of Pediatrics, 97:668–676, 1980.

Townsend, M, Feeny, DH, Guyatt, et al. Evaluation of the burden of illness for pediatric asthmatic patients and their parents. Annals of Allergy, 67:403–408, 1991.

Varray, AL, Mercier, JG, Terral, CM, & Prefaut, CG. Individualized aerobic and high intensity training for asthmatic children in an exercise readaptation program: Is training always helpful for better adaptation to exercise? Chest, 99:579–586, 1991.

Voy, RO. The U.S. Olympic Committee experience with exercise-induced bronchospasm, 1984. Medicine and Science in Sports and Exercise, 18:328–330, 1986.

Wantanabe, H. The effect of disodium cromoglycate against bronchial hyperresponsiveness in asthmatic children. Journal of Asthma, 29:117–120, 1982.

Weiss, KB, Gergen, PJ, & Hodgson, TA. An economic evaluation of asthma in the United States. New England Journal of Medicine, 326:862–866, 1992.

Wennergren, G, Engstrom, I, & Bjure, J. Transcutaneous oxygen and carbon dioxide levels and a clinical symptom scale for monitoring the acute asthmatic state of infants and children. Acta Paediatrica Scandinavica, 75:465–469, 1986.

Chapter 27

Thoracic Surgery

BETSY A. HOWELL, PT, MS

INTRODUCTION

Approximately 8 to 10 in 1000 children born each year have congenital heart defects (Callow, 1989). The impact a congenital heart defect has on a child varies greatly depending on the type of defect as well as the individual child. For example, 2 children, each diagnosed with a ventricular septal defect, may have entirely different histories. One child may go undiagnosed for several years, whereas the other child may require surgery in infancy. Formerly, the majority of congenital heart defects were repaired when the child was at least 1 year old, often older. More of these surgeries are now performed during infancy, which is likely to affect how children with congenital heart defects grow and develop. Physical therapists involved with this population need to closely monitor and document the nature and extent of developmental differences that may result from earlier surgical repair. To prepare therapists for this task, this chapter de-

scribes congenital heart defects; surgical repairs, including heart and heart-lung transplantation; acute and chronic physical impairments secondary to heart defects and surgery; profound cyanosis or neurologic complications; and physical therapy for the population of children with cardiac defects.

CONGENITAL HEART DEFECTS

The cause of congenital heart defects is not known; however, the occasional presence of more than 1 child with congenital heart disease in the same family suggests a possible genetic component. Approximately 10% of children with congenital heart defects also have other physical malformations (Noonan, 1981). Heart defects are associated with Down syndrome, Turner's syndrome, Williams syndrome, Marfan's syndrome, and the Vater association. Infants of diabetic mothers also have an increased incidence of congenital heart disease (Clarke et al., 1991).

Diagnosis of cardiac problems may occur at birth and be followed by further evaluation at that time. Some infants with severe cyanotic disease are not diagnosed before they are discharged to home, but several weeks later they may be diagnosed with a heart defect when they present with symptoms of septic shock. Other cardiac defects may not be diagnosed until much later, even as late as adolescence. For example, coarctation of the aorta is occasionally diagnosed during a sports physical examination when a large difference between upper and lower extremity blood pressure or an abnormally high upper extremity blood pressure is observed.

The infant with a congenital heart defect often presents with abnormal respiratory signs, including a labored breathing pattern and an increased respiratory rate. The infant may be diaphoretic and tachycardiac. Edema around the eyes and decreased urine output (evidenced by dry diapers) may also be observed. Eating problems result from difficulty in coordinating sucking and swallowing with breathing at an increased rate. Irritability that is difficult to assuage may be noted. These symptoms of congestive heart failure can lead to the diagnosis of a cardiac defect or provide evidence of the worsening of a known defect.

Congenital heart defects are usually classified as acyanotic or cyanotic. In acyanotic lesions, the child is pink and has normal oxygen saturation. If there is mixing or shunting of blood within the heart, the blood shunts from the left side of the heart to the right side, so oxygenated blood goes to the lungs as well as to the body. Common acyanotic lesions include atrial septal defects, ventricular septal defects, patent ductus arteriosus, coarctation of the aorta, pulmonary stenosis, and aortic stenosis.

In cyanotic defects, blood is typically shunted from the right side of the heart to the left side. Unoxygenated blood is then returned to the body, resulting in arterial oxygen saturation levels 15 to 30% below normal values. Common cyanotic lesions include tetralogy of Fallot, transposition of the great arteries, tricuspid atresia, pulmonary atresia, truncus arteriosus, total anomalous pulmonary venous return, and hypoplastic left-heart syndrome.

Type and timing of intervention depend on the defect and the age of the child. Some defects are repaired immediately, whereas others require a staged procedure, with the first several surgeries being palliative rather than corrective. Some acyanotic defects are not repaired until the child is several years old. Less impairment of growth and weight gain, however, occurs when surgery is per-

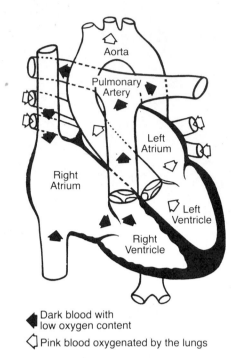

FIGURE 27–1. Normal anatomic relationships of heart structures. (From Driscoll, DJ. Evaluation of the cyanotic newborn. The Pediatric Clinics of North America. 37[1]:5, 1990.)

formed in the first 2 years of life (Rosenthal, 1983; Suoninen, 1971). Acyanotic and cyanotic defects are described in the next two sections and may be compared with normal anatomy of the heart (Fig. 27–1).

ACYANOTIC DEFECTS

Atrial Septal Defect

Atrial septal defect, one of the most common congenital heart defects, is an abnormal communication between the left and right atria (Fig. 27–2). The defect is classified by its location on the septum. Blood is generally shunted from the left atrium to the right atrium. This defect has traditionally been repaired when a child is between 4 and 6 years old because of slow progression of damage to the heart and lungs. If a child presents with more severe symptoms, the defect is repaired sooner (Mee, 1991). Some adults presenting with signs of heart failure are found to have a previously undiagnosed atrial septal defect. As medical technology advances, late diagnoses should become rare.

FIGURE 27–2. Atrial septal defect. (Reprinted with permission of Ross Laboratories, Columbus, OH 43216, © 1970 Ross Laboratories.)

Surgical repair has traditionally been made through a median sternotomy incision; however, a right thoracotomy approach has also been used primarily for cosmetic reasons. The defect is usually sutured together, or a patch closure is used when necessary (Kopf & Laks, 1991). The timing of surgery depends on the age of the child, when the diagnosis is confirmed, and how symptomatic the child is, but it typically occurs during the first 5 years of life.

Ventricular Septal Defect

Ventricular septal defect is the most common congenital heart defect (20–30% of all children with congenital defects) (Graham et al., 1989). It can be present alone or in association with other defects such as the tetralogy of Fallot and transposition of the great arteries. Ventricular septal defect alone is discussed here. A ventricular septal defect is a communication between the ventricles that allows blood to be shunted between them, generally from left to right (Fig. 27–3). The increase in blood flow through the right ventricle to the lungs may lead to pulmonary hypertension. In severe cases, in which pulmonary pressures exceed systemic pressures, shunting switches from right to left, which is often labeled Eisenmenger's syndrome (Graham et al., 1989). A large defect may lead to early left

ventricular failure. An infant with a large ventricular septal defect presents with signs of severe respiratory distress, diaphoresis, and fatigability, especially during feeding, when the infant's endurance is stressed (Giboney, 1983). The infant's weight is dramatically affected in this situation. A child this severely affected has a much earlier surgical repair than a child who is asymptomatic.

Small defects may close spontaneously. Defects that compromise the clinical status of the patient must be surgically closed. The timing of surgery varies, depending on the child's tolerance of the defect. A child with a larger defect undergoes surgery earlier to diminish the negative effects on growth and the pulmonary system. Surgical intervention is through a mediastinal approach and usually requires a synthetic patch closure (Arciniegas, 1991). The mortality for surgical closure of a ventricular septal defect without other associated defects is very low (1%) (Arciniegas, 1991).

Patent Ductus Arteriosus

The ductus arteriosus is a large vessel that connects the main pulmonary artery to the descending aorta (Fig. 27–4). It usually closes soon after birth but dilates (remains patent) in response to hypoxia or prostaglandins E_1 and E_2 (Levitsky & del Nido, 1991). The ability to maintain patency of the

FIGURE 27–3. Ventricular septal defect. (Reprinted with permission of Ross Laboratories, Columbus, OH 43216, © 1970 Ross Laboratories.)

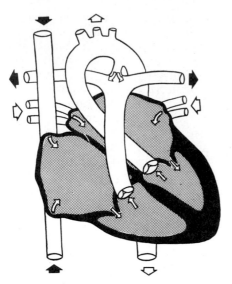

FIGURE 27–4. Patent ductus arteriosus. (Reprinted with permission of Ross Laboratories, Columbus, OH 43216, © 1970 Ross Laboratories.)

ductus arteriosus becomes important in certain cyanotic heart defects to be discussed later. A high incidence of patency is found in premature infants because of respiratory distress syndrome and the resulting hypoxia. Surgical repair is generally performed by a left thoracotomy incision. The ductus is ligated and sutured.

Coarctation of the Aorta

Coarctation of the aorta is defined as a narrowing or closing of a section of the aorta (Fig. 27–5). Patent ductus arteriosus was observed in approximately 23% of diagnosed cases of coarctation of the aorta (Waldhausen et al., 1991). Infants with a severe narrowing may develop left ventricular failure (Girlando, 1988). Early repair is necessary when a child is severely symptomatic. The child or adult without symptoms may go undiagnosed until a routine physical examination reveals an abnormally high upper extremity blood pressure.

Surgical intervention is the primary method of treating coarctation of the aorta. Access to the aorta is through a left thoracotomy, after which the aorta is repaired with an end-to-end anastomosis, subclavian flap, or a patch aortoplasty (Waldhausen et al., 1991). The operative mortality for surgical repair is low (3%) (Waldhausen et al., 1991).

Pulmonary Stenosis

Pulmonary stenosis is a narrowing of the right ventricular outflow tract and is classified by the location of the narrowing relative to the pulmonary valve. It often occurs in association with other heart defects. Timing of surgery depends on the severity of the narrowing and the degree of functional compromise.

Surgery is performed through a median sternotomy; the actual surgical procedure depends on the site of narrowing. A valvotomy may be performed, or in severe cases, the valve may need to be replaced (Moulton & Malm, 1991). Mortality varies with the age of the child at the time of repair. Children older than 2 years have a low mortality rate (.5%), whereas the rate for those younger than 1 year increases to 10% (Moulton & Malm, 1991).

Aortic Stenosis

Aortic stenosis is a narrowing of the left ventricular outflow tract and is classified by its relation to the aortic valve (supravalvular, valvular, or subvalvular) (Fig. 27–6). An aortic valvotomy is performed through a median sternotomy in infants and children with severe stenosis. In severe cases, a valve replacement may be necessary if a valvotomy

FIGURE 27–5. Coarctation of the aorta. (Reprinted with permission of Ross Laboratories, Columbus, OH 43216, © 1970 Ross Laboratories.)

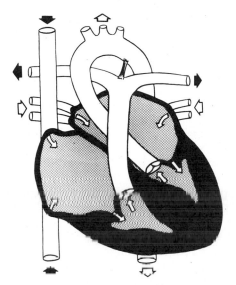

FIGURE 27–6. Aortic stenosis. (Reprinted with permission of Ross Laboratories, Columbus, OH 43216, © 1970 Ross Laboratories.)

cannot be performed (Weldon et al., 1991). Mortality rate around the time of surgery is 6% (Weldon et al., 1991).

CYANOTIC DEFECTS

Tetralogy of Fallot

The tetralogy of Fallot is the most common cyanotic cardiac defect, accounting for almost 50% of all cyanotic lesions. The primary abnormalities that occur in the tetralogy of Fallot are a ventricular septal defect, right ventricular outflow tract obstruction, an aorta that overrides the right ventricle, and hypertrophy of the right ventricle (Laks & Breda, 1991a) (Fig. 27–7). Clinical manifestations of the defect depend on severity of the obstruction of the right ventricular outflow tract. With increasing severity, an increase in cyanosis is observed that becomes more marked when the child is overexerted or upset. Clubbing of the nailbeds occurs and becomes more apparent after the first 6 to 8 months. The height and weight of the child are often affected. Cyanotic or blue episodes occur, which are thought to be caused by an abrupt decrease in pulmonary blood flow and are characterized by dyspnea, syncope, and deepening cyanosis (Laks & Breda, 1991a; Page, 1986). The cyanotic

episodes are typically relieved by squatting or by bringing the knees to the chest. These maneuvers are believed to increase systemic vascular resistance and ultimately to increase pulmonary blood flow. Oxygen or morphine or both may also need to be administered (Laks & Breda, 1991a).

Surgical intervention depends on the patient's symptoms and overall clinical picture. Early palliation may be necessary if an infant is severely involved and would probably not survive corrective surgery. The palliative procedure used most often is a Blalock-Taussig (BT) shunt performed through a thoracotomy. The BT shunt involves an anastomosis of the subclavian artery to the pulmonary artery, providing increased pulmonary blood flow while the infant gains more time to grow before undergoing corrective surgery. Mild growth retardation may occur in the upper extremity on the side of the shunt, but it has not been viewed as a major problem (Page, 1986). Another important consequence of early palliation is continued cyanosis until complete repair is performed.

Corrective surgery involves closing the ventricular septal defect and relieving the right outflow tract obstruction. After surgical repair, an exercise stress test is warranted before the initiation of an exercise program because of a 14% incidence of ventricular arrhythmias at rest and a 30% incidence during exercise (Garson et al., 1980). With advances in

FIGURE 27–7. Tetralogy of Fallot. (Reprinted with permission of Ross Laboratories, Columbus, OH 43216, © 1970 Ross Laboratories.)

surgical technique, mortality rates for surgical repair (5%) have been drastically reduced (Laks & Breda, 1991a).

Transposition of the Great Arteries

In transposition of the great arteries, the pulmonary artery arises from the morphologic left ventricle, and the aorta arises from the right ventricle (Callow, 1989) (Fig. 27–8). In the absence of other defects, the systemic blood returns to the body unoxygenated and pulmonary blood returns to the lungs fully oxygenated. This situation is obviously not compatible with life unless the ductus arteriosus remains patent. Immediate intervention, usually with the infusion of prostaglandin E_1, is necessary to keep the ductus arteriosus open. An atrial septostomy is performed by a cardiac catheterization to keep the child alive until surgical intervention occurs.

The type of surgical intervention used for correction of transposition of the great arteries depends largely on the surgeon's preference. In some institutions, a Mustard or Senning technique is used to redirect the venous return to the atria, either by baffles or flaps of atrial wall, respectively (de Leval, 1991; Trusler, 1991). These techniques leave the right ventricle as the pumping chamber for the systemic system.

The Rastelli procedure is a surgical technique used when a severe left ventricular outflow tract obstruction and a ventricular septal defect coexist. Repair usually occurs when the child is between 4 and 6 years old. A conduit diverts blood from the left ventricle through the ventricular septal defect and right ventricle to the aorta, a right ventricle to pulmonary artery conduit is formed, and any previous shunts are eliminated (Williams, 1991). Reoperation for conduit enlargement is not uncommon. Depression of right ventricular function over time has been reported in some patients whose defects were corrected with these procedures (Jarmakani & Canent, 1974; Nakazawa et al., 1986).

The preferred technique, when anatomically possible, is the arterial switch procedure. Surgery during the first 2 to 4 weeks of life is preferred so that the left ventricle meets the systemic demands. Surgical repair occurs through a median sternotomy and involves transecting the aorta and pulmonary artery. The coronary arteries are excised with a wide button of aortic tissue and reimplanted in the old pulmonary arterial vessel; the great vessels are then switched and anastomosed so that the aorta connects to the left ventricle and the pulmonary artery connects to the right ventricle. The arterial switch procedure produces results that are free of the dysrhythmias and right ventricular failure associated with the techniques described above (Callow, 1989). Survival rates at major centers in which this technique is performed have been good (>90%) (Castaneda & Mayer, 1991).

Tricuspid Atresia

Tricuspid atresia is the failure of development of the tricuspid valve, resulting in a lack of communication between the right atrium and right ventricle. Usually, an atrial septal defect or a ventricular septal defect or both exists to allow pulmonary blood flow (Fig. 27–9). The right-to-left shunt allows mixing of unoxygenated and oxygenated blood, causing the child to be cyanotic. The right ventricle is frequently underdeveloped.

Surgical repair is staged, with the initial operation shunting blood from the body to the lungs with a BT shunt through a thoracotomy. If, however, the ventricular septal defect is large and too much blood is going to the lungs, a band may be placed around the pulmonary artery to decrease blood flow to the lungs. The child remains cyanotic for several years.

The next stage of surgical repair is often the Fontan procedure (or a modification thereof) performed through a median sternotomy in which the right atrium is attached to the pulmonary artery or directly to the right ventricle, using a conduit or

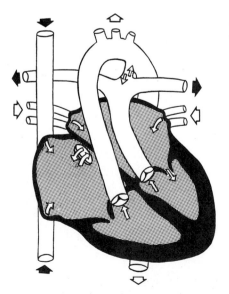

FIGURE 27–8. Transposition of the great arteries. (Reprinted with permission of Ross Laboratories, Columbus, OH 43216, © 1970 Ross Laboratories.)

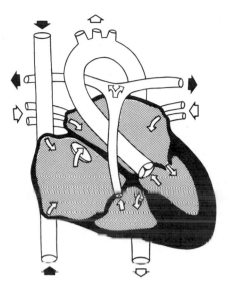

FIGURE 27–9. Tricuspid atresia. (Reprinted with permission of Ross Laboratories, Columbus, OH 43216, © 1970 Ross Laboratories.)

baffle. The ventricular septal defect may be surgically closed (Laks & Breda, 1991b). It is not uncommon to have significant chest tube drainage for weeks after the Fontan surgery, thereby increasing the length of hospital stay.

In some institutions, a bidirectional Glenn procedure performed before the Fontan procedure leads to an improved outcome. In the Glenn procedure, the superior vena cava is anastomosed to the right pulmonary artery. The child remains cyanotic but gains time for growth before undergoing the Fontan operation. Operative mortality has decreased from 15 to 30% to less than 5% with improved surgical technique and patient selection (Laks & Breda, 1991b).

Pulmonary Atresia

Pulmonary atresia occurs when the pulmonary valve fails to develop, resulting in obstruction of blood flow from the right heart to the lungs. Blood flow to the lungs is initially maintained by a patent ductus arteriosus. An atrial septal or ventricular septal defect may also be present, allowing shunting of the blood from the right heart to the left heart and ultimately back to the body. The size of the right ventricle may vary, impacting later surgical decisions. Early intervention involves maintaining patency of the ductus arteriosus to increase blood flow to the lungs until surgery can be performed. An atrial septostomy is usually performed during

the initial cardiac catheterization. A BT shunt is frequently performed as soon as possible.

Later surgery involves ligating the previous shunt, closing the atrial septal defect, and opening the pulmonary valve by a valvulotomy, infundibular graft, or right ventricle-to-pulmonary artery conduit. If the ventricle is poorly developed, the Fontan procedure may be performed to provide communication through a conduit between the right atrium and pulmonary artery (Puga, 1991). Children remain cyanotic during their early developmental years until the Fontan operation is performed. Surgical mortality is nearly 10% (Puga, 1991).

Truncus Arteriosus

Truncus arteriosus occurs when the aorta and pulmonary artery fail to separate in utero and form a common trunk arising from both ventricles (Fig. 27–10). Four grades of the condition are differentiated, depending upon the location of the pulmonary arteries. Early surgical intervention is necessary. Surgical repair is through a median sternotomy and involves removing the pulmonary arteries from the truncus, closing the ventricular septal defect, and connecting the pulmonary arteries to the right ventricle by an extracardiac baffle. Mortality is lower in patients operated on in the first 6 months of life (9% vs 18% for later repair) (Milgalter & Laks, 1991; Peetz et al., 1982).

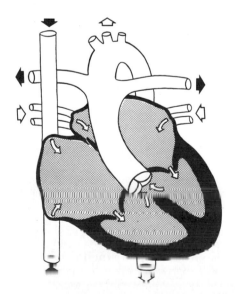

FIGURE 27–10. Truncus arteriosus. (Reprinted with permission of Ross Laboratories, Columbus, OH 43216, © 1970 Ross Laboratories.)

Total Anomalous Pulmonary Venous Return

Total anomalous pulmonary venous return occurs when the pulmonary veins fail to communicate with the left atrium and instead connect to the coronary sinus of the right atrium or to one of the systemic veins. The ductus arteriosus often remains patent (Fig. 27-11). The increase in flow through the right side of the heart and into the lungs may lead to congestive heart failure. Anastomosis of the pulmonary veins to the left atrium through a median sternotomy is usually performed as soon as possible. Postoperative ventilation may be difficult because of stiffness and wetness of the lungs from the previous excessive blood flow (Byrum et al., 1982; Hammon & Bender, 1991). Mortality continues to improve but remains nearly 30% for infants (Hammon & Bender, 1991).

Hypoplastic Left-Sided Heart Syndrome

Hypoplastic left heart syndrome, the most common form of a univentricular heart, is marked by hypoplasia or absence of the left ventricle and hypoplasia of the ascending aorta, often coexisting with severe aortic valve hypoplasia. A patent ductus arteriosus provides systemic circulation until surgical intervention. Without surgical intervention, death is certain; however, the surgical mortality rate is still high (40%) (Bailey & Gundry, 1990).

Three options are available to parents of infants diagnosed as having hypoplastic left heart syndrome. One option is no surgical intervention. As a second option, the child's name may be placed on a waiting list for a heart transplant, or as a third, the child may undergo a series of palliative procedures. The initial surgical procedure (Norwood I) involves enlarging the atrial septal defect, transecting the main pulmonary artery and anastomosing it to the aorta, and reconstructing the aortic root. A BT or central shunt is placed to allow pulmonary blood flow. The second stage is a bidirectional Glenn procedure anastomosing the superior vena cava to the pulmonary arteries and ligating the BT shunt. The Fontan procedure may be performed several months to a few years later. This procedure provides continuity between the right atrium and pulmonary artery, and the pulmonary venous return is separated from the systemic system. As a result, the right ventricle pumps fully oxygenated blood to the body (Johnson, AB, & Davis, 1991; Norwood, WI, 1991a, 1991b). Heart transplantation is also offered as a second-stage possibility. The postoperative stay is usually lengthy, and children often have difficulty in being weaned from the ventilator. Although infants who survive the first stage may die (10%) before reaching the second stage, surgical interventions continue to lower mortality (Bailey & Gundry, 1990).

Heart Transplantation

Cardiac transplantation is a viable option for children with end-stage heart failure secondary to congenital malformations or for children with cardiomyopathy. Introduction of cyclosporine to control rejection has increased survival rates to 60% after 5 years. The previous indication for transplantation in children was largely cardiomyopathy (62%). Since 1988, however, the number of transplants for congenital heart defects has surpassed that of cardiomyopathy (Kriett & Kaye, 1991; Pennington et al., 1991). The increase is at least partly related to the fact that cardiac transplantation is being offered more frequently as an option for children with hypoplastic left heart syndrome. As a result, a greatly increased number of children under 1 year of age have received a cardiac transplant (Bailey et al., 1988; Bove, 1991; Pennington et al., 1991; Starnes et al., 1992). Starnes and associates (1992) have observed a 74% 1- and 2-year survival

FIGURE 27-11. Total anomalous pulmonary venous return. (Reprinted with permission of Ross Laboratories, Columbus, OH 43216, © 1970 Ross Laboratories.)

rate in infants under 1 year of age undergoing cardiac transplantation.

Surgery is performed through a median sternotomy and involves removal of the recipient heart with residual atrial cuffs remaining. The atria are reanastomosed with the donor heart, and then the great arteries are connected (Haas et al., 1991). Severing of the vagus nerve and the cervical and thoracic sympathetic cardiac nerves leaves the heart denervated (Clough, 1990; Kent & Cooper, 1974). An intrinsic control system exists within the heart, so it is not dependent on innervation for function. Cardiac impulse formation occurs because of spontaneous depolarization of the sinoatrial node (Kent & Cooper, 1974). The sinus node firing rate is faster than the usual heart rate in resting humans, so the heart rate of an individual after transplantation is faster than normal (Uretsky, 1990).

Several other influences on myocardial contractility remain, including the Frank-Starling effect, the Anrep effect, and the Bowditch effect. The Frank-Starling effect is the increase in cardiac output by an increase in stroke volume after an increased input or venous return (Kent & Cooper, 1974). This is an important effect that helps the body meet its early oxygen needs for exercise after transplantation. With the Anrep effect retained, the cardiac muscle increases its contractile force when the aortic pressure rises (afterload). The Bowditch effect describes an augmented contractile force of the heart with an increase in heart rate (Clough, 1990; Kent & Cooper, 1974). The transplanted heart has an increased sensitivity to circulating catecholamines (epinephrine and norepinephrine). Epinephrine increases the heart rate and the force of myocardial contraction, and norepinephrine increases the peripheral vascular resistance (Clough, 1990). The hormonal release takes several minutes to have an effect on the heart's rate and contractility, so it is generally advised that patients perform several minutes of warm-up exercises before vigorous exercise. It also takes several minutes for the body to reduce the hormones to normal levels, so a cool-down period at the end of exercise is also advised. The resting heart rate is higher than usual in transplant recipients, and the peak heart rate is lower, both should be taken into account when transplant patients are exercising (Uretsky, 1990).

Antirejection treatment begins with triple therapy of cyclosporine, azathioprine (Imuran), and prednisone. The use of steroids is discontinued as soon as possible and only reinstituted if rejection occurs (Bailey et al., 1988; Pennington et al., 1991). The use of steroids should be taken into consideration when the weight and height percentiles of transplant recipients are reviewed. The majority of

children increase their weight rather dramatically without a concomitant increase in height (Fricker et al., 1990; Pennington et al., 1991). Cyclosporine has been noted to cause hypertension, hyperplasia of the gastrointestinal mucosa, hirsutism, and gingival hyperplasia (Haas et al., 1991). The immunosuppressive medications also accelerate atherosclerosis, even in children, as well as decrease the body's ability to fight infections.

Rejection is an ongoing issue in all transplant patients. Signs and symptoms of rejection range from fever, malaise, poor appetite, weight gain, tachycardia, tachypnea, and low urine output to poor perfusion, complete heart block, pulmonary edema, and shock (Haas et al., 1991). Severe rejection has been observed in several adolescent transplant recipients after missing just one dose of cyclosporine.

Several complications are fairly common in the pediatric heart transplant population. Hypertension and seizures have been observed in a number of patients. Seizures are believed to be caused by high cyclosporine levels; however, they do not generally recur once the patient is on a therapeutic dose of anticonvulsants (Fricker, 1990; Pennington et al., 1991). Other central nervous system disturbances have been observed in children, ranging from lethargy and confusion to localized neurologic defects and behavioral disturbances. Central nervous system dysfunction occurs more frequently in children than in adults; fortunately, the impairment is usually transient (Haas et al., 1991).

Conditions Requiring Lung and Heart-Lung Transplantation

More than 200 heart-lung transplantations take place each year, with a small proportion of those being in children. In 1990, 214 single-lung and 60 double-lung transplants were reported (Kriett & Kaye, 1991). Primary pulmonary hypertension and Eisenmenger's syndrome are the indications for over 50% of the heart-lung transplants being done, with a small percentage performed for congenital heart disease and about 30% performed for cystic fibrosis. Primary pulmonary disease is the usual diagnosis of lung transplant recipients; however, some transplants occur secondary to lung failure caused by congenital heart defects. Lung transplants in these cases are usually associated with cardiac repair. Previous thoracotomy is no longer considered a contraindication for heart lung or lung transplantation; however, it does increase the risk of perioperative bleeding (Whitehead et al., 1990). The mortality rate for children has been reported at nearly 30% in the first year after transplant and less than 10% later (Wilkinson, 1989).

The surgical procedure for a heart-lung transplantation is performed through a median sternotomy. The recipient heart and then lungs are removed. The donor organs are placed inside the chest cavity with the trachea anastomosed several rings above the carina. The right atrial anastomosis is performed and followed by anastomosis of the aorta (Bonser & Jamieson, 1990). Because of the risk of tracheal dehiscence, an omentum wrap around the suture line is typically used (Griffith et al., 1987).

The surgical procedure for a single-lung transplantation is performed through a thoracotomy incision. The removal of diseased lung is followed by the placement of the donor lung. The bronchial anastomosis is completed with an omentum wrap and followed by anastomosis of the pulmonary artery (Bolman et al., 1991).

When both lungs are transplanted, pulmonary innervation is lost (Jamieson et al., 1984). An early study observed bronchial hyperresponsiveness to inhaled methacholine, which was thought to be caused by denervation hypersensitivity (Glanville et al., 1989). Since that time, however, the postganglionic cholinergic nerve responses have been observed to be intact, as demonstrated by a normal bronchoconstrictor response to a stimulant. Airway hypersensitivity, therefore, is most likely a result of intact postganglionic cholinergic nerve response instead of denervation hypersensitivity (Stretton et al., 1990). Hypersensitivity was not observed during exercise (Glanville et al., 1989).

Because secretions below the tracheal anastomosis in the denervated lung do not excite the cough reflex, percussion, postural drainage, and breathing exercises are required to aid expectoration (Bonser & Jamieson, 1990). A certain amount of atelectasis is observed in all patients, especially those whose transplanted lungs need to be compressed to fit into the thoracic cage (Jamieson et al., 1984). Pulmonary edema is also frequently observed in the early postoperative period. Positive end expiratory pressure is often used with mechanical ventilation to reduce atelectasis and pulmonary edema (Whitehead et al., 1990).

The diagnosis of rejection is made based on clinical signs and symptoms suggesting a deterioration in function. Chest radiographic findings and pulmonary function test results are noninvasive indicators. If necessary, a transbronchial biopsy is performed when patients are breathless and febrile and have rales and wheezes on auscultation (Hutter et al., 1988).

Pulmonary infection occurs in most transplant recipients, usually repeatedly. Obliterative bronchiolitis is also a frequent posttransplant complication that has been reported to affect 71% of long-term survivors (Glanville et al., 1990; Starnes et al., 1991). The acute phase of obliterative bronchiolitis is characterized by varying degrees of bronchiolar obstruction by plugs of granulation tissue; in the chronic phase, the bronchioles are partially to completely occluded (Aziz & Jamieson, 1991). Severe damage may necessitate retransplantation. With improvements in immunosuppression, obliterative bronchiolitis is becoming less frequent in adults; the same progress is anticipated in children.

The education of parents and children about the implications and ramifications of a heart, heart-lung, or lung transplantation must be thorough and frank, including discussion of the implications of being on a waiting list and the extent of the postoperative care after transplantation. Geographic and social dislocation may occur during assessment and during the wait for a transplant (Warner, 1991). Warner stresses that families must be aware that, although transplantation is a last resort, it still may not be the answer. Compliance prior to transplantation may be an indicator of posttransplant compliance. Noncompliance is a contraindication for transplantation because rigid adherence to the immunosuppressive regimen is imperative. Missed doses of cyclosporine can result in death.

Technologic Support

Mechanical ventilation is common after open-heart surgery in the pediatric patient but should not deter the physical therapist from beginning treatment. The use of high-frequency jet ventilation in the period after open-heart surgery in pediatric patients may, however, militate against early physical therapy. High-frequency jet ventilation introduces a small tidal volume at a very rapid rate. Its use allows delivery of oxygen and removal of carbon dioxide at reduced mean airway and peak inspiratory pressures and is often used in unstable patients for whom physical therapy is contraindicated (Norwood & Civette, 1991). The three main advantages of high-frequency ventilation over conventional approaches to ventilation are improvement in the ventilation/perfusion ratio, less reduction of cardiac output, and minimized barotrauma (McWilliams, 1987).

Nasal intermittent positive pressure ventilation has been used for short periods in the pediatric surgical patient who has had difficulty in remaining extubated. This type of ventilation provides respiratory support through a preset tidal volume or inspiratory time, resulting in improved arterial blood gas tensions, improved alveolar ventilation, and decreased work of breathing (Bott et al., 1992).

Extracorporeal membrane oxygenation may be used for cardiovascular support in children after open-heart surgery. Indications for biventricular support by extracorporeal membrane oxygenation in the early postoperative period include progressive hypotension, increased ventricular filling pressures, poor peripheral perfusion, decreased urine output, and decreased mixed venous oxygen saturation (Weinhaus et al., 1989). Extracorporeal membrane oxygenation is especially effective in treating conditions with right heart failure and has also been used as a support while waiting for a heart, heart-lung, and lung transplantation (Weinhaus et al., 1989). The extracorporeal membrane oxygenation pump takes over oxygenation and perfusion of the child's body while the heart and lungs are "rested."

FIGURE 27-12. Child on first day after cardiac surgery.

MANAGEMENT OF ACUTE IMPAIRMENT

Education

The majority of acute impairments after thoracic surgical procedures occur in the immediate or early postoperative period. Rockwell and Campbell (1976) described a preoperative program to assist in minimizing postoperative complications and to educate the parents of children 3 to 12 years of age. Education is facilitated through an audiotape and puppet show as well as by a coloring book that shows the child what will happen after surgery. Preoperative programs probably benefit the parents as much as the child in alleviating some anxiety about the surgery. Preoperative education for the child younger than 5 years is also described by Page (1986). The program lists concepts that may be helpful in teaching and preparing the child and family for surgery. A doll is used to educate the child about placement of tubes and incisions; pictures are used for parents. Preparing children before the surgery should assist in obtaining their cooperation after surgery as well as minimize their fears.

Pulmonary Management

The primary area to be addressed after heart repair is the pulmonary status of the patient. Numerous articles describe pulmonary complications and

physical therapy in the postoperative pediatric patient (Ali et al., 1974; Bartlett, 1980, 1984; Bartlett et al., 1973a, 1973b; Gamsu et al., 1976; Krastins et al., 1982; Thoren, 1954; Van De Water et al., 1972; Vraciu & Vraciu, 1977). Although intervention varies with the age of the child, the primary goals are to mobilize secretions, increase aeration, and increase general mobility (Fig. 27-12).

Mucus transport is slowed after surgery and can lead to atelectasis (Gamsu et al., 1976). Atelectasis also occurs secondary to an altered breathing pattern, prolonged positioning in supine, and possible diaphragmatic dysfunction in the early postoperative period (Bartlett, 1984). In early studies by Bartlett (1980; Bartlett et al., 1973a) lack of deep breaths was observed as a causative factor in atelectasis. The yawn maneuver or prolonged inspiration with normal or increased inflation prevented atelectasis (Bartlett et al., 1973b). Bartlett (1984) observed that a collapsed lung expands only after the normal lung is fully inflated. This is achieved with prolonged inspiration. The restriction in ventilation has also been attributed to incoordination and reduction of rib expansion after sternotomy (Locke et al., 1990).

Incentive spirometry is an effective tool for reducing the occurrence of atelectasis in the pediatric population (Krastins et al., 1982). The primary emphasis with incentive spirometry or any other respiratory intervention should be on prolonged inspiration. When the inspiration is held for at least 3 seconds, arterial oxygen tension improves (Ward et al., 1966). Huckabay and Daderian (1990) observed an increase in compliance with breathing exercises after surgery when children were given a choice and some control regarding breathing exer-

FIGURE 27–13. Two-year-old child blowing bubbles on first day after repair of an atrial septal defect.

cises. With young children, tools such as bubble blowing or blowing on a windmill can be used (Rockwell & Campbell, 1976) (Fig. 27–13). Although these are expiratory maneuvers, a child often takes in a large inspiration before exhaling. Other respiratory techniques can also be performed to mobilize secretions as well as increase aeration, such as percussion and postural drainage, vibration, segmental expansion, and assisted cough techniques (Hussey, 1992) (Fig. 27–14).

The lack of pulmonary innervation in lung and heart-lung transplant recipients further impedes the removal of secretions. During treatment, it should be taken into consideration that secretions below

the tracheal anastomosis do not elicit the cough reflex. This can be particularly challenging in the young child who is extubated and unable to follow commands to cough.

Segmental expansion techniques may be performed to reduce postoperative complications and increase segmental aeration (Vraciu & Vraciu, 1977). This technique is performed by placing a hand over a particular segment and allowing it to move with the ventilator or respiratory cycle. Gentle pressure may be applied to the chest wall during exhalation at the end of the expiratory phase just before the inspiratory phase. This facilitates air flow to the specific segment (Massery, 1987). When a specific lobe or segment has decreased aeration, this technique, used in conjunction with gentle sustained pressure on the opposite upper lobe, may increase aeration to the affected area. When the patient is side-lying, gentle rocking may also stimulate segmental expansion and relax the patient (Massery, 1987). This technique is particularly effective when the child is upset or does not tolerate percussion or other treatment techniques. It may also decrease the respiratory rate and is especially useful with infants who cannot respond to verbal relaxation instructions. Segmental expansion techniques are also beneficial when the patient is having excessive bleeding after surgery and use of other more vigorous techniques is contraindicated (Johnson, BA, 1991). The author has used this technique with lung transplant recipients who have been unable to cooperate or follow commands for deep breathing and coughing and found it to work well in decreasing atelectasis and increasing oxygen saturation. Segmental expansion techniques performed before other respiratory techniques may further enhance their benefit.

Percussion may need to be performed to assist in removal of excess secretions. Percussion is defined as a rhythmical clapping with cupped hands over the involved lung segment performed throughout the respiratory cycle, with the goal of mechanically dislodging pulmonary secretions (Imle, 1981). Vibration also assists in mobilization of secretions. It is performed by creating a fine oscillating movement of the hand on the chest wall just before expiration and continuing until the beginning of inspiration (Imle, 1981).

Both percussion and vibration techniques can be performed in conjunction with postural drainage. Optimal positions are described and pictured in Frownfelter's text on chest physical therapy (Crane, 1987). Positioning must be used with caution in the postoperative patient; use of the Trendelenburg position, for example, is often contraindicated after open-heart surgery. It is important to confirm with

FIGURE 27–14. Child undergoing percussion on first day after cardiac surgery.

the nurse or the physician whether it is even suitable for the child to be flat in bed. Despite limitations, percussion and vibration can be performed in the positions available. It has been the author's experience that children respond well to both percussion and vibration, even on the first postoperative day. Encouraging the child to tell you if the treatment hurts—because it should not be painful—often facilitates cooperation. It may also be helpful to coordinate the treatment with administration of pain medications. Percussion may be contraindicated when platelets are low, pulmonary artery pressures are too high, or the child becomes too agitated with treatment. Vibration can generally be safely used instead. Blood pressure and intracardiac pressures should be closely monitored throughout the treatment because they are indicators of intolerance to treatment. Parameters, set on an individual basis, are usually established by the physician.

A counter-rotation technique described by Massery (1987) for altering respiratory rate in the neurologically impaired patient has also been safely used in the pediatric patient after open-heart surgery through a median sternotomy only. The technique has been used by the author to slow the respiratory rate as well as increase expansion of the lateral segment. It generally relaxes patients as well as increases their tidal volume. When the technique is used in the postoperative cardiac patient, extreme caution must be exercised to avoid disturbing chest tubes and other intravenous lines. This treatment is recommended only after intracardiac lines have been removed. The sternal incision has not been a problem; since it is stable, it does not undergo any mobilization during application of this technique.

The techniques just described not only facilitate increased lung expansion but also mobilize secretions. Once mobilized, secretions act as an irritant in the airway when the child takes a deep breath and a spontaneous cough usually occurs (Bartlett, 1984). The child may need some assistance in removing excess secretions, owing either to lack of cooperation or to inability to cooperate secondary to age. This may be accomplished by coughing or airway suctioning.

If the child is intubated, suctioning is done to clear secretions and maintain patency of the tube. Children who have cyanotic heart defects, such as hypoplastic left heart syndrome, tend to desaturate during suctioning. It is extremely important to hyperventilate these patients with oxygen and a resuscitation bag before and after suctioning and to monitor their oxygen saturation as well as other hemodynamic parameters (Boutros, 1970; Fox, WW, et al., 1978; Hussey, 1992; Rosen, 1962).

During suctioning, normal sterile saline may be instilled through the endotracheal tube to thin the thickened secretions. If the child is not intubated and is unwilling to cough, nasal pharyngeal suctioning may be performed to stimulate a cough as well as clear secretions. If the child is able to drink, a small sip of water or juice may also stimulate a cough. During coughing, a blanket or soft stuffed animal may be used to help splint the incision and minimize discomfort (Johnson, BA, 1991).

Pain

Postoperative pain can be detrimental to the child's recovery. It is important that pain medications be given regularly, not only to reduce anxiety (which further increases pain from splinting) but also to encourage deeper breathing. A child in pain does not take deep breaths, even spontaneously. Morphine, a commonly used postoperative narcotic, depresses spontaneous sighing; patients receiving morphine should be encouraged to voluntarily take deep breaths (Egbert & Bendixon, 1964).

Other techniques now being used to manage postoperative pain include the administration of epidural morphine, and patient-controlled analgesia (Asantila et al., 1986; Wilson, 1991). Both have proved effective in management of postoperative pain, especially in thoracotomy patients. Proper pain management is also extremely important in mobilizing the patient.

Early Mobilization

Postoperative immobility can lead to a variety of problems, including reduced ventilation and perfusion distribution (Peters, 1979), shallow breathing (Risser, 1980; Scheidegger et al., 1976), fever (Chulay et al., 1982), retention of secretions (Pairolero & Payne, 1991), fluid shifts (Rubin, 1988), and generalized discomfort from immobility. The child should be mobilized as soon as possible to minimize these deleterious effects.

Range of motion exercise should be initiated as soon as possible. It may not be possible to attain normal range of motion immediately because of discomfort or intravenous or arterial lines, but any movement helps to mobilize the patient. Range of motion exercise is extremely important for the child with a thoracotomy incision since this incision tends to produce more guarding than does a median sternotomy. Passive to active assisted range of shoulder motion to 90° of flexion is usually tolerable. Discomfort often occurs when the arm is returned to a neutral position. The therapist may apply gentle resistance to the arm as the child attempts to return the arm to a neutral position because contraction of the arm muscles tends to minimize discomfort (Johnson, BA, 1991).

The child's position should be changed regularly to avoid retention of secretions in the dependent portion of the lung (Pairolero & Payne, 1991). Regular turning has been observed to decrease postoperative fevers (Chulay et al., 1982). It also assists in decreasing postoperative chest wall immobilization, which is thought to decrease ventilation (Peters, 1979). The supine position alone contributes to airway closure (Dean, 1985; Risser, 1980) and a shift in blood volume to the dependent side (Rubin, 1988).

Arterial oxygen saturation is also affected by body position because of ventilation and perfusion matching (Dean, 1985). The supine position tends to decrease ventilation, which affects ventilation and perfusion matching and may ultimately decrease oxygen saturation. Positioning the patient effectively can reduce the pulmonary dysfunction that occurs most commonly when perfusion is greater than ventilation (Dean, 1985). The prone position has been observed to be associated with a significantly higher arterial oxygen tension than the supine position (Fox, MD, & Molesky, 1990) as well as an increased tidal volume and improved lung compliance (Dean, 1985). This position can be especially beneficial in preventing respiratory difficulty in a child who is extubated.

The side-lying position has been observed to be a better position for improving oxygenation than is the supine position (Banasik et al., 1987; Dean, 1985). In studies, adult patients became better oxygenated when the "good" lung was in the dependent position (Banasik et al., 1987; Todd, 1990). In children, however, the opposite was observed, namely, improved gas exchange with the good lung uppermost (Davies et al., 1985). It has been observed in lung transplant recipients that regional differences in blood flow distribution produced by position changes may lead to significant changes in oxygenation. Positioning the patient in side-lying, with the best lung dependent, may improve ventilation and perfusion matching (Todd, 1990). The best lung may or may not be the transplanted lung in the early postoperative period; thus, tolerance to having the transplanted lung dependent should be confirmed with the surgeons before placing the patient in this position.

Early ambulation after surgery reduces both pulmonary and circulatory complications (Webber, 1991). It has been observed to be as effective as deep breathing exercises in minimizing complications in adults (Dull & Dull, 1983). Ambulation was observed to be beneficial in returning respiratory function toward normal by inducing more frequent and deeper sigh respirations (Scheidegger et al., 1976). Activity and mobility have been clinically observed to minimize chest tube output. At our center, children ambulate as soon as atrial lines and groin lines are removed and the child is extubated. Children often ambulate for the first time with any or all of the following: central venous pressure line, peripheral intravenous line, arterial line, chest tubes, temporary pacemakers, and oxygen (Fig. 27–15). The first walk is often only for 5 to 10 feet and may be difficult for the patient. Anxiety often plays as great a role in the perceived difficulty as does the discomfort. It may be beneficial for the patient to receive some pain medication before the first walk. Parents are also anxious, so the benefits of early ambulation should be explained to them ahead of time, with emphasis on the problems that can occur by remaining in bed.

Medical Complications

Several medical complications can affect postoperative function. Secondary to phrenic nerve palsy, some children may have a paralyzed diaphragm after surgery that affects their early postoperative course as well as their long-term respiratory status and endurance. The paralyzed diaphragm may persist but is seldom permanent (Markland et al., 1985; Morriss & McNamara, 1975). Infants have horizontal ribs and lack the normal bucket handle movement, relying primarily on use of the dia-

FIGURE 27–15. Child ambulating on first day after repair of an atrial septal defect.

phragm for respiration. Paralysis of the diaphragm by unilateral or bilateral phrenic nerve palsy can cause further respiratory problems, including difficulty in weaning from the ventilator (Hussey, 1992).

Peroneal nerve palsy is another complication of surgery, usually caused by improper positioning of the lower extremity during surgery. The resultant drastic alteration in the child's gait must be addressed as soon as possible. An ankle-foot orthosis can improve gait and should only be necessary for a short period of time.

Postoperative neurologic impairments can occur subsequent to prolonged surgical time, usually related to length of hypothermic arrest, low cardiac output, or arrhythmias after surgery (Ferry, 1990; Wells et al., 1983). Neurologic consequences can also be the result of an air embolus, a prolonged hypotensive period (van Breda, 1985), or complications of long-term cyanosis (Amitta et al., 1984). The child who has suffered a neurologic insult requires early intervention as well as long-term physical therapy. A child with severe extensor tone may benefit from inhibitive casts on the lower extremities as well as hand splints to decrease the effects of increased tone and maintain range of motion. Parent education concerning the impact of a neurologic insult should begin as soon as the diagnosis is confirmed, including information on handling and positioning the child with increased tone, appropriate stimulation, use of adaptive equipment, and long-term follow-up.

The following case history describes a typical course of surgeries, with complications that resolved, in a child with cyanotic heart disease.

CASE HISTORY: DAVID

David was born with severe cyanotic congenital heart disease. He was diagnosed with total anomalous pulmonary venous return, transposition of the great arteries, hypoplastic left ventricle syndrome, atrial-ventricular septal defect, and pulmonary atresia. He had two surgeries performed within the first month of life. At 10 days of age, he had ligation of the ductus arteriosus and a modified BT shunt. At 4 weeks of age, he required repair of his right pulmonary artery. Then, at 4 months of age, he underwent surgery to repair his total anomalous pulmonary venous return. After this surgery, it took approximately 4 weeks to wean him from the ventilator, owing to a left phrenic nerve palsy. He was discharged to home on nasogastric feedings, which continued until he was 1 year old. He advanced from nasogastric feedings to baby food and liquid from a "tippy" cup.

David experienced some delay in achieving developmental milestones. He sat independently at 9 months of age. At 16 months of age, David had a bidirectional Glenn procedure and his BT shunt taken down. He did well after this surgery and was discharged to home within 1 week of his surgery date. He developed well over the next 18 months, with marked improvement in his activity level. For instance, David crawled at 17 months of age and then walked at 19 months.

At 3 years of age, David had a Fontan procedure performed, which he tolerated well until seizures occurred on the third postoperative day. A computed tomography scan revealed a right frontal lobe infarct, and increased tone and briskness of reflexes were noted on his left side. He was irritable and difficult to console. Initially, David demonstrated left-sided neglect and a decrease in his protective reactions to the left. Within 1 week, his tone was only minimally increased and he was able to use his left extremities with cueing. Within 2 weeks, his protective reactions were symmetric, and he was shifting his weight and using either extremity readily. His ambulation was typical of a child after surgery, with slight balance problems and the use of a wide base of support. He did have difficulty coming to a standing position from sitting without support, which resolved within 4 weeks.

David's parents are attentive and recognize tasks that are difficult for him. They have continued home exercises to encourage use of his left extremities and have had better cooperation from him than have the therapists. He continues to be followed for re-evaluation several times a year to monitor his progress and update his home program.

Age-Specific Disabilities in the Immediate Postoperative Period

The infant who undergoes surgery within the first few days of life suffers immediate disruption of all aspects of normal newborn life. The infant is often sedated, restrained, and intubated, all of which interferes with being held, bundled, and fed. Parents need education about the areas of stimulation that are withdrawn from their child during this time and instruction in ways to compensate for this deprivation. Often, the infant may be so sick that the parents have not had time to interact with the child from the time of birth. The fact that their child is born with a congenital anomaly may further impede the attachment process (Loeffel, 1985). The therapist assists the process by involving the parents in treatment as soon as possible.

Toddlers who have cardiac surgery often recover very quickly and with few impairments. Anxiety over being left alone during the hospitalization may be the biggest problem interfering with function in this age group (Loeffel, 1985). The child may feel abandoned and react by becoming passive and apathetic or, conversely, by becoming aggressive. These behaviors are more frequently observed in the child who is in the hospital for the first time, such as the child with an atrial septal defect. They are rarely observed in children who have experienced numerous hospitalizations and surgical procedures, such as children with cyanotic heart disease.

Toddlers tend to be limited more by their parents' restrictions than by their own physical limitations (Clare, 1985; Loeffel, 1985). Activity guidelines should be reviewed with parents on an ongoing basis; showing them by example may be even more helpful. Although it is beneficial to explain to the parents ahead of time what their child will experience, it may be helpful to wait to tell the toddler what is happening as it is happening.

Adolescents who have cardiac surgery may need to be encouraged to move and may need to be assisted to become active. The parents are often more reluctant than the child about early mobilization, including ambulation. They should be reassured that it is beneficial for their child to move as soon as possible. Adolescents may choose to assert their independence and try to do everything for themselves, or they may choose to become totally dependent on their parents and hospital staff. Whichever situation occurs, young persons benefit from early education about how to move and what they should be doing. This helps them to realize what is expected of them. They should be informed of what they need to do and not given a choice when the task is not optional (van Breda, 1985).

CHRONIC DISABILITIES AND FUNCTIONAL LIMITATIONS

Various disabilities as well as functional limitations occur as a result of primary impairments incurred by children with congenital heart defects. The disabling process may start very early secondary to poor attachment between parent and infant (Goldberg, S, et al., 1990b). Poor attachment can lead to poor social development. This disability is further compounded by the overprotection and excessive activity restrictions imposed by some parents. Parents have stated that they were afraid to permit activity in their child with congenital heart disease (Gudermuth, 1975). If this attitude is allowed to persist, the child's developmental and

functional level will surely suffer. It has also been observed that maternal perceptions of their child's disease severity was a stronger predictor of emotional adjustment than was disease severity (DeMaso et al., 1991). Emotional maladjustment may contribute to the poor self-esteem that is often noted in children with congenital heart defects. The limitations resulting from decreased activity, delayed development, poor self-esteem, overprotection by parents, as well as physical illness, may all lead to poor peer interactions. This may further limit a child with congenital heart disease from interacting with society. These issues should be addressed with parents and the child as early as possible to try to limit the effect on developmental progression and functional capabilities. Subsequent sections elaborate on various aspects of the disabling process across childhood.

Infancy

In children with congenital heart disease, several contributing factors can lead to impairment and functional limitations in infancy. Common problems include poor feeding, poor growth, and developmental lag. If the child does not have surgery immediately or only a palliative surgery is performed, there can be tremendous parental frustration and anxiety concerning their child's health. Parents must constantly watch for signs and symptoms of congestive heart failure in their infant. These signs include the onset of rapid breathing, changes in behavior, edema, excessive sweating, fatigue, vomiting, and poor feeding (Clare, 1985; Zahr & Boisvert, 1990). Parental anxiety, however, does not necessarily relate to disease severity (DeMaso et al., 1991).

Parental frustration and stress can impair early attachment to the infant. It has been observed during the period of 1 year that securely attached infants showed greater improvements in health than did insecurely attached infants (Goldberg, S, et al., 1991). When compared with healthy infants and infants with cystic fibrosis, infants with congenital heart disease were the least attached to their mothers (Goldberg, S, et al., 1990b). Parents of infants diagnosed with congenital heart defects reported more stress than parents of healthy children and parents of children diagnosed with cystic fibrosis (Goldberg, S, et al., 1990a). Normal attachment may be difficult, particularly with the very sick infant who is frequently hospitalized. The health care team should begin working with the parents as early as possible on how they can interact with their infant and how important it is for them to do so as part of the normal bonding process.

It is not uncommon for infants with congenital heart disease to be poor feeders, which further increases parental stress. An infant expends most of his energy during eating; therefore, this may be the only time when the heart cannot provide adequate systemic oxygenation (Bruning & Schneiderman, 1983). Decreased ventilation is observed during feeding, creating a decrease in the partial pressure of oxygen and an increase in the partial pressure of carbon dioxide (Mathew, 1988; Mathew et al., 1985). This decrease in ventilation may seriously compromise the child with congenital heart disease. An increase in metabolic rate observed in children with congenital heart disease further compounds the problem. Not only do they not eat well, but they also require more calories to thrive (Gingell & Hornung, 1989).

Watching their child failing to thrive can be devastating to parents and can further increase their anxiety about feeding their child and trying to encourage adequate caloric intake (Gingell & Hornung, 1989). Rejection of the feeding by an infant has been observed to be the least enjoyable aspect of feeding for mothers (Gudermuth, 1975). The prolonged feeding time can be frustrating to parents as well as make them feel inadequate (Bruning & Schneiderman, 1983; Loeffel, 1985). If alternative feeding methods are used, such as nasogastric or gastrostomy tube feedings, parents should be educated not only in how to administer the feeding but also in how to interact with their child during the feeding (Loeffel, 1985). They should be encouraged to hold and nurture their child during supplemental feedings. It may be helpful to tell parents that providing this time for normal, nonstressful interaction may improve the parent-infant attachment and may ultimately improve the health of their infant.

It is also important to inform the parents that the overall time that supplemental feedings are necessary varies with each child. Some parents have stated that they were able to remove supplemental feedings within 1 week of leaving the hospital; others have stated that it took months for their child to take enough by mouth to be able to discontinue supplemental feedings. Many parents have stated to this author that their infant ate better at home, where it was possible to eat on demand and to have a more routine day.

Physical therapy assessment is sometimes needed to observe the infant feeding and parental interaction. There may be other problems unrelated to the poor endurance exhibited by the infant with congenital heart disease. If oral motor dysfunction

exists, it should be addressed with parents as soon as possible. Some parents need assistance in how best to handle and support their child during feeding. It can also be beneficial for the parents to observe that their child does not feed well for anyone.

Poor growth is closely associated with poor feeding. It has been observed that infants with cyanotic heart disease have poor growth in height and weight, whereas infants with acyanotic heart disease, specifically those with a large left-to-right shunt, are severely underweight secondary to the marked increase in metabolism (Gingell & Hornung, 1989). Parents should be informed that their child may not grow and gain weight as well as other children. The child's growth improves after surgery but may not achieve normal parameters. This lack of catch-up growth is especially remarkable in children with cyanotic defects with a right-to-left shunt (Gingell & Hornung, 1989; Rosenthal, 1983).

Functional limitations, especially delayed achievement of basic motor skills, can be observed in the infant with cardiac disease. Decreased nutritional status and cardiac function may leave the infant too weak to expend the energy required for normal motor activity (Loeffel, 1985). Some cyanotic children preferentially scoot around on their buttocks and, even after extensive intervention at home, do not crawl. They often go on to walking without ever crawling (Johnson, BA, 1991), probably owing to the increased energy expenditure associated with use of both upper and lower extremities in crawling. Cyanotic children also tend to have an internal mechanism that only permits them to do what they are physically capable of doing, given their oxygen saturation (Clare, 1985). They often rest without cueing and can rarely be pushed beyond what they are willing to do. Intervention may or may not improve the child's functional abilities; however, it may do a great deal to relieve parental anxiety. Education should be focused on what the child is doing normally, such as using normal movement patterns, instead of on developmental lag based solely on age. Intervention should include parental education concerning areas the parent can work on with the child throughout the day, rather than in one focused block of time.

The presence of congestive heart failure is significantly associated with mental and motor developmental delay. Infants with congestive heart failure scored less well than expected on the Bayley Scales of Infant Development as early as at 2 months of age (Aisenberg et al., 1982). This information is useful when working with parents to help them understand that their child is demonstrating typical developmental skills for a child with congenital heart disease. This does not mean that intervention does not improve the situation. Parents should be encouraged to work with their child on developmental tasks that are challenging. If functional limitations are minimized early, the effect of reparative surgery may be dramatic.

Neurologic impairment and functional limitations may also occur from external forces related to the surgical repair. Discrepancy exists among research study findings regarding the effect of deep hypothermia and circulatory arrest on the psychomotor and intellectual development of infants (Blackwood et al., 1986; Brunberg et al., 1973; Haka-Ikse et al., 1978; Messmer et al., 1976; Settergren et al., 1982; Stevenson et al., 1974). It was observed in one group of infants that immediate neurologic problems were prevalent but transient; only 1 of 23 infants had any residual deficit (Brunberg et al., 1973). Messmer and associates (1976) observed no delay in psychomotor and intellectual development in infants after deep hypothermia. In another study, the researchers did not observe neurologic impairment after surgery but they did observe mild developmental delays, most profoundly in cyanotic infants (Haka-Ikse et al., 1978). In light of this controversy, therapists should realize the potential for problems. Parents should be advised that their child might take longer than usual to accomplish developmental milestones. They should be educated about how they can facilitate normal development but that intervention will not make their child progress any faster than their capabilities allow.

Preschool Period

The preschool child with chronic disabilities caused by congenital heart disease has grown up in the medical environment. This may help to alleviate some of the child's and the parents' anxieties. However, parental anxieties can be exacerbated during this period as they begin to realize the impact their child's cardiac disease has on growth and development. The child's symptoms could be worsening, and another surgery may soon be needed. The parents' response and interaction during this period is important; it should be recognized that parents already have the tendency to be overprotective of their child and that this may increase during the preschool period.

The emotional adjustment of the child has been observed to be affected by the mother's *perception* of the severity of their illness more than by its *actual* severity (DeMaso et al., 1991). If the mother perceives the child's disease to be more severe than

it is and limits the child accordingly, the child's physical and social development may suffer. In acyanotic children, it has been observed that the intelligence quotient (IQ) was lower when associated with poorer adjustment, greater dependence, and greater maternal pampering and anxiety (Rasof et al., 1967). Functional limitations may be out of proportion compared with what the child is actually capable of doing. Intervention may need to be initiated to instruct parents on what activities the child is capable of performing as well as how the child self-limits activity without parental intervention.

Children with congenital heart disease have been observed to have some developmental delay—especially those children with cyanotic disease. (Feldt et al., 1969; Rasof et al., 1967). Cyanotic children scored significantly lower than acyanotic and normal children in all subscales of the Gesell Developmental Schedules, and on Stanford-Binet and Cattell intelligence tests (Rasof et al., 1967). Cyanotic children were observed to sit and walk later than acyanotic and normal children and were slower in speaking phrases than were children without disabilities (Feldt et al., 1969; Rasof et al., 1967; Silbert et al., 1969). Curtailment of physical activity in the child with severe cardiac dysfunction interferes with the active manipulation of objects needed for the adequate development of early sensorimotor processes (Rasof et al., 1967; Silbert et al., 1969). This lack of opportunity may affect IQ scores and psychologic development.

Educating parents about what they should be allowing their child to do is as important as teaching them precautions pertaining to their child. Children were observed to have significant gross motor advances during the second year of life when parental warmth was combined with a decrease in parental restrictions. It was also observed that children with congenital heart disease performed better on IQ tests when their parents attempted to accelerate their child's development (Rasof et al., 1967). Parents should also be taught that children with cardiac disease, particularly cyanotic disease, limit their own activity and stop and rest when needed (Clare, 1985; Silbert et al., 1969). Early sensorimotor training by the parents or a professional may not improve the child's physical performance, but it could benefit psychologic development (Silbert et al., 1969).

Children with Down syndrome were observed to score higher on developmental tests and achieve feeding milestones earlier if parents followed through appropriately with therapy instructions (Cullen et al., 1981). Parents may find great satisfaction in knowing they can assist their child tremendously if they interact with their child, allow him or her to play, and impose appropriate discipline when necessary (Loeffel, 1985).

School-Aged Period

The relationship between lack of opportunity to perform early developmental tasks due to incapacitating cardiac disease and later IQ scores tends to disappear as children grow older (Rasof et al., 1967; Silbert et al., 1969). This finding may be due to 1) different testing methods for older children, 2) surgical intervention, 3) reduction of early parent overprotectiveness, and 4) the child's experiences in early years (Linde et al., 1967; Rasof et al., 1967). Intelligence testing for children younger than 2 years relies heavily on sensorimotor function, whereas testing for older children relies more on verbal abilities and reasoning (Linde et al., 1966). This difference should be taken into consideration when evaluating test results on children with cardiac defects.

Surgical intervention that corrects a cyanotic defect plays an important role in the child's development. Improvement in IQ has been reported after surgery (Linde et al., 1970; O'Dougharty et al., 1985). Self-confidence, social confidence, and general adjustment have also improved after surgery (Linde et al., 1970). If decreased experiences are a factor in developmental performance, then a child who is no longer limited by disease should develop more normally.

Parental overprotectiveness can continue to prove more limiting to a child's development than the defect itself. Acyanotic children have been found to be more overprotected relative to the severity of their disease than cyanotic children (Linde et al., 1966). Maternal guilt is related to maternal anxiety as well as to overprotectiveness. Parental restriction generally begins with the advice of the physician and proceeds from there (Bergman & Stamm, 1967; Clare, 1985; Kong et al., 1986). Social and emotional maladjustment in children with cardiac disease can be due to maternal maladjustment and guilt (Kong et al., 1986). Psychosocial or therapy intervention by professionals could be beneficial to preserving a more normal parent-child interaction. Some improvement in maternal interaction and attitude has been noted after surgical correction of the child's cardiac defect (O'Dougharty et al., 1985).

School adjustment and poor interaction have been observed to be altered in children with congenital heart disease. In a study by Youssef (1988), school absenteeism was high in these children and

was proportional to the severity of their disease. Teachers have noted that children with congenital heart disease had more school problems, and more behavior problems were observed in boys. Those children with more behavior problems had a lower self-esteem and more depression (Youssef, 1988). After surgical intervention, some of these problems may be alleviated; the child should miss less school and have an improved physical status and an increased activity level (Linde et al., 1970). Children may need professional intervention after surgical repair, however, to teach them how much they are capable of doing.

Physicians must make an accurate diagnosis of the child's cardiac disease and give appropriate activity guidelines. Restrictions should be considered radical rather than conservative advice (Bergman & Stamm, 1967). It has been observed that normal children misdiagnosed with a cardiac defect suffer from the overprotectiveness of parents as a result of physician-imposed activity restrictions (Bergman & Stamm, 1967). Intervention should focus on both the child's functional limitations (or inability to perform a task) and the parental restrictions placed on the child.

Adolescence

Adolescents who have congenital heart disease and physical limitations show increased feelings of anxiety and impulsiveness (Kramer et al., 1989). Early professional intervention to assist the parents and child to cope best with the child's physical limitations may be helpful.

A delay in the onset of puberty in adolescents with congenital heart disease may further complicate their social development. The body structure of the adolescent with congenital heart disease was found to be noticeably different from that of normal adolescents. The weight and height were markedly less with the presence of cardiac disease. Adolescents with heart disease had head, neck, and shoulder measurements similar to those of healthy adolescents, but the thorax, trunk, pelvis, and lower extremities were significantly smaller. The anterior-posterior diameter of the pelvis was so reduced that it appeared almost flat (Angelov et al., 1980). Physical differences of this magnitude can only make adolescents with heart disease feel even more different and intensify their low self-esteem.

Intervention that encourages the adolescent to participate in physical activities including guidelines on how to participate, may improve peer interaction and ultimately self-esteem. Education regarding physical activity and an opportunity to participate may be all the adolescent needs. Children who participated in an exercise program were observed to have improvement in their self-esteem as well as in their strength. Parents were found to be less restrictive and had less anxiety about their child after a formal exercise program (Donovan et al., 1983).

Physical activity is important for all children, including children with congenital heart disease. The defect and surgical intervention as well as possible alterations in response to exercise must be understood before prescribing an exercise program for a child with congenital heart disease. The American Heart Association has published an extensive review of exercise testing in the pediatric age group, including recommendations for those with various congenital heart defects (James et al., 1982).

Cardiac rehabilitation programs for children with cardiac disease have shown significant and beneficial changes in hemodynamics as well as improvement in exercise endurance and tolerance (Balfour et al., 1991; Bar-Or, 1985; Goldberg, B, et al., 1981; Koch et al., 1988; Mathews et al., 1983; Perrault & Drblik, 1989; Ruttenberg et al., 1983). Improvement from physical training allowed adolescents to function at nearly normal activity levels (Goldberg, B, et al., 1981). The psychologic improvements were as noticeable and important as the physical improvements (Donovan et al., 1983; Koch et al., 1988; Mathews et al., 1983).

The child who has a heart transplant can also participate in an exercise program; however, the cardiovascular response is different from usual. The transplanted heart is denervated, and therefore the cardiac response of increased contractility and increased rate is no longer controlled by nerve stimulation. The increase in cardiac output necessary to meet the demand of increased activity during exercise is first enhanced by an increase in stroke volume and then later by an increase in heart rate due to catecholamines (Clough, 1990; Kent & Cooper, 1974). Adolescents who have undergone heart transplantation are able to achieve an increase in cardiac output in response to exercise; however, they do not achieve the same peak workloads or maximal oxygen consumption as do normal adolescents (Christos et al., 1992).

During the early phase of rehabilitation, many children with transplanted hearts are so debilitated that they are unable to perform at an intensity that would raise their heart rate. The dyspnea index used as part of the Stanford heart transplant protocol is helpful in monitoring the child's physical tolerance during activity (Sadowsky et al., 1986). The child counts out loud to fifteen. The goal initially is to attempt to do this on one breath. At first, it may take three breaths to count to fifteen while at rest. Exercise should only increase the number of breaths to reach fifteen by one or two breaths and should not be resumed until return to resting base line. Most children progress quickly, usually reaching fifteen on one breath within 1 week of beginning exercise. The dyspnea index is an easily used mechanism for self-monitoring of exercise tolerance at home (Johnson, BA, 1991).

The patient who has had a heart-lung transplant has similar responses to exercise as patients with heart transplants for an increased ventilatory response to exercise (Banner, N, et al., 1988; Banner, NR, et al., 1989; Sciurba et al., 1988). The dyspnea index is again useful with these patients.

Heart, heart-lung, and lung transplant recipients have experienced marked rehabilitation after transplantation (Bolman, 1991). The quality of life improves, with most children functioning at an age-appropriate level without developmental delays (Dunn et al., 1987; Lawrence & Fricker, 1987; Niset et al., 1988).

▌SUMMARY

This review of congenital heart defects, surgical and therapeutic intervention, and developmental consequences provides therapists with a foundation for treating this patient population. As surgical intervention occurs earlier and corrective techniques are performed sooner, it will be increasingly important to evaluate and monitor developmental progression. Children with congenital heart defects cannot be made to perform a developmental task that they do not have the energy to perform. The physical therapist plays an integral role in the "habilitation" and rehabilitation of children with congenital heart disease. A major part of this role involves parent education concerning typical developmental sequences in children with cardiac conditions and appropriate parent-child interaction.

References

Aisenberg, RB, Rosenthal, A, Nadas, AS, & Wolff, PH. Developmental delay in infants with congenital heart disease. Pediatric Cardiology 3:133–137, 1982.

Ali, J, Weisel, RD, Layug AB, Kripke, BJ, & Hechtman, HB. Consequences of postoperative alterations in respiratory mechanics. American Journal of Surgery, 128:376–382, 1974.

Amitia, Y, Blieden, L, Shemtove, A, & Neufeld, H. Cerebrovascular accidents in infants and children with congenital cyanotic heart disease. Israel Journal of Medical Sciences, 20:1143–1145, 1984.

Angelov, G, Tomova, S, & Ninova, P. Physical development and body structure of children with congenital heart disease. Human Biology 52:413–421, 1980.

Arciniegas, E. Ventricular septal defect. In Baue, AE, Geha, AS, Hammond, GL, Laks, H, & Naunheim, KS (Eds.), Glenn's Thoracic and Cardiovascular Surgery (5th ed.). Norwalk, CT: Appleton & Lange, 1991, pp. 1007–1016.

Asantila, R, Rosenburg, PH, & Scheinin, B. Comparison of different methods of postoperative analgesia after thoracotomy. Acta Anaesthesiologica Scandinavica, 30:421–425, 1986.

Azia, S, & Jamieson, S. Combined heart and lung transplantation. In Baue, AE, Geha, AS, Hammond, GL, Laks, H, & Naunheim, KS (Eds.), Glenn's Thoracic and Cardiovascular Surgery (5th ed.). Norwalk, CT: Appleton & Lange, 1991, pp. 1623–1638.

Bailey, LL, Assaad, AN, Trimm, RF, Nehlsen-Cannarella, SL, Kanakriyeh, MS, Haas, GS, & Jacobson, JG. Orthotopic transplantation during early infancy as therapy for incurable congenital heart disease. Annals of Surgery, 203:279–283, 1988.

Bailey, LL, & Gundry, SR. Hypoplastic left heart syndrome. In Gillette, PC (Ed.), The Pediatric Clinics of North America. Philadelphia: WB Saunders, 1990, pp. 137–150.

Balfour, IC, Drimmer, AM, Nouri, S, Pennington, DG, Hemkins, CL, Harvey, LL. Pediatric cardiac rehabilitation. American Journal of Diseases of Children, 145:627–630, 1991.

Banasik, JL, Bruya, MA, Steadman, RE, & Demand, JK. Effect of position on arterial oxygenation in postoperative coronary revascularization patients. Heart and Lung, 16:652–657, 1987.

Banner, N, Guz, A, Heaton, R, Innes, JA, Murphy, K, & Yacoub, M. Ventilatory and circulatory responses at the onset of exercise in man following heart or heart-lung transplantation. Journal of Physiology, 399:437–449, 1988.

Banner, NR, Lloyd, MH, Hamilton, RD, Innes, JA, Guz, A, & Yacoub, MH. Cardiopulmonary response to dynamic exercise after heart and combined heart-lung transplantation. British Heart Journal, 61:215–223, 1989.

Bar-Or, O. Physical conditioning in children with cardiorespiratory disease. In Terjung, RL (Ed.), Exercise and Sport Science Review. New York: Macmillan, 1985, pp. 305–334.

Bartlett, RH. Pulmonary pathophysiology in surgical patients. Surgical Clinics of North America, 60:1323–1338, 1980.

Bartlett, RH. Respiratory therapy to prevent pulmonary complications of surgery. Respiratory Care, 29:667–677, 1984.

Bartlett, RH, Brennan, ML, Gazzaniga, AB, & Hanson, EL. Studies on the pathogenesis and prevention of postoperative pulmonary complications. Surgery, Gynecology and Obstetrics, 137:925–933, 1973a.

Bartlett, RH, Gazzaniga, AB, & Geraghty, TR. Respiratory maneuvers to prevent postoperative pulmonary complications. Journal of the American Medical Association, 224:1017–1021, 1973b.

Bergman, AB, Stamm, SJ. The morbidity of cardiac nondisease in schoolchildren. New England Journal of Medicine, 276:1008–1013, 1967.

Blackwood, MJ, Haka-Ikse, K, & Steward, DJ. Developmental outcome in children undergoing surgery with profound hypothermia. Anesthesiology, 65:437–440, 1986.

Bolman, RM, Shumway, SE, Estrin, JA, & Hertz, MI. Lung and heart-lung transplantation. Annals of Surgery, 214:456–470, 1991.

Bonser, RS, & Jamieson, SW. Heart-lung transplantation. Clinics in Chest Medicine, 11:235–246, 1990.

Bott, J, Keilty, SE, Brown, A, & Ward, EM. Nasal intermittent positive pressure ventilation. Physiotherapy, 78:93–96, 1992.

Boutros, AR. Arterial blood oxygenation during and after endotracheal suctioning in the apneic patient. Anesthesiology, 32:114–118, 1970.

Bove, EL. Transplantation after first-stage reconstruction for hypoplastic left heart syndrome. Annals of Thoracic Surgery, 52:701–707, 1991.

Brunberg, JA, Reilly, EL, & Doty, DB. Central nervous system consequences in infants of cardiac surgery using deep hypothermia and circulatory arrest. Circulation, 49 & 50(suppl II):60–67, 1973.

Bruning, MD, & Schneiderman, JU. Heart failure in infants and children. In Michaelson, CR (Ed.), Congestive Heart Failure. St. Louis, MO: Mosby, 1983, pp. 467–484.

Byrum, CJ, Dick, M, Behrendt, DM, & Rosenthal, A. Repair of total anomalous pulmonary venous connection in patients younger than 6 months old. Circulation, 66(suppl I):208–214, 1982.

Callow, LB. A new beginning: Nursing care of the infant undergoing the arterial switch operation for transposition of the great arteries. Heart and Lung, 18:248–257, 1989.

Castaneda, A, & Mayer, JE. Arterial switch operation for transposition of the great arteries. In Baue, AE, Geha, AS, Hammond, GL, Laks, H, & Naunheim, KS (Eds.), Glenn's Thoracic and Cardiovascular Surgery (5th ed.). Norwalk, CT: Appleton & Lange, 1991, pp. 1227–1235.

Christos, SC, Katch, V, Crowley, DC, Eakin, BL, Lindauer, AL, & Beekman, RH. Hemodynamic responses to upright exercise of adolescent cardiac transplant patients. Journal of Pediatrics, 121:312–316, 1992.

Chulay, M, Brown, J, & Summer, W. Effect of postoperative immobilization after coronary artery bypass surgery. Critical Care Medicine, 10:176–179, 1982.

Clare, MD. Home care of infants and children with cardiac disease. Heart and Lung, 14:218–222, 1985.

Clarke, CF, Beall, MH, & Perloff, JK. Genetics, epidemiology, counseling, and prevention. In Perloff, JK, & Child, JS (Eds.), Congenital Heart Disease in Adults. Philadelphia: WB Saunders, 1991, pp. 141–165.

Clough, P. The denervated heart. Clinical Management, 10:14–17, 1990.

Crane, LD. The neonate and child. In Frownfelter, DL (Ed.), Chest Physical Therapy and Pulmonary Rehabilitation. Chicago: Year Book Publishers, 1987, pp. 666–697.

Cullen, SM, Cronk, CE, Pueschel, SM, Schnell, RR, & Reed, RB. Social development and feeding milestones of young Down syndrome children. American Journal of Mental Deficiency, 85:410–415, 1981.

Davies, H, Kitchman, R, Gordon, I, & Helms, P. Regional ventilation in infancy. New England Journal of Medicine, 313:1626–1628, 1985.

Dean, E. Effect of body position on pulmonary function. Physical Therapy, 65:613–618, 1985.

de Leval, MR. Senning operation. In Baue, AE, Geha, AS, Hammond, GL, Laks, H, & Naunheim, KS (Eds.), Glenn's Thoracic and Cardiovascular Surgery (5th ed.). Norwalk, CT: Appleton & Lange, 1991, pp. 1211–1216.

DeMaso, DR, Campis, LK, Wypij, D, Bertram, S, Lipshitz, M, & Freed, M. The impact of maternal perceptions and medical severity on the adjustment of children with congenital heart disease. Journal of Pediatric Psychology, 16:137–149, 1991.

Donovan, EF, Mathews, RA, Nixon, PA, Stephenson, RJ, Robertson, RJ, Dean, F, Fricker, FJ, Beerman, LB, & Fischer, DR. An exercise program for pediatric patients with congenital heart disease: Psychological aspects. Journal of Cardiac Rehabilitation, 4:476–480, 1983.

Dull, JL, & Dull, WL. Are maximal inspiratory breathing exercises or incentive spirometry better than early mobilization after cardiopulmonary bypass? Physical Therapy, 63:655–659, 1983.

Dunn, JM, Cavarocchi, NC, Balsara RK, Kolff, J, McClurken, J, Badellino, MM, Vieweg, C, & Donner, RM. Pediatric heart transplantation, at St. Christopher's Hospital for Children. Journal of Heart Transplantation, 6:334–342, 1987.

Egbert, LD, & Bendixon, HH. Effect of morphine on breathing pattern. Journal of the American Medical Association, 188:485–488, 1964.

Feldt, RH, Ewert, JC, Stickler, GB, & Weidman, WH. Children with congenital heart disease. American Journal of Diseases of Children, 117:281–287, 1969.

Ferry, PC. Neurologic sequelae of open-heart surgery in children. American Journal of Diseases of Children, 144:369–373, 1990.

Fox, MD, & Molesky, MG. The effects of prone and supine positioning on arterial oxygen pressure. Neonatal Network, 8:25–29, 1990.

Fox, WW, Schwartz, JG, & Shaffer, TH. Pulmonary physiotherapy in neonates: Physiologic changes and respiratory management. Journal of Pediatrics, 92:977–981, 1978.

Fricker, FJ, Trento, A, & Griffith, BP. Pediatric cardiac transplantation. In Brest, AN (Ed.), Cardiovascular Clinics. Philadelphia: FA Davis, 1990, pp. 223–235.

Gamsu, G, Singer, MM, Vincent, HH, Berry, S, & Nadel, JA. Postoperative impairment of mucous transport in the lung. American Review of Respiratory Disease, 114:673–679, 1976.

Garson, A, Gillette, PC, Gutgesell, HP, & McNamara, DG. Stress-induced ventricular arrhythmia after repair of tetralogy of Fallot. American Journal of Cardiology, 46:1006–1012, 1980.

Giboney, GS. Ventricular septal defect. Heart and Lung, 12:292–299, 1983.

Gingell, RL, & Hornung, MG. Growth problems associated with congenital heart disease in infancy. In Lebenthal, E (Ed.), Textbook of Gastroenterology and Nutrition in Infancy (2nd ed.). New York: Raven Press, 1989, pp. 639–649.

Girlando, RM, Belew, B, & Klara, F. Coarctation of the aorta. Critical Care Nurse, 8:38–50, 1988.

Glanville, AR, Baldwin, JC, Hunt, SA, & Theodore, J. Long-term cardiopulmonary function after human heart-lung transplantation. Australian and New Zealand Journal of Medicine, 20:208–214, 1990.

Glanville, AR, Gabb, GM, Theodore, J, & Robin, ED. Bronchial responsiveness to exercise after human cardiopulmonary transplantation. Chest, 96:281–286, 1989.

Goldberg, B, Fripp, RR, Lister, G, Loke, J. Nicholas, JA, & Talner, NS. Effect of physical training on exercise performance of children following surgical repair of congenital heart disease. Pediatrics, 68:691–699, 1981.

Goldberg, S, Morris, P, Simmons, RJ, Fowler, RS, & Levison, H. Chronic illness in infancy and parenting stress: A comparison of three groups of parents. Journal of Pediatric Psychology, 15:347–358, 1990a.

Goldberg, S, Simmons, RJ, Newman J, Campbell, K, & Fowler, RS. Congenital heart disease, parental stress, and infant-mother relationships. Journal of Pediatrics, 119:661–666, 1991.

Goldberg, S, Washington, J, Morris, P, Fischer-Fay, A, & Simmons, RJ. Early diagnosed chronic illness and mother-child relationships in the first two years. Canadian Journal of Psychiatry, 55:726–733, 1990b.

Graham, TP, Bender, HW, & Spach, MS. Ventricular septal defect. In Adams, FH, Emmanouilides, GC, & Riemenschneider, TA (Eds.), Moss's Heart Disease in Infants, Children, and Adolescents. Baltimore: Williams & Wilkins, 1989, pp. 189–208.

Griffith, BP, Hardesy, RL, Trento, A, Paradis, IL, Duquesnoy, RJ, Zeevi, A, Dauber, JH, Dummer, JS, Thompson, ME,

Gryzan, S, & Bahnson, HT. Heart-lung transplantation: Lessons learned and future hopes. Annals of Thoracic Surgery, 43:6–16, 1987.

Gudermuth, S. Mothers' reports of early experiences of infants with congenital heart disease. Maternal—Child Nursing Journal, 4:155–164, 1975.

Haas, GS, Bailey, L, & Pennington, DG. Pediatric cardiac transplantation. In Baue, AE, Geha, AS, Hammond, GL, Laks, H, & Naunheim, KS (Eds.), Glenn's Thoracic and Cardiovascular Surgery (5th ed.). Norwalk, CT: Appleton & Lange, 1991, pp. 1297–1317.

Haka-Ikse, K, Blackwood, MA, & Steward, DJ. Psychomotor development of infants and children after profound hypothermia during surgery for congenital heart disease. Developmental Medicine and Child Neurology, 20:62–70, 1978.

Hammon, JW, & Bender, HW. Anomalous venous connection: Pulmonary and systemic. In Baue, AE, Geha, AS, Hammond, GL, Laks, H, & Naunheim, KS (Eds.), Glenn's Thoracic and Cardiovascular Surgery (5th ed.). Norwalk, CT: Appleton & Lange, 1991, pp. 971–993.

Huckabay, L, & Daderian, AD. Effect of choices on breathing exercises post-open heart surgery. Dimensions in Critical Care Nursing, 9:190–201, 1990.

Hussey, J. Effects of chest physiotherapy for children in intensive care after surgery. Physiotherapy, 78:109–113, 1992.

Hutter, JA, Despins, P, Higenbottam, T, Stewart, S, & Wallwork, J. Heart-lung transplantation: Better use of resources. American Journal of Medicine, 85:4–11, 1988.

Imle, PC. Percussion and vibration. In MacKenzie, CF, Ciesla, N, Imle, PC, & Klemic, N (Eds.), Chest Physiotherapy in the Intensive Care Unit. Baltimore, Williams & Wilkins, 1981, pp. 81–91.

James, FW, Blomqvist, CG, Freed, MD, Miller, WW, Moller, JH, Nugent, EW, Riopel, DA, Strong, WB, & Wessel, HU. Standards for exercise testing in the pediatric age group. Circulation, 66:1377A–1397A, 1982.

Jamieson, SW, Stinson, EB, Oyer, PE, Reitz, BA, Baldwin, J, Modry, D, Dawkins, K, Theodore, J, Hunt, S, & Shumway, NE. Heart-lung transplantation for irreversible pulmonary hypertension. Annals of Thoracic Surgery, 38:554–562, 1984.

Jarmakani, JM, & Canent, RV. Preoperative and postoperative right ventricular function in children with transposition of the great vessels. Circulation, 49 & 50(suppl II):39–45, 1974.

Johnson, AB, & Davis, JS. Treatment options for the neonate with hypoplastic left heart syndrome. Journal of Perinatal and Neonatal Nursing, 5:84–92, 1991.

Johnson, BA. Postoperative physical therapy in the pediatric cardiac surgery patient. Pediatric Physical Therapy, 2(1):14–22, 1991.

Kent, KM, & Cooper, T. The denervated heart: A model for studying autonomic control of the heart. New England Journal of Medicine, 291:1017–1021, 1974.

Koch, BM, Galioto, FM, Vaccaro, P, Vaccaro, J, & Buckenmeyer, PJ. Flexibility and strength measures in children participating in a cardiac rehabilitation exercise program. Physician and Sports Medicine, 116:139–147, 1988.

Kong, SG, Tay, JS, Yip, WC, & Chay, SO. Emotional and social effects of congenital heart disease in Singapore. Australian Paediatric Journal, 22:101–106, 1986.

Kopf, GS, Laks, H. Atrial septal defects and cor triatriatum. In Baue, AE, Geha, AS, Hammond, GL, Laks, H, & Naunheim, KS (Eds.), Glenn's Thoracic and Cardiovascular Surgery (5th ed.). Norwalk, CT: Appleton & Lange, 1991, pp. 995–1005.

Kramer, HH, Aswiszus, D, Sterzel, U, van Halteren, A, & Clafen, R. Development of personality and intelligence in children with congenital heart disease. Journal of Child Psychiatry, 30:299–308, 1989.

Krastins, IR, Corey, ML, McLeod, A, Edmonds, J, Levison, H, & Moles, F. An evaluation of incentive spirometry in the management of pulmonary complications after cardiac surgery in a pediatric population. Critical Care Medicine, 10:525–528, 1982.

Kriett, JM, & Kaye, MP. The registry of the international society for heart and lung transplantation: Eighth official report —1991. Journal of Heart and Lung Transplantation, 10:491–498, 1991.

Laks, H, & Breda, MA. Tetralogy of Fallot. In Baue, AE, Geha, AS, Hammond, GL, Laks, H, & Naunheim, KS (Eds.), Glenn's Thoracic and Cardiovascular Surgery (5th ed.). Norwalk, CT: Appleton & Lange, 1991a, pp. 1179–1201.

Laks, H, & Breda, MA. Tricuspid atresia. In Baue, AE, Geha, AS, Hammond, GL, Laks, H, & Naunheim, KS (Eds.), Glenn's Thoracic and Cardiovascular Surgery (5th ed.). Norwalk, CT: Appleton & Lange, 1991b, pp. 1259–1272.

Lawrence, KS, & Fricker, FJ. Pediatric heart transplantation: Quality of life. Journal of Heart Transplantation, 6:329–333, 1987.

Levitsky, S, & del Nido, P. Patent ductus arteriosus and aortopulmonary septal defects. In Baue, AE, Geha, AS, Hammond, GL, Laks, H, & Naunheim, KS (Eds.), Glenn's Thoracic and Cardiovascular Surgery (5th ed.). Norwalk, CT: Appleton & Lange, 1991, pp. 1017–1025.

Linde, LM, Rasof, B, & Dunn, OJ. Mental development in congenital heart disease. Journal of Pediatrics, 71:198–203, 1967.

Linde, LM, Rasof, B, & Dunn, OJ. Longitudinal studies of intellectual and behavioral development in children with congenital heart disease. Acta Paediatrica, 59:169–176, 1970.

Linde, LM, Rasof, B, Dunn, OJ, & Rabb, E. Attitudinal factors in congenital heart disease. Pediatrics, 38:92–101, 1966.

Locke, TJ, Griffiths, TC, Mould, H, & Gibson, GJ. Rib cage mechanics after median sternotomy. Thorax, 45:465–468, 1990.

Loeffel, M. Developmental considerations of infants and children with congenital heart disease. Heart and Lung, 14:214–217, 1985.

Markland, ON, Moorthy, SS, Mahomed, Y, King, RD, & Brown, JW. Postoperative phrenic nerve palsy in patients with open-heart surgery. Annals of Thoracic Surgery, 39:68–73, 1985.

Massery, M. Respiratory rehabilitation secondary to neurological deficits: Treatment techniques. In Frownfelter, DL (Ed.), Chest Physical Therapy and Pulmonary Rehabilitation. Chicago: Year Book Publishers, 1987, pp. 538–544.

Mathew, OP. Respiratory control during nipple feeding in preterm infants. Pediatric Pulmonology, 5:220–224, 1988.

Mathew, OP, Clark, ML, Pronske, ML, Luna-Solarzano, HG, & Peterson, MD. Breathing pattern and ventilation during oral feeding in term newborn infants. Journal of Pediatrics, 106:810–813, 1985.

Mathews, RA, Nixon, PA, Stephenson, RJ, Robertson, RJ, Donovan, EF, Dean, F, Fricker, FJ, Beerman, LB, & Fischer, DR. An exercise program for pediatric patients with congenital heart disease: Organizational and physiologic aspects. Journal of Cardiac Rehabilitation, 3:467–475, 1983.

McWilliams, BC. Mechanical ventilation in pediatric patients. Clinics in Chest Medicine, 8:597–607, 1987.

Mee, RB. Current status of cardiac surgery in childhood. Progress in Pediatric Surgery, 27:148–169, 1991.

Messmer, BJ, Schallberger, Y, Gattiker, R, & Senning, A. Psychomotor and intellectual development after deep hypothermia and circulatory arrest in early infancy. Journal of Thoracic and Cardiovascular Surgery, 72:495–501, 1976.

Milgalter, E, & Laks, H. Truncus arteriosus. In Baue, AE, Geha,

AS, Hammond, GL, Laks, H, & Naunheim, KS (Eds.), Glenn's Thoracic and Cardiovascular Surgery (5th ed.). Norwalk, CT: Appleton & Lange, 1991, pp. 1079–1987.

Morriss, JH, & McNamara, DG. Residua, sequelae and complications of surgery for congenital heart disease. Progress in Cardiovascular Diseases, 18:1–25, 1975.

Moulton, AL, & Malm, JR. Pulmonary stenosis, pulmonary atresia, single pulmonary artery and aneurysm of the pulmonary artery. In Baue, AE, Geha, AS, Hammond, GL, Laks, H, & Naunheim, KS (Eds.), Glenn's Thoracic and Cardiovascular Surgery (5th ed.). Norwalk, CT: Appleton & Lange, 1991, pp. 1131–1163.

Nakazawa, M, Okuda, H, Imai, Y, Takanashi, Y, & Takao, A. Right and left ventricular volume characteristics after external conduit repair (Rastelli procedure) for cyanotic congenital heart disease. Heart and Vessels, 2:106–110, 1986.

Niset, G, Coustry-Degre, C, & Degre, S. Psychosocial and physical rehabilitation after heart transplantation: 1-year follow-up. Cardiology, 75:311–317, 1988.

Noonan, JA. Syndromes associated with cardiac defects. In Engle, MA (Ed.), Pediatric Cardiovascular Disease. Philadelphia: FA Davis, 1981, pp. 97–115.

Norwood, SH, & Civette, JM. Ventilatory assistance and support. In Baue, AE, Geha, AS, Hammond, GL, Laks, H, & Naunheim, KS (Eds.), Glenn's Thoracic and Cardiovascular Surgery (5th ed.). Norwalk, CT: Appleton & Lange, 1991, pp. 45–66.

Norwood, WI. Hypoplastic left heart syndrome. Annals of Thoracic Surgery, 52:688–695, 1991a.

Norwood, WI. Hypoplastic left heart syndrome. In Baue, AE, Geha, AS, Hammond, GL, Laks, H, & Naunheim, KS (Eds.), Glenn's Thoracic and Cardiovascular Surgery (5th ed.). Norwalk, CT: Appleton & Lange, 1991b, pp. 1123–1130.

O'Dougharty, M, Wright, FS, Loewenson, RB, & Torres, F. Cerebral dysfunction after chronic hypoxia in children. Neurology, 35:42–46, 1985.

Page, GG. Tetralogy of Fallot. Heart and Lung, 15:390–400, 1986.

Pairolero, PC, & Payne, WS. Postoperative care and complications in the thoracic surgery patient. In Baue, AE, Geha, AS, Hammond, GL, Laks, H, & Naunheim, KS (Eds.), Glenn's Thoracic and Cardiovascular Surgery (5th ed.). Norwalk, CT: Appleton & Lange, 1991, pp. 31–43.

Peetz, DJ, Spicer, RL, Crowley, DC, Sloan, H, & Behrendt, DM. Correction of truncus arteriosus in the neonate using a nonvalved conduit. Journal of Thoracic and Cardiovascular Surgery, 83:743–746, 1982.

Pennington, DG, Noedel, N, McBride, LR, Naunheim, KS, & Ring, WS. Heart transplantation in children: An international survey. Annals of Thoracic Surgery, 52:710–715, 1991.

Perrault, H, Drblik, SP. Exercise after surgical repair of congenital cardiac lesions. Sports Medicine, 7:18–31, 1989.

Peters, RM. Pulmonary physiologic studies of the perioperative period. Chest, 76:576–585, 1979.

Puga, FJ. Surgical treatment of pulmonary atresia with ventricular septal defect. In Baue, AE, Geha, AS, Hammond, GL, Laks, H, & Naunheim, KS (Eds.), Glenn's Thoracic and Cardiovascular Surgery (5th ed.). Norwalk, CT: Appleton & Lange, 1991, pp. 1165–1177.

Rasof, B, Linde, LM, Dunn, OJ. Intellectual development in children with congenital heart disease. Child Development, 38:1043–1053, 1967.

Risser, NL. Preoperative and postoperative care to prevent pulmonary complications. Heart and Lung, 9:57–67, 1980.

Rockwell, GM, & Campbell, SK. Physical therapy program for the pediatric cardiac surgical patient. Physical Therapy, 56:670–676, 1976.

Rosen, M, & Hillard, EK. The effects of negative pressure during tracheal suction. Anesthesia and Analgesia, *41*:50–57, 1962.

Rosenthal, A. Care of the postoperative child and adolescent with congenital heart disease. In Barness, LA (Ed.), Advances in Pediatrics. Chicago: Year Book Publishers, 1983, pp. 131–167.

Rubin, M. The physiology of bedrest. American Journal of Nursing, *88*:50–56, 1988.

Ruttenberg, HD, Adams, TD, Orsmond, GS, Conlee, RK, & Fisher, AG. Effects of exercise training on aerobic fitness in children after open heart surgery. Pediatric Cardiology, *4*:19–24, 1983.

Sadowsky, HS, Rohrkemper, KF, & Quon, SYM. Rehabilitation of Cardiac and Cardiopulmonary Recipients. An introduction for Physical and Occupational Therapists. Stanford, CA: Stanford University Hospital, 1986.

Scheidegger, D, Bentz, L, Piolino, G, Pusterla, C, & Gigon, JP. Influence of early mobilisation on pulmonary function in surgical patients. European Journal of Intensive Care Medicine, *2*:35–40, 1976.

Sciurba, FC, Owens, GR, Sanders, MH, Bartley, BP, Hardesty, RL, Paradis, IL, & Costantino, JP. Evidence of an altered pattern of breathing during exercise in recipients of heart-lung transplants. New England Journal of Medicine, *319*:1186–1192, 1988.

Settergren, G, Ohqvist, G, Lundberg, S, Henze, A, Bjork, VO, & Persson, B. Cerebral blood flow and cerebral metabolism in children following cardiac surgery with deep hypothermia and circulatory arrest. Clinical course and follow-up of psychomotor development. Scandinavian Journal of Thoracic Cardiovascular Surgery, *16*:209–215, 1982.

Silbert, A, Wolff, PH, Mayer, B, Rosenthal, A, & Nadas, AS. Cyanotic heart disease and psychological development. Pediatrics, *43*:192–200, 1969.

Starnes, VA, Marshall, SE, Lewiston, NJ, Theodore, J, Stinson, EB, & Shumway, NE. Heart-lung transplantation in infants, children, and adolescents. Journal of Pediatric Surgery, *26*:434–438, 1991.

Starnes, VA, Oyer, PE, Bernstein, D, Baum, D, Gamberg, P, Miller, J, & Shumway, NE. Heart, heart-lung, and lung transplantation in the first year of life. Annals of Thoracic Surgery, *53*:306–310, 1992.

Stevenson, JG, Stone, FE, Dilliard, DH, & Morgan, BC. Intellectual development of children subjected to prolonged circulatory arrest during hypothermic open heart surgery in infancy. Circulation, *49 & 50*(suppl II):54–59, 1974.

Stretton, CD, Mak, JCW, Belvisi, MG, Yacoub, MH, & Barnes, PJ. Cholinergic control of human airways *in vitro* following extrinsic denervation of the human respiratory tract by heart-lung transplantation. American Review of Respiratory Disease, *142*:1030–1033, 1990.

Suoninen, P. Physical growth of children with congenital heart disease. Acta Paediatrica. Supplement, *225*:7–50, 1971.

Thoren, L. Post-operative pulmonary complications. Acta Chir Scandinavia, *107*:193–205, 1954.

Todd, TR. Early postoperative management following lung transplantation. Clinics in Chest Medicine, *11*:259–267, 1990.

Trusler, GA. The Mustard procedure. In Baue, AE, Geha, AS, Hammond, GL, Laks, H, & Naunheim, KS (Eds.), Glenn's Thoracic and Cardiovascular Surgery (5th ed.). Norwalk, CT: Appleton & Lange, 1991, pp. 1203–1209.

Uretsky, BF. Physiology of the transplanted heart. In Brest, AN (Ed.), Cardiovascular Clinics. Philadelphia: FA Davis, 1990, pp. 23–55.

van Breda, A. Postoperative care of infants and children who require cardiac surgery. Heart and Lung, *14*:205–207, 1985.

Van De Water, JM, Watring, WG, Linton, LA, Murphy, M, & Byron, RL. Prevention of postoperative pulmonary complications. Surgery, Gynecology and Obstetrics, *135*:229–233, 1972.

Vraciu, JK, & Vraciu, RA. Effectiveness of breathing exercises in preventing pulmonary complications following open heart surgery. Physical Therapy, *57*:1367–1371, 1977.

Waldhausen, JA, Myers, JL, & Campbell, DB. Coarctation of the aorta and interrupted aortic arch. In Baue, AE, Geha, AS, Hammond, GL, Laks, H, & Naunheim, KS (Eds.), Glenn's Thoracic and Cardiovascular Surgery (5th ed.). Norwalk, CT: Appleton & Lange, 1991, pp. 1107–1122.

Ward, RJ, Danziger, F, Bonica, JJ, Allen, GD, & Bowes, J. An evaluation of postoperative maneuvers. Surgical Gynecology & Obstetrics, *66*:51–54, 1966.

Warner, JO. Heart-lung transplantation: All the facts. Archives of Disease in Childhood, *66*:1013–1017, 1991.

Webber, BA. Evaluation and inflation in respiratory care. Physiotherapy, *77*:801–804, 1991.

Weinhaus, L, Canter, C, Noetzel, M, McAlister, W, & Spray, TL. Extracorporeal membrane oxygenation for circulatory support after repair of congenital heart defects. Annals of Thoracic Surgery, *48*:206–212, 1989.

Weldon, CS, Behrendt, DM, & Haas, GS. Congenital malformations of the aortic valve and left ventricular outflow tract. In Baue, AE, Geha, AS, Hammond, GL, Laks, H, & Naunheim, KS (Eds.), Glenn's Thoracic and Cardiovascular Surgery (5th ed.). Norwalk, CT: Appleton & Lange, 1991, pp. 1089–1106.

Wells, FC, Coghill, S, Caplan, HL, & Lincoln, C. Duration of circulatory arrest does influence the psychological development of children after cardiac operation in early life. Journal of Thoracic and Cardiovascular Surgery, *86*:823–831, 1983.

Whitehead, B, James, I, Helms, P, Scott, JP, Smyth, R, Higenbottam, TW, McGoldrick, J, English, TAH, Wallwork, J, Elliott, M, & de Leval, M. Intensive care management of children following heart and heart-lung transplantation. Intensive Care Medicine, *16*:426–430, 1990.

Wilkinson, JL. Heart and heart/lung transplantation in children. Australian Paediatric Journal, *25*:111–118, 1989.

Williams, WH. Rastelli's operation for "anatomic" repair of transposition of the great arteries with ventricular septal defect and left ventricular outflow tract obstruction. In Baue, AE, Geha, AS, Hammond, GL, Laks, H, & Naunheim, KS (Eds.), Glenn's Thoracic and Cardiovascular Surgery (5th ed.). Norwalk, CT: Appleton & Lange, 1991, pp. 1217–1226.

Wilson, RS. Anesthesia for thoracic surgery. In Baue, AE, Geha, AS, Hammond, GL, Laks, H, & Naunheim, KS (Eds.), Glenn's Thoracic and Cardiovascular Surgery (5th ed.). Norwalk, CT: Appleton & Lange, 1991, pp. 19–29.

Youssef, NM. School adjustment of children with congenital heart disease. Maternal–Child Nursing Journal, *17*:217–302, 1988.

Zahr, LK, & Boisvert, J. Hypoplastic left heart syndrome repair. Dimensions in Critical Care Nursing, *9*:88–96, 1990.

Section Five

Special Settings and Special Considerations

ROBERT J. PALISANO, PT, ScD
Section Editor

Chapter 28

The Burn Unit

MERILYN L. MOORE, PT

Burn-related injuries are listed as the leading cause of accidental death in children younger than the age of 2 and the second leading cause of accidental death in children younger than the age of 14 (Warden et al., 1988). Data accumulated by the National Burn Information Exchange, a voluntary registry established in 1964 (Feller, 1982), show that a disproportionately high number of burn accidents occur during the first 4 years of life and that boys are affected more often than girls. This age group alone incurs 52% of all pediatric burns.

During the first 2 years of life, 95% of the burn injuries occur indoors and the etiologic agent is a hot liquid in 80% of the patients (Feller, 1980). As the child gets older, the proportion of indoor injuries progressively declines and scalds become less frequent. During adolescence, 60% of the injuries occur outdoors and only 20% occur as a result of scalding (Green, 1984). The depth and extent of the burn also increase as the child gets older.

A retrospective study of 70 patients with burns admitted to a pediatric hospital identified associated familial risk factors (Boucher et al., 1993) including recent immigration, current separation or divorce, and familial concerns requiring intervention by the child protective agency. Four percent of children came from families who had pre-

vious involvement with the child protective agency, and in a further 5% the families were investigated after the burn injury.

During the past 20 years, great strides have been made in the management of thermal injuries. In 1968, patients sustaining burns on more than 35% of the body had a 50% survival rate. In 1988, the 50% survival rate applied to those victims with burns on more than 70% of their total body surface (Warden et al., 1988).

The improvement in the survival rate of pediatric patients is equally encouraging. In 1949, Bull and Squire reported a 50% mortality rate in children younger than 14 years of age with burns of 51% of the total body surface area. Forty-three years later Herndon and Rutan (1992a) reported a 50% mortality rate in children younger than 15 years of age with burns of greater than 95% of the total body surface area. This drastic change in the mortality rate after thermal injuries can be attributed to four primary changes in burn care, based on intensive basic science and clinical research: 1) resuscitation and prevention of hypovolemic shock, 2) support of the hypermetabolic response to burn trauma, 3) control of infection, and 4) early excision of the burn wound (Herndon & Rutan, 1992a)

With increased survival, the treatment of children with burns is concerned not only with prevention of infection but also with the psychological and social outcome of the patient. Pediatric survivors often must live with permanent disfigurement and physical disabilities. Another outcome of quality care assessment studies on data collected by the National Burn Information Exchange is marked reduction in length of hospitalization (Feller & Jones, 1984). With reduced mortality and reduced length of hospitalization, rehabilitation takes on added importance.

Roles and responsibilities of various members of the burn team overlap, thus changing the traditional role of the physical therapist. The purpose of this chapter is to provide a guide to better understanding of potential problems of the child who is burned and to outline resources available to the physical therapist providing quality care on the burn unit.

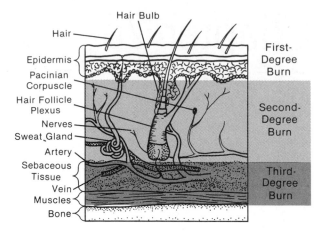

FIGURE 28–1. Degrees of burn. (Redrawn with permission from Duran-Coleman, LA. Rehabilitation of the burn survivor. Progress Report Journal, *4*[3]:5, 1992.)

CLASSIFICATION AND PATHOPHYSIOLOGY OF BURNS

Burn injuries occur when energy is transferred from a heat source to the body. If heat absorption exceeds heat dissipation, cellular temperature rises above the point at which cell survival is possible. Tissue damage begins at temperatures of 40°C and increases logarithmically as the temperature rises. At 45°C, denaturation of tissue proteins ensues and leads to cellular necrosis (Carvajal, 1990). The extent of injury is related to 1) heat intensity, 2) duration of the exposure, and 3) tissue conductance (Achauer & Martinez, 1985).

Burns may be categorized into four types, ac-

cording to the primary mechanism of injury: thermal, radiation, electrical, or chemical (Bayley, 1990). Thermal injuries include burns caused by contact with hot liquids (spills or immersion scalds), hot solid objects, or flames and make up approximately 95% of all burns treated (Solem, 1984). Chemical and electrical injuries comprise about 5% of burns admitted to a regional burn center. Radiation injuries are extremely rare.

Burn injuries are classified as first, second, or third degree according to the depth of tissue damage. A summary of burn classification characteristics is provided in Figure 28–1 and Table 28–1. Some authors describe deeper full-thickness damage as fourth-degree burns, involving not only the entire thickness of the skin but also subadjacent structure such as subcutaneous fat, fascia, muscle,

TABLE 28–1. **CLASSIFICATION OF BURNS**

		Second Degree		
Criterion	**First Degree**	**SUPERFICIAL**	**DEEP**	**Third Degree**
Depth	Superficial epidermis	Epidermis and a small part of the dermis	Epidermis and a deeper portion of the dermis	Total destruction of the epidermis and dermis; may involve deeper tissue, muscle, or subcutaneous fat
Sensation	Painful	Increased sensitivity to pain and temperature	Increased sensitivity to pain and temperature	No pain or temperature sensation
Color	Bright red	Red	Marbled-white edematous appearance	White, brown-black charred appearance
Texture	Edematous	Normal or firm	Firm	Firm or leathery
Blisters	Some, blanches with pressure	Large, thick-walled, will usually increase in size	Large, thick-walled, will usually increase in size	None, or if present will not increase in size

From Duran-Coleman, LA. Rehabilitation of the burn survivor. Progress Report Journal, 4(3):5, 1992.

or bone. Burns involving tendon, muscle, or bone are most common on digits, hands, feet, and over bony prominences such as the iliac crest, patella, anterior tibia, and cranium, since these areas have only a thin covering of subcutaneous tissue (Solem, 1984).

Because skin varies in thickness in different parts of the body, application of the same intensity of heat for given periods of time results in different burn depth. Thus in the young child in whom dermal papillae and appendages have yet to develop fully, deeper burns result from heat of the same intensity that produces a moderate second-degree burn in the adult. The skin is thickest on the back and on the palm of the hands and is thinnest on the inner arm. Burned parts involving the thickest areas of skin regenerate faster.

Certain burn patterns are indicative of possible abuse (Doane, 1989), for example, burns of the buttocks, feet, and perineum when the backs of knees and anterior hip areas are not burned. This typically occurs when a child is placed in a tub of hot water. The child flexes into a protective position by curling up the knees and hips.

The extent of burn injury can be estimated in several ways. One approach is referred to as the "rule of nines" (Mikhail, 1988), which divides the body surface into areas, each representing 9% or a multiple of 9% of body surface area. This method is particularly unreliable in children younger than 15 years of age since it underestimates burned areas of the head and neck and overestimates burned areas of the legs (Solem, 1984). Another method, the Berkow chart (Feller & Jones, 1974), is modeled after Lund and Browder's work (1944), which recognizes that the proportion of body surface covering specific body parts changes with age. For example, the head and neck of an infant constitute 20% of the body surface compared with 9% in the adult.

Thermal destruction of the skin initiates a chain of physiologic changes in the local wound as well as severe multiple systemic responses in almost all organ systems. The total amount of cell death and extracellular destruction is dependent on local chemical responses to the initial insult, and the systemic response to burn injury (Dimick, 1984). Important clinically apparent local responses include loss of the ability to regulate evaporative water loss, impairment of the body's first line of defense against infection, and the loss of massive amounts of body fluids through open wounds. The systemic effects of the burn injury on other organs are well described in the literature (Achauer & Martinez, 1985; Dimick, 1984). It is the physiologic changes occurring in the skin and subadjacent tissues that are addressed in the primary physical impairment section of this chapter.

THE BURN UNIT AND TEAM APPROACH TO CARE

Appropriate treatment decisions can be made after calculation of the severity of the burn by following the American Burn Association treatment guidelines. Patients with minor burns may be treated as outpatients. Moderately severe *uncomplicated* burns may be treated in a community hospital by an experienced surgeon or physician. Burns that should be referred to a burn unit include larger second-degree burns (greater than 25% in adults or 20% in children); all third-degree burns greater than 10%; burns of difficult areas such as the hands, face, eyes, ears, feet and perineum; and burns with associated injuries including inhalation or electrical injuries, fractures, or other trauma. A survey of 73 burn units suggests that there is significant variation in some aspects of burn care (Alexander et al., 1993). The director's experience and training appear to play the most important role in determining each center's preferences.

The burn unit is much like other intensive care units, but it also has unique characteristics. As in other units, it is a place characterized by high technology, specially trained staff, a team approach, and isolation, which may lead to a dehumanizing situation in which the patient is viewed in a fragmented and anatomic manner. The need for compassion, empathy, guidance, interest, and support is paramount. On the other hand, significant differences exist between the burn unit and other acute care units. The sights and smells characteristic of burn injury make for an obvious difference from other emergency care settings. Isolation of both staff and patient from the outside world is often more pronounced in the burn unit primarily because of fear of infection. There is also the constant issue of pain management. Patients in burn centers stay longer than in other intensive care units, or indeed, any other hospital units. This results in a much more intense and prolonged patient–staff interaction.

The fact that the staff functions as a multidisciplinary team is also more apparent in the burn center. The team approach to burn care was developed in specialized burn treatment facilities established over the past 20 years. Presently burn teams usually consist of physicians and nursing personnel, physical therapists and occupational therapists, clinical nutritionists, social workers, psychiatrists or psychologists, child life specialists or recreational therapists, school teachers, and, when available, orthotists, prosthetists, and medical sculptors. The team must never lose sight of the child and the family as being the center around which all disci-

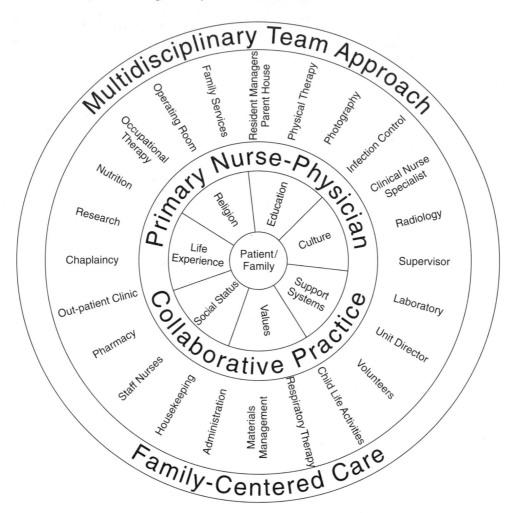

FIGURE 28-2. Model of family-centered care approach. The primary nurse and physician work together with the direct care providers and the support services to form the multidisciplinary team. (From Warden, GD, Brinkerhoff, C, Castellani, D, & Rieg, LS. Multidisciplinary team approach to the pediatric burn patient. Quality Review Bulletin, *14*:219–226, 1988.)

plines and activities revolve. Throughout the hospital stay, factual information and alternative courses of action are provided to the child and the family to facilitate decision-making. A model of a family-centered care approach is illustrated in Figure 28-2 (Warden et al., 1988).

The burn team approach is based on a mutual respect and appreciation of each burn team member's contribution to the overall care of the patient and the development of a decision-making process that relies on the input of the child and participating family (on wound round and individually with staff) and all professional team members. Discussions at burn team conferences not only lead to improved patient care but also provide an opportunity for members to gain insights from the experiences of other team members who are caring for the same patient. Daily pressures the team must face include viewing mutilations and disfigurement, inflicting pain, dealing with emergency situations, and confronting death.

Medical Management of Burns

When a child is admitted to the appropriate facility, an estimate of the depth and surface area of the burn and the child's overall condition is first made. These decisions determine the need for immediate lifesaving measures, such as endotracheal intubation, ventilatory support, and intravenous fluid therapy (Hartford, 1984).

Shock is usual in children with burns affecting more than 12% of the surface area but can occur when the surface area is smaller if the burn is full thickness and when the child is younger than 1 year of age (Solomon, 1985). An intravenous line and urinary catheter are placed and fluid delivery is begun. Until the capillary leak stops, intravenous fluid therapy is necessary to maintain the circulation and perfusion of tissues. After fluid resuscitation has been started and a detailed history and physical examination completed, attention is directed to care of the burn.

Escharotomy, incision through the burn, may be necessary to relieve the pressure caused by progressive edema in the extremities with circumferential deep burns. It is usually done when the tissue pressure exceeds 40 mm Hg. The incisions are made along the medial and lateral aspects of the limb. As the tissues are released, the subcutaneous fat bulges through the incision, tissue tension is relieved, and effective circulation is restored. Among patients with deep burns or high-voltage electrical injury involving muscle, fasciotomy may be necessary to relieve elevated pressure in fascial compartments unrelieved by simple escharotomy.

As soon as the patient's condition is stabilized, the wounds are assessed for the purpose of developing a plan for wound closure. Necrotic tissue produced by the burn must be removed, either by daily mechanical debridement during wound care or, in deeper burns, by surgical excision either directly to fascia or tangentially (i.e., shaving sequential levels until viable tissue is exposed), and closure must be accomplished with autogenous split-thickness skin grafts.

Aggressive and thorough wound care is important to help delineate wounds before early surgical intervention, to protect and promote good granulation tissue until grafting, or to promote rapid healing in wounds that are healing without surgical intervention. There are three types of cleansing techniques: 1) local care of a particular wound or area (using a sterile container of water and cleansing agents at bedside or any convenient area); 2) spray hydrotherapy or nonsubmersion (using a shower head to allow the water to run intermittently over the burn wounds with the patient on a stretcher suspended over a tank or tub); and 3) submersion, which may or may not include agitation of the water (submerging the patient or burned extremity in a tub, tank, or whirlpool of water for up to 20 minutes). The choice depends on the depth of injury, extent and location of the wound, and medical condition of the patient (Head, 1984).

Most burn wound protocols call for daily or twice-daily dressing changes (Bayley, 1990). Various topical burn creams and solutions are available. No single topical agent has been demonstrated to be universally effective for burn care. Each has advantages and disadvantages, and the effectiveness of even a single agent may decrease after time. Different agents may be used on the same patient either concurrently, on different burned areas, or sequentially as the wound and its bacterial flora change. Each topical agent is applied with gauze dressings (type used is needs-specific). Gauze should be wrapped distally to proximally on burned extremities, and no two burn surfaces should be allowed to touch (i.e., fingers and toes should be wrapped separately, and burned ears should not touch the burned head). Such attention to detail helps to prevent webbing caused by raw surfaces growing together (Bayley, 1990) Wrapping digits individually also facilitates active and functional movements (Puddicombe & Nardoner, 1990).

Excision may be initiated a few days after the burn or as soon as the patient is hemodynamically stable and edema has decreased (Heimbach, 1987). An autograft is immediately placed, or a temporary biologic or synthetic dressing is used until autografting can be done in a subsequent operation. Surgical excision is advantageous in contributing to decreased complications from invasive burn wound sepsis and a shorter time period from injury to wound closure and hospital discharge (Bayley, 1990).

Unless of small size, all full-thickness wounds require skin grafts. Wounds of partial-thickness depth that do not heal spontaneously in a reasonable time, may, if donor skin is available, be closed with a skin graft. Split-thickness skin grafts are used almost exclusively. This implies that the grafts are cut through a partial-thickness of depth of skin, leaving epidermal regenerative cells that cause re-epithelialization of the donor site. Full-thickness skin grafts and flaps are occasionally used in primary repair of specific burn wounds (e.g., very deep electrical burns) but are primarily used later in some reconstructive procedures.

Skin grafts may be cut from virtually any area of the body except the face and hands. The foot as a skin donor source is generally impractical. The scalp is a superior donor site. It has excellent blood supply with deep, closely placed hair follicles that are able to effect re-epithelialization in 4 or 5 days. Regrowth of scalp hair hides the donor site. Donor sites of the torso and extremities heal more slowly.

In the majority of instances, wounds of the hands, face, and neck take precedence for skin grafts. However, when there is limited donor skin consideration must be given to covering larger areas to try to reduce the size of the wound to first preserve the patient's life. The next priority for skin grafts after the hands, face, and neck is the skin over joints.

Skin grafts must be undisturbed in order to take. Fibrin causes initial adherence. The cells of the graft are nourished by tissue fluid until inosculation (anastomosis) of blood vessels between the wound and the graft establishes a nutritive blood flow in the graft. Inosculation occurs in about 2 days. Joints must be held immobile until the take of the skin graft is ensured. This is usually accomplished by splinting, or by the use of skeletal traction in specific instances (Fig. 28–3).

In most cases there is enough tensile strength between the graft and the wound to permit active range of motion (ROM) on the fourth and certainly by the sixth day after skin grafting. Gentle passive ROM can be added on the sixth or seventh day.

Early massive excision of the burn wound has increased the median lethal dose to 98% of total body surface area burn but represents the problem of wound closure (Herndon & Rutan, 1992b). Autograft substitutes must be used for a large burn. Alternate methods of wound closure that are currently used include biologic dressings, biosynthetic dressings, artificial skin, and cultured skin.

Biologic dressings consist of viable or once-viable tissues used to temporarily cover wounds in place of conventional dressings or leaving the wound exposed. Frequently used materials are partial-thickness grafts from living or recently deceased humans (hemografts or allografts), partial-thickness skin grafts from pigs (heterografts or xenografts), or amnion from the human placenta. All biologic dressings, viable and nonviable, can be used for

short-term, several-day, wound coverage (Hartford, 1984). In a large burn, biological dressings can be lifesaving by providing temporary wound closure until completion of autografting. Biologic dressings may also be effectively employed to protect wounds that have been covered by widely meshed graft. Used in this way, the wounds between the autografts are closed as well.

Problems with availability, sterility, and cost have led to the search for synthetic skin substitutes, which may eventually replace biologic dressings as temporary wound coverings (Bayley, 1990). The most popular currently is Biobrane, a knitted elastic flexible nylon fabric that is bonded to a thin Silastic semipermeable membrane coated with products of dermal collagen. Sterile and semi-transparent, Biobrane has an indefinite shelf-life, allows the passage of some topical agents, and is cheaper than homograft or pig skin. Biobrane has been used to cover clean partial-thickness burns, temporarily to close excised full-thickness burns, and to dress meshed autograft and donor sites.

Dermagraft is a newly developed dermal substitute in early stages of clinical trials (Economou et al., 1993). It consists of polyglycolic acid mesh impregnated with viable human neonatal fibroblasts. Fibroblasts secrete native human collagen, growth factors, and other matrix proteins, forming a living, three-dimensional dermal tissue. It may be potentially useful as a synthetic dermal graft in large-area, full-thickness burns.

There is an ever-increasing number of other strictly synthetic dressings on the market with use in burn care (Bayley, 1990). These thin, transparent

FIGURE 28–3. Positioning in the burn intensive care unit. A 16-year-old adolescent with severe burns is positioned in a Clinitron air-fluidized bed. Note bilateral calcaneal and tibial traction with additional right footsplint attachment, arm-trough attachment to the bed for shoulder positioning and hand elevation, and a splint applied to the anterior neck.

elastic materials are used to cover clean partial-thickness wounds and donor sites. Occlusive and waterproof, these dressings are moisture, vapor, and air permeable. This allows for the exchange of gases necessary for healing but still provides for protection of the wound from microbial contamination. The use of such materials creates an environment that virtually eliminates pain and decreases healing time (Hartford, 1984).

Recently, confluent sheets of epidermal cells (cultured epidermal autograft) have been grown successfully from a small partial-thickness skin graft or biopsy of the patient's own unburned skin (Clugston et al., 1991; Desai et al., 1991; Herndon & Rutan, 1992b). Cultured keratinocyte sheets lack a dermal component, however, and this is a potentially serious deficiency for achieving a successful replacement for full-thickness skin losses. Investigations are aimed at improving the engraftment and ultimate survival of cultured epidermal autograft.

Clinical and scientific research continues to improve the potential for recovery of severely burned children. Two examples of treatments that have contributed to improved recovery are the clinical use of propranolol and growth hormone. Baron and Herndon (1993) reported safe administration of propranolol to 43 children with massive burns (Mean percentage of total body surface area burn = 60 ± 18%). Cardiac work was reduced by more than 70 beats per minute, and patient anxiety decreased. Herndon and colleagues (1990) and Gilpin and associates (1993) demonstrated a significant decrease in length of hospital stay as a result of increased healing rates of donor sites when recombinant human growth hormone was administered.

PRIMARY PHYSICAL IMPAIRMENT

Burn Scar

Regeneration of epithelial elements in partial-thickness injury to resurface the area comes from the epithelial cells lining every hair follicle and sweat gland. Healing of partial-thickness burns usually takes 14 days, but if the burn is sufficiently deep these burns may take 21 days for complete healing. As the epithelium grows, the normal pigmentation gradually and progressively returns. As the regenerated epithelium differentiates and forms the keratin layer of the skin once again, the epithelium becomes reinvolved in the temperature regulatory process by maintaining and conserving the core body temperature.

A significant basic pathophysiologic consequence of burn injury is a loss of capillary integrity leading to edema formation, which is a result of the outpouring of protein-rich intravascular fluid into the interstitium. This process occurs at all areas of partial-thickness burns and at areas adjacent to and subadjacent to full-thickness burns. As the patient voluntarily limits movement at the injured part because of pain, and as a result of direct damage to the lymphatic systems, this edema fluid accumulates and persists in tissue spaces around tendons, joints, and ligaments. New collagen fibers form in this protein-rich edema fluid and eventually organize into unyielding adhesions and thickened support structures whose normal elasticity is lost.

Healing of deep dermal wounds also results in the replacement of normal integument with a mass of metabolically highly active tissues lacking the normal architecture of the skin (Parks et al., 1977). Several theories have been formulated to explain the processes involved in burn scar hypertrophy and contracture (Howell, 1984). Several different processes appear to be at work in the healing wound. These processes include the following: mass production of large amounts of fused highly disorganized collagen; replacement of the normal dermal elastic ground substance with inelastic chondroitin sulfate A; involuntary contraction of myofibroblasts; and inflammatory response with increased vascularity and localized lymphedema.

The bonds between the twisted collagen and firm inelastic ground substance, coupled with the simultaneous contraction of the myofibroblasts, contribute to the "heaped up" appearance of the hypertrophic scar. In addition, underlying voluntary skeletal muscle contraction reinforces the compaction of the collagen. The intensity and duration of the vascular response provides a visible clue to the likelihood of hypertrophic scarring and contracture formation (Larson et al., 1979). The hyperemia of the scar tissue signifies ongoing change within the closed wound. As long as this clinical characteristic persists, scar maturation has not been completed and hypertrophy is a possibility. The darker a patient's skin, the more predisposed that patient is toward hypertrophic scarring. Also, children are more susceptible to the development of hypertrophic scarring than adults (Deitch et al., 1983; Sullivan, 1990).

The active phase of scarring gradually subsides and will usually be completed in 1½ to 2 years after the burn (Bayley, 1990; Dimick, 1984). In this regard, clinical reports indicate more rapid maturity for sheet graft compared with that reported for meshed grafts (Schwanholt et al., 1993). If appropriate measures are instituted during this active period, the scar tissue loses its redness and softens. Linares and co-workers (1973) have shown that "pressure induces loosening of collagen bundles and encourages parallel orientation of the collagen bundles to the skin surface with the disappearance of the dermal nodules." With the application of pressure there is a coincident restructuring of the collagen mass and a decrease in vascularity and cellularity. Larson and colleagues (1974) reported that at least 25 mm Hg pressure must be achieved to provide histologically and clinically significant pressure. As much as 40 mm Hg pressure may be needed in the extremities and trunk to overcome normal capillary opening pressure (Parke et al., 1977).

The position of comfort for most patients is that of flexion of the joints, and they will assume this position if allowed to do so. Maintenance of a flexed posture permits new collagen fibers in the wound to fuse together, resulting in contracture formation. Eventually the scar will mature, becoming a solid mass of fused collagen. The resulting mass of collagen will have a Swiss-cheese appearance as a result of continuing reabsorption of the collagen. The contracture, however, will remain because of fusion of some of the collagen fibers into the shortened position. Other several long-term disabilities occur as a result of skin grafting required for third-degree burns. When the skin is transplanted to the area of third-degree burn, no hair follicles or sweat glands are included. Therefore, these grafted areas do not have the specialized skin appendages. Without these, the grafted area has none of the normal body oils, resulting in excessively dry skin. Another problem for patients with extensive skin grafting is created by the absence of sweat glands in grafted skin. The grafted areas are unable to dissipate the core body temperature if it is too high. Patients are cautioned about this problem and warned to avoid environments with high heat and humidity because they may have trouble dissipating excessive core body temperature.

Patients frequently report having other abnormal or odd sensations in their burn wounds, which are probably a result of regeneration of nerve endings into the burned areas. As the nerve endings grow through the areas of burned tissue, they frequently meet an obstruction that may cause an area of hypersensitivity, characterized by unusual or odd sensations. Small neuromas may occur in scattered areas throughout the burned area, causing hypersensitivity.

Scar formation is a natural sequela in the healing process of burned skin. It cannot be prevented, although current research suggests the potential for therapeutic use of interferons to downregulate collagen production and inhibit wound contraction (Ghahary et al., 1993; Nedelec et al., 1993).

Musculoskeletal Complications

In addition to burn scarring, many musculoskeletal complications are associated with immobility and inactivity during the acute phase of rehabilitation of the patient with burns. They include peripheral nerve involvement, exposed tendons and joints, heterotopic bone formation, amputations, and problems associated with cultured epithelial autografts.

Peripheral nerve damage occurs in 15% (Henderson et al., 1971) to 29% (Helm et al., 1977) of patients resulting from 1) electrical injury by passage of current through the nerve (Hunt, 1984), 2) edema with elevated tissue pressure (Rorabeck & Clark, 1978), 3) metabolic abnormalities and nutritional deficiencies (Collins et al., 1979), and 4) localized nerve compression or stretch injury from improper dressings or positioning (Helm, 1984).

Heterotopic bone formation around joints may cause a disabling complication in 2 to 3% of patients with burns who are hospitalized (Evans, 1966). The most common site of heterotopic calcification following burn injury is the elbow. The calcification is usually located posteriorly and medially with a bony bridge between the olecranon of the ulna and the medial epicondyle and intercondylar portion and posterior shaft of the humerus. Heterotopic bone formation is rare in children but may be evident in the adolescent population. Treatment consists of continuing physical therapy efforts at remobilization of the joint. Heterotopic bone disappears spontaneously in about one half of the cases. If excision is indicated, heterotopic ossification usually does not re-form after removal, and functional and often normal ROM is restored.

The patient with associated limb amputation presents a number of unique rehabilitative problems to the physical therapist. Some of these situations are described by Ward and associates (1990a) as intolerance of the stump to pressure or manipulation because of remaining open wounds or fragility of newly healed skin grafted areas on the residual limb or as delayed gait or functional training because of wounds on other body surface areas. There is also an increased risk of developing joint contractures because of hypertrophic scarring and the inevitable loss of muscle strength from bedrest after surgery. Nevertheless, despite these problems, it appears that most patients with burns who require limb amputation can achieve successful prosthetic use (Ward et al., 1990b).

The functional difficulties experienced by therapists working with severely burned patients who were grafted with cultured epithelial autografts have been outlined by Egan (1992). Cultured cells grow into very fragile skin that is highly susceptible to cuts and bruises and lacks tensile strength. These problems have persisted in patients grafted with cultural skin for as long as 2 years after initial treatment. Cultured skin also lacks any pigmentation and so is "blotchy white" and very susceptible to sunburn. Scarring occurs less often with cultured skin, but its fragility and lack of pigmentation present functional and cosmetic challenges, particularly to patients with black skin.

PHYSICAL THERAPY GOALS AND PROCEDURES

Assessment and Plan

The purposes of the therapist's initial assessment are to determine the child's status, identify the rehabilitation needs, and anticipate the patient's potential problems. The first task is to ascertain the immediate postinjury status of the patient. The information necessary to make this determination includes an assessment of the circumstances of the injury; the duration, type, and extent of the burn; preexisting medical and rehabilitation problems; concurrent injuries; and ROM estimates. The developmental status of young children before the burn injury must be ascertained. The level of achievement of school-aged children, both physically and scholastically, should also be established to set realistic functional goals.

Identifying the rehabilitation needs of the child requires thorough assessment as well as an understanding of the implications of different types of burns and their locations. The expected clinical course and approximate length of stay of the patient should be estimated initially to anticipate potential emotional, physiologic, and rehabilitation problems.

Physical therapy assessment in the postacute stage should consist of the following: burn scar assessment (color, firmness, and flexibility), ROM of joints adjacent to burned areas, pain, gait, and functional ability. Goals of the therapy program at this stage are based on the child's status, the effectiveness of the treatment procedures performed during the acute care period or after previous reconstructive operations, and the compliance of patient and family. Goals must be discussed with the child who is old enough to understand and in every case with the family.

Once the child has been assessed, an individualized program plan is established in collaboration with the patient or the family and other members of the burn care team. The program plan includes specific short- and long-term goals and the methods to achieve these goals. The program plan is developed with the primary focus on the prevention of deformities. The program plan and the implementation methods vary with the stages of wound recovery. Throughout implementation, the program plan is coordinated closely with that of other team members, since outcome standards are multidisciplinary. Success depends not on an individual discipline but rather on the cooperation and knowledge of each team member.

The deforming effects of burn scar contractures can be decreased by use of the following therapeutic procedures: proper patient positioning and splinting, ROM and graded resistive exercises, early ambulation, application of elastic pressure garments (with various silicone or foam inserts), and patient and family education regarding skin care and the rehabilitation program. Other modalities such as continuous passive motion, fluidotherapy, and paraffin all aid in increasing skin pliability and desensitizing the healed burn area. Rehabilitative interventions, such as static and dynamic splinting, serial casting, and stretching exercises, to prevent or treat burn scar contractures should be based on sound biomechanical principles such as creep, stress relaxation, successive elongation, strain rate, and hysteresis (Richard et al., 1993). Table 28–2 outlines application of these principles to management of burn scar contracture. The treatment plan should also include play activities and training in functional activities to facilitate the development of coping behavior. The child should be allowed as much self-care as is possible, depending on the stage of recovery. Participation in dressing changes, decision-making when confronted with equal alternatives, and personal hygiene must be encouraged to give the individual a sense of control.

Positioning and Splinting

One of the many benefits of an early positioning program is reduction of edema in the extremities, allowing return to functional movement. Elevating the extremities allows reduction of edema, utilizing the pull of gravity. Proper positioning can help maintain ROM and counteract contracture by maintaining proper flexibility of connective tissue and skin.

Positioning must be individualized to the child's need. A series of positions should be designed for each involved joint, whereby the child alternates positions every 2 to 4 hours, since static positioning is not well tolerated. When skin grafts or biologic

TABLE 28-2. **BIOMECHANICAL BASIS FOR PHYSICAL MANAGEMENT OF BURN PATIENTS**

Mechanical Principles	Definition	Clinical Application
Creep	A progressive elongation that occurs when tissue is stretched and the stretching force is kept constant	Dynamic splinting Tissue expanders Ilizarov external fixators
Stress relaxation	A progressive reduction in force required to maintain tissue at a given length	Serial casting Static splinting
Successive elongation	Repeated stretching of tissue until a steady state of tissue length is achieved	Continuous passive motion Repeated stretching
Strain rate	Amount of tissue elongation per unit time	Low- versus high-velocity stretching
Hysteresis	The delayed return of elongated tissue to its original resting length	Splinting and positioning required after exercise to maintain tissue elongation

Data from Richard, RL, Staley, MJ, Miller, SF, Warden, GD, & Finley, RK, Jr. Biomechanical basis for physical management of burn patients. Poster presented at the meeting of the American Burn Association, Cincinnati, March 1993.

dressings are required, accurate positioning contributes to good wound coverage.

Children usually have difficulty understanding the long-range benefits of positioning procedures. Often, splinting is the most appropriate and effective method for proper positioning, especially during unsupervised periods and during sleep, when positions that contribute to deformity are often assumed. When the child is able to be active during the day, night splinting may be indicated to maintain ROM gained during the day.

When voluntary movement is impaired, as in the presence of peripheral neuropathies, the area must be continuously splinted to avoid contracture formation. Twenty-four-hour splinting is also indicated to maintain slack on exposed tendons until wound closure occurs.

Clarke and colleagues (1990) noted that the typical burned hand in the child results from a different pattern of injury and responds differently to therapeutic intervention when compared with the adult hand. Scald burns are most common in pediatric hand burns. In addition, children develop less stiffness in response to immobilization. Normal hand function can therefore be achieved in the majority of cases. However, deep flame injuries to the hand present a specific challenge to the rehabilitation team. The challenge is to manage the short lever arm available in the application of treatment modalities. In the young child this is further complicated by the lack of muscle strength to oppose the force of the contracting burn scar and by the inability to understand and cooperate in the treatment process. In addition, the young child tends to form more scar tissue.

These potential problems can be managed with the full participation of the burn team, the child, and the family. Warden and associates (1993) demonstrated that even severe hand burns necessitating partial amputations or those with exposed joints and tendons during the initial acute hospitalization can have functional results when the appropriate principles of care are used.

Factors to consider in splinting include construction, correct fit, application, and adjustment. A pliable, light-weight, low-heat thermoplastic material is desirable. Bulky dressings should be minimized since they interfere with the fit of the splint and compromise alignment. Splints must be checked at least once daily and necessary adjustments made. Pain, numbness, tingling, inflammation, or maceration of good tissue indicates a malfitting or improperly applied splint, which can cause pressure necrosis of burned and unburned areas. Immediate adjustment is mandatory to prevent further damage.

Splints are also used to reduce existing contracture and, therefore, preclude or minimize the need for extensive reconstructive surgery. Children who are developing contractures or scar bands over the volar aspect of the hand, wrist, elbow, posterior knee, or dorsum of the ankle and foot are fitted with conforming splints to oppose contracture formation by producing a softening and flattening effect on the scar band, which then allows increased skin excursion. Frequently, these splints are worn at night only, and the child is encouraged to move actively during the day. As the contracture resolves, the splint is remolded progressively until proper alignment of the part is achieved. The anterior neck is one area where a conforming splint worn at all times except for bath, meals, and exercise can be effective in maintaining ROM and normal contour (Fig. 28-4).

Specific splints for various joints are described in detail by Willis (1970), Pullium (1984), and Richard and Staley (1993). More recent studies describe innovative splint designs. The "T-shirt" splint,

A   B

FIGURE 28–4. *A,* Neck contracture. When conforming pressure is not applied to healing areas of deep dermal burn, unsightly and debilitating ropelike scar bands can form, as illustrated at the anterior neck of this young teenager. *B,* Conforming neck splint. Contouring of the chin angle and neck can be maintained with constant pressure of a conforming splint, as illustrated in this contrasting picture.

named for its appearance, is one method for treating the problem of severe contracture causing rounding of the shoulders, concavity of the chest wall, kyphotic posturing, and decreased shoulder ROM from deep burns of the neck, chest, and axillae (Gilliam et al., 1993). A modified ankle-foot orthosis consisting of a footplate and two supports, one on the medial and one on the lateral aspect of the leg, was described by Bennett and co-workers (1993). Using this design allows the calcaneal region to be free of pressure, decreasing the risk of skin breakdown.

Dynamic splinting is the most effective method of correcting contractures involving the extensor surfaces of the wrist, hand, and posterior elbow. The proximity of the extensor tendons to the burned surface may result in scar adhesions forming around or attaching to the tendon. Dynamic splints that apply elastic tension in opposition to

the contracture but allow controlled resisted motion force excursion of the tendon through the scar formation.

Dynamic orthoses, such as Dynasplint and Ultraflex Systems, have been reported as an additional form of effective splinting in burns (Richard, 1986; Richard et al., 1988). The splints are three-point pressure, spring-loaded orthoses designed to deliver a low-load, prolonged stretch to healing connective tissue. Pediatric sizes are available.

Serial casting may be a successful alternative when low-force dynamic splinting cannot be sized small enough for a child or when patient compliance is unreliable. The goal in serial casting is gradual realignment of the collagen in a parallel and lengthened state by constant circumferential pressure from the cast, which cannot be removed by the patient. When casts are applied well and padded appropriately, there is little risk of pressure areas, because the casts are conforming and do not slip distally. Following serial casting for 7 days, the more traditional methods of treatment (paraffin, massage, ROM exercise, and splinting) are continued to preserve the increased movement. Casts also delay or eliminate the need for surgical correction (Bennett et al., 1989). Serial casting has been shown to be highly effective in increasing ROM of the burned foot (Ridgway et al., 1991) and the burned hand (Harris et al., 1993). The fabrication and use of removable digit casts to improve ROM at the proximal interphalangeal joint have also been described (Torres-Gray et al., 1993).

When optimal positioning is not possible, such as when air-fluidized beds are used, severe fixed ankle and foot deformities may occur over a prolonged time period. The typical deformities include ankle plantar flexion and varus (equinovarus) and forefoot adduction and supination. External fixators have been introduced in burn management. A clinical report by Metzger and co-workers (1993) describes the use of Brooker and Hoffman fixators, which can be used to arrest further deformity but do not allow for correction; and Ilizarov fixators, which allow a multidimensional application of force to achieve anatomically correct positioning (Fig. 28–5). The use of fixators, and the Ilizarov fixator in particular, is superior to splinting because of the propensity for formation of decubiti when rigid splints are used.

Exercise and Activities

The child who has been burned tends to avoid movement, or, at best, moves rigidly and slowly. Planned exercise programs, therefore, are needed to prevent undesirable burn wound healing sequelae.

FIGURE 28–5. Ilizarov external fixator on lower extremity. Gradual shortening of the anterior rods with simultaneous lengthening of the posterior rods results in correction of an equinus deformity by stretching scar tissue and the Achilles tendon.

Although therapists hold primary responsibility for implementation of these programs, optimal physical restoration will largely depend on the combined and concentrated efforts of all team members, the child, and the family.

Many factors influence the therapist's ability to provide adequate exercise for children with burn injuries. Pain, surgical procedures, wound complications, and the child's and the family's adjustment to the injury affect therapy. The therapist's skill in timing the initiation of exercise and in choosing the type of exercise and the timely transferral of care to the child and family are important to the level of function attained and the duration of the rehabilitation program.

Although children recovering from burns share common problems, each patient has unique requirements for physical therapy and needs a customized exercise program. Specific exercises for common problems encountered by burn patients have been published (Nothdurft et al., 1984; Richard & Staley, 1993). Therapists often need to be creative with specific exercises, and written instructions are needed for older children and parents to perform exercise in the absence of the therapist. Hayes-Lundy and associates (1993) performed a pilot study to test the usefulness of a computer-generated exercise program called PTEX to create customized exercise programs for patients. Patients given PTEX programs performed their exercises with an 88% success rate, compared with a 54% success rate for patients given handwritten programs.

The type and intensity of exercise progresses according to the child's recovery status. Goals and type of exercise needed for each stage of recovery are outlined in Table 28–3. During the emergent or resuscitative period, emphasis of treatment is placed on positioning and splinting. However, if the patient is alert, he or she may be able to engage in some movement activities such as bed mobility and positioning of extremities for dressing applications. Exercise is initiated for most patients as soon as adequate signs of burn shock resuscitation have been observed, generally within the first 24 to 72 hours after injury. Escharotomies do not preclude exercise. Exercises that would compromise or dislodge lines and airways are withheld and emphasis is placed on positioning.

As the child makes the transition from the emergent phase to the acute phase of burn rehabilitation, the physical treatment program must also change to meet the patient's needs. The acute phase generally refers to the time period after emergent care through wound coverage, when the foundations of scarring are just beginning to form. Functional impairment is a major threat during this period.

TABLE 28–3. **EXERCISE GOALS FOR EACH STAGE OF RECOVERY**

Stage	Exercise Goals	Methods
Emergent	1. Edema resolution 2. Maintenance of joint mobility 3. Prevention of respiratory complications	Slow, gentle active or active-assistive ROM 2–4 times/day
Acute	1. Stretch healing skin 2. Maintain full joint ROM 3. Preserve coordination of multiple joint movements 4. Promote functional independence 5. Minimize muscular atrophy	ROM exercises, functional activities, ambulation
Postacute/ rehabilitation	1. Increase joint ROM 2. Prevent/correct contracture 3. Strengthen and recondition 4. Maximize functional abilities	ROM/ADL/ambulation programs, incorporating stretching, coordination, strengthening, endurance, and conditioning

Exercises are performed with each isolated joint through appropriate planes of motion. Multiple joint movements are then encouraged, emphasizing gentle sustained stretch for each burned area. Multiple vigorous repetitions of movement should be avoided. Active and active-assistive ROM with terminal stretch aids in maintaining joint mobility and tissue pliability as well as minimizing loss of strength. Many patients will lose ROM if left to do exercises on their own, despite verbal encouragement. This is particularly true with children.

Compared with adults, children exhibit increased pain reactions during exercise, often owing to fear and apprehension. Coordinating administration of pain medications with the nursing staff before exercise sessions greatly enhances the quality of exercise and amount of cooperation offered by the patient. It is also helpful for patient relaxation to initiate the exercise treatment with nonpainful or less painful exercises and gradually progress to the more painful exercises.

Other specific management techniques used for pain control include anesthesia, hypnosis, and behavioral modification. The reinforcement given by way of reward for lack of negative response to pain proved to be a successful management technique (Varni et al., 1980). Behavioral techniques such as desensitization, modeling, operant conditioning, and environmental manipulation have also been used successfully. The importance of pain management cannot be overemphasized. Any safe and effective method should be used.

Play and group activities are fun and allow children increased control. Play is perhaps the best method to elicit desired active movement in young children. A report by Mahaney (1990) describes the loss of a severely burned child's ability to play and outlines the critical importance of play in the development of cognition, affectivity, and social learning (areas related to coping behavior). In addition, im-

plementing music therapy techniques during exercise sessions may provide an organizing structure within which rehabilitative and developmental gains can occur. Use of empathy, empowerment of caregivers, modeling, and coaching techniques encourages a positive working alliance with caregivers and allows for successful transfer of the intervention to the family (Badger et al., 1993).

If pain control, relaxation, and exercise techniques have failed to maintain joint range, ROM exercise performed while the patient is under anesthesia is sometimes recommended to determine the extent of joint restriction and as an adjunct to routine exercise sessions (Nicosia et al., 1979). This is a particularly beneficial procedure when assessing whether the child's fear, apprehension, or manipulative behavior are interfering with achieving the goals of exercise sessions.

After grafting, exercise to the grafted area is discontinued for approximately 5 days to encourage incorporation of the graft into the wound bed. Proper patient positioning is stressed at this time. Exercise is also withheld to joints proximal and distal to the grafted area, which, if exercised, might influence graft stability. Active and active-assistive ROM exercises to all other nongrafted areas are continued. On removal of staples or sutures, if the graft appears stable, exercise to the grafted area can be resumed with approval from the attending physician. It is wise for the therapist to observe dressing changes to identify areas of graft slough and possible tendon exposure.

It is typical that ROM decreases during the immobilization period after grafting. A general theory is that approximately 25% of the motion is lost during the postgraft stage (Artz et al., 1979). However, the patient who maintains essentially normal ROM during the pregrafting phase has a good prognosis to regain ROM. With most patients, full joint motion is expected 7 to 10 days after grafting.

As healing progresses, either spontaneously or after grafting, functional strengthening is introduced into the exercise program. Even if the child has open wounds and bandages, minimal manual resistance by the therapist is begun for initial strengthening. Resistance to isotonic contraction can be applied gently, or the child is asked to maintain a position and then resistance is applied.

The postacute rehabilitative phase begins when the catabolic state reverses and there are few unhealed burn areas. This is the difficult and lengthy phase of wound contracture and hypertrophic scarring in which physical function and appearance can be altered significantly. A child who heals initially with full ROM has the potential to develop severe deformities during the post-acute period as the healed skin matures and hypertrophic scarring develops. Sustained stretching is one of the most effective exercise techniques for lengthening bands of scar tissue and increasing ROM. Active-assistive ROM with the therapist applying mild manual stretching at the extremes of motion is well tolerated. Skin should be stretched to the point of blanching. Holding the stretch for counts of 10 or 15 is recommended at the terminal point of stretch as tolerated. Whenever possible, overall patterns of motion are emphasized since scar tissue may cause profound limitations of motion when multiple joints are involved.

Coordinated movement is generally diminished after burn injury. It is essential that substitution patterns be recognized and altered before they become deeply ingrained as conditioned responses. Coordination exercises are extremely beneficial in eliminating the mechanical robot-like postures and movements frequently characteristic of patients with burns. In children, the application of neurodevelopmental treatment techniques provides a holistic means to address the goal of increased ROM by enhancing postural stability, mobility, and achievement of age-appropriate developmental milestones. By using this approach, Burne and colleagues (1993) have shown that therapeutic technique can be more easily incorporated into the child's home life through parent teaching, focusing on every-day activities, and including the family's goals and lifestyle.

Careful integration of conditioning with all other postacute rehabilitation exercise programs enhances the patient's restoration to a normal lifestyle. When possible, conditioning exercise incorporates activities enjoyable to the child, such as bicycling, dancing, or swimming, and provides the child not only with a sense of physical well-being but also with an opportunity for social interaction.

Ambulation

The ability to move about has a significant impact on the restoration of independence. Children begin ambulation as soon as the physical condition warrants, usually by 48 to 72 hours after injury, when vital signs are stable and fluid resuscitation is complete. With proper precautions and necessary staff participation, children in the burn unit are assisted in ambulation to the limits of their physical endurance. Technical maneuvers and precautions have been developed by Hollowed and associates (1993) that ensure safety during ambulation. Beginning ambulation while the patient is still intubated has proved to be effective in reducing pulmonary complications and has increased the survival rate in patients with acute burns from 88% to 95%. The more involved case may require greater planning. Transferring a child to a tilt table sometimes is the only way to progress the patient to weight bearing.

For nongrafted lower extremity burns, ambulation is initiated once the child is medically stable unless tendons or joint capsules are exposed, severe swelling or cellulitis is present, or the soles of the feet are severely burned. Mild to moderate burns of the feet do not preclude early ambulation. Dressings with extra padding and foam-soled slippers will protect the wounds and aid in reducing the discomfort of bearing weight. To avoid venous stasis in lower extremities and discomfort associated with upright positions, elastic bandages are applied from toe to groin before standing, and full weight bearing is encouraged. A figure-of-eight wrap is used, since this provides an even distribution of pressure and better support for the extremity than do circular wraps.

Assistive devices such as walkers, crutches, and canes are *not* encouraged, and use of a normal gait pattern is emphasized. However, young children frequently show regression in walking, particularly if they had been ambulating only a few weeks before the burn injury. Knowing what the child wants to play with or walk to may be the key to initiating ambulation (Johnson, 1984a). Toys such as hot wheels or tricycles can be great incentives. For the younger or smaller child, a circular walker allows the child to move around independently, but close supervision is needed for safe activity.

When to initiate ambulation after grafting is controversial. A prospective study by Schmitt and associates (1991) indicated a significant reduction (mean of 4.1 days) in length of hospital stay when patients who ambulated on postoperative day 7 were compared with patients who ambulated on postoperative day 11. Results of a study by Kowalske and colleagues (1993) found no difference in graft take or time to complete wound closure following lower extremity skin grafting between early (postoperative day 3/4) and late (postoperative day 7/8/9) ambulators. Increased skin graft loss was, however, seen in patients whose physical conditions prohibited ambulation on the randomly assigned day.

Obviously the patient with a less complicated burn can master the progression of walking with few problems. In fact, Unna's boot, a zinc oxide–calamine gelatin bandage, has been used with small wounds to allow patients to ambulate within 48 hours after grafting (Harnar et al., 1982). Turner and co-workers (1993) reported the efficacy of a modified Linton dressing in promoting wound healing of lower leg burns and continued ambulation.

Pressure Garments and Inserts

Hypertrophic scarring remains a major problem for the recovering patient. The mainstay of treatment is controlled pressure to the involved areas with Coban or Ace bandages and presized or custom-fit elastic garments. Inserts of rubber, foam, or gel materials have been used to improve the response to pressure. The use of pressure for the treatment of hypertrophic scars or keloids and severe contractures became a standard treatment in every burn facility from the early 1970s. Historically, the use of controlled pressure originated and was promoted by the clinical and basic sciences approach developed by the wound healing team of the Shriners Burns Institute at Galveston, Texas (Linares et al., 1993).

The following guidelines on the characteristics of burn treatment can help the therapist select methods of pressure: 1) healing time of the burn, 2) size of the unhealed areas, 3) fragility or condition of the healed skin, 4) location of the burn, and 5) treatment cost (Johnson, 1984b). Briefly, all patients whose burns require 14 to 21 days to heal and who have areas grafted with split-thickness grafts should have prophylactic pressure therapy. Lower extremity burns may require pressure not only to minimize scarring but also to minimize persistent edema and discoloration. Pressure should be applied as early as possible. The type of pressure, however, will depend on the fragility of the newly healed skin and remaining open areas.

Signs that the pressure program has been successful can be seen as early as 24 to 48 hours after the initial application. Immediately after the removal of the garment, evidence of clinically significant pressure includes blanching of scar tissue, flattening of the scar, increased softness, decreased edema, minimal blistering, and no tingling or numbness. If any of these effects are not observed, the therapist should consider the following reasons: 1) fit of garment—if the patient has gained or lost over 10 pounds, this may be enough to decrease the pressure garment's effectiveness; and 2) condition of a garment—the wear life of pressure garments for the average patient is 3 months. If the garment loses its stretch and does not cause blanching of the scar, it has lost its effectiveness and new garments must be made.

When isolated areas of hypertrophy remain, sufficient pressure has not been applied. Areas where this commonly occurs include the sternum, face, volar aspect of the hand, angle of the mandible, web spaces, and across the flexor surfaces of the joint. Pressure garments frequently need to be supplemented by inserts in these areas to exert the needed pressure (Fig. 28–6). Characteristics to be considered in choosing the composition of the insert include its texture, flexibility, compressibility, and ability to conform. For effectiveness, an insert

FIGURE 28–6. Custom-fit pressure garments. Extra pressure is often needed to further enhance effectiveness of the garments as illustrated by the silicone face pad and/or the elastic band and application of conforming hand splints with elastic wraps over elastic gloves.

must be worn for the same amount of time as the pressure garment (23 hours per day).

A thorough knowledge of properties of all available inserts is required to provide an effective pressure program. No single material suffices for all the situations in which an insert is indicated. Information regarding the qualities of various materials for pressure inserts is described by Alston and associates (1981), Perkins and colleagues (1987), and Ainsworth and co-workers (1993). Many patients and therapists report difficulties when using silicone or other types of inserts under garments. The most common problems include irritation of skin from the pad, limited joint motion, sweating, annoying odor, and movement of the insert. One resourceful method used to apply a silicone elastomer pad beneath a pressure garment was described by Van den Kerckhove and colleagues (1991). Elastomer is molded on the patient between layers of Tubi-Grip. Another system for making a custom pocket has been described by Taylor (1993). Extra material in the form of a pocket can be stitched into the external vascular support to keep an insert from shifting its position and provide a soft, breathable, contact layer to the skin.

There appears to be consensus in the literature that silicone pads are especially effective in diminishing the thickness of the scar. Some authors suggest that this happens only in the body areas where high pressure was maintained (Van den Kerckhove et al., 1991). Others have reported that silicone products induce a positive effect on burn scars without pressure (Bowering et al., 1992). Good results can be obtained even with old scars (Quin, 1987; Van den Kerckhove et al., 1991).

Caution and close monitoring of pressure garments is essential particularly when used in the young growing child. Two studies suggest serious complications in children with head and neck burns. Fricke and colleagues (1992) demonstrated changes in growth direction of the mandible and maxilla after consistent application of the total face mask. In addition, Chester and associates (1993) claim that the most common cause of obstructive sleep apnea is excessive pressure on the mandible by compression garments, particularly chin straps.

Compliance with wearing correctly applied pressure garments for effective scar control is crucial for burn survivors. External pressure support is prescribed to be used 23 hours a day until the remodeling phase of healing is complete. Spurr and Shakespeare (1990) list the difficulties that arise with a pressure garment program. Pressure garment therapy is long lasting, inconvenient for patients, and relatively expensive. There is no guarantee that the child and parents will comply with the advice given

to wear the garments. One study of adult patient compliance with pressure therapy determined that total compliance was less than 50% (Greenspan et al., 1993). Factors affecting compliance included patient's reported perception of the burn and garment, understanding of the pressure program and its effect, psychosocial influences, garment-specific factors, and the level of functional independence related to the burn and garment use. The identification of factors that affect garment use is therefore critical in formulating strategies to improve the compliance of burn survivors.

An example of garment design modification to enhance compliance for children who wear diapers has been reported (Schwartz et al., 1993). Pediatric patients in diapers are difficult to fit with external vascular support garments. Soft diapers under a leotard decrease the amount of compression applied to buttock scars. Although the healing wound, donor site, or graft remains active, the scar tissue remains painful or pruritic whenever the garment is removed. If the infant excoriates the scars when the garment is off, the scars become thicker and more painful. The discomfort of frequent diaper changes stresses parents, contributing to poor compliance with garment application. A three-piece leotard was designed with detachable legs and an open crotch. The "brief" portion of the garment can be replaced without removing the stocking portions, and the open crotch allows ready diaper change without removing any portion of the garment. Repetitive shearing over fragile epithelium is minimized, and caregiver participation is enhanced, with subsequent optimal cosmetic and functional outcomes for the toddler.

There is some indication that the introduction of colored pressure garments may contribute to better compliance. A study by Thompson et al. (1992) suggested that colored garments may lead to social acceptance of the patient, which in turn could increase the child's self-esteem.

As scar tissue approaches maturity, the hyperemia fades and the scar flattens and becomes more pliable and soft. When these qualities persist for several weeks after removal of the pressure garments, the scar tissue is mature, and the garments and inserts may then be discontinued.

Other Modalities

Numerous modalities, each having a specific physiologic effect, are available in rehabilitation. Only the more commonly accepted modalities that have proved effective for the management of problems existing in the burn population will be addressed. These are paraffin, ultrasound, continuous passive motion, and fluidotherapy.

The combination of paraffin with sustained stretch usually begins late in the acute phase of rehabilitation after major healing has occurred, and it is generally continued throughout the patient's rehabilitation. The use of paraffin is particularly indicated when a painful and contracting scar limits joint ROM. The superficial heat and lubrication reduce scar pain and improve scar extensibility (Head & Helm, 1977; Nothdurft et al., 1984). The paraffin mixture is used when it reaches a temperature of 46°C to 48°C or when a light skim covers the top of the mixture. Caution is suggested for newly healed scar tissue, which will blister easily if the standard paraffin bath temperature is used. Pouring or patting of the paraffin is done after the patient is positioned with the affected part in a sustained maximum stretch. The treatment time is 20 to 30 minutes. Patients report decreased joint pain, and objective measurements show a 5 to 10° increase in ROM after paraffin treatment. Claims that the results last up to 4 hours have been documented (Head & Helm, 1977).

Application of topical ultrasound directly to burn scars produces a rise in deep tissue temperature that is reported to increase extensibility of collagen and decrease pain associated with stretching (Belenger et al., 1969; Rozanova, 1979; Wright & Haase, 1971). However, a randomized blinded study by Ward and associates (1993) compared results of patients who received standard burn physical therapy and topical ultrasound with patients who received standard care alone. Statistical analysis revealed no differences in ROM or perceived pain between the two groups. Furthermore, there was no discernible trend toward subjective or objective improvements with ultrasound treatment.

Continuous passive motion has been shown to be beneficial in the rehabilitation of the thermally injured patient (Covey, 1988). This modality is limited to older children and adolescents, since infant and pediatric-sized units are yet to be developed. In addition to the general effects of continuous passive motion (including delivery of a specific arc of motion at a specific speed and constant control of rate and degree of motion, which fosters patient relaxation and increased ROM), the autorange or continuous passive motion unit can be adjusted to maintain the contractured extremity at the end of its available range for a regulated amount of time. Continuous passive motion should be used as an adjunct and not as a replacement for the traditional manual therapy techniques.

The fluidotherapy unit can be considered when seeking a thermotherapeutic agent to decrease pain or increase ROM in a body part, particularly a foot or a hand (Nothdurft et al., 1984). This high-intensity superficial heat modality consists of a dry whirlpool of finely divided solid particles suspended in a heated air stream. The use of fluidotherapy with burns is not well documented. The burn patient's skin durability and sensation must be evaluated before submersion in the unit. Periodic monitoring of the patient's skin responses while undergoing each treatment is imperative. The combination of the dry heat with the massaging solid particles, the allowance for active exercise while undergoing each treatment, and the fact that this unit can be used in the presence of open wounds (with protection of thin plastic or rubber gloves) are advantages of this modality for the management of distal extremity problems in the older child or adolescent patient.

Family Education

It is crucial that the child's family understand the daily care that will be required at home. There may be extensive technical and medical information for parents to absorb, and it is best if the family begins early in the child's hospitalization to be instructed in all aspects of care and to ask questions, discuss treatments, and watch demonstrations. Some centers have found it helpful to create manuals to be reviewed with family members before discharge (Bochke, 1993; Reed & Heinle et al., 1993). In this way parents have a chance to absorb written material and to practice the child's care under supervision of the health care providers before the discharge actually takes place. Thus, when they arrive home with the child, they will feel more confident about their ability to carry out the required therapy. Special patient and family problems such as illiteracy, low learning levels, foreign languages, and deafness have also been addressed with customized guides, including pictorial guides, laminated flipcharts, card file system, audio tapes, video tapes, and photographic guides (Walling et al., 1993).

Indirect Services

Indirect services such as management, supervision, quality assurance, consultation, and research are also important components of the physical therapist's role in burn care (as have been described for occupational therapists by Kohlman-McChonny et al., 1985). Management is concerned with the delivery of effective care in a cost-efficient manner. The quality and appropriateness of physical therapy services are monitored through the use of quality assurance programs, including participation in accreditation procedures. Technologic advances in the treatment of burn injuries offer ongoing opportunities for collaborative research to improve the quality of care of the child with burn injuries.

Outpatient Therapy and Follow-Up

Perhaps the most difficult problem that a therapist faces during home care is the tendency for the child to manipulate his or her parents and thereby fail to carry out the prescribed home programs. This is particularly true if the parents feel guilty about the burn accident. Some children take advantage of feelings of guilt or sympathy and will resist therapy at home, even if they were cooperative while in the hospital. In conjunction with this, some parents also perceive their child to have more problems than the child or his or her teacher reports. Results of a study by Meyer and associates (1993) suggest that troubled parents may overestimate the difficulties of their child. Shelby and associates (1993) have identified additional family factors. Parents of children who sustained burns reported more depression or anxiety than spouses of adults who were burned. Higher somatic symptom reporting was associated with fewer social resources, higher anxiety, and depression. Lower somatic symptoms were seen in parents reporting high hardiness, esteem, and perceived family social support.

Most children, therefore, continue to require daily therapy from professionals when they make the transition into postacute rehabilitation, although professional therapy should serve a secondary role. A study by Housinger and co-workers (1992) clearly demonstrated that pediatric outpatient rehabilitation can only be expected to succeed in the presence of dedicated efforts by parents. Duration of sessions varies according to involvement and the child's tolerance. Moderate to major burns require anywhere from 1 to 5 hours of treatment per day, including rest periods. As the child demonstrates increased independence and goals are achieved, sessions are reduced to 2 to 3 times a week and eventually to weekly rechecks. Although therapy is demanding and crucial during this time period, children should also be allowed time for other activities to make the transition to a normal lifestyle. Reybons (1992) stresses that leisure and recreation activities provide an opportunity for burn survivors to re-establish control over leisure time.

After discharge from the burn unit, settings for postacute rehabilitation are quite variable. In acute hospitals, the patient may continue to be seen in outpatient therapy settings. Burn centers sometimes transfer daily therapy care of children who travel from great distances to a community hospital and then follow the patient periodically in an outpatient burn clinic. Some burn centers have rehabilitation beds or "step down units" that continue medical care until the patient is better able to handle the home situation. Other centers have transitional units, in which children and their families assume responsibility for care in a protective environment (Daugherty et al., 1993). Children with complicated injuries, amputations, large body surface area burns, or neurologic involvement may need several months in a designated rehabilitation center for proper care.

In most cases it is desirable for the child to return to the burn facility for follow-up outpatient clinic visits. Frequent checkups will allow the burn team to monitor the child's progress, see if the program is being followed, and alter the treatments when necessary. The checkups also enable the staff to detect any problems that may develop and to change the therapy program as necessary. As healing occurs, many questions regarding skin care will arise during therapy sessions and at outpatient clinic follow-up visits.

Some of the more common problems include skin breakdown, maceration, dryness, itch, sun intolerance, and impaired thermoregulation. Other issues addressed at clinic visits include physical activity level, continued use and fit of pressure garments and splints, maturation of scars, implementation of cosmetics use, and plan for further surgical procedures. If the family does not live near the primary care facility, local follow-up care can be arranged. In all cases, however, it is important that family members be encouraged to contact the hospital whenever they have concerns or questions. With open communication, the development of subsequent problems can be minimized.

CHRONIC FUNCTIONAL LIMITATIONS

Persistent cutaneous inflexibility may result in tightening of underlying muscles, tendons, ligaments, joint capsule, fascia, and bone. Chronic limitation of motion, therefore, may continue to affect the physical ability of a child and become more noticeable with growth. Reconstructive procedures are often required after growth spurts and until bony growth is complete (Dado & Angelats, 1990). Aesthetically pleasing and good functional results may therefore be more difficult to achieve in children compared with adults. The child will require further intervention by the physical therapist after each reconstructive procedure for management of the new grafts.

Typical Disabilities Identified

In an article by Kraemer and colleagues (1988), the incidence of surgical release of contractures was 4 times higher in children than in adults, even though burn wound size was similar in both populations. Areas associated with the highest incidence of contracture formation were the hand and the central body regions (head, neck, and axilla). Central body region contractures, plus contractures at sites that had been previously fascially excised, had the poorest outcome after surgical reconstruction. The review also concluded that reconstructive surgery should be delayed, when possible, until the burn scars have matured (consistent with findings by Parks and associates [1978], Huang and colleagues [1978], and Alexander and co-workers [1981]). However, the study by Kraemer and colleagues (1988) also suggests that early contracture release can be successfully performed in patients with severe contractures that significantly limit function.

The potential problems of each body area are listed in Table 28–4. Surgical and rehabilitative goals for correction of chronic problems vary according to the age and stated needs of each child. Consideration of length, sensibility, mobility, stability, strength, and, to a lesser extent, appearance dictate the reconstructive needs (Kurtzman & Stern, 1990). The emphasis on function versus appearance is different for children of each age group.

One of the more challenging areas requiring reconstruction after burn injury is the neck. High rates of contracture recurrence have also been documented. A study of pediatric burn patients by Waymack (1986) revealed recurrence rates of 81% after Z-plasty releases and of 62% with split-thickness skin grafts. However, the use of a neck hyperextension splint for over 1 year after skin grafting decreased the recurrence rate to 17%. Perineal contractures are also a frequent problem in the pediatric population. Pisarski and co-workers (1993) list several procedures for correction but report a high recurrence rate (46%), even with postoperative pressure garments, splints, and exercise.

One form of reconstructive procedure that has been developed and refined in the past decade is that of scalp tissue expansion for the treatment of burn alopecia (scalp baldness). The procedure is

TABLE 28–4. POTENTIAL IMPAIRMENTS

Body Area	Impairment
Face	Facial disfigurement (contractures of eyelids, nose, mouth, ears, and adjacent facial skin)
	Inability to close eyes
	Loss of facial expression
	Teeth malalignment
	Drooling and inability to close lips
Neck	Lower lip eversion
	Loss of normal cervical spine ROM
	Limited visual fields
	Difficulties in anesthesia
Trunk	Protraction of shoulders
	Kyphosis
	Functional scoliosis
	Decreased respiratory function
	Breast entrapment
	Peroneal banding
Axilla	Type 1: either anterior or posterior contracture
	Type 2: anterior and posterior contracture with sparing of dome
	Type 3: anterior and posterior contracture and axillary dome
Hands	Metacarpophalangeal extension deformities
	Wrist extension deformities
	Proximal interphalangeal flexion deformities
	Interdigital web contractures
	Clawing of fourth and fifth digits
	Thumb contractures (adduction > opposition > flexion and extension)
Arms and legs	Antecubital banding and flexion
	Posterior popliteal banding
	Anterior hip banding and flexion
	Medial and lateral malleolar scarring
Foot and ankle	Hyperextension of metatarsophalangeal joints
	Equinovarus
	Cavus foot
	Rockerbottom deformity

illustrated in Figure 28–7. Normal hair-bearing scalp skin is stretched by gradual expansion with saline solution of a balloon placed under the skin. The balloon is removed, and the extra hair-bearing skin is attached as a flap to the area of excised alopecia skin. Choucair and Donelan (1993) report good results in the majority of patients with minimal complications to the point that a significant number of patients are now undergoing repeat expansion of previously expanded hair-bearing scalp.

In one study the health care worker's perception of burn scars was compared with that of the patient (Prothman et al., 1993). Of scar variables, including color, texture, dryness, lack of hair, lack of stretch, wrinkles, height, and mesh appearance, only inter-rater scores for vascularity correlated positively with patient scores for scar appearance. Patients most often stated that nothing bothered them about the scar. However, when problems were reported,

FIGURE 28–7. Scalp tissue expander series. *A,* Deep dermal burns of the scalp leave areas of alopecia, as shown in this picture of a young girl. Excision and primary closure is impossible for such a large area. *B,* Gradual expansion of normal hair-bearing skin is achieved with insertion of tissue expanders placed under the skin and expanded over a period of weeks or months with injections of saline solution. *C,* An excellent cosmetic result, after removal of the expanders and scarred scalp tissue and flap replacement with the expanded hair-bearing scalp skin.

the scar variables that were most unattractive to the patient were often different from those that bothered the staff. This must be considered when planning reconstructive surgery.

Older children appear to have a much more difficult time accepting the residual scar. When faced with the burden of coping with disfigurement resulting from a burn injury, the adolescent's sense of self-esteem may be diminished. Providing adolescents the opportunity to learn makeup techniques that lessen the impact of their scars is an effective intervention for enhancing self-perception and

their perception of how others view them. This was demonstrated in a study of 115 patients attending reconstructive makeup clinics (Beattie et al., 1993).

Assessment of Performance in Life Roles

Several factors are to be considered in the child's return to school and potential for future employment. These include 1) preinjury status, 2) changes in physical ability resulting from the burn injury, 3) disfigurement, and 4) the need for long-term and periodic treatment. Physical therapists, as part of the burn team, are often involved in the return-to-school process, both in assessment of the child's abilities (including treatment suggestions for school therapists or physical education specialist) and in preparing the teachers and students for the child's new abilities and needs (by means of individualized videotapes and, when necessary, on-site school visits). Reybons (1992) has summarized the problems a burn survivor may experience in community reintegration as follows:

- Architectural barriers: stairs, ramps, escalators, doors
- Physical barriers: decreased ROM, contractures, decreased fine motor skills, decreased endurance, loss of hands
- Social barriers: facial disfigurement, feelings of "invasion of privacy," decreased initiation of contact with strangers

Over the long term, most patients do well and report a minimal impact of the burn injury in their lives and a satisfactory quality of life (Tarnowski et al., 1989). A 5-year study of physical and psychological outcome after burns (Sheffield et al., 1988) resulted in the following significant findings:

1. Ten to 15% of patients have postburn courses complicated by psychiatric problems, noncompliance, and limited ROM.

2. Patients who are more physically or psychologically impaired, or both, require longer follow-up treatment.

3. Noncompliant patients believe that the impact of the event on their lives is greater than others and report diminished quality of life.

A study reported by Blakeney and associates (1993) examined the psychological adjustment of a group of children who survived the most severe burn injuries and the impact of such injury on the families. The conclusions were that children with burns affecting more than 80% total body surface area develop positive feelings about themselves and appear no more troubled than a comparable group of children without burns. One of these children is pictured in Figure 28–8. The impact on the families is significant, however, and must be considered of consequence in the rehabilitation of the child.

❙ SUMMARY

Physical therapy for children with burns should begin at the time of injury and may extend for several years beyond the initial hospitalization. In the physical treatment of burns there is no single

FIGURE 28–8. Functional outcomes. Rehabilitated 9-year-old child after severe burns and triple-extremity amputations, independently riding her bicycle with the aid of a left myoelectric hand, a right below-knee prosthesis and a left above-knee prosthesis.

best treatment method. As each child presents with unique problems, specific treatment techniques are incorporated into an individualized rehabilitation program developed by the team, the child, and the family. The recovery process is long and often complicated, but successful rehabilitation, based on a comprehensive psychological, social, and physical view of the child is extremely gratifying.

References

Achauer, BM, & Martinez, SE. Burn wound pathophysiology and care. Critical Care Clinics, 1(1):47–58, 1985.

Ainsworth, P, Blache, C, Dyess, DL, & Luterman, A. Silipos gel, a new and improved gel insert for treatment of hypertrophic scarring. Paper presented at the meeting of the American Burn Association, Cincinnati, March 1993.

Alexander, JW, MacMillan, BG, & Martel, L. Surgical correction of postburn flexion contractures of the fingers in children. Plastic and Reconstructive Surgery, 68:218–224, 1981.

Alexander, J, Fakhry, S, Smith, D, Meyer, AA, & Peterson, HD. Regional and institutional variation in burn care. Paper presented at the meeting of the American Burn Association, Cincinnati, March 1993.

Alston, DW, Kozerefski, P, Quan, PE, & Luterman, A. Materials for pressure inserts in the control of hypertrophic scar tissue. Journal of Burn Care and Rehabilitation, 1:40–43, 1981.

Artz, C, Moncrief, J, & Pruitt, B (Eds.). Burns: A Team Approach. Philadelphia: WB Saunders, 1979

Badger, K, Gaboury, T, & Warden, GD. A collaborative effort: Music therapy and occupational/physical therapy in pediatric burn rehabilitation. Poster presented at the meeting of the American Burn Association, Cincinnati, March 1993.

Baron, P, & Herndon, DN. Chronic propranolol administration safely decreases cardiac work and anxiety in massively burned pediatric patients. Paper presented at the meeting of the American Burn Association, Cincinnati, March 1993.

Bayley, EW. Wound healing in the patient with burns. Nursing Clinics of North America, 25(1):205–222, 1990.

Beattie, DM, Chedekel, DS, & Krawczyk, T. Utilization of a reconstructive makeup clinic for self-image enhancement in burned adolescents. Paper presented at the meeting of the American Burn Association, Cincinnati, March 1993.

Belenger, M, Vanderelst, E, & Toussaint, JP. New contributions to treatment of localized burns of the hand. Annales de Chirurgie Plastique, 9:199, 1969.

Bennett, GB, Helm, P, Purdue, GF, & Hunt, JL. Serial casting: A method for treating burn contractures. Journal of Burn Care and Rehabilitation, 10:543–545, 1989.

Bennett, MB, Epp, J, Boaz, M, Mani, M, & Varghese, G. An alternate to traditional ankle foot orthoses. Poster presented at the meeting of the American Burn Association, Cincinnati, March 1993.

Blakeney, P, Meyer, W, Moore, P, Murphy, L, Robson, M, & Herndon, D. Psychosocial sequelae of pediatric burns involving 80% or greater total body surface area. Paper presented at the meeting of the American Burn Association, Cincinnati, March 1993.

Bochke, I, Frauenfeld, A, Hartlieb, D, Zwicker, M, & Inkson, T. Patient and family education in burn care: Development of a series of teaching books by a multidisciplinary team. Poster presented at the meeting of the American Burn Association, Cincinnati, March 1993.

Boucher, G, Drzewiecki, A, & Schnurr, RG. Familial stress factors related to childhood burns. Paper presented at the meeting of the American Burn Association, Cincinnati, March 1993.

Bowering, KD, Davey, RB, & Wallis, KA. The use of contact media in a burn scar management program. Video produced by the Adelaide Children's Hospital Educational Resource Center, Adelaide, Australia, 1992.

Bull, JP, & Squire, JR. A study of mortality in a burn unit: Standards for the evaluation of alternative methods of treatment. Annals of Surgery, 130(2):160, 1949.

Burne, BA, Hackencamp, TB, Pfabe-Wiggans, S, & Sprecht, D. The application of neurodevelopmental treatment in pediatric burns. Poster presented at the meeting of the American Burn Association, Cincinnati, March 1993.

Carvajal, HF. Burns in children and adolescents: Initial management as the first step in successful rehabilitation. Pediatrician, 17:237–243, 1990.

Chester, CH, Candlish, S, & Zuker, RM. Prevention of obstructive sleep apnea in children with burns of the head and neck. Paper presented at the meeting of the American Burn Association, Cincinnati, March 1993.

Choucair, RJ, & Donelan, MB. Secondary tissue expansion in the treatment of burn alopecia. Paper presented at the meeting of the American Burn Association, Cincinnati, March 1993.

Clarke, HM, Wittpenn, GP, McLeod, AME, Candlish, SE, Guernsey, CJ, Weleff, DK, & Zuker, RM. Acute management of pediatric hand burns. Hand Clinics, 6:221–232, 1990.

Clugston, PA, Snelling, CFT, Macdonald, IB, Maledy, HL, Boyle, JC, Germann, E, Courtemanche, AD, Wirtz, P, Fitzpatrick, DJ, Kester, DA, Foley, B, Warren, RJ, & Carr, NJ. Cultured epithelial autografts: Three years of clinical experience with eighteen patients. Journal of Burn Care and Rehabilitation, 12:533–539, 1991.

Collins, WF, Burns, RO, & Johns, TR. Common neuromuscular disorders and injuries to the peripheral and cranial nerves and spinal cord. Archives of Neurology, 36:771–781, 1979.

Covey, M. Application of CPM devices with burn patients.

Journal of Burn Care and Rehabilitation, 9:496–497, 1988.

Dado, DV, & Angelats, J. Management of burns of the hands in children. Hand Clinics, 6:711–721, 1990.

Daugherty, MB, DeSerna, C, Barthel, P, & Warden, GD. Moving patients and families toward independence: Establishing a transitional unit. Poster presented at the meeting of the American Burn Association, Cincinnati, March 1993.

Deitch, EA, Wheelaham, TM, Rose, MP, Clotier, J, & Coltes, J. Hypertrophic burn scars: Analysis of variables. Journal of Trauma, 23:895–898, 1983.

Desai, MH, Mlakar, JM, & McCauley, RL, Abdullah, KM, Rutan, R, Hall-Waymack, J, Robson, M, & Horndon, D. Lack of long-term durability of cultured keratinocyte burn-wound coverage: A case report. Journal of Burn Care and Rehabilitation, 12:540–545, 1991.

Dimick, AR. Pathophysiology. In Fisher, SV & Helm, PA (Eds.), Comprehensive Rehabilitation of Burns. Baltimore: Williams & Wilkins, 1984, pp. 16–27.

Doane, CB. Children with severe burns. In Pratt, PN, & Allen, AS (Eds.), Occupational Therapy for Children. St. Louis: CV Mosby, 1989, pp. 524–534.

Economou, TP, Kealey, GP, Lewis, RW, III, & Rosenquist, MD. An experimental study to determine the effects of dermagraft on skin graft viability in the presence of bacterial wound contamination. Paper presented at the meeting of the American Burn Association, Cincinnati, March 1993.

Egan, M. Cultured skin grafts: Preserving lives, challenging therapists. OT Week, July 23, 1992, pp. 12–15.

Evans, EB. Orthopedic measures in the treatment of severe burns. Journal of Bone and Joint Surgery (American), 48:643, 1966.

Feller, I. Prevention of burns in 1 and 2 year olds. NBIE Newsletter vol. 1, No. 2, 1980.

Feller, I. Burn epidemiology: Focus on youngsters and the aged. Journal of Burn Care and Rehabilitation, 3:285, 1982.

Feller, I, & Jones, CA. Nursing the Burned Patient. Ann Arbor, MI: Institute for Burn Medicine, 1974, p. 5.

Feller, I, & Jones, CA. Introduction: Statement of the problem. In Fisher, SV, & Helm, PA (Eds.), Comprehensive Rehabilitation of Burns. Baltimore: Williams & Wilkins, 1984, pp. 1–8.

Fricke, N, Dutcher, K, Omnell, L, Engrav, L, & Hollender, L. Effects of pressure garment wear on facial and dental development. Paper presented at the meeting of the American Burn Association, Salt Lake City, April 1992.

Ghahary, A, Shen, YJ, Liu, G, & Tredget, EE. Increased expression of fibronectin mRNA in human hypertrophic scar tissues and its regulation by interferon-2b. Paper presented at the meeting of the American Burn Association, Cincinnati, March 1993.

Gilliam, KS, Hatler, B, Adams, S, & Helm, P. T-shirt splint for prevention of burn scar contracture of the neck, chest, and axillas. Poster presented at the meeting of the American Burn Association, Cincinnati, March 1993.

Gilpin, DA, Herndon, DN, Rutan, RL, & Barrow, RE. Recombinant human growth hormone accelerates wound healing in children with large cutaneous burns. Paper presented at the meeting of the American Burn Association, Cincinnati, March 1993.

Green, A. Epidemiology of burns in childhood. Burns, 10:368–371, 1984.

Greenspan, B, Johnson, J, Gorga, D, Goodwin, CW, & Nagler, W. Compliance with pressure garment use in burn survivors. Paper presented at the meeting of the American Burn Association, Cincinnati, March 1993.

Harnar, T, Engrav, L, Marvin J, Heimbach, D, Cain, V, & Johnson, C. Dr. Paul Unna's boot and early ambulation after skin grafting the leg. Journal of Plastic and Reconstructive Surgery, 69:359–360, 1982.

Harris, LD, Hatler, B, Adams, S, Gilliam, KS, & Helm, P. Serial casting and its efficacy in the treatment of the burned hand. Paper presented at the meeting of the American Burn Association, Cincinnati, March 1993.

Hartford, CE. Surgical management. In Fisher, SV, & Helm, PA (Eds.), Comprehensive Rehabilitation of Burns. Baltimore: Williams & Wilkins, 1984, pp. 28–63.

Hayes-Lundy, C, Ward, S, Mills, P, & Saffle, J. Use of computer-generated exercise programs to augment therapy programs. Poster presented at the meeting of the American Burn Association, Cincinnati, March 1993.

Head, MD. Wound and skin care. In Fisher, SV, & Helm, PA (Eds.), Comprehensive Rehabilitation of Burns. Baltimore: Williams & Wilkins, 1984, pp. 148–176.

Head, MD, & Helm, PA. Paraffin and sustained stretching in the treatment of burn contracture. Burns, 4:136–139, 1977.

Heimbach, DM. Early burn excision and grafting. Surgical Clinics of North America, 67:93, 1987.

Helm, PA. Neuromuscular considerations. In Fisher, SV, & Helm, PA (Eds.), Comprehensive Rehabilitation of Burns. Baltimore: Williams & Wilkins, 1984, pp. 235–241.

Helm, PA, Johnson, ER, & Carlton, AM. Peripheral neurological problems in the acute burn patient. Burns, 3:123–125, 1977.

Henderson, B, Koepke, GH, & Feller, I. Peripheral polyneuropathy among patients with burns. Archives of Physical Medicine and Rehabilitation, 52:149–151, 1971.

Herndon, DN, Barrow, RE, Kunkel, KR, Broemeling, L, & Rutan, RL. Effects of recombinant human growth hormone on donor-site healing in severely burned children. Annals of Surgery, 212:424–429, 1990.

Herndon, DN, & Rutan, RL. Have we improved burn care? In Carlson, RW, & Reines, HD (Eds.), Critical Care State of the Art (Vol. 13). Anaheim, CA: Society of Critical Care Medicine, 1992a, pp. 389–406.

Herndon, DN, & Rutan, RL. Use of dermal templates and cultured cells for permanent skin replacement. Wounds, 4(2):50–53, 1992b.

Hollowed, KA, Gunde, MA, Lewis, MS, & Jordon, MH. Ambulation of intubated burn patients. Poster presented at the meeting of the American Burn Association, Cincinnati, March 1993.

Housinger, T, Morress, C, Dinkler, T, & Warden, GD. Outpatient therapy: Its efficacy in pediatric burns. Paper presented at the meeting of the American Burn Association, Salt Lake City, April 1992.

Howell, JW. Posthospitalization care. In DiGregorio, VR (Ed.), Rehabilitation of the Burn Patient. New York: Churchill Livingstone, 1984, pp. 151–172.

Huang, TT, Blackwell, SJ, & Lewis, SR. Ten years' experience in managing patients with burn contractures of axilla, elbow, wrist, and knee joints. Plastic and Reconstructive Surgery, 61:70–76, 1978.

Hunt, JL. Electrical injuries. In Fisher, SV, & Helm, PA (Eds.), Comprehensive Rehabilitation of Burns. Baltimore: Williams & Wilkins, 1984, pp. 249–266.

Johnson, CL. Ambulating patients after lower extremity grafting. Journal of Burn Care and Rehabilitation, 5:114–115, 1984a.

Johnson, CL. Physical therapists as scar modifiers. Physical Therapy, 64(9):1381–1387, 1984b.

Kohlman-McGourty, L, Givens, A, & Buddingh-Fader, P. Roles and functions of occupational therapy in burn care delivery. American Journal of Occupational Therapy, 39:791–794, 1985.

Kowalske, K, Purdue, G, Hunt, J, & Helm, P. Early ambulation following skin grafting of lower extremity burns: A randomized controlled trial. Paper presented at the meeting of the American Burn Association, Cincinnati, March 1993.

Kramer, MD, Jones, T, & Deitch, EA. Burn contractures: Inci-

dence, predisposing factors, and results of surgical therapy. Journal of Burn Care and Rehabilitation, 9:261–265, 1988.

Kurtzman, LC, & Stern, PJ. Upper extremity burn contractures. Hand Clinics, 6:261–279, 1990.

Larson, DL, Abston, S, Willis, B, Linares, HA, Dobrkovsky, M, Evans, EB, & Lewis, SR. Contracture and scar formation in the burn patient. Clinics in Plastic Surgery, 1:653, 1974.

Larson, DL, Huang, T, Dobrkovsky, M, Bauer, PS, & Parks, DH. Prevention and treatment of scar contracture. In Artz, CP, Moncrief, JA, Pruitt, B (Eds.), Burns: A Team Approach. Philadelphia: WB Saunders, 1979, pp. 466–491.

Linares, HA, Kischer, CW, Dobrkovsky, M, & Larson, DL. On the origin of the hypertrophic scar. Journal of Trauma, 13:70–75, 1973.

Linares, HA, Larson, DL, & Willis-Galstaum, BA. Historical notes on the use of pressure in the treatment of hypertrophic scars or keloids. Burns, 10:17–21, 1993.

Lund, CC, & Browder, NC. The estimation of areas of burns. Surgery, Gynecology and Obstetrics, 79:352, 1944.

Mahaney, NB. Restoration of play in a severely burned three-year-old child. Journal of Burn Care and Rehabilitation, 11:57–63, 1990.

Metzger, DJ, Cioffi, WG, Martin, S, McManus, WF, & Pruitt, BA. Ilizarov technique in the management of joint deformity in thermally injured patients. Paper presented at the meeting of the American Burn Association, Cincinnati, March 1993.

Meyer, W, Blakeney, P, Moore, P, Murphy, L, Robson, M, & Herndon, D. Parental well-being and behavioral adjustment of pediatric burn patients. Paper presented at the meeting of the American Burn Association, Cincinnati, March 1993.

Mikhail, NJ. Acute burn care: An update. Journal of Emergency Nursing, 14:1, 1988.

Nedelec, B, Shen, YJ, Ghahary, A, Scott, P, & Tredget, EE. Inhibition of wound contraction in hypertrophic scar fibroblasts by interferon alpha-2b. Paper presented at the meeting of the American Burn Association, Cincinnati, March 1993.

Nicosia, J, Stein, E, & Stein, J. The advantages of physiotherapy for burn patients under anaesthesia. Burns, 6:202–204, 1979.

Nothdurft, D, Smith, PS, & LeMaster, JE. Exercise and treatment modalities. In Fisher, SV, & Helm, PA (Eds.), Comprehensive Rehabilitation of Burns. Baltimore: Williams & Wilkins, 1984, pp. 96–147.

Parks, DH, Bauer, PS, & Larson, DL. Late problems in burns. Clinics in Plastic Surgery, 4:547, 1977.

Parks, DH, Evans, EB, & Larson, DL. Prevention and correction of deformity after severe burns. Surgical Clinics of North America, 58:1279–1289, 1978.

Perkins, K, Davey, RB, & Wallis, K. Current materials and techniques used in a burn scar management program. Burns, 13:406–410, 1987.

Pisarski, GP, Greenhalgh, DG, & Warden, GD. The management of perineal contractures in the pediatric burn patient. Paper presented at the meeting of the American Burn Association, Cincinnati, March 1993.

Prothman, J, Engrav, L, & Cain, V. Evaluating appearance of burn scars: Patient vs. health care worker perceptions. Paper presented at the meeting of the American Burn Association, Cincinnati, March 1993.

Puddicombe, BE, & Nardone, MA. Rehabilitation of the burned hand. Hand Clinics, 6:281–292, 1990.

Pullium, GF. Splinting and positioning. In Fisher, SV, & Helm, PA (Eds.), Comprehensive Rehabilitation of Burns. Baltimore: Williams & Wilkins, 1984, pp 64–95.

Quin, KJ. Silicone gel in scar treatment. Burns, 13:133–140, 1987.

Reed, L, & Heinle, J. Meeting the challenge of education for a diversified patient population in a burn treatment center. Design of 2 patient handbooks. Poster presented at the meeting of the American Burn Association, Cincinnati, March 1993.

Reybons, MD. Community re-entry and leisure: Reuniting a lifestyle with a burn survivor. Progress Report, 4(3):20–22, 1992.

Richard, RL. Use of the Dynasplint to correct elbow flexion burn contracture: A case report. Journal of Burn Care and Rehabilitation, 7:151–152, 1986.

Richard, RL, Jones, LM, Miller, SF, & Finlay, RK, Jr. Treatment of exposed bilateral Achilles tendons with use of the Dynasplint. Physical Therapy, 68:989–991, 1988.

Richard, RL, & Staley, M. Burn Care and Rehabilitation Principles and Practice. Philadelphia: FA Davis, 1993.

Richard, RL, Staley, MF, Miller, SF, Warden, GD, & Finley, RK, Jr. Biomechanical basis for physical management of burn patients. Poster presented at the meeting of the American Burn Association, Cincinnati, March 1993.

Ridgway, CL, Daugherty, MB, & Warden, GD. Serial casting as a technique to correct burn scar contractures. Journal of Burn Care and Rehabilitation, 12:67–72, 1991.

Rorabeck, CH, & Clark, KM. The pathophysiology of the anterior tibial compartment syndrome: An experimental investigation. Journal of Trauma, 18:299, 1978.

Rozanova, EP. The use of ultrasonics for the prevention of contractures after burns. Orthopedia Traumatologia, 34:13, 1979.

Schmitt, MA, French, L, & Kalil, ET. How soon is safe? Ambulation of the patient with burns after lower-extremity skin grafting. Journal of Burn Care and Rehabilitation, 12:33–37, 1991.

Schwanholt, C, Ridgway, C, Greenhalgh, D, Staley, M, Gaboury, T, Morress, C, Walling, S, & Warden, G. A prospective study of burn scar maturation in pediatrics: Does age matter? Paper presented at the meeting of the American Burn Association, Cincinnati, March 1993.

Schwartz, K, Rivers, E, Timming, R, Solem, L, & Ahrenholz, D. Improved outcomes for pediatric patients through the use of specialty three piece external vascular support leotards. Poster presented at the meeting of the American Burn Association, Cincinnati, March 1993.

Sheffield, CG, III, Irons, GB, Mucha, P, Malec, JF, Ilstrup, DM, & Stonnington, HH. Physical and psychological outcome after burns. Journal of Burn Care and Rehabilitation, 9:172–177, 1988.

Shelby, J, Groussman, M, Addison, C, Burgess, Y, Sullivan, J, & Saffle, J. Stress resiliency in close relatives of thermally injured patients. Paper presented at the meeting of the American Burn Association, Cincinnati, March 1993.

Solem, LD. Classification. In Fisher, SV, & Helm, PA (Eds.), Comprehensive Rehabilitation of Burns. Baltimore: Williams & Wilkins, 1984, pp. 9–15.

Solomon, JR. Pediatric burns. Critical Care Clinics, 1(1):159–173, 1985.

Spurr, ED, & Shakespeare, PG. Incidence of hypertrophic scarring in burn-injured children. Burns, 16:179–181, 1990.

Sullivan, T. Rating the burn scar. Journal of Burn Care and Rehabilitation, 11:256–260, 1990.

Tarnowski, KJ, Rasnake, LK, Linscheid, TR, & Mulick, JA.

Behavioral adjustment of pediatric burn victims. Journal of Pediatric Psychology, 14:607–615, 1989.

Taylor, A. Pockets stitched into external vascular supports improve management of hypertrophic scars. Poster presented at the meeting of the American Burn Association, Cincinnati, March 1993.

Thompson, R, Summers, S, Dobbs, R, & Wheeler, T. Color-pressure garments: Perceptions from the public. Paper presented at the meeting of the American Burn Association, Salt Lake City, April 1992.

Torres-Gray, D, Johnson, J, Greenspan, B, Goodwin, CW, & Nagler, W. The fabrication and use of removable digit casts to improve range of motion at the proximal interphalangeal joint. Poster presented at the meeting of the American Burn Association, Cincinnati, March 1993.

Turner, D, Leman, C, & Jordan, M. Ambulatory treatment of lower leg burns using the Linton compression dressing. Poster presented at the meeting of the American Burn Association, Cincinnati, March 1993.

Van den Kerckhove, E, Boeckx, W, & Kochuyt, A. Silicone patches as a supplement for pressure therapy to control hypertrophic scarring. Journal of Burn Care and Rehabilitation, 12:361–369, 1991.

Varni, JW, Bessman, CA, Russo, DC, & Cataldo, MF. Behavioral management of chronic pain in children: A case study. Archives of Physical Medicine and Rehabilitation, 61:375–379, 1980.

Walling, S, Walling, R, & Warden, GD. The development of home program instructional guides to accommodate the special needs of patients and families. Poster presented at the meeting of the American Burn Association, Cincinnati, March 1993.

Ward, S, Hayes-Lundy, C, Reddy, R, Brockway, C, Mills, P, & Saffle, J. Evaluation of topical therapeutic ultrasound to improve response to physical therapy and lessen scar contracture following burn injury. Paper presented at the meeting of the American Burn Association, Cincinnati, March 1993.

Ward, RS, Hayes-Lundy, C, Schnebly, WA, Reddy, R, & Saffle, JR. Rehabilitation of burn patients with concomitant limb amputation: Case reports. Burns, 16(5):390–392, 1990a.

Ward, RS, Hayes-Lundy, C, Schnebly, WA, & Saffle, JR. Prosthetic use in patients with burns and associated limb amputations. Journal of Burn Care and Rehabilitation, 11:361–364, 1990b.

Warden, GD, Brinkerhoff, C, Castellani, D, & Rieg, LS. Multidisciplinary team approach to the pediatric burn patient. Quality Review Bulletin, 14:219–226, 1988.

Warden, GD, Lang, D, & Housinger, TA. Management of pediatric hand burns with tendon, joint and bone injury. Paper presented at the meeting of the American Burn Association, Cincinnati, March 1993.

Waymack, JP. Release of burn scar contractures of the neck in paediatric patients. Burns, 12:422–426, 1986.

Willis, B. The use of orthoplast splints in the treatment of the acutely burned child. American Journal of Occupational Therapy, 24:187–191, 1970.

Wright, ET, & Haase, KH. Keloids and ultrasound. Archives of Physical Medicine & Rehabilitation, 52:280, 1971.

Chapter 29

The Special Care Nursery

LINDA KAHN-D'ANGELO, PT, ScD

This chapter describes the history and organization of the special care nursery and discusses which neonates and infants are at risk for central nervous system (CNS) dysfunction or developmental delay. Both a theoretic basis for and a discussion of physical therapy assessment, goals, and intervention for infants in the special care nursery are presented.

The gestational and pathophysiologic conditions considered in this chapter are prematurity, hypoxic-ischemic encephalopathy, fetal alcohol syndrome, fetal abstinence syndrome, exposure to human immunodeficiency virus (HIV) infection, neonatal seizures, birth injuries related to the CNS, and spina bifida. The follow-up of the special care nursery graduate is addressed, and a case history is used to illustrate and integrate the material presented in this chapter.

HISTORY OF THE SPECIAL CARE NURSERY

Modern neonatal care was born with the development of the first incubator by Couveuse in France in 1880 (Hodgman, 1985). The first text on the premature infant, *The Nursling*, authored by Budin, a student of Couveuse, was published in 1900. Dr. Martin Cooney, who was one of Budin's students, used these principles of treatment for the premature infant and in a bizarre entrepreneurial twist exhibited them to the public for a fee (Silverman, 1979). The main principles of treatment were support of body temperature, control of nosocomial infection, minimal handling, and provision of special nursing care. Interestingly, nurseries were quiet, and lights were dimmed at night. This exhibition was seen in Chicago by Dr. Julius Hess, who applied these principles in the late 1940s and achieved a neonatal mortality rate for preterm infants of 20%, which was respectable for the time. In response to the increased survival of these premature infants, use of these principles spread across the United States.

During the 1950s a number of cities developed centers for the care of premature infants and a number of states developed maternal mortality committees that gathered data to be used as a basis for planning activities directed at preventing maternal mortality. During the 1960s, Arizona, Massachusetts, and Wisconsin promulgated standards for maternity units and developed regional perinatal care centers. Reports from several professional organizations, including the American Medical Association, the American College of Obstetricians and Gynecologists, the American Academy of Pediatrics, and the Academy of Family Physicians, along with reports on data collected in the three states mentioned earlier, stimulated the development of the regional organization of perinatal services (Fanaroff & Graven, 1992).

By the late 1960s ill full-term infants were also being treated in the premature nursery. Advances in microlaboratory techniques for biochemical determinations from minute quantities of blood and the development of miniaturized monitoring equipment, prolonged ventilatory support systems, and means to conserve body heat improved the care of the neonate with serious illness (Fanaroff & Graven, 1992). Expansion of neonatal pharmacology, widespread use of phototherapy for manage-

ment of hyperbilirubinemia, and methods of delivery of high caloric solutions parenterally when oral feeding was not possible also improved the chances for survival of the very sick neonate. In 1975, the emergence of the new subspecialties of neonatology and perinatology provided specialists in the field of caring for infants in the high-technology nursery.

During the past 2 decades there has been considerable progress in the treatment of critically ill neonates and children. The remarkable improvement in survival and quality of life for these patients unquestionably resulted from nationwide development of regional intensive care units in which an organized, highly specialized, multidisciplinary approach became the standard of care. The number of neonates needing close supervision and expert cardiorespiratory and metabolic support is large enough to make such units an essential component of a perinatal health care delivery system (Sarnaik & Preston, 1985). Currently, there are 700 neonatal intensive care units (NICUs) in the United States, which is a 30- to 40-fold increase since the 1960s. It is well recognized that the increase in the number of NICUs is matched by a significant drop in neonatal and perinatal mortality of low birth weight (LBW) infants (Lubchenco et al., 1974; McDonald, 1981; Teberg et al., 1977). Long-term outcome of the very low birth weight (VLBW) infant, however, has come under scrutiny with the suspicion that the typical nursery stay of several weeks may have a significantly detrimental effect on later behavioral performance (Hodgman, 1985).

Organization of Special Care Nursery Services

Special care units are designed to meet a wide range of special needs, from the monitoring of apparently well infants at risk of serious illness to the intensive treatment of acutely ill infants. This range of services requires that the special care nursery be arranged for graduated care for the infant population (Whaley & Wong, 1991).

Because it is not economically feasible for every institution to have a functioning NICU these services are organized on a regional basis. A regionalized system consists of facilities in a designated geographic area that provide three prescribed levels of care. The characteristics of these facilities, according to Fanaroff and Graven (1992) and Whaley and Wong (1991), are as follows:

Level I: a facility designed to provide management of normal maternal and newborn care but able to identify high-risk pregnancies and high-risk neonates early and to implement emergency care in the event of complications. These are usually small community hospitals removed from urban areas but vital to health care in the region.

Level II: a facility that serves larger communities, usually located in urban or suburban areas, and provides a full range of maternity and newborn care. It is equipped to manage a majority of maternal and neonatal complications, depending on the resources and services available. A level II facility includes both a normal newborn nursery and a transitional care nursery and usually provides in-house anesthesia, electronic fetal monitoring, short term assisted ventilation, continuous neonatal monitoring, 24-hour blood gas determination, diagnostic radiography and ultrasonography, and nutritional and respiratory therapy.

Level III: an NICU that offers the full range of maternal and newborn services of a level II facility and also has the capacity to provide care for the most complex neonatal complications. At least one full-time neonatologist is on the staff as well as pediatric surgeons, geneticists, radiologists, anesthesiologists, and hospital epidemiologists. Chorionic villus sampling, neonatal surgery capability, extracorporeal oxygenation capability, and pediatric subspecialists in cardiology and genetics may also be available.

Regional Perinatal Center: a level III facility that also has responsibility for coordination and management of special services, including transportation, outpatient and inpatient consultation and diagnostic services for levels I and II, specialized nursing services, and outreach education programs for institutions, health care professionals, and the public within the region.

The Neonatal Intensive Care Unit Environment

The NICU is a busy, often crowded place, where the atmosphere is frequently high pressured (Pelletier & Palmeri, 1985). The amount and complexity of the equipment can be overwhelming to a newcomer. Each tiny patient lies in an incubator, open warmer, or crib, surrounded by and connected to ventilators and monitors, including heart, apnea, and oxygen monitors and infusion pumps (Fig. 29–1). Phototherapy lights, diagnostic transilluminators, and portable radiographic, electroencephalographic, and ultrasonographic units are also present in an NICU.

NICUs were designed to decrease neonatal morbidity and mortality. In an attempt to meet this goal, the NICU provides the neonate with a habitat

FIGURE 29–1. Infant surrounded by typical NICU equipment. (From Crane, L. Physical therapy for the neonate with respiratory disease. In Irwin, S. & Tecklin, JS [Eds]. Cardiopulmonary Physical Therapy [2nd ed.] St. Louis. CV Mosby, 1990, p. 400.)

for growth starkly different from the intrauterine environment. The intrauterine environment is replaced by bright lights, high noise levels, and the intrusive medical procedures characteristic of high-technology treatment (Campbell, 1986; Gottfried, 1985).

LIGHTING

Typically, the ambient illumination within the NICU consists of daylight and artificial fluorescent lighting (Moseley et al., 1988). The American Academy of Pediatrics recommends a minimum light intensity of 100 foot-candles at the infant's level for adequate visualization by staff (Weibley, 1989). This same level of illumination may contribute to retinopathy of prematurity (ROP) (Glass et al., 1985; Kretzer & Hittner, 1986). No diurnal rhythmicity of light exists in the NICU, which some investigators believe may interfere with the infant's development of normal biologic rhythms. Glass and colleagues (1985) studied the effects of draping sunglass-filtering material over half of the incubators. As a result of this study, an editorial in the journal that published the study recommended immediate diurnal cycling and dimming of lights (Weibley, 1989).

SOUND

In the intrauterine environment, auditory stimuli include sound levels at about 85 dB consisting of rhythmic swooshing and bubbling sounds punctuated by the steady pulse of the maternal heartbeat (Gottfried, 1985; Gottfried & Hodgman, 1984). In the NICU, the infant is surrounded by noise on a level comparable with that of auto traffic and, at times, heavy machinery. Highly exaggerated noise levels are present from trash receptacles, addressograph machines, centrifuges, telephones, and monitor alarms (Hilton, 1987). These harsh sounds can cause some infants to become hypoxic as part of a startle response (Thomas, 1989). Sound levels within the incubator are identical to those of the unit. The environment inside the incubator is characterized by continuous white noise and nonspeech sounds. Harsh mechanical noises penetrate clearly, but speech sounds are indistinct and deflected (Newman, 1981). This lack of distinctness and the deflection of speech sounds may have negative effects on later interactive behavior if the infant learns to look away from the speaker to locate him or her. Drugs commonly used in the nursery are known from animal studies to potentiate noise-induced hearing loss (Perlstein, 1992). The American Academy of Pediatrics has recommended that noise levels be reduced to less than 70 dB, that manufacturers of incubators reduce the noise levels of motors below 58 dB, and that physicians limit the use of ototoxic drugs in neonates (Peabody & Lewis, 1985; Perlstein, 1992). Auditory evoked potential tests are typically done in every nursery before a neonate is discharged to establish risk for hearing loss.

MEDICAL PROCEDURES

In the NICU, the infant is placed on a flat mattress and is exposed to a dry, cool, air-filled environment. In the uterine environment the 28- to 32–week fetus sleeps 80% of the time. In contrast, premature infants were found to be disturbed an average of 132 times per day (Korones, 1976). The mean duration of undisturbed rest was 4 to 10 minutes.

Tactile input often heralds medical or technical events and causes sustained arousal, which exacts a physiologic toll on the infant. Unable to make sense of life-sustaining efforts, the infant begins to respond negatively to touch (Gottfried & Hodgman, 1984).

WHO IS THE AT-RISK NEONATE/INFANT?

The meaning of the designation "high-risk infant" differs according to the area of expertise of the professional using the term. The neonatologist defines risk as related to morbidity or mortality, whereas psychologists, physical therapists, occupational therapists, and speech therapists may define the at-risk infant as one who has a high probability of manifesting developmental delay as a result of exposure to any one of a number of medical factors (Rosetti, 1986; Wilhelm, 1984). High-risk infants are classified according to birth weight, gestational age, and pathophysiologic problems (Whaley & Wong, 1991). Problems related to physiologic status are closely associated with the maturity of the infant and hypoxic episodes during the perinatal period as well as with fetal exposure to alcohol and drugs and with HIV infection.

PREMATURITY AND LOW BIRTH WEIGHT

Infants born prematurely or who are small for gestational age (SGA) are divided into two major categories: LBW, from 1501 to 2500 g, and VLBW, below 1501 g. Over 40,000 VLBW infants are born each year, and half of neonatal deaths occur in VLBW infants (Semmler, 1989). These high-risk infants are a heterogeneous group, comprising infants born preterm (less than 37 weeks' gestation) and those born at term but of reduced weight (Kleigman, 1992). Black mothers are twice as likely as white mothers to deliver VLBW infants (Semmler, 1989). VLBW infants have an increased incidence of neurologic sequelae, delayed development, and lower intellectual and language abilities (Teberg, 1977).

SGA infants are those whose birth weights are below the 10th percentile of published norms or whose ponderal index (ratio of birth weight to the cube root of the infant's length at birth) is low (Als et al., 1976). Term SGA infants demonstrate developmental problems such as behavioral and learning disorders at follow-up, and preterm SGA infants may have an even greater percentage of abnormal developmental outcomes than term SGA neonates (Kahn-D'Angelo, 1987).

The Clinical Assessment of Gestational Age in the Newborn Infant was developed by Dubowitz and colleagues in 1970, and this assessment is the tool most often used to assess gestational age. This tool includes 10 neurologic and reflex items and 11 external or superficial criteria that are scored on a 4-point scale, and it is commonly administered by physicians or nurses in the newborn unit. The accuracy of gestational age is determined within a variation of ±2 weeks on each assessment, with a 95% confidence level. This test was standardized on 167 infants whose mothers were sure of the date of their last menstrual period. It has been used in the assessment of growth in early infancy and, in conjunction with the neurologic examination, to assess differences in development between twins, preterm infants with intraventricular hemorrhage (IVH), and the effects of eclampsia, placental abruption, and intrauterine growth retardation (Francis et al., 1987). The determination of gestational age is crucial for infants in the special care nursery to interpret neurologic and behavioral findings relative to the correct gestational age. Although gestational age is usually determined by physicians or nurses in the NICU, the physical therapist should be familiar with the Clinical Assessment of Gestational Age in the Newborn Infant and how gestational age is determined.

MEDICAL COMPLICATIONS AND TREATMENT IN PREMATURITY

Respiratory Distress Syndrome

Respiratory distress syndrome (RDS), or hyaline membrane disease, is the most common single cause of respiratory distress in neonates. The principal factors in the pathophysiology of RDS are pulmonary immaturity and deficiency of surfactant. Low surfactant production results in increased surface tension, alveolar collapse, diffuse atelectasis, and decreased lung compliance. These factors cause an increase in pulmonary artery pressure that leads to extrapulmonary right-to-left shunting of blood and ventilation-perfusion mismatching (Carlo & Chatburn, 1988; Sweeney & Swanson, 1990; Walsh et al., 1988). Prematurity is the single most important risk factor for development of RDS. Perinatal complications such as asphyxia, maternal diabetes, and delivery by caesarean section may increase the incidence or severity of RDS.

Treatment of infants with RDS depends on the severity of the disorder and includes oxygen supplementation, assisted ventilation, surfactant administration, and extracorporeal membrane oxygenation (ECMO). Continuous distending pressure ventilators, either positive or negative pressure, are used in the management of RDS. The positive pressure ventilator is used more often; the negative-pressure ventilator assists ventilation by creating a negative pressure around the thorax and abdomen. Nasal and nasopharyngeal prongs are used for these ventilators (Carlo et al., 1992; Crane, 1990). (See Chapter 24 for a more detailed description of ventilators.)

Synthetic and combined natural and synthetic preparations of surfactant are being used in the treatment of RDS. Surfactant therapy appears to improve oxygenation of ventilated preterm infants within several hours of treatment. Surfactant is administered through an endotracheal tube in several doses; the infant is placed in different positions for each dose to enhance distribution throughout the lung. The resultant increase in arterial oxygen tension (Pao_2) is thought to be caused by an improved match between ventilation and perfusion (Martin & Fanaroff, 1992). Mortality from RDS is reduced, as is the incidence of air leaks, when multiple doses of surfactant are administered. Surfactant use has not, however, resulted in a decrease in bronchopulmonary dysplasia (BPD), IVH, or patent ductus arteriosus.

The prognosis of infants with RDS varies with the severity of the original disease (Carlo & Chatburn, 1988). Mortality is about 10% and is the leading cause of neonatal mortality and morbidity. Infants who do not require assisted ventilation recover without sequelae, but the clinical course of the very immature infant may be complicated by air leaks and BPD. Infants who survive severe RDS often require frequent hospitalization for upper respiratory tract infections and have an increased incidence of neurodevelopmental sequelae.

ECMO is a technique of cardiopulmonary bypass

modified from techniques developed for open-heart surgery that are used to support heart and lung function (Whaley & Wong, 1991). In newborns with respiratory failure, the immature lungs are allowed to rest and recover to avoid the damaging effects of artificial ventilation. Because of the need for systemic heparinization and the resultant risk of systemic and intracranial hemorrhage, ECMO is reserved for use with infants of at least 34 weeks' gestational age, weight more than 2000 g, no evidence of intracranial bleeding, less than 10 days' assisted ventilation, and reversible lung disease (Stork, 1992). ECMO is now used with considerable frequency in support of neonates with severe but reversible respiratory failure, including complicating meconium aspiration, congenital diaphragmatic hernia, sepsis, persistent fetal circulation, and RDS (Martin & Fanaroff, 1992).

Bronchopulmonary Dysplasia

Infants with BPD or chronic lung disease include those who, after requiring mechanical ventilation during the first week of life, remain dependent on oxygen for more than 28 days and have persistent areas of increased densities on chest radiographs (Carlo & Chatburn, 1988). The overall incidence varies from 15 to 50% of infants weighing less than 1500 g and requiring ventilation, depending on diagnostic criteria and the neonatal population being studied.

Pathophysiologic features of BPD include interstitial fibrosis resulting from absorption of intraalveolar exudate by the alveolar wall during the resolution of RDS. Alveolar collapse may cause parts of the lung to become airless and solid. These nonaerated regions form scars of condensed lung tissue and become fibrotic. Mucosa of the bronchioles becomes dysplastic and inflamed, and there is hypertrophy of the smooth muscle of bronchioles and arterioles. Pulmonary function testing reveals severe maldistribution of ventilation in these infants. They have increased airway resistance, decreased dynamic compliance, and a large increase in the work of breathing.

Prematurity, barotrauma from high pressures used in assisted ventilation, and pulmonary oxygen toxicity are accepted as key causal components of BPD (Bancalari, 1992). Also, the endotracheal tube itself hinders drainage of tracheal secretions and increases both dead space and resistance to air flow. Other factors that may contribute to the pathogenesis of BPD are infection, pulmonary edema resulting from a patent ductus arteriosus or excessive fluid administration, and increased airway resistance.

Medical treatment of BPD includes respiratory support, fluid management, infection control, and bronchodilator therapy. Respiratory support includes use of mechanical ventilation only when needed and the use of the lowest peak airway pressure necessary to maintain adequate ventilation. Duration of mechanical ventilation should be limited (Bancalari, 1992). Intermittent mandatory ventilation, which allows the infant to breathe spontaneously between a set number of mechanical breaths per minute, may also be used (Carlo & Chatburn, 1988; Platzker, 1988).

Because infants with BPD are prone to developing cor pulmonale, congestive heart failure, and pulmonary edema, chronic diuretic therapy is instituted. The infant or child with BPD must also be closely monitored for infections, especially those caused by bacteria and fungi. If bronchospasm is a factor, inhaled bronchodilator, dexamethasone, or theophylline therapy may be required (Bancalari, 1992; Davis et al., 1990).

Chest physical therapy is a component of the care of an infant with BPD for airway clearance problems caused by submucosal and peribronchial smooth muscle hyperplasia, oxygen therapy, and the presence of frequent lower respiratory tract infections (Crane, 1987, Dean, 1987; Hazinski & Pacetti, 1988).

The incidence of developmental disability, such as mental retardation and cerebral palsy, in infants and children with BPD has been reported to be 29 to 34% (Robertson et al., 1991; Skidmore et al., 1990; Vidyasagar, 1985; Vohr et al., 1991). The important predictors for these disabilities are intracranial hemorrhage and periventricular echodensity, rather than the severity of the BPD itself (Luchi et al., 1991).

Periventricular Leukomalacia

Periventricular leukomalacia is the principal ischemic lesion of the premature infant (Volpe, 1987). The lesion is caused by a reduction in cerebral blood flow in the highly vulnerable periventricular region of the brain where the arterial "end zones" of the middle, posterior, and anterior cerebral arteries meet. Major systemic hypotension with resuscitative difficulties after birth may be a major factor. Contributory roles may be played by a patent ductus arteriosus and severe apneic spells (McMenamin et al., 1984; Sweeney & Swanson,

1990). Periventricular leukomalacia often occurs later than in the first week of life.

Serial ultrasonography, computed tomography, magnetic resonance imaging, and positron emission tomography are useful diagnostic tools for periventricular leukomalacia (Sinha et al., 1990). With the increased availability of high-resolution cranial ultrasonography, ultrasonographic white matter echodensities and echolucencies in LBW infants suggest later disabilities, especially cerebral palsy, more accurately than any other antecedent (Leviton & Paneth, 1990; Miller & Murray, 1992). Serial ultrasonographic studies are important because the evolution of periventricular echodensity is related to prognosis. Early periventricular echodensity that resolves during the first weeks of life is not correlated with later major disabilities; development of cysts as a result of dissolution of brain tissue secondary to infarction, however, is correlated with later cerebral palsy and cognitive deficits (Mantovani & Powers, 1991). Cerebral palsy occurs in infants who develop bilateral cysts larger than 3 mm in diameter in the parietal or occipital areas in more than 90% of the cases.

Medical management includes maintenance of adequate ventilation. The area affected includes the white matter through which long descending motor tracts travel to the spinal cord from the motor cortex. Because the motor tracts involved in the control of leg movements are closest to the ventricles, and therefore more likely to be damaged, spastic diplegia is the most common clinical sequela (Fig. 29–2). If the lesion extends laterally, the arms may be involved, with resulting spastic quadriplegia. Visual deficits may also result from damage to the optic radiations (Catto-Smith et al., 1985; Papile, 1992).

Periventricular-Intraventricular Hemorrhage

Periventricular-intraventricular hemorrhage is one of the most common types of acute perinatal brain injury in the neonatal period and is second only to RDS as a major cause of death in preterm infants (Volpe, 1987). Periventricular-intraventricular hemorrhage is characteristic of the premature infant of less than 32 weeks of gestational age and weighing less than 1500 g. An inverse relationship exists between gestational age and incidence of periventricular-intraventricular hemorrhage. The average incidence is 40% in preterm infants of less than 35 weeks of gestational age. Most hemorrhages occur within the first 2 postnatal days, and virtually all occur within 1 week of birth (Papile, 1992). This lesion involves bleeding into the subependymal germinal matrix, which is a gelatinous area that contains a rich vascular network supplied mainly by Heubner's artery, a branch of the anterior cerebral artery. This matrix is prominent from 26 to 34 weeks of gestation and is usually gone by term. The vessels that traverse the matrix are primitive in appearance, with a single layer of endothelium without smooth muscle, elastin, or collagen, and the area is devoid of supportive stroma. The site of origin of this lesion is from these primitive capillaries. In a small number of preterm infants, hemorrhage may occur from the choroid plexus or roof of the fourth ventricle (Fig. 29–3). This type of hemorrhage is precipitated by systemic hypertension and perturbations in arterial pressure and blood flow to the immature subependymal vascular bed (Bada et al., 1990; Fok et al., 1990; Takashima et al., 1989).

Neuropathologic complications of IVH are hydrocephalus, germinal matrix destruction, cyst formation, and accompanying hypoxic-ischemic lesions. A 4-level grading scale based on ultrasound scan has been developed by Papile to classify hemorrhages (Papile et al., 1983). Grade I is isolated germinal matrix hemorrhage. Grade II is IVH with normal-sized ventricles that occurs when hemorrhage in the subependymal germinal matrix ruptures through the ependyma into the lateral ventricles. Grade III includes IVH with acute ventricular dilation, and grade IV involves hemorrhage into the periventricular white matter.

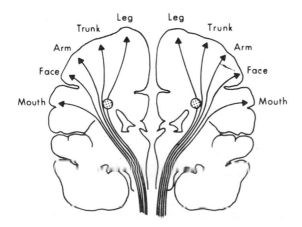

FIGURE 29–2 Diagram of corticospinal tracts. Dotted circular areas indicate periventricular leukomalacia that would be expected to affect descending fibers for control of the lower extremity. (From Volpe, JJ. Neurology of the Newborn [2nd ed]. Philadelphia, WB Saunders, 1987, p. 311.)

FIGURE 29–3. Coronal section of the cerebrum showing intraventricular hemorrhage. (From Volpe, JJ. Neurology of the Newborn [2nd ed]. Philadelphia: WB Saunders, 1987, p. 314.)

Ultrasonography, computed tomography, and positron emission tomography are useful for diagnosis. Treatment includes support of cerebral perfusion by maintaining arterial blood pressure and avoidance of cerebral hemodynamic disturbances caused by rapid volume expansion, pneumothorax, increased arterial blood pressure, and hypoxemia. Serial imaging to monitor ventricular size and ventriculostomy or shunting for hydrocephalus are also important treatment components (Volpe, 1987). Prophylactic treatment with phenobarbital, indomethacin, pancuronium (a neuromuscular blocking agent), ethamsylate (to reduce capillary bleeding), and vitamins E and K is under investigation. When hemorrhage has occurred, medical management includes maintenance of cerebral perfusion through control of blood pressure and decrease in intracranial pressure through lumbar puncture and ventricular drainage.

The risk of major neurologic disability in LBW preterm infants increases with each higher grade of IVH (McMenamin et al., 1984). Grades I, II, and III result in a 15, 30, and 40% incidence of neurologic sequelae, respectively (Volpe, 1987). The most decisive determinant of neurologic impairment, such as spastic diplegia or quadriplegia with intellectual impairment, is hemorrhagic intracerebral involvement (grade IV), which results in a 90% incidence of major neurologic sequelae (Catto-Smith et al., 1985; Koeda et al., 1990; Volpe, 1987; Yokochi et al., 1991). Dubowitz and Dubowitz (1981a, b) have noted that a tight popliteal angle (130° or less in infants of up to 31 weeks' gestation,

and 110° or less at 32 to 35 weeks' gestation) is a sign of IVH.

Necrotizing Enterocolitis

Necrotizing enterocolitis (NEC) is an acute inflammatory disease of the bowel that occurs most frequently during the first 6 weeks of life in premature infants weighing less than 2000 g (Whaley & Wong, 1991). Although the precise cause of the disease is not known, several factors appear to play a role in the pathogenesis of NEC. These factors include intestinal ischemia, infectious agents and toxins, and enteral alimentation. Diagnosis is made by physical examination, laboratory studies, and radiography. Vomiting, abdominal distention, bloody stools, and lethargy are signs of this condition. Medical care of infants with NEC includes parenteral alimentation, gastric suction, and administration of broad-spectrum antibiotics (Cressinger et al., 1992). Laboratory findings include anemia, leukopenia, and electrolyte imbalance. Breath hydrogen measurements have been found to be 99% effective in detecting absence of the disease and are suggested as an aid to diagnosis of NEC (Cheu et al., 1989). Abdominal radiographs are performed every 6 to 8 to hours to detect progressive intestinal obstruction or possible perforation. Surgical intervention is indicated when there is radiographic evidence of fixed, dilated intestinal loops accompanied by intestinal distention (Cressinger et al., 1992). Surgical procedures include intestinal decompression by nasogastric tube placement or gastrostomy, resection of necrotic bowel, and diversion of the proximal fecal stream by ileostomy, jejunostomy, or colostomy.

NEC is the most common cause of death in neonates undergoing surgery. The average mortality rate after surgery is 30 to 40%. Stricture formation, which is abnormal narrowing of the intestines, occurs in 25 to 35% of the survivors of medical or surgical treatment and presents as failure to thrive, feeding abnormalities, diarrhea, or bowel obstruction (Cressinger et al., 1992).

Retinopathy of Prematurity (ROP)

ROP is a developmental vascular retinopathy that occurs in the incompletely vascularized retina of premature infants (Phelps, 1992). It is characterized by severe vascular constriction and followed by hypoxia of the immature vasculature of the retina. Subsequently, there is vascular proliferation of retinal capillaries into the hypoxic area. New vessels proliferate toward the lens; and the aqueous humor and then the vitreous humor become turbid. The retina becomes edematous, and hemorrhages separate the retina from its attachment. The outcome of the disease ranges from normal vision to total loss of vision if there is advanced scarring from the retina to the lens resulting in retinal detachment (Whaley & Wong, 1991). ROP was called retrolental fibroplasia in the early 1940s and was virtually eliminated with the severe restriction of oxygen use between 1950 and 1970. The condition has recurred as one of the major causes of disability in preterm infants as a result of the increased survival of VLBW infants. The incidence of ROP increases with lower gestational age or birth weight. Hyperoxia, shock, asphyxia, hypothermia, vitamin E deficiency, and light exposure have been implicated as possible pathogenic factors (Kretzer & Hittner, 1986).

Prevention and treatment include oxygen administration at Pao_2 between 50 and 70 mm Hg, administration of vitamin E (which is still under investigation), and surgery such as laser photocoagulation, cryotherapy, vitrectomy, and scleral buckling (Kretzer & Hittner, 1986). Outcome of surgery ranges from complete recovery or mild myopia to blindness, depending on the extent of the disease, which is rated in stages 1 through 4 based on fundoscopic examination. 1—demarcation line separating the posterior vascularized retina from the anterior nonvascularized retina, 2—intraretinal ridge formation, 3—intraretinal ridge plus fibrovascular proliferation, and 4—retinal detachment

(Kingham, 1986). Whether there is "plus" disease for each of the above stages (e.g., 3+) is also determined. Plus disease occurs when the retinal arteries and veins become tortuous and dilated as a result of shunting from arterioles to veins in the peripheral retina with active ROP (White et al., 1991).

Hyperbilirubinemia

Hyperbilirubinemia, or physiologic jaundice, is the accumulation of excessive amounts of bilirubin in the blood. Bilirubin is one of the breakdown products of hemoglobin from red blood cells. This condition is seen commonly in premature infants who have immature hepatic functions, an increased hemolysis of red blood cells as a result of high concentrations of circulating red blood cells, a shorter life span of red blood cells, and possible polycythemia from birth injuries (Whaley & Wong, 1991). Treatment of hyperbilirubinemia has as its main goal the prevention of kernicterus, which is the deposition of unconjugated bilirubin in the brain, especially in the basal ganglia and hippocampus. LBW infants of less than 2000 g receive phototherapy at 24 hours of life for 96 hours, regardless of bilirubin concentration. Phototherapy is administered by banks of eight to ten fluorescent lamps placed 12 to 16 inches above the unclothed infant in an open radiant warmer or incubator (Gartner & Lee, 1992). The infant's eyes are shielded by patches to avoid retinal damage. Studies show that on/off cycles of more than 1 hour are as effective as continuous treatment. A new technique of fiberoptic phototherapy uses light from a halogen lamp transmitted through a fiberoptic bundle to a blanket that is wrapped around the infant (Gartner & Lee, 1992).

If phototherapy is not effective in reducing the total serum bilirubin concentrations to acceptable levels, exchange transfusion is done. In this technique, approximately 85% of the infant's red blood cells are replaced. Human trials are underway to test tin mesoporphyrin to reduce hyperbilirubinemia. This is a synthetic heme analogue that limits the rate of degradation of heme to bile (Gartner & Lee, 1992).

HYPOXIC-ISCHEMIC ENCEPHALOPATHY OF THE FULL TERM INFANT

Hypoxic-ischemic encephalopathy (HIE) designates clinical and neuropathologic findings of an encephalopathy that occurs in a full term infant who has experienced a significant episode of perinatal asphyxia (Brann & Schwartz, 1992a; Volpe, 1987). The relative importance of antepartum, intrapartum, and postnatal hypoxic-ischemic insults is difficult to determine. Major signs of HIE include seizures; abnormalities in state of consciousness, tone, posture, reflexes, respiratory pattern, and autonomic function; and tenseness of the anterior fontanelle. Conditions associated with increased risk for fetal asphyxia are altered placental exchange, reduced maternal blood flow to the placenta, and decreased maternal oxygen saturation. Altered placental exchange may result from abruption, placenta previa, postmaturity, prolapsed umbilical cord, umbilical cord around the neck, intrauterine growth retardation, and placental insufficiency. Maternal hypotension may reduce the blood flow to the placenta, and maternal hypoventilation, hypoxia, or cardiopulmonary disease may decrease maternal oxygenation. Intrapartum insults include those related to traumatic delivery, prolonged labor, and acute placental or cord problems. Prolonged partial asphyxia from any cause sets into motion a spiral of cytotoxic edema, with impaired cerebral blood flow, which leads to cerebral necrosis or ulegyria (Fig. 29–4).

Therapeutic care of an infant at significant risk for development of HIE includes careful monitoring by serial neurologic assessments, detection of reduced cerebral perfusion pressure, assessment of the structural status of brain with computed tomography or ultrasonography, and electroencephalography or evoked potential tests (Brann & Schwartz, 1992a). Treatment of HIE remains controversial because of a lack of complete understanding of the biologic processes that maintain cellular homeostasis and neurologic function. The goals of treatment of HIE are elimination of the original cause of hypoxia and the alleviation of tissue ischemia.

Volume expansion with the use of pressor agents to increase blood pressure is used to maintain cerebral blood flow. Partial exchange transfusion may be done if the infant's hematocrit is low to decrease hyperviscosity and enhance tissue oxygenation. Sodium bicarbonate and glucose are administered to treat severe, persistent metabolic acidosis and hypoglycemia, respectively. The use of barbiturates is being studied because they reduce the energy requirements of the brain and have been shown to decrease intracranial pressure in adults.

Sarnat and Sarnat (1976) identified three stages of encephalopathy after asphyxia. Stage 1 lasts less than 24 hours and is characterized by hyperalertness and low threshold Moro and stretch reflexes, with normal muscle tone and electroencephalogram. The duration for stage 2 is approximately 5 days; clinical signs include lethargy, mild hypotonia, strong distal flexion, hyperactive stretch reflexes, weak suck and Moro reflexes, strong tonic neck reflex, and multifocal seizures. Stage 3 is stupor, which lasts from a few hours to 4 weeks, with flaccidity alternating with decerebrate posturing, absent reflexes, response only to strong noxious stimuli, rare seizures, and an isopotential electroencephalogram.

When the infant with hypoxic-ischemic insult has a normal neurologic examination by 1 week of age, sequelae are minimal. Those who continue to have an abnormal neurologic examination by 3 weeks of age, however, are at risk to develop major neurologic sequelae (Harper & Yoon, 1987). The neurologic sequelae of HIE include motor deficits with or without mental retardation and seizures or both. Neuropathologic classifications of HIE include selective neuronal necrosis, status marmoratus, parasagittal cerebral injury, and focal ischemic brain necrosis (Volpe, 1987).

FIGURE 29–4. Model for production of cerebral edema. Decreased blood pressure (BP) leads to decreased cerebral blood flow (CBF) and ischemia. (From Campbell, SK: Clinical decision making: Management of the neonate with movement dysfunction. In Wolf, SL [Ed.], Clinical Decision Making in Physical Therapy. Philadelphia: FA Davis, 1985, p. 299.)

Selective Neuronal Necrosis

Selective neuronal necrosis, the most common type of HIE, is the death of neurons in a widespread but characteristic pattern. The major sites of neuro-

TABLE 29–1. SELECTIVE NEURONAL NECROSIS IN NEONATAL HYPOXIC-ISCHEMIC ENCEPHALOPATHY—MAJOR SITES

Cerebral cortex—hippocampus > supralimbic cortex
Diencephalon—thalamus, hypothalamus, and lateral geniculate body
Basal ganglia—caudate, putamen, and globus pallidus
Midbrain—inferior colliculus, oculomotor and trochlear nuclei, red nucleus, substantia nigra, and reticular formation
Pons—motor nuclei of trigeminal and facial nerves, dorsal > ventral cochlear nuclei, reticular formation, and pontine nuclei
Medulla—dorsal motor nucleus of vagus nerve, nucleus ambiguus, inferior olivary nuclei, cuneate and gracilis nuclei
Cerebellum—Purkinje cells, dentate, and other roof nuclei.

From Volpe, JJ. Neurology of the Newborn (2nd ed.). Philadelphia: WB Saunders, 1987, p. 213.

nal necrosis include the hippocampus of the cerebral cortex and parts of the diencephalon, basal ganglia, pons, medulla, and cerebellum (Table 29–1, Fig. 29–5). (Cabañas et al., 1991). Although the reasons for the vulnerability of these areas are not clear, putative mechanisms include circulatory, metabolic, and excitotoxic amino acid action on the synaptic terminals that contain excitatory amino acids. Clinical findings with this type of neuropathologic condition include stupor, coma, seizures, hypotonus, and oculomotor, sucking, and tongue movement problems. Long-term sequelae include mental retardation, spastic quadriparesis, seizure disorder, ataxia, bulbar and pseudobulbar palsy, hyperactivity, and impaired attention.

Status Marmoratus

Status marmoratus is neuronal loss, gliosis, and hypermyelinization of the basal ganglia and thalamus. Effects are not noted in full form until the latter part of the first year of life, although injury occurs in the perinatal period (Volpe, 1987). The cause of this lesion is unclear, but there is a correlation with perinatal asphyxia. Neonatal findings are unknown at this time, but long-term clinical sequelae include choreoathetosis, mental retardation, spastic quadriplegia, and dystonia.

Parasagittal Cerebral Injury

Parasagittal cerebral injury results in a lesion of the cerebral cortex and subcortical white matter. This injury is usually bilateral and symmetric, with the parietal-occipital regions most affected (Volpe, 1987). The areas of necrosis are the border zones between the end fields of the major cerebral arteries. Clinical signs in the neonatal period include proximal limb weakness, especially in the upper extremities. Long-term sequelae include spastic quadriparesis and specific intellectual deficits such as delay in development of language, visuospatial abilities, or both.

Focal Ischemic Brain Necrosis

The category of focal ischemic brain necrosis includes large, localized areas of neuronal death in the distribution of the major blood vessels in the cerebral cortex and subcortical white matter. The focal ischemic brain necrosis occurs perinatally as the result of cerebrovascular insufficiency secondary to malformation of vessels, arterial obstruction due to thrombi or emboli, or systemic circulatory insufficiency near the end of the second trimester. Resolution of neuronal necrosis results in the formation of cavities. Neurologic features during the neonatal period include hemiparesis, quadriparesis, and stereotyped and nonhabituating reflex responses. This lesion results in spastic hemiparesis in the case of a limited focal lesion, mental retardation, and seizure disorder (Volpe, 1987).

FIGURE 29–5. CT scan of selective cortical neuronal necrosis of a 4-week-old infant who experienced severe perinatal asphyxia. Note cortical atrophy and white matter injury. (From Volpe, JJ. Neurology of the Newborn [2nd ed]. Philadelphia: WB Saunders, 1987, p. 245.)

NEONATAL SEIZURES

Neonatal seizures are the most frequent and distinct neurologic signs that occur in the neonatal period (Brann & Wiznitzer, 1992). Most occur between the second and fifth days of life, and 85% occur in the first 15 days of life. A seizure during the neonatal period is a medical emergency, since it may indicate a life-threatening disease or disorder that can produce immediate and irreversible brain damage. Neonatal seizures may also result in decreased DNA content and brain cell number.

The causes of neonatal seizures include asphyxia, the most frequent cause in full-term infants, intracranial hemorrhage, subarachnoid bleeding secondary to asphyxia, birth trauma, and IVH in preterm infants (Volpe, 1987). Infectious causes include sepsis, meningitis, and TORCH infections. Hypoglycemia and congenital cerebral malformations are also causes.

Clinical manifestations of seizures in neonates differ greatly from those in older infants and children because of the immaturity of the brain. Clinical signs in the neonate include facial, oral, lingual, and ocular movements and autonomic manifestations such as apnea and changes in blood pressure, heart rate, and pupil size (Table 29–2). Abnormal movements and alteration of tone in the trunk and extremities, including rowing and bicycling movements, are also clinical signs of neonatal seizure (Mizrahi & Kellaway, 1987). Treatment includes administration of anticonvulsants such as phenobarbital, phenytoin, and diazepam to control seizures and intravenous glucose for hypoglycemia.

Neonatal seizures are one of the strongest predictors of later motor or intellectual deficit. Approximately 29% of all infants with neonatal seizures later exhibit mental retardation, motor impairment, or both. Seizures that occur in conjunction with perinatal asphyxia, severe IVH, intracranial infection, and prematurity with prolonged hypoglycemia have poor prognoses, with possible permanent neurologic sequelae such as cerebral palsy or mental retardation. Seizures that occur with subarachnoid hemorrhage without asphyxia or as a result of metabolic disorders have good prognoses if treatment begins early.

FETAL ALCOHOL SYNDROME

Chronic alcohol exposure in utero may result in a multitude of symptoms at birth, including withdrawal symptoms of irritability, tremors, apnea, and seizures (Volpe, 1987; Whaley & Wong, 1991). When severe, phenobarbital or paregoric (morphine) may be used to control withdrawal symptoms (Harper & Yoon, 1987). Alcohol rapidly crosses the placenta and the blood–brain barrier of the fetus, and there is a dose-dependent relationship between maternal alcohol intake in the first weeks of pregnancy and the occurrence of features of the fetal alcohol syndrome (FAS).

The full manifestation of FAS is characterized by a triad of symptoms composed of growth deficiency, cardiac defects, and CNS dysfunction with mental retardation and dysmorphology including facial, genital, and joint abnormalities (Barbour, 1990). Approximately 89% of infants born with full FAS will demonstrate developmental delay (Volpe, 1987).

In utero alcohol exposure is related to a wide continuum of effects ranging from full FAS to partial FAS, also referred to as fetal alcohol effects, to more subtle effects, such as neurologic disorders without dysmorphology (Scott et al., 1991). These subtle neurologic effects include hyperactivity, delayed language development, fine and gross motor problems, slowed reaction time, and problems with judgement and comprehension (Autti-Rämö & Granström, 1991; Scott et al., 1991). Long-term effects of prenatal alcohol exposure include deficits in several areas of intellectual functioning, including information processing, short-term memory, encoding, and preacademic skills (Coles et al., 1991; Little et al., 1989). Streissguth (1986) reported that 24% of children born to binge drinkers and 15% born to nonbinge drinkers were receiving special education services at 7.5 years of age.

FETAL ABSTINENCE SYNDROME

Maternal use of narcotics during pregnancy leads to the development of dependency on that drug by the fetus. The most commonly used drugs are heroin, methadone, and cocaine, and there is often maternal use of several drugs during pregnancy (Finnegan, 1988). The fetus experiences withdrawal

TABLE 29–2. **CHARACTERISTICS OF SUBTLE SEIZURES IN PREMATURE AND FULL-TERM INFANTS**

Ocular-tonic horizontal deviation of eyes ± jerking; and sustained eye opening with ocular fixation
Eyelid blinking or fluttering
Sucking, smacking, drooling, and other oral-buccal-lingual movements
"Swimming," "rowing," and "pedaling" movements
Apneic spell

From Volpe, JJ. Neurology of the Newborn (2nd ed.). Philadelphia: WB Saunders, 1987, p. 134.

when the mother is withdrawn from her drug or drugs or when the fetus is delivered. Symptoms of withdrawal are similar to those of withdrawal from alcohol and include irritability, tremors, seizures, apnea, increased muscle tone, inability to sleep, hyperactive deep tendon reflexes, incoordination, ineffective sucking and swallowing, and shrill crying (Hayford et al., 1988; Dixon, 1989). Premature delivery, meconium aspiration, and abruptio placentae are common complications of labor and delivery (Chasnoff, 1988). Disturbances in the behavioral organization and interactive abilities of these neonates make early bonding and attachment difficult (Hume et al., 1989). Follow-up studies indicate growth retardation and long-term intellectual impairment as well as learning difficulties in children exposed to drugs in utero (Bauman & Levine, 1986; Davis & Templer, 1988; Free et al., 1990; Hume et al., 1989; Lewis et al., 1989).

EXPOSURE TO HUMAN IMMUNODEFICIENCY VIRUS

The risk of developing HIV infection of infants born to women with a positive HIV titer is estimated to be 30 to 75% (Pizzi & Hinds-Harris, 1990). Infants are often asymptomatic at birth, and the infection may not become evident until the child is 12 to 18 months old, with the median age at onset of symptoms being 9 months. Infection early in fetal development may lead to microcephaly and facial anomalies. The mortality rate for infants infected early in fetal development is especially high. Infants exposed to HIV should be monitored for signs of infection, such as failure to thrive, weight loss, temperature instability, and diarrhea, and assessed for opportunistic infections such as herpes simplex virus infection, cytomegalovirus infection, lymphoid interstitial pneumonia, and viral, fungal, or protozoal infections. Because neonates with HIV infection are usually asymptomatic, they are not admitted to the NICU unless there are problems unrelated to HIV. It should be noted, however, that infants who were seropositive exhibited significantly lower scores on the Bayley Scales of Infant Development than seronegative infants (Aylward et al., 1992).

BIRTH INJURIES RELATED TO THE NERVOUS SYSTEM

Birth injuries are those sustained during labor and delivery and represent an important cause of neonatal morbidity (Mangurten, 1992). The most common traumatic lesions related to the nervous system include caput succedaneum, linear skull fracture, and brachial plexus injury.

Caput Succedaneum

Caput succedaneum is hemorrhagic edema caused by compression of a portion of the scalp from the pressure of the uterus or vaginal wall during a vertex delivery. The clinical manifestation is a soft swelling usually a few millimeters thick. The edema is external to the periosteum and crosses suture lines. The lesion steadily resolves over the first days of life, and no intervention is necessary.

Linear Skull Fracture

Linear skull fractures are relatively common in newborns and are caused by direct compression of the head during a prolonged labor and delivery and use of forceps during delivery. Uncomplicated linear skull fractures are diagnosed by radiographs and require no treatment.

Brachial Plexus Injuries

Brachial plexus injury or palsy is a paralysis involving the muscles of the upper extremity after mechanical trauma to the spinal roots of the fifth cervical (C-5) through the first thoracic (T-1) nerves during birth. Brachial plexus injuries are classified into three types: Erb's or upper arm paralysis (involving C-5 and C-6), Klumpke's or lower arm paralysis (involving C-8 and T-1), and Erb-Klumpke or whole arm paralysis. Most cases of brachial plexus injury follow a prolonged and difficult labor. The infant is frequently of high birth weight, sedated, and hypotonic, rendering the arm vulnerable to separation of bony segments, overstretching, and soft tissue injury (Mangurten, 1992; Scoles, 1992; Shepherd, 1991). Traction on the shoulder during delivery of the head in a breech presentation, and lateral traction of the head and neck while delivering the shoulders in a vertex presentation can injure the C-5 and C-6 roots. More forceful traction may result in paralysis of the whole arm. Forceful elevation and abduction of the arm, stretching the lower plexus under and against the coracoid process of the scapula, may be the cause of the less common Klumpke or lower palsy.

The birth trauma that injures the brachial plexus may also injure the facial nerve or cause fractures of the clavicle or humerus; it may also cause subluxation of the shoulder or torticollis or a hemiparalysis of the diaphragm by injuring the phrenic nerve at C-4.

In most infants with brachial plexus injury, the nerve sheath is torn and the nerve fibers are compressed by hemorrhage and edema. Clinical manifestations include a characteristic arm position of adduction, internal rotation with extension of the elbow, pronation of the forearm, and flexion of the wrist (Fig. 29–6). Passive abduction of the extremity results in it falling limply. The Moro, biceps, and radial reflexes are absent; grasp is intact.

Treatment of brachial plexus injury includes rest for 7 to 10 days after injury to allow hemorrhage and edema to decrease. During this time, partial immobilization is accomplished by positioning the limb gently across the upper abdomen (Volpe, 1987). Physical therapy begins after the initial period of immobilization. The goals of treatment are to maintain range of motion (ROM) by gentle passive exercising, to stimulate muscle function as neural regeneration occurs, and to encourage active movement (Fig. 29–7) (see Shepherd, 1991, for a comprehensive physical therapy assessment and treatment plan). Splinting is controversial, and continuous splinting in the "Statue of Liberty" splint is no longer recommended because it results in formation of abduction contractures and subsequent hypermobility of the shoulder. Intermittent splinting of the wrist and stabilization of the fingers is recommended by some health care professionals for lower arm palsy (Mangurten, 1992).

SPINA BIFIDA

Spina bifida includes a continuum of congenital anomalies of the spine that range from failure of fusion of the posterior vertebral arch or arches to open spinal defects such as myelomeningocele (Edwards & Derechin, 1988) (see Chapter 22 for a full discussion of myelodysplasia). When an open defect is present, early closure of the back lesion is performed during the first 24 to 48 hours after birth to prevent infections such as meningitis and to prevent trauma to the exposed tissue and stretching of the other nerve roots. There are proponents, however, for the delay of sac closure to allow for further assessment of neurologic function, intellectual potential, and extent of complications. These proponents also believe that delaying closure results in improved tolerance of the procedure, allows for

FIGURE 29–6. Four-week-old infant with partial paralysis of right arm as a result of brachial plexus injury. (From Shepherd, RB. Brachial plexus injury. In Campbell, SK [Ed.], Pediatric Neurologic Physical Therapy. New York: Churchill Livingstone, 1991, p. 107.)

FIGURE 29–7. Therapist attempting to elicit activity in the deltoid muscle by encouraging hand-to-face movement. (From Shepherd, RB. Brachial plexus injury. In Campbell, SK [Ed.], Pediatric Neurologic Physical Therapy. New York: Churchill Livingstone, 1991, p. 112.)

better epithelialization of the sac, and permits easier mobilization of skin for closure (Charney et al., 1985). If prophylactic antibiotics are administered during the delay, infection rates are low. The most prudent course seems to be prompt closure after rational decision-making by the parents and physicians (Volpe, 1987). The object of sac closure is to replace the neural tissue into the vertebral canal, cover the spinal defect, and achieve a flat and watertight closure of the sac (Huttenlocher, 1987).

Hydrocephalus is a common complication of myelodysplasia and occurs in approximately 90% of neonates after sac closure. Ventriculoperitoneal shunting is performed when there are clinical or diagnostic signs of hydrocephalus. Clinical signs include full anterior fontanelle and split cranial sutures. Serial computed tomography or ultrasonography are tools used to diagnose hydrocephalus.

Physical Therapy Assessment and Treatment

Physical therapy assessment of the neonate with myelodysplasia in the special care nursery may be done before or after closure of the back or both. This assessment is important to evaluate skeletal alignment, ROM, the level of motor and sensory functioning, reflex development, and behavioral organization. The neonate with myelomeningocele may present with joint deformities as the result of imbalance of muscle action and positioning in utero. Intermittent taping, positioning, ROM exer-

cising, and splinting are techniques used by the physical therapist to treat joint deformities. Intermittent taping is more adaptable to the nursery setting and is reported to be more effective than ROM exercises to improve mobility (Sweeney & Swanson, 1990). A thorough knowledge of arthrokinematic principles and techniques is necessary to position the joint in a corrected position before taping. Skin protection solution is put under the tape, and adhesive removal solution is used when tape is removed. The therapist who performs taping must carefully observe skin condition and vascular tolerance when developing a taping schedule. Positioning may also help to improve or maintain skeletal alignment, such as prone positioning to maintain hip joint ROM. Splinting or serial casting may also be used to improve skeletal alignment (Schneider & Gabriel, 1990).

Range of Motion

ROM testing of the newborn with spina bifida is indicated to identify impairments and, if necessary, to take advantage of the neonatal period of hyperplasticity of ligaments, resulting from transplacental transfer of relaxin and estrogen from the mother (Hensinger, 1977; Sweeney & Swanson, 1990). The therapist must be aware of normal neonatal physiologic flexion of the hips and knees and the possibility of hip dislocation. Because of the latter, it is recommended that hip adduction be tested only to the neutral position. ROM exercises should be performed slowly and gently to avoid fractures of paralyzed lower extremities. Common limitations in muscle extensibility for neonates with spina bifida include tightness of hip flexors, hip adductors, and dorsiflexors or everters of the ankle (Mazur & Menelaus, 1991; Tappit-Emas, 1989). ROM exercises should be done with hands placed close to the joint being moved with a brief hold at the end of the range (Tappit-Emas, 1989).

Manual Muscle Testing

Muscle testing is performed by the physical therapist to determine the level of cord functioning. Obviously, conventional methods of muscle testing are not appropriate for the neonate. Schneider and Gabriel (1990) offer some strategies for determining muscle function that include carefully considering the state of the infant, "tickling," holding the extremities in positions such as hips and knees flexed, and holding a limb in an antigravity position to stimulate the infant to move or hold a limb. Movements of the extremities may be observed, and contractions may be palpated. Gentle resistance may be given to elicit a stronger response (Tappit-Emas, 1989). Muscle strength may be graded as present, absent, or trace. Repeated assessment is recommended to obtain as accurate a picture as possible of muscle function.

Sensory Testing

Sensory testing should be performed when the neonate is in a quiet, awake state. The skin is stroked with a pin or other sharp object to determine the neonate's reaction to pain, such as facial grimacing. The therapist begins at the anal area, the lowest sacral innervation level, and strokes across buttocks, down the posterior thigh and leg, up the anterior surface of the leg and thigh, and across the abdominal musculature to determine reaction to pain (Schneider & Gabriel, 1990). The neonate's response should be recorded for each dermatome.

Reflex and Behavioral Assessment

The physical therapist may also include reflex and behavioral testing such as the Brazelton Neonatal Behavioral Assessment Scale in the evaluation of the neonate with spina bifida (Brazelton, 1984). The purpose of this part of the assessment is to evaluate reflex activity such as sucking and swallowing and to determine the current status of the infant's organization of physiologic response to stress, state control, motor control, and social interaction (Schneider & Gabriel, 1990). The physical therapist notes the strengths as well as the problems the neonate is having. When performing a reflex or behavioral assessment, it is important to ascertain that the neonate's performance is not affected by CNS-depressant drugs.

PAIN

The neonate's ability to perceive pain has become a focus of clinical and research attention (Pigeon, et al., 1989). Previously, it was assumed that the neonate's nervous system functioned at a decorticate level, with insufficient myelinization of pain tracts and centers to perceive, feel, or remember pain (Franck, 1987; Whaley & Wong, 1991). Increased knowledge of the capabilities of the newborn brain and advances in neonatal pharmacology have fostered a concern for the importance of protecting the neonatal CNS from stresses in the NICU environment. Evidence exists that pain pathways, cortical and subcortical centers of pain perception, and neurochemical systems associated with pain transmission and modulation are intact and functional in the neonate. Slow conduction speed is the result of less myelinization, but it is balanced by shorter interneuronal distances traveled by painful nerve impulses (Anand & Hickey, 1987).

Although it is difficult to assess pain in the neonate, the physical therapist working with neonates and infants in the special care nursery should be aware of the methods used to assess pain and be able to perform the nonpharmacologic procedures to alleviate pain. Both physiologic and behavioral responses of the neonate to nociceptive or painful stimuli have been identified. Physiologic manifestations of pain include increased heart rate, blood pressure, and respirations, with evidence of decreased oxygenation. Skin color and character when pain is present include pallor or flushing, diaphoresis, and palmar sweating. Other indicators of pain are increased muscle tone, dilated pupils, and laboratory evidence of metabolic or endocrine changes (Whaley & Wong, 1991). Neonatal behavioral responses to nociceptive input include sustained and intense crying; facial expression of grimaces, furrowed brow, quivering chin, or eyes tightly closed; motor behavior such as limb withdrawal, thrashing, rigidity, flaccidity, and fist clenching; and changes in state (Pigeon et al., 1989). An infant may, however, be experiencing pain when lying quietly with closed eyes (Shapiro, 1989).

Nonpharmacologic methods to alleviate pain include decreasing stimulation, swaddling, nonnutritive sucking, tactile comfort measures, rocking, containment, and music (Franck, 1987; Whaley & Wong, 1991). Morphine and fentanyl are the two most commonly used analgesics in the NICU.

THEORETIC FRAMEWORK FOR NEONATAL PHYSICAL THERAPY

The theoretic basis for neonatal physical therapy may be described in general and specific conceptual frameworks. The general model of the disabling process developed by the National Center for Medical Rehabilitation Research (National Advisory Board on Medical Rehabilitation Research, 1993) describes pathophysiologic condition, impairment, functional limitation, disability, and societal limitation as being the dimensions of a disability. The infant in the special care nursery is at risk for disability that includes the interaction of all of these dimensions. High-risk neonates frequently demonstrate impairments in muscle tone, ROM, elicited reflexes, and automatic postural reactions. Functional limitations may include problems in feeding, visual and auditory responsiveness, and motor abilities, such as head control and movement of hands to mouth. Neonates may also demonstrate limitations such as the inability to breathe and feed by natural means. The combination of pathologic condition such as IVH and seizures and impairments creates for some infants an increased risk of long-term functional limitation or disability. Physical therapy assessment aims to determine the presence of and risk for each of these dimensions. The goal of physical therapy is to prevent or minimize impairment and functional limitations and thereby decrease the risk of long-term disability. Outcome assessment can be done by documenting the attainment of physical therapy goals and objectives through scientific methods such as a single-case study (see Chapter 7; Campbell, 1985; Heriza & Sweeney, 1990a, 1990b).

A theoretic framework more specific to neonatal physical therapy described by Sweeney and Swanson (1990) incorporates concepts of pathokinesiology, neonatal behavioral organization, and crisis intervention. Neonatal behavioral organization concepts of this model are those proposed in Als's "synactive" model of behavioral organization (1986). This model describes a synactive process of the four subsystems of autonomic, motor, state and attentional, and interactive behaviors of the neonate to determine physiologic stability and the organization of motor, state, and interactive function.

The synactive model is useful when trying to determine the risk-benefit ratio as well as the tolerance of a neonate to developmental assessment and intervention procedures. For example, a neonate who reacts to assessment procedures with autonomic and visceral stress signals such as gagging, tremors, or irregular respirations is demonstrating physiologic instability resulting from a negative interaction of subsystems. These reactions indicate a higher risk than benefit from this developmental assessment. The neonate who reacts to the same assessment with smooth respiration, pink color, well-regulated tone, and smooth movements is tolerating the procedure with a beneficial interaction of subsystems. Determination of the risk-benefit ratio and tolerance of the neonate to developmental assessment and intervention is an important part of the theoretic framework proposed by Sweeney and Swanson (1990).

Models, such as the two presented, that address characteristics of the infant and the environment provide a theoretic framework for the development of guidelines for intervention and treatment strategies. These models and guidelines also allow for generation of hypotheses that may be examined through clinical research. Physical therapists who work in special care nurseries should base their intervention strategies on current knowledge of neonatal development and intervention (Fetters, 1986).

The pathophysiologic status associated with the medical conditions described in this chapter has the potential to cause many different interactions of disabling dimensions, including interaction of impairments in posture, movement, skeletal alignment, ROM, state organization, and respiration, with functional limitations and disability associated with developmental delays. The physical therapist who has expertise in neonatal care has much to offer as a member of a developmental team in the prevention and treatment of impairments that occur in high-risk neonates. It has been recommended that physical therapists working in the NICU complete continuing education in neonatal medicine, fetal development, assessment and development in early infancy, parental education, early intervention, and interdisciplinary interaction in the specialized setting of the special care nursery, as well as a supervised preceptorship in such a nursery (Campbell, 1985; Sweeney & Swanson, 1990). Knowledge of current theories of motor control and early motor learning also form important bases for the physical therapy neonatology specialist. For additional information on preparation for providing service in the NICU the reader is referred to the American Physical Therapy Association, Section on Pediatrics, policy statement on competencies for the physical therapist in the NICU (Scull & Dietz, 1989).

Chest Physical Therapy Assessment

Chest physical therapy assessment of an infant in the special care nursery includes observation, inspection, and auscultation (Crane, 1990; Parker, 1985). Observation and inspection include assessing signs of respiratory distress, chest configuration, skin color, breathing patterns, coughing, and sneezing. Signs of respiratory distress include retractions, nasal flaring, expiratory grunting, inspiratory stridor, use of accessory respiratory muscles (manifested by head bobbing), and bulging of intercostal muscles during expiration (Fig. 29–8). Abnormal chest configurations include barrel-shaped chest and pectus excavatum. Cyanosis around lips and mouth is a significant sign of hypoxemia.

Irregularity of respiration is normal in a neonate, and respiratory rates should be counted over a period of 60 seconds. Sneezing is more frequent than coughing, and along with the gag reflex is an airway protective mechanism. Auscultation of the neonatal chest is important for the determination of the type of treatment, the area to be treated, and to

FIGURE 29–8. Observation and scoring of respiratory retractions. (Reproduced with permission from Silverman, WA, & Andersen, DH. Controlled clinical trial of water mist on obstructive respiratory signs: Death rate among premature infants. Pediatrics, *17*:1–10, 1956. Copyright 1956.)

FIGURE 29–9. Auscultation of infant's lungs with neonatal stethoscope. (From Crane, L. Physical therapy for the neonate with respiratory disease. In Irwin, S, & Tecklin, JS [Eds.], Cardiopulmonary Physical Therapy. St. Louis: CV Mosby, 1990, p. 402.)

document the results of bronchial drainage techniques (Fig. 29–9). Nevertheless, auscultation of an infant is a gross assessment because of the thin chest wall, proximity of structures, and easy transmission of sounds. Specific location of the sound does not always correlate to underlying lung segment, and auscultatory findings must be correlated with radiologic evidence. Palpation of the mediastinum and the trachea in the suprasternal notch is performed to ascertain if there is subcutaneous emphysema, edema, or rib fracture (Crane, 1986, 1987, 1990).

Acute Chest Physical Therapy

Chest physical therapy is indicated for RDS, meconium aspiration syndrome, neonatal pneumonia, and BPD (Crane, 1990; Hough, 1991). All these conditions involve problems with airway clearance of secretions. The primary goal of chest physical therapy for neonates and infants in the special care nursery, therefore, is to improve airway clearance and thereby improve ventilation and decrease the work of breathing. Because ill neonates respond to many procedures with hypoxemia and increased oxygen consumption (Long et al., 1980; Yeh et al., 1984), chest physical therapy procedures should be performed only when clearly indicated. The therapist must be constantly aware of the effects of this type of therapy on heart rate, oxygenation, blood pressure, and state control. The chest physical ther-

apy procedures appropriate for infants include positioning, chest percussion, vibration, and airway suctioning.

POSITIONING

Positioning is indicated to enhance ventilation-perfusion ratios and to drain bronchopulmonary segments. The prone position has been shown to have advantageous effects of improving oxygenation, lung compliance, state of alertness, and vital signs, whereas the semierect positions may also improve oxygenation (Martin et al., 1979; Wagoman et al., 1979). Traditional positioning for postural drainage may need to be modified because of precautions and contraindications to certain positions (Table 29–3). For example, the prone position is contraindicated by an untreated tension pneumothorax, and the head-down Trendelenburg position is contraindicated when there is IVH of grades II to IV, acute congestive heart failure, or cor pulmonale (Crane, 1990). The time necessary for effective drainage of a lung area is a minimum of 3 to 5 minutes. Areas of greatest involvement should be treated first.

Chest percussion and vibration are used with postural drainage to facilitate the loosening and movement of secretions and mucus plugs in the conducting airway. Percussion and vibration may be used separately or together, as indicated by the condition and tolerance of the infant. Once again,

TABLE 29-3. PRECAUTIONS AND CONTRAINDICATIONS FOR POSTURAL DRAINAGE IN A NEONATE

Position	Precaution	Contraindication
Prone	Umbilical arterial catheter Continuous positive airway pressure in nose Excessive abdominal distention Abdominal incision Anterior chest tube	Untreated tension pneumothorax
Trendelenburg position (head down)	Distended abdomen SEH/IVH* (grades I and II) Chronic congestive heart failure or cor pulmonale Persistent fetal circulation Cardiac dysrhythmias Apnea and bradycardia Infant exhibiting signs of acute respiratory distress Hydrocephalus Less than 28 weeks' gestational age	Untreated tension pneumothorax Recent tracheoesophageal fistula repair Recent eye or intracranial surgery Intraventricular hemorrhage (grades III and IV) Acute congestive heart failure or cor pulmonale

*Subependymal hemorrhage/intraventricular hemorrhage.
From Crane, L. Physical therapy for the neonate with respiratory disease. In Irwin, S, & Tecklin, JS (Eds.), Cardipulmonary Physical Therapy (2nd ed.). St. Louis: CV Mosby, 1990, p. 406.

there are precautions and contraindications for these techniques (Tables 29-4 and 29-5).

Several hand positions and a variety of devices can be used for percussion. All hand positions use a cupping gesture and include the full hand, four or three fingers, or the thenar and hypothenar eminences (Figs. 29-10 through 29-12). The therapist must avoid percussing over the liver, spleen, and kidneys and limit the areas percussed to within the

TABLE 29-4. PRECAUTIONS AND CONTRAINDICATIONS FOR CHEST PERCUSSION OF A NEONATE

Precautions	Contraindications
Poor condition of skin Coagulopathy Presence of a chest tube Healing thoracic incision Osteoporosis and rickets Persistent fetal circulation Cardiac dysrythmias Apnea and bradycardia Signs of acute respiratory distress Increased irritability during treatment Subcutaneous emphysema Bronchospasm, wheezing, rhonchi Subependymal hemorrhage/intraventricular hemorrhage Prematurity (less than 28 weeks' gestational age)	Intolerance to treatment as indicated by low TcPO$_2$ values Rib fracture Hemoptysis

From Crane, L. Physical therapy for the neonate with respiratory disease. In Irwin, S, & Tecklin, JS (Eds.), Cardiopulmonary Physical Therapy (2nd ed.). St. Louis: CV Mosby, 1990, p. 408.

borders of the lungs (Crane, 1990). Devices used for percussion include baby bottle nipples and small anesthesia masks. Vibration may be administered by manual vibratory motion transmitted through the therapist's fingers to the infant's chest wall or by mechanical vibrators such as an electric toothbrush with padded bristles (Table 29-5).

SUCTIONING

Airway suctioning is usually needed to help the infant clear the secretions loosened by bronchial drainage (Crane, 1987, 1990). Therapists working with infants with pulmonary dysfunction should know how to suction or how to assist. It is recommended that suctioning be done by two caregivers (Crane, 1986, 1990). Deep tracheal suctioning is most effective and safe when performed through an artificial airway such as a nasotracheal or tracheostomy tube (Crane, 1990; Hubbell & Webster, 1986). A recommended procedure for suctioning includes first hyperventilating the infant with a self-inflating bag and then increasing the oxygen concentration by 10 to 20%. The catheter is then wet in sterile saline, inserted with no suction into the airway until resistance is met, and then retracted slightly; the catheter is then slowly turned while being withdrawn, and intermittent suction is applied for 10 seconds.

DEVELOPMENTAL PHYSICAL THERAPY ASSESSMENT

The general purposes of the developmental physical therapy evaluation are to identify the presence or risk of impairment that requires immediate at-

FIGURE 29–10. Chest percussion using three fingers with middle finger tented. (From Crane, L. Physical therapy for the neonate with respiratory disease. In Irwin, S, & Tecklin, JS [Eds.], Cardiopulmonary Physical Therapy. St. Louis: CV Mosby, 1990, p. 411.)

tention and to determine when there is risk of impairment or functional limitation that requires close monitoring. The physical therapist who is a member of an NICU developmental team is most involved with assessment and prevention or treatment of postural, neuromotor, orthopaedic, and feeding impairments. The therapist is also concerned with the assessment of the risk for functional limitations in development and parent–infant attachment. During assessment procedures, the therapist must be aware of signs that the infant

is undergoing stress, such as hypoxemia, excessive increase in heart rate, gagging, choking, and gasping. The therapist may need several brief sessions to fully assess the infant who is medically fragile (Sweeney, 1986). If the infant is too fragile for formal assessment, observation during other procedures may be useful (Als, 1984). Assessment instruments specifically relevant to the needs of the premature infant include the Neurological Assessment of the Preterm and Full-Term Newborn Infant (Dubowitz & Dubowitz, 1981a, 1981b), the Assessment of Premature Infant Behavior (APIB) (Als et al., 1982), the Neonatal Individualized Developmental Care and Assessment Program (NIDCAP) (Als, 1984), and the Neurobehavioral Assessment for Preterm Infants (NAPI) (Korner et al., 1991). Cioni and Prechtl (1990) have also developed a systematic analysis of the quantitative and qualitative characteristics of general movements from sequential videorecordings. Finally, a new assessment tool for infants from 32 weeks' postconceptual age to 3.5 months of age after term, the Test of Infant Motor Performance (TIMP), is under development (Campbell et al., 1993; Kolobe et al., 1992).

Neurological Assessment of the Preterm and Full-Term Newborn Infant

The Neurological Assessment of the Preterm and Full-Term Newborn Infant is a systematic, quickly administered, neurologic and neurobehavioral as-

FIGURE 29–11. Palmar view of three fingers cupped for percussion with middle finger tented. (From Crane, L. Physical therapy for the neonate with respiratory disease. In Irwin, S, & Tecklin, JS [Eds.], Cardiopulmonary Physical Therapy. St. Louis: CV Mosby, 1990, p. 409.)

FIGURE 29–12. Manual chest vibration. (From Crane, L. Physical therapy for the neonate with respiratory disease. In Irwin, S, & Tecklin, JS [Eds.], Cardiopulmonary Physical Therapy. St. Louis: CV Mosby, 1990, p. 412.)

sessment developed by Dubowitz and Dubowitz (1981a, b; Dubowitz, 1988). The test was developed to document changes in neonatal behavior in the preterm infant after birth, to compare preterm neonates with full-term neonates, to detect deviations in neurologic signs, and to document patterns of resolution in neurologic deficits (Sweeney, 1986). The test includes multiple neurobehavioral items of the Brazelton Neonatal Behavioral Assessment Scale (NBAS) (1984) using the six behavioral states. The neurobehavioral items include habituation to light and sound while sleeping, auditory and visual orientation responses, quality and duration of alertness, defensive reaction to cloth over face, peak of excitement, irritability, and consolability.

TABLE 29–5. **PRECAUTIONS AND CONTRAINDICATIONS FOR VIBRATION OF A NEONATE**

Precaution	Contraindications
Increased irritability/crying during treatment	Untreated tension pneumothorax
Persistent fetal circulation	Intolerance to treatment as indicated by low TcPO$_2$ values
Apnea and bradycardia	
	Hemoptysis

From Crane, L. Physical therapy for the neonate with respiratory disease. In Irwin, S, & Tecklin, JS (Eds.), Cardiopulmonary Physical Therapy (2nd ed.). St. Louis: CV Mosby, 1990, p. 408.

The 15 neurologic items were taken from the Clinical Assessment of Gestational Age by Dubowitz and colleagues (1970), the Neurological Examination of the Newborn (Prechtl & Beintema, 1964), and the neurological examination of the full-term infant and the abnormal inventory protocol by Saint-Anne Dargassies (1977). The Neurological Assessment of the Preterm and Full-Term Newborn Infant was tested on more than 500 infants during a 2-year period. The test takes 15 minutes or less to administer. Scoring is done by looking at patterns of response rather than by determining a summary or total score.

In a prospective study of the predictive validity of the Neurological Assessment of the Preterm and Full-Term Newborn Infant, Dubowitz and colleagues (1984) found that 91% of premature infants who were classified as normal at 40 weeks of gestation were normal according to detailed neurologic assessment and the Griffiths Mental Development Scale at 1 year. Sixty-five percent of infants classified as abnormal at 40 weeks' gestation, including those with cerebral palsy, dystonia, global delays, clumsiness, and hearing or visual deficit, were considered abnormal at 1 year.

Although reliability has not been determined, this examination has great potential for physical therapists who work in the NICU because of its brief administration time and systematic method of recording. Caution must be used when administering this assessment because it has been documented that medically stable preterm infants demonstrated an increase in heart rate during and after this examination (Sweeney, 1986).

The Assessment of Premature Infant Behavior

The APIB (Als et al., 1982) is a refinement and extension of the Brazelton NBAS (Brazelton, 1984). The APIB is appropriate for at-risk infants and healthy full-term infants (Als, 1986). The APIB provides an integrated profile of the infant's functioning when varying developmental demands are made. It was designed to structure a comprehensive observation of a preterm infant's autonomic, adaptive, and interactive responses to graded handling and environmental stimuli. This assessment is derived from a synactive theory and is focused on assessing the organization and balance of the infant's physiologic, motor, and behavioral state; attention and interaction; and self-regulating subsystems (Als et al., 1987; Sweeney & Swanson, 1990). It presents graded sequences of increasingly vigorous environmental inputs or packages, moving from distal stimulation during sleep to mild tactile stimulation, to medium stimulation paired with vestibular stimulation (Als, 1986). Items that address social interaction and attention are administered when the infant is in specified behavioral states. This allows identification of tasks that stress the infant and tasks that are tolerable. From these data, developmentally appropriate goals are established as well as supportive strategies to keep the infant stimulated at an appropriate level.

Administration of the APIB is lengthy and may be more appropriate for clinical research than for clinical practice. Specific clinical training with a preceptor is advised to learn to safely and reliably administer, score, and interpret the test. The validity of the APIB has been documented by identification of stable, reproducible behavioral patterns in preterm and full-term infants and by the correlation between behavioral patterns identified by the APIB with electrophysiologic patterns demonstrating hemispheric differences between full-term and preterm infants (Als, 1986).

Neonatal Individualized Developmental Care and Assessment Program

The Neonatal Individualized Developmental Care and Assessment Program (NIDCAP) was developed to provide developmental observation and assessment training for neonatal health care professionals and includes Naturalistic Observation of Newborn Activity (Als, 1984). This involves systematic observation—without the observer manipulating or interacting—of the preterm or full-term infant in the nursery or home during environmental inputs, caregiving routines, and manipulations. A behavior observation check sheet based on the concepts of the APIB includes environmental characteristics such as light, sound, and positioning apparatus and items on respiration, color, motor, state, face, extremity movement, attention, posture, and the response to manipulation. The self-regulatory balance of the infant is recorded, with some of the signs of stress being irregular respirations, color other than pink, tremors, startles and twitches, and visceral signs including spitting up, gagging, hiccoughing, grunting, and gasping. Other signs of stress that can be recorded include flaccidity, frequent extensor movements of extremities, arching, tongue thrusts, finger splaying and fisting, fussing, yawning, and eye averting. Physiologic signs include heart rate below 120 or above 160 beats per minute, respiratory rate below 40 or above 60, and transcutaneous Po_2 below 55 or above 80 mm Hg. Suggestions for caregiving modifications that may reduce stress for the infant are developed from the summary. These suggestions may pertain to lighting, noise level, activity level, bedding, aids to self-regulation, interaction, timing of manipulations, and transition facilitation. Training in the NIDCAP including the observational training and the APIB is conducted in the NICU at Brigham and Women's Hospital in Boston, Massachusetts, and at Wake Medical Center in Raleigh, North Carolina.

The Neurobehavioral Assessment for Preterm Infants

The Neurobehavioral Assessment for Preterm Infants (NAPI) was developed by Korner and colleagues (1991) to assess longitudinally the neurobehavioral development of preterm infants. It assesses the neurobehavioral dimensions of motor development, alertness and orientation, scarf sign, popliteal angle, irritability, percent of asleep ratings, and vigor of crying. Test-retest reliability coefficients for these dimensions range from .60 to .85, and the mean inter-rater reliability is .85.

Quantitative and Qualitative Analysis of General Movement from Sequential Videotapes

Ferrari and colleagues (1990) have developed a method of systematic analysis of qualitative chan-acteristics of general spontaneous movements from sequential videorecordings. These authors used videorecordings to document the early evolution of different types of cerebral palsy in infants with brain lesions. An evaluation sheet is used to describe general movement characteristics such as amplitude, speed, character (cramped or floppy), sequencing, fluency, and subtle distal movements to arrive at a global evaluation. Cramped synchronized movement and lack of fluency and complexity are indicative of the development of cerebral palsy, whereas the occurrence of rotational components superimposed on extension and flexion of the limbs is an indication of normal development.

Test of Infant Motor Performance

The Test of Infant Motor Performance (TIMP) is under development for infants from 32 weeks' postconceptual age to 3.5 months post term (Campbell et al., 1993; Kolobe et al., 1992). The construct underlying the development of this test is postural alignment and selective control necessary for functional movements in early infancy. Spontaneous and elicited movements are assessed with separate subscales. This test is the first designed specifically for use by physical therapists and occupational therapists (see Chapter 1).

Full-Term Infant Assessments

Assessment instruments for at-risk full-term infants include the Neurological Examination of the Full-Term Newborn Infant (Prechtl, 1977), the Neonatal Behavioral Assessment Scale (Brazelton, 1984), and the Neonatal Neurobehavioral Examination (Morgan, 1988). These assessments may be used with preterm infants once they reach 38 weeks' conceptual age, but criteria for scoring are based on the development of full-term infants.

THE NEUROLOGICAL EXAMINATION OF THE FULL-TERM NEWBORN INFANT

The Neurological Examination of the Full-Term Newborn Infant was developed by Prechtl and Beintema to identify abnormal neurologic signs in the newborn period (Prechtl, 1977; Prechtl & Beintema, 1964). This examination was standardized on 1500 neonates who were born at between 38 and 42 weeks' gestational age. Prechtl reported interrater reliability coefficients to be in the range of .80 to .96. The test includes an observation period and a screening examination to determine if the full

30-minute assessment of posture, tone, reflexes, and spontaneous movement is required. Prechtl's examination includes observation of behavioral state changes, threshold of reactions to stimuli, and intensity of responses. Different patterns of findings led Prechtl to identify four clinical syndromes. The comatose syndrome includes absent or minimal arousal to pain or other stimuli and abnormal respiratory patterns. The apathetic syndrome consists of a very high stimulatory threshold for response and frequently occurs before manifestation of the hemisyndrome, which includes three symmetric findings. The hyperexcitable syndrome includes instability of behavioral states, prolonged crying, tremor, hypertonus, increased deep tendon reflexes, and hyperkinesis.

Bierman-van Eedenburg and co-workers (1981) and Njiokiktjien and Kurver (1980) have attempted to analyze the predictive ability of this examination. In the first study a high rate of false-positive findings was reported. In the latter report, the suboptimal group differed significantly on a few of the behavioral and neurologic items when infants were evaluated at 21 to 23 months of age, suggesting that subtle neurologic differences were maintained across time. Harris and Brady (1986) pointed out that these investigators did not examine predictive validity in the true statistical sense through the use of correlation coefficients.

NEONATAL BEHAVIORAL ASSESSMENT SCALE

Brazelton and associates (1984) developed the NBAS to document individual differences in the behavior of full-term infants and to score the infant's available responses and effect on his or her environment (Als, 1977). The NBAS assesses interactive ability, motor behavior, behavioral state organization, and physiologic organization. Interactive ability items include response to auditory and visual animate and inanimate stimuli, consolability, and alertness. Motor items include observation of hand-to-mouth activity, head control during pull-to-sit, response to cloth over face, and reflex items taken from Neurological Examination of the Full-Term Newborn Infant (Prechtl, 1977). Behavioral state items include the infant's ability to cycle through the various states and to habituate to auditory, visual, and tactile stimuli during sleep states. Clusters of behavior indicative of problems with interactive, motor, and organizational behavior have been described (Brazelton et al., 1987). This assessment tool has also been used as a parent teaching intervention and, when used as such, may lead to positive effects in the infant–parent interaction and later cognitive and fine motor development (Francis et al., 1987).

The NBAS has not been formally standardized. Inter-rater reliability has been reported to be .85 to 1.00 (Francis et al., 1987). Recommended training includes viewing a training film that describes the scale, observation of a demonstration examination performed by a certified examiner, practice training in examining at least 20 infants and then determining reliability with a certified examiner to a set criterion for certification (Brazelton et al., 1987). Certification for use of the Brazelton NBAS in research is offered in many university health science centers or university-affiliated child development centers including the Children's Hospital in Boston, Massachusetts.

NEONATAL NEUROBEHAVIORAL EXAMINATION

The Neonatal Neurobehavioral Examination was designed to characterize the various aspects of neurobehavioral aptitude at a given conceptual age with objective, numerical scores (Morgan et al., 1988). The authors stated that a quantitative rather than a qualitative assessment would be valuable in identification of infants at risk for developmental disabilities and would also provide a research tool for evaluating early treatment protocols. The test was constructed from items taken from the work of Brazelton (1984) and Dubowitz and Dubowitz (1981a). The 27 assessment items are organized into sections on tone and motor patterns, primitive reflexes, and behavioral responses. Interestingly, the response decrement items of the Brazelton scale were not included because the authors believed that high-risk infants must habituate themselves to noxious sounds and lights because they are continuously exposed to them in an NICU. A 3-point scoring system is used for each item, with the highest total score being 81 and the lowest possible score being 27.

The test was standardized on 54 healthy full-term infants at 2 days of age and on 298 high-risk infants at 37 to 40 weeks' conceptional age (gestational age at birth plus chronologic age) or at discharge, whichever came first. Scores fell into three clusters for the high-risk infants, which correlated with conceptual age and not with severity of illness or gestational age at birth. No reliability or predictive validity data were reported by the authors.

Oral-Motor Assessment

Oral motor assessment should also be included in the neonatal therapist's repertoire. Two useful

oral-motor assessments are the Neonatal Oral-Motor Assessment Scale (NOMAS) (Braun & Palmer, 1985/1986) and the Nursing Child Assessment Feeding Scale (NCAFS) (Barnard & Eyres, 1979). The NOMAS assesses components of nutritive and nonnutritive sucking. Variables assessed during sucking include rate, rhythmicity, jaw excursion, tongue configuration, and tongue movement. A pilot study determined cutoff scores for oral-motor disorganization and dysfunction. The NCAFS assesses parent–infant feeding interaction and evaluates responsiveness of parents to their infant's cues, signs of distress, and social interaction during feeding.

High-Risk Profiles

Assessment may lead to identification of the infant as having one of three basic high-risk profiles as described by Sweeney and Swanson (1990). These profiles include the irritable hypertonic infant, the lethargic hypotonic infant, and the disorganized infant with fluctuating tone and movement.

The irritable hypertonic infant is often in a state of overstimulation, with poor self-quieting abilities. Extensor patterns of posture and movement predominate, with little antigravity flexion available. Movement is disorganized and tremulous, with poor midline orientation. Feeding is difficult as a result of increased tone in the oral musculature. Visual tracking is also difficult.

The hypotonic infant is lethargic even at feeding time. Crying is weak and of short duration. Hypotonicity is noted in the trunk, intercostal, and neck accessory musculature, with decreased respiratory capacity. An infant who fits this profile demonstrates paucity of movement, weak and uncoordinated sucking, and poor interactive capability.

Sweeney (1986) describes the disorganized infant as demonstrating fluctuating tone and irritability when overstimulated. An infant who fits this profile remains passive when left alone but responds well to swaddling. When calm, the infant interacts and feeds well; but when distracted and overstimulated, the infant becomes hypertonic and irritable.

NEONATAL PHYSICAL THERAPY DEVELOPMENTAL TREATMENT

The goals of physical therapy for neonates may include interventions aimed at reducing impairment, such as improving muscle tone, preventing limitations in ROM, and developing normal movement and postural adaptation; those aimed at preventing functional limitations, such as improving oral-motor control for sucking; and those aimed at promoting cognitive and affective development as well as parent–infant attachment (Campbell, 1985; Sweeney & Swanson, 1990). Parents, primary nurses, and other caregivers should be involved in the development of these goals. Specific intervention strategies, whether direct or by consultation, include modification of the environment, positioning, promotion of normal movement, and modulation of sensory input (e.g., oral-motor stimulation, hydrotherapy, and the use of water mattresses). Parent education regarding the development and input appropriate for neonates is an important aspect of intervention (Gottwald & Thurman, 1990).

The design for an intervention plan should include the establishment of individualized programs based on needs, including the medical status, postconceptional age, and behavioral abilities of each infant. These individualized programs should include the provision of social interaction stimuli during alert periods, avoidance of handling during quiet sleep periods, and immediate termination or alteration of stimulation producing avoidance responses (Campbell, 1985). Avoidance responses include vomiting, sneezing, coughing, hiccoughing, gagging, sighing, respiratory changes, or changes in tone (Als, 1986). While the neonate is in the NICU, the environment should be modified to avoid over-stimulation by decreasing light, noise, and activity levels (Avery & Glass, 1989; Field, 1990). There should be contingent tactile and kinesthetic responses by the caregiver to stress signals by the neonate to alleviate stress, if possible, or to help the infant prepare for, or adapt to, stress-producing stimuli. Once the neonate is moved to a transitional or growing unit, contingent sensorimotor stimulation can be added to the environmental modifications.

Positioning

Positioning has already been mentioned in relation to improving oxygenation. Positioning is also important to promote state organization, stimulate the flexed midline positions typical of the full-term infant, and maintain ROM (Sweeney & Swanson, 1990). The premature infant does not have the opportunity to develop physiologic flexion and may demonstrate hypotonia (Fig. 29–13). The preterm infant must also contend with ventilatory and infusion equipment, which often exaggerates extension of the neck, trunk, and extremities. Hypotonic extended limbs may also be fixed to padded boards to protect intravenous lines (Fetters, 1986). Prolonged hyperextension may lead to neck extensor muscle contracture (Sweeney & Swanson, 1990) (Fig. 29–14).

The prone position, with head in midline and

FIGURE 29–13. Characteristic hypotonic posture with minimal movement against gravity in a premature infant at 4 months of age. (From Sweeney, JK, & Swanson, MW. At-risk neonates and infants: NICU management and follow-ups. In Umphred, DA [Ed.], Neurological Rehabilitation [2nd Ed.]. St. Louis: CV Mosby, 1990, p. 218.)

FIGURE 29–14. Neck hyperextension posture exaggerated by position of the endotracheal tube. (From Sweeney, JK, & Swanson, MW. At-risk neonates and infants: NICU management and follow-ups. In Umphred, DA [Ed.], Neurological Rehabilitation [2nd Ed.]. St. Louis: CV Mosby, 1990, p. 201.)

elevation of the head at 30°, has the beneficial effects of decreasing intracranial pressure, gastroesophageal reflux, and aspiration and increasing stomach emptying (Semmler, 1989; Wolfson et al., 1992). Many different methods are used for placing the infant in prone and side-lying positions, including diaper rolls, sandbags or intravenous bags, customized foam inserts, buntings and nests (Semmler, 1989; Sweeney & Swanson, 1990) (Figs. 29–15 through 29–17). The desired posture includes neck flexion or chin tucking, trunk flexion, shoulder protraction, posterior pelvic tilt, and symmetric flexion of legs. When supine positioning is used, the head is positioned in midline and blanket

FIGURE 29–15. Positioning in flexion using a long blanket roll reinforced by a sand or intravenous bag. (From Sweeney, JK, & Swanson, MW. At-risk neonates and infants: NICU management and follow-up. In Umphred, DA [Ed.], Neurological Rehabilitation [2nd Ed.], St. Louis: CV Mosby, 1990, p. 201.)

FIGURE 29–16. Sidelying positioning to reduce extension posturing. (From Sweeney, JK, & Swanson, MW. At-risk neonates and infants: NICU management and follow-ups. In Umphred, DA [Ed.], Neurological Rehabilitation [2nd Ed.]. St. Louis: CV Mosby, 1990, p. 200.)

rolls may be placed along the infant's sides and under the shoulder girdle for support as well as under the knees. Supported semi-erect positions while the infant is swaddled may also be beneficial to elicit the alert state, head righting, and visual and auditory tracking.

Hammocks and water mattresses are also used in conjunction with positioning. Water mattresses are soft, and the surface intermittantly oscillates, pro-viding gentle vestibular and proprioceptive stimu-lation. Water mattresses have proved effective in decreasing apnea, reducing position-induced head flattening, and improving skin conditions (Deiriggi, 1990; Piecuch, 1988; Sweeney & Swanson, 1990; Taylor & Dalbec, 1989). Positions should be changed throughout the day, especially for infants with respiratory problems involving increased se-cretions (Crane, 1987).

FIGURE 29–17. Use of anterior roll and pacifier promotes flexed position. (From Sweeney, JK, & Swanson, MW. At-risk neonates and infants: NICU management and follow-ups. In Um-phred, DA [Ed.], Neurological Rehabili-tation [2nd Ed.]. St. Louis: CV Mosby, 1990, p. 200.)

Contingent Sensorimotor Stimulation

Psychologists and nurses have studied the effect of supplemental stimulation on weight gain, visual responsiveness, growth, development, and sensorimotor functions (Fetters, 1986; Field, 1980; Heriza, 1989). Most of these studies have involved the relatively healthy premature infant weighing more than 1000 g at birth. Little research has been published on the effects of supplemental stimulation of the sicker, VLBW, or asphyxiated newborn (Campbell, 1985). The majority of supplemental stimulation studies used predetermined, packaged, nonindividualized treatments (Harris et al., 1988). A few studies of sensory stimulation interventions have been individualized and based on behavioral cues from the infant (Als, 1986; Fetters, 1986; Heriza, 1989).

The physical therapy goals of contingent sensorimotor interaction in the special care nursery include improving behavioral organization, facilitating the normal development and integration of sensory systems, and enhancing development of motor behavior and interactive abilities as well as parent–infant attachment. Sensory input must be provided in a graded manner that is contingent on the infant's behavioral cues. Gradual introduction of unimodal sensory stimulation may be necessary at first to allow the infant to maintain state control. Once the infant is able to maintain state control, multimodal stimuli may be used.

The therapist must know how to use various types of techniques to aid the infant's state organization, self-consolation, and orienting, such as encasement, swaddling, and firm tactile input to the soles of the feet. Constant vigilance must be practiced to weigh the costs and benefits of any assessment and intervention. The therapist must be constantly aware of changes in heart rate, blood pressure, and oxygen levels as well as state control or organization changes during and after assessment and intervention.

By using the high-risk infant assessment profiles of Sweeney and Swanson (1990) as a point of reference, it is obvious that different strategies of intervention should be used for infants who fit each profile. The lethargic hypotonic infant needs stimulation to reach the alert state and facilitation of proximal neck and trunk musculature, whereas the hypertonic, irritable infant needs calming to the alert state and inhibition of increased tone.

Als (1986) found that infants who were dependent on a respirator and at high risk for BPD improved self-regulation capabilities after a series of procedures were implemented. These procedures included inhibition through firm tactile input to the soles of the feet, encasement of the infant's trunk and back of the head in the caregiver's hand, the tactile input of a finger to squeeze or suck, and nonnutritive sucking of a finger or a "suckel." By contrast, sensory inputs such as rocking, stroking, and talking were not well tolerated by infants.

Methods of calming an irritable hypertonic infant include swaddling, that is, wrapping the infant in a blanket or using a bunting. If swaddling is done with flexed, midline extremity positioning, there may be facilitation of flexor tone, increased hand-to-mouth awareness, and decreased jittery and disorganized movements. Vestibular stimulation in a horizontal position with the infant swaddled has a calming effect.

Procedures used to promote an alert state include positioning in supported sitting, swaddling, and using a bunting or tactile containment. In the more robust infant, carefully graded, arrhythmic vestibular input, such as quick rocking in the upright position, and light touch may be used for state arousal. Once the alert state is reached and can be maintained, sensory input such as visual or auditory stimuli may be added one at a time and modified as indicated by the infant's response. Visual stimuli include the therapist's face, a black-and-white bull's-eye target, and a red ball. Auditory stimuli include classical instrumental music, calling the infant's name, and a soft rattle (Brazelton et al., 1987; Collino & Kuck, 1991). Once it has been determined that the infant can maintain an alert state and can fixate on an object, visual tracking may be attempted.

Early movement experiences such as hand-to-mouth contact, shoulder protraction and retraction, pelvic tilt, movement of extremities against gravity, and holding of the head in midline may also be facilitated (Campbell, 1985). Hand-to-hand, hand-to-knee, and hand-to-foot activity may also be encouraged to provide tactile stimulation and flexion input.

Oral-Motor Therapy

The infant in the special care nursery often exhibits feeding difficulties related to neurologic immaturity, abnormal muscle tone, depressed oral reflexes, or prolonged use of endotracheal tubes for mechanical ventilation (Sweeney & Swanson, 1990). Decreased tongue mobility, tongue thrusting, poor seal on nipple due to weak lip closure, weak suckling, or hypersensitivity of the oral area may also have a negative impact on feeding (Semmler, 1989).

Nonnutritive sucking should be encouraged early

with the immediate aim of self-consolation and the long-term goal of normal oral-motor development. Achieving a quiet alert state and positioning the infant in supported sitting with semiflexion of the neck may also enhance feeding behavior. Methods of tactile stimulation of facial muscles and intraoral structure and external support to the infants' cheeks have been described (Anderson, 1986; Harris, 1986; Soltesz & Brockway, 1989; Sweeney & Swanson, 1990).

FOLLOW-UP ASSESSMENT AND CARE OF THE SPECIAL CARE NURSERY GRADUATE

Follow-up assessment and care of infants admitted to special care nurseries varies from state to state and with the particular problems or risk factors of each infant. Primary medical follow-up care is usually provided by a community pediatrician in private practice, a hospital, or a community-based organization. An interdisciplinary program such as an early intervention program also provides assessment, monitoring, and direct treatment as well as a support group for parents (Hack, 1992; Leonard, 1988). Results of the assessments of the follow-up clinic and early intervention program will determine if specialized services are necessary beyond the provision of general recommendations for development and parent education. Specialized referral for nutrition, audiology, and ophthalmology needs will also be made if necessary. Since many early intervention programs have waiting lists for physical therapy and occupational therapy, these services may be provided by the community visiting nurse association or other home care agencies.

Most graduates of the special care nursery return periodically to a follow-up clinic affiliated with the level III facility. Clinics vary in their criteria for follow-up care. Follow-up studies have indicated that factors such as birth weight, gestational age, Apgar scores, time on a ventilator, IVH, seizures, and environmental factors such as maternal drug or alcohol use are useful criteria.

The physical therapist has a role in the follow-up care of infants who were admitted to the special care nursery as a team member of the early intervention program, visiting nurse association, or follow-up clinic. As a team member, the therapist plays an important role in the assessment and monitoring of sensorimotor development and pulmonary status with the goals of preventing or decreasing the risk of impairment or functional limitation as well as providing continued parent education and anticipatory guidance (Platzker et

al., 1988; Resnick et al., 1987; Rothberg, 1991; Thom, 1988). Interventions such as positioning, sensory stimulation, and facilitation of movement are also provided when necessary by early intervention programs or community therapists. The therapist also augments parent education to maximize follow-through of intervention strategies and initiates referrals to other professionals when appropriate.

CASE HISTORY

The following hypothetical case history of a neonate with a cluster of problems typically seen in the special care nursery illustrates physical therapy assessment and treatment in the NICU. Several other excellent case histories are available in the literature (Campbell, 1985; Fiterman, 1987; Heriza, 1989).

CASE HISTORY: THOMAS

Thomas was born at 28 weeks' gestation with a birth weight of 1260 g (2 lb, 12.5 oz). Maternal complications included severe preeclampsia and excessive weight gain during the last month of pregnancy. Thomas had Apgar scores of 2 and 5 at 1 and 5 minutes, respectively, and he was blue and limp at birth. He did not respond to bagging and was treated with ventilation for 2 weeks after birth. Perinatal medical problems included asphyxia, RDS, hyperbilirubinemia, and a grade II IVH.

Thomas was referred to physical therapy at 3 weeks' chronologic age because of irritability and hypertonicity. The physical therapist performed a chart review and spoke with the primary nurse before observing Thomas during routine nursing care using the Naturalistic Observation of Newborn Activity (Als, 1984). He demonstrated a low tolerance to handling and was frequently in a state of overstimulation with signs of stress such as irregular respiration, startling, and grunting. The therapist also noted that Thomas's parents visited him daily.

The physical therapist also used the Neurological Assessment of the Preterm and Full-Term Newborn Infant (Dubowitz & Dubowitz, 1981b) because of its ease of administration and scoring and its inclusion of behavioral, movement, muscle tone, and reflex sections. Findings included poor habituation to light and rattle stimuli, with posture and movement that were predominantly in extension, tremulous, and disorganized. The therapist also noted that Thomas showed poor midline orientation and limited antigravity movement into flexion. Visual tracking was impaired, and frequent consoling by the examiner was needed. The therapist also spoke with both parents and found that they were anxious and apprehensive of interacting with their son but were highly invested in him and willing to learn how to respond appropriately to him.

The therapist developed a treatment plan that included swaddling, positioning, and sensory input in response to the infant's cues. Swaddling, or using a bunting with the infant in a flexed, midline extremity position, provided neutral warmth and an organizing effect on state and movement. Positioning Thomas prone with his head elevated 30° promoted the development of flexor tone and posture, decreased intracranial pressure, and maintained ROM. When he was placed supine, a roll inserted under his knees promoted flexion. Use of a hammock facilitated a flexed position, and a water mattress also helped to reduce irritability.

Appropriate sensory inputs included the use of a "suckel" or appropriately sized pacifier along with swaddling, bunting, or hand containment techniques. Stimulation to maintain an alert state included swaddling and gentle vestibular rocking in a horizontal position. Once Thomas was able to maintain an alert state, the therapist began using unimodal stimuli such as the visual stimulus of her face or voice only to engage visual and auditory tracking. She also used a black, white, and red picture to facilitate visual tracking.

The therapist taught many of these techniques to the parents, who became more and more comfortable in interacting with Thomas once they learned how to read his cues (Harrison, 1989). The therapist also recommended several books for the parents to read, including those by Harrison & Kositsky (1983) and Manginello and DiGeronimo (1991).

The therapist was constantly monitoring Thomas's physiologic and state responses to her interaction with him. She also communicated daily with the primary nurse and several times a week with the parents. The therapist continued to treat Thomas when he was transferred to the step-down facility, and she assisted in his discharge planning, which included referrals to a local visiting nurses association and early intervention program, as well as the hospital's premature infant follow-up clinic.

Acknowledgments

Special thanks and acknowledgment are extended to Patricia Carvajal, PT, Rehabilitation Clinical Specialist at Brigham and Women's Hospital, Boston, Massachusetts, for her willingness to share her expertise.

References

Als, H. Neonatal Individualized Developmental Care and Assessment Program (NIDCAP). Boston: Children's Hospital, 1984.

Als, H. A synactive model of neonatal behavioral organization: Framework for the assessment of neurobehavioral develop-ment in the premature infant and for support of infants and parents in the neonatal intensive care environment. Physical and Occupational Therapy in Pediatrics, 6(3/4):3–54, 1986.

Als, H, Lester, BM, & Brazelton, TB. Dynamics of the behavioral organization of the premature infant: A theoretical perspective. In Field, TM (Ed.), Infants Born at Risk. New York: Spectrum Publications, 1987, pp. 173–192.

Als, H, Lester, BM, Tronick, E, & Brazelton, TB. Towards a research instrument for the assessment of preterm infants' behavior (APIB). In Fitzgerald, HE, & Yosman, MW (Eds.), Theory and Research in Behavioral Pediatrics, vol. 1. New York: Plenum Press, 1982, pp. 35–63.

Als, H, Tronick, E, Lester, B, & Brazelton, TB. The Brazelton Neonatal Behavioral Assessment Scale. Journal of Abnormal Psychology, 5:215–231, 1977.

Als, H, Tronick, E, Adamson, L, & Brazelton, TB. The behavior of the full-term yet underweight newborn infant. Developmental Medicine and Child Neurology, 18:590–602, 1976.

Anand, KJ, & Hickey, P. Pain and its effects in the human neonate & fetus. New England Journal of Medicine, 317:1321–1329, 1987.

Anderson, J. Sensory intervention with the preterm infant in the neonatal intensive care unit. American Journal of Occupational Therapy, 40(1):19–26, 1986.

Autti-Rämö, I, & Granström, ML. The effect of intrauterine alcohol exposition in various durations on early cognitive development. Neuropediatrics, 22:203–210, 1991.

Avery, GB, & Glass, P. The gentle nursery: Developmental intervention in the NICU. Journal of Perinatology, 9(2):204–206, 1989.

Aylward, EH, Butz, AM, Hutton, N, Joyner, ML, & Vogelhut, JW. Cognitive and motor development in infants at risk for human immunodeficiency virus. American Journal of Diseases of Children, 146:218–222, 1992.

Bada, HS, Korones, SB, Perry, EH, Arheart, KL, Ray, JD, Pourcyrous, M, Magill, HL, Runyan, W, III, Somes, GW, & Clark, FC. Mean arterial blood pressure changes in premature infants and those at risk for intraventricular hemorrhage. Journal of Pediatrics, 117(4):607–614, 1990.

Bancalari, E. Neonatal chronic lung disease. In Fanaroff, AA, & Martin, RJ (Eds.), Neonatal-Perinatal Medicine: Diseases of the Fetus and Infant. St. Louis: Mosby–Year Book, 1992, pp. 861–875.

Barbour, BG. Alcohol and pregnancy. Journal of Nurse-Midwifery, 35(2):78–85, 1990.

Barnard, KE, & Eyres, SJ. Feeding scale. In Child Health Assessment (DHEW Publication No. HRA 79–25), Hyattsville, MD: U.S. Department of Health, Education, and Welfare, Health Resources Administration, Bureau of Health Manpower, Division of Nursing, 1979.

Bauman, P, & Levine, S. The development of children of drug addicts. International Journal of Addiction, 21(8):849–863, 1986.

Bierman-van Eedenberg, M, Jurgens-van der Zee, AD, & Olinga, AA. Predictive value of neonatal neurological examination: A follow-up study at 18 months. Developmental Medicine and Child Neurology, 2:296–305, 1981.

Boome, RS, & Kaye, JC. Obstetric traction injuries of the brachial plexus. Journal of Bone and Joint Surgery (British), 70:571–576, 1988.

Brann, AW, Jr, & Schwartz, JF. Assessment of neonatal neurologic function. In Fanaroff, AA, & Martin, RJ (Eds.), Neonatal Perinatal Medicine: Diseases of the Fetus and Infant. St. Louis: Mosby–Year Book, 1992a, pp. 691–699.

Brann, AW, Jr, & Schwartz, JF. Birth injury. In Fanaroff, AA, & Martin, RJ (Eds.), Neonatal-Perinatal Medicine: Diseases of the Fetus and Infant. St. Louis: Mosby–Year Book, 1992b, pp. 703–718.

Brann, AW, Jr, & Schwartz, JF. Developmental anomalies and

neuromuscular disorders. In Fanaroff, AA, & Martin, RJ (Eds.), Neonatal-Perinatal Medicine: Diseases of the Fetus and Infant. St. Louis: Mosby–Year Book, 1992c, pp. 734–752.

Brann, AW, Jr, & Schwartz, JF. Birth injury. In Fanaroff, AA, & Martin, RJ (Eds.), Neonatal-Perinatal Medicine: Diseases of the Fetus and Infant. St. Louis: Mosby–Year Book, 1992b, pp. 703–718.

Braun, MA, & Palmer, MM. A pilot study of oral-motor dysfunction in "at-risk" infants. Physical and Occupational Therapy in Pediatrics, 5(4):13–25, Winter 1985/1986.

Brazelton, TB. Neonatal Behavioral Assessment Scale (2nd ed.). Clinics in Developmental Medicine, No. 88. Philadelphia: JB Lippincott, 1984.

Brazelton, TB, Nugent, NK, & Lester, BM. Neonatal Behavioral Assessment Scale. Osofsky, JD (Ed.), Handbook of Infant Development (2nd ed.). New York: John Wiley & Sons, 1987, pp. 780–817.

Budin, P. Le Nourisson. Paris: Octave Doin, 1900. (English translation by Maloney, WJ. The Nursling. London: Caxton Publishing, 1907.)

Cabañas, F, Pellicer, A, Pérez-Higueras, A, Garcia-Alix, A, Roche, C, & Quero, J. Ultrasonographic findings in thalamus and basal ganglia in term asphyxiated infants. Pediatric Neurology, 7:211–215, 1991.

Campbell, SK. Clinical decision making: Management of the neonate with movement dysfunction. In Wolf, SL (Ed.), Clinical Decision Making in Physical Therapy. Philadelphia: FA Davis, 1985, pp. 295–324.

Campbell, SK. Organizational and educational considerations in creating an environment to promote optimal development of high-risk neonates. Physical and Occupational Therapy in Pediatrics, 6(3/4):191–204, 1986.

Campbell, SK, Osten, E, Kolobe, THA, & Fisher, A. Development of the Test of Infant Motor Performance. Physical Medicine and Rehabilitation Clinics of North America, 4(3):541–550, 1993.

Carlo, WA, & Chatburn, RL. Assisted ventilation of the newborn. In Carlo, WA, & Chatburn, RL (Eds.), Neonatal Respiratory Care. Chicago: Year Book Medical Publishers, 1988, pp. 320–346.

Carlo, WA, Martin, RJ, & Fanaroff, AA. Assisted ventilation and the complications of respiratory distress. In Fanaroff, AA, & Martin, RJ (Eds.), Neonatal-Perinatal Medicine: Diseases of the Fetus and Infant. St. Louis: Mosby–Year Book, 1992, pp. 820–833.

Catto-Smith, AG, Yu, VYH, Bajuk, B, Orgill, AA, & Astbury, J. Effect of neonatal periventricular haemorrhage on neurodevelopmental outcome. Archives of Disease in Childhood, 60:8–11, 1985.

Charney, EB, Weller, SC, Sutton, LN, Bruce, DA, & Schut, LB. Management of the newborn with myelomeningocele: Time for a decision-making process. Pediatrics, 75:58–64, 1985.

Chasnoff, IJ. Drug use in pregnancy: Parameters of risk. Pediatric Clinics of North America, 35:1403–1412, 1988.

Cheu, HW, Brown, DR, & Rowe, M. Breath hydrogen excretion as a screening test for the early diagnosis of necrotizing enterocolitis. American Journal of Diseases of Children, 143:156–159, 1989.

Cioni, G, & Prechtl, HFR. Preterm and early postterm motor behaviour in low-risk premature infants. Early Human Development, 23:159–191, 1990.

Coles, CD, Brown, RT, Smith, IE, Platzman, KA, Erickson, S, & Falek, A. Effects of prenatal alcohol exposure at school age. Neurotoxicology and Teratology, 13:357–367, 1991.

Collins, SK, & Kuck, K. Music therapy in the neonatal intensive care unit. Neonatal Network, 9(6):23–26, 1991.

Crane, LD. Cardiorespiratory management of the high-risk neonate: Implications for developmental therapists. Physical and Occupational Therapy in Pediatrics, 6(3/4):255–282, 1986.

Crane, LD. The neonate and child. In Frownfelter, DL (Ed.), Chest Physical Therapy and Pulmonary Rehabilitation (2nd ed.). Chicago: Year Book Medical Publishers, 1987, pp. 666–698.

Crane, LD. Physical therapy for the neonate with respiratory disease. In Irwin, S, & Tecklin, JS (Eds.), Cardiopulmonary Physical Therapy. St. Louis: CV Mosby, 1990, pp. 389–415.

Cressinger, KD, Ryckman, FC, Flake, AW, & Balistreri, WF. Necrotizing enterocolitis. In Fanaroff, AA, & Martin, RJ (Eds.), Neonatal-Perinatal Medicine: Diseases of the Fetus and Infant. St. Louis: Mosby–Year Book, 1992, pp. 1068–1074.

Davis, DD, & Templer, DI. Neurobehavioral functioning in children exposed to narcotics in utero. Addictive Behaviors, 13:275–283, 1988.

Davis, JM, Sinkin, RA, & Aranda, JV. Drug therapy for bronchopulmonary dysplasia. Pediatric Pulmonology, 8:117–125, 1990.

Dean, E. The intensive care unit: Principles and practice of physical therapy. In Frownfelter, DL (Ed.), Chest Physical Therapy and Pulmonary Rehabilitation. Chicago: Year Book Medical Publishers, 1987, pp. 377–442.

Deiriggi, PM. Effects of waterbed flotation on indicators of energy expenditure in preterm infants. Nursing Research, 39:140–146, 1990.

Desmond, MM, & Thurber, SD. Historical perspectives. In Ballard, RA (Ed.), Pediatric Care of the ICN Graduate. Philadelphia: WB Saunders, 1988, pp. 3–11.

Dixon, SD. Effects of transplacental exposure to cocaine and methamphetamine on the neonate (specialty conference). Western Journal of Medicine, 150:436–442, 1989.

Dubowitz, L. Neurologic assessment. In Ballard, RA (Ed.), Pediatric Care of the ICN Graduate. Philadelphia: WB Saunders, 1988, pp. 59–85.

Dubowitz, L, & Dubowitz, V. The Neurological Assessment of the Preterm and Full-Term Newborn Infant. London: William Heinemann Medical Books, 1981a.

Dubowitz, L, & Dubowitz, V. The Neurological Assessment of the Preterm and Full-Term Newborn Infant. Clinics in Developmental Medicine, No. 79. Philadelphia: JB Lippincott, 1981b.

Dubowitz, L, Dubowitz, V, & Goldberg, C. Clinical Assessment of Gestational Age in the Newborn Infant. Journal of Pediatrics, 77:1–10, 1970.

Dubowitz, L, Dubowitz, V, Palmer, PG, Miller, G, Fawer, CL, & Levene, MI. Correlation of neurologic assessment in the preterm newborn infant with outcome at 1 year. Journal of Pediatrics, 105:452–456, 1984.

Edwards, MSB, & Derechin, ME. Neurosurgical problems in the infant. In Ballard, RA (Ed.), Pediatric Care of the ICN Graduate. Philadelphia: WB Saunders, 1988, pp. 196–204.

Fanaroff, AA, & Graven, SN. Perinatal services and resources. In Fanaroff, AA, & Martin, RJ (Eds.), Neonatal-Perinatal Medicine: Diseases of the Fetus and Infant. St. Louis: Mosby–Year Book, 1992, pp. 12–21.

Ferrari, F, Cioni, G, & Prechtl, HFR. Qualitative changes of general movements in preterm infants with brain lesions. Early Human Development, 23:193–231, 1990.

Fetters, L. Sensorimotor management of the high-risk neonate. Physical and Occupational Therapy in Pediatrics, 6(3/4): 217–230, 1986.

Field, T. Supplemental stimulation of preterm neonates. Early Human Development, 4:301–314, 1980.

Field, T. Alleviating stress in newborn infants in the intensive care unit. Clinics in Perinatology, 17(1):1–9, 1990.

Finnegan, L. Management of maternal and neonatal substance abuse problems. National Institute on Drug Abuse Research Monograph Series, 90:177–189, 1988.

Fiterman, C. Physical therapy in the NICU. In Connolly, BH, & Montgomery, PC (Eds.), Therapeutic Exercise in Developmental Disabilities. Chattanooga, TN: Chattanooga Corporation, 1987, pp. 29-41.

Fok, TF, Davies, DP, & Ng, HK. A study of periventricular haemorrhage, post-haemorrhagic ventricular dilatation and periventricular leucomalacia in Chinese preterm infants. Journal of Paediatric Child Health, 26:271-275, 1990.

Francis, PL, Self, PA, & Horowitz, FD. The behavioral assessment of the neonate: An overview. In Osofsky, JD (Ed.), Handbook of Infant Development (2nd ed.). New York: John Wiley & Sons, 1987, pp. 723-779.

Franck, LS. A national survey of the assessment and treatment of pain and agitation in the neonatal intensive care unit. Journal of Gynecological and Neonatal Nursing, Nov/Dec: 387-393, 1987.

Free, T, Russell, F, Mills, B, & Hathaway, D. A descriptive study of infants and toddlers exposed prenatally to substance abuse. Maternal Child Nursing, 15:245-249, 1990.

Gartner, LM, & Lee K-Sun. Unconjugated hyperbilirubinemia. In Fanaroff, AA, & Martin, RJ (Eds.), Neonatal-Perinatal Medicine: Diseases of the Fetus and Infant. St. Louis: Mosby-Year Book, 1992, pp. 1075-1103.

Glass, P, Avery, GB, Siva Subramanian, KN, Keys, MP, Sostek, AM, & Friendly, DS. Effect of bright light in the hospital nursery on the incidence of retinopathy of prematurity. New England Journal of Medicine, 313:401-404, 1985.

Gottfried, AW. Environment of newborn infants in special care units. In Gottfried, AW, & Gaiter, JL (Eds.), Infant Stress Under Intensive Care. Baltimore: University Park Press, 1985, pp. 23-54.

Gottfried, AW, & Hodgman, J. How intensive is newborn intensive care? An environmental analysis. Pediatrics, 74:292-294, 1984.

Gottwald, SR, & Thurman, SK. Parent-infant interaction in neonatal intensive care units: Implications for research and service delivery. Infants and Young Children, 2(3):1-9, 1990.

Hack, M. Follow-up for high-risk neonates. In Fanaroff, AA, & Martin, RJ (Eds.), Neonatal-Perinatal Medicine: Diseases of the Fetus and Infant. St. Louis: Mosby-Year Book, 1992, pp. 753-758.

Harper, RG, & Yoon, JJ. Handbook of Neonatology (2nd ed.). Chicago: Year Book Medical Publishers, 1987.

Harris, MB. Oral-motor management of the high-risk neonate. Physical and Occupational Therapy in Pediatrics, 6(3/4): 231-254, 1986.

Harris, SR, & Brady, DK. Infant neuromotor assessment instruments: A review. Physical and Occupational Therapy in Pediatrics, 6(3/4):121-154, 1986.

Harris, SR, Atwater, SW, & Crowe, TK. Accepted and controversial neuromotor therapies for infants at high risk for cerebral palsy. Journal of Perinatology, 8:3-12, 1988.

Harrison, H, & Kositsky, A. The Premature Baby Book: A Parent's Guide to Coping & Caring in the First Years. New York: St. Martin's Press, 1983.

Harrison, LL. Teaching stimulation strategies to parents of infants at high risk. Maternal Child Nursing, 14:125, 1989.

Hayford, SM, Epps, RP, & Dahl-Regis, M. Behavior and development patterns in children born to heroin-addicted and methadone-addicted mothers. Journal of the National Medical Association, 80:1197-1200, 1988.

Hazinski, MF, & Pacetti, AS. Nursing care of the infant with respiratory disease. In Carlo, WA, & Chatburn, RL (Eds.), Neonatal Respiratory Care. Chicago: Year Book Medical Publishers, 1988, pp. 154-235.

Hensinger, RN. Orthopedic problems of the shoulder & neck. Pediatric Clinics of North America, 24:889, 1977.

Heriza, CB. The neonate with cerebral palsy. In Scully, R, & Barnes, ML (Eds.), Physical Therapy. Philadelphia: JB Lippincott, 1989, pp. 1238-1257.

Heriza, CB, & Sweeney, JK. Effects of NICU intervention of preterm infants: I. Implications for neonatal practice. Infants and Young Children, 2(3):31-47, 1990a.

Heriza, CB, & Sweeney, JK. Effects of NICU intervention on preterm infants: II. Implications for movement research. Infants and Young Children, 2(4):29-41, 1990b.

Hilton, A. The hospital racket: How noisy is your unit? American Journal of Nursing, Jan: 59-61, 1987.

Hodgman, JE. Introduction. In Gottfried, AW, & Gaiter, JL (Eds.), Infant Stress Under Intensive Care. Baltimore: University Park Press, 1985, pp. 1-6.

Hough, A. Physiotherapy in Respiratory Care. San Diego, CA: Singular Publishing, 1991, pp. 194-203.

Hubbell, KM, & Webster, HF. Respiratory management of the neonate. In Streeter, NS (Ed.), High-Risk Neonatal Care. Rockville, MD: Aspen Publications, 1986, pp. 107-162.

Hume, RF, Jr., O'Donnell, KJ, Stanger, CL, Killam, AP, & Gingras, JL. In utero cocaine exposure. Observations of fetal behavioral state may predict neonatal outcome. American Journal of Obstetrics and Gynecology, 161:685-690, 1989.

Huttenlocher, PR. The nervous system. In Behrman RE, Vaughn, VC, & Nelson, WE (Eds.), Nelson Textbook of Pediatrics (13th ed.). Philadelphia: WB Saunders, 1987, pp. 1274-1330.

Kahn-D'Angelo, L. Is the small for gestational age, term infant at risk for developmental delay? Physical and Occupational Therapy in Pediatrics, 7(3):69-73, 1987.

Kennell, JH, & Klaus, MH. Care of the parents. In Carlo, WA, & Chatburn, RL (Eds.), Neonatal Respiratory Care. Chicago: Year Book Medical Publishers, 1988, pp. 212-235.

Kingham, JD. Classification of retinopathy of prematurity. In McPherson, AR, Hittner, HM, & Kretzer, FL (Eds.), Retinopathy and Prematurity. Toronto: BC Decker, 1986, pp. 17-26.

Kleigman, R. Bioethics of the mother, fetus and newborn. In Fanaroff, AA, & Martin, RJ (Eds.), Neonatal-Perinatal Medicine: Diseases of the Fetus and Infant. St. Louis: Mosby-Year Book, 1992, pp. 22-35.

Koeda, T, Suganuma, I, Kohno, Y, Takamatsu, T, & Takeshita, K. MR imaging of spastic diplegia: Comparative study between preterm and term infants. Neuroradiology, 32(3):187-190, 1990.

Kolobe, THA, Campbell, SK, Osten, ET, Girolami, GL & Lenke, M. Development of the Test of Infant Motor Performance (Abstract). Pediatric Physical Therapy, 4:4, 1992.

Korner, AF, Constantinou, J, Dimiceli, S, Brown, BW, Jr., & Thom, VA. Establishing the reliability and developmental validity of a neurobehavioral assessment for preterm infants: A methodological process. Child Development, 62:1200-1208, 1991.

Korones, SB. Disturbance and infants' rest. In Moore, T. (Ed.), Iatrogenic Problems in Neonatal Intensive Care, Report of the 69th Ross Conference on Pediatric Research. Columbus, OH: Ross Laboratories, 1976.

Kretzer, FL, & Hittner, HM. Human retinal development: Relationship to the pathogenesis of retinopathy of prematurity. In McPherson, AR, Hittner, HM, & Kretzer, FL (Eds.), Retinopathy and Prematurity. Toronto: BC Decker, 1986, pp. 27-52.

Leonard, CH. High-risk infant follow-up programs. In Ballard, RA (Ed.), Pediatric Care of the ICN Graduate. Philadelphia: WB Saunders, 1988, pp. 17-23.

Leviton, A, & Paneth, N. White matter damage in preterm newborns: An epidemiologic perspective. Early Human Development, 24:1-22, 1990.

Lewis, KD, Bennett, B, & Schmeder, NH. The care of infants menaced by cocaine abuse. Maternal Child Nursing, 14:324-329, 1989.

Little, RE, Anderson, KW, Ervin, CH, Worthington-Roberts, B, & Clarren, SK. Maternal alcohol use during breast-feeding and infant mental and motor development at one year. New England Journal of Medicine, 321:425-430, 1989.

Long, JG, Philip, AGS, & Lucey, JF. Excessive handling as a cause of hypoxemia. Pediatrics, 65:203–207, 1980.

Lubchenco, LO, Bard, H, Goldman, AL, Coyer, WE, McIntyre, C, & Smith, DM. Newborn intensive care and long-term prognosis. Developmental Medicine and Child Neurology, 16:421–431, 1974.

Luchi, JM, Bennett, FC, & Jackson, JC. Predictors of neurodevelopmental outcome following bronchopulmonary dysplasia. American Journal of Diseases of Children, 145:813–817, 1991.

Manginello, FP, & DiGeronimo, TH. Your Premature Baby. New York: John Wiley & Sons, 1991.

Mangurten, HH. Birth injuries. In Fanaroff, AA, & Martin, RJ (Eds.), Neonatal-Perinatal Medicine: Diseases of the Fetus and Infant. St. Louis: Mosby–Year Book, 1992, pp. 346–371.

Mantovani, JF, & Powers, J. Brain injury in premature infants: Patterns on cranial ultrasound, their relationship to outcome, and the role of developmental intervention in the NICU. Infants and Young Children, 4(2):20–32, 1991.

Martin, RJ, & Fanaroff, AA. The respiratory distress syndrome and its management. In Fanaroff, AA, & Martin, RJ (Eds.), Neonatal-Perinatal Medicine: Diseases of the Fetus and Infant. St. Louis: Mosby–Year Book, 1992, pp. 810–819.

Martin, RJ, Herrell, N, Rubin, D, & Fanaroff, A. Effect of supine and prone positions on arterial oxygen tension in the preterm infant. Pediatrics, 63:528–531, 1979.

Mazur, JM, & Menelaus, MB. Neurologic status of spina bifida patients and the orthopedic surgeon. Clinical Orthopedics, 264:54–64, 1991.

McDonald, AD. Survival and handicap in infants of very low birthweight. Lancet, 2:194–198, 1981.

McMenamin, JB, Shackelford, GD, & Volpe, JJ. Outcome of neonatal intraventricular hemorrhage with periventricular echodense lesions. Annals of Neurology, 15:285–290, 1984.

Medical News & Perspectives. Individualized care, as well as intensive care, may reduce morbidity among premature infants. Journal of the American Medical Association, 264:2611–2614, 1990.

Miller, MJ, & Murrary, GS. Noninvasive diagnostic techniques. In Fanaroff, AA, & Martin, RJ (Eds.), Neonatal-Perinatal Medicine: Diseases of the Fetus and Infant. St. Louis: Mosby–Year Book, 1992, pp. 700–702.

Mizrahi, EM, & Kellaway, P. Characterization and classification of neonatal seizures. Neurology, 37:1837–1844, 1987.

Morgan, AM, Koch, U, Lee, V, & Aldag, J. Neonatal Neurobehavioral Examination. Physical Therapy, 68:1352–1358, 1988.

Moseley, MJ, Thompson, JR, Levene, MI, & Fielder, AR. Effects of nursery illumination on frequency of eyelid opening and state in preterm neonates. Early Human Development, 18:13–26, 1988.

National Advisory Board on Medical Rehabilitation Research. Research Plan for the National Center for Medical Rehabilitation Research (NIH Publication No. 93-3509). Rockville, MD: National Institutes of Health, 1993.

Newman, LF. Social and sensory environment of low birth weight infants in a special care nursery. Journal of Nervous and Mental Disease, 169:448–455, 1981.

Njiokiktjien, C, & Kurver, P. Predictive value of neonatal neurological examination for cerebral function in infancy. Developmental Medicine and Child Neurology, 22:736–747, 1980.

Northway, WH, Jr., Moss, RB, Carlisle, KB, Parker, BR, Popp, RL, Pitlick, PT, Eichler, I, Lamm, RL, & Brown, BW, Jr. Late pulmonary sequelae of bronchopulmonary dysplasia. New England Journal of Medicine, 323:1793–1799, 1990.

Papile, LA. Periventricular-intraventricular hemorrhage. In Fanaroff, AA, & Martin, RJ (Eds.), Neonatal-Perinatal Medicine: Diseases of the Fetus and Infant. St. Louis: Mosby–Year Book, 1992, pp. 719–728.

Papile, L, Munsick-Bruno, G, & Schaefer, A. Relationship of cerebral intraventricular hemorrhage and early childhood neurological handicaps. Journal of Pediatrics, 193:273–277, 1983.

Parker, A. Chest physiotherapy in the neonatal intensive care unit. Physiotherapy, 71(2):63–65, 1985.

Peabody, JL, & Lewis, K. Consequences of newborn intensive care. In Gottfried, AW, & Gaiter, JL (Eds.), Infant Stress Under Intensive Care. Baltimore: University Park Press, 1985, pp. 199–226.

Pelletier, JM, & Palmeri, A. High risk infants. In Clark, PN, & Allen, AS (Eds.), Occupational Therapy for Children. St. Louis: CV Mosby 1985, pp. 292–311.

Perlstein, PH. Physical environment. In Fanaroff, AA, & Martin, RJ (Eds.), Neonatal-Perinatal Medicine: Diseases of the Fetus and Infant. St. Louis: Mosby–Year Book, 1992, pp. 401–419.

Phelps, DL. Retinopathy of prematurity. In Fanaroff, AA, & Martin, RJ (Eds.), Neonatal-Perinatal Medicine: Diseases of the Fetus and Infant. St. Louis: Mosby–Year Book, 1992, pp. 1391–1395.

Piecuch, R. Cosmetics: Skin scars, and residual traces of the ICN. In Ballard, RA (Ed.), Pediatric Care of the ICN Graduate. Philadelphia: WB Saunders, 1988, pp. 50–56.

Pigeon, HM, McGrath, PJ, Lawrence, J, & MacMurray, SB. Nurses' perceptions of pain in the neonatal intensive care unit. Journal of Pain Symptom Management, 4:179–183, 1989.

Pizzi, M, & Hinds-Harris, M. Infants and children with HIV infection: Perspectives in occupational and physical therapy. Physical and Occupational Therapy in Pediatrics, 10(4):103–123, 1990.

Platzker, ACG. Chronic lung disease of infancy. In Ballard, RA (Ed.), Pediatric Care of the ICN Graduate. Philadelphia: WB Saunders, 1988, pp. 129–156.

Platzker, ACG, Lew, CD, Cohen, SR, Thompson, J, Ward, SLD, & Keens, TG. Home care of infants with chronic lung disease. In Ballard, RA (Ed.), Pediatric Care of the ICN Graduate. Philadelphia: WB Saunders, 1988, pp. 289–294.

Prechtl, H. The Neurological Examination of the Full-Term Newborn Infant (2nd ed.). Clinics in Developmental Medicine, No. 63. Philadelphia: JB Lippincott, 1977.

Prechtl, H, & Beintema D. The Neurological Examination of the Newborn Infant. Clinics in Developmental Medicine, No. 12. London: Heinemann Educational Books, 1964.

Resnick, MB, Eyler, FD, Nelson, RM, Eitzman, DV, & Bucciarelli, RL. Developmental intervention for low birth weight infants: Improved early developmental outcome. Pediatrics, 80:68–74, 1987.

Robertson, CM, Etches, PC, Goldson, E, & Kyle, JM. Eight-year school performance, neurodevelopmental, and growth outcome of neonates with bronchopulmonary dysplasia: A comparative study. Pediatrics, 89:365–372, 1991.

Rossetti, LM. High-Risk Infants: Identification, Assessment, and Intervention. Boston: Little, Brown, 1986.

Rothberg, AD, Goodman, M, Jacklin, LA, & Cooper, PA. Six-year follow-up of early physiotherapy intervention in very low birth weight infants. Pediatrics, 88:547–552, 1991.

Saint-Anne Dargassies, S. Neurological Development in the Full-Term and Premature Neonate. New York: Excerpta Mcdica, 1977.

Sarnaik, AP, & Preston, G. The organization of a pediatric critical care service. In Vidyasagar, D, & Sarnaik, AP (Eds.), Neonatal and Pediatric Intensive Care. Littleton, MA: PSG Publishing Co, 1985, pp. 339–344.

Sarnat, HB, & Sarnat, MS. Neonatal encephalopathy following

fetal distress: A clinical and electroencephalographic study. Archives of Neurology, 33:696, 1976.

Schneider, JW, & Gabriel, KL. Congenital spinal cord injury. In Umphred, DA (Ed.), Neurological Rehabilitation (2nd ed). St. Louis: CV Mosby, 1990, pp. 423–484.

Scoles, PV. Neonatal musculoskeletal disorders. In Fanaroff, AA, & Martin, RJ (Eds.), Neonatal-Perinatal Medicine: Diseases of the Fetus and Infant. St. Louis: Mosby–Year Book, 1992, pp. 1396–1403.

Scott, KG, Urbano, JC, & Boussy, CA. Long-term psychoeducational outcome of prenatal substance exposure. Seminars in Perinatology, 15:317–323, 1991.

Scull, S, & Dietz, J. Competencies for the physical therapist in the neonatal intensive care unit (NICU). Pediatric Physical Therapy, 1:11–14, 1989.

Semmler, CJ. A Guide to Care and Management of Very Low Birth Weight Infants: A Team Approach. Tucson, AZ: Therapy Skill Builders, 1989.

Shapiro, C. Pain in the neonate: Assessment and intervention. Neonatal Network, 8(1):7–21, 1989.

Shepherd, RB. Brachial plexus injury. In Campbell, SK (Ed.), Pediatric Neurologic Physical Therapy (2nd ed.). New York: Churchill Livingstone, 1991, pp. 101–130.

Silverman, WA. Incubator-baby side shows. Pediatrics, 64:127–141, 1979.

Sinha, SK, D'Souza, SW, Rivlin, E, & Chiswick, ML. Ischaemic brain lesions diagnosed at birth in preterm infants: Clinical events and developmental outcome. Archives of Disease in Childhood, 65:1017–1020, 1990.

Stjernqvist, K, & Svenningsen, NW. Neurobehavioural development at term of extremely low-birthweight infants. Developmental Medicine and Child Neurology, 32:679–688, 1990.

Stork, EK. Extracorporeal membrane oxygenation. In Fanaroff, AA, & Martin, RJ (Eds.), Neonatal-Perinatal Medicine: Diseases of the Fetus and Infant. St. Louis: Mosby–Year Book, 1992, pp. 876–882.

Streissguth, AP. The behavioral teratology of alcohol: Performance, behavioral, and intellectual deficits in prenatally exposed children. In West, JR (Ed.), Alcohol and Brain Development. New York: Oxford University Press, 1986, pp. 3–44.

Sweeney, JK. Physiologic adaptation of neonates to neurological assessment. Physical and Occupational Therapy in Pediatrics, 6(3/4):155–170, 1986.

Sweeney, JK, & Swanson, MW. At-risk neonates and infants: NICU management and follow-up. In Umphred, DA (Ed.), Neurological Rehabilitation. St. Louis: CV Mosby, 1990, pp. 183–238.

Takashima, S, Mito, T, Houdou, S, & Ando, Y. Relationship between periventricular hemorrhage, leukomalacia and brainstem lesions in prematurely born infants. Brain Development, 11:121–124, 1989.

Tappit-Emas, E. Spina bifida. In Tecklin, JS (Ed.), Pediatric Physical Therapy. Philadelphia: JB Lippincott Company, 1989, pp. 106–140.

Taylor, KJ, & Dalbec, S. Use of a pressure-reducing cushion in a neonatal setting. Journal of Enterostomal Therapy, 16:137, 138, 1989.

Teberg, A, Hodgman, JE, Wu, PYK, & Spears, RL. Recent improvements in outcome for the small premature infant. Clinical Pediatrics, 16:307–313, 1977.

Thom, VA. Physical therapy: Follow-up of the special-care infant. In Ballard, RA (Ed.), Pediatric Care of the ICN Graduate. Philadelphia: WB Saunders, 1988, pp. 86–93.

Thomas, KA. How the NICU environment sounds to a preterm infant. Maternal Child Nursing, 14:249–251, 1989.

Vidyasagar, D. The organization of a neonatal intensive care unit. In Vidyasagar, D, & Sarnaik, AP (Eds.), Neonatal and Pediatric Intensive Care. Littleton, MA: Publishing Sciences Group, 1985, pp. 344–347.

Vohr, BR, Coll, CG, Lobato, D, Yunis, KA, O'Dea, C, & Oh, W. Neurodevelopmental and medical status of low-birthweight survivors of bronchopulmonary dysplasia at 10 to 12 years of age. Developmental Medicine and Child Neurology, 33:690–697, 1991.

Volpe, JJ. Neurology of the Newborn (2nd Ed.). Philadelphia: WB Saunders, 1987.

Wagoman, MJ, Shutack, JG, & Moomjian, AS. Improved oxygenation and lung compliance with prone positioning of neonates. Journal of Pediatrics, 94:787–791, 1979.

Walsh, MC, Carlo, WA, & Miller, MJ. Respiratory diseases of the newborn. In Carlo, WA, & Chatburn, RL (Eds.), Neonatal Respiratory Care. Chicago: Year Book Medical Publishers, 1988, pp. 260–288.

Weibley, TT. Inside the incubator. Maternal Child Nursing, 14:96–100, 1989.

Whaley, LF, & Wong, DL. Nursing Care of Infants and Children (4th ed). St. Louis: Mosby–Year Book, 1991.

White, GL, Jr., Trainor, SF, Kivlin, JD, & Wood, SD. Identification and treatment of retinopathy of prematurity: An update and review. Southern Medical Journal, 84:475–478, 1991.

Wilhelm, IJ. The neurologically suspect neonate. In Campbell, SK (Ed.), Pediatric Neurologic Physical Therapy (2nd ed.). New York: Churchill Livingstone, 1991, pp. 67–100.

Wolfson, MR, Greenspan, JS, Deoras, KS, Allen, JL, & Shaffer, TH. Effect of position on the mechanical interaction between the rib cage and abdomen in preterm infants. Journal of Applied Physiology, 72:1032–1038, 1992.

Yeh, TF, Lilien, LD, Leu, ST, & Pildes, RS. Increased O_2 consumption and energy loss in premature infants following medical care procedures. Biology of the Neonate, 46:157–162, 1984.

Yokochi, K, Aiba, K, Horie, M, Inukai, K, Fujimoto, S, Kodama, M, & Kodama, K. Magnetic resonance imaging in children with spastic diplegia: Correlation with the severity of their motor and mental abnormality. Developmental Medicine and Child Neurology, 33:18–25, 1991.

Chapter 30

Family-Centered Intervention

JOYCE W. SPARLING, PT, OT, PhD
THUBI H.A. KOLOBE, PT, PhD
LINDA EZZELLE, PT, MS

Family members are knowledgeable about the functional performance of their child with special needs. Because research is now providing support for this observation (Bricker & Squires, 1989b; Brooks-Gunn & Lewis, 1979), and the federal government is mandating recognition of the importance of families in the care of children (Public Law 94-142, 1975; Public Law 99-457, 1986; Public Law 102-119, 1991), the role of the developmental therapist continues to be redefined. Not only do therapists require an understanding of the scientific basis of a child's disorder, but they now need to comprehend the scientific sociocultural context within which the child performs. Although therapeutic intervention has been extended to include interaction with the caretaker as well as the child, this interaction is often based on beliefs developed only on the basis of empirical data. Results of the systematic study of families and the interaction process have not been included in physical therapy educational curricula and, therefore, have not been applied by physical therapists in intervention.

Research in allied health fields supports this professional lack of knowledge of families. According to one survey (Cochrane et al., 1990), physical therapists reported that they are not conversant with the scientific basis of practice related to the family. Representatives of 87% of responding entry-level and postprofessional programs believed that they needed further course instruction in family-centered intervention. This result is not unique to the profession of physical therapy but is also characteristic of occupational therapy (Humphry & Link, 1990) and speech and language pathology (Crais & Leonard, 1990). Information has been requested to assist in clarifying parental and therapeutic roles and communication styles, in determining the timing of and strategies to be used in family intervention, and in assessing the context for this intervention. Understanding the issues of contemporary family life, such as stressors related to single-parenting, dual careers, poverty, or cultural diversity, is central to effective interaction with families. Pediatrics instruction requires a reorientation for families and children to benefit fully from intervention.

The purpose of this chapter is to describe the scientific as well as the clinical rationale for assisting therapists in interacting with contemporary families for the benefit of the child. This approach to the child with special needs identifies the family,

Supported in part by the Research and Training Branch of the Maternal and Child Health Bureau, grant 149 and grant MCJ-IL 170590, U.S. Department of Health and Human Services, Health Resources and Services Administration.

including the child, as the unit of health and education (Sparling, 1991a). In this model, the informational, educational, and health needs of the family are addressed in concert with those of the child even though the individual is the "ultimate target" of intervention (U.S. Department of Health and Human Services, 1990). To employ this model, health care professionals are challenged to extend their knowledge base to include research on family interaction, stressors, cultural diversity, and support and to apply their new understanding to intervention with families. Conversely, special educators are challenged to understand more about the child's physical impairment to interact effectively with the family and other members of the intervention team.

Given the changing demographics in the United States, the contemporary family unit is described in this chapter so that the contextual stressors that families and their children may experience can be recognized. Contextual support in terms of the family, community, and society is presented as a mediator of these stressors. An enumeration of physical therapy and caregiver competencies leads into a delineation of the intervention process with contemporary families.

THE CONTEMPORARY FAMILY AND CHANGE

The contemporary family consists of "those significant others who profoundly influence the personal life and health of the individual over an extended period of time" (Sparling & Sekerak, 1992b, p. 71) (Fig. 30–1). Because parents are interactive with their child in utero (Cranley, 1993), this definition applies to families of fetuses as well as neonates, infants, and school-aged children. Efforts to categorize family behaviors and conditions have been depicted in models developed by psychologists and those in related fields. These models assist us in understanding more about family interaction, but most require specialized training for application to a specific family (Ackerman, 1984; Beavers et al., 1985; Epstein et al., 1983; Morris, 1990; Olson, 1986; Reiss, 1981). Some categorize families according to interaction styles and attitudes that are based on a complexity of assumptions related to demographic variables and stressor conditions. These models do not always address the continuum of family characteristics and interactions and the unique ways in which individual families interact with their children at different periods in their life.

Because of the innumerable variables involved in family functioning, each family exhibits a different composite of concerns and needs. To express this point more vividly, the initial physical therapy decision-making process will be described for two families who could be placed in a similar functional category according to Olson's Circumplex Model (Olson, 1986) but who in reality functioned very differently. The Olson model describes 16 types of family systems characterized on dimensions of adaptability and cohesion. Either low or high scores on these two dimensions describe families who function in the extreme. The two children for whom physical therapy was requested for develop-

FIGURE 30–1. A contemporary family consisting of cousins, grandparents, and an uncle.

mental delay were 6 months of age, had no siblings, and lived in a single-parent family that included a maternal grandmother. One family lived in the rural south, while the other lived in the urban north. In both situations the mothers were in their late teens and had dropped out of school before the birth of their sons.

On initial assessment at 6 months of age, Charles was 2 months delayed in gross motor skills, did not explore his environment, and had a "flat" affect. During physical therapy sessions, the mother was quiet and hesitant to interact with the therapist. The grandmother assumed primary responsibility for decision-making regarding Charles. Six weeks after the initiation of physical therapy, Charles' grandmother contacted the home health agency to report the disappearance of Charles and his mother. The grandmother contacted the police and stated that she intended to find her daughter and fight for the custody of her grandson. Approximately 2 weeks after this contact, Charles' mother called the agency and stated that she and her son were living with Charles' father, who was providing emotional and financial support. She requested that their whereabouts not be shared with the grandmother. In addition, the mother requested that home intervention be resumed. During these interventions, both parents were present and were attentive and interactive. After several visits, Charles' mother revealed that as a child she had not had a close relationship with her own mother and characterized her original family by behaviors that Olson might label as "low" in cohesion and "high" on the dimension of adaptability. Her present nuclear family appeared "connected" on cohesion and "structured" on adaptability, placing them in a "balanced" category. After the move, and with support of his father, Charles demonstrated steady progress in the development of gross motor skills, testing within a low normal range at 16 months of age when physical therapy was terminated. At this time, his social progress was dramatic, as evidenced by babbling, laughing, and age-appropriate toy play.

In contrast, Greg's family provided a different developmental context. Greg was referred to and assessed at an urban early intervention center at 6 months of age with a diagnosis of tetralogy of Fallot and developmental delays. Greg lived with his mother, Maria, his uncles, and his grandmother. Since birth, Greg's grandmother reportedly had made most of the decisions regarding his operations and other medical interventions and had accompanied Maria and Greg to the initial evaluation. At the individualized family service plan (IFSP) meeting, Greg's mother attended alone and explained to the team that her mother wanted her to establish relationships with the team and believed that this would not happen if she were present as she had been in the past. Although Maria expressed her developmental goals for

Greg and identified some of the areas with which she needed help, she was often hesitant. After the team reassured her that the IFSP could be changed after she discussed the contents with Greg's grandmother, she became more relaxed. These behaviors suggest that the family was moving from an enmeshed family functioning at one extreme to a more balanced or "flexibly connected" family.

This greater balance was noted during the next 6 months as the grandmother drove Maria and Greg to the center, sometimes participating in the sessions and sometimes dropping them at the center and running errands. During one of the meetings, Greg's grandmother expressed her desire to have her daughter return to school. To make this possible she offered to help look after Greg daily during school hours. The team in turn agreed to schedule one morning appointment every month to enable the grandmother to participate in Greg's therapy session. Maria showed more independence and began to participate in other center activities, such as attending parent groups once a month. In these activities she displayed confidence in managing Greg's needs, while Greg's grandmother and a friend continued to be available to her for support. Nine months later, Greg was enrolled in a child care center for children of teenage mothers who were returning to school and Maria had returned to school and continued to take turns with her mother in bringing Greg to the center.

These young children and their families initially appeared to be similar, could be described or labeled with similar categorical terms, yet were very different. They varied on numerous characteristics, including reciprocity, degrees of dependence, and confidence in making choices. Attempts to categorize these families according to categorical variables, therefore, were thwarted just as are attempts to categorize children with special needs. As complex systems that change over time, families have different structures and developmental histories; as a result, families function differently and require different intervention approaches. According to Brazelton (1982), the success of intervention with a family is directly related to the interventionist's perception of that family as a unique unit.

A model that considers uniqueness and the volatility of contemporary life, yet provides a direction for intervention, has been described by Gottman (1991). This model is based on chaos theory, which has been derived from the application of mathematical equations to the observation of natural events. Rather than types of marital and family systems, Gottman has emphasized change in families. Change can be described as "regulated" or "chaotic." Regulated change occurs in families that experience consistent behavioral cycles or expected patterns of adaptation. When these families move into disequilibrium because of a stressor or group of stressors, they resort to fixed patterns of behavior to return them to equilibrium. Families experiencing chaotic change exhibit behavior that is "deviation amplifying" (p. 259) in that small stressors create major upheavals within the family system. Normative events, which are adapted to in a regulated family, can cause major disruption within a family experiencing chaotic change. The "extreme sensitivity to initial conditions" (p. 259) characterizing families who experience chaotic change, warns the interventionist and provides a perspective regarding the families' extreme response to seemingly insignificant factors. Gottman's interpretation is consistent with the emphasis in current research on family interaction and the amelioration of stress through social support, as intimated in the cases of Charles and Greg.

Research and clinical observation suggest that a family's perception of stressor events and the social support that is available during periods of change interact with a family's typical pattern of response. These factors describe a complexity of behavior that obfuscates attempts to develop simple solutions to family dilemmas and intervention. The confluence of stressors and support in contemporary families defines the uniqueness of each family and demands an individual approach to addressing a family's needs, concerns, and priorities. Bricker (1989) has outlined these factors in a global perspective appropriate for guiding intervention with contemporary families experiencing change themselves and change in relation to their children with special needs. This model (shown in Fig. 30–2)

emphasizes the importance of stressors and social support in early intervention. These factors are central to contemporary intervention within an ecologic perspective. Therapists performing within this perspective emphasize child-oriented goals that will enhance the child's functioning within the current environment (Olson & Kwiatkowski, 1992). The way in which stressors and support interact, therefore, will provide an initial framework for discussion.

FAMILY STRESSORS

All contemporary families experience unique stressors. Families react to these stressors according to the family's perception of them, the number of stressful events they are experiencing simultaneously, the family's resources for managing the stressors, and characteristics of the stressor events themselves (McCubbin & Patterson, 1982). Unlike McCubbin and Patterson, who categorized responses to stress in terms of either good or bad adaptation, Boss (1985) has described outcomes more realistically in terms of a continuum. To study this continuum of adjustment, Petersen and Wikoff (1987) assessed 105 mothers of children with a disability on a combination of home environment and family adjustment variables. Using canonical correlation techniques, the investigators determined that the mere presence of a child with a disability in the family was not sufficient to elicit maladaptation. The number of child-related stressors and the amount and quality of family resources, such as social support, were the most significant variables in the adjustment of the family. This study suggests that the interventionist needs to be aware of the real and perceived stressors and the unique resources or support available to each family unit, because these factors relate to adaptation and to the potential involvement of the family in the health care of the child.

Adaptation appears to be a continuous variable depending on the unique combination of these stressors and resources. Major contemporary stressors are often sociocultural and are related to the structure of families, such as families with single parents and dual careers, to the poverty level of families, or to the developmental transitions experienced by families.

Families with Single Parents

The statistics related to paternal- and maternal-headed families with a single parent describe these families as one of the most common family units

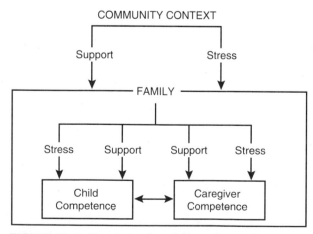

FIGURE 30–2. Transactional model in environmental context. (Redrawn from Bricker DD. Early Intervention for At-Risk and Handicapped Infants, Toddlers, and Preschool Children [2nd ed.]. Palo Alto, CA: VORT Corporation, 1989. Copyright © 1989 Diane D Bricker by permission of VORT Corp.)

with which therapists will interact (U.S. House of Representatives, 1989). The total number of single-parent–headed families in the United States has increased from 9% in the 1960s to 24% in the 1980s (Burns, 1992). This trend exists in other industrialized societies and appears to be related to changes in divorce laws and marriage attitudes. Because of divorce, separation, or a parent having never been married, or being widowed, approximately 50% of children in the United States will at one time or another live in a single-parent family. At least 20% of these family units live in poverty, suggesting an at-risk status for future generations. To meet these challenges, policies to promote further educational opportunities for these parents have been created to alleviate their poverty and enhance their self-esteem. These programs have proven successful (Burns, 1992), but access to them requires availability of child care, which presents a barrier for single parents.

In a review of the United States census data from 1969 to 1972, McHanahan (1983) noted that single mothers experience more chronic life strains, more major life events, and greater withdrawal of social and psychologic supports than their married male counterparts. This study did not report single-male–headed family data because, according to the author, there were so few in the early 1970s. Recent statistics reveal that the number of single-father–headed households in the United States is markedly increasing. The U.S. House of Representatives Report (1989) estimates a 142% increase from 1970 to 1988 in children living with fathers only. This figure suggests that study and concern for male-headed families with a single parent should be supported and problems of single fathers identified (Sparling, 1992a). Hamner (1985) has described some of these problems as loss of self-esteem, loneliness, difficulty in creating meaningful social relations, and extensive role responsibilities, including work and child care.

Other reviews (Sparling, 1991a) document these worrisome trends related to children and their families in the United States and suggest the need for "two-generational" intervention (Smith, 1991) in which the focus is on the caretaker as well as the child. This approach becomes particularly relevant in intervention with children with special needs (Gallagher, Beckman, & Cross, 1983) as well as with families with single parents. Sharing information and facilitating the education of single mothers and siblings may have an impact on the family with a child with a developmental disability in addition to providing direct therapeutic services for the child (Fig. 30–3). The case of John depicts some of the stressors experienced by a single-parent family.

John is a 4-year-old child with sickle cell anemia. He sustained a left cerebrovascular accident and after 3 weeks was discharged from the hospital with home health care referrals for physical therapy, occupational therapy, and speech therapy. John lived with his mother and five siblings, who ranged in age from infancy to 13 years. The family occupied a small four-room home that was poorly lit and without air conditioning. No toys were in the home. The mother was unemployed. At the time of initial assessment, John demonstrated a right hemiplegia and had difficulty in

FIGURE 30–3. A sibling is participating in the intervention program.

understanding speech. He was cruising and taking a few steps with hands held, and he was feeding himself with his left hand. John's mother was concerned with his limitations but was not present during therapy sessions, leaving the older siblings to baby-sit. She did not interact with goal setting or suggestions for home activities. John's brothers and sisters, however, were present during therapy and eager to interact with the physical therapist. Following initial one-on-one activities with John, the therapist interacted with him and his siblings in their yard. Activities included games involving balance, bilateral upper extremity coordination, and unilateral stance. The brothers and sisters were encouraged to participate, were eager to help their brother, and appeared excited with his progress. Requiring little encouragement, they played games with John outside the therapy sessions and were extremely effective in carrying out home activities. Under their tutelage, John made steady progress in gross motor skills, progressing to independent ambulation.

Although John's mother could have been labeled noncompliant, she also could have been in need of respite care, a major problem for single caretakers. In the case of John, some respite care for the mother was achieved effectively by siblings and the therapist, offering support rather than working to achieve compliance with an exercise regimen. With this emphasis, the intervention became appropriate to the needs of the whole family, with John and his siblings learning together. In this family, a potential effect is described of child impairment on siblings' behaviors. This effect has been recorded by Powell and Ogle (1985), who have described strategies for parents to use to promote effective interaction with the siblings of a child with an impairment.

Families with Dual-Career Parents

Families with dual careers as well as single parents are also becoming more prevalent. Dual-career families are a modification of the nuclear family and are characterized by both parents pursuing a career and maintaining a family, often including children (Gilbert, 1985). These families may include part-time workers as well as full-time workers who share family responsibilities. Although having dual careers may enhance financial status and self-esteem, these families also may experience family and work role conflicts, energy depletion, time constraints on the pursuit of interaction and the maintenance of social support systems, and cultural discrepancies related to role responsibilities (Farber, 1988). Evening or weekend meetings and written as well as verbal information may be necessary intervention accommodations for these families. The therapist may become involved in helping to establish household schedules and task responsibilities to fit in needed health-related activities. The identification of support persons with similar interests, the provision of respite care, and the facilitation of role sharing are major mediating variables in the adaptation of these families.

Although they may not perceive their work in terms of careers, families living at the poverty level may also have two working parents and experience many similar stressors. Breslau and associates (1982) conducted a study on the impact of child disability on the participation of women in the labor force. Based on information from 369 families with children with impairments such as cerebral palsy and myelodysplasia and a comparison group of 456 families with children without impairment, these investigators reported a differential effect of the child on labor-force participation according to race and income. Those mothers of two-parent working families with low incomes and who were black were affected the most. They either dropped out of the labor force because of the poor income it provided or the severity of their child's needs or had to work longer hours at a low-paying job to meet their basic survival requirements.

The impact of long work hours on families living in poverty is described by Farran and Ramey (1980) in reporting the results of a longitudinal study with mothers living in poverty and middle-class mothers. Between 6 and 20 months of age, children become more mobile and verbal, placing an added stress on their mothers. During this period, low-income mothers in this study tended to withdraw from interaction while middle-class mothers engaged in more interaction. Results of developmental testing revealed a negative effect on developmental performance of children of the mothers with a low income. Whether withdrawal resulted from increased fatigue related to longer work hours, as suggested by Breslau and associates (1982), is unknown. It does appear that availability of the caretaker for interaction is a major factor in learning. Intervention studies suggest that low-income mothers could benefit from training in ways to access the health care system and develop communication skills (Cosper & Erickson, 1985).

Poverty

An interaction effect exists for families with single parents or two workers and families living in poverty. In 1990, nearly 14% of the total United States population was officially designated as poor, a dramatic increase over the previous 30 years. At present, approximately 40% of our nation's poor are children (Sidel, 1992). In 1959, 23% of those living in poverty were single mothers while, in 1990, nearly 52% of those living in poverty in this country were single-mother families. These conditions are worse for African-American and Latino women. Nearly 74% of poor African-American families are headed by a woman, while 47% of poor Latino families are headed by a woman with no male present (Sidel, 1992). Follow-up data suggest that those children who are vulnerable at birth as a result of poverty and single-parent status are more likely than those not living in these conditions to require special education placement (Goldberg, 1990). When poverty and minority status coincide with motor involvement, structuring appropriate intervention becomes even more complex.

Transitions

Children without developmental delays and their families experience life-cycle transitions that affect child development and family functioning. Children with disabilities and their families experience additional transition challenges. Supreme among these are transitions related to the receipt of services from various agencies in the United States, as described in the provisions of PL 102-119 (Parts H and B) (1991) and PL 94-142 (1975). These agencies vary in philosophy, funding regulation, and staffing patterns, facts that may be the source of confusion and stress for the family (Dunn et al., 1989). Transitions and change related to them create uncertainties and stress and require the assumption of new roles (Turnbull & Turnbull, 1986). Concerns about the appropriateness of a setting, adaptation of the child to the setting, and the child's ability to cope with being separated from the family, making friends, being accepted, and receiving appropriate education and related services all contribute to stress during transitions. Families experiencing contemporary stressors of other types may be particularly vulnerable to changes in service delivery settings, a situation described in the case of Gertrude.

Gertrude is a 14-year-old girl with myelomeningocele and hydrocephalus. She lives with her parents, two older brothers (aged 17 and 15.5 years), and one younger sister (aged 10). Gertrude's mother, Lisa, is a homemaker and the children's primary caregiver. Gertrude is in a special class studying at the ninth grade level. Since 3 months of age, she has been receiving weekly physical therapy in the schools and weekly physical and occupational therapy in a children's reha-

bilitation center. Gertrude ambulates with crutches and bilateral ankle-foot orthoses. Her therapeutic program consists mainly of strengthening and endurance exercises. In addition, the condition of her feet is monitored and adaptive equipment is provided.

Until a year ago, Lisa had been a very capable mother, had a good relationship with Gertrude, was active in the parents' group, and sometimes volunteered at Gertrude's school. When Gertrude graduated from junior high school a year ago, her parents wanted her to be mainstreamed into a regular classroom near her home despite the fact that the school principal and teacher did not believe that Gertrude would benefit from being placed in a regular classroom. During that summer, Gertrude's attitude changed, her relationship with her mother deteriorated, and her interaction with her siblings was minimal. She often refused to come to therapy and walked less. At this time the mother reported behavior problems in Gertrude's younger sister and requested counseling for her. Following several sessions, the psychotherapist on the team requested that all services be temporarily discontinued because the parents were experiencing marital discord, in addition to the crises with Gertrude's siblings. After several sessions with the family and with Gertrude, the psychotherapist reported that Gertrude expressed that she did not want to change schools and lose her friends. Her younger sister, although close to Gertrude, apparently did not want her to come to her school because she thought the other children would make fun of her. After the team agreed that Gertrude would stay at her old school for as long as she wanted, Gertrude's attitude became more positive, her interactions with therapists and her sister improved, and she resumed regular therapy.

Gertrude's situation demonstrates the need for an individualized transition plan for each child and family. Such a specific plan including implementation steps must be described in each child's IFSP. To meet this federal mandate, families need support in developing their own strategies for managing transitions (Turnbull & Turnbull, 1986). The family and child in collaboration with professionals should explore transitional options as early as possible in the process. Some anxiety can be alleviated by giving families appropriate information to come to an understanding about the transition, to allay their fears about making inappropriate decisions, and to assist them in becoming effective advocates for their children. For Gertrude, the professionals overlooked the importance of including siblings and children in decision-making and involving the whole family in the transition process. As the process develops, communication among professionals in various agencies or environments must occur. To facilitate communication, therapists need explicit knowledge of other community agencies, sensitivity to family and community diversities, a belief in the collaborative decision-making process, and time to support and advise families until the child is established in a new program.

Other Stressors

Besides contemporary family stressors related to poverty and family structure, there may be stressors that relate to the frequent cultural and cognitive differences between service providers and service recipients (Kolobe, 1992). An example of these stressors can be found in the survey research of Tellerman and Medio (1988). Of 230 pediatricians of the American Academy of Pediatrics, 68% were influenced positively by mothers who followed pediatric recommendations, 60% were influenced by mothers who communicated clearly, 58% by mothers who kept appointments, and 56% by mothers who understood the recommendations made by the pediatrician. These data indicate that pediatricians are predominantly influenced by mothers who are compliant and who have a certain level of communicative and cognitive skills. If these results can be generalized to therapists, it may be that those families who are unable to communicate effectively with their middle-class therapists, teachers, and physicians may not receive the services intended under the U.S. public laws.

Stressors that relate directly to the daily care of the child with special needs include severity of child disability (Blacher, 1984), home programs, housing barriers and needs, appointments with special services, and sibling responsibilities (Hinojosa, 1990). Factors enabling mothers to adapt to these stressors described by Hinojosa included a father who provided companionship, who understood the stressors the mother was experiencing, and who supported the mother. Therapeutic support for these mothers was provided to such an extent that "instead of expecting compliance with a strict program, therapists could concentrate on assisting mothers with ways to adapt their lives so that they can meet their children's needs with minimal dislocation to themselves" (Hinojosa, 1990, p. 156). Support for family members appears to be an important mediating variable in adaptation, yet generic support is not easily described. The unique constellation of stressors experienced by contemporary families requires a combination of support ranging from financial and intellectual support to social support. Awareness of these dimensions of support for mediating unique stressors could direct therapists in accomplishing more effective intervention.

Cultural Considerations

Each family's perception of stressors and the family's ability to cope, adapt, or access resources are strongly influenced by the family's cultural background. Cultures tend to preserve their value system, particularly through childrearing practices (Brown, 1981). From the first days of life, the parents' caretaking behaviors shape their children into the culture to which they belong (Lynch & Hanson, 1992). Examples of childrearing practices that are influenced by culture are use of visual and auditory stimuli, provision of stimulation to calm an infant, feeding infants on demand, picking infants up when they cry, use of praise and punishment, and expectations regarding self-help (Clark, 1981). Cultural diversity in these childrearing practices may be altered by some of the factors of contemporary families as previously discussed.

The concept of cultural identity must be considered when interacting with families. Families become more or less enculturated as situations demand, and cultural pluralism is a view that is gaining acceptance (Anderson, 1986; Chan, 1990; Green, 1982; Hammer, 1989; Lynch, 1987; Lynch & Hanson, 1992; McGoldrick et al., 1982). Unlike the melting-pot view, cultural pluralism views children and their families as different-but-equal. Some families may practice both the dominant and nondominant cultures (bicultural or multicultural), choose to maintain their cultural roots, or assimilate values of the dominant culture (Green, 1982). These differences are supposed to contribute strength and not weakness to various communities (Green, 1982). Other concepts associated with and often mistaken for culture are ethnicity, minority, and race, but defining culture in terms of ethnicity, race, and minority status overlooks the variations within groups and often results in stereotyping of families (Green, 1982; Lynch & Hanson, 1992; McGoldrick et al., 1982).

Family-centered intervention is a cross-cultural encounter of the culture of the professional and that of the family (Hanson, 1992). This cross-cultural encounter is particularly crucial when one considers the demographics of families in the United States. It is estimated that by the year 2000, 38% of U.S. children younger than 18 will be non-white (Research and Policy Committee of the Committee for Economic Development, 1987). As cited in Hanson (1992), there will be 2.4 million more Latino children, 1.7 million more African-American children, 483,000 more children of other races, and 66,000 more white children than there were in 1985. Also according to Hanson (1992), as of July 1988, 18.5 million of the nearly 64 million children in the United States were younger than the age of 5. Using a conservative estimate of 3%, 555,000 of these 18.5 million children will have identified disabilities. This means that the number of children from nondominant cultures who require services will increase and the programs serving the children and their families will continue to be predominantly staffed by professionals from the dominant culture, resulting in cultural mismatch. According to Green, "it is when individuals confront others with different cultures that a sense of cultural distinctiveness becomes important" (Green, 1982, p. 12). For some contemporary families, intervention services and outcome proposed by professionals from the larger culture may be inconsistent with the family's expectations.

Each family's view about the cause of the disability will influence the choice of intervention. In some cases, professional help (such as early intervention) may be sought as a last resort. The family's definition of criteria for problem resolution has to also be taken into consideration when working with culturally diverse families. Resolution for some families may be when the intervention and the family's understanding of it match (Mead, 1956; Green, 1982; Taft, 1977).

The family of an 18-month-old child, Ricky, with congenital rubella syndrome was referred to a community-based early intervention center. Ricky's mother (Elsa) spoke Spanish only, and his father was bilingual. The child had been receiving intervention at an outpatient center of a large hospital since he was 3 months of age. He received weekly physical therapy and speech therapy as well as other medical interventions. During the evaluation session at the center, Elsa reported that the child had not responded to these treatments and that she did not follow through with home programs because the child was very irritable and often threw up food. Asked if she had communicated her observations to the therapists and physicians she said "no." Asked if she was going to continue with therapy there, she said "yes," because her child needed more therapy. Ricky was very irritable during the arena assessment, even with Elsa handling the child under the directions of the team members. Following the session, the team met with Elsa to discuss the family's major concerns and priorities, to share their observations with Elsa, and to develop an interim IFSP. Because of his irritability and poor sleeping and eating behaviors, home-based intervention was agreed on, with monthly physical, occupational, and speech therapies, and weekly visits by a parent–infant educator. The educator was always accompanied by one of the professionals. At the 3 months review, the team expressed that the child's progress was very slow and too much professional time was expended on the family (the family lived 45 to 60 minutes from the center). A physical therapy consultant

working with the team on family-centered interventions advised the team to focus only on caretaking tasks (which is what was listed by the family as "major concerns") in the child's IFSP. The therapist also recommended that the team select an older, more experienced Mexican-American educator to work with the family for 3 months. The temporary plan was discussed with the family, and they gladly embraced it. By the end of the second month, Ricky had made tremendous progress in all areas of development. His mother was in charge of the home program and chose to discontinue outpatient therapy at the hospital. She initiated introduction of semi-solid and chunky foods and proudly related Ricky's improved sleeping and eating habits, social interactions, and motor abilities to the therapist consultant and the team. She highly praised the parent–infant educator.

What was different about this second situation? Many factors obviously contributed to the success of the intervention, among which may be the facts that 1) the parent–infant educator was from the same ethnic group and country as the parents; 2) the therapists and teacher were European-Americans; 3) none of the therapists and teacher had children of their own; and 4) the parent–infant educator spoke the mother's language and shared some of the mother's cultural values in childrearing practices. The educator, although not a health care professional, helped the mother regain her pride as a mother, as opposed to teaching her activities that her son rejected and that created tension between them and feelings of inadequacy. These services were presented to the family in a way that was culturally acceptable to them.

Culturally sensitive interventions with contemporary families require an awareness of one's individual and professional culture (Lynch & Hanson, 1992). According to the authors, "when we (professionals) are out of touch with our own culture and its influence on us, it is impossible to work effectively with people whose cultures differ from our own. Only when we examine the value, beliefs, and patterns of behavior that are a part of our own cultural identity can we distinguish truth from tradition" (Lynch, 1992, p. 21). Brownlee (1978) suggested that "outside health workers who have poor understanding of their own culture, that of the society where they are working and the differences between them, are likely to give assistance that may actually do more harm than good. . . . When intervention fails, the tendency is to fault the professional's skills and knowledge; seldom is the appropriateness of the intervention for the intended families questioned" (p. 1). Therapists need to be aware of where the power is within each contemporary family; in many families, the father is the decision-maker. When learning about cultures, it is better to seek knowledge from members of that culture because most of the cultural practices are passed on verbally, through modeling and social interactions. Therapists may also consult with professionals from other ethnic and cultural backgrounds who are able to articulate the diverse lifestyles of their communities (Green, 1982). Language can be a barrier to cross-cultural communication, but speaking the same language does not guarantee effective communication (Lynch, 1992). Intervention is a reciprocal process between families and therapists, a process in which both parties teach and learn.

▌ SUPPORT

Social support refers to mutually rewarding personal interactions from which an individual derives feelings of being needed, valued, and esteemed. The need for professional social support has been well documented even before the birth of a child. Professional support offered through prenatal exercise classes has been shown to be related to the amount of medication requested during labor and the request by mothers for breast feeding (Bennett et al., 1985). In an earlier study (Sosa et al., 1980), mothers who had a support person with them during labor had significantly fewer perinatal problems and interacted more with their child after birth than mothers without support.

Social support is a dynamic need of special children and their families that varies throughout the life course. Darling (1979) has described the shift in type of support as the child matures from professional support, to family support, to support from friends. Previous study has suggested that the caretakers of younger children rely on spouse interaction (Flynt et al., 1992) and physician information for support, while caretakers of older children rely more on friends and community members (Darling, 1979). The following situation describes the changing characteristics of support.

Patsy and her husband had three daughters for whom they provided love and support. As the children reached the ages of 7, 9, and 12, Patsy was anxious to have another child in the family. Because of her age and religious beliefs, Patsy decided to adopt a child and became thoroughly involved with a 3-month-old infant who had been subjected to abuse by the infant's biologic family. The infant, Suzanne, became a member of Patsy's family and was included in all family activities. As Suzanne developed, it became clear that she was

visually impaired and severely mentally retarded. Patsy was devoted to her and collaborated effectively with the early intervention teams assigned to the case. In addition to her other disabilities, Suzanne experienced petit mal seizures, so Patsy was in constant attendance, even sleeping in the room with the child. To obtain some respite care, Patsy sought the assistance of her other children, because her husband was not as supportive of these needs. The children were expected to come home after school and care for Suzanne through dinner time. When the father lost his job, Patsy went to work, leaving Suzanne in a child care center during the day and at home with the other children the rest of the day. The responsibility for Suzanne rested as much with her adopted siblings as with her adopted parents. The long-term effects of the provision of support by these siblings are unknown.

In addition to personal support in mediating stressors, support may be financial, intellectual, or religious (Heifitz, 1987). Not only is support offered in different ways and perceived to have different meanings by families, but the theoretical foundation of the concept of support is differentially construed by a variety of professionals. Stewart (1989) describes five social support theories that can be clinically applied and, therefore, are germane to our discussion. Attribution theory relates to motives for helping, the process of gaining or giving support, and the negative as well as positive aspects of support. Coping theory refers to the cognitive aspects of support and its costs to those involved. Equity theory describes the reciprocal nature of support, while loneliness theory emphasizes the affective aspects of support and social-comparison theory addresses the effects of peer support.

Combining these perspectives, Stewart proposes several major concepts to enhance intervention. Health care professionals and persons providing support need to be in agreement about their intervention approach if the intervention is to be effective. Team members need to understand that support can foster adaptation to stress and prevent health disorders and that therapists have a role in understanding the sources of, if not in providing, support. Therapists can ascertain whether their patients have a social network that mediates potential loneliness and ultimately helps in modifying their health problems. According to Stewart, recognition by a health care professional of the reciprocal role of social support may encourage the professional to share information and offer support to decrease the patient's sense of isolation.

The reciprocal nature of support is reminiscent of the transactional approach described in Bricker's model (see Fig. 30-2), in which stressors and the support needed to mediate them are major intervention determinants for the child, caregiver, family, and community. In this model, individual child and caregiver competencies are expressed through a decision-making process. The outcome of this process defines to some large degree the competency of the family as it meets its own and society's demands within a unique community context. To provide intervention without considering these factors diminishes the potential effectiveness of the intervention.

PHYSICAL THERAPY COMPETENCIES

Specific professional competencies are suggested for effective practice by pediatric physical therapists, and specific educational practices are mandated by federal law. According to the literature on professional competencies, physical therapists can and should provide family-centered care (Chiarello et al., 1992; Effgen et al., 1991; Harris, 1990; Kolobe, 1991; Phillips, 1990; Sparling, 1992b). Physical therapists should be able to interpret the results of assessments for parents, consider the family's needs and concerns in establishing short-term and long-term objectives for their child, and work collaboratively in implementing and evaluating these program objectives. The therapist guides families in establishing and prioritizing their health and educational objectives. To adequately support the child and family, the therapist may, and in some cases should, discuss cultural, socioeconomic, ethical, historical, and personal values and attributes of the caretaking family and its membership related to the child. Developing a partnership between professional and parent is a stated competency for pediatric physical therapists and is one that continues to be influential in the family's adaptation process (Featherstone, 1980). Recognition of family stressors and a commitment to facilitating the process of obtaining support to alleviate these stressors is a logical and necessary component of pediatric physical therapy practice. Fundamental to the enactment of these family competencies is an understanding of the laws supporting family-centered intervention as described in Chapters 31 and 33.

CAREGIVER COMPETENCIES

A major component of family-centered intervention is the sharing of information to enhance the decision making process. The physical therapist no longer is the sole decision-maker but is now challenged to empower (Dunst et al., 1989) the parent

FIGURE 30–4. Family-centered intervention allows parents to choose activities that are enjoyed by the whole family.

or other caregivers to collaborate in and even direct the decision-making process (Fig. 30–4). Through this process of learning more about his or her child, the caregiver grows in self-esteem and confidence even to the point of becoming the service coordinator for the child (Lash, 1992). This level of competency describes a caregiver who coordinates services to support the developmental and educational needs of the child. This level of involvement is not appropriate for all parents or caregivers. As in the case of John, some parents will elect not to be involved at all. The appropriateness of variations in involvement for individual family members is in keeping with the intent of the federal law and suggests a continuum rather than a hierarchy of involvement. Components of this continuum are depicted in Figure 30–5. Although this is only a skeleton describing caregiver involvement, use of this model rather than a hierarchic model (Simeonsson & Bailey, 1990) emphasizes that caregivers have a right to select the way in which they will be involved. The model also suggests a responsibility

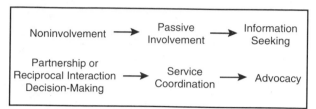

FIGURE 30–5. Continuum of caregiver involvement.

of the caregiver to define the level of his or her own involvement and in this way acts as a contract.

The families we have already discussed fit well within this continuum of involvement. Although initially noninvolved, Charles' parents became partners with the therapist, seeking information and making joint decisions based on that information. John's mother was noninvolved, letting her other children assume therapeutic caretaking. Suzanne's foster mother moved from partnership, to actual service coordination for her child, to advocacy roles, and then returned to more passive or attentive involvement as her daughters assumed caretaker roles. In the case of Ann, presented below, involvement was initiated through the parent's search for information but quickly developed into skilled decision-making on the part of the parent.

Ann was a 9-month-old infant with global developmental delay. A physical therapy referral was made because Ann's mother and the home interventionist noted a delay in gross motor activities. The majority of the initial physical therapy assessment involved observation of Ann playing on the floor. The mother offered information only when requested, appearing polite but uncomfortable with the interview. After the assessment in which Ann was identified to be performing at a 3- to 4-month gross motor level, physical therapy was recommended once a week. The mother stated that she would prefer a visit every other week with sessions coinciding with those of the home interventionist with whom she was familiar. After three visits were made at this frequency, a fourth visit was made by the therapist alone as a result of scheduling difficulties. At this session, the mother noted the improved performance of her child with appropriate handling and asked for a physical therapy session in addition to the usual special education visit. During these sessions, Ann's mother became more interactive, asking questions and offering information, while admitting that she was not likely to carry out formal exercises. The therapist, therefore, showed her simple activities that could be encouraged during play or bath time. By 18 months of age, Ann was taking two to three independent steps and her mother

requested decreasing therapy to monthly visits. These consultative visits were maintained during Ann's transition to a development preschool. According to the involvement continuum, Ann's family revealed confidence in the decision-making process, enabling them with guidance to determine the direction and amount of intervention appropriate for their family situation. Involvement was terminated when a successful transition was made to a preschool setting.

Ann's situation suggests the relationship between caretaker involvement, therapeutic role enactment, and intervention success. The physical therapist enabled the mother to determine her degree and kind of involvement, and thereby the therapist maintained contact with the family over the critical period in the child's development from 9 to 24 months of age. The therapist was flexible and confident in her support of the changing needs of the primary caretaker and family while focusing on the motor development of the child. Whether the family chose to be the designated "service coordinator" for the child is unknown, but independent decision-making was consistent and appeared to be related to the success of the intervention.

THE INTERVENTION PROCESS

Intervention with children who have special needs is determined by federal law and available resources. Within the law, the child with special needs is recognized as a system that is embedded within the larger family, sociocultural, and health care systems. All four systems are characterized by and respond to intrinsic and extrinsic stressors, many of which relate to available resources. The role of the pediatric physical therapist, therefore, is not a simple one and can no longer be a unilateral one with the therapist assessing child needs and providing child treatment. Pediatric physical therapists are challenged to extend their expertise beyond the target child to include factors that we now know have an impact on child outcome. This knowledge, and the law it has helped to create, mandate a different kind of intervention and an even greater professional responsibility than existed previously. Advocacy, collaboration, inclusion, prevention, problem solving, and process are the current by-words related to child intervention. The major steps of this complex process can be outlined in terms of the major intervention areas of assessment, program development, implementation, and evaluation. Although the steps are logical, somewhat inclusive, and supported by law, they will never be enacted exactly as stated, because those who are the focus of the intervention and those enacting the intervention are each different, develop differently, and perform differently. These steps are simply guidelines to encourage continued dialogue about the intervention process and in doing so ultimately elevate the child with special needs to a higher level of function and to an equal status with other members of society.

Eleven major steps of the early intervention process with families are described. Activities within these steps are construed as essential to intervention and at times necessitate that the physical therapist will assume aspects of another discipline's role to provide appropriate and comprehensive intervention. This concept is antithetical to therapists' typical disciplinary training and to cultural emphasis on the rights of the individual. If the maternal and child health goals for the United States as expressed in Healthy Children 2000 (U.S. Department of Health and Human Services, 1990) are to be met, however, and intervention is to be provided to children in the rural and urban areas, then flexibility, adaptability, and accountability must become professional characteristics. The eleven process areas are listed below:

1. Identification of caretakers
2. Determination of caretaker involvement with the child
3. Determination of the appropriate setting and timing for intervention
4. Initial observation of child with the caretaker
5. Assessment of the stressors and support of the child and family
6. Formal assessment of the child
7. Assessment of the community context
8. Development of the IFSP
9. Treatment of the child
10. Evaluation of treatment regimen and caregiver concerns
11. Evaluation of community involvement

Traditionally, physical therapists have competently fulfilled the demands of steps 6 and 9 and informally observed and questioned the family. In response to the increase in results of systematic research related to child and family development, and to the goals for children for the year 2000, the other steps are now suggested as essential intervention concerns that, if not addressed by another team member, must be addressed by the physical therapist. These steps have the potential to assist parents in extending their knowledge of their child's functional ability and to enable therapists to provide more appropriate intervention.

Identification of Caretakers, Their Involvement, and the Intervention Setting. The caretakers of a child are identified before any intervention, thereby emphasizing their importance in the intervention process. No preconceived ideas can be held about the caretaker role, since this role might be filled by foster parents, biologic parents, youthful or aging grandparents, or siblings. In the case of John, the siblings were the major caretakers related to movement development and were the family members with whom the therapist needed to interact. In the case of Ann, the therapist had to review the situation and adjust intervention strategies to meet the needs of a more independent caretaker.

Determination of Caretaker Involvement with the Child. Caretaker involvement has been a major concern since 1975 with the enactment in the United States of Public Law 94-142 and its mandated opportunity for caretaker involvement in intervention with his or her children. A continuum of involvement already has been described (see Fig. 30-5) to emphasize the various needs of caregivers. An understanding that all caregivers do not want to, or cannot, participate directly in the care of their child can be determined through sensitive contextual observation and caregiver interview. Determination of the family's involvement with the child must be undertaken only with the family's permission. Awareness of the conditions of intervention may facilitate a successful initial contact and extend future interaction with the family and the child.

Professional involvement is another concern. To conduct a comprehensive assessment and develop an appropriate intervention plan for the child, best practice dictates a team approach. According to Dunn and colleagues (1989), a team can consist of only a therapist and a caretaker. Ideally, the makeup of a team should reflect the unique needs of each family. Further information on team models can be found in Chapters 18 and 31.

Determination of the Appropriate Setting and Timing for Intervention. Having identified the person or family members with whom intervention will occur, and the amount of involvement, the time and setting for assessment and intervention will in most cases be automatically achieved. In the case of John, the major setting was the playground with the siblings. With Ann, the setting was initially the home whenever the special educator was present. The setting changed and became the preschool in which Ann was enrolled. In the following case, the setting was determined by family needs to include the father.

The college-educated parents of a 4-week-old girl with Down syndrome were referred for consultation because the Parents and Children Together (PACT) interventionist had a waiting list for initial assessment. A variety of times for meeting were offered the mother, but having just moved to town she had difficulty obtaining babysitting for her other young child. When an evening appointment in the home was suggested, the mother was immediately enthusiastic, saying she wanted her husband involved and this would permit him to be present at the initial consultative meeting.

The family was in the initial stages of adaptation. They had chosen not to have prenatal assessment and then been informed in the neonatal period that they had a child with Down syndrome. The family's immediate need was for information about the impairment, early intervention and its long-term benefits, and future therapeutic demands and school placement for the two children. The home with the father present was the most efficient and supportive setting. Meeting the setting and scheduling needs of the family permitted the initiation of joint family-therapist decision-making related to the child.

The setting of the initial interview may determine the future success of intervention. In the ideal situation, the setting most convenient for the family should be selected and should take into consideration family stressors such as babysitting needs, as well as the potential for obtaining a child's optimal performance. Intervention settings may be mandated by the child's age and may include prenatal exercise classes, home, pediatric follow-up clinic, or preschool. Appropriateness for the family as well as efficiency should dictate the selection of the initial setting. Although cost and safety are involved in determination of intervention setting, initial interaction is appropriate and cost-effective in the family-selected setting for children who are developmentally delayed (Schraeder et al., 1990) or have a chronic health problem (Larson, 1980). Evaluation in the home may provide additional information for developing an intervention plan. Type of floor surface, limited space, and curbs and steps may need to be considered as barriers to the use of adaptive equipment and wheelchairs and need to be addressed in the IFSP.

Initial Observation of Child with the Caregiver. The parable of three youths and their transition from scholarly to clinical wisdom, as paraphrased by Patton (1990), is particularly applicable to the belief in the expenditure of clinical time devoted to observation and interview.

Three youths were sent into the world for six months to observe human interactions. Upon returning to their mentor after six months, the youths reported on their observations. The first youth stated that he learned that all people behave the same: they come to the market place, conduct business and pleasurable interactions and leave. The second youth stated that he understood that life was simple in its organization: all people were in search of the basic necessities of life and their activities reflected this search. The third youth reported that he was uncertain in his knowledge: he kept wondering about the people he saw, where they came from, where they were going and why, and what they were trying to achieve. In reporting this information, he believed he had failed in his observation of the human condition. Instead, his mentor informed him that he had learned the most of the three youths. In observing and asking questions about his observations, he had learned the most about the meaning of another person's experience (Patton, 1990, pp. 277–278).

The approach used by the third youth is suggested as appropriate in the therapeutic intervention with families. By presenting themselves to families first as understanding listeners and keen observers of their child's functional activities, therapists communicate to the caregivers the fact that their concerns are central to intervention.

Effective interaction with the family unit in a therapeutic context is characterized by the ability to observe in an unbiased manner, ask pertinent questions, and listen. Observation is a well-developed skill of therapists, a skill that needs to be extended to include the observation of interactions and their effect on the developing child. Farran and colleagues (1986) have developed an assessment of the caregivers' involvement with their child. Learning the components of the assessment through the film that accompanies it and practicing its use can facilitate the therapist's awareness and knowledge of interaction elements.

Through attention to the caregivers' comments and questions, the therapist can identify concerns while observing the spontaneous behavior of the child, a process that conserves rather than expends time. In the home interview with the parents of the 4-week-old infant with Down syndrome, the child's age-appropriate patterns of movement and posture were noted in her initial antigravity neck flexion, homolateral reaching and arm extension, initial attempts at moving from prone to sidelying, and difficulty with tongue retraction. A reciprocal exchange of sounds with the father was so powerful that the sibling, mother, and therapist felt a momentary exclusion and at the same time a respect for the child's and father's interactive ability. Their enjoyment and skill in interaction suggested a technique to enhance intervention.

Determination of some unique needs of members of the family can also be accomplished during the initial interview. At the end of the interaction, these concerns can be summarized and prioritized, but initially the concerns need expression without imposing an order on them. In the hour-long interview with the family of the child with Down syndrome, the need for the father to take a time-out from the interview and from the realities of his new responsibilities was clear and was afforded him by the changing of diapers. The need of the mother for specific information was identified by her questions about the process of motor development. Essential stressors and resources for managing them were observed by the therapist but not verbalized by the family.

Previous research has suggested the prenatal period as a time of adaptation with prenatal exercise classes (Cranley, 1993) or high-risk clinics (Sparling et al., 1988) offering initial support and an opportunity to develop rapport between therapist and parent before the needed attendance to the child's needs in the neonatal period. Postnatal interaction with a first-time parent must take into consideration that the parents' expectations of a normal child have not been met. Cowan and co-workers (1991) have identified five domains critical in facilitating the adaptation to parenthood. These areas include assessment of each individual in the family, parental relationships especially related to communication and division of labor, caregiver relationship with the child, intergenerational relationships, and relationships with other family and community members. This perspective is consistent with the ecologic view that is fundamental to family-centered intervention. The long-term benefits that accrue from the therapeutic understanding of the milieu of the child can be dramatic, albeit time consuming.

The interview process related to early intervention has been described by several authors (Patton, 1990; Sullivan, 1970; Winton & Bailey, 1988). Depending on the designation of the service coordinator, who may be the caretaker (Lash, 1992) or even the therapist, the physical therapist may be in a position to conduct initial interviewing. This potential suggests that each therapist should gain an understanding of and experience in interviewing family members to develop skill in ascertaining their changing concerns and needs.

Specific behaviors essential to effective interviewing have been identified by Winton and Blow (1991). These include nonverbal behaviors such as the maintenance of eye contact, attempts to elicit and explore parental concerns and interests, questions and comments that are nonjudgmental and understandable, provision of relevant and well-timed information, and attention to parental solutions and strategies. The way in which questions are asked can determine the information obtained. Winton and Bailey (1988) have described three major types of questions, each of which can be used to obtain different kinds of information. One type is the linear question that is used to obtain specific information or a "yes" or "no" response. A second type is an open-ended question that is used to facilitate elaboration on an issue. A third type is circular, in which every response facilitates or dictates an additional response. At times the therapeutic use of silence is more helpful than questioning. Realini and associates (1992) have developed a scale to assess the use of silence in a medical interview. This tool is extremely helpful in recognizing the importance of silence and the ways in which silence can be used to enhance the therapeutic interview.

Observation of interactive skills and asking questions to learn of family concerns and needs are skills seldom taught in therapeutic programs. Listening to the concerns of the caretaker and, when indicated, to other family members becomes a major role of the contemporary developmental therapist. Therapeutic agendas may be more readily accepted by the caregiver if the agendas are responsive to the unique concerns and characteristics of the family as well as the child.

Assessment of the Stressors and Support of the Child and Family. A 10-step caretaker decision tree has been outlined to assist with infant intervention (Sparling, 1992b). The steps in this approach, shown in Figure 30–6, could be duplicated with caretakers of toddlers and school-aged children. The process consists of asking questions about the family unit. These questions may be asked directly of the caretakers or may act as thought questions for the therapist. For example, question 3 asks,

Question 1	Does this at-risk child need assessment?
Question 2	Does the family choose to be involved?
Question 3	Are you concerned about family membership and intergenerational factors?
Question 4	Are you concerned with family routines, roles, and resources?
Question 5	Are you concerned about family environments?
Question 6	Are you concerned about family characteristics basic to interaction?
Question 7	Are you concerned about family/child behaviors in interaction?
Question 8	Are you concerned about motor behaviors as yet unobserved?
Question 9	Are you concerned about mediating variables?
Question 10	Are you concerned about changes in these behaviors over time?

FIGURE 30–6. Decision making model for therapists during initial parent interview. (From Sparling, JW. Assessment of family resources and needs. In Wilhelm, IJ [Ed.], Physical Therapy Assessment in Early Infancy. New York, Churchill Livingstone, 1993, pp. 71–104.)

"Are you concerned about family membership and intergenerational factors?" If the response is yes, the therapist might interview the parent in more detail using the genogram (Hartman, 1978). The genogram is a depiction of three generations of family members, including gender, health problems, and other significant data related to the child and family. This specific approach proved extremely helpful with a child with infantile autism and his single mother. Interview of the single mother from 32 weeks of gestation when maternal diabetes was diagnosed to the child's fourth birthday enabled the mother to gain support while the physician and therapist gained information relative to a potential genetic component of the child's diagnosis (Sparling, 1991b). Knowledge of the father's lineage and its potential effect on her son was one of the many stressors she had been experiencing during the adaptation to her son's disorder. An open-ended question related to this factor permitted a discussion of the inadequate support the mother was now receiving from relatives because of this factor and enabled her to address an additional need for community support in terms of preschool placement. Assessment of the family's stressors and support is undertaken only with the family's permission and participation.

Although assessment of stressors and support is not the focus of the physical therapist's education, these "avenues of influence" (Humphrey, 1989) often have a direct impact on the motor performance of the child. In this case, the mother had dreamed of having a son who would be a professional football player. Having been thwarted in this dream, she was initially reluctant to be involved in establishing a motor program for her child. Sharing the dimensions and need for such a program could only be addressed after she had expressed her own concerns and needs for support.

Numerous family-oriented assessments measure aspects of social support. Through assessment of support, the therapist can determine specific areas that are stressful for the caretaker. Berrera (1981) has developed the 40-item Inventory of Socially Supportive Behaviors (ISSB). Although this assessment has been responded to by pregnant adolescents, it is applicable to other populations. The assessment describes the supportive behavior, requests how often the behavior has been performed for the individual in the last week, and then asks who provided the support. By using this assessment, the extent of support for the individual or family can be readily determined.

The Family Routines Inventory (Gallagher et al., 1983) can be conducted as a family interview. Family members can score it separately, or it can be used as the focus of a family interview. Determin-

ing caretakers' perceptions of family roles and responsibilities relates directly to the balance of work assumed by family members and to the perceived dimensions of caregiving in the family.

The Family Needs Survey (Bailey & Simeonsson, 1988) includes eight items related to social support. In assessing 34 two-parent families receiving home-based intervention services with this survey, the authors found that 74% of the mothers and 50% of the fathers wanted information about other parents who had a child with a similar condition to their child. Although over 60% of mothers wanted to communicate with these parents, only 27% of the fathers wanted to pursue interaction with these parents. At times, a brief assessment such as this may help the therapist to clarify unique family needs or the readiness for interaction of individual family members.

Formal Assessment of the Child in a Community Context. The child's initial assessment provides a window through which professionals gain an understanding of the child's developmental abilities and needs. In family-centered intervention, professionals and the family negotiate and agree on the type of assessment, the format of assessment, and the location and time of assessment (Leviton et al., 1992). In addition, most states require that at least one developmental test, which includes all areas of development, be used for every child during the initial assessment, to determine the child's functional levels. Therapists have to be competent, therefore, in the administration and scoring of tests required by their states.

Assessment of the child's physical abilities must be expanded to include three levels of functioning. Level I describes the assessment of impairment that includes the child's motor control during movement, passive and active range of motion, amount of force created by specific muscles, sensory perception, and biomechanical alignment of the body during movement and static postures. Level II describes the assessment of function that may include attributes such as the child's ability to perform purposeful transitional movements and the child's endurance and speed and energy requirements in performing age-appropriate gross motor activities. Level III describes the assessment of the child's environment that may include factors related to family interaction and the community in which the family resides. In family-centered assessment, the therapist extends the evaluation beyond level II to include the extent to which motor skills exhibited by the child foster or hinder caregiving or limit the child's ability to integrate into environments in which children without disabilities develop and function. In addition, assessment helps to determine the activities the child enjoys, the way these activities fit into the family's interaction patterns and daily life, and potential benefits the child can gain from other community resources such as a swimming program or gymnastic program at the local YMCA. The therapist, therefore, must be knowledgeable about community resources available to children.

One type of assessment that is consistent with family-centered intervention is arena assessment. This approach permits professionals and caretakers to observe the spontaneous behavior of the child under different situations and is consistent with the transdisciplinary approach (Linder, 1990). In the arena assessment model, a facilitator may serve as a primary tester while other members of the team observe and score discipline-specific aspects of the assessment (Wolery & Dyk, 1984). The physical therapist is expected to assess sensorimotor areas and may serve as a facilitator of the assessment, depending on the child's primary area of need. Other members of the team may assist the facilitator during the assessment. Parents may also serve as facilitators, particularly if the child is hesitant to participate in the process.

The arena model has been rated by parents as superior to assessment within the interdisciplinary model (Wolery & Dyk, 1984). In a study comparing these two approaches to assessment, the majority of the parents rated the arena model as more thorough and accurate in describing their child's abilities and as less time consuming than assessment within the interdisciplinary approach. Professionals rated the arena model as more effective, more conducive to team interaction, and more appropriate for small children and all children with severe disabilities than for older children with mild disabilities. Professionals rated both approaches as equal in efficiency.

Advantages of the arena model have been summarized by Wolery and Dyk (1984). They include reduction of the number of professionals handling the child, reduction of redundant testing and parent questioning, provision of a more holistic view of the child, increase in team interaction and learning, greater consensus on the outcome of the assessment than when each discipline tests the child independently, and decrease in child fatigue. The arena approach requires active observation by all team members, provides an opportunity for a team member to clarify test items or child responses for the family members, and permits the family to administer items to achieve the child's best response. More detailed qualitative assessment of the child's functional status or control of movement and posture can be obtained through additional observation or standardized assessment as described for infants by Wilhelm (1992), in Chapters 1 and 2,

and in chapters on specific impairments in disabling conditions in this text.

In addition to observational and standardized assessment of sensorimotor development, the physical therapist may be responsible for noting other health care needs such as cardiorespiratory status, growth parameters, and state control. Consultation with other team members, such as the nurse, will be essential to a comprehensive assessment of the child.

Assessment of the Community Contexts. In the past 30 years, the rise in poverty in the United States and the increased number of single-parent households, divorces, and nonmarital pregnancies speak to a decrease in children's economic and even emotional well-being. One in five children live in poverty, a rate suggesting future economic problems for American families and their children (Eggebeen & Lichter, 1991). Curtailed adult educational and socioeconomic achievements are often concomitants of these high poverty rates. The combination of these factors leads to higher infant mortality rates (Tresseras et al., 1992) and potentially to lower health status of the children who do survive.

Identification of the contexts in which children live, such as those related to decreased nutrition, clothing, and shelter, can make an intervention program more realistic. When these basic needs are not addressed, exercise regimens appear to be superfluous and are seldom sustained, resulting in the professional's designation of parental noncompliance (Coy, 1989; Hunt et al., 1989). The home program model described by Rainforth and Salisbury (1988) emphasizes embedding program goals and regimens into existing family routines, thus decreasing the potential for noncompliance.

Although details of these family conditions are within the practice domain of the social worker, physical therapists unconcerned about these basic needs cannot provide realistic intervention for such children. There are well-known assessments to evaluate the contexts in which children live (Caldwell & Bradley, 1984; Harms & Clifford, 1980). Efforts have been made to make these assessments unbiased according to ethnicity and other social factors. Observation and interview in addition may be essential assessments of the environment.

Development of the IFSP. Although the IFSP for children between birth and 3 years of age is mandated by federal law, each family of a child with special needs requires a service plan specifically developed to address the child's needs. The principle underlying an IFSP is that families have diverse needs based on their individual structure, values, and coping styles. For intervention to be meaningful for the child, therefore, the individuality of their contemporary family needs to be determined

(Kjerland & Kovach, 1987). To help delineate individual needs and concerns and assist in the IFSP process, parents and professionals must function as a collaborative team (McGonigel et al., 1991) (Fig. 30–7).

To ensure equal partnership in the development of an IFSP, the family should be provided with information that will enable them to make informed decisions and choices. This information may result from the initial arena assessment or may be shared with the family in the form of a postevaluation interpretive conference. However the information is shared, it should be available a few weeks before the IFSP meeting, enabling the family to decide on whom they want to invite to the meeting and which professionals should be present to address the parents' concerns. During goal setting, family goals related to the child must receive the most attention. Consideration of family goals represents a shift from therapists' traditional decision-making roles of determining the child's needs, appropriate services, and family responsibilities.

Developing an IFSP for each child and family is a challenge to professionals providing family-centered intervention. Several issues, some of which have been outlined by Olsen and Kwiatkowsky (1992), contribute to this challenge.

1. The IFSP must include the developmental levels of the child. As mentioned earlier, various states have interpreted this mandate differently, causing some confusion for the physical therapist in meeting the federal mandate.

2. The IFSP must include the statement of the family's resources, priorities, and concerns related to enhancing the child's development. One ap-

proach to this challenge is suggested in Figure 30–6. The way in which family information is incorporated into the IFSP provides an additional challenge.

3. A statement of outcomes to be achieved by the child and family must also be included in the IFSP. Establishing goals for the child suggests an ecologic perspective, while establishing goals for the family suggests a systems perspective and establishing goals for the family and child to alleviate sources of stress suggests a stress-support perspective. These perspectives are complementary, and an understanding of them must be available to the therapist interacting with contemporary families. At any one time, one perspective may need to be emphasized. As depicted in Figure 30–8, the system consists of the focal child and a mother, father, and grandparent. The motor needs of the son will be the focus of the therapist's attention, but the lack of interaction of the son with parents, as shown by the absence of arrows, must be a major stressor within the system and will have some bearing on the success of intervention. Intervention, therefore, must address the child's needs, the lack of interaction of parents and son, and the stress that results from the way in which this family is functioning.

4. Specific services required to meet the child and family needs must be identified in the IFSP. Availability of personnel resources reflects the current staffing patterns of the program or agency as opposed to the needs of the child and family. In some cases, the most appropriate place to intervene with the child may be in the home, particularly with medically fragile infants. Children and families who receive home-based intervention, however, often receive less frequent and less intensive inter-

FIGURE 30–7. A parent and a therapist collaborate during the 6-month review of a child's IFSP.

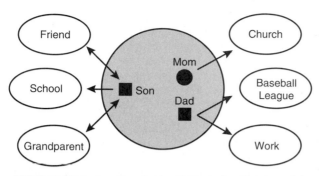

FIGURE 30-8. Ecomap. Arrows indicate the direction of the interaction: there is no interaction among family members but much interaction of members with external activities. (From Sparling JW. Assessment of family resources and needs. In Wilhelm, IJ [Ed.], Physical Therapy Assessment in Early Infancy. New York: Churchill Livingstone, 1992.)

vention because of extensive travel times and lack of staff availability. Involvement in advocacy at a local, state, and national level may be the only way to address this problem. This is particularly important because the efficacy of physical therapy may well depend on the extent to which goals stated in IFSPs have been met.

Treatment of the Child. One of the historical questions related to treatment is parent participation. An early paper by Farber and Lewis (1975) suggested that parents are requested to participate in the education of their child because school personnel have abrogated their responsibility in this area. The authors suggest that it is simply an economic necessity to have parents provide services or treatment. This argument is not as tenable as it was in 1975 because of the passage of the federal laws mandating parental involvement. With the shortage of physical therapists, however, similar questions arise about the extent of caretaker responsibility.

In contrast, physical therapists have historically questioned the quality of "treatment" offered by someone other than a therapist. The now famous study by Palmer and associates (1988) brought into question not only the kind and amount of physical therapy but also the way in which it was provided by the parent in consultation with the therapist. The concept of compliance is a related issue. Caretakers can be under stress and for a variety of reasons often cannot maintain the regimens established by therapists. To intimate noncompliance in such cases suggests that therapists are performing as experts and parents are passive recipients of their authoritative instruction. This situation is not the intent of the federal legislation related to children with special needs.

The way in which information is shared with caretakers, whether written or verbal, and the way treatment goals are collaboratively established with caretakers (Bazyk, 1989) often determines the success of physical therapy. Similarly, the physical therapist's skill is a treatment factor, as are the models under which treatment is provided. Therefore, parent–professional collaboration with a skilled and knowledgeable therapist will have far-reaching intervention outcomes.

Evaluation of Treatment Regimen and Caregiver Concerns. One of the most significant evaluations of a child's progress can be made by persons who live with the child. As a result of intervention, families know how much easier it is for the child to transfer or to achieve a standing posture. They know how the child performs during functional activities. One way in which to record these data is for the caregiver to keep a diary. For some, this is an additional stressor, while for others it is a release. For Ann's mother, keeping a diary might have given her a mechanism to monitor the course of intervention. In addition, the therapist's ongoing evaluation of the child should include an assessment of the barriers limiting progress. These barriers may include an overzealous and autonomous therapist, an incorrigible caregiver, or a team in conflict. Through evaluation, differing cultural perspectives of the players may be delineated and unique barriers to change eliminated. To support change, large data sets need to be established to obtain valid information about the duration and effectiveness of treatment, the need for equipment to support treatment, and the effectiveness of caregiver involvement in treatment.

Evaluation of Community Involvement. Within the systems and the ecologic perspectives, the community and its service systems are critical to family intervention (Cantor, 1989). Requirements for third-party payment directly affect the receipt of treatment and equipment necessary for the child to learn. Team interaction, selection of treatment priorities, and elimination of duplication of services enable limited professional services to be extended to more children. In this time of health care personnel shortage, duplication of services must be avoided. For example, oral-motor intervention cannot be construed as the domain of physical therapy, occupational therapy, and speech and language pathology and, therefore, offered by all to one child. In contrast, all team members need to be vigorous advocates for the health and welfare of the children they serve.

Community support consists of formal support from local, state, and federal agencies and private foundations. Public support for centralized education offers the child and family opportunities for group as well as individualized learning, preparation for adult living, establishment of social relationships, and effective use of resources. In addition, the use of public resources for the child with special needs extends a message to the community about civil rights and the need for acceptance of individual differences. To determine the components of support and whether communities are providing that support, the Massachusetts Human Services Research Institute is developing an assessment (Family Support Bulletin, 1992, pp. 11–14). Use of this chart might be an effective way to access caregiver opinions of service at different times in a family's receipt of those services.

PREVENTION

The basic principle underlying physical therapy interventions with children and their families is prevention. Prevention is one of the best ways to minimize the impact of disability on children and families. A prevention program entails early identification of the child's and the family's needs and early referral to appropriate community resources. Consistent with federal laws on early intervention, prevention programs must be comprehensive and geared toward the child and family's environment. A prenatal prevention program may be indicated to address this country's horrifying statistics related to our maternal and child health population (U.S. Department of Health and Human Service, 1990). For infants who are biologically at risk, prevention programs are initiated in the nursery. Follow-up prevention programs are located in hospitals and staffed primarily by health care professionals. High-risk follow-up clinics serve as a link between the hospital and the community.

The role of the physical therapist in the prevention program is that of an evaluator, consultant, advisor, and educator (Fig. 30–9). The physical therapist must be trained in the administration of comprehensive screening tests that assess all areas of the child's development, such as the Infant Monitoring Questionnaire (Bricker & Squires, 1989a and b), and may include assessment of potential or real family stressors. A role of therapists in hospital and community-based programs is to develop better communication with other service providers to ensure that families obtain appropriate services, including information on motor and functional development and early warning signs of developmental difficulties. Sharing this information with families of infants in the neonatal intensive or intermediate care units can be challenging but must be done in a nonthreatening manner. Providing advice includes the sharing of information on appropriate resources and phone numbers of a parent liaison in the local community or the local interagency coordinating council. If indicated, the therapist should develop an IFSP with the family, including goals of the prevention program, timeliness for periodic screenings, criteria for termination of the prevention program, or initiation of early intervention.

The following case situation describes a prevention program delivered in the context of a family support model (Kaplan-Sanoff et al., 1991). Edu-

FIGURE 30–9. Therapist showing parents various ways of handling their premature infant, a process aimed at prevention.

cating the family about children's developmental sequences, the family's close observation of children in the home, and the availability of another child for comparison led to collaboration of the therapist and the parents in the development of the IFSP (Beckwith & Parmalee, 1986). The children's case also demonstrates the importance of periodic screening and developmental testing as part of a prevention program.

Kim and Karen are identical twins born at 29 weeks' gestational age to a 23-year-old mother. Both infants were on ventilators during the first 1.5 weeks of life. Kim developed respiratory complications requiring an additional 1 week on the ventilator. Both infants had a history of intraventricular hemorrhages and bronchopulmonary dysplasia; Kim also developed retinopathy of prematurity. Physical therapy was requested and initiated for Kim at 34 weeks' gestational age for motor "disorganization" and inability to sustain alert interactive states.

Therapy focused on adapting Kim's environment through positioning, tactile stimulation, handling, decreasing external stimuli such as light by covering the crib, and playing the parents' talking tapes. Kim's mother visited the infants daily and reportedly was very involved in the infants' care. Kim was discharged at 44 weeks' gestational age, 3 weeks after Karen. On discharge, Kim was referred to an early intervention program that encouraged participation of siblings in therapy. Although the parents had tentatively arranged for the twins' grandmother to take care of Karen on "therapy days," the family was asked if Karen could attend Kim's intervention sessions and they agreed. During weekly therapy sessions the therapist noted that Karen, although more advanced than Kim, displayed mild motor coordination problems. After discussing this with the family, the parents decided to closely monitor and observe Kim at home.

At Kim's 6-month review of the IFSP with the whole family, the physical therapist inquired whether the family wanted the intervention team to assess Karen to make sure that her needs were also being addressed. The family agreed. A team evaluation determined that Karen demonstrated language and perceptuomotor delays for her adjusted age. The findings were discussed with the family, and speech therapy and special education services were initiated for both infants.

▌ CONCLUSION

The challenge for early interventionists is to determine strategies for providing the best practice given less than adequate health care and educational resources. This challenge is complicated by

characteristics of contemporary family life that involve change. Experiencing conditions necessitating change, however, can facilitate interaction and foster the development of decision-making skills. In other words, the therapist can use these contemporary stressors to help develop problem-solving skills, one of the long-term goals of intervention. In this approach, the therapist identifies the stressors and determines the support perceived by families, while addressing the functional limitations of the child based on an understanding of the pathophysiology of the child's diagnosis. This marriage of pathophysiologic and sociocultural knowledge is critical for the physical therapist based on research related to motor development and functional independence (Campos et al., 1982; Cassidy, 1986; Cintas, 1992; Clydesdale et al., 1990) and education (Bricker, 1989). In keeping with this perspective, Haley and Baryza (1990) have challenged physical therapists to develop a hierarchy of psychosocial factors to accompany their motor outcome model that is initiated at the level of spontaneous movement and terminates in motor skills and adaptive motor function.

Recognizing the importance of the immediate family and larger sociocultural environments for the developing child supports effective early intervention. Family and contextual variables that support child motor outcome goals vary over the course of development. One factor may take precedence over another at any one time, but at no time can child, family, or sociocultural variables be excluded from the therapist's considerations. Unless physical therapists search for family-oriented outcomes related to movement, that is, adaptive motor activities that have functional meaning for the family, therapists will not be engaging in best practice for children and their families.

References

Ackerman, NJ. A Theory of Family Systems. New York: Gardner Press, 1984.

Anderson, L. Ethnicity and illness experience: Ideological structures and the health care delivery system. Social Sciences and Medicine, 22:1277–1283, 1986.

Bailey, DB & Simeonsson, RJ. Assessing needs of families with handicapped infants. Journal of Special Education, 22(1): 117–127, 1988.

Bazyk, S. Changes in attitudes and beliefs regarding parent participation and home programs: An update. American Journal of Occupational Therapy, 43;723–728, 1989.

Beavers, R, Hampson, R, & Hulgus, Y. Commentary: The Beavers system approach to family assessment. Family Process, 24:398–405, 1985.

Beckwith, L, & Parmalee, A. EEG patterns of preterm infants, home environment and later IQ. Child Development, 57:777–789, 1986.

Bennett, A, Hewson, D, Booker, E, & Holliday, S. Antenatal preparation and labor support in relation to birth outcomes. Birth, *12*(1):9–16, 1985.

Berrera, M, Jr. Social support in the adjustment of pregnant adolescents. In Gottlieb, BH (Ed.), Social Networks and Social Support. Beverly Hills: Sage, 1981, pp. 69–96.

Blacher, J. A dynamic perspective on the impact of a severely handicapped child on the family. In Blacher, J (Ed.), Severely Handicapped Young Children and their Families. New York: Academic Press, 1984, pp. 3–50.

Boss, P. Family stress: Perception and context. In Sussman, MB, & Sternmetz, S (Eds.), Handbook on Marriage and the Family. New York: Plenum Press, 1985, p. 704.

Brazelton, TB. Early intervention: What does it mean? In Fitzgerald, HE, Lester, BM, & Yogman, MW (Eds.), Theory and Research in Behavioral Pediatrics (vol. 1). New York: Plenum Press, 1982, pp. 1–34.

Breslau, N, Salkever, D, & Staruch, KS. Women's labor force activity and responsibilities for disabled dependents: A study of families with disabled children. Journal of Health and Social Behavior, *23*:169–183, 1982.

Bricker, D. Early Intervention for At-risk and Handicapped Infants, Toddlers and Preschool Children (2nd ed.). Palo Alto, CA: VORT Corporation, 1989.

Bricker, D, & Squires, J. Low cost system using parents to monitor the development of at-risk infants. Journal of Early Intervention, *13*(1):50–60, 1989a.

Bricker, D, & Squires, J. The effectiveness of parental screening of at-risk infants: The infant monitoring questionnaires. Topics in Early Childhood Special Education, *9*(3):67–85, 1989b.

Brooks-Gunn, J, & Lewis, M. Parents of handicapped infants: Their role in identification, assessment, and intervention. Paper presented at the Ira Gordon Memorial Conference, Chapel Hill, NC, 1979.

Brown, MS. Culture and childrearing. In Clark, AL (Ed.), Culture and Childrearing. Philadelphia, PA: FA Davis, 1981, pp. 3–35.

Brownlee, AJ. Community, Culture, and Care: A Cross-cultural Guide for Healthworkers. St. Louis, MO: CV Mosby, 1978.

Burns, A. Mother-headed families: An international perspective and the case of Australia. Social Policy Report, *6*(1):1–23, 1992.

Caldwell, BM, & Bradley, RH. Manual for the Home Observation for Measurement of the Environment (Rev. Ed.). Little Rock: University of Arkansas, 1984.

Campos, J, Svejda, M, Campos, R, & Bertenthal, B. The emergence of self-produced locomotion: Its importance for psychological development. In Bricker, D (Ed.), Intervention with At-risk and Handicapped Infants. Baltimore, MD: University Park Press, 1982, pp. 195–216.

Cantor, MH. Social care: Family and community support systems. Annals of the American Academy of Political and Social Science, *503*:99–112, 1989.

Cassidy, J. The ability to negotiate the environment: An aspect of infant competence as related to quality of attachment. Child Development, *57*:331–337, 1986.

Chan, SQ. Early intervention with culturally diverse families of infants and toddlers with disabilities. Infants and Young Children, *3*(2):78–87, 1990.

Chiarello, L, Effgen, S, & Levinson, M. Parent-professional partnerships in evaluation and the development of individualized family service plans. Pediatric Physical Therapy, *4*:64–69, 1992.

Cintas, HM. The relationship of motor skill level and risk-taking during exploration in toddlers. Pediatric Physical Therapy, *4*:165–170, 1992.

Clark, AL. Childrearing in matrix America. In Clark, AL (Ed.), Culture and Childrearing. Philadelphia: FA Davis, 1981, pp. 37–54.

Clydesdale, TT, Fahs, IJ, Kilgore, KM, & Splaingard, ML. Social dimensions to functional gain in pediatric patients. Archives of Physical Medicine and Rehabilitation, *71*:469–472, 1990.

Cochrane, CG, Farley, BG, & Wilhelm, IJ. Preparation of physical therapists who work with handicapped infants and their families: Current status and training needs. Physical Therapy, *70*:372–380, 1990.

Cosper, M, & Erickson, M. The psychological, social and medical needs of lower socioeconomic status mothers of asthmatic children. Journal of Asthma, *22*:145–148, 1985.

Cowan, CP, Cowan, PA, Heming, G, & Miller, NB. Becoming a family: Marriage, parenting, and child development. In Cowan, PA, & Hetherington, M (Eds.), Family Transitions. Hillsdale, NJ: Lawrence Erlbaum Associates, 1991, pp. 79–109.

Coy, JA. Autonomy-based informed consent: Ethical implications for patient noncompliance. Physical Therapy, *69*:826–833, 1989.

Crais, ER, & Leonard, CR. PL 99-457: Are speech-language pathologists prepared for the challenge? Journal of the American Speech-Language and Hearing Association, *32*:57–61, 1990.

Cranley, M. The origins of the mother–child relationship: A review. Physical and Occupational Therapy in Pediatrics, *12*(2/3):39–51, 1993.

Darling, RB. Families against Society: A Study of Reactions to Children with Birth Defects. Beverly Hills, CA: Sage, 1979, p. 78.

Dunn, W, Campbell, PH, Oetter, PL, Hall, S, Berger, E, & Strickland, LR. Guidelines for Occupational Therapy Services in Early Intervention and Preschool Services. Rockville, MD: American Occupational Therapy Association, 1989.

Dunst, CJ, Trivette, CM, Gordon, NJ, & Pletcher, LL. Building and mobilizing informal family support networks. In Singer, GHS, & Irwin, LK, (Eds.), Support for Caregiving Families: Enabling Positive Adaptation to Disability. Baltimore, MD: Paul H. Brookes, 1989, pp. 121–141.

Effgen, SK, Bjornson, K, Chiarello, L, Sinzer, L, & Phillips, W. Competencies for physical therapists in early intervention. Pediatric Physical Therapy, *3*:77–80, 1991.

Eggebeen, DJ, & Lichter, DT. Race, family structure, and changing poverty among American children. American Sociological Review, *56*:801–817, 1991.

Epstein, NB, Baldwin, LM, & Bishop, DS. The McMaster Family Assessment Device. Journal of Marriage Family Therapy, *9*:171–177, 1983.

Farber, R. Integrated treatment of the dual-career couple. American Journal of Family Therapy, *16*(1):46–57, 1988.

Farber, B, & Lewis, M. The symbolic use of parents: A sociological critique of educational practice. Journal of Research in Development and Education, *8*(2):34–43, 1975.

Farran, DC, Kasari, C, Comfort, M, & Jay, S. Parent–Caregiver Involvement Scale (PCIS). Greensboro, NC: University of North Carolina, 1986.

Farran, DC, & Ramey, CT. Social class differences in dyadic involvement during infancy. Child Development, *51*:254–257, 1980.

Featherstone, H. A Difference in the Family: Life with a Disabled Child. New York: Basic Books, 1980.

Flynt, SW, Wood, TA, & Scott, RL. Social support of mothers of children with mental retardation. Mental Retardation, *30*:233–236, 1992.

Gallagher, J, Beckman, P, & Cross, A. Families of handicapped children: Sources of stress and its amelioration. Exceptional Children, *50*:10–19, 1983.

Gilbert, LA. Men in Dual Career Families: Current Realities and Future Prospects. Hillsdale, NJ: Lawrence Erlbaum Associates, 1985.

Goldberg, S, Morris, P, Simmons, JM, & Levison, J. Chronic illness in infancy and parenting stress: A comparison of three groups of parents. Journal of Pediatric Psychology, 15:347–358, 1990.

Gottman, JM. Chaos and regulated change in families: A metaphor for the study of transitions. In Cowan, PA, & Hetherington, M, (Eds.), Family Transitions. Hillsdale, NJ: Lawrence Erlbaum Associates, 1991, pp. 247–272.

Green, JW. Cultural Awareness in the Human Services: Ethnicity and Social Services. Englewood Cliffs, NJ: Prentice-Hall, 1982, pp. 3–27.

Haley, SM, & Baryza, MJ. A hierarchy of motor outcome assessment. Self initiated movements through adaptive motor function. Infants and Young Children, 3:1–14, 1990.

Hammer, MR. Intercultural communication competence. In Asante, MK, & Gudykunst, WB (Eds.), Handbook of International and Intercultural Communication. Newbury Park, CA: Sage, 1989, pp. 247–260.

Hamner, TJ, & Turner, PH. Parenting in Contemporary Society. Englewood Cliffs, NJ: Prentice-Hall, 1985.

Hanson, MJ. Ethnic, cultural, and language diversity in intervention settings. In Lynch, EW, & Hanson, MJ (Eds.), Developing Cross-cultural Competence: A Guide for Working with Young Children and their Families. Baltimore, MD: Paul H. Brookes, 1992, pp. 1–18.

Harms, T, & Clifford, RM. Early Childhood Environment Rating Scale. New York: Teachers College Press, 1980.

Harris, SR. Efficacy of physical therapy in promoting family functioning and functional independence for children with cerebral palsy. Pediatric Physical Therapy, 2:160–164, 1990.

Hartman, A. Diagramming assessment of family relationships. Social Casework, 59:465–476, 1978.

Heifetz, LJ. Integrating religious and secular perspectives in the design of disability services. Mental Retardation, 25:127–131, 1987.

Hinojosa, J. How mothers of preschool children with cerebral palsy perceive occupational and physical therapists and their influence on family life. Occupational Therapy Journal of Research, 10:144–163, 1990.

Humphry, R. Early intervention and the influence of the occupational therapist on the parent–child relationship. American Journal of Occupational Therapy, 43:738–742, 1989.

Humphry, R, & Link, S. Entry level preparation of occupational therapists to work in early intervention programs. American Journal of Occupational Therapy, 44:828–833, 1990.

Hunt, LM, Jordan, B, Irwin, S, & Browner, CH. Compliance and the patient's perspective: Controlling symptoms in everyday life. Culture, Medicine and Psychiatry, 13:315–334, 1989.

Kaplan-Sanoff, M, Parker, S, & Zuckerman, B. Poverty and early childhood development: What do we know and what should we do? Infants and Young Children, 4(1):68–76, 1991.

Kjerland, L, & Kovach, J. Structure for Program Responsiveness to Parents. Eagan, MN: Project Dakota, 1987.

Kolobe, THA. Family-focused early intervention. In Campbell, SK (Ed.), Pediatric Neurologic Physical Therapy (2nd ed.) New York: Churchill Livingstone, 1991, pp. 397–432.

Kolobe, THA. Working with families of children with disabilities. Pediatric Physical Therapy, 4:57–63, 1992.

Larson, CP. Efficacy of prenatal and postpartum home visits on child health and development. Pediatrics, 66:191–197, 1980.

Lash, M. Families as service coordinators. Rehab Update, Fall 1992, pp. 4–5.

Lovitun, A, Mueller, M, & Kauffman, C. The family centered

consultation model: Practical application for professionals. Infants and Young Children, 4(3):1–8, 1992.

Linder, TW. Transdisciplinary Play-based Assessment: A Functional Approach to Working with Young Children. Baltimore, MD: Paul H. Brookes, 1990.

Lynch, EW. Families with different cultures. In Bristol, M, & Kasari, C (Eds.), The Family Support Network Series: Monograph One. Moscow, ID: Family Support Network Project, University of Idaho, 1987, pp. 80–88.

Lynch, EW. Developing cross-cultural competence. In Lynch, EW, & Hanson, MJ (Eds.), Developing Cross-cultural Competence: A Guide for Working with Young Children and their Families. Baltimore, MD: Paul H. Brookes, 1992, pp. 35–64.

Lynch, EW, & Hanson, MJ. Developing Cross-cultural Competence: A Guide for Working with Young Children and their Families. Baltimore, MD: Paul H. Brookes, 1992.

McCubbin, H, & Patterson, JM. Systematic Assessment of Family Stress, Resources and Coping. St. Paul: University of Minnesota, 1982, pp. 7–15.

McGonigel, MJ, Kaufmann, RK, & Johnson, BH (Eds.). Recommended Practices for the Individualized Family Service Plan. Bethesda, MD: Association for the Care of Children's Health, 1991.

McHanahan, SS. Family structure and stress: A longitudinal comparison of two-parent and female-headed families. Journal of Marriage and the Family, 65:345–357, 1983.

McGoldrick, M, Pearce, J, & Giordano, J. Ethnicity and Family Therapy. New York: Guilford Press, 1982, pp. 3–30.

Mead, M. Understanding cultural patterns. Nursing Outlook, 4:260–262, 1956.

Morris, TM. Culturally sensitive family assessment: An evaluation of the Family Assessment Device used with Hawaiian-American and Japanese-American families. Family Process, 29:105–116, 1990.

Olson, DH. Circumplex model VII: Validation studies and FACES III. Family Process, 25:337–351, 1986.

Olson, J, & Kwiatkowski, K. Theoretical approaches: Foundations for quality service. In Olson, J, Kwiatkowski, K (Eds.), Planning Family Goals: A Systems Approach to the IFSP. Tucson, AZ: Communication Skill Builders, 1992, pp. 13–41.

Palmer, FB, Shapiro, BK, Wachtel, RC, Allen, MC, Hiller, JE, Harryman, SE, Mosher, BS, Meinert, CL, & Capute, AJ. The effects of physical therapy on cerebral palsy. New England Journal of Medicine, 318:803–808, 1988.

Patton, MQ. Qualitative Evaluation and Research Methods (2nd ed.). Newbury Park, CA: Sage, 1990, pp. 277–368.

Petersen, P, & Wikoff, RL. Home environment and adjustment in families with handicapped children: A canonical correlation study. Occupational Therapy Journal of Research, 7:67–82, 1987.

Phillips, WE. Stress and coping in the family of the child with cerebral palsy: The role of the physical therapist. Pediatric Physical Therapy, 2:166–168, 1990.

Powell, TH, & Ogle, PA. Brothers & Sisters: A Special Part of Exceptional Families. Baltimore, MD: Paul H. Brookes, 1985.

Public Law 94-142, Education for All Handicapped Children Act, 1975.

Public Law 99-457, Education of the Handicapped Act Amendments of 1986, 20 CSC Secs. 1400-1485, 1986.

Public Law 102-119, Individuals with Disabilities Education Amendments of 1991.

Rainforth, B, & Salisbury, CL. Functional home programs: A model for therapists. Topics in Early Childhood Special Education, 7(4):33–45, 1988.

Realini, A, Kalet, A, & Sparling, J. Silence in the medical interaction: II. A means of encouraging patient participation in the interaction. Paper presented at the American Academy of

Family Physicians 44th Annual Scientific Assembly, San Diego, CA, October 15–18, 1992.

Reiss, D. The Family's Construction of Reality. Cambridge, MA: Harvard University Press, 1981.

Research and Policy Committee of the Committee for Economic Development. Children in Need: Investment Strategies for the Educationally Disadvantaged. New York, NY: Committee for Economic Development, 1987.

Schraeder, BD, Heverly, MA, & Rappaport, J. The value of early home assessment in identifying risk in children who were very low birth weight. Pediatric Nursing, 16:268–272, 1990.

Sidel, R. Women and children first: Towards a US family policy. American Journal of Public Health, 82:664–665, 1992.

Simeonsson, RJ, & Bailey, DB. Family dimensions in early intervention. In Meisels, SJ, & Shonkoff, JP (Eds.), Handbook of Early Childhood Intervention. New York: Cambridge University Press, 1990, p. 428.

Smith, S. Two-generation program models: A new intervention strategy. Social Policy Report, 5(1):1–4, 1991.

Sosa, R, Kennell, J, Klaus, M, Robertson, S, & Urrutia, J. The effect of a supportive companion on perinatal problems, length of labor, and mother–infant interaction. New England Journal of Medicine, 303:597–600, 1980.

Sparling, JW. The cultural definition of the family. Physical and Occupational Therapy in Pediatrics, 11(4):17–29, 1991a.

Sparling, JW. Brief report: Infantile autism: A prospective report from pregnancy to four years. Journal of Autism and Developmental Disabilities, 21(2):229–236, 1991b.

Sparling, JW, Berger, B, & Biller, M. Fathers: Myth, reality and PL 99-457. Infants and Young Children, 4(3):9–19, 1992a.

Sparling, JW. Assessment of family resources and needs. In Wilhelm, IJ, (Ed.), Physical Therapy Assessment in Early Infancy. New York: Churchill Livingstone, 1992b, pp. 71–104.

Sparling, JW, Seeds, JW, & Farran, DC. The relationship of obstetrical ultrasound to parent and infant behavior. Obstetrics and Gynecology, 72:902–907, 1988.

Sparling, JW, & Sekerak, DK. Embedding the family perspective in an entry level physical therapy curriculum. Pediatric Physical Therapy, 4:116–122, 1992.

Stewart, MJ. Social support: Diverse theoretical perspectives. Social Science and Medicine, 28:1275–1282, 1989.

Sullivan, HS. The Psychiatric Interview. New York: WW Norton, 1970.

Taft, R. Coping with unfamiliar cultures. In Warren, N (Ed.), Studies in Cross Cultural Psychology. San Diego, CA: Academic Press, 1977, pp. 121–153.

Tellerman, K, & Medio, F. Pediatricians' opinions of mothers. Pediatrics, 81:186–189, 1988.

Tresserras, R, Canela, J, Alvarez, J, Sentis, J, & Salleras, L. Infant mortality, per capita income, and adult illiteracy: An ecological approach. American Journal of Public Health, 82:435–437, 1992.

Turnbull, A, & Turnbull, H. Families, Professionals, and Exceptionality: A Special Partnership. Columbus, OH: Merrill Publishing, 1986.

U.S. Department of Health and Human Services. Healthy Children 2000: National Health Promotion and Disease Prevention Objectives Related to Mothers, Infants, Children, Adolescents, and Youth. Washington, DC: Public Health Service, 1990.

U.S. House of Representatives. U.S. Children and their Families: Current Conditions and Recent Trends, 1989. Washington, DC: U.S. Government Printing Office, 1989.

U.S. House of Representatives Select Committee on Children, Youth, and Families: U.S. Children and their Families: Current Conditions and Recent Trends, 1989 (3rd ed.). Washington, DC: U.S. Government Printing Office, 1989.

Wilhelm, IJ, (Ed.). Physical Therapy Assessment in Early Infancy. New York: Churchill Livingstone, 1992.

Winton, PJ, & Bailey, DB. The family-focused interview: A collaborative mechanism for family assessment and goal-setting. Journal of the Division of Early Childhood, 12:195–207, 1988.

Winton, PJ, & Blow, C. Family Interview Performance Rating Scale. Chapel Hill, NC: Frank Porter Graham Child Development Center, 1991.

Wolery, M, & Dyk, L. Arena assessment: Description and preliminary social validity data. TASH, 9:231–235, 1984.

Chapter 31

The Educational Environment

SUSAN K. EFFGEN, PT, PhD

Almost from the start of physical therapy in the United States, physical therapists have worked in educational environments. The Civil Rights Movement of the 1960s and federal legislation of the 1970s, however, marked the beginning of major changes in all services to children with special needs. In this chapter the history of the delivery of physical therapy in educational environments is reviewed along with a discussion of federal legislation and significant court cases that have changed how all children with special needs are educated and receive physical therapy. The focus is on key issues related to physical therapy in educational environments such as inclusionary education, models of team interaction, service delivery models, the individualized educational plan (IEP), the individualized family service plan (IFSP), and treatment strategies. Management issues and critical issues facing school-based physical therapists are also discussed.

BACKGROUND

Although the history of physical therapy in the United States is traced to "reconstruction aides"

serving the injured of World War I, it can also be traced to the service of "crippled children." These children were served in hospitals and special settings. Special schools and classes began to appear early in the twentieth century in cities such as Boston, Chicago, and Detroit. The children had a variety of disabilities. The most common diagnoses were poliomyelitis and spastic paralysis (Cable et al., 1938; Givins, 1938), followed by cardiac disorders, "obstetrical arms," bone and joint tuberculosis, clubfeet, and osteomyelitis (Batten, 1933; Cable et al., 1938; Mulcahey, 1936). By the 1930s, numerous articles had been published describing the delivery of physical therapy in these special schools (Batten, 1933; Mulcahey, 1936; Sever, 1938; Vacha, 1933).

The role of physical therapy in schools has continued to expand throughout the century. Epidemics of poliomyelitis increased the need for physical therapists and special schools. After the vaccine for poliomyelitis was discovered in the 1950s, the need for special schools was temporarily reduced. Books such as *Karen* (Dahl, 1947), which described the needs of an intellectually normal child with cerebral palsy, increased public awareness of the needs of these children; and school services started to expand to include more children with neurologic impairments.

Historically placed in special schools, the majority of these children had normal or nearly normal intelligence. Many schools required children to be toilet-trained, and some required children to be independent ambulators. This trend to serve only those with physical disabilities and normal intelligence continued in many areas of the United States until schools were mandated in 1975 to serve all children with special needs by the enactment of Public Law (PL) 94-142, the Education for All Handicapped Children Act.

FEDERAL LEGISLATION AND LITIGATION

A number of social and political events paved the way for the enactment of PL 94-142, the Education for All Handicapped Children Act. In 1954, the historic Supreme Court decision regarding segregated schools, *Brown* v. *Board of Education of Topeka*, was decided. Separate but equal schools were found inherently unequal. This Court decision was to end the segregated education of African-American children. The principles and grounds of this case could equally apply to segregated schools for those with disabilities. The call for social equality had begun and would eventually include those with disabilities. President Kennedy's personal experience with those with disabilities helped lead him to establish a President's Panel on Mental Retardation in 1961. Television documentaries exposed institutions in New York, and Blatt and Kaplan's book, *Christmas in Purgatory: A Photographic Essay on Mental Retardation* (1966), raised national concern for the care and treatment of those with disabilities. Wolfensberger (1971) was an influential proponent of deinstitutionalization and normalization. Cruickshank (1980, p. 65) noted that "as is usually the case with major changes in social policy, the normalization trend is not based on empirical data showing greater effectiveness or efficiency of the changes proposed by its advocates." The normalization trend was, rather, an emphasis on civil rights of individuals, a prevailing anti-institutional attitude—especially governmental institutions—and a commitment "to the democratic, the individualistic, and the humanitarian" (Cruickshank, 1980, pp. 65–66). The federal Developmental Disabilities Assistance and Bill of Rights Act of 1975 (PL 94-103) included a provision that states had to develop and incorporate a "deinstitutionalization

and institutional reform" plan (Braddock, 1987, p. 71). Advocacy groups had gained power, and they used the judicial system to win their rights.

The *Pennsylvania Association for Retarded Citizens* (PARC) v. *Commonwealth of Pennsylvania* (1971) was the historic, decisive court case establishing the uncompromising right to an education for all children with disabilities. This was a class-action suit filed on behalf of 14 specifically named children and all other children who were in a similar "class" to those with trainable mental retardation. In Pennsylvania, these children were excluded from public school if a psychologist or mental health professional certified that a child could no longer profit from attendance at school. The local school board could refuse to accept or retain a child who had not reached the mental age of 5 years. Children who were classified as trainable mentally retarded, therefore, were unable to get a public education in Pennsylvania. The court sided with the children.

In *PARC* v. *Commonwealth of Pennsylvania*, the court found that all children, between 6 and 21 years of age, regardless of degree of disability, were to be given a "free and appropriate public education (FAPE)." Children with disabilities were to be educated with children without disabilities in the least restrictive environment (LRE). The educational system was ordered to stop applying exclusionary laws; parents were to become involved in the child's program; and re-evaluations were to be done. This landmark court case established many important principles that were later incorporated into the Education for All Handicapped Children Act.

Simultaneous with *PARC* v. *Commonwealth of Pennsylvania*, other important court cases were being decided. *Mills* v. *Board of Education of the District of Columbia* (1972) was filed on behalf of all children excluded by the public schools for a disability of any kind, including behavioral problems. The major result of this case was that all children, no matter how severe their mental retardation, behavioral problem, or disability, were educable and must be provided for suitably by the public school system.

In the *Maryland Association for Retarded Citizens* v. *Maryland* (1972) court case it was found that children have the right to tuition subsidies, the right to transportation, and the right to be educated with children who are not disabled. These cases and others across the nation began to establish the right of all children to a "free and appropriate public education." It was in this climate that PL 94-142 was enacted.

PL 94-142 Education for All Handicapped Children Act

PROVISIONS

On November 29, 1975, PL 94-142, the Education for All Handicapped Children Act, was passed by the U.S. Congress. The law included the elements won in individual court cases across the nation and provided for a "free and appropriate public education" for all children with disabilities from the age of 6 to 21 years (age 5 years if this is the age a state begins to provide public education to children without disabilities). The major provisions of PL 94-142 concern the concepts zero reject, education in the least restrictive environment, right to due process, nondiscriminatory evaluation, IEP, parent participation, and the right to related services, which include physical therapy.

Zero Reject

All children are to receive an education, including children with severe or profound disabilities. Children with severe or profound disabilities were initially to receive priority for service since they were most likely not receiving any service at that time. These children were institutionalized, in day-training centers without qualified special education teachers, or at home not receiving any services.

Least Restrictive Environment

Public agencies are to ensure

(1) That to the maximum extent appropriate, children with disabilities, including children in public or private institutions or other care facilities, are educated with children who are nondisabled; and
(2) That special classes, separate schooling or other removal of children with disabilities from the regular educational environment occurs only when the nature or severity of the disability is such that education in regular classes with the use of supplementary aids and services cannot be achieved satisfactorily.

(*FEDERAL REGISTER,* SEPTEMBER 29, 1992, p. 44823.)

Attendance at a special school to receive related services was definitely not in keeping with the spirit of the law. Therefore, related service personnel, such as physical therapists, needed to determine ways of delivering services in the regular educational environment.

Right to Due Process

Parents were given significant rights under PL 94-142. They had the right to an impartial hearing, the right to be represented by counsel, and the right to a verbatim transcript of a hearing and written findings. They could appeal and get an independent evaluation. Later, under PL 99-372, Handicapped Children's Protection Act [1986, 20 USC 1415 (e) (4), (f)], they would be able to get reimbursed for legal fees if they prevailed in a court case.

Nondiscriminatory Evaluation

Several court cases at this time had noted the discriminatory nature of the testing and placement procedures used in many school systems. Nondiscriminatory tests were to be used, and no one test could be the sole criterion used for placement. Nondiscriminatory testing is critical in the cognitive and language domain; however, physical therapists should also be careful to determine that their tests are not biased. When possible, standardized tests that have been normed on different racial and cultural groups should be used.

Individualized Educational Plan

Every child receiving special education must have an individualized educational plan (IEP). This is the comprehensive plan outlining the specific special educational and related services the child is to receive. It includes annual goals and objectives. The IEP is developed annually at an IEP meeting attended by the child's parents, a representative of the local educational agency, the child's teacher, and an individual involved in the child's evaluation. Physical therapists are not required to attend this meeting, but good practice dictates they attend meetings for the children they serve. How to develop an IEP is addressed later in this chapter.

Parent Participation

Active participation of parents is encouraged under PL 94-142. Parents are the individuals responsible for the continuity of services for their child and should be the child's best advocates. Parents are major decision-makers in the development of the IEP. They must give permission for an evaluation, they can restrict the release of information, they have access to their child's records, and they can request due process hearings.

Related Services

Related services, such as transportation, speech pathology, audiology, psychological services, physical therapy, occupational therapy, recreation, and medical and counseling services are to be provided "as may be required to assist a handicapped child to benefit from special education" (PL 99-142, 89 Stat 775). This quotation from the law has been interpreted in many different ways. Physical therapy "to assist a handicapped child to benefit from special education" in some school systems is limited to only those activities that help the child write or sit properly in class. Other school systems more appropriately interpret the law to mean physical therapy that can help the child explore the environment, perform activities of daily living, improve function in school, prepare for vocational training, and improve physical fitness so as to be better prepared to learn. In some school systems, this also includes management of impairment that might restrict achievement of independent function.

Just as important as the law are the regulations under which the law is carried out. After Congress passes a law and the president signs it, congressional staff write the rules and regulations that govern how that law is to be enforced. The regulations for PL 94-142 were developed with many participants. The willing participation of many sectors of the public and private community was necessary for the smooth implementation of this law (Martin, EW, 1989). The diverse and extensive initial input into the regulations probably accounted for the continued public support for the law and the public outcry when attempts were made to weaken the regulations early in the Reagan administration (Martin, EW, 1989).

CASE LAW

A law as comprehensive and complex as PL 94-142 was bound to lead to some controversy. All possible situations could not be anticipated, and some issues were even expected to be resolved by the courts. As a result, there have been a number of significant court cases that have helped define the scope of PL 94-142.

Related Services

Tatro v. *Texas* (1980) was one of the early major cases involving PL 94-142. Amber Tatro had spina bifida and required clean intermittent catheterization several times during the school day. Amber's parents wanted assistance with catheterization at school. The school officials refused, saying catheterization was a medical procedure and Amber could not attend school unless her parents handled the procedure. The parents then initiated what turned out to be a 10-year legal battle. During the legal process, they were told that although catheterization was necessary to sustain Amber's life, it was

not necessary to benefit from education; the school system, therefore, was not obligated to provide the service. After a complicated course though the court system, the case was heard by the U.S. Supreme Court. Amber attempted to attend the Supreme Court proceedings, only to discover that the Supreme Court was not readily accessible.

The Supreme Court found that clean intermittent catheterization was a related service that enabled the child to benefit from special education.

A service that enables a handicapped child to remain at school during the day is an important means of providing students with the meaningful access to education that Congress envisioned. The Act makes specific provision for services, like transportation, for example, that do no more than enable a child to be physically present in class.

(MARTIN, R, 1991, P. 45; *TATRO* V. *TEXAS*, 1980, at 891.)

This case is important to physical therapists. The realm of related services was expanded, as was the meaning of "required to benefit from special education."

Best Possible Education

Rowley v. *Board of Education of Hendrick Hudson Central School District* (1982) involved Amy Rowley, who was deaf. Amy attended a regular school. She had a special tutor, her teachers were trained in basic sign language, she was provided with a sound amplifier to use in class, and the school installed telecommunications devices for the deaf in her home to facilitate communication with her parents. After experimenting with an interpreter in class, the school system decided she did not need the service. Her parents believed she needed the interpreter and went through due process to continue to have the interpreter. A district court held that Amy was not receiving a free and appropriate public education because she did not have "an opportunity to achieve her full potential commensurate with the opportunity provided to other children." The school system appealed, and the case eventually went to the U.S. Supreme Court. The 1982 Supreme Court decision held that Congress did not intend to give handicapped children a right to the best possible education, i.e., education that would "maximize their potential"; it rejected the standard used by the lower courts that handicapped children are entitled to an educational opportunity "commensurate with the education available to nonhandicapped children"; and set two standards, namely, that a state is required to provide meaningful access to an education for each handicapped child and that sufficient supportive and related services must be provided to permit the child to benefit educationally from special education instruction.

When the Supreme Court applied these standards in *Rowley* v. *Board of Education of Hendrick Hudson Central School District* it found that Amy did not need interpreter services because she was making "exemplary progress in the regular education system" with the help of the extensive special services her school was providing.

The Court was careful to point out that merely passing from grade to grade does not mean a child's education is appropriate. The services that constitute an appropriate education must be based on each child's individual needs Although Amy was not found to require an interpreter, other children may require this service, based on their individual needs.

The *Rowley* decision has had significant impact on the provision of related services, including physical therapy. Unfortunately, in some school systems the *Rowley* decision has been used to limit the amount of physical therapy provided on the premise that schools are not obligated to provide the "best services." What must be remembered is that Amy was receiving extensive services and was making "exemplary progress in the regular education system." Therapists must recognize that this "exemplary progress" may be a reason to terminate physical therapy unless significant educational need for physical therapy can be thoroughly substantiated.

Extended School Year (ESY)

As children with special needs began to benefit from 9-month educational programs, some parents realized that their children were regressing during the summer and that it took several months to regain those lost skills when these children returned to class in the fall. Since the U.S. Congress had realized that more than the traditional 12 years of schooling might be necessary for children with disabilities to reach their potential, then perhaps it could be inferred that if a child lost ground during the summer, extended school year services might be necessary (Martin, 1991).

Several court cases sought to clarify this issue. In both *Battle* v. *Commonwealth of Pennsylvania* (1981), and *Georgia Association of Retarded Citizens* v. *McDaniel* (1981), parents sought to extend the school year. In Pennsylvania, it was found that the state's policy of defining a school year as 180 days could not be used to prevent the provision of an extended school year. In Georgia, the court

ruled that an extended school year must be based on individual cases. The child must show significant regression, the extended year must be part of the IEP, and an extended year does not mean 5 days a week for 52 weeks but must be based on a program to facilitate attainment of goals.

Eligibility for extended school year services must now be based on several criteria. These include "individual need, nature and severity of the disability, educational benefit, regression and recoupment, self-sufficiency and independence, and failing to meet short-term goals and objectives" (Rapport & Thomas, 1993, p. 16). The possibility of receiving services for the entire year has many implications for physical therapy. The children most likely to require extended school year services are usually those with the most serious disabilities, often requiring physical therapy. One criterion used to qualify for extended school year services is documentation of regression during vacation and the length of time it takes to recoup or relearn former skills. It is therefore vital for physical therapists to do comprehensive, objective assessments before and after all school breaks. Documentation of regression, especially during short breaks, might enable a child to receive physical therapy during the summer. Using the child's status at the end of the summer as the basis for extended school year physical therapy services might be confounded if parents obtain private physical therapy and other services during the summer and regression is prevented.

An ethical dilemma can arise for some physical therapists over the extended school year concept. Some school therapists provide private physical therapy during the summer and might prefer that the school system not provide the service. Others might not want the obligation of having to provide services during the summer, either through the school or privately, and this could influence their documentation. Therapists must be very careful to recognize this potential conflict of interest.

PL 99-457 Education of the Handicapped Act Amendments of 1986 and PL 102-119 Individuals with Disabilities Education Act Amendments of 1991 (IDEA)

On October 8, 1986, PL 99-457, the Education of the Handicapped Act Amendments of 1986 was enacted. This act was an extension of PL 94-142 to serve infants, toddlers, and preschoolers with disabilities and their families. There were four major parts, or titles, to this original law. Title I, Handicapped Infants and Toddlers became known, by its area of insertion, as Part H. Title II is Handicapped Children Aged 3 to 5, Title III is Discretionary Programs, and Title IV is Miscellaneous. PL 99-457 is also discussed in Chapter 33 on medicolegal issues. A discussion of family-centered intervention is presented in Chapter 30.

On October 7, 1991, PL 94-142 and PL 99-457 were reauthorized and amended as PL 102-119, the Individuals with Disabilities Education Act Amendments of 1991, or IDEA. The first two titles of the law have a significant impact on the delivery of all early intervention services, including physical therapy, to children younger than 5 years of age.

TITLE I—INFANTS AND TODDLERS WITH DISABILITIES

It is therefore the policy of the United States to provide financial assistance to States—
(1) to develop and implement a statewide, comprehensive, coordinated, multidisciplinary, interagency program of early intervention services for infants and toddlers with disabilities and their families,
(2) to facilitate the coordination of payment for early intervention services from Federal, State, local, and private sources (including public and private insurance coverage), and
(3) to enhance its capacity to provide quality early intervention services and expand and improve existing early intervention services being provided to infants and toddlers with disabilities and their families. . . . "(1) The term "infants and toddlers with disabilities" means individuals from birth to age 2, inclusive, who need early intervention services because they—
(A) are experiencing developmental delays, as measured by appropriate diagnostic instruments and procedures in one or more of the following areas: cognitive development, physical development . . ., communication development . . ., social or emotional development, or . . . adaptive development or
(B) have a diagnosed physical or mental condition which has a high probability of resulting in developmental delay. Such term may also include, at a State's discretion, individuals from birth to age 2, inclusive, who are at risk of having substantial developmental delays if early intervention services are not provided.
(2) The term "early intervention services" are developmental services which—
(A) are provided under public supervision,
(B) are provided at no cost except where Federal or State law provides for a system of payments by families, including a schedule of sliding fees,
(C) are designed to meet the developmental needs of an infant or toddler with a disability in any one or more of the following areas:
(i)   physical development,
(ii) cognitive development,
(iii) communication development,
(iv) social or emotional development, or
(v)   adaptive development,
(D) meet the standards of the State, including the requirements of this subchapter,
(E) include—
(i)   family training, counseling, and home visits,
(ii)   special instruction,
(iii) speech pathology and audiology,
(iv)   occupational therapy,
(v)   physical therapy,
(vi)   psychological services,
(vii) . . . service coordination services,
(viii) medical services only for diagnostic or evaluation purposes,
(ix)   early identification, screening, and assessment services,
(x)   health services necessary to enable the infant or toddler to benefit from the other early intervention services,
(xi)   social work services,
(xii) vision services,
(xiii) assistive technology devices and assistive technology services, and
(xiv) transportation and related costs that are necessary to enable an infant or toddler and the infant's or toddler's family to receive early intervention services,
(F) are provided by qualified personnel, including—
(i)   special educators,
(ii)   speech and language pathologists and audiologists,
(iii) occupational therapists,
(iv)   physical therapists,
(v)   psychologists,
(vi)   social workers,
(vii) nurses,
(viii) nutritionists,
(ix)   family therapists,
(x)   orientation and mobility specialists, and
(xi)   pediatricians and other physicians,
(G) to the maximum extent appropriate, are provided in natural environments, including the home, and community settings in which children without disabilities participate . . .

(PL 99-457, 100 stat 1145–1147; PL 102-119, 105 stat 595-596, SEC 1471–1472.)

The law describes many of the details of comprehensive early intervention services. Each child must have a multidisciplinary assessment of his or her unique needs and the identification of needed services. A written individualized family service plan (IFSP) must be developed by the multidisciplinary team, including the parent or guardian. The IFSP must be evaluated once a year and reviewed at 6-month intervals or more often, based on the needs of the child and family.

The assessment and IFSP must be completed by a multidisciplinary team. For children with problems in physical development, the physical therapist should be a member of the team. The development of appropriate, expected major outcomes, goals, and objectives involving the motor domain is the responsibility of physical therapists in collaboration with the other members of the multidisciplinary team, including the family. The law states that the responsibility of early intervention personnel including physical therapists is to help identify the "specific early intervention services necessary to meet the unique needs of the infant or toddler and the family." Furthermore, the law states that identification of the "frequency, intensity, and method of delivering services," (PL 99-457, 100 Stat 1150) must be based on sound professional judgment coupled with the realistic estimation of the capabilities of the family and the resources of the community. Title I provides for a comprehensive service delivery system for infants and toddlers with disabilities and their families. The IFSP and the role of physical therapy in early intervention are discussed later in this chapter and in Chapter 30.

TITLE II—CHILDREN AGED 3 TO 5 WITH DISABILITIES

Title II of PL 102-119 and PL 99-457 provide for special education and related services for children 3 to 5 years of age with disabilities. This may include 2-year-old children who will reach age 3 during the school year. As in Title I, the children include those

"experiencing developmental delays, as defined by the State and as measured by appropriate diagnostic instruments and procedures, in one or more of the following areas: physical development, cognitive development, communication development, social or emotional development, or adaptive development."

(PL 102-119, 105 stat 587)

The children need not fit into a specific diagnostic category, as required for school-aged children in PL 94-142.

Children 3 to 5 years of age are to have IEPs, as

are school-aged children; however, in the reauthorization, PL 102-119, the state has the option of allowing the use of IFSPs for preschool-aged children. The use of IFSPs is supported by the Council for Exceptional Children, Division of Early Childhood Education (1990), and the American Physical Therapy Association, Section on Pediatrics (1991). Many professionals believe the problems of preschoolers and their families are more similar to those of infants and toddlers than they are to those of school-aged children.

A major concern about using an IEP, besides the lack of family focus, is the issue of whether physical therapy is considered a related service, as it is in PL 94-142. If physical therapy falls under the category of related services, then it must be provided "to assist a child with a disability to benefit from special education" (*Federal Register*, September 29, 1992, p. 44803). Physical therapists should encourage the use of IFSPs; and if an IEP is used, they should encourage a more liberal interpretation to allow the provision of physical therapy as provided in early intervention.

Least Restrictive Environment

Early intervention services to infants and toddlers with disabilities and special education services and related services to preschool-aged children are to change from "segregated to integrated environments." This is a continuation of the mandate "not to remove the children from natural environments." The Rules and Regulations of PL 99-457 note, however, that the least restrictive environment for an infant might include the hospital setting. With the majority of mothers of young children working, early intervention services need to be provided in a variety of child care settings. It is, however, frequently a problem to place infants and toddlers with disabilities in appropriate child care settings serving children without disabilities. The provision of early intervention services in child care settings can also be difficult because of the professional travel involved, the possible disruptive nature of providing intervention in a setting not accustomed to having professionals coming in and out, and the absence of parents.

Transition

Transition is an important issue in PL 102-119. Early intervention personnel, as well as school personnel, are to plan for the successful transition to the next level of service. Transition plans must be included in the IFSP and IEP.

Assistive Technology

The inclusion of assistive technology devices and assistive technology services is new to PL 102-119.

An assistive technology device means any item, piece of equipment, or product system whether acquired commercially off the shelf, modified, or customized, that is used to increase, maintain, or improve the functional capabilities of children with disabilities. . . Assistive technology services means any service that directly assists a child with a disability in the selection, acquisition, or use of assistive technology device.

(*FEDERAL REGISTER*, SEPTEMBER 29, 1992, P. 44801.)

The assistive technology services include evaluation, purchasing, selecting, and coordinating with other therapies. This is an important area for physical therapists, who frequently provide assistive devices to minimize disability. Therapists adapt seating so children can function better and safely in the classroom. They assist other team members in devising the most functional communication systems along with providing access to switching devices and computers. Ambulation devices are frequently necessary to allow the child to ambulate throughout the school. Power mobility devices also allow the child with severe impairments and functional limitations to independently access the school building and grounds and, thereby, minimize disability. The law allows for continued provision and expansion of these assistive technology services. The extent of services and the purchasing of devices will vary among school systems until there are further federal directives. For additional information, the reader is referred to Chapter 23 on assistive technology.

PL 101-336 Americans With Disabilities Act (ADA)

The Americans with Disabilities Act (PL 101-336) was signed into law on July 26, 1990, and became effective January 26, 1992. It "extends to individuals with disabilities comprehensive civil rights protection similar to those provided to persons on the basis of race, sex, national origin, and religion under the Civil Rights Act of 1964" (*Federal Register*, July 26, 1991, p. 3540). The regulations cover employment; public service, including public transportation, public accommodations, and telecommunications; and miscellaneous provisions. Although the law is not specific in reference to issues related to children in school, its provisions

have direct impact. Public buildings, including schools, need to be accessible, and children should be able to use public transportation to get to school, work, and social activities. Children with disabilities should expect to be able to use the skills learned at school in an accessible workplace. The Americans with Disabilities Act is discussed in Chapter 33 on medicolegal issues.

▌EDUCATIONAL MILIEU

Physical therapists are not new to special educational environments but have only recently begun serving children with disabilities in the regular education setting. Educational administrators and teachers may not be familiar with the role of physical therapy, just as the physical therapist may not be familiar with the educational milieu. Hence, there is the need for open communication and collaboration. Physical therapists must take the time to develop relationships and to understand the written and unwritten rules of the educational environment. With experience, teachers and therapists can learn to create an excellent working environment for themselves and an effective educational setting (Steed, 1991).

Least Restrictive Environment

Education of all children in the least restrictive environment, no matter how severe their disability, is what the federal laws and "best practices" indicate we must strive to achieve (Meyer et al., 1991; PL 102-119; Rainforth et al., 1992; Taylor, 1988). The conceptual framework for the least restrictive environment started in the 1960s to offer children with disabilities a range of service opportunities. Reynolds (1962) advocated a continuum of placement options from most restrictive to least restrictive. Deno (1970) termed this the "cascade" of educational placements. The cascade of environments, from most to least restrictive, includes the residential setting, home-bound services, special schools, special classes in regular schools, regular classes with resource assistance, and being educated in regular classes in the neighborhood school with children without disabilities. Terminology used to describe least restrictive environment has evolved from "mainstreaming," to "integrated," to "inclusion"; the difference is more than merely a change in language.

The least restrictive environment is not necessarily as widely accepted as one might assume. Regular educators are often concerned about having children with special needs placed in their classrooms without appropriate support services. Administrators are often concerned about the cost to the regular education system. Parents sometimes believe that segregated environments have better services for their child. Taylor (1988), an advocate for total integration, now finds that we are "Caught in the Continuum." His thought-provoking article outlines some of the pitfalls in the concept of least restrictive environment. His major concerns are as follows (Taylor, 1988, pp. 45–48):

1. "The LRE principle legitimates restrictive environments." A continuum legitimizes each segment of the continuum and therefore still allows restrictive placement.

2. "The LRE principle confuses segregation and integration on the one hand with intensity of services on the other." The principle assumes that the most segregated settings offer the most intensive services. These are, however, very separate issues. "In fact, some of the most segregated settings have provided the least effective services."

3. "The LRE principle is based on a readiness model." The assumption is that an individual must be "ready" or "graduate" to the next level of the LRE. "The irony is that the most restrictive placements do not prepare people for the least restrictive placements. Institutions do not prepare people for community living, segregated day programs do not prepare people for competitive work, and segregated schooling does not prepare students for integrated schooling."

4. "The LRE principle supports the primacy of professional decision making." Taylor believes "integration is ultimately a moral and philosophical issue, not a professional one."

5. "The LRE principle sanctions infringements on the people's rights." "The question implied by LRE is not whether people with developmental disabilities should be restricted but to what extent" (Turnbull, 1981, p. 17).

6. "The LRE principle implies that people must move as they develop and change." Individuals who make progress are forced to constantly move to lesser and lesser restrictive environments. This can be disruptive to the development of friendships and a sense of stability.

Taylor (1988) proposes that a commitment to integration, specifically for those individuals with severe disabilities, requires a shift in focus:

1. *From the development of facilities and programs into which people must fit to the provision of services and supports necessary for people with severe disabilities to participate fully in community life;*

2. *From neighborhoods to typical homes, from regular school buildings to regular classes, and from vocational models to typical jobs and activities;*

3. *From professional judgment as a basis for determining community involvement to personal choice;*

4. *From a presumption in favor of integration to a mandate to provide opportunities for integration;*

5. *From a conditional ("to the extent necessary, appropriate, feasible") to an unconditional commitment to integration;*

6. *From requiring individuals to change in order to participate in the community to requiring service systems to change;*

7. *From restrictions applied categorically as a condition for receiving service to opportunities available to nondisabled people;*

8. *From disability labels as a factor in determining community participation to a recognition of common human needs;*

9. *From independence to community belonging; and*

10. *From placing people in the community to helping them become part of the community.*

(TAYLOR, 1988, P. 51)

These shifts in focus, which are already occurring in some parts of the United States, present some challenges for physical therapists. Therapists must be prepared to work in regular local schools. A problem related to working in the regular schools is the lack of peer contact and therefore professional discussions and peer review. The therapist might also have to travel far to see a single child and bring equipment to the school or arrange for storage. It might take a long time to get to know the staff and where things are at each individual school. Scheduling services and times to meet with teachers is difficult. Physical therapists and teachers must work together in these times of change so that best practices and effective service can be achieved in an integrated environment at the local school.

Models of Team Interaction

There has been an evolution in the concept of team interaction during the past 2 decades. The hierarchy of team interaction is presented in Table 31–1. The unidisciplinary model is not a team model and should rarely if ever be used in school settings. The multidisciplinary model involves several professionals doing independent evaluations and then meeting to discuss their evaluations and

TABLE 31–1. MODELS OF TEAM INTERACTION

Type of Model	Description
Unidisciplinary	Professional works independently of all others.
Intradisciplinary	Members of the same profession work together without significant communication with members of other professions.
Multidisciplinary	Professionals work independently but recognize and value the contributions of other professions. "Little or no interaction or ongoing communication occurs among professionals." (Thurman & Wilderstrom, 1990, p. 225). However, the Rules and Regulations (*Federal Register*, June 22, 1989, p. 26313) for PL 99-457 redefines multidisciplinary to mean "the involvement of two or more disciplines or professions in the provision of integrated and coordinated services, including evaluation and assessment."
Interdisciplinary	Individuals from different disciplines work together cooperatively to evaluate and develop programs. Emphasis is on teamwork. Role definitions are relaxed.
Transdisciplinary	Professionals are committed "to teaching, learning and working with others across traditional disciplinary boundaries." (Rainforth et al., 1992, p. 13). Role release occurs when a team member assumes the responsibilities of other disciplines for service delivery.
Collaborative	The team interaction of the transdisciplinary model is combined with the integrated service delivery model. Services are provided by professionals across disciplinary boundaries as part of the natural routine of the school and community.

determine goals, objectives, and a plan of action. The meaning of multidisciplinary has changed since 1986 because of its usage in PL 99-457. In the law, the term *multidisciplinary* is used to describe an interdisciplinary model. Since *multidisciplinary* was a statutory term, it could not be changed. Therefore, a new definition was presented in the Rules and Regulations for PL 99-457: "Multidisciplinary means the involvement of two or more disciplines or professions in the provision of integrated and coordinated services, including evaluation and assessment activities" and the development of the IFSP (*Federal Register*, June 22, 1989, p. 26313). This is consistent with the definition of an interdisciplinary model. Therefore, there is frequently confusion when using the term *multidisciplinary*.

The definition and application of the transdisciplinary model is also ambiguous. For some, the continuous sharing of information across disciplines is sufficient for a transdisciplinary model. For others, there must be complete role release. Role release involves not merely the sharing of information but also the sharing of performance competencies. Team members teach each other specific interventions so that all can provide greater consistency and frequency in meeting the child's needs.

A new concept identified as a model of team interaction is *family centered*. This concept, however, is not a model of team interaction but is the theoretic construct around which the team works. The family and the child are the reason for the team's existence, and the team must function to meet the family's concerns and priorities.

As the team process has developed, the use of the terms *collaboration* and *collaborative teams* has appeared. The defining characteristics of collaborative teamwork, as conceptualized by Rainforth and colleagues (1992), are presented in Table 31–2. These researchers believe that significant benefits are gained because of the "diverse perspectives, skills, and knowledge available from the variety of disciplines represented on the educational team. This creates a tremendous resource of problem solving

TABLE 31–2. DEFINING CHARACTERISTICS OF COLLABORATIVE TEAMWORK

1. Equal participation in the collaborative teamwork process by family members and the educational service providers on the educational team
2. Equal participation by all disciplines determined to be necessary for students to achieve their individualized educational goals
3. Consensus decision making about priority educational goals and objectives related to all areas of student functioning at school, at home, and in the community
4. Consensus decision making about the type and amount of support required from related services personnel
5. Attention to motor, communication, and other embedded skills and needs throughout the educational program and in direct relevance to accomplishing priority educational goals
6. Infusion of knowledge and skills from different disciplines into the design of educational methods and interventions
7. Role release to enable team members who are involved most directly and frequently with students to develop the confidence and competence necessary to facilitate active learning and effective participation in the educational program
8. Collaborative problem solving and shared responsibility for student learning across all aspects of the educational program

From Rainforth, B, York, J, & MacDonald, C. Collaborative Teams for Students with Severe Disabilities, 1992, p. 16. Paul H Brookes Publishing Co., P.O. Box 10624, Baltimore, MD 21285-0624.

and support" (Rainforth et al., 1992, p. 21). Collaborative teams are of vital importance when working with children having multiple disabilities or with those who are severely or profoundly disabled.

When joining a team, physical therapists are encouraged to ask for a clarification and a definition of terms regarding models or expectations of team interaction. All individuals should have the same understanding to avoid miscommunication and conflict.

Models of Service Delivery

There is an array of models of physical therapy service delivery. Unfortunately, there is also an array of confusing and conflicting terms used to describe the various models. The Iowa State Department of Education (David & Randall, 1988) defined direct, integrated, and consultative models along dimensions that are important for service delivery (Table 31–3). Monitoring (Effgen, 1989;

TABLE 31–3. PHYSICAL THERAPY SERVICE DELIVERY MODELS IN EDUCATIONAL SETTINGS

	Direct	Integrated	Consultative	Monitoring	Collaborative
THERAPIST'S PRIMARY CONTACT	Pupil	Pupil, teacher, parent, aide	Teacher, parent, aide, pupil	Pupil	Entire team, pupil
ENVIRONMENT FOR SERVICE DELIVERY	Distraction-free environment (may need to be separate from learning environment) Specialized equipment needed	Learning environment and other natural settings Therapy area if necessary for a specific child	Learning environment and other natural settings	Learning environment Therapy area if necessary for a specific child	Learning environment and other natural settings
METHODS OF INTERVENTION	Educationally related functional activities Specific therapeutic techniques that cannot safely be delegated Emphasis on acquisition of new motor skills	Educationally related functional activities Positioning Emphasis on practice of newly acquired motor skills in the daily routine	Educationally related activities Positioning Adaptive materials Emphasis on adapting to learning environment and generalization of acquired skills	Emphasis on making certain child maintains status to benefit from special education	Educationally related activities
AMOUNT OF ACTUAL SERVICE TIME	Regularly scheduled sessions, generally at least weekly	Routinely scheduled Flexible amount of time depending on needs of staff or pupil	Intermittent or as needed, depending on needs of staff or pupil	Intermittent, depending on needs of pupil, may be as infrequent as once in 6 months	Ongoing intervention Discipline-referenced knowledge shared among team members so relevant activities occur throughout the day
IMPLEMENTER OF ACTIVITIES	PT	PT, PTA, teacher, parent, aide, OT, COTA	Teacher, parent, aide	PT	Team
INDIVIDUALIZED EDUCATION PLAN OBJECTIVES	Specific to therapy programs as related to educational needs	Specific to educational program	Specific to educational program	Specific to being able to maintain educational program	Organized around life domains in an ecologic curriculum

Adapted from David, K., & Randall, K. Iowa Guidelines for Educationally Related Physical and Occupational Therapy Services. Des Moines, IA. Department of Education, 1988.
COTA = certified occupational therapist assistant; OT = occupational therapist; PT = physical therapist, PTA = physical therapist assistant.

Lindsey et al., 1980) and the collaborative models (Rainforth et al., 1992) are also forms of service delivery.

DIRECT MODEL

In the direct model, the therapist is the primary service provider to the child. This is the traditional model used to provide physical therapy. Direct therapy is given when specific therapeutic techniques cannot be safely delegated and when there is emphasis on acquisition of new motor skills. Rarely, if ever, should direct therapy be given without working with the child's teachers and parents. It is not unusual for a child to receive direct therapy for a specific goal while other models of service delivery are used to achieve other goals. A combination of several models of service delivery is consistent with the integrated service delivery model.

INTEGRATED MODEL

The integrated model is the second model described in Table 31–3. There have been a number of different definitions of *integrated*. The Iowa State Department of Education defines the integrated model as one in which the therapist's contact is not only the child but also the teacher, aide, and family; service delivery is in the learning environment, and the method of intervention is educationally related functional activities, with an emphasis on practice of newly acquired motor skills. The implementer of the activities may be the teacher, aide, another professional, parent, or the physical therapist. As seen in Table 31–3, this model may also include direct and consultative services.

Dunn (1991) further classified the integrated model as consisting of peer integration, functional integration, practice integration, and comprehensive integration. Peer integration occurs when a child with a disability functions in a classroom or at a social event with children without disabilities. Functional integration occurs when a child can use a therapeutic strategy or newly acquired skill in the natural environment. Encouragement of functional integration is the rationale behind providing therapy in the natural environment, especially when the objectives involve fluency (refinement of skills) and generalization of the ability to perform the skills in multiple environments with different trainers and equipment. Practice integration involves the collaboration of professionals to meet a child's individual needs. Comprehensive integration combines all the areas of integration and is the level toward which we must strive.

The integrated model of service delivery can, and

frequently does, include direct physical therapy services provided by a physical therapist. The therapist, however, must collaborate with all other key individuals serving the child. Goals and objectives should be jointly developed, and all individuals serving the child should be instructed in how to achieve these objectives within their capability. Direct services, if best for the child, are provided in the least restrictive environment. Only when it is in the best interests of the child should the therapy session be in a restrictive environment, such as a treatment room. Common examples of when therapy might be best in a more restrictive environment are when the child is taking mainly academic courses, when extensive equipment is required, or when the child is highly distractable.

CONSULTATIVE MODEL

In the consultative model, the therapist's contacts are the teacher, aide, parent, and child. The service is provided in the learning environment, and the method of intervention is educationally related activities for the school-aged child or early intervention services, as needed, for the younger child. Activities are implemented by all personnel except the therapist. The therapist meets with, and demonstrates activities to, all appropriate staff. The responsibility for the outcome is with the consultee —the individuals, usually the teachers, receiving the consultation (Dunn, 1991).

Consultation may be child-specific, as outlined in Table 31–3, but might also include programmatic consultation involving issues related to safety, transportation, architectural barriers, equipment, documentation, continuing education, and for improvement of the program's quality (Lindsey et al., 1980). Programmatic consultation should be the first activity of a therapist at the beginning of each academic year or should occur the first time a therapist goes to a new school. Issues related to safety, transportation, and positioning are frequently more important than child-specific goals and objectives. Once the environment is safe, the child is properly positioned throughout the day, and a safe means of mobility is determined, then the specific therapeutic program can be initiated.

MONITORING MODEL

In the monitoring model of service delivery the therapist remains responsible for the outcome of the intervention. Staff are instructed as appropriate, but the therapist, although not proving direct intervention, maintains regular contact with the child to check on status. Monitoring is important for follow-up of children who have musculoskeletal, neurologic, or cardiopulmonary impairments that might deteriorate over time or functional limitations that would then require direct, integrated, or consultative intervention. Monitoring allows the therapist to check on the need for modifications in adaptive equipment, orthoses, and prostheses. Monitoring is also an important way of checking to determine if a child is progressing as necessary for transition to the next level of educational or vocational services. Monitoring is an important element of transition from direct or integrated services to no services. Monitoring gives the family, child, and therapist a sense of security that the child is being observed. Also, if the child should require physical therapy service, it generally allows more rapid receipt of services because physical therapy is already listed on the IEP.

COLLABORATIVE MODEL

Not everyone would consider the collaborative model a model of service delivery; however, since it is defined as a combination of transdisciplinary team interaction and an integrated service delivery model, it should be discussed as part of service delivery (Rainforth et al., 1992). As noted in Tables 31–1 and 31–3, services in a collaborative model are provided by all team members, as in an integrated model, but the degree of role release and crossing of disciplinary boundaries is greater. The team assumes responsibility for developing a consensus on the goals and objectives and the implementation of the program activities. The activities are educationally relevant and are implemented in the natural routine of the school and community. In the collaborative model, the amount of service delivery or practice in an activity should, theoretically, be greater than in other models because the entire team is carrying out the activities. In practice, this might not be the case because of the varied levels of skill of the implementors, insufficient "natural" opportunities to practice an activity, competition among activities, and the difficulty of some activities (Prieto, 1992; Soccio, 1991). Individual state practice acts may also prohibit physical therapists from having professionals from other disciplines carry out certain therapeutic activities.

▌ PROGRAM DEVELOPMENT

Evaluation and Assessment

Determination of eligibility for services and measurement of outcomes of services is based on comprehensive evaluation and ongoing assessment. Federal Rules and Regulations specifically define the terms *evaluation* and *assessment*. "Evaluation means the procedures used . . . to determine whether a child has a disability and the nature and extent of special education and related services that the child needs. The term means procedures used selectively with an individual" (*Federal Register*, September 29, 1992, p. 44819). "Assessment means the ongoing procedures used by appropriate qualified personnel throughout the period of a child's eligibility" (*Federal Register*, June 22, 1989, p. 26320). These definitions of evaluation and assessment in the *Federal Register* probably reflect their use in school system practice; however, they are not consistent with the definitions in the American Physical Therapy Association's Standards for Tests and Measurements in Practice (American Physical Therapy Association, Task Force on Standards, 1991b) used in this text.

The evaluation is used to determine eligibility for services, and, therefore, it is of utmost importance that it be comprehensive and objective. Selection of standardized tests should be based on professional judgment and dictated by the characteristics of the individual child. Therapists should work with school personnel to identify appropriate tests. The child's functional abilities should be assessed in the natural environment. This means that the therapist must see the child in the classroom, hallway, and other school settings. For infants, toddlers, and preschoolers, the therapist should visit the child at home, in the child care center, or at preschool. If it is not feasible to assess the child in these natural environments, every attempt must be made to make the evaluation setting as close to the natural environment as possible. The evaluation should also include a full assessment of all body systems: musculoskeletal, neurologic, and cardiopulmonary. Impairment of any of these systems can cause functional limitations. These limitations frequently must be remediated before the child can improve in functional abilities. The IEP or IFSP includes the objectives related to attainment of the functional activities.

The evaluation is critical in determining eligibility for services and the type of services and, later, in comparing the success of services and the need for extended school year programming. In school-aged children, a motor delay or disability does not necessarily qualify a child for special education and related services. The children must first have an educational need for special education. The categories that qualify school-aged children for special education are presented in Table 31–4. Once the child meets the criteria for special education in one of

TABLE 31–4. **FEDERAL DEFINITIONS OF CHILDREN WITH DISABILITIES**

Disability	Definition
Developmental delay	The term "children with disabilities" for children aged 3 through 5 may, at a State's discretion, include children—Who are experiencing developmental delays, as defined by the State and as measured by appropriate diagnostic instruments and procedures, in one or more of the following areas: physical development, cognitive development, communication development, social or emotional development, or adaptive development, and Who, for that reason, need special education and related services. . . .
Autism	means a developmental disability significantly affecting verbal and nonverbal communication and social interaction, generally evident before age 3, that adversely affects a child's educational performance. Other characteristics often associated with autism are engagement in repetitive activities and stereotyped movements, resistance to environmental change, or change in daily routines, and unusual responses to sensory experiences. The term does not apply if a child's educational performance is adversely affected primarily because the child has a serious emotional disturbance.
Deaf-blindness	means concomitant hearing and visual impairments, the combination of which causes such severe communication and other developmental and educational problems that they cannot be accommodated in special education programs solely for children with deafness or children with blindness.
Deafness	means a hearing impairment that is so severe that the child is impaired in processing linguistic information through hearing, with or without amplification, that adversely affects a child's educational performances.
Hearing impairment	means an impairment in hearing, whether permanent or fluctuating, that adversely affects a child's educational performance but that is not included under the definition of deafness.
Mental retardation	means significantly subaverage general intellectual functioning existing concurrently with deficits in adaptive behavior and manifested during the developmental period that adversely affects a child's educational performance.
Multiple disabilities	means concomitant impairments (such as mental retardation–blindness, mental retardation–orthopaedic impairment, etc) the combination of which causes such severe educational problems that they cannot be accommodated in special education programs solely for one of the impairments. The term does not include deaf-blindness.
Orthopaedic impairment	means a severe orthopedic impairment that adversely affects a child's educational performance. The term includes impairments caused by congenital anomaly (e.g., clubfoot, absence of some member, etc.), impairments caused by disease (e.g., poliomyelitis, bone tuberculosis, etc.), and impairments from other causes (e.g., cerebral palsy, amputations, and fractures or burns that cause contractures).
Other health impairment	means having limited strength, vitality or alertness, due to chronic or acute health problems such as a heart condition, tuberculosis, rheumatic fever, nephritis, asthma, sickle cell anemia, hemophilia, epilepsy, lead poisoning, leukemia, or diabetes that adversely affects a child's educational performance.
Serious emotional disturbance	is defined as follows: The term means a condition exhibiting one or more of the following characteristics over a long period of time and to a marked degree that adversely affects a child's educational performance— A) An inability to learn that cannot be explained by intellectual, sensory, or health factors; B) An inability to build or maintain satisfactory interpersonal relationships with peers and teachers; C) Inappropriate types of behavior or feelings under normal circumstances; D) A general pervasive mood of unhappiness or depression; or E) A tendency to develop physical symptoms or fears associated with personal or school problems; ii) The term includes schizophrenia. The term does not apply to children who are socially maladjusted, unless it is determined that they have a serious emotional disturbance.
Specific learning disability	means a disorder in one or more of the basic psychological processes involved in understanding or in using language, spoken or written, that may manifest itself in an imperfect ability to listen, think, speak, read, write, spell, or to do mathematical calculations. The term includes such conditions as perceptual disabilities, brain injury, minimal brain dysfunction, dyslexia, and developmental aphasia. The term does not apply to children who have learning problems that are primarily the result of visual, hearing, or motor disabilities, of mental retardation, of emotional disturbance, or of environmental, cultural, or economic disadvantage.
Speech and language impairment	means a communication disorder such as stuttering, impaired articulation, a language impairment, or a voice impairment that adversely affects a child's educational performance.
Traumatic brain injury	means an acquired injury to the brain caused by an external physical force, resulting in total or partial functional disability or psychosocial impairment, or both, that adversely affects a child's educational performance. The term applies to open- or closed-head injuries resulting in impairments in one or more areas, such as cognition; language; memory; attention; reasoning; abstract thinking; judgment; problem-solving; sensory, perceptual, and motor abilities; psychosocial behavior; physical functions; information processing; and speech. The term does not apply to brain injuries that are congenital or degenerative, or brain injuries induced by birth trauma.
Visual impairment including blindness	means an impairment in vision that, even with correction, adversely affects a child's educational performance. The term includes both partial sight and blindness.

From Federal Register, September 29, 1992, pp. 44801–44802.

these categories, their related service needs can be considered and determined at the IEP meeting. No matter how great the need for physical therapy, the child must first be eligible for special education.

The need for related services must be based on the individual needs of the child. All related services are to be provided "as may be required to assist a child with a disability to benefit from special education." (*Federal Register*, September 29, 1992, p. 44803). There can be no set criteria to determine educational needs for physical therapy. Flexible guidelines might be developed, but they cannot be exclusionary. Several school systems, however, have attempted to develop exclusionary criteria. One such criterion is the use of prerequisite skills that must be demonstrated before the child is considered likely to benefit from related services (Rainforth, 1991). Performance discrepancy criteria, also called cognitive referencing, has been attempted by some systems, including the state of Louisiana (Carr, 1989). In this system, "The criteria do not allow for the treatment of children whose cognitive scores are below their motor scores" (Carr, 1989, p. 506). The foundation for this decision is a belief that a "positive correlation exists between the development of cognition and motor skills" (Simunds, 1992, p. 1). In this case, the child most appropriate for physical therapy is a child with normal intellectual skills but delay in motor skills. Children whose level of cognition and motor skills are similar would not be eligible for services. Aside from the legal and ethical questions regarding cognitive referencing, one study has not supported its use (Cole et al., 1991). In this study, children with equivalent motor and cognitive skills made significantly greater improvement on a perceptual test after at least 6 months of physical therapy and/or occupational therapy than did the group of children with cognitive skills that were higher than their motor skills.

The Individuals with Disabilities Education Act Amendments of 1991 limit related services to only those children requiring special education. Section 504 of another federal law, the Rehabilitation Act of 1973 (PL 93-112), however, might be used to broaden a student's eligibility for related services in school (National Information Center for Children and Youth with Disabilities, 1991). State educational agencies that receive federal funds are not allowed to exclude qualified individuals with disabilities from participation in any program offered by the agency. This includes public schools. The definition of "qualified handicapped person" under Section 504 is broader than it is in PL 102-119. Under Section 504

"handicapped persons means any person who (i) has a physical or mental impairment which substantially limits one or more major life activities. . . . Major life activities means functions such as caring for one's self, performing manual tasks, walking, seeing, hearing, speaking, breathing, learning, and working."

(*FEDERAL REGISTER*, Sec. 1043, (j), 1988.)

Thus, it is possible that a child who does not require special education but who is a "qualified handicapped person" might be able to receive all the aids and services necessary to receive a free and appropriate public education (National Information Center for Children and Youth with Disabilities, 1991).

A specified amount of delay or impairment in physical or motor development qualifies infants and toddlers for early intervention services and, if appropriate, physical therapy. The amount of delay a child must display is determined by each individual state. States use standards such as the following (Garwood & Sheehan, 1989):

- 20% or 25% delay in one or more developmental areas
- 1.5 standard deviation below the mean in at least one area or 1 standard deviation below the mean in two areas
- moderate or severe delay or substantial likelihood of becoming delayed
- moderate or severe sensory impairment
- delay in months as follows
  - 1 year of age: 3 months' delay
  - 1.5 years of age: 4.5 months' delay
  - 2 years of age: 6 months' delay
  - 3 years of age: 9 months' delay
- 15% below chronologic age in two or more areas

Infants might qualify for early intervention services in one state and not another. In addition, eligibility can easily be influenced by the tests used. The criteria on some tests are far more rigorous than on others, and a child is likely to score lower on a more rigorous test than on either a less rigorous test or one that allows scoring by parent report (Long, 1992).

In addition to the comprehensive assessment of the child, early intervention programs must conduct family assessments to determine the resources, priorities, and concerns of the family related to enhancing the development of their child. The physical therapist, due to the interrelationship of the child and family evaluation, might be required to participate in or perform a family assessment.

The therapist should become knowledgeable in family assessment tools and seek appropriate training (Chiarello et al., 1992; Sparling, 1993).

Developing Goals and Objectives

To develop appropriate goals and objectives, desired outcomes must first be identified (McEwen & Shelden, 1992). Determining a desired outcome might be as simple as merely asking the child, or it might require several multidisciplinary meetings. Outcome statements do not need to be measurable, but they should be functional. Once the desired outcome is identified, the goals that are necessary to achieve the outcome must be expressed. Goals are written to be achieved in 1 year. McEwen and Shelden (1992) indicated that goals should be measurable, although others (Montgomery, 1987; Wilson, 1991) indicated that goals may be global statements that are not necessarily measurable. After the desired outcomes and goals are identified, the measurable objectives must be developed.

All objectives must contain a statement of the behavior to be achieved, under what conditions, and the criteria to be used (Effgen, 1991; Mager, 1962). It is common to first develop long-term objectives. In educational environments these objectives are for 1 year and are referred to as "short-term instructional objectives." These "objectives are developed based on a logical breakdown of the major components of the annual goals, and can serve as milestones for measuring progress towards meeting the goals" (*Federal Register*, September 29, 1992, p. 44838). Once a major objective is developed, it can be broken down into short-term objectives. Short-term objectives are based on a task analysis of the major, or long-term, objective. When possible, each short-term objective should be functional and educationally relevant; however, there are situations in which some of the short-term objectives might not be functional but are vital to achieving the long-term objective. The recognition and listing of all these non–educationally relevant objectives is important to document progress. Achievement of these objectives indicates progression toward the educationally relevant, functional objective. Teachers would agree that reading is a very important goal of education; however, few teachers would negate the importance of the child's first knowing the nonfunctional, although prerequisite, alphabet. The situation is the same in physical therapy. Sitting is an important functional skill; however, without the prerequisite trunk muscle strength and hip range of motion, independent sitting is impossible.

An example of a desired outcome and the objec-

TABLE 31–5. EXAMPLE OF DESIRED OUTCOME AND OBJECTIVES INVOLVED IN A SPECIFIC TASK

Outcome Statement
I want to be able to climb the steps to get into school.

Functional Long-Term Objective or Measurable Goal That Is Educationally Relevant
Jonathan will be able to walk up and down the school stairs independently without using the railing.

Functional Short-Term Objectives That Are Educationally Relevant
(If part of the IEP, would be called short-term instructional objectives or, if not in IEP, would be part of the instructional plan.)
1. Jonathan will be able to climb up 8 stairs at school with minimal assistance using a railing.
2. Jonathan will be able to climb up 8 stairs at school with minimal assistance without using a railing.
3. Jonathan will be able to climb down 8 stairs at school with minimal assistance using a railing.
4. Jonathan will be able to climb down 8 stairs at school with minimal assistance without using a railing.
5. Jonathan will be able to climb up 8 stairs at school without assistance or a railing.
6. Jonathan will be able to climb down 8 stairs at school without assistance or a railing.

Short-Term Objectives That May or May Not Be Considered Educationally Relevant
(These objectives are necessary to achieve the educationally relevant objectives and would be part of the instructional plan, not IEP.)
1. Jonathan will progress from 30° to 50° of active right-knee flexion.
2. Jonathan will progress from a poor to a fair muscle-strength grade in his left quadriceps.
3. Jonathan will achieve 90° of active right-knee flexion.
4. Jonathan will achieve a good muscle-strength grade in his left quadriceps.

tives involving independent stair climbing is given in Table 31–5. To climb stairs independently—a very functional, educationally relevant task—a child should have 90° of knee flexion and good strength in the quadriceps muscles. The educationally relevant objectives go in the child's IEP, and the other short-term objectives, which may or may not be considered educationally relevant, might go in the teacher's or therapist's plan. Documentation of achievement of each objective is important to report to both the child and family. Many small gains should be recognized and rewarded in lieu of waiting, perhaps forever, for the achievement of the major long-term objective.

When doing a task analysis and developing the short-term objectives, several variables should be considered: 1) changes in the behavior itself, 2) changes in the conditions under which the behavior is performed, and 3) changes in the criteria expected for ultimate performance (Effgen, 1991). Changes in the behavior may reflect maturation of the behavior itself, progressing from basic skills to more complex skills, or increasing levels of functional activity. Changes in conditions may be from simple to complex, such as walking in an empty hallway to walking in a hallway filled with students. Progression of criteria may be qualitative or quantitative. The criterion might include the qualitative measure of hip extension during midstance—which helps to make gait more efficient—or a more direct quantitative measure of the walking speed. Use of quantitative criteria, such as judgment by three of four trials or 80% of the time, should be considered carefully. Successfully crossing the street only 80% of the time can be fatal! Selection of the behavior, conditions, and criteria for judging attainment of each objective for each individual child must be based on sound professional judgment. Books or other materials that provide lists of potential objectives should not replace the judgment of the professional.

In addition to the task variables, consideration should be given to the "hierarchy of response competence" outlined by Alberto and Troutman (1990). Skill must first be acquired; it is then refined as fluency or proficiency develops. The skill must then be maintained and finally generalized to multiple environments, trainers, and equipment. *Acquisition, fluency, maintenance, and generalization* of behaviors are the terms used by educators. Use of this terminology is important when there is a need to convey the rationale for providing services past the acquisition phase.

Therapists are also encouraged to consider the prompting system used as a strategy to achieve an objective and as a variable in writing the criteria for judging attainment of the objective. A systematic delivery of levels of prompting assistance may be implemented in two ways. One is the "system of maximum prompts," and the other is the "system of least prompts" (Alberto & Troutman, 1990; Effgen, 1991). The prompts are usually a verbal or visual cue, model, prompt or partial assistance, or guide or "put through." In the "system of maximum prompts," the therapist first provides maximum assistance and then a guide and then, gradually over successive sessions, reduces the amount of assistance as the child achieves more independence. This is a common technique used by therapists, and it allows for maximal success during learning. This system is best suited for the initial acquisition of a skill, when it is important to avoid unsafe movement, and for a complex series of tasks such as some activities of daily living.

The "system of least prompts" starts by providing the least amount of assistance, usually a verbal or visual cue, and then progresses to a model, prompt, guide, or maximal assistance as necessary. This approach allows the child to display his or her best effort before the therapist prematurely pro-

vides unnecessary assistance. The "system of least prompts" is best for skills under some initial control or those in which the child is developing fluency or generalization to new settings, individuals, or equipment.

Individualized Education Plan

The individualized education plan (IEP) is the document that guides the program of special education and related services for the school-aged child of 5 to 21 years of age. It is also the document used in many states for the educational program of preschoolers aged 3 to 5 years. The IEP, as discussed previously, is developed at a meeting of the child's parents and members of the educational team. The physical therapist is not required by law to attend but has a professional obligation to participate when decisions regarding physical therapy are being made. The physical therapy contribution to the IEP must relate to the educational needs of the child. Measurable behavior objectives called short-term instructional objectives or IEP objectives in the Federal Rules and Regulations (*Federal Register*, September 29, 1992, p. 44838) must be developed. In the vast majority of situations, the objectives should be functional, with implementation integrated in the child's overall program.

The IEP for each child must include the following:

1. *A statement of the child's present levels of educational performance;*
2. *A statement of annual goals, including short-term instructional objectives;*
3. *A statement of the specific educational and related services to be provided to the child and the extent that the child will be able to participate in regular educational programs;*
4. *The projected dates for initiation of services and the anticipated duration of the services; and*
5. *Appropriate objective criteria and evaluation procedures and schedules for determining, on at least an annual basis, whether the short term instructional objectives are being achieved.*

(*FEDERAL REGISTER*, SEPTEMBER 29, 1992, P. 44815.)

"The IEP sets forth in writing a commitment of resources necessary to enable a child with a disability to receive needed special education and related services" (*Federal Register*, September 29, 1992, p. 44833). It is also a "management tool" and a "compliance/monitoring document" and

serves as an evaluation device for use in determining the extent of the child's progress towards meeting the projected outcomes. IDEA does not require that teachers or other school personnel be held accountable if a child with a disability does not achieve the goals and objectives set forth in the IEP.

(*FEDERAL REGISTER*, SEPTEMBER 29, 1992, P. 44833.)

The Federal Rules and Regulations for PL 102-119 (*Federal Register*, September 29, 1992, p. 44838) address a number of common questions regarding the content of the IEP. "The goals and objectives in the IEP are not intended to be as specific as the goals and objectives that are normally found in daily, weekly, or monthly instructional plans." Therapists should interpret this to mean that the annual goals, written as specific "short term instructional objectives," are included in the IEP.

"On the other hand, the objectives in classroom instructional plans deal with more specific outcomes that are to be accomplished on a daily, weekly, or monthly basis. Classroom instructional plans generally include details not required in an IEP, such as the specific methods, activities, and materials."

It is probably difficult for most therapists to consider a year "short term." However, in the educational life of a child, 1 year is relatively short term. Therapists working in schools also need to recognize that their objectives are "instructional plans" that will need to be written daily, weekly, or monthly, depending on the child and the frequency with which the child is seen by the therapist. Physical therapists should document achievement of these instructional objectives, whether or not the school administration requests this information.

Determining which "short-term instructional objectives" become part of the IEP, versus part of the therapist's instructional plans, and the amount of services written in the IEP is critical. The IEP objectives and the stated frequency of services cannot be changed without initiating another IEP meeting. "However, as long as there is no change in the overall amount [of time], some adjustments in scheduling the services should be possible (based on the professional judgment of the service provider) without holding another IEP meeting" (*Federal Register*, September 29, 1992, p. 44839). This clarification is helpful because it allows therapists to choose between blocked and distributed practice or group and individual sessions as long as the overall amount of time for service delivery for the individual child does not change.

Individualized Family Service Plan

The IFSP is developed for infants and toddlers and their families and, in some states, for preschool-aged children and their families. The IFSP differs from the IEP in its conceptual framework. The family is central to the development of the young child and is therefore central to the IFSP. The philosophy of family-centered early intervention is consistent with current theories of infant development and family functioning.

The IFSP is developed by a multidisciplinary team, including the parent or guardian. Physical therapy is one of the early intervention services, and therefore the need for physical therapy is based on the disability or delay in physical development. In early intervention, physical therapy is not a related service that is provided based only on the educational needs of the child.

The IFSP must be in writing and contain

"1. a statement of the infant's or toddler's present levels of physical development, cognitive development, communication development, social and emotional development, and adaptive development based on acceptable objective criteria,

"2. a statement of the family's resources, priorities, and concerns relating to enhancing the development of the family's infant or toddler with disabilities,

"3. a statement of the major outcomes expected to be achieved for the infant and toddler and the family, and the criteria, procedures, and schedule used to determine the degree to which progress toward achieving the outcomes is being made and whether modifications or revisions of the outcomes or services are necessary,

"4. a statement of specific early intervention services necessary to meet the unique needs of the infant or toddler and the family, including the frequency, intensity, and the method of delivering services,

"5. a statement of the natural environments in which early intervention services shall appropriately be provided,

"6. the projected dates for initiation of services and the anticipated duration of such services,

"7. the name of the service coordinator from the profession most immediately relevant to the infant's, toddler's, or family's needs who is otherwise qualified to carry out all applicable responsibilities under this part,

"8. the steps to be taken supporting the transition of the toddler with disabilities to services

provided under part B (for school-aged children) to the extent that such services are considered appropriate.

(PL 99-457, 100 stat 1150; PL 102-119, 105 stat 597.)

The contents of the IFSP must be fully explained to the parents, and informed written consent must be obtained before providing early intervention services. If the parents do not consent to some aspects of the services, then the early intervention services to which there is consent are provided (PL 102-119, 105 Stat 597).

Service Coordinator

A service coordinator must be named to facilitate the development, implementation, and evaluation of the IFSP. Service coordination, previously referred to as case management, "is recognized as one of the most essential, if not the essential service, in community programs. It is viewed as a means of overcoming the complexity and fragmentation of our service system" (Miller, 1983, p. 7). The service coordinator implements the IFSP and coordinates planning with other agencies and individuals. The service coordinator assists the child and family in obtaining the rights, procedural safeguards, and services provided by the state's early intervention program. Service coordination activities include

(1) Coordinating the performance of evaluations and assessments;
(2) Facilitating and participating in the development, review, and evaluation of individualized family service plans;
(3) Assisting families in identifying available service providers;
(4) Coordinating and monitoring the delivery of available services;
(5) Informing families of the availability of advocacy services;
(6) Coordinating with medical and health care providers; and
(7) Facilitating the development of a transition plan to pre-school services, if appropriate.

(*FEDERAL REGISTER,* JUNE 22, 1989, P. 26311; PL 102-119, 105 stat 595.)

The identity of the service coordinator is to be decided at the local level. A physical therapist, with the appropriate training, may wish to assume the role of service coordinator.

INTERVENTION

The federal emphasis in the United States on individually determining what is best for each child is appropriate. The form and content of the intervention is dictated by the IEP and IFSP. The objectives, frequency, location, and intensity of service are decided at the IEP and IFSP meetings, as discussed previously. The therapist, family, and rest of the intervention team must then decide on the best intervention strategies.

"Best practices" indicate that most, if not all, intervention should occur in the natural environment (American Physical Therapy Association, Section on Pediatrics, 1987; Association for Those with Severe Handicaps, 1986; Effgen & Klepper, 1994; Rainforth et al., 1992). In the school setting, the therapist should first ensure that the child is properly positioned on the bus and in the classroom. The safety of the aisles for ambulation or wheelchair mobility should be assessed. Architectural barriers must be evaluated, and appropriate actions taken to eliminate or lessen them. The teachers and family must be consulted regarding their problems or concerns. They should be instructed in proper handling, positioning, and use of body mechanics.

Direct intervention, if indicated, should then start in the classroom or home. This is accomplished easily with preschoolers and those in special classes for children with severe or profound disabilities (Giangreco et al., 1989). It is more difficult for children whose educational programs consist primarily of academic subjects. Physical therapy in the algebra class or the reading room, after the initial consultation, is generally inappropriate. Common sense must prevail. Perhaps therapy can be given during gross motor time in a preschool or during physical education. This is not always appropriate, however, because this might be the only time the child has to engage in free play and physical activity. Taking this opportunity away from the child might affect motivation, cooperation, and the development of important social skills that occur during these activities. Therefore, it is not always an easy task to determine the best natural environment for delivering services.

In the integrated service delivery model, collaborative team model, and family-centered intervention, the teachers, staff, and parents are usually participants in the delivery of some aspects of the therapeutic program. Their involvement may be as simple as using proper carrying techniques, or as complicated as facilitating the proper reciprocal creeping pattern. These individuals must first be instructed in proper positioning and use of any adaptive equipment and then in how to encourage selected gross motor activities. It is probably best to have classroom staff encourage activities at the fluency or generalization stage of motor development. Frequently, motor activities at the initial acquisition stage are too difficult for untrained individuals, are unsafe without experienced guidance, or may result in undesired movement.

Selection of which activities to teach others is a professional decision that must be based on characteristics of the individual child, the specific activity, and the capabilities and interest of the other individuals. In a series of three single-subject design studies, Prieto (1992) found that when teachers are properly instructed in gross motor activities the frequency with which they encourage children to perform those activities generally increases. Soccio (1991) performed a single-subject design study to examine the frequency of opportunities to practice specific gross motor skills during physical therapy and group early intervention classes. There was no difference in the number of opportunities to practice head control when direct physical therapy was compared with integrated group sessions for a child with severe disabilities. However, 2 children with cerebral palsy had more opportunities to practice standing and ambulation activities during direct, individual physical therapy sessions than during integrated group sessions in the classroom. The results suggest that the opportunity to practice certain motor activities in the classroom varies based on the type of movement and the class routines.

The specific type of treatment provided depends on the needs of the individual child and the education, training, and experience of the therapist. There is no one accepted treatment approach. Information provided throughout this text should assist the therapist in providing "state of the art" physical therapy. Physical therapy in an educational setting should be based on sound professional judgment and guided by the IEP or IFSP. If the appropriate treatment cannot be provided for a school-aged child because it is not educationally relevant and is not related to the objectives in the IEP, the therapist has a *professional obligation* to inform the parents. Once the parents are aware of the limitations of school-based physical therapy, they might obtain additional therapy elsewhere. Physical therapy for infants based on the IFSP, as noted before, need not be educationally relevant and can therefore be as comprehensive as required to meet the individual needs of the child and the family.

Physical therapists in educational settings need not write the daily notes required in other settings. In the United States, however, they must comply with their individual state practice acts. They must be careful to record objectively the child's status before and after both short and long school breaks, including those that occur when a child is absent for surgery or an illness. This is important in determining the need for extended school year services. A simple but comprehensive system of data collection using self-graphing data collection sheets is recommended (Alberto & Troutman, 1990; Effgen, 1991). One example of recording prompting needed to achieve a motor skill is provided in Figure 31–1. Extensive documentation is also necessary to support the need to increase, decrease, or terminate treatment. Physical therapy is not a lifelong activity such as learning. Both therapists and parents must recognize that, after a period of no change in status, physical therapy should be terminated or the child placed on a monitoring service delivery system. A continued desire for ambulation or similar activity is not sufficient reason for continued therapy after due diligence in trying to achieve an objective.

Therapists should strive to achieve the competencies for physical therapists in early intervention (Effgen et al., 1991) or school-based physical therapy (American Physical Therapy Association, 1990) that have been developed and endorsed by the Section on Pediatrics of the American Physical Therapy Association. They are an excellent resource for therapists working in these settings, both for identifying minimal standards for practice as well as for encouraging professional growth. The competencies may also be shared with administrators to help define the role of physical therapy as well as the resources necessary for effective service delivery. The therapist should continually read, participate in continuing education, take graduate courses, and engage in dialogue with colleagues. Therapists working in school systems and early intervention settings must be aware of the potential for professional isolation and seek opportunities for developing improved competence. Employers must support therapists' efforts at maintaining their professional skills (Effgen, 1988).

MANAGEMENT OF PHYSICAL THERAPY SERVICES

An important factor in successful management and service delivery in an educational environment is recognition and understanding of the significance of the team process. The physical therapist is part of the educational or early intervention team. Physical therapists must focus on collaboration with mem-

Trials

	7/24	7/25	7/26	7/27	7/28
Verbal Cue	1 2 3 4 5 6	1 2 3 4 5 6	1 2 3 4 5 6	1 2 3 4 5 (6)	1 2 (3)(4)(5)(6)
Gesture	1 2 3 4 5 6	1 2 3 4 5 6	1 2 3 4 5 6	1 2 (3)(4)(5) 6	1 (2) 3 4 5 6
Model	1 2 3 4 5 6	1 2 3 4 5 6	1 2 3 4 5 6	1 2/3 4 5 6	1/2 3 4 5 6
Prompt	1 2 3 4 5 6	1 2 3 (4)(5)(6)	(1)(2)(3)(4)(5)(6)	(1)(2) 3 (4) 5 6	(1) 2 3 4 5 6
Guide	(1)(2)(3)(4)(5)(6)	(1)(2)(3) 4 5 6	1 2 3 4 5 6	1 2 3 4 5 6	1 2 3 4 5 6
Incorrect	1 2 3 4 5 6	1 2 3 4 5 6	1 2 3 4 5 6	1 2 3 4 5 6	1 2 3 4 5 6
Date	7/24	7/25	7/26	7/27	7/28
Objective/task	Creep to swing	Creep to swing	Creep to swing	Creep to swing	Creep to swing
Cue(s)	Verbal cue: "Creep to the swing." Gesture—wave forward Model—therapist creeps Prompt—tap abdominal muscles Guide—support at abdomen and assist with arm and leg movement Use "least to maximum" prompting system.	Same as 7/24	Same as 7/24, except prompt was a quick tap to the abdominal muscles and triceps	Same as 7/26	Same as 7/26
Criterion and Conditions	Independently creep to swing, 12 feet away, with abdomen off the floor and elbows straight, 3 times	Same as 7/24	Same as 7/24	Same as 7/24	Same as 7/24
Comments	Required much assistance, did not appear interested in task.	Placed toy in swing, which appeared to stimulate interest; had difficulty with elbow extension.	Continues to have difficulty with elbow extension, especially on right.	Elbow extension improved bilaterally.	Ready to creep further distances; still concerned about ability to maintain elbow extension.

FIGURE 31–1. Self-graphing data collection sheet. (Adapted from Alberto, PA, & Schofield, P. Instructional interaction pattern for the severely handicapped. Teaching Exceptional Children, *12*:16–19, 1979. Copyright 1979 by The Council for Exceptional Children. Reprinted with permission. From Effgen, SK. Systematic delivery and recording of intervention assistance. Pediatric Physical Therapy, *3*:63–68, 1991.)

bers of all other disciplines and recognize their vital importance in the total well-being of the child. They cannot work in isolation if they expect maximal effectiveness. The team, including the child and family, must decide on the most appropriate services at each phase in the child's life. Therapists must be willing and have the support necessary to increase and decrease services as appropriate for each individual child.

Just as team leaders or case managers are needed in intervention teams, so too a manager or director of physical therapy is needed in school settings. The majority of directors of physical therapy in school

systems across the nation are not physical therapists or, indeed, any type of therapist (Effgen & Klepper, 1994). This has serious implications. To understand professional roles and responsibilities and how to nurture a professional, one must understand the profession. Many of the problems currently encountered in school systems could probably be prevented if therapists were supervised by other experienced therapists. Therapist managers understand the profession and are able to professionally and appropriately address management issues.

Therapists new to a system must receive orientation, mentoring, and in-service education. The roles and responsibilities of each therapist and all support staff should be defined clearly in a detailed job description that complies with federal and state laws. Therapists want to be introduced to the entire team of professionals with whom they will be working at all sites. They want to know whom to ask for equipment, space, and other items necessary for successful intervention. These introductions should be part of a planned orientation program. Therapists need to know when the teams meet at each school, how referrals are received and handled, how meetings are planned, how caseloads are determined, how to plan for personal continuing education, what and where the program's written policies are and how they can be changed, how peer review or quality improvement is done, and what the emergency procedures are, to name but a few issues. None of these are unusual requests; they can easily and cost-effectively be done in any system.

Once the therapist is properly introduced and oriented to the system, administrators must understand that therapists are not generally concerned about receiving tenure and a lifelong position. Employment is readily available for therapists, and they can and frequently do change positions. Therefore, administrators and therapists must talk to each other before problems arise and the therapist seeks other employment. Frequent areas of discontent are the lack of continuing education opportunities, insufficient peer contact, lack of an identified place to work, lack of time allotted for administrative tasks and meetings, and too much travel (Effgen & Klepper, 1994). More time and effort should be spent in retention of physical therapists so there is not so great a need for recruitment.

A system for obtaining referrals from physicians, if dictated by state law, must be developed. The referral allows the therapist to evaluate and then determine and provide appropriate treatment for the child. Most physical therapy state practice acts in the United States allow a therapist to evaluate without a referral, and 30 states (American Physical Therapy Association, 1993) allow therapists to evaluate and treat without a referral. Depending on the complexity of the child's medical problems and the need for pertinent information, a therapist might still want a referral no matter what the individual state law. Collaboration with physicians and all members of the child's medical and educational team encourages optimal service delivery.

A method must be developed for determination of therapy caseloads, and a rational system must be created for determining who should receive treatment and how much treatment should be given. This can be a very difficult task. The Florida Department of Exceptional Student Education (1987) developed a matrix that combines "Clinical Judgment Factors" and a "Therapy Profile," to determine the amount of physical therapy or occupational therapy a specific child receives. The Therapy Profile has the following sections: Developmental Skills, Range of Motion, Gross Motor, Muscle Tone, Muscle Strength, Activities of Daily Living, Adaptive Equipment, Positioning, Fine Motor, Oral Motor, Perceptual Motor, and Gait. Points are awarded based on the degree of function. The Clinical Judgment Factors are Chronological Age, Expected Response to Educationally Relevant Therapy, Extent of Direct Previous Therapy, Extent to Which Physical Management Needs Met in Other Programs, Priority of Direct Educationally Relevant Therapy Needs in Relation to Other Educational Programming, and Immediacy of Need. This system has provided Florida with a rational approach to determining who receives therapy and how much therapy they receive. It provides needed documentation to support complex, sensitive decisions regarding allocating services.

The American Occupational Therapy Association (1980) and the Georgia Alliance of School Occupational and Physical Therapists (Effgen, 1984) have published systems for determining therapy caseloads. These two systems suggest that each therapist can see from 15 to 40 children per week. The large variance is suggested because of different amounts of time required for travel, administration, meetings, construction of equipment, and consultation. The degree of need for therapy and the other support services available also affect the number of children who can be served. Children with critical needs for therapy require more intense, perhaps daily, therapy than do those with lesser needs. A therapist whose caseload includes only children having extensive needs for therapy is able to serve fewer children than a therapist whose caseload includes all children having minimal needs. Therapists who must travel a great deal or attend many meetings have much less time for direct student contact. For comparison, the average staff physical therapist in hospital-based pediatric physical therapy departments has 4 to 6.5 hours per day of charged care in an 8-hour work day (Tolley, 1993). There is no reason to expect as many contact hours from school-based therapists who work less than 8 hours per day.

CRITICAL ISSUES

Shortage of Physical Therapists

The shortage of qualified pediatric physical therapists is an overriding issue facing most school-based physical therapy. This issue affects almost every aspect of service delivery. The reasons for the shortage are numerous and include the low pay in schools, professional isolation, challenge of other areas of practice, and difficulty in working with children. Solutions are numerous and sometimes complex, but one of the easiest is often neglected. The best way to train and then recruit new physical therapists is to have them at a specific facility on clinical affiliations while they are students. Therefore, if a therapist is practicing in a school setting without an active student affiliation program, the therapist is part of the problem and not contributing to a solution. School systems must also recognize that therapists need to be recruited. This is a new concept for many educators, who have more than enough applications to fill other positions. It takes time, effort, and a plan to recruit qualified physical therapists.

Service Delivery System

The shortage of therapists also affects the type of service delivery system used and the roles assumed by all personnel. The literature supports an integrated service delivery model (Dunn, 1991; Rainforth et al., 1992). The advantages of more frequent practice in the natural setting with the support of all personnel is obvious. An appropriately administrated integrated therapy program, however, requires more, not less, staff. Training all personnel in a truly integrated transdisciplinary or collaborative model requires a great deal of time for training and meetings (Giangreco et al., 1989; Rainforth et al., 1992; York et al., 1990). There are those, however, who incorrectly think these models can be used to decrease the time required for physical therapy. Instead of having a therapist provide the required treatment, unqualified staff might provide "activities" without adequate supervised instruction or a teacher might be forced to squeeze one more task, for which he or she is not properly trained, into a busy agenda. Instead of providing the therapy in a room with necessary equipment, a

classroom or hallway is used in the name of natural environment. Models come and go, and rarely is there sufficient empirical data to support any service delivery system. Educators and therapists alike must step back and ask if they are truly meeting the needs of each child.

Professional Roles

The roles of all personnel are affected by the shortage of physical therapists. In systems in which there is full staffing, professionals jointly decide on the specific role of the various professionals. Overlap of professional roles is acknowledged, and divisions of responsibility are made that are best suited to the needs of the child, system, and professional staff (Fairfax, 1992).

There is no one accepted model of specific professional roles. In general, the overlap in physical therapy and occupational therapy and education is greatest when professionals from these disciplines are serving young children. For older children there is less overlap in professional roles. Areas of frequent overlap between occupational therapy and physical therapy include programs for strength and endurance, body awareness, classroom positioning and adaptations, and enhancement of motor experience (Fairfax, 1992). Areas of overlap between physical therapists and educators might include advanced gross motor skills, endurance training, and writing. In systems in which there is a critical shortage of physical therapists, the breadth of roles assumed by other staff members increases based on need and not necessarily on professional skill. Professionals concerned about their roles and the roles assumed by other staff members should carefully review their state practice acts.

Educationally Relevant Physical Therapy

Educationally relevant versus non–educationally relevant physical therapy is a frequent topic of debate, as discussed previously. In school systems committed to the comprehensive provision of services to children with disabilities and with adequate therapy staffing, the definition of educationally relevant physical therapy is frequently broad based and depends on the individual needs of the child addressed at the IEP meeting.

Having goals and objectives that are mutually agreed on by the entire educational team helps to make physical therapy more educationally relevant. The educational system was never meant to provide for all the child's therapy needs. In addition, therapy takes time away from other educational and social opportunities that are vital to the total well-being of the child.

Least Restrictive Environment

As more children are educated in the least restrictive environment, therapists must be willing to travel to meet the needs of those students. Unfortunately, travel to many schools is not the most time- and cost-effective method of service delivery. Therapists and administrators must be creative in their approach to serving children in their local schools, as they have been in Iowa (Neitopski et al., 1990) and Vermont. Giangreco and co-workers (1993b) developed Choosing Options and Accommodations for Children (COACH): A Guide to Planning Inclusive Education, which has been used extensively and successfully in Vermont. This educational planning tool has received national validation for use with children who are both deaf and blind and have multiple disabilities (Giangreco, et al., 1993a).

Reimbursement for Services

The cost of providing related services in educational environments and physical therapy in early intervention settings is a serious concern of program administrators. PL 94-142 and PL 99-457 provided some federal funding, but it has never been sufficient to cover the full spectrum of services needed by children in special education and early intervention programs. Physical therapists have traditionally earned more than do their counterparts in education, and this has led to some resentment. Many therapists are unwilling to accept a low-paying position in a school system but will accept a more financially rewarding contract with the school system. Although contract therapists might be excellent, they do not provide a long-term commitment to the system.

To cover the costs of physical therapy, some school systems are attempting to charge third-party payers. This is a serious concern because of the lifetime cap on many insurance policies and the possibility of losing insurance if bills are too high. Parents are not required to have their insurance company pay for services that are part of a free and appropriate public education. Parents must not be intimidated into thinking their child will not receive services if they choose not to have their insurance company pay. Medicaid has approved procedures allowing school systems to bill Medicaid directly for physical therapy. As new federal policies develop for the provision of health care services to children, it is likely that the funding of physical therapy for children will change.

▌SUMMARY

In the United States, physical therapy is mandated as part of federally sponsored programs to serve infants, toddlers, children, and youth with disabilities. For school-aged children, physical therapy is a related service of the educational program for those children who require special education. Physical therapy is part of the early intervention services provided to infants who have disabilities or delay in physical development.

The provision of physical therapy in an educational environment is a challenging and somewhat unusual setting for the physical therapist. It is not the "high-tech," health-focused environment of the modern hospital setting or the therapy-focused environment of the rehabilitation setting. In the educational environment, the therapist is a member of a team of professionals for whom therapy may or may not carry a high priority in the overall goals and objectives for an individual child. The educational needs of the child have the highest priority.

The therapist must learn to understand the educational milieu to provide the best possible services and be satisfied in the work environment. The federal, state, and local laws and rules and regulations that govern services in the educational environment must be understood and respected. Rules and regulations are meant to help serve the child and family, not hinder service provision.

Therapists who work in the educational environment have a true picture of the everyday lives of the children they serve. They see at first hand the struggles these children face. Daily, they are asked to solve complex problems to make life better for these children and their families. It is a rewarding and wonderful environment in which to work for those who are willing and able to adjust to its unique demands.

References

Alberto, PA, & Schofield, P. Instructional interaction pattern for the severely handicapped. Teaching Exceptional Children, 12:16–19, 1979.

Alberto, PA, & Troutman, AC. Applied Behavior Analysis for Teachers (3rd ed.). Columbus, OH: Merrill, 1990.

American Occupational Therapy Association. Guidelines for Occupational Therapy Services in the Public Schools (2nd ed.). Rockville, MD: American Occupational Therapy Association, 1980.

American Physical Therapy Association. Physical Therapy Practice in Educational Environments. Alexandria, VA: American Physical Therapy Association, 1990.

American Physical Therapy Association. Practice Department Report. Alexandria, VA: American Physical Therapy Association, 1993.

American Physical Therapy Association, Section on Pediatrics. TASH Position Statement. On the Provision of Related Services to Persons with Severe Handicaps. Alexandria, VA: American Physical Therapy Association, 1987.

American Physical Therapy Association, Section on Pediatrics. Report of the Section on Pediatrics of the American Physical Therapy Association to the Senate Committee on Labor and Human Resources and the House of Representatives Committee on Education and Labor on Reauthorization of Part H of the Education of the Handicapped Act. Alexandria, VA: American Physical Therapy Association, 1991.

Association for Those with Severe Handicaps. Position Statement of the Related Services Subcommittee of the TASH Critical Issues Committee. Seattle, WA: The Association for Those with Severe Handicaps, 1986.

Batten, HE. The industrial school for crippled and deformed children. Physical Therapy Review, 13:112–113, 1933.

Battle v Commonwealth of Pennsylvania, 629 F2d 280 (3rd Cir 1981).

Blatt, B, & Kaplan, F. Christmas in Purgatory: A Photographic Essay on Mental Retardation. Boston: Allyn & Bacon, 1966.

Braddock, D. Federal Policy Toward Mental Retardation and Developmental Disabilities. Baltimore: Paul H Brookes, 1987, p. 71.

Brown v Board of Education of Topeka, 347 US 483 (1954).

Cable, OE, Fowler, AF, & Foss, HS. The crippled children's guide of Buffalo, New York. Physical Therapy Review, 16:85–88, 1938.

Carr, SH. Louisiana's criteria of eligibility for occupational therapy services in the public school system. American Journal of Occupational Therapy, 43:503–506, 1989.

Chiarello, L, Effgen, SK, & Levinson, M. Parent professional partnership in evaluation and development of individualized family service plans. Pediatric Physical Therapy, 4:64–69, 1992.

Cole, KN, Mills, PE, & Harris, SR. Retrospective analysis of physical and occupational therapy progress in young children: An examination of cognitive referencing. Pediatric Physical Therapy, 3:185–189, 1991.

Council for Exceptional Children, Division of Early Childhood Education. Statement of the International Division for Early Childhood of the Council for Exceptional Children to the Congress of the United States with Respect to Reauthorization of Part II and Amendments to Part B of the Education of the Handicapped Act Regarding Services to Children from Birth to Age Six Years. Reston, VA: Council for Exceptional Children, 1990.

Cruickshank, WM. Psychology of Exceptional Children and Youth (4th ed.). Englewood Cliffs, NJ: Prentice-Hall, 1980, pp. 65–66.

Dahl, B. Karen. New York: Random House, 1947.

David, K, & Randall, K. Iowa Guidelines for Educationally Related Physical and Occupational Therapy Services. Des Moines, IA: Department of Education, 1988.

Deno, E. Special education as developmental capital. Exceptional Children, 37:229–237, 1970.

Dunn, W. Integrated related services. In Meyer, LH, Peck, CA, & Brown, L. (Eds.), Critical Issues in the Lives of People with Severe Disabilities. Baltimore: Paul H Brookes, 1991, pp. 353–378.

Effgen, SK. Southeastern Region V. focus: Determining school therapy caseloads based upon severity of need for services. Totline, 10(2):16–17, 1984.

Effgen, SK. Preparation of physical therapists and occupational therapists to work in early childhood special education settings. Topics in Early Childhood Special Education, 7(1):10–19, 1988.

Effgen, SK. Physical therapy in schools. In Tecklin, JS (Ed.), Pediatric Physical Therapy. Philadelphia: JB Lippincott, 1989, pp. 287–302.

Effgen, SK. Systematic delivery and recording of intervention assistance. Pediatric Physical Therapy, 3:63–68, 1991.

Effgen, SK, Bjornson, K, Chiarello, L, Sinzer, L, & Phillips, W. Competencies for physical therapists in early intervention. Pediatric Physical Therapy, 3:77–80, 1991.

Effgen, SK, & Klepper, S. Survey of physical therapy practice in educational settings. Pediatric Physical Therapy, 6:15–21, 1994.

Fairfax County Public Schools. PT/OT, Education's Helping Hands. Fairfax, VA: Fairfax County Public Schools, 1992.

Federal Register, Part II, Department of Education, 34 CRF Parts 300 and 301, Assistance to States for the Education of Children with Disabilities Program and Preschool Grants for Children with Disabilities, Final Rule; Vol. 57, No. 189, September 29, 1992.

Federal Register, Part III, Department of Education, 34 CFR Part 303, Early Intervention Program for Infants and Toddlers with Handicaps; Final Regulations, June 22, 1989.

Federal Regulations, Section 104, 3(j), 1988.

Florida Department of Exceptional Student Education. OT/PT Reporting System. Evaluation Protocols for Occupational and Physical Therapists in Public School. Tallahassee, FL: Department of Exceptional Student Education, 1987.

Garwood, SG, & Sheehan, R. Designing a comprehensive early intervention system: The challenge of Public Law 99-457. Austin, TX: Pro-ed, 1989.

Georgia Association of Retarded Citizens v McDaniel, 511 F Supp 1263 (Northern District of Georgia, 1981).

Giangreco, MF, Cloninger, CJ, Dennis, RE, & Edelman, SW. National expert validation of COACH: Congruence with exemplary practice and suggestions for improvement. Journal of the Association for Persons with Severe Handicaps, 18:109–120, 1993a.

Giangreco, MF, Cloninger, CJ, & Iverson, V. Choosing Options and Accommodations for Children: A Guide to Planning Inclusive Education. Baltimore: Paul H Brookes, 1993b.

Giangreco, MF, York, J, & Rainforth, B. Providing related services to learners with severe handicaps in educational settings: Pursuing the least restrictive option. Pediatric Physical Therapy, 1:55–63, 1989.

Givins, EV. The spastic child in the classroom. Physical Therapy Review, 18:136–137, 1938.

Lindsey, D, O'Neal, J, Haas, K, & Tewey, SM. Physical therapy services in North Carolina's schools. Clinical Management in Physical Therapy, 4:40–43, 1980.

Long, TM. The use of parent report measures to assess infant development. Pediatric Physical Therapy, 4:74–77, 1992.

Mager, RF. Preparing Instructional Objectives. Belmont, CA: Fearon, 1962.

Martin, EW. Lessons from implementing PL 94-142. In Gallagher, JJ, Trohanis, PL, & Clifford, RM (Eds.), Policy Implementation & PL 99-457: Planning for Young Children with Special Needs. Baltimore: Paul H Brookes, 1989, pp. 19–32.

Martin, R. Extraordinary Children, Ordinary Lives: Stories Behind Special Education Case Law. Champaign, IL: Research Press, 1991, pp. 45–63.

Maryland Association for Retarded Citizens v Maryland, Equite No. 100/182/77676 (Cir Ct Baltimore County, 1972).

McEwen, I, & Shelden, M. Writing functional goals: A means to integrate related services in special education. Paper presented at conference of The Association for Persons with Severe Handicaps Annual Convention, San Francisco, November 1992.

Meyer, LH, Peck, CA, & Brown, L (Eds.). Critical Issues in the Lives of People with Severe Disabilities. Baltimore: Paul H Brookes, 1991.

Miller, GE. Case management: The essential service. In Sanborn, CJ (Ed.), Case Management in Mental Health Services. New York: Haworth, 1983, p. 7.

Mills v Board of Education of the District of Columbia, 348 F Supp 866 (D DC 1972).

Montgomery, PC. Treatment planning: Establishing behavioral objectives. In Connolly, BH, & Montgomery, PC. (Eds.), Therapeutic Exercise in Developmental Disabilities. Chattanooga, TN: Chattanooga Corporation, 1987, pp. 21–26.

Mulcahey, AL. Detroit schools for crippled children. Physical Therapy Review, 16:63–64, 1936.

National Information Center for Children and Youth with Disabilities. Related services for school-aged children with disabilities. News Digest, National Information Center for Children and Youth with Disabilities, Vol. 1, Issue 2, p. 8, 1991.

Nietopski, SH, Nietopski, J, & Maurer, S. A comprehensive state education agency plan to promote the integration of students with moderate/severe handicaps. Journal of the Association for Persons with Severe Handicaps, 15(2):106–113, 1990.

Pennsylvania Association for Retarded Citizens v Commonwealth of Pennsylvania, Civil Action No. 71-42, 334 F Supp 1257 (ED Pa 1971), 343 F Supp 279 (ED Pa 1972).

Prieto, GM. Effects of physical therapist instruction on the frequency and performance of teacher assisted gross motor activities for students with motor disabilities. Unpublished master's thesis, Hahnemann University, Philadelphia, 1992.

Public Law 93-112, Rehabilitation Act (1973), 29 USC Section 794.

Public Law 94-103, Developmental Disabilities Assistance and Bill of Rights Act (1975). US Statutes at Large 89, pp 486–507.

Public Law 94-142, Education of All Handicapped Children Act (1975), 89 Stat 773–796.

Public Law 99-372, Handicapped Children's Protection Act (1986), 20 USC §1415(e) (4), (f).

Public Law 99-457, Education of the Handicapped Act Amendments of 1986, 100 Stat 1145–1177.

Public Law 101-336, Americans with Disabilities Act (1990), 42 USC Sec 12101.

Public Law 102-119, Individuals with Disabilities Education Act Amendments of 1991, 105 Stat 587–608.

Rainforth, B. OSERS clarifies legality of related services eligibility criteria. TASH Newsletter, 17:8, 1991.

Rainforth, B, York, J, & MacDonald, C. Collaborative Teams for Students with Severe Disabilities. Baltimore: Paul H Brookes, 1992.

Rapport, MJ, & Thomas, SB. Extended school year: Legal issues and implications. Journal of the Association for Persons with Severe Handicaps, 18(1):16–27, 1993.

Reynolds, M. A framework for considering some issues in special education. Exceptional Children, 28:367–370, 1962.

Rowley v Board of Education of Hendrick Hudson Central School District, 458 US 176 (1982).

Sever, JW. Physical therapy in schools for crippled children. Physical Therapy Review, 18:298–303, 1938.

Simunds, EE. Judicial interpretation of related services guidelines: A commentary. Alexandria, VA: American Physical Therapy Association, Section on Pediatrics, 1992.

Soccio, CA. Direct-individual versus integrated-group models of physical therapy service delivery. Unpublished master's thesis, Hahnemann University, Philadelphia, 1991.

Sparling, JW. Assessment of family resources and needs. In Wilhelm, IJ (Ed.), Physical Therapy Assessment in Early Infancy. New York: Churchill Livingstone, 1993, pp. 71–104.

Steed, CM. Professional relationship between physical therapist and teacher in a public school system. Unpublished master's thesis, Hahnemann University, Philadelphia, 1991.

Task Force on Standards for Measurement in Physical Therapy. Standards for tests and measurements in physical therapy practice. Physical Therapy, 71:589–622, 1991.

Tatro v Texas, 625 F2d 557 (1980); on rem'd 516 F Supp 968 (1981); aff'd 703 F2d 823 (1983); SCt No. 83-558 (aff'd July 5, 1984).

Taylor, SJ. Caught in the continuum: A critical analysis of the least restrictive environment. Journal of the Association for Persons with Severe Handicaps, 13(1):41–53, 1988.

Thurman, SK, & Widerstrom, AH. Infants and Young Children with Special Needs (2nd ed.). Baltimore: Paul H Brookes, 1990.

Tolley, B. Productivity expectations for hospital-based pediatric physical therapists. Pediatric Physical Therapy, 5:16–21, 1993.

Turnbull, R, Ellis, JW, Boggs, EM, Brookes, PO, & Biklen, DP (Eds.). Least Restrictive Alternatives: Principles and Practices. Washington, DC: American Association on Mental Deficiency, 1981.

Vacha, VB. History of the development of special schools and classes for crippled children in Chicago. Physical Therapy Review, 13:21–26, 1933.

Wilson, JM. Cerebral Palsy. In Campbell, SK (Ed.), Clinics in Physical Therapy: Pediatric Neurologic Physical Therapy (2nd ed.). New York: Churchill Livingstone, 1991, pp. 301–360.

Wolfensberger, W. Will there always be an institution? The impact of new service models. Mental Retardation, 9:31–38, 1971.

York, J, Rainforth, B, & Giangreco, MF. Transdisciplinary teamwork and integrated therapy: Clarifying the misconceptions. Pediatric Physical Therapy, 2:73–79, 1990.

Chapter 32

Private Practice Pediatric Physical Therapy: A Quest for Independence and Success

VENITA S. LOVELACE-CHANDLER, PT, PCS, PHD
BENJAMIN R. LOVELACE-CHANDLER, PT, PCS, PHD

During the 1960s and 1970s, many physical therapists, including members of the American Physical Therapy Association (APTA), were opposed to therapists who chose to practice in the private enterprise arena and described private practice therapists as "unethical, dishonest, and unprofessional" (Guglielmo, 1988). More recently, a strong, independent private sector has been accepted as an ideal rather than an abomination in physical therapy (Carlson, 1987). A profession is defined by autonomy, public image, and income more than specialty or discipline (Wood, 1986), and society's value of a professional service is judged by the extent of private practice (Cooper, 1982). In 1976, of approximately 18,000 active members, a mere 1138 or 6% of the membership of the APTA chose to belong to the Private Practice Section (Walker, 1977); by 1992, the section membership had increased only to 8% of the total APTA active membership (personal communication, Bryant, 1993). Although this percentage translates to approximately 4300 members and probably represents only a portion of the therapists in private practice, the growth of this practice setting has been slow and may be hindering the development of professionalism within physical therapy.

If the extent of private practice is a measure of professionalism, then pediatric physical therapists may have cause for concern regarding the extent of professionalism within pediatric services. The number of physical therapists who limit their private practices to pediatrics, although unknown, is perceived to be extremely small. Of 1609 respondents to a 1992 survey on private practice (Private Practice Section, 1992), only 26.6% indicated that pediatric services were among the services offered by their practices; 96.1% indicated the inclusion of orthopaedic services. Additionally, sports, neurologic, industrial wellness, wound healing, hand rehabilitation, and geriatric services were offered more frequently than pediatric services. Even more alarming, 10 of 13 clinical service areas were predicted to expand in the private practices to a greater extent than the expansion of pediatric services, with only cardiopulmonary and mental health services predicted to have less growth.

The motivators for establishing a private practice include greater patient contact, larger income, independence, fulfilling community or client needs, and prestige (Cole, 1986; Smoyak, 1986; Wood, 1986), and pediatric physical therapists should be interested in pursuing these goals. Our experience in pediatric private practice was initiated with motivations for independence in decision making and the desire to reduce the length of the chain of command. Each of us had held more than one employed physical therapy administrative position, yet neither of us had been satisfied with the control that existed at that level of authority. In every instance, a higher administrator determined staffing patterns, equipment purchases, funding for continuing education, and often the types and amount of physical therapy services to be offered. Frequently, services were selected for productivity rather than to address the best interests of clients or families, and rates were established to recover costs elsewhere in the institution rather than to reflect the costs of providing physical therapy. Often, we had been thwarted in efforts to design services that were based on our philosophy of best practice.

In 1982, one of us was in an employed administrative position re-experiencing these same negative factors when the decision was made to begin a private practice. The practice was established as a sole proprietorship with the therapist/owner who provided treatment and a spouse/therapist who volunteered as business manager, bookkeeper, and billing specialist. We selected a sole proprietorship, the legal title for a business with one owner (Wood, 1986), because the organizational structure is simple, the paperwork is minimal, and governmental restrictions are few. For example, our practice was opened by merely ordering business cards!

In our case, the spouse was satisfied in an employed position and was willing to provide financial security during the first 2 years of the practice. Health, dental, and life insurance were available through a family plan with the spouse's employer. The spouse had 2 years of experience as an insurance filing clerk and the willingness to work part time for the practice. With sufficient resources and the desire to be independent in professional practice, the business was established and has flourished. Even during difficult periods, the owner experienced enormous control, independence, and job satisfaction, and both of us were delighted with the financial gain that exceeded expectations.

More physical therapy practitioners must seek the private practice setting if increased recognition as a profession is to be achieved, and pediatric physical therapists must be among those practitioners who accept the risks and rewards that accompany the professional status of private practice. A paucity of material related to pediatric private practice is available in the physical therapy literature and may help to explain the small number of pediatric private practitioners. This chapter is written for the physical therapist who may be consider-

ing developing a pediatric private practice or for the student who may wish to learn about a possible work setting, that of the full-time independent pediatric practitioner. The purposes of this chapter are to define the private practitioner, including characteristics and responsibilities, provide information on risk management concepts for establishing and maintaining a private practice, cite the current trends in private practice, and provide insight into the uniqueness of a private practice limited to pediatric service provision through a description of one experience.

Existing research findings and general information on topics related to private practice in any health care profession, but particularly in physical therapy, have been used to address the purposes of the chapter. Most published information describes private practice services for adults. In this chapter, the information from literature on other professions and the information relating to adult services has been extrapolated for application in private practice pediatric physical therapy, and no evidence can be offered for the appropriateness of this extrapolation. We hope that the chapter will provide informative reading and direction for the pediatric physical therapist beginning a private practice and will allow the reader to avoid many of the mistakes and problems of our early years. Certainly, a revelation to us in preparing this chapter was the quantity of information available to the therapist interested in private practice relative to how little we knew as beginners. Our intent is for the entrepreneurial pediatric therapist or student to be encouraged and to use the information of this chapter in a quest for the independence and success available in private practice.

THE PRIVATE PRACTITIONER

History and Definition

Although the origin of physical therapy private practice is difficult to ascertain, evidence exists that a few therapists were engaged in such practices in the 1950s and that these therapists exchanged information regarding the private practice setting during a meeting at the 1954 Annual Conference of the APTA (Dicus, 1991). In 1955, the APTA responded to a request from private practice therapists by establishing a steering committee to make recommendations on the advisability of creating a Self-Employed Section. The committee members perceived defining who constituted a self-employed therapist as one of the most difficult problems in the development of the section. Dicus (1991) noted that this difficulty in clearly delineating the private practitioner resulted in such problems as uncertainty regarding the philosophy of the section, a lack of common ground among members, diversity in educational needs, and misunderstanding of governmental regulations. The problems persisted during the section's formative years and during the evolution into the current Private Practice Section (PPS) (renamed in 1975) (Reuss, 1991).

Frazian (1985) notes that the definition of private practice is still disputed. Between the purely staff therapist, employed by an institution, and the purely independent therapist, owner of a practice or corporation, are innumerable therapists who are establishing lifestyles and professional private practices to meet the needs of society and themselves. Examples of the variety of private practices include performing a few hours of home health care services in addition to a full-time employed position, working part time in an employed position and part time as owner of a practice, and providing numerous hours through several contractual arrangements. Contracting denotes assuming responsibility for providing clinical services in a particular setting for a fixed payment (Bernstein, 1986). Contractors are self-employed and have differing financial processes in regard to income tax, Social Security tax, and retirement funds, but little difference may be noted in the actual provision of clinical services by employees or contractors.

Although Brown (1992) questions the use of the term *private practice* and alludes to every physical therapist as an independent practitioner with a high level of decision-making ability and professionalism, the guidelines in this chapter are directed to a very specific practitioner whom we have defined as follows: *The private practice physical therapist has autonomy, uses minimal bureaucracy, practices according to professional values, and takes risks to achieve financial and professional independence and success.*

Autonomy. A frequent misconception is that any therapist contracting for services is a private practitioner (Faust & Meaker, 1991). Private practice is more than having a contract with an agency or facility. The first requirement of self-employment is the ability to function in an autonomous manner as a businessperson. When one giant corporation enters into a business relationship with another corporation, autonomous practice is absent, and this arrangement is no more a private practice than the per diem therapist who engages in a contractual relationship with a large health care institution. Pediatric physical therapists must be willing to assume autonomy in managing the practice, designing and offering services, implementing marketing strategies, billing for services, establishing relationships with children and families, and consulting with other professionals and agencies.

Minimal Bureaucracy. Private practice is characterized by low levels of internal bureaucracy as opposed to the management style of a typical corporation (Faust & Meaker, 1991). Private practitioners are free to choose a streamlined bookkeeping system and may have less paperwork than that required by agencies. Within the boundaries established by licensure laws, the rules and standards for continuing education, promotion, supervision and delegation, and collegial consultation can be established without approval from other administrative bodies. Decisions regarding equipment purchases, budgeting, and secretarial support are made by the owner, often the sole practitioner, but may in larger practices include input from other appropriate employees. Pediatric therapists must be willing to exercise independent decision making and must understand that supervisors, department directors, and administrators are usually not available to assist (or resist) the private practitioner's decisions.

Professional Practice. Professional values and norms direct the behavior of the private practice organization. Corporations, including health agencies, often use marketing forces and business perspectives to determine organizational structure and behavior. Although knowledge and use of business principles are essential to survival in private practice, the services must be offered in a manner in which professional standards are paramount and supersede financial considerations. Wood (1986) suggests that private practice is more a philosophy than a work setting and that professional success can be achieved without financial success, but we believe that financial success in private practice cannot be achieved without quality services. The pediatric physical therapist in private practice will find that the business will be successful only when professionalism and quality coexist with financial concerns to offer the consumer a service worth purchasing.

Risk Taking. The great risks involved in initiating a private practice, including costs and the potential for mistakes, have been cited by several authors (Cole, 1986; Flower, 1986; Kooper & Sullivan, 1986; McClain et al., 1992; Parish, 1986; Walker, 1977; Wood, 1986; Woody, 1986). Many practicing therapists are not interested in management and avoid the business responsibilities and attention to detail required in private practice (Deaton, 1992b; Walker, 1977). Many small businesses with marketable services or products fail because the initial financial resources are exhausted before income can be produced (Walker, 1977) or because business responsibilities have been mismanaged.

One characteristic of private practice is the personal assumption of risk and the realization that service delivery within private enterprise carries the opportunity to fail (Wood, 1986). Possibilities for risking and failing include financial, professional, personal and family, and legal aspects. Pediatric private practitioners must have sufficient general knowledge of business management to understand basic principles and to seek qualified counsel when needed. Although many risks will be present at the onset of the practice, additional risks will accompany expansion in an established practice, whether the expansion involves purchasing equipment, hiring additional personnel, or changing office space (Cole, 1986). Three concepts regarding risks should be considered before beginning a private practice: 1) risk taking involves the possibility of either negative or positive outcome; 2) risk management fosters positive outcome and allows entering risky situations with hope as opposed to avoiding risky situations for fear of negative results; and 3) methods for minimizing risks have been identified and are available for use by new private practitioners (McFadden & Hanschu, 1985).

Personal and Professional Characteristics

Although Walker (1977) advocates that only well-seasoned, experienced physical therapists should consider entering private practice, a setting he considers unsuited for the novice, physical therapy will not achieve increased recognition as a profession until more practitioners seek the private practice setting. New graduates and other therapists may enter this arena if personal characteristics and professional skills are compatible with private practice. The person drawn to private practice is attracted primarily by the opportunity to be self-governed and by the desire to be one's own boss (Cole, 1986). The private practitioner is focused on self-control, independence, self-governance, and diversity of tasks. Expertise or specialization is necessary to the success of a practice. Wood (1986) offers the following two very direct statements that should be carefully considered by the therapist interested in private practice: "If you don't have anything to market, stay out of the marketplace" (p. 6), and "it is impossible to be too blunt with yourself when assessing your skills and expertise" (p. 7).

Walker (1977) suggests that the physical therapist in private practice must possess the following seven traits:

1. The therapist needs good physical and mental health to sustain the long hours, work stress, coping mechanisms, and interference with routine often associated with a new private practice.

2. The ability to develop strong relationships with clients, physicians, and other health care personnel is essential to the business aspects of the practice, and the ability to maintain a supportive relationship with family and friends is essential to personal well-being.

3. Self-discipline, including adherence to a self-imposed schedule, timely devotion to business details, and self-initiation skills, are crucial to the private practitioner. The therapist who functions best when responsible to someone else's schedule and goals should remain in an employed position.

4. An interest in business management and such subjects as accounting, bookkeeping, and economics is necessary for financial success. The ability to handle personal finances and to promptly manage personal bank accounts, tax files, real estate issues, insurance coverage and claims, and savings accounts might provide insight into the probability of successful business management.

5. Good oral and written communication skills are important to successful interaction with clients, physicians, third-party payers, and other health care personnel. Private practitioners must be comfortable with face-to-face professional contacts with the intent of securing referrals, with technical report writing to enhance reimbursement, and with difficult situations such as collecting payment from clients.

6. Professional training and experience must be adequate for the services to be marketed. Self-advancement and self-directed learning are essential to building a successful private practice.

7. Dedication and determination to address the problems as well as the promises of a private practice are necessary for successful risk management.

The Committee on Private Practice of the American Speech-Language-Hearing Association (ASHA) (1991) provides 13 personal characteristics that should be considered when initiating a private practice. These characteristics include necessary experience, an established reputation, good clinical skills, an affinity for the work, willingness and ability to work long hours for a few years, handling a challenge, learning what is not known, acceptance of no or low income for a period of time, desire for a private practice, family support, stress management, strong self-image, and a network or support system. Physical therapy private practitioners also will find these characteristics to be essential.

Cole (1986), writing about speech-language pathology and audiology but offering advice applicable to any private practitioner, cautions that individuals should examine their professional practice attitudes and personal characteristics in relation to the roles that must be assumed as business owner, manager, and clinician. The business aspects of owning and managing a private practice are often shocking to therapists who consider their work as a service to be given to clients. Therapists must be willing to regard services as a product to be sold for a profit but realize that most of the time and energy for the first year or more will be devoted to building the practice without experiencing any profit.

All health care professionals who engage in private practice probably do so for similar professional reasons. Smoyak (1986) noted that private practice offers psychiatric nurses the advantages of maximal autonomy for patients and professionals with little bureaucratic red tape and interference with professional judgment. The author offers the following comment:

Patients, if they can afford it, or have insurance that will allow it, can freely select the practitioner of their choice, using such criteria as age, sex, race, credentials, style, location, availability, cost, educational background, and recommendation of others. Theoretically, this freedom to select the therapist may increase the probability that the treatment will be helpful. Similarly, the therapist's freedom to concentrate on specific treatments and kinds of patients should enhance their clinical skills. A fee-for-service system, with practitioners earning income by hours spent in treating patients, tends to maximize productivity and minimize time spent on paperwork, meetings, and other nonincome functions. (p. 22)

Parsons (1986) refers to private practitioners as "heroes" and "politicians" who develop expertise through specialization and let others know about their expertise through marketing. The individual practitioner is able to use specialization for visibility and as a means for special clarity about capabilities and limitations. For example, the practice may be limited to a specific age range, such as infants and toddlers, preschoolers, or adolescents, or to a diagnostic category, such as developmental disabilities or orthopaedics. The therapist learns how therapy is viewed by different segments of the community where the practice will be established and markets the service in a manner that is meaningful to the community. The service must be competent and be sought by clients. The ability to develop referral sources depends on others' perceptions of the therapist's competence, which is influenced by professional visibility and charisma. Building a caseload requires offering unique services, accepting third-party payment, providing flexible scheduling, meeting with physicians and other health care professionals, being competent, giving

speeches, meeting local health needs, cultivating personal referral sources, and achieving professional visibility. Speaking to community groups, giving workshops, publishing, and participating in professional activities increase visibility. In our practice, treatments were donated to clients who had no funding to establish relationships with physicians who were sending referrals to pediatric centers that required reimbursement. Calling the physicians regarding client issues, writing thorough evaluations, and providing follow-up letters to referral sources allowed for the rapid expansion of the referral base. After only 1 month, client referrals were sufficient to meet operating costs of the practice and to provide a very minimal salary.

The Small Business Administration (SBA) is a federal funding entity that provides support to owners of small businesses. The SBA provides a list of basic survival skills needed to run a business (Roussel & Epplin, 1987). These skills include a working knowledge of basic recordkeeping; financial management; personnel management; market analysis; breakeven analysis; product or service knowledge; federal, state, and local taxes; legal structure; and communication skills. Of these basic skills, the typical therapist will possess service knowledge and communication skills.

Deaton (1992a), a frequent speaker at the annual meetings of the PPS, recently complimented the "nerve" of therapists. He indicated the respect he had for the body of knowledge required to skillfully practice physical therapy. Students study for many years in prerequisite coursework and intense physical therapy coursework. As new graduates, these therapists enter a complex health care system with a maze of administrative, reimbursement, social, and clinical issues. Therapists survive the maze, providing quality services to a wide variety of clients with diverse pathologies. As if this feat were not adequate, an increasing number of therapists decide to enter the private enterprise arena. The skills required to be a successful business owner are not possessed nor even known!

Deaton's description certainly fit our business adventure. The owner and spouse possessed several but not all of the professional characteristics recommended as essential. Clinical skills in the area of pediatrics were varied and advanced. We both had 11 years of pediatric experience, master's degrees that included coursework in pediatric physical therapy, doctoral degrees in health education, and certification in specific clinical techniques such as neurodevelopmental treatment. The owner had administrative experience from serving as a physical therapy department director in an outpatient pediatric physical therapy center, as director of physical therapy at a residential facility for 1200 clients with developmental disabilities, and as the director of rehabilitation at an urban children's medical center. An interest in business management, accounting, bookkeeping, and economics was absolutely lacking, and the business aspects of owning and managing the practice were shocking to us. We were anxious to implement our philosophy of care and anticipated the outstanding services that we would offer children and families, but we never considered cash flow problems, third-party payers who provided reimbursement but only after months of delay, families who received payment from third-party payers and spent the funds on personal expenditures, parents who were offended when asked for payment, and funding agencies who refused to reimburse for outpatient services provided by a private practitioner in an office or home when identical outpatient services were reimbursable if provided in a hospital or center by the same practitioner.

The spouse had 2 years of experience in insurance processing, and all billing was done in evening hours. In retrospect, only one client who was expected to pay failed to do so. Our collection rate was incredible, but the toll on personal lives, marriage, and children cannot be overestimated. If we had been aware of the business aspects of private practice and our obvious deficiencies in management, the practice would still have been initiated but we would have sought assistance from others earlier and would not have considered ourselves as failures because of the reimbursement, tax, accounting, and recordkeeping problems. Physical therapists who desire to enter private practice in pediatrics must develop business skills or purchase business services from others if professional and personal satisfaction is to be optimal.

Jayaratne and colleagues (1991) found that although the need for a continuous supply of clients and concerns over the business aspects of a private practice may produce stress in social workers, the private practice setting created less strain than agency settings. Social workers in private practice reported fewer psychological and health strains, higher levels of performance, and better feelings about their life circumstances. These authors suggested that individuals who seek private practice may differ from employed individuals by being healthier from the beginning, having characteristics that foster health, serving kinds of clients that produce less stress in the practitioner, or experiencing different psychosocial aspects of business in the private practice arena. We believe that the private practice environment has afforded more happiness and better mental health for the owner than any previous employed position. The spouse has been able to experience many of the rewards of the practice through a sense of accomplishment, less marital stress, and greater financial gains. In addition to the personal and professional characteristics listed previously, the private practice pediatric physical therapist may need the ability to accept the improved health, happiness, and well-being available in a private practice.

Personal and Professional Responsibilities

Statements of ethical principles and conduct have been developed by the APTA (1982, 1987). Although these statements apply universally to members of that association and may be adopted by nonmember physical therapists and physical therapist assistants, ethical behavior is situational, and specific circumstances may determine the manner in which the ethical principles are applied. We have perceived that employed therapists have greater ethical expectations of private practitioners than of themselves or other employed therapists. Flower (1986) determined that speech-language pathologists and audiologists perceive private practice as entailing unique ethical considerations and responsibilities that are more challenging than the ethical concerns of employed therapists, suggesting that increased expectations for private practitioners are not unique to the profession of physical therapy. He suggests that although private practitioners may engage in unethical practices such as treating clients with dubious prognoses, maintaining clients endlessly in treatment programs, making recommendations without regard for economic impact, and failing to obtain informed consent, employed therapists commit the same unprofessional behaviors. Ethical considerations remain similar regardless of the delivery system, and personal and professional responsibilities for quality services at reasonable cost are not limited to the private practice environment.

Wood (1986) notes that certain aspects of professional morality underlie the spirit of ethical principles and that these aspects include professional responsibility, integrity, and competence. Institutions frequently provide administrative leadership that reduces individual professional responsibility, or at least perceived responsibility, and institutions are able to compensate for limited professional competence in one practitioner through supervision by or use of other practitioners. In institutions, several therapists may collaborate on difficult ethical decisions and produce a superior decision, but poor ethical decisions by one therapist may also be concealed and the therapist protected by other staff members. Concerns regarding ethical practice should be heeded by physical therapists because sheltering and protection are not usually available to private practitioners in any profession.

Flower (1986) suggests six areas of frequent ethical dilemmas for private practitioners that, if monitored appropriately, produce ethical practices. The six areas include professional competence (practitioner and employees), confidentiality and informed consent, fees and financial activities, marketing and advertisement, relationships, and product recommendation and dispensing. The reader is referred to Flower's work for a comprehensive discussion of each area.

We suggest that the private practice pediatric physical therapist may ethically treat any patient who seeks services, with the methods known by the therapist, unless a misfit between the need and the skills exists. A single practitioner may be more limited in treatment strategies than therapists in a hospital or group practice, and a practitioner should seek advice or make referral to another therapist if other strategies are warranted. Private practitioners are cautioned that pride, an unwillingness to limit a practice or admit deficiencies, and fear of economic loss may prevent a practitioner from admitting shortcomings. Economic motives also may reduce cost-effective or relevant treatment.

The Code of Ethics of the APTA (1987) and the guides for conduct (APTA, 1982, 1989a, 1989b) are valuable resources for all private practitioners. Additionally, the Section on Pediatrics of the APTA offers documents to assist pediatric practitioners in offering ethical and appropriate services (Scull & Deitz, 1989; Task Force on Early Intervention, 1991), and the Section publication *Pediatric Physical Therapy* is a valuable source for articles, commentaries, and other information of use to private practitioners. Adhering to the regulations regarding state licensure and pursuing development through continuing education will assist in maintaining ethical and competent practice.

RISK MANAGEMENT IN ESTABLISHING A PRIVATE PRACTICE

Starting a Practice

Walker (1977) notes that no clear-cut "how to" methods exist for establishing a professional office, but several common considerations and general investigative procedures must be followed. Mistakes will be made, costs will vary, and the risks are great, but so are the rewards. Knowledge of the process might lessen the mistakes, risks, and costs, thereby increasing the rewards for the pediatric therapist beginning a private practice.

Sims (1992) suggests identifying and building the practice desired by the individual therapist, not the practice everyone else thinks should be built. Pediatric private practitioners need to determine if services will be provided to children from birth to 21 years of age or a specific segment of the pediatric population and to children with all types of disabilities or only a specific disability. A subspecialty practice within the broader pediatric specialty may be appropriate. Remember that the practitioner must possess the skills and expertise for the planned practice and that a niche in the marketplace must exist if success is to be obtained.

Our practice was envisioned as an office-based practice that would provide services for young children with developmental disabilities, probably from birth to 12 years of age. The office practice never flourished as well as desired, and in the early years, few infants and toddlers were referred. A niche in the marketplace did not exist for office services for young children because most families could obtain this type of physical therapy service from a variety of outpatient treatment centers that also provided social services, educational classes for preschoolers, and other therapies. Our business became particularly successful because services were provided at schools, child care centers, or client homes as was necessary to provide ecologically based services to children. Our niche, or rather gulf, in the marketplace developed by addressing special situations such as contracting with school districts to relieve the shortage of school-based therapists, serving the children of working parents in the everyday environment of the child, providing treatment to clients receiving educational services at home, and traveling to the homes of families without transportation or to small, nearby towns where several families resided but where no services were available. Contracts with school districts sustained the practice at first, but the school districts wanted employees rather than autonomous practitioners, and the relationships died a natural death as the practice grew with individual clients.

During the first 2 years, our practice was not the business we had "wanted," but autonomy, low bureaucracy, and our philosophy of care were present. Within a few years, the practice was shaped into the desired business, but even during the early years the practice was limited to clients younger than 21 years of age. The owner declined adult clients, even though numerous referrals were received for adults with neurologic involvement. Success was the result of blending the wishes of the owner with the needs in the marketplace.

Selecting a Legal Structure

Every business organization must have a legal structure (Hampton, 1986). Numerous potential legal structures exist and should be considered by the therapist initiating a private practice. The tax obligations, financial advantages, applicable laws and liabilities, and employer/employee benefits available for each legal entity are determined by federal and state regulations. An attorney and an accountant, both with expertise in small businesses, should be consulted to determine the legal form most appropriate for the planned practice. The county clerk and the state licensing board can provide information about the legal forms available in a specific geographic location (ASHA, 1991). Generally, an individual practice consists of a single therapist providing services for a fee through a small business, a partnership has two or more co-owners, and professional and technical staff members of the same professional group employed and directed by one therapist constitute an associate private practice (McClain et al., 1992). The specific legal form for each of these organizational patterns may vary. For example, a single practitioner may be a sole proprietor or the owner of a corporation.

The three common and most appropriate legal structures for a professional practice are sole proprietorship, partnership, and corporation (Hampton, 1986; Parish, 1986; Wood, 1986). As indicated previously, the sole proprietorship is the simplest form of legal structure. Additionally, this form is used by more than half of all business organizations, and almost half of all sole proprietorships are service organizations (Hampton, 1986).

Partnerships have two or more owners who enter into business together (Hampton, 1986). Parish (1986) notes that a partnership is similar to a marriage and that this form of legal structure requires partners who are personally compatible and possess complementary abilities. One partner needs controlling interest in the business or final decisions may be difficult to achieve. If the partnership is split equally among partners, then disputes are resolved only by compromise or defeat. When disputes cannot be resolved, then dissolution of the partnership may be required and also may be similar to a marriage that ends in divorce. A buy-sell agreement established at the initiation of the partnership indicates the mechanism for dissolving the partnership by allowing one partner to buy the percentage of the business held by other partners or to sell the partner's percentage to other partners or someone else. Comprising less than 10% of all organizations, partnerships are the least common legal structure for businesses (Hampton, 1986).

Corporations form the most complex type of legal structure, and an attorney will be needed to prepare the "Articles of Incorporation" (Parish, 1986). The corporation is a legal entity, and the owner who incorporates a company becomes an employee of the corporation. Income tax is paid on the profits of the corporation separately from the individual taxes paid by the owner/employee. Income levels that exceed $50,000 may indicate the need for a corporate structure to maximize tax benefits (Sullivan, 1986). Several types of corporations exist (Hampton, 1986), and an attorney or accountant can assist in determining the correct type for the planned business. Costs of incorporating a business range from $500 to $1500, according to the geographic location and the type of corporate structure (Sullivan, 1986). About 20% of all businesses are corporations, but the vast majority of business income is generated by this type of legal structure (Hampton, 1986).

For 6 years, our business was operated as a sole proprietorship, but we incorporated the practice during the seventh year. A lawyer advised that incorporation would assist in several of the tax complications relating to contracting with other therapists and would provide better liability protection for the owner. In a sole proprietorship, our home and cars could be taken to settle a business debt in the event of litigation, and we believed that our personal assets had to be safe from the liabilities of the business. The private practice pediatric therapist should seek advice from a lawyer, a tax consultant, and a financial advisor to determine the most suitable organizational structure for the proposed practice.

Hampton (1986) suggests that the private practitioner will have the final decision regarding the legal structure of the business and that the decision will be based on personal or professional needs. In our experience, we did not have the expertise to determine the best legal structure and were forced to rely on an accountant we trusted. Our accountant has changed the type of corporation once since we incorporated to better reflect the financial status of our business. Parish (1986) warns that the complexity of the tax structure for corporations requires that accountants and attorneys will be needed for the foreseeable future. We are unable to intelligently read our incorporation documents or our corporate tax forms even though the spouse had tax preparation experience and filed all tax documents for the sole proprietorship without assistance from an accountant. We accept the premise that changes in the practice in subsequent years and changes in tax law may require adjustment in the legal structure of the business. Periodic review of the status of

TABLE 32–1. **CHARACTERISTICS OF THE THREE MAJOR LEGAL STRUCTURES OF A BUSINESS**

Sole Proprietorship	Partnership	Corporation
Easiest to initiate, sell, or dissolve; taxed on business profits that are considered personal income; owner personally liable for the debts; owner's personal assets at risk if sued (Parish, 1986)	Two or more people share costs and profits; each partner is liable; each partner is taxed personally; should involve written agreement that describes control of business, key-man, insurance, time, functions and duties of each partner, division of profits and loss; buy-sell agreement needed; all partners liable for the actions of each other (Parish, 1986)	Identity separate from the owner; owner may be an employee; business is taxed separately from the owner as an employee (Parish, 1986)
Simplest, most common form of legal structure; more than 70% of all business organizations are sole proprietorships, but only 8% of total gross income of businesses is from sole proprietorship (Hampton, 1986)	May restrict liability by being a limited partner if one partner has unlimited liability; written agreement not required but recommended (Hampton, 1986)	Variations in type of corporation (Hampton, 1986)
Owner has full responsibility for conducting business; owner reaps the profits; can minimize liability risks through careful financial management (Sullivan, 1986)	Each partner carries risk of personal property; allows for maximizing assets to start the business; capital costs may be divided among partners; the impact of debt, illness, or lack of ability in a particular aspect of the business is reduced (Sullivan, 1986)	Personal assets are protected unless personal negligence of the officers; owners personally guarantee loans for the corporation; state laws for corporation may differ from federal tax law (Sullivan, 1986)
Subject to the fewest governmental restrictions; provides the greatest autonomy; owner pays self-employment tax; usually use social security number as business taxpayer identification number; must pay quarterly tax estimates; fringe benefits are not always deductible; employees may be hired or contracts with other practitioners may be developed on an as-needed basis (Wood, 1986)	Partners share control and authority; one partner's reputation extends to other partners; partners must compromise; philosophies of all partners must agree for successful partnership; any number of persons can form a partnership; the overhead costs for several or all partners may be less than for each practitioner separately; individual goals may change, leading to partner-incompatibility; several types of partnerships (Wood, 1986)	Close governmental regulations; expensive to form because of legal and filing fees; adaptable to both small and large practices; deductible fringe benefits may be available to corporate employees; may enhance image of the business; the act of incorporating helps produce guidelines for dealing with problems (Wood, 1986)

any pediatric private practice is recommended. Table 32–1 provides the features of each of the three common organizational structures (Hampton, 1986; Parish, 1986; Sullivan, 1986; Wood, 1986).

Developing a Business Plan

A business plan is the key to obtaining financing and to business success and should be developed as soon as the type of practice has been determined (Sims, 1992). A fundamental task in business planning is to set goals and objectives toward which the practice will be moving. Formulating strategies and establishing alternative courses of action to achieve the goals must be accomplished and must include the financial, physical, and human resources necessary for goal attainment (Tillman & Parke, 1991).

PLANNING FOR FINANCIAL RESOURCES

The financial aspects of the business plan include the initial or start-up costs for the entire practice (Sims, 1992). All expected expenses should be arranged within a monthly, quarterly, and yearly spending budget. Projected revenues for the practice should be compiled using the same time periods. Reviewing the resulting statistics and writing a short narrative on how the pediatric practice fits into the physical therapy market in the projected area will prepare the therapist to discuss the plan with other persons. Bankers, accountants, and businesspersons are able to review the plan for realism and feasibility. Two forms of the financial plan might be designed (Driskell, 1988). The short form should be designed to impress the lender and to give the lender an overview of the business. The long form complements the short form by providing detailed information to allow the practitioner to answer all questions. The two forms have the same format, but more detail is included in the longer form. The lender will need information on physical therapy in general, licensure and legal considerations, and the growth of physical therapy services. Include the types of services you will offer, referral sources, the available market, and information on your education and work experience. Provide the same information for other staff you intend to use. Explain how the loan will be used and the proposed method of repayment.

Seek help from professionals when designing the financial plan. Aydelotte and associates (1988) inferred that nurse entrepreneurs in private practice who sought assistance from sources other than nurses made higher incomes than nurses who sought assistance from other nurses when initially establishing a practice. These authors suggested that further research is needed to determine if assistance from sources other than nurses leads to higher income levels for private practice nurses. However, the inference is sufficient to suggest that expertise in business is critical to accurate development of a financially sound business plan and that physical therapists may not possess the knowledge necessary for financial planning for a pediatric private practice.

Therapists with a written plan and an understanding of the financial risk should apply for the needed capital from a bank. Aydelotte and associates (1988) found that nurses who used sources of venture capital other than personal savings received higher gross income than nurses who used individual savings. No explanation was offered by the authors, but the possibility exists that true entrepreneurial ventures and subsequent income might be restricted if only existing savings are considered in planning. However, the loan application for a novice businessperson may be denied by the bank, and the plan and presentation may need to be adjusted before proceeding to the next bank (Sims, 1992). The banker may want a financial projection for 1 to 5 years, which is a difficult task for many new private practitioners. Nevertheless, adequately capitalizing for the needs of the practice at the beginning and adhering to a budget will minimize financial pressures (Walker, 1977).

A supply of money must flow into the business if the business is to continue. The business plan should include obtaining enough income to cover salaries for 4 to 6 months. The bank will assist in establishing a line of credit so only the amount of money needed for expenses will be borrowed. The base of referrals is the financial foundation to a practice, and time will be required to establish a referral base in a community. Be innovative in marketing the services of the practice, and do not rely on referrals from one or two sources to maintain the practice. A maximum of 5% of referrals from any one source will avoid financial pressures should the source terminate referrals. Initially, the private practitioner may need to accept referrals from any source, but the goal of diversity among referral sources should be sought as the practice develops (Sims, 1992).

While speaking to a group of students regarding private practice, Finch (1982) remarked that if he terminated his practice of approximately 15 years, he could still receive an income for 2 to 3 years from his outstanding accounts. Cash flow may be very slow in the initial stages of a practice, and numerous accounts will require several months or more for collection. We experienced very minimal cash flow for the first 2 years of the practice, and accounts receivable mounted. We now average $125,000 to $150,000 in accounts receivable at any given time. A major third-party payer once delayed payment of a large account for 3 years. We have found that many insurance companies will require numerous requests before payment is sent. Learn how to bill and collect for your services by recognizing what different insurance companies require for claim submission as well as what each will pay when billed. A universal billing form (Form HCFA-1500) is acceptable to many insurance companies and is available for purchase. (Refer to Appendix I for an address for ordering the universal billing form.) The Health Care Finance Administration in cooperation with the American Medical Association periodically reviews and modifies the form, and the practitioner should be aware of the need to obtain the most recently approved form.

Medicaid is a federally funded program administered by a state agency to provide reimbursement for medical services for low-income clients and includes physical therapy services. Many pediatric clients will have Medicaid funding, and billing for these clients can be accomplished through electronic billing on a computer. The state provides the necessary software and inservice training on electronic billing, and this method is superior in processing and collection. Presently, insurance companies accept electronic billing only when the billing is accomplished through a clearinghouse for a fee, but direct electronic billing to all third-party payers is expected to be available in the near future.

Our practice was opened with no established referral base. Miraculously, four clients were referred after contact with pediatricians and orthopaedists and formed the income source for the first few weeks. The owner moonlighted on weekends at a general hospital to pay the costs of the business for the first 4 months. Contracts with school districts and other agencies were negotiated, and additional clients were referred to the office. Several contracts with state-supported child care centers for children with developmental disabilities have been maintained for more than 10 years. These centers value the quality of services provided by the business and have been receptive to funding increases whenever necessary.

The determination of fees to be charged for services may be simple or complex. The fee schedule may be based on the general fee structure of other service providers in the geographic area, but if the private practitioner has lower overhead costs than agencies or other providers, then the fees may be appropriately lower. Major insurance companies will have established "usual and customary" rates, and payment for pediatric physical therapy services will be based on those rates regardless of the established fees of the practice. Practitioners should only charge for services rendered, should establish fees commensurate with the costs of providing the services, should disclose the schedule of fees, and should learn to discuss fees with potential clients or their caretakers (Bernstein, 1986).

PLANNING FOR PHYSICAL RESOURCES

Office space is an important consideration when preparing the business plan. The space should meet the needs of both clients and staff and provide for the placement of needed equipment so that an efficient flow can occur (Sims, 1992). Walker (1977) suggests listing space and utility requirements and drawing a tentative floor plan before shopping for office space. He notes that the needs of the practice will change and growth should be anticipated. A private office might be considered a luxury at first but will become a necessity as the practice grows. A waiting area is nonproductive space but will be necessary to meet the needs of clients and families. Restrooms also are a necessity, and local and state codes may determine whether employees and clients may use the same restroom facilities and whether the space may be generic for both genders. Remember to note parking and accessibility needs when planning or selecting space. Water supply, storage closets and cabinets, cleaning and maintenance, utility costs, convenience for the targeted market, and the option to extend the lease are other important considerations in acquiring space.

We chose to rent a two-room office with a 3-year lease. The rent was satisfactory and the location was one of convenience to the owner's home, but no market survey or other consideration was given

to the location as a marketing tool to acquire clients. No lawyer reviewed the lease, and although the specifics of the lease were adequate, the time frame proved too long for our needs. We were unaware of the advice to allow for growth, and we desired larger space before the lease expired. Luckily, the company that held the lease was able to offer us an office with more space at a nearby location. Because the move was profitable for the company, we were allowed to terminate the first lease with no penalty.

For the initial office, a handmade divider separated the waiting area from the "office" in one room, and the second room was used for treatment. We shared restroom space with another office. This arrangement was never satisfactory because of the need to modify the restroom for pediatric clients. Private practices for adult clients may have individual treatment rooms, partitioned areas within a larger treatment area, or a large gym area with no cubicles. In a pediatric office, the treatment area for infants and toddlers might be separate from treatment areas for older children, but our experience has not indicated the need for numerous treatment rooms or cubicles. We eventually needed a room for a billing office, a room for staff desks, and a room for casting. The space we selected at that time also had three additional rooms that were used for treatment, but one large space would have been adequate. Although individual treatment areas provide privacy for clients and diversity of design to meet specific client needs, the requirements for additional electrical wiring, ventilation, lighting, decorating, and equipment increase costs. If the tentative floor plan is drawn to scale and incorporates the planned use of the space for ambulation, exercise, play, or other activities, then the practitioner should be able to identify space requirements. A realtor will be helpful in locating suitable space, in negotiating the price, and in arranging for structural changes in the space if warranted for the practice, and a lawyer should be used to review the lease.

Some practitioners interested in private practice will find themselves in an employed position with a contract that prohibits competing with the employer in a certain geographic area or for a specific period of time following employment, and this restriction may limit the choice of locations. Burch and Iglarsh (1988) suggest that at least 5 miles and probably 7½ to 10 miles should exist between the practice location and other competitors and that this distance usually satisfies legal issues regarding competition clauses. Pediatric therapists with no legal encumbrances to geographic location will want to consider the distance between the private practice and other pediatric service providers. Pediatric therapists, however, may have a smaller percentage of a market area as potential clients than other specialists and may need to draw from a larger geographic base. The uniqueness of the private practice environment may allow competition with other pediatric service providers.

Our practice was initiated in a city with a population of approximately 200,000 persons and with two established pediatric outpatient agencies and a children's hospital that provided outpatient services. At the time we established the service, no other pediatric private practices existed, but we were not certain that a city of that size could support a practice limited to pediatrics. As indicated previously, we had to revise our practice goals to accommodate the marketplace, but the practice was very successful. Over the next several years, numerous physical therapists engaged in pediatric private practice activities of several varieties, and occupational therapists also established practices limited to pediatrics. Although we changed locations twice since the practice was begun, the market for our practice continues to be the entire city (which now has a population of approximately 250,000 persons), surrounding smaller towns, and a few sites in other areas of the state. The current office is located in close proximity to several pediatric physician offices, but these offices do not form a strong referral base for the practice. Proximity to other providers and to a physician referral base are suggestions for the locations of adult practices in larger cities or states, but we are unable to determine if these suggestions apply to pediatric practices.

Equipment needs include both office equipment and physical therapy equipment. Office equipment may cost up to $10,000 (Sims, 1992), and estimates for physical therapy equipment offered to us by private practitioners engaged in orthopaedic practice varied from $100,000 to $300,000. Pediatric private practitioners are able to initiate a practice with much less funding. The specific disabilities of the clients who will be served will influence the selection of physical therapy equipment, but an office that provides play-based therapy for clients who are developmentally challenged might require only mats, therapeutic balls, bolsters, mirrors, toys, and a standing/ambulation area. Bernstein (1986) notes that crayons, dolls, blocks, and brand-name toys may serve the needs of younger children, but games and more sophisticated entertainment are required for older children.

An office practice providing services to pediatric clients with orthopaedic or other disabilities would have specific equipment needs, and equipment requirements are mandated by at least one major funding source for pediatric clients. If the practice provides services for clients funded by Medicaid, you will need to be Medicare-certified, which is interpreted to mean that all physical therapy treatments could be provided by the practice. Each state has enormous latitude in deciding how the regulations will be interpreted and which services will be reimbursable. Heat, cold, electrotherapy, and other physical agents may be required by the specific official who inspects the office for compliance with Medicare requirements. The state agency should be contacted to obtain a list of the requirements for certification before final equipment costs are determined. Even if you do not see clients with diagnoses that would require physical agents, you must be able to provide those services if you are seeking Medicaid reimbursement for any clients.

For our initial office, waiting area and office furniture consisted of a small desk and desk chair, four chairs discarded from our home, a phone and answering machine, the room divider, and a table with a lamp. The treatment room was carpeted and consisted of a mat placed on the floor, a large wall mirror, and numerous toys. Wall decorations were handmade and were appropriate for an infant's room. The initial cost for these items was only several hundred dollars, but the office was not certified for Medicaid clients at that time.

The current office contains a large, carpeted treatment room with floor mat, therapeutic balls, bolsters, shelves, and toys. One small treatment room contains a floor mat, a large mirror, shelves, and toys, and the other small treatment room contains a platform mat and large mirror. The hall and large treatment room provide ambulation areas as does the outdoor sidewalk and lawn areas in good weather. The practice is housed in a building with another health care professional, and the waiting room is shared. The casting room contains a sink and cabinets; the billing office has a desk, desk chair, side chair, telephone, and computer; and the staff office contains several desk areas, a reception area with a window opening into the waiting room, telephone, lamp, computer, typewriter, copier, and other office equipment. Although the equipment assets of the practice now total several thousand dollars, these assets were obtained over numerous years, and the typical pediatric practice will never experience equipment costs in the hundred thousand dollar range.

PLANNING FOR HUMAN RESOURCES

A practitioner may employ other therapists and staff or contract for other services if needed. The solo practitioner will have difficulty attending continuing education programs, taking vacation time, or using sick leave unless help is available. Burch and Iglarsh (1988) recommend finding a therapist who can be trusted with the practice to offer relief to the solo practitioner. Employing or contracting with other therapists and support staff requires an understanding of laws and regulations for personnel. The services of the lawyer and tax consultant for the practice can be used to determine the best plan for obtaining the services of other persons.

Planning for needed support staff must be as deliberate as planning for other aspects of the business (Sims, 1992). Office staff must have the equipment necessary to accomplish the required tasks, must be clearly informed of the job responsibilities, and must be given time to learn the equipment and the management systems for the practice. Some practices choose to use a medical billing and collecting firm to manage accounts receivable if the staff do not have expertise in billing.

An administrative assistant may provide the expertise in business management not typically possessed by the physical therapist owner. Private practices have differing needs, and the administrative assistant may be an on-the-job trained office manager or a certified public accountant and financial planner (Wilson, 1992). The owner must determine the needs of the practice, seek an administrative assistant with the skills necessary to meet needs, and relinquish the responsibilities and tasks to the administrative assistant. The administrative assistant may have responsibility for any task that is not directly treatment related, but all administrative assistants should have experience with preparation and collection of accounts receivable. Lynch (1992) suggests that the administrative assistant should mirror the practitioner/owner in personality, image, competence, and commitment. The Private Practice Section (PPS) has supported the development of the Private Practice Physical Therapy Administrative Assistants group, which has bylaws and publishes a newsletter. This group meets at annual meetings of the PPS and provides excellent information and support for administrative assistants and private practitioners.

Salaries for yourself and other staff, if used, must be determined, and salaries will be the major expense of a service business. A friend with a long-standing adult orthopaedic private practice suggested establishing a 3-year goal for the owner to reach the salary that was abandoned to start the practice. The first-year salary for the owner for our practice was set at $15,000, the amount necessary to supplement the spouse's salary for our personal expenses. As previously noted, the spouse provided

billing services and no other staff were employed. The telephone answering machine served as receptionist when a client was being treated. All bills and the salary as established were paid, and the net loss for the first year was $97.00. During the second year, an additional therapist was hired as an independent contractor, and the salary available to the owner exceeded the salary originally determined to be the 3-year goal. The salary level for the owner grew at a rapid rate, and competitive salaries were soon offered to numerous other therapists.

The decision will have to be made to keep the practice small or to allow growth. Over a 10-year period of time, our practice expanded to include 14 employees. A half-time secretary was eventually hired, followed by a full-time secretary during the ninth year, and an administrative assistant and a half-time secretary during the tenth year. In retrospect, the administrative assistant should have been employed earlier and responsibilities for billing should have been delegated from the beginning. Currently, eight physical therapists, three physical therapist assistants, two speech-language pathologists, and one part-time occupational therapist are employed by the practice. Several sources offer suggestions for recruiting and retaining quality staff in a physical therapy private practice (Deaton & Gutterud, 1992; McNeil, 1990, 1991).

RISK MANAGEMENT IN MAINTAINING A PRIVATE PRACTICE

For a new practice, resource development and availability may be of primary importance in business planning. As the practice matures, the practitioner will need to continually assess the strengths and weaknesses of the practice, to take advantage of change, and to exhibit management control (Dillon & Duke, 1991). Management control involves using resources in an effective manner to accomplish the goals and objectives of the practice. Dillon and Duke (1991) suggest the use of critical success factors, the crucial components of a business, to achieve success. The owner should identify the specific key components and measure performance by focusing on these components through information gathering and reporting. Deaton (1992a) noted that therapists in private practice often use computer programs to collect and produce lengthy reports that do not highlight the crucial components of the business. For example, information on the number of units of service for each referring physician would not be useful in a practice in which the therapists determine the frequency and type of treatment procedures to be provided. Information on the number of units of service generated each month would be useful in determining peak service months and in planning for vacations and staffing.

Dillon and Duke (1991) provide several questions that may assist the owner in identifying the critical success factors for the practice. Measurable indicators for each critical success factor must be determined and used for management control. Indicators should allow comparison to a desired level of performance, use staff input to enhance compliance and cooperation, be reliable, provide timely information, and allow for simple identification of problem areas.

We did not employ risk management concepts using critical success factors or any other type of control processes when the business was initiated, nor for the first several years. Experience in accounts receivable collection enhanced success, but luck was a primary factor in maintaining the practice. Eventually, we realized the need to gather information on the number of patients treated in each facility and at the office; the collection rate for different insurance companies; the cost of each employee including vacation time, sick time, and continuing education time and expenses; the revenue generated by each employee; and the cost of supplies and casting materials. We perceived this information as comprising the critical success factors for our business; and as control over these crucial components was established and maintained, the profit for the practice increased significantly. As when planning a practice, the financial, physical, and human resources should be considered in maintaining a successful practice.

Maintaining Financial Resources

Private practitioners must establish effective collection practices and be effective in determining when to refer an account to an attorney or collection agency for assistance in bringing the account current. Keeping accounts receivable current is an important but difficult task. As previously mentioned, many accounts will be outstanding for lengthy periods of time. Prompt and consistent billing of new charges and reminders of outstanding charges will allow for continual collections after the first year or so of practice. The owner must establish standards by which credit is extended to clients and by which sufficient information is obtained to enable collection of an account should delinquency occur. In addition to the demographic information obtained from clients at the initiation of treatment,

the owner or staff responsible for billing should find out where the individual responsible for payment of the charges is employed and where banking is done. If possible, a copy of the bank account number should be obtained by copying one of the checks (Merry, 1992) and the insurance or Medicaid card should be copied. Figure 32–1 provides an example of the form we used to gather client information. Merry (1992) provides suggestions on contracts with clients, collecting debt, terminating services for clients with delinquent accounts, and using an attorney to collect accounts. He notes that failure to implement and follow collection practices will be costly to a private practice. Newell (1988) provides samples of a payment policy statement, a reminder letter, and a final notice letter as well as suggestions for collecting accounts by telephone.

We require the party responsible for payment to authorize payment of benefits to the practice (see Fig. 32–1). This necessitates that all billing be done by the practice rather than having clients submit claim forms, but we are comfortable with the collection rate obtained through the use of assignment of benefits to the practice. Occasionally, an insurance company will reimburse the client for services, but if an authorization for payment to the practice is on file, the insurance company will pay the practice and assume responsibility for recovery of the payment from the client.

Financial resources may be compromised by unethical staff. Deaton (1992a) asked a large audience of private practice physical therapists to indicate the incidence of stealing by staff. Over 50% of the practitioners indicated that staff had taken funds from the practice. In our practice, we believe that one staff member managed to divert several thousand dollars into a personal account. Staff are able to bill for relatives who never received services and for fictitious clients using a false address. A second bank account may be established for deposits. The owner may never know that the false billing has occurred. An accountant will be able to assist in planning to prevent stealing and in designing safeguards for the owner who is not competent in the business aspects of the practice.

Our practice referral base is largely through the state system of case management coordinators, and over 50% of our clients have Medicaid funding. Despite awareness of the recommendation that no more than 5% of referrals should occur from one referral source, we are unable to alter our referral base. Many pediatric therapists will find that current laws and regulations ensure services to infants and toddlers through mechanisms funded by the state, and that referral source will form a substantial portion of the revenue for a practice. We expe-

CLIENT:

| ADDRESS: | PHONE #: | SS #: | DATE OF BIRTH: | SEX: Male _____ Female _____ | DIAGNOSIS: |

PHYSICIAN:

| PHYSICIAN'S ADDRESS: | PHYSICIAN PHONE #: | PARENT'S NAMES and SS #: Father: SS#: Mother: SS #: | PARENT'S ADDRESS: | PARENT'S PHONE #: Home: Work: |

INSURANCE INFO: Primary Insurance Company:

| Employer: | Employee: | ID #: | Group #: | OTHER INSURANCE: Secondary Insurance Company: | Employer: | Employee: | ID #: |

ASSIGNMENT OF BENEFITS

I authorize payment of medical benefits be paid directly for services rendered.

_____
Signature

AUTHORIZATION FOR TREATMENT

I authorize treatment be given as ordered by my physician.

_____
Signature

AUTHORIZATION TO RELEASE MEDICAL INFORMATION

I authorize release of any medical information to another physician or insurance company to assist in treatment or claim processing.

_____
Signature

FIGURE 32–1. Example of a client information sheet and assignment form for a private practice.

rienced a severe cash flow problem in the tenth year of business when the state funding for Medicaid was jeopardized by low state revenues. Very quickly, the state owed more than $100,000, and the business experienced the only true threat to continuation. The funds were eventually paid in full, but we learned that a successful business could be at risk if a major funding source was eliminated.

Likewise, if the business continues to grow, cash flow problems will recur. Employees will often be paid several months before the funds generated by the employees are received. Each owner will have to determine the desire for growth and the tolerance for cash flow difficulties. An established practice will be able to maintain an ongoing line of credit with the bank and to pay bills and employees while experiencing growth. Dobrin (1991) cautions that the banking industry has problems that transcend the profession of physical therapy and that loans for growth may be difficult to obtain unless an existing base of clients is evident.

Maintaining Physical Resources

Although physical resources, particularly office space and location, may change with growth of the practice, few pediatric therapists will have yearly purchases of expensive equipment as is the case for therapists engaged in practice areas using ever-advancing, high-technology equipment. Pediatric assessment instruments, inhibitive casting supplies, and new innovations in ambulation equipment have resulted in expenditures in the area of physical resources that have required management control. A platform mat, an additional floor mat, therapeutic balls and bolsters, and equipment for therapists traveling to numerous locations have been purchased, but all the initial equipment is still in use after 10 years of practice, and few major equipment expenses have occurred. Toys and expendable play supplies represent the largest portion of expenses for the practice beyond salaries, mileage reimbursement, and continuing education.

Maintaining Human Resources

A challenge for private practitioners is attracting and retaining qualified physical therapists (Deaton & Gutterud, 1992). McNeil (1990) suggests that the gap between supply and demand is increasing at an intimidating rate and that private practices experience employee turnover of up to 40% annually. New and experienced therapists and assistants are seeking the best employment offer, and owners must offer a salary and benefit package that is competitive (Deaton & Gutterud, 1992). McNeil (1990) notes that modeling, having a defined philosophy of management, gaining credibility with employees, and offering opportunities for growth and development are some key points in reducing turnover in physical therapy private practices.

Most of the therapists and physical therapist assistants in our practice work in relative isolation, meeting only weekly for a staff conference or for supervisory sessions between therapists and assistants. This isolation is common in private practice but presents a particular challenge for pediatric therapists who are accustomed to center-based practices. New graduates in our practice have fewer adjustment difficulties with the isolated treatment environments than do experienced therapists, and this phenomenon was a surprise to the owner who was hesitant to employ new graduates in a private practice with so many isolated activities. One explanation for the success with new graduates may be that educational programs are preparing graduates for diverse practice environments. All of the new graduates employed in recent years have held the entry-level master of science degree. New graduates receive orientation and mentoring on a planned basis, and all therapists and assistants have access to their co-workers by telephone. Social activities are included in the weekly staff meetings to promote a sense of belonging and collegiality.

Student affiliation agreements are maintained with one physical therapist assistant and four physical therapist educational programs. Students participate in all aspects of the practice and serve as a source for recruitment as well as motivators for the staff. Students often provide inservice presentations and perform unique projects that stimulate therapists, assistants, and clients.

Continued education and opportunities for growth are of primary importance in our practice. Information regarding specialized skills, such as inhibitive casting or family-guided services, are shared freely among practitioners either through consultation or inservice education. The practice supports graduate or other formal education experiences, and tuition reimbursement is available to therapists and physical therapist assistants who seek further academic education. Achievement of recognized specialization is fostered, and two therapists in addition to the owner and co-therapist have become certified pediatric specialists.

Attracting therapists who would travel to multiple locations, including some potentially unsafe home environments, was also a challenge for our practice. We have attempted to balance this challenge with the practical benefit of reimbursing mileage costs and with philosophical advantages. Each therapist is offered the opportunity to provide services within a philosophy of private practice including maximal autonomy, self-governance, reduced bureaucracy, and independence in exercising professional judgment. Each assistant is afforded similar opportunity within the constraints of supervision and delegation. The result has been an excellent retention rate with only three therapists and one assistant leaving the practice for other opportunities during the 10 years of the practice.

TRENDS IN PRIVATE PRACTICE

Issues identified by the Private Practice Section of the APTA as potentially harmful to private practitioners include continuing difficulty with referral for profit and physician-owned physical therapy services, the rapid growth of non–physical therapist corporate-owned practices, and cost-containment measures that provide inequitable constraints on physical therapists. The Private Practice Section has acknowledged that physical therapists need to take a proactive stance in dealing with these issues. Pediatric physical therapy is not exempt from these concerns, and many pediatric therapists are not reimbursed for services or are reimbursed at a lower rate if services are provided in a private practice setting rather than in an established pediatric facility.

Most therapists, including those in private practice, do not have a business background, and the Private Practice Section offers a quarterly publication, *Physical Therapy Today*, to provide information on business as well as clinical issues. The annual meeting of the Private Practice Section is designed to provide additional educational opportunities for private practitioners, and regional meetings are held each year.

The Section on Pediatrics of the APTA has recognized some movement toward private practice among section members. The movement appears to be primarily for increased autonomy and because of disenchantment with practice settings in which pediatric therapists perceive themselves as "revenue generators" for a facility rather than as caregivers for clients (Dasch & Finney, 1991).

Current trends indicate the need for physical therapists to move into environments such as health maintenance organizations, preferred provider arrangements, and point-of-service plans and less often into individual practice settings. One projection is that physical therapist–owned practices using a group mode will be more common as the base for practice than the solo mode (Moffat,

1991). Faust and Meaker (1991) suggest that a group private practice can have the three key elements of private practice: 1) high autonomy, 2) strong professional identity, and 3) low bureaucracy. These authors note that therapists tend to distance themselves from the important topics of reimbursement, business, and administration. "The therapy company," a group practice, might allow several therapists to combine resources to address these business needs and to meet the essential practice roles of clinical services, management, administration, and professional activities.

Moffat (1991) also recommends using the skills of the physical therapist assistant to complement practice and to free therapists to maximize their own skills. Assistants have traditionally been encouraged to seek general hospital experiences (Infante et al., 1976; Larson & Davis, 1975; Physical Therapy Assistant Program, 1975), but settings providing specialized health care have been suggested as appropriate for employment of the assistant (Lovelace-Chandler & Lovelace-Chandler, 1979).

The private practice arena offers numerous opportunities for appropriate use of physical therapist assistants. Understanding the academic preparation of the assistant and adhering to the ethical guidelines of the APTA (1982, 1989a) and the legal restrictions of the state are important prerequisites to determining the appropriate functions for assistants in any practice arena. Our philosophy includes the belief that no treatment techniques performed in the duties of the practice are inconsistent with the qualifications of the assistant. Tasks related to treatment are delegated only after a therapist performs the initial client evaluation and establishes a treatment plan. We previously noted that individual patients' differences, unique circumstances, individual assistants' competencies, and acute or severe problems might restrict the delegation of tasks (Lovelace-Chandler & Lovelace-Chandler, 1979). In that article, we suggested how to develop a job description for the physical therapist assistant for any particular setting, how to determine the incoming skills of the individual assistant, and how to provide education or remediation if skills were lacking. Thirteen tasks that we deemed as appropriate for delegation to assistants treating clients with developmental disabilities were included. We have experienced a general reluctance on the part of pediatric physical therapists to use the skills of the physical therapist assistant. The pediatric therapist in private practice needs to recognize that effective use of assistants is essential to providing high-quality services at the lowest cost.

Health care reforms will require more emphasis

on prevention and on health restoration (Moffat, 1991). The low level of bureaucracy of private practice provides the unique opportunity to quickly respond to shifts in public policy and to play a major role in prevention. Pediatric therapists must assume responsibility for accident prevention among clients and families. Ecologically appropriate safety education needs to be provided to families and caregivers for all of the child's environments and to older children who can assume responsibility for accident prevention. For example, clients in wheelchairs need to learn to use the device for independent mobility without compromising the safety of themselves or those around them, and private practitioners can educate clients, parents, siblings, and other children in the school setting. Additionally, private practice therapists might contract with the state child care licensing agency or the state insurance carrier to provide training in appropriate lifting and handling techniques to personnel in state-supported child care centers for children with impaired mobility.

The promotion of patient and family education is important in all aspects of therapy (Moffat, 1991), but pediatric therapists must be particularly responsive to the legislative mandates for family-guided care. Private practitioners must seek methods that allow reimbursement for educational activities with clients. Group practices might include health educators, case managers, or other persons expert in client and family education.

Economic trends of the 1990s and beyond may hinder growth for private practitioners. Dobrin (1991) suggests that physical therapists may counteract this trend by marketing in a concerted manner to promote the practice. Brown and Morley (1986) suggest that four factors are essential to developing a marketing plan:

1. Determine the needs and wants of your clients (in the case of pediatric physical therapy, the needs and wants of the families) and examine your practice from the viewpoint of the client. Another professional may serve as a consultant and may be able to assume the client's viewpoint more accurately than you. A consumer survey may be effective in determining the perspectives of families and of older clients served by your practice.

2. The practice must be coordinated in conducting the marketing program. The marketing philosophy and basic principles should be shared with and accepted by all staff.

3. Ethical methods of marketing are a necessity. The responsibilities and ethics of the professional transcend the quest for economic survival. A good marketing plan will reinforce and enhance the socially responsible principle of providing high-qual-

ity, cost-effective care that is in the best interest of the client and family.

4. The marketing plan must be executed in a cost-effective manner. The public will not begrudge efforts to increase profit through marketing if the profits are viewed as reasonable and the service meets health care needs. Momberg (1988) recommends that physical therapists spend 5% to 10% of any anticipated increased profits on advertising. The higher percentage is expended during the initial aspects of establishing the business or in marketing a new service, and the lower percentage is recommended for ongoing advertising.

Trzecki (1988) recommends the VIP method of *v*isibility, *i*mage, and *p*romotion for marketing physical therapy services. When conducted correctly, promotion highlights visibility and enhances image. Money directed to marketing is directed away from client services (Barone, 1988), and only the amount needed to market the practice in a dignified and professional manner should be expended. The ethics of marketing is unquestioned if the practitioner believes that the practice offers the highest quality of services and that these services are equal to or exceed the quality of services provided by competitors (Brown & Morley, 1986). Failure to market the services would deprive potential clients of access to quality care. Dignity and responsibility for marketing and advertisement rests with the individual practitioner. "Communicate your passion, caring and expertise and your market will break down your doors" (Barone, 1988, p. 47). Numerous resources exist to assist the pediatric private practitioner in planning marketing strategies (Abeln, 1993; Adams, 1993; Baum, 1992; Davidson, 1987; Dohallow, 1993; Klehfoth, 1993; Nosse & Friberg, 1992; Patin & Adams, 1991; Schunk, 1989; Schunk & Jaffe, 1993).

THE UNIQUE PHILOSOPHY OF PEDIATRIC PHYSICAL THERAPY

Any practitioner considering a private practice limited to pediatric physical therapy must be cognizant of the uniqueness of pediatrics as a specialty. Cherry (1991) has summarized the philosophy, the scientific components, and the quantitative and qualitative differences that must be considered in selecting treatment techniques that meet the needs of children. Albeit evolved from the philosophy and techniques of the wider field of physical therapy, pediatric physical therapy is distinguished by a distinct philosophy. Inherent in this philosophy are the beliefs that a child is viewed as a whole person existing in the context of the family and with natural ecologic settings, that the developmental characteristics of children require unique knowledge of existing and future development, and that children require advocacy.

An appreciation of the child as a whole person, a holistic approach, would dictate that pediatric physical therapists use transdisciplinary communication and collaboration. The private practitioner could screen for impairments in related areas such as cognitive, biologic, psychosocial, and speech/language performance that could influence or be influenced by motor performance or the specific physical concern. If the screenings suggested the need for referral, the practitioner must be prepared with knowledge of community resources and an attitude of client sharing. The pediatric therapist may choose a joint practice with professionals from appropriate fields or an arrangement that allows consultation as indicated.

The natural ecologic settings for children are the home and school (Cherry, 1991). Other frequent settings include child care centers, churches or other religious environments, and settings where leisure activities are enjoyed. Therapists in private practice must be willing to determine the ecologic settings for the children in their practice and to provide services within those settings, using the natural activities of the settings as the treatment strategies. Private practitioners must be willing to view family members, in addition to the child, as clients with wishes and needs, and be responsive to those wishes and needs. Otherwise services will be sought from facilities or practitioners who identify and implement family goals. Family-focused therapy became prominent in the United States after the passage of PL 99-457, and the private practitioner has numerous resources available to assist in service design using family theory (see Chapter 30).

Developmental science, pediatric medical pathology, and assessment and management of developmental risk factors form the scientific bases of pediatric physical therapy, and knowledge in these areas must be added to the knowledge base required for any area of physical therapy practice. Treatment techniques for children may be adapted from adult treatment or may be specific to the young client (Cherry, 1991). Private practitioners wishing to offer services to children must possess the unique knowledge and skills necessary for the practice of pediatrics.

RECOMMENDATIONS FOR BEST PRACTICE IN PEDIATRIC PRIVATE ENTERPRISE

The following recommendations are offered to summarize our beliefs regarding best practice in

private practice physical therapy. We have not always followed these recommendations, but the business would probably have been more successful if we had done so. You will be able to determine which recommendations meet your philosophy of care and your needs regarding the financial, physical, and human resources of the practice.

1. Possess advanced skill in the specialty area of pediatrics. Although recognized specialization such as that awarded by the American Board of Physical Therapy Specialists (ABPTS) should not be a requirement for initiating a pediatric practice, any clinician who is not acquiring the skills essential to that credential should not be in pediatric private practice.

2. Gain knowledge of all appropriate laws, regulations, policies, and position statements that affect pediatric physical therapy. Federal laws have greatly influenced the practice of pediatric physical therapy in recent years, and state laws and regulations determine which pediatric therapy services are allowable and will be reimbursed. State and city laws and regulations affect the operation of the business.

3. Have business skills available to the business. The owner/therapist does not need to have knowledge of accounting, taxes, bookkeeping, and management, but this knowledge must be accessible to the business through the use of lawyers, accountants, bankers, and billing specialists. Business sense is required to achieve business cents (translate dollars).

4. Provide services that are needed in the marketplace. The trends in health care cost containment and private practice service provision will increase competition among health care providers. Pediatric therapists must be responsive to the needs and wants of clients and families.

5. Identify the quantity of services you can provide. Do not exceed that quantity, or quality will suffer.

6. Design the appropriate setting if an office practice is used. The space and decor should reflect the clients you serve. Employ staff who mirror your philosophy and image.

7. Purchase the correct supplies. Experienced pediatric therapists will know that diapers, tissues, crayons, toys, games, holiday decorations, and stickers are more important purchases for the pediatric practice than massage lotion, but vendors who serve practices for adults will not be able to recommend the correct supplies for new pediatric practitioners.

8. Know how to play with the clients you serve. New graduates may not have knowledge of play activities commensurate with their knowledge of therapeutic techniques. Seek continuing education

or consultation for this and any other area of service provision in which you are lacking.

9. Understand the ecologic settings for children. The work of children is their play, and children function within the context of family life, preschool, or school. Design the practice to fit into the lives of children and families.

10. Offer family-guided physical therapy in the private enterprise arena. Understand the context of the family and the advocacy role of the family. Develop cultural competence for the families you serve. Learn about the language, food, holiday, religious, child-rearing, and discipline preferences of your clients. Accept the closeness you will develop with families and children. In private practice, professional distance is reduced. Demonstrate affection or even love for your clients. Aloofness and professional demeanor are inconsistent with the intimacy found in most private practices. Families may tolerate inappropriate behaviors from institutions, but private practitioners will be held more responsible for correct interactions.

SUMMARY

The private practice pediatric physical therapist has autonomy, uses professional values, and takes risks with a minimum of bureaucracy to achieve independence and success. The roles of owner, business manager, and clinician must coexist, and the private practitioner must seek services from such resources as accountants, bankers, lawyers, realtors, and other therapists to augment the knowledge and skills required of those roles. Personal and professional characteristics and responsibilities have been suggested by numerous authors, and possession or development of these attributes will diminish risk and liability. A private practice is established and maintained through selection of an appropriate legal structure and consideration of the necessary financial, physical, and human resources. Societal trends offer private practitioners the opportunity for creative business activities when services are envisioned through the unique philosophy of pediatric physical therapy and with regard for best practices. Professionalism in pediatric physical therapy will be enhanced as an increased number of therapists enter the private practice arena.

References

Abeln, SH. A payer-based marketing approach. Physical Therapy Today, *16*(1):25–29, 1993.

Adams, C. Preproduced marketing tools. Physical Therapy Today, *16*(1):42–44, 1993.

American Physical Therapy Association. Code of Ethics. Alexandria, VA: APTA, 1987.

American Physical Therapy Association. Guide for Conduct of the Affiliate Member. Alexandria, VA: APTA, 1989a.

American Physical Therapy Association. Guide for Professional Conduct. Alexandria, VA: APTA, 1989b.

American Physical Therapy Association. Standards of Ethical Conduct for the Physical Therapist Assistant. Alexandria, VA: APTA, 1982.

American Speech-Language-Hearing Association. Considerations for establishing a private practice in audiology and/or speech-language pathology. ASHA, *33*(suppl 3):10–21, 1991.

Aydelotte, MK, Hardy, MA, & Hope, KL. Nurses in Private Practice: Characteristics, Organizational Arrangements, and Reimbursement Policy. Kansas City, MO: American Nurses' Foundation, 1988.

Barone, DL. Being market-wise. Physical Therapy Today, *11*(3):46–47, 1988.

Baum, N. Marketing Your Clinical Practice Ethically, Effectively, Economically. Gaithersburg, MD: Aspen Publishers, 1992.

Bernstein, DK. Part-time private practice in speech-language pathology and audiology. In Butler, KG (Ed.), Prospering in Private Practice: A Handbook for Speech-Language Pathology and Audiology. Gaithersburg, MD: Aspen Publishers, 1986, pp. 13–46.

Brown, S. Sorry—I'm not in private practice. Clinical Management, *12*(1):14–15, 1992.

Brown, SW, & Morley, AP. Marketing Strategies for Physicians: A Guide to Practice Growth. Oradell, NJ: Medical Economics Books, 1986.

Burch, EA, & Iglarsh, A. A conversation about starting a private practice. Physical Therapy Today, *11*(4):37–42, 1988.

Carlson, T. Tom Carlson, 1987 Robert G. Dicus award winner. Whirlpool, *10*:35–37, 1987.

Cherry, DB. Pediatric physical therapy: Philosophy, science, and techniques. Pediatric Physical Therapy, *3*(2):70–75, 1991.

Cole, PR. Private practice: Personal prerequisites and potential. In Butler, KG (Ed.), Prospering in Private Practice: A Handbook for Speech-Language Pathology and Audiology. Gaithersburg, MD: Aspen Publishers, 1986, pp. 3–11.

Cooper, E. The state of the profession and what to do about it. ASHA, *24*:931–936, 1982.

Dasch, D, & Finney, M. The future and specialty practice. Clinical Management, *11*(6):26–33, 1991.

Davidson, JP. Advanced marketing techniques: Becoming your own press agent. Whirlpool, *10*(1):38–42, 1987.

Deaton, WC. Do you know where your practice is tonight? Paper presented at the 1992 Private Practice Section Annual Conference and Exposition, Dallas, TX, November 11–15, 1992a.

Deaton, WC. Running your practice by the numbers. Physical Therapy Today, *15*(2):31–35, 1992b.

Deaton, WC, & Gutterud, SR. Attracting and retaining quality staff: Using fringe benefits and incentive compensation. Physical Therapy Today, *15*(3):44–47, 1992.

Dicus, RG. Origins of the self-employed section. Physical Therapy Today, *14*(4):19–20, 22, 1991.

Dillon, RD, & Duke, PJ. Planning for success. Clinical Management, *11*(5):28–32, 1991.

Dobrin, J. Private practice: Big, small, or not at all. Physical Therapy Today, *14*(3):52, 54, 56, 1991.

Dohallow, J. A physical therapist's guide to marketing a private practice. Physical Therapy Today, *16*(1):46–48, 1993.

Driskell, C. Planning for success: Developing a business plan to secure financing. Physical Therapy Today, *11*(1):40–41, 1988.

Faust, L, & Meaker, MK. Private practice occupational therapy in the skilled nursing facility: Creative alliance or mutual exploitation? American Journal of Occupational Therapy, 45:621–627, 1991.

Finch, J. Private practice physical therapy: Presentation for physical therapy students. Conway, AR, 1982.

Flower, RM. Ethical concerns in private practice. In Butler, KG (Ed.), Prospering in Private Practice: A Handbook for Speech-Language Pathology and Audiology. Gaithersburg, MD: Aspen Publishers, 1986, pp. 101–123.

Frazian, BW. Tidal surge and private practice: The historic eighties. In Cromwell, FS (Ed.), Private Practice in Occupational Therapy. New York: Haworth Press, 1985, pp. 7–13.

Guglielmo, FX. The 1988 Robert G. Dicus award recipient. Physical Therapy Today, 11(4):18–24, 1988.

Hampton, D. Establishing and equipping an audiology private practice. In Butler, KG (Ed.), Prospering in Private Practice. A Handbook for Speech-Language Pathology and Audiology. Gaithersburg, MD: Aspen Publishers, 1986, pp. 135–148.

Infante, MS, Speranza, KA, & Gillespie, PW. An interdisciplinary approach to the education of health professional students. Journal of Allied Health, 5(4):13–22, 1976.

Jayaratne, S, Davis-Sacks, ML, & Chess, WA. Private practice may be good for your health and well-being. Social Work, 36(3):224–229, 1991.

Klehfoth, K. Public relations: The key to a profitable small practice. Physical Therapy Today, 16(2):34, 36, 1993.

Kooper, JD, & Sullivan, CA. Professional liability: Management and prevention. In Butler, KG (Ed.), Prospering in Private Practice: A Handbook for Speech-Language Pathology and Audiology. Gaithersburg, MD: Aspen Publishers, 1986, pp. 59–79.

Larson, CW, & Davis, ER. Following up the physical therapist assistant graduate: A curriculum evaluation process. Physical Therapy, 55:601–606, 1975.

Lovelace-Chandler, V, & Lovelace-Chandler, B. Employment of physical therapist assistants in a residential state school. Physical Therapy, 59(10):1243–1246, 1979.

Lynch, R. Selection of an administrative assistant. Physical Therapy Today, 15(2):50–51, 1992.

McClain, L, McKinney, J, & Ralston, J. Occupational therapists in private practice. American Journal of Occupational Therapy, 46:613–618, 1992.

McFadden, SM, & Hanschu, B. Risk taking in occupational therapy. In Cromwell, FS (Ed.), Private Practice in Occupational Therapy. New York: Haworth Press, 1985, pp. 3–6.

McNeil, LL. The people part of practice management. Physical Therapy Today, 13(1):34–35, 37–38, 40, 1990.

McNeil, LL. Employee turnover: Do we have a problem? Physical Therapy Today, 14(3):57–60, 1991.

Merry, TR. Ten commonly asked questions in dealing with accounts receivable: What every private practice owner would like to ignore but can't. Physical Therapy Today, 15(1):59–62, 64–65, 1992.

Moffat, M. Beyond 2000: Who will you be? Clinical Management, 11(6):8–9, 1991.

Momberg, WA. Budgeting your advertising dollars. Physical Therapy Today, 11(3):48, 1988.

Newell, D. Collecting accounts receivable by telephone. Physical Therapy Today, 11(2):28–31, 1988.

Nosse, LJ, & Friberg, DG. Management Principles for Physi-

cal Therapists. Baltimore: Williams & Wilkins, 1992, pp. 177–191.

Parish, R. Constraints and commitments: An introduction to the financial aspects of private practice. In Butler, KG (Ed.), Prospering in Private Practice: A Handbook for Speech-Language Pathology and Audiology. Gaithersburg, MD: Aspen Publishers, 1986, pp. 81–99.

Parsons, L. Planning and initiating a private practice in nursing psychotherapy. In Durham, JD, & Hardin, SB (Eds.), The Nurse Psychotherapist in Private Practice. New York: Springer, 1986, pp. 75–86.

Patin, S, & Adams, C. The marketing plan: An integrative tool for the future. Physical Therapy Today, 14(3):68, 70, 72, 1991.

Physical Therapy Assistant Program. Physical therapy assistant program evaluation. Charlotte, NC: Central Piedmont Community College, 1975.

Private Practice Section. 1992 profile of a private practice physical therapist. Physical Therapy Today, 15(3):60–69, 1992.

Reuss, R. The maturation of the private practice section. Physical Therapy Today, 14(4):24–26, 28–32, 34–36, 38–48, 1991.

Roussel, FJ, & Epplin, R. Thinking About Going into Business? Management Aid Number 2.025. Fort Worth, TX: U.S. Small Business Administration, 1987.

Schunk, C. The referral within: Marketing to your peers. Physical Therapy Today, 12(4):52–53, 1989.

Schunk, C, & Jaffe, RL. Teamwork: The marketing management tool. Physical Therapy Today, 16(1):31–32, 34, 37, 40, 1993.

Scull, S, & Deitz, J: Competencies for the physical therapist in the neonatal intensive care unit (NICU). Pediatric Physical Therapy, 1(1):11–14, 1989.

Sims, D. Wishing you continued success. Physical Therapy Today, 15(1):7–11, 1992.

Smoyak, SA. The nurse psychotherapist as unique practitioner. In Durham, JD, & Hardin, SB (Eds.), The Nurse Psychotherapist in Private Practice. New York: Springer, 1986, pp. 21–23.

Sullivan, CA. Business and management aspects of private practice in speech-language pathology and audiology. In Butler, KG (Ed.), Prospering in Private Practice: A Handbook for Speech-Language Pathology and Audiology. Gaithersburg, MD: Aspen Publishers, 1986, pp. 149–165.

Task Force on Early Intervention, Section on Pediatrics, APTA. Competencies for physical therapists in early intervention. Pediatric Physical Therapy, 3(2):77–80, 1991.

Trzecki, KJ. Considering marketing? Be a VIP. Physical Therapy Today, 11(3):42–45, 1988.

Walker, RC. Over My Shoulder: Reflections on Beginning a Private Practice in Physical Therapy. Cedar Rapids, IA: RC Walker, 1977.

Wilson, FD. Administrative assistants: What role should they play? Physical Therapy Today, 15(2):47–49, 1992.

Wood, ML. Private Practice in Communication Disorders. Boston: College-Hill Publications, 1986.

Woody, RH. Legal issues for private practitioners in speech-language pathology and audiology. In Butler, KG (Ed.), Prospering in Private Practice: A Handbook for Speech-Language Pathology and Audiology. Gaithersburg, MD: Aspen Publishers, 1986, pp. 47–57.

Appendix I

Resources for Information for the Pediatric Private Practitioner

American Physical Therapy Association
1111 N. Fairfax Street
Alexandria, VA 22314
1-800-999-APTA

Private Practice Section, APTA
1101 17th Street, NW, Suite 1000
Washington, DC 20036
(202) 457-1115

Pediatric Section, APTA
(same address and telephone as the APTA)

Consult the "U.S. Government" section in the telephone directory for the Small Business Administration (SBA) Office nearest you or call: 1-800-U ASK SBA.

A free SBA list of publications and videotapes may be obtained from

Small Business Directory
P.O. Box 1000
Ft. Worth, TX 76119

The Universal Billing Form (HCFA-1500) may be purchased at the following address:

American Medical Association
c/o The Order Department
P.O. Box 2964
Milwaukee, WI 53201

Information on specialization in pediatrics may be obtained from

The American Board of Physical Therapy
Specialties
(same address and telephone as the APTA)

Chapter 33

Medicolegal Issues in the United States

WENDY E. PHILLIPS, PT, PCS, MA, MS
MICHAEL L. SPOTTS, JD

INTRODUCTION

The implementation of federal legislation along with increased litigation related to patient care and outcome in a rapidly evolving medical system increases the likelihood of an interaction between pediatric physical therapists and the legal system. A conceptual understanding of public laws, such as the Education of the Handicapped Act Amendments of 1986 (PL 99-457) and the Americans with Disabilities Act of 1990 (PL 101-336), is required of the practicing clinician or student who will be working with children and adolescents with disabilities and their families. Similarly, a familiarity with the process of litigation as it is relevant to issues, such as medical malpractice and petitions for the determination of appropriate medical treatment, is useful.

The purpose of this chapter is to provide an overview of the two U.S. public laws, PL 99-457 and PL 101-336, just mentioned. Also provided is an overview of the process of litigation as it is relevant to pediatric patients, using case histories as examples. The physical therapist's responsibility in reporting cases of child abuse and neglect is also included along with related ethical issues. The clinical implications of the federal legislation discussed are presented in several chapters of this book, particularly Chapter 31 on the educational environment and Chapter 30 on family-centered intervention.

Public Law 99-457

The 1986 amendments to the Education of the Handicapped Act provide for the development of comprehensive, coordinated, multidisciplinary, interagency programs of early intervention services for infants and toddlers and their families. At the present time, states which have received funding should have programs in place. This law specifies the focus of services provided, the disciplines involved, and the format for the delivery of services. The clinician involved in the provision of physical therapy services to the birth through 2 years, inclusive, population needs to become familiar with the law's specifications related to physical therapy. This chapter reviews those sections of the law that are particularly relevant to the practice of physical therapy.

PL 101-336

In an attempt to rectify past discrimination against individuals with physical and mental disabilities with respect to housing, employment, and other areas, the Americans with Disabilities Act was developed. Although a superficial review of the act may suggest that its focus is the adult population, various provisions are directly or indirectly applicable to families with children with disabilities.

For example, parents are protected from discrimination with respect to employment hiring practices based on their status as parents of a child with a disability. The act ensures that a parent cannot be denied health insurance for the family because of the child's condition. These and other provisions of the act that may affect children and families served by the pediatric physical therapist are discussed.

Child Abuse and Neglect

Although specific laws with respect to child abuse and neglect vary in the United States from state to state, the purpose is consistent: to provide for the protection of children whose health and welfare are adversely affected and further threatened by the conduct of those responsible for their care and protection. The law dictates that certain persons, including hospital or medical personnel, report all suspected cases of abuse and neglect to the appropriate state agency. Failure to report a suspected case of abuse or neglect results in a misdemeanor charge.

Physical abuse, sexual abuse, and neglect are all conditions that by law must be reported. Child and adult behaviors associated with physical and sexual abuse may not be easily identified by the physical therapist. For example, the behaviors associated with child sexual abuse, including enuresis, nightmares, a decline in academic performance, secretiveness, and helpless behavior, may not routinely be identified as possibly related to suspected child sexual abuse. This section includes a description of

child and adult behavior that may be associated with abuse as well as a general protocol for the documentation and reporting of suspected abuse. Appropriate referrals to other professionals in situations of suspected abuse are also considered.

Litigation

Although litigation is an unsavory topic to many pediatric physical therapists, it has become a fact of the operation of the U.S. health care system. As the number of lawsuits increases, so does the probability that the pediatric physical therapist's assessment or treatment documentation may be subpoenaed for use in court.

There are various reasons for an emphasis on objective and comprehensive documentation, including determination of progress and change and the evaluation of the effectiveness of treatment. When records may be reviewed or interpreted by persons who do not share the physical therapist's vocabulary and who are not familiar with specific treatment techniques, use of objective data and standardized, norm-referenced measures are essential. With the use of a case history format, the usefulness and relevance of various forms of treatment documentation are considered, including those of a case history in which a physical therapist's documentation was important in determining the outcome of the case.

Medical Technology

Technologic advances in medical treatment have increased the rate of survival of infants and children who are medically fragile. Increasingly, differences of opinion among medical professionals or between parents and medical professionals regarding the choice of medical treatment and the continuation or deceleration of medical support have been decided in the courts. An estimate of a child's present functional status or future outcome may be a consideration in the determination of a plan of appropriate medical care. Estimated functional outcome may be determined by the clinical opinion of the physician, psychologist, or physical therapist.

Formulation of an opinion or a functional prognosis for a child with a central nervous system deficit or congenital anomaly may not be a familiar task for the pediatric physical therapist. Should an opinion be requested, the pediatric physical therapist will require skills, including the ability to draw from past experience with similar cases and from the results of outcome-focused research studies, and in the presentation of the results of the assessment, which may include the use of standardized measures. A case history is presented as an illustration.

A related issue involves the pediatric physical therapist's ability to identify any personal values and beliefs that may affect objectivity in the formulation of an opinion regarding a child's functional abilities and outcome. A consideration of the relationship between belief systems and decision-making as well as the influence of the therapist's ethical standards is included.

EDUCATION OF THE HANDICAPPED ACT AMENDMENTS OF 1986 (PL 99-457)

Background and Purpose

The purpose of the federal Education of the Handicapped Act Amendments of 1986 was to extend the educational and related services already provided to school-aged children to infants and toddlers and their families. The government's motivation for the development and enactment of the law was related to the prevention of disabilities. Early intervention was considered a means of preventing developmental delay, minimizing the need for special education and institutionalization, and preventing stress experienced by families of disabled infants and toddlers.

Directing action toward the goal of prevention, the federal government adopted a policy to provide financial assistance to stated programs whose focus was the following:

"1) To develop and implement a statewide comprehensive, coordinated and multidisciplinary interagency program of early intervention services for infants and toddlers with disabilities and their families,

"2) To facilitate the coordination of payment for early intervention services from Federal, State, local and private sources (including public and private insurance coverage), and

"3) To enhance a program's capacity to provide quality early intervention services and expand and improve existing early intervention services being provided to infants and toddlers with disabilities and their families."

(20 USCS 1471, SEC. 671 (B)).

The focus of this part of the chapter is on a review of those aspects of the law that are particu-larly relevant to the practice of pediatric physical therapy and on a discussion of the potential implications of the enactment of the law related to the practice of pediatric physical therapy.

Title I — Handicapped Infants and Toddlers

DEFINITIONS

"1) The infant and toddler population is defined as a group "from birth through age two inclusive who need early intervention services because they

"A) are experiencing developmental delays as measured by appropriate diagnostic instruments and procedures in one or more of the following areas: Cognitive development, physical development, language and speech development, psychosocial development, or self-help skills; or

"B) have a diagnosed physical or mental condition which has a high probability of resulting in developmental delay. Such term may include, at a State's discretion, individuals from birth [through] age 2, inclusive, who are at risk for having substantial developmental delays if intervention services are not provided."

(20 USC 1472, SEC. 672).

The criteria for eligibility for early intervention services related to the use of "appropriate diagnostic instruments" may be interpreted as either a mandate or a recommendation for the use of standardized measures for assessment purposes (20 USC 1472 sec. 672). In this case, the pediatric physical therapist involved in the evaluation of infants and toddlers for the purpose of the determination of eligibility for early intervention services may need to be competent in the administration of standardized, norm-referenced measures. The pediatric physical therapist who selects and administers a measure appropriate for this population requires skills and knowledge in the area of test construction and theory, including the concepts of reliability and validity, standardization procedures, and norm-referencing, as well as a basic understanding of statistical theory as related to assessment of a given infant's performance in comparison with that of other similar infants in the general population. A need for skills and knowledge in those areas is reflected in the Competencies for Physical Therapists in Early Intervention developed by the American Physical Therapy Association Task Force on Early Intervention (Effgen et al., 1991).

REQUIREMENTS FOR A STATEWIDE SYSTEM

Guidelines for both the general requirements and the minimal components of a statewide system of intervention emphasize the family as the focal unit for the early intervention services. This focus differs from prior legislation, that is, the Education of All Handicapped Children Act (PL 94-142, 1975), in which services were mainly focused on the child.

The family focus of intervention services is evident in the criteria for the development of the Individualized Family Service Plan (IFSP). In addition to addressing the results of an evaluation of the infant or toddler's performance in several areas of development, the IFSP must include an assessment of a family's strengths and needs. The family is to be considered in the determination of which Early Intervention services are to be provided, and in the projection of major outcomes related to intervention.

A shift from a focus on achieving child-centered goals to an emphasis on the family as the unit of intervention may require an alternative framework for the conceptualization of the child and family and the areas of focus of the early intervention services. Foster and Phillips (1992) have argued that a systemic model in which the interrelationships among child, family, professionals, and affiliated agencies and institutions are considered may increase the effectiveness of problem solving and the development of a plan for intervention with young children and their families. Family-centered intervention is presented in Chapter 30.

PROCEDURAL SAFEGUARDS

The procedural safeguards established by PL 99-457 guarantee parental rights related to the provision of services to their child. Provisions to ensure confidentiality are also stated. A grievance procedure whereby parents who have an administrative complaint may have their controversy heard in a state or federal court is outlined. The right of confidentiality concerning personally identifiable information and the parental right to examine a child's record are stated.

The rights of children whose parents or guardians are not known or not available are protected, as are the parents' rights to be informed of any pending change in a plan for an evaluation or placement of their child. The parental right to receive written notice in his or her primary language is stated. Should a complaint be pending or should a proceeding be in process, the child's right to continue to receive early intervention services is guaranteed.

Knowledge of the provisions of PL 99-457 that protect the rights of parents of infants and toddlers who are receiving early intervention services helps the pediatric physical therapist to act as an advocate for families, particularly when working with families who are indigent and disenfranchised. The pediatric physical therapist's role as advocate for the rights of parents is included in the Competencies for Physical Therapists in Early Intervention. Specifically, Competency 7.5 states, "The physical therapist possesses skills necessary to advocate the right of parents to be decision makers in the early intervention process, and provide them with the information and options needed for informed decisions" (Effgen et al., 1991, p. 79).

STATE INTERAGENCY COORDINATING COUNCILS

The requirement for the establishment of a coordinating council of 15 members, which includes parents, professionals involved in the provision of early intervention services, and representatives of state and related agencies, is made. The purpose of the council is to advise the lead agency of the state in establishing guidelines for the performance of the programs of early intervention, to advise the lead agency of needed amendments, and to submit to the governor of the state an annual report on the status of the early intervention programs in the state.

Considering the requirements for the composition of the coordinating council and its stated purpose, the council members may be able to be resources for the pediatric physical therapist who is interested in the status of early intervention programs. Reciprocally, the pediatric physical therapist may be in a position to provide council members with useful feedback regarding experiences with early intervention programs and their adequacy in serving the targeted population.

FUNDING

Early intervention services are defined as developmental and are to be provided at no cost to families except when federal or state law provides for a system of payments that includes sliding fees. Because early intervention programs do not (by definition) generate capital for their operation, they are necessarily dependent on external sources of funding. The relatively high proportion of children and families living in poverty who are dependent on an already overextended public assistance and insurance system and the general effects of the present economic conditions, including the decrease in available governmental revenues, may make the implementation of early intervention programs particularly difficult. Whether or not early intervention programs are able to coordinate funding from secondary sources in order to provide services to families may ultimately determine their ability to be effective.

ELIGIBILITY FOR FUNDING

The plan for the establishment of early intervention programs provided funding during a period of planning beginning in 1986. States making an application for funding for the first 2 years of grants provided evidence of a plan for the development of a statewide system of early intervention. In the third and fourth years, states receiving funding were required to demonstrate that a plan or a policy for the development of an early intervention program had been adopted. By the third and fourth years, multidisciplinary assessments were to be conducted, individualized family service plans (IFSPs) developed, and case management services provided. States not able to provide assessment, IFSP development, and case management services by the third and fourth years but able to provide evidence of a good-faith effort to do so could receive continued funding as long as a plan for the development of these services was outlined. For the fifth and subsequent years, states receiving funding needed to provide evidence that the required services were being provided. Appropriations for funding for all sections of PL 99-457 began in 1986, to be available through 1991. The law was amended in October 1990 (PL 101-476) to extend funding and support and was reauthorized the following year as the Individuals with Disabilities Education Act (IDEA) Amendments of 1991 (PL 102-119). After the fifth year, the specific amounts of funding were not included.

The law states that sufficient funds are to be found such that funding for early intervention services for infants, toddlers, and young children is not withdrawn or reduced. When the specific time frame for approved funding and the recommendation for the identification of alternative sources in federal agencies are considered, the stability of adequate long-term funding for the programs developed under this law is of concern. The longevity of federally initiated early intervention programs may be dependent in part on the programs' ability to creatively access alternative funding sources.

Title II — Handicapped Children Aged 3 to 5

Title II of PL 99-457 specifies the allocation of federal monies to support preschool programs for children aged 3 to 5. Eligibility requirements for states applying for these funds are outlined. Funding amounts were originally delineated for 1987 through 1989 and were increased in 1990 (PL 101-476) and 1991 (PL 102-119). The cap on the amount of funding available per child increased from $300 per child in 1987 to $1000 per child in 1990. An additional lump sum of $12 million was allocated for 1991 to be shared by the 50 states. The increase in funding allocations between 1987 and 1990 was expected to be related to an increase in the special education services, including physical therapy, available to preschool-aged children.

Title III — Discretionary Programs

REGIONAL RESOURCE AND FEDERAL CENTERS

Title III of PL 99-457 provides for the establishment of regional resource centers and federal centers. Such centers were to be established jointly between the government and institutions of higher education, public agencies, and private, nonprofit organizations. The purpose of the regional resource centers is related to problem solving concerning 1) providing high-quality special education and related services to infants, children, and their families; 2) assisting in developing and replicating successful programs for the targeted families; 3) gathering and disseminating information to state educational agencies; 4) coordinating with other centers on relevant projects; 5) improving training activities for professionals working with infants and children with disabilities and their families; and 6) providing training for agencies and institutions regarding techniques and approaches for the submission of applications for grants, contracts, and cooperative agreements. In addition, one national coordinating center was to be established for the purpose of assisting the regional resource centers in the delivery of technical assistance that is consistent with the national priorities.

EXPERIMENTAL, OUTREACH, AND DEMONSTRATION PRESCHOOL PROGRAMS

Title III also provided support for the development of experimental, outreach, and demonstration preschool programs. Such demonstration programs are to facilitate intellectual, emotional, physical, mental, social, speech and language, and self-help skill development. Demonstration programs must also facilitate parent participation and community awareness.

PROGRAMS FOR CHILDREN WITH SEVERE DISABILITIES

Title III of PL 99-457 provides guidelines for activities related to educational services for children with severe disabilities. Grants and contracts to be funded concern the research needed to identify and meet the needs of children with severe disabilities, the demonstration of new and improved methods that contribute to the education and adjustment of these children, the training of personnel who work with the targeted population, and the dissemination of information about effective methods and practices. Physical therapy care of students with severe disabilities is presented in Chapter 18 on mental retardation.

POSTSECONDARY EDUCATION

PL 99-457 established funding priorities for the purpose of the development of models for postsecondary, vocational, technical, and continuing or adult education for individuals with disabilities. Funding priority is to be given to regional model centers for the deaf and to centers for individuals with other disabilities. One of the emphases for the funded projects is the development of postsecondary education programs to facilitate the inclusion of individuals with disabilities.

SECONDARY EDUCATION AND TRANSITIONAL SERVICES FOR YOUNG PERSONS

The emphasis of this section of Title III is on facilitating the strengthening and coordination of special education–related services for young persons with disabilities who are currently in school or have recently left school to facilitate transition to postsecondary education, vocational training, and employment. An emphasis is also placed on improving vocational and life skills of disabled individuals. Projects to be funded need to emphasize strategies for the transition to independent living and vocational training; demonstration models for the provision of services; demographic studies that provide information on the individuals who will receive services; research on the development of exemplary models; or development of evaluative procedures, curriculum development, and physical education and recreation therapy for the targeted population. This section of the law mandates that both students with disabilities and their parents participate in these projects.

GRANTS FOR PERSONNEL TRAINING

PL 99-457 makes available grants to institutions for the training of personnel who will work with children with disabilities, including those in the fields of special education, speech and language pathology, adaptive physical education, and related services to infants and preschool-aged children in educational settings, including physical therapy. Grants are to be made with projected shortages of personnel in mind. Grants to institutions may be made for the purpose of training in new approaches and technologies as well as for the preparation of staff to work with the these children. Grants may also be used to train parents to work with professionals to enable them to participate more effectively in obtaining educational services for their children. Agencies applying for grants must address the needs of families of children with disabilities and must include parents as well as professionals on their committees.

GRANTS FOR TRAINEESHIPS

Support is provided for projects that encourage students to seek careers and employment in the various fields that relate to education of children and adolescents with disabilities. Projects may address the collection of data that will help determine the current and projected needs for special education and related services personnel, the dissemination of information to high school counselors regarding these professions, and the available sources of financial assistance. Emphasis is also placed on the establishment of a network among higher educational institutions to address supply and demand issues.

This section of PL 99-457 provides some practical strategies for addressing personnel shortages; however, the results of efforts are not likely to be experienced for at least 4 to 6 years after their implementation. The limited number of existing programs to train physical therapists also affects the ability of such strategies to increase the number of physical therapists available to work in early intervention settings.

RESEARCH AND DEMONSTRATION PROJECTS IN EDUCATION

This section of the law provides financial assistance to agencies and educational institutions in supporting special education and related services personnel in research that improves special education services available to targeted populations and that increases the related knowledge base. An emphasis is placed on research that assists in the development of improved techniques, devices, and curricula; facilitates the application of new technology; and develops models for the delivery of early intervention services. Also included is support for the dissemination of knowledge and the development of instruments, including tests and scales.

PANELS AND EXPERTS

The law provides support for the creation of panels of experts whose purpose is the critical evaluation of submitted proposals and projects. Panels are to be composed of experts in the areas of special education and relevant disciplines as well as individuals with disabilities and parents of children with disabling conditions. The emphasis on a panel composed of laypersons as well as professionals is consistent with other sections of PL 99-457, the objectives of which are to facilitate cooperative relationships among parents, individuals with disabilities, and professionals.

TECHNOLOGY, EDUCATIONAL MEDIA, AND MATERIALS

Support to higher educational institutions is made in the form of grants and contracts for the purpose of advancing the use of technology and media for the education of students with disabilities and the provision of early intervention services. Funded projects are to facilitate the effective use of media with targeted populations, the development and marketing of new materials, and the dissemination of information related to media and technology. Assistive technology is discussed in Chapter 23.

QUALIFIED PERSONNEL

The establishment and maintenance of standards for personnel to work in early intervention programs is supported by this section of PL 99-457. Established standards are to be consistent with state requirements for licensure, certification, or registration. Determination of the highest educational requirements for each profession is to be made. This section may affect the practice of pediatric physical therapy since each state determines the educational level required for work with the infant and toddler population. For example, one state may elect to require a bachelor's degree for practice, and another may require a master's degree. Although it is unlikely that a graduate degree will be required during a time of severe personnel shortage, the re-

quirement of a master's degree may be one possible interpretation of the law.

EVALUATION

Support for program evaluations in early intervention as well as projects to determine the efficacy of early intervention services is found in the last section of PL 99-457, which was enacted in 1986. Outcome variables are not, however, related to functional or qualitative changes in children receiving services, nor are they related to families' perception of the effectiveness of early intervention. Change, according to this section, is to be determined based on descriptive data, including the number of children receiving services, the number of children moving to regular education classrooms, and the number of special education and related service personnel required to staff programs. Funds expended for early intervention services are to be considered as well as funding for studies that include outcome variables. At least one longitudinal study to determine educational and occupational outcome for students receiving early intervention services is to be conducted. The outcome of intervention with children and families from ethnic minority groups is to be an objective of evaluative studies.

Recent Amendments

Amendments to PL 99-457 made in October 1990 include updates, results of program evaluations, and appropriations for funding after 1989. The rapidly changing population of the United States with respect to ethnic minorities and their expected impact on the special education population is addressed. Recommendations in this area include recruitment of more staff members from ethnic minority groups and attempts to increase the number of individuals from ethnic minority groups who participate in grant competitions. The needs of children with limited proficiency in English are also addressed.

PL 99-457 was again amended in October of 1991. One of the main emphases of this amendment was to update the text of the law related to use of people-first language of recipients of benefits. These changes were also applied to related previously enacted laws.

Funding increases are outlined, including specific instructions concerning funding for Native American infants and children living on reservations. The application of a tracking system as well as the development of an advisory board composed of persons providing services to this population, parents, and tribal organization representatives is detailed. This amendment also extends services to infants and their families who are part of the military system.

An emphasis on including infants at risk for disability in programs is stated. Outreach programs for low-income groups, ethnic minority groups, and those in rural settings are articulated. Facilitating the inclusion of infants and toddlers with disabilities in programs with a majority of infants who do not have disabilities is included.

The designation of funding for tracking and referral systems for infants and toddlers at risk as well as for personnel training is also outlined in this amendment. The development of a formula for the determination of future funding levels is considered.

At the time of this writing, 23 states and U.S. territories have fully implemented PL 99-457 and are providing multidisciplinary services to infants and their families. Seventeen additional states have applied for full application. Twelve states are using grant extensions to prepare further for applications for full implementation.

States have the option to decide not to fully implement PL 99-457, even after receiving funding for 5 or more years of preparations. States that decide not to fully implement the law are ineligible for further federal funding and are not obligated to provide services to all eligible infants and families.

For states that developed their own early intervention programs before passage of PL 99-457, a decision not to fully implement the program may not necessarily limit the resources available to families. If states with limited resources before passage of PL 99-457 decide not to fully implement the law, infants and families may find themselves with few or no resources at all. Which of the remaining states decide to implement the law should be determined by the mid-1990s.

TITLE II AMENDMENTS

Ethnic Minority Groups

The needs of Native American children receiving special education services are considered in the 1990 amendments, exemplifying a shift toward consideration of the particular needs of children of ethnic minority groups. A mandate for a plan that describes service provision for this population was made. The preparation of adequate personnel who are themselves members of ethnic minority groups is also addressed in the amendments. The gathering of data that describe the adequacy of the personnel pool in 1990–1991 will address personnel needs in general as well as provide an estimate of the number of persons from ethnic minority groups involved in early intervention and special education.

Evaluation

The evaluation of program effectiveness continues to be a priority. The number of children leaving special education to move into regular education programs continues to be considered an important outcome variable. New priorities related to developing program evaluation procedures include 1) criteria and procedures for the assessment of children from ethnic minority groups, 2) a system of personnel recruitment, 3) practices that allow the inclusion of children with disabilities in educational settings, 4) effective allocation and use of human and fiscal resources, 5) interagency coordination to manage the distribution of resources, and 6) strengthened communication between parents and school. These priorities reflect a move toward the conservation of resources, both human and fiscal. An emphasis continues to be placed on longitudinal studies involving students who have participated in early intervention to determine its effectiveness.

TITLE III—DISCRETIONARY PROGRAMS

Amendments to PL 99-457 in this section include priorities for training agencies and institutions in submitting applications for grants, contracts, and cooperative agreements and priorities for providing technical assistance to children from ethnic minority backgrounds and for providing assistance to state educational agencies through regional resource centers. Provisions for services to children who are deaf and blind are also given. The development, improvement, and demonstration of new and existing methods for use with this population is an objective of this section.

An emphasis is placed on providing technical assistance to programs that seek to include children with disabilities. Support is also to be given to extended school year programs. A continued funding objective is for programs that facilitate the transition from secondary school to vocational programs. The establishment of working relationships between the private sector (employers) and families of students is emphasized as a possible strategy for preparing students with disabilities for employment.

TITLE IV—MISCELLANEOUS

Title IV of PL 99-457 is concerned with the training of personnel who will be involved in the education of disabled individuals. Support is to be made available to institutions of higher learning that train personnel to work with infants and young children and their families and is particularly to be directed at training members of ethnic minority groups. Supervisory boards of demonstration projects are to include parents and professionals who are members of ethnic minority groups. Continuing support is made for clearinghouses and for their role as sources of information for professionals working with the targeted populations.

Priorities for research determined by this amendment include projects related to the synthesis and interpretation of current knowledge related to the infant and toddler population and to increasing the knowledge base. Projects related to knowledge and skills required to work with the targeted population, efficacy of current strategies, improvement of curricula, and development of new measurement instruments are priorities. Increasing the knowledge base regarding minority families and those with limited English language skills is emphasized.

Pediatric physical therapists working in the field of early intervention are likely to be affected by the 1990 amendments, particularly those related to the new and revised research priorities. Both measurement and efficacy research, areas that have been the focus of pediatric physical therapy research, continue to be supported by the amendments. Another area of impact is the new emphasis placed on providing effective and appropriate services to children and families who are from different ethnic backgrounds. As a result of the priorities, physical therapists may begin to seek additional training in working with families and children from varied cultural and linguistic backgrounds. Projects that address the determination of the special needs of children and families from different ethnic groups will be supported, as will those that prepare early intervention personnel to be more effective in their work with these families.

Impact of PL 99-457 on Pediatric Physical Therapy Practice

PL 99-457 is likely to have wide-ranging effects on the practice of physical therapy with infants, young children, and their families. Possibly the greatest impact will be on the focus of services. The emphasis of early intervention services is on the family, in contrast to the previous model, in which the child was the focus of services, with the family considered only as a support system for the child. In accordance with PL 99-457, the needs of the child in the context of the family are a primary consideration in the development of goals and in treatment planning.

The primary role of parents and families is also evident in established priorities and requirements related to research, expert panels, and special projects. Research projects related to efficiency and efficacy of early intervention services must address family as well as child outcomes. Projects overseen by a supervisory board must include parents, individuals with disabilities, or both. In this way, parents have the opportunity to provide feedback that influences the direction of projects and research to better address their own perceived needs and concerns.

The focus of early intervention services as defined by PL 99-457 encourages pediatric physical therapists to develop new models for the conceptualization of their working relationship with families and will likely affect treatment and research models as well. The recent emphasis on effective intervention with families and children from varied cultural and linguistic backgrounds other than English will also influence the context of the practice of physical therapy with children. Changes in the context in which pediatric physical therapists practice with infants and toddlers related to PL 99-457 are notable at the present time and are likely to continue to evolve in the future.

CASE HISTORIES

In this section, three case histories involving legal issues related to PL 99-457 are presented. These cases include situations in which pediatric physical therapists may be involved in advocacy on behalf of families of infants and toddlers with special needs. Each case is presented with subsequent comments by an attorney.

CASE HISTORY: ASHLEY

Mrs. Gee requested an evaluation for her 6-month-old daughter Ashley to determine whether she might be eligible for early intervention services. Ashley, who was the product of a 24-week gestational pregnancy, experienced multiple neonatal complications including a grade III–IV intracranial hemorrhage, severe bronchopulmonary dysplasia, and retinopathy of prematurity. She was hospitalized for the first 4 months of her life, and as a result the family incurred substantial medical expenses. Ashley's father was laid off from work, and the medical bills were a source of considerable stress for the family. Mrs. Gee sought the early intervention services, in part because she would not have to incur further medical bills.

Mrs. Gee was interviewed by the early intervention team coordinator, and then Ashley was evaluated by a physical therapist and a special education teacher. Because Ashley did not perform at a level 2 standard deviations below the mean for her age on assessments of motor and cognitive performance, the team recommended no intervention at that time. Mrs. Gee continued to have concerns regarding Ashley's development and wondered if she could request a reconsideration of Ashley's case.

Response

Related to this case, PL 99-457 requires the development of an IFSP. The law requires the family plan to include a multidisciplinary assessment of the unique strengths and needs of the child. From the multidisciplinary assessment, appropriate services are to be identified and made available. The assessments performed by the physical therapist and special education teacher may be considered to have fulfilled this requirement. The conclusion, however, that Ashley would not be eligible for services based solely on the results of her performance on standardized measures of cognitive and motor development may not have been completely correct.

According to PL 99-457, one of the criteria under which an infant may be considered for services is the presence of a medical condition or diagnosis that places an infant at risk for developmental problems. Ashley's medical history of delivery at 24 weeks' gestational age, with neonatal complications including a grade III–IV intraventricular hemorrhage, places her at great risk for cognitive and motor developmental problems. Although Ashley does not yet demonstrate frank motor or cognitive deficits on standardized tests, her medical history should make her eligible for early intervention services.

The law states, however, that the child's needs are not the only criterion taken into consideration when developing the IFSP. The law requires that the parents be allowed to direct the assessment of resources. The parents act to determine the priorities, and their concerns must be considered in the development of this plan. The assessment team must identify the support needed as well as the resources available to enhance the parents' capacity to meet the developmental needs of their child.

In this case, the key area related to the IFSP is the requirement that the resources of the family must be considered in the development of the plan. In the Gees' case, Mrs. Gee's concern regarding her child's

development, the hospital bills, and lack of family income must be taken into consideration. The team must consider the family's overall capacity to meet the needs of this child.

CASE HISTORY: RYAN

The Johnson family had received early intervention services for their son Ryan for the previous 8 months through the special education department of their neighborhood school. Ryan, a 20-month-old child with a diagnosis of spastic diplegic cerebral palsy, had received occupational therapy and cognitive training since his initial enrollment in the program. When Ryan began pulling to stand, his family requested services from the team physical therapist to help with preambulation activities.

The staff at the early intervention program listened to the Johnsons' requests but refused to alter Ryan's program of occupational therapy and cognitive training. The Johnsons wanted to pursue the matter formally but hesitated to do so because of their fear that the services Ryan was receiving might be compromised.

Response

The federal courts have heard cases similar to the Johnson case. The courts have decided that parents do not have the right under the Education of All Handicapped Children Act (PL 94-142) to compel a school district to provide specific programs or employ a specific methodology in providing education for their child who has a disability.

The courts have also held that if there is a rigid rule under which special education officials refuse even to consider providing physical therapy, there may exist a conflict with the child's procedural right to an individualized educational program (Hampton & Newberger, 1985). If a rigid rule is involved, the Johnsons may have a chance at a favorable change in their son's program.

The Johnsons may request that their child be reassessed but cannot compel the school system to provide physical therapy. If, however, the Johnsons discover that the school system is not providing physical therapy for any of their early intervention students, then there may be a course of action. Regardless of the outcome, the Johnsons are protected from any alteration or interruption of their existing program as a response to their request for re-evaluation and from any challenge of their son's program.

CASE HISTORY: JOSÉ

The Sanchez family immigrated to the United States several years ago. Initially, they lived in a community with a large number of other Mexican immigrant families. In their community, they were able to socialize and conduct business in Spanish with other individuals who shared similar experiences. Recently, the family relocated to a small community several hours away where Mr. Sanchez had been offered a better job. Although the family enjoyed the benefits of a better paying job in their new community, they felt isolated in their neighborhood, which included few Spanish-speaking families.

When Mrs. Sanchez suspected a motor problem in her youngest child, José, she went to the local Early Intervention Program for help. Although Mrs. Sanchez's English skills were limited, she was able to communicate with the program coordinator sufficiently to arrange an evaluation for José. After the evaluation, the program coordinator met with Mrs. Sanchez to schedule an IFSP meeting. Mrs. Sanchez related that she could communicate in English well enough to participate in the meeting, but she believed that her husband, his sister, and her mother would need an interpreter. The program coordinator had not had such a request in the past and wondered whether, since Mrs. Sanchez had some English fluency, an interpreter were really necessary.

Response

In drafting PL 99-457, Congress took into account the fact that the population for whom English is not the primary language is the fastest growing group in the country. In certain areas, students with limited proficiency in English make up almost half of all students entering kindergarten. Congress found that there has been a discrepancy in the level of referral and placement of children with limited proficiency in English in special education. The U.S. Department of Education has found that services provided to students with limited English proficiency often fail to respond primarily to the child's academic needs. Congress recognized that these trends pose special challenges for special education in the referral, assessment, and services for these students.

Under 20 USCS §1412 (5)(C), the state is required to use testing materials and procedures that are not socially or culturally discriminatory. The materials and procedures must be administered in the child's native language or mode of communication whenever it is possible. In the case of José, the state must provide an interpreter to explain the test and procedures.

PL 101-476 also supports work that facilitates the provision of services that are effective for families of various cultures. For a family of the Sanchezs' cultural background, the extended family is as essential to family functioning as is the nuclear family in other cases; efforts may, therefore, be made to support the extended family structure, including an interpreter for the IFSP meeting.

AMERICANS WITH DISABILITIES ACT OF 1990 (PL 101-336)

Although the Americans with Disabilities Act is frequently considered to be most closely related to employment and public access for individuals with disabilities, sections of the law are particularly relevant to families of children with disabilities. The purpose of this section is to summarize sections of this law that are useful to pediatric physical therapists in their role as advocates for families of children with disabilities. Illustrative case examples are included.

Employment

The Americans with Disabilities Act prevents an employer from denying an employment opportunity or benefit because of an individual's association with a person who has a disability. The law protects a parent from being denied a job because she or he has a child with a disability. An employer cannot assume that because of the disabled child's needs, the parent may be unavailable or unreliable with respect to job requirements.

The law also prohibits discrimination related to health insurance benefits that are offered as a fringe benefit of employment. An employer cannot deny a job or refuse to hire a parent of a child with a disability because the employer anticipates an increase in insurance costs because of the nature of the child's disability, nor can an employer subject an employee who has a child with a disability to different terms or conditions of insurance. Although the parent of a child with a disability is protected from discrimination in the areas of hiring and insurance, the employer is not obligated to modify work schedules to facilitate child care.

The Americans with Disabilities Act also protects parents from discrimination related to association with other individuals with disabilities or to working with organizations associated with persons with disabilities. For example, a parent who does volunteer work for a service organization for acquired immunodeficiency syndrome cannot be discriminated against in employment opportunities or in benefits of employment such as health insurance.

Enforcement Provisions

Parents who believe that they have been discriminated against related to hiring or insurance can file a charge with the Equal Employment Opportunity Commission (EEOC). Parents may also file a charge if they believe that retaliation has occurred as a result of filing a charge or opposing a discriminatory practice.

The EEOC investigates charges of discrimination. If the EEOC believes that discrimination has occurred, an attempt at resolution will be made. If conciliation fails, the EEOC will file suit or issue a "right to sue" letter to the person who filed the charge. Remedies for violations of the Americans with Disabilities Act related to employment include hiring, reinstatement, promotion, the payment of back pay and front pay, and restoration of benefits, including health insurance.

Charges of discrimination by employers of more than 25 persons occurring on or after July 26, 1992, may be filed as of that date. For employers of fewer than 15 persons, charges of discrimination occurring on or after July 26, 1994, may be filed beginning July 26, 1994. Charges of discrimination must be filed with the EEOC within 180 days of the alleged discriminatory act.

Transportation

The Americans with Disabilities Act protects individuals with disabilities from discrimination with respect to participation in any public services, programs, or activities. Public transportation, including buses and rapid rail systems, is included under the rubric of "public services." According to the law, new buses and rail cars purchased after July 26, 1990 as well as stations constructed after this date must be accessible to individuals with disabilities who may require wheelchairs or other assistive devices for mobility or who may have a visual impairment.

Public transportation services for individuals with disabilities must be available on a schedule that is comparable to that provided for persons without a disability. Available transportation may include transportation that is accessible to a person who does or does not require a wheelchair lift for transportation. The law provides for assistance with transportation to regular public transportation stops for those who are unable to reach these stops without assistance. The law also provides for transportation of an accompanying assistant for the individual with a disability as long as the assistant's seat is not needed for another person with a disability.

Parents of children with disabilities who live in areas served by public transportation should expect increased availability of accessible transportation services. Bus service, for example, should be available on the same schedule as service for persons without a disability. Public transportation service may also become available at a family's residence, should a child be unable to get to a regular transportation stop independently. On intercity and commuter rail systems, at least one rail car per train must be accessible to individuals with disabilities.

Physical Structures

The Americans with Disabilities Act also protects individuals with disabilities from discrimination related to limited access to public accommodations. Public accommodations may include hotels, restaurants, food and retail stores, and shopping malls. Recreational facilities, such as amusement parks, zoos, and museums, are also included. Educational facilities, such as nurseries, elementary or secondary schools, and public and private undergraduate and graduate colleges and universities, must also be accessible. Such public accommodations were to be made accessible as of January 1, 1992.

Families of children with disabilities may expect greater access to structures in their communities related to education, shopping, and recreation. Greater access for persons who require assistance or devices for mobility should facilitate the integration of these individuals into all areas of the community.

CASE HISTORY: ANNA

Ms. Jones is the single parent of a child, Anna, who has Down syndrome. Ms. Jones is a licensed ultrasound technologist and worked until the birth of her daughter. She planned to return to work 3 months after her daughter's birth; however, because of the medical complications Anna experienced, Ms. Jones decided to remain at home, forfeiting her past position. By the time Anna was 8 months old, she was doing well medically, and Ms. Jones applied for a job with a small, private company that contracted out ultrasonography services to local hospitals and physicians' offices.

During the employment interview, the personnel director commented favorably on Ms. Jones' excellent work record and references from her past employer. He inquired regarding the reason that Ms. Jones decided not to return to her old position. When Ms. Jones related the circumstances of her daughter's birth and disability, the tone of the interview changed. The personnel director questioned Ms. Jones regarding her ability to meet her daughter's medical needs and the demands of a full-time job and interjected his personal experience with a family in his neighborhood who had a child with a disability. In that family, the mother's decision to remain at home was considered a necessity.

Ms. Jones believed when she left the interview that she would probably not be offered the job. Her suspicion was confirmed when she received a letter stating that the job was offered to another qualified applicant. Ms. Jones was puzzled when the company continued to advertise the position. She contacted the personnel director again and was able to convince him of her ability to handle both the job and the care of her daughter. After considerable negotiation, she was offered the position under the stipulation that she accept a lower amount of health insurance coverage than the company's other employees and pay a slightly higher rate. Ms. Jones questioned the personnel manager's right to make such an offer and wondered if she should seek the opinion of an employment rights specialist.

Response

Ms. Jones should seek the opinion of an employment rights specialist. Under the employment component of the Americans with Disabilities Act, the actions of this employer are illegal. In a hiring situation, it is illegal even to consider a dependent who has a disability. This act attempts to level the playing field for parents of children with disabilities. Questions as to the health of dependent children are not related to the job and, therefore, are prohibited under this act.

Second, Ms. Jones is entitled to exactly the same benefits as the company's other employees. It is illegal under this act to require Ms. Jones to contribute more for health insurance or to provide her with less coverage. The employer cannot pass the extra cost of the insurance on to the parent.

CHILD ABUSE AND NEGLECT

The subject of child abuse and neglect is discussed more openly and freely at the present time than in the past. A possibly related phenomenon is the increase in the number of reported cases of child abuse (De Jong et al., 1983; Hampton & Newberger, 1985). Because pediatric physical therapists may be involved in the treatment of children who are at risk for or have experienced child abuse or neglect, a review of the signs of abuse as well as the physical therapist's responsibility with respect to reporting suspected abuse is provided in the following section.

Neglect

Child abuse and neglect are defined by the Child Abuse Prevention and Treatment Act of 1974 (PL 93-247) as "the physical or mental injury, sexual abuse, negligent treatment or maltreatment of a child under the age of eighteen by a person who is responsible for the child's welfare under circumstances which indicate that the child's health and welfare are harmed or threatened hereby" (PL 93-247, p. 247). Child abuse and neglect may occur in various forms, including, but not limited to, severe physical injury that may be fatal or life threatening.

Child neglect occurs when a child's basic needs are not being met by an adult who is responsible. Neglectful situations may involve inadequate or unstable shelter or inadequate or inappropriate nutrition. Neglect may also occur related to lack of needed medical or dental care. Concerning medical neglect, the pediatric physical therapist may be the member of the health care team who observes and documents a pattern of missed appointments or noncompliance with instructions that results in a deterioration in the child's status. In such a situation, the physical therapist is responsible for reporting the suspected neglect to the proper authorities.

A difficulty in the determination of neglect is related to willfulness. Neglect need not be a willful act on the part of the adult responsible (Newberger et al., 1987). Neglect may be related to a parent's inability to meet a child's needs because of extreme environmental stresses or may be related to a parent's limited knowledge base concerning appropriate stimulation and behavior management for children.

Neglect that is not willful may be distressing to report from the physical therapist's perspective. Filing a report may be associated with blaming the parents for the child's situation. An important consideration in a case of nonwillful neglect is the ultimate effect on the child: If the child is not thriving because nutritional, medical, or other physical or emotional needs are not being met, intervention is needed. Examples of situations in which neglect may be present are listed in Table 33–1.

TABLE 33–1. **SIGNS AND SITUATIONS ASSOCIATED WITH CHILD NEGLECT**

Evidence of poor nutrition
  Reports of hunger
  Nutritionally inadequate diet
Evidence of poor hygiene
  Soiled clothing
  Soiled skin, body odors
  Skin breakdown in diaper area
  Dental caries
Lack of compliance with medical or therapy appointments
  Excessive cancellations
  Frequent "no shows"
  Lack of follow-through with home program instructions
    resulting in a decline in the child's status

Physical Abuse

The constellation of symptoms associated with physical child abuse have been collectively named the battered child syndrome (Kempe et al., 1962). The associated physical injuries may be detected by a child's pediatrician, an emergency department physician, or school nurse. The physical manifestations include injury to bone and soft tissue as well as affective changes. Signs and symptoms associated with the battered child syndrome are listed in Table 33–2.

Because a child's clothing is routinely removed during physical therapy sessions, signs of physical abuse may be more readily and naturally observed during treatment than in other settings, such as the school classroom. When symptoms are observed, the suspected abuse must be reported to the proper authorities. The fact that symptoms commonly associated with abuse may also be related to other medical conditions or common childhood accidents deserves careful consideration. A differential diagnosis can be made only by a physician. Questionable symptoms require further investigation by a physician.

Sexual Abuse

The signs of sexual abuse that may be observed by the pediatric physical therapist are likely to be manifested behaviorally. Psychosomatic or behavioral illnesses, behavioral alterations, and acting-out behaviors may accompany sexual child abuse (Gommes-Schwartz et al., 1985). Somatization, or the expression of emotional conflicts as symptoms of physical illness, frequently occurs in association with sexual child abuse (Rosenfeld, 1982; Rosenfeld & Sarles, 1987). The occurrence of behavioral disorders such as anorexia nervosa or bulimia and enuresis or encopresis may signal sexual abuse. Abdominal pain without an organic cause is an example of psychosomatic problems that may be associated with sexual abuse. Behavioral changes such as an alteration in school performance, atypical shyness, and extroverted or hostile behavior may be associated with sexual abuse (Rosenfeld, 1982; Rosenfeld & Sarles, 1987).

Psychosomatic and behavioral problems, however, may be associated with problems other than sexual abuse, and such symptoms and signs require further evaluation by a professional such as a medical social worker, psychologist, or physician. Sexual acting-out behavior, sexual aggression toward other children, or an overly sophisticated knowledge of sexual activities and practice are salient signs of sexual abuse.

Child sexual abuse accommodation syndrome (Summitt, 1982) describes the behaviors associated with a child's attempt to adapt to sexual abuse that occurs over time. As a young child attempts to cope with feelings of disbelief, rejection, helplessness, and self-blame associated with victimization by sexual abuse, long-lasting behavioral changes may be noted. Secrecy; helplessness; entrapment and accommodation; delayed, conflicted, and unconvincing disclosure of incidents; and retraction of reported abuse are all behaviors associated with child sexual abuse accommodation syndrome.

A pediatric physical therapist who observes a child behaving in a manner that may be associated with ongoing sexual abuse should give such behavior careful consideration. Secrecy regarding relationships with certain adults or conflicting reports about incidents that are suspicious may be indicators of a child's victimization by sexual abuse. A pediatric physical therapist who suspects sexual abuse may work together with a social worker, psychologist, or physician to further evaluate the child's situation and make necessary reports to the appropriate authorities.

Legal Obligation to Report

A review of state laws in various geographic regions of the United States reveals that health care professionals, including physical therapists, are unequivocally required to immediately report suspected child abuse to the proper agency (III Illinois Annotated Statutes; Official Code of Georgia, Annotated). Each state or county has established a protocol for the reporting of suspected abuse. Protocols describe the routing of reports of abuse, the consideration of factors in the determination of the child's risk status, and a plan for removal from the home, if necessary (California Penal Code). Protocols are available for examination through county departments of family and children's services and agencies such as state councils on child abuse.

Failure to report suspected child abuse is a misdemeanor in most states. Associated penalties in-

TABLE 33–2. **SIGNS AND SYMPTOMS OF PHYSICAL ABUSE: BATTERED CHILD SYNDROME**

Bony fractures
Soft tissue injuries
Burns
Hematomas
Welts
Internal injuries
Contusions

clude monetary fines, imprisonment, or both. Failure to report suspected abuse may also result in the revocation or suspension of a professional license or the denial of licensure renewal.

Many state statutes protect an individual who reports suspected abuse from civil action related to a lack of substantiation of the report (Official Code of Georgia, Annotated). Such a statute frees the individual making the report from undue concern over retaliation on the part of the accused party should the report be unconfirmed. Alternately, state statutes also address the situation in which individuals knowingly make false reports of abuse (23 Illinois Annotated Statutes). A consideration of the repercussions for failure to report suspected abuse reflects the seriousness of this crime and its effect on children.

Physical therapists, as well as other professionals involved in the care of children, must be aware of their legal obligations with respect to child abuse and neglect. Because of the frequent contact of pediatric physical therapists with children over time, therapists are in a position to note physical and behavioral changes. Together with other health care team members, such as social workers and psychologists, pediatric physical therapists can help protect children from abusive environments.

The following case example taken from the experience of one of the authors (WP) is presented as an illustration of issues related to the reporting of suspected child abuse by health care professionals in general and pediatric physical therapists specifically.

CASE HISTORY: JERRY

Amy, a pediatric physical therapist working in an early intervention program, makes routine home visits to infants and their families. A considerable proportion of Amy's caseload is with indigent families. One of Amy's patients is Jerry, an 18-month-old infant with spina bifida. Jerry's defect is extensive and at the upper thoracic level of his spine. Jerry demonstrates some functional use of his upper extremities but no volitional movement in his lower extremities.

Jerry lives with his parents, Mr. and Mrs. Smith, and two older siblings. Mrs. Smith was in junior high school when her eldest child was born. She is now 18 years old. Mrs. Smith has attempted to complete her high school education, but her course work has been interrupted by Jerry's frequent hospitalizations. In a conversation with Amy, Mrs. Smith related that she does not receive much support from Mr. Smith, who believes that Jerry will somehow eventually recover from his disability. She also told Amy about Mr. Smith's history

of substance abuse and her own history of having been abused during her childhood. At the present time, Mrs. Smith appears listless, and Amy believes that Mrs. Smith is depressed.

On her visits to Jerry's house, Amy has been concerned about Jerry's care. He has not usually been bathed and dressed by the time she visits at 1 o'clock in the afternoon. His diaper is usually wet, and his pajamas smell of urine. He often acts hungry and weak. Mrs. Smith frequently reports that she has fed Jerry "a few bites from her own plate," but not a full meal of his own.

One occasion when Amy worked with Jerry in his own bedroom, she noticed that one of the railings of his crib was missing, leaving an open space. Amy was also concerned because on one of her visit days, she had met Mrs. Smith walking home from the store and Mrs. Smith reported that Jerry was not at home and said that Amy should not come in. Amy believed that she had heard Jerry's voice inside the home.

During Amy's most recent visit to Jerry's home, she discovered a small decubitus ulcer forming in the sacral region of Jerry's spine. Amy was concerned about Jerry's health and safety but at the same time did not want to blame Mrs. Smith. Amy believed that Mrs. Smith was probably doing the best she could, considering her depression, her lack of resources, and lack of support from Jerry's father. Amy decided that she needed to try to determine her responsibility in informing an outside agency about her concerns for Jerry's welfare.

Response

The state laws usually require that all cases of suspected abuse and neglect be reported immediately to the proper authorities. The key word here is "suspected" abuse and neglect. The law does not require a case of neglect to be proven before it is reported. It requires that any information that would tend to indicate that a child is abused or neglected be reported.

It is important that the physical therapist document specific findings and report a case to the authorities. Many states make failure to report a case of suspected abuse or neglect a misdemeanor punishable by up to 12 months in jail.

LITIGATION

Although litigation is an area in which pediatric physical therapists may not wish to be involved, issues related to medical malpractice are permeating all areas of the health care system. Medically related lawsuits are increasing rapidly in our society. Pediatric physical therapists need to be aware of the process of litigation and of how they may willingly or unwillingly be involved. In this section issues relevant to litigation are presented from an attorney's perspective to make the pediatric physical therapist aware of how components of practice, such as medical documentation, fit in the scheme of medically related litigation.

O'Sullivan (1975) has outlined the process of review of the medical record in preparation for the presentation of a medical malpractice case in court. Consistency in chart records is considered to be a primary point of evaluation of a medical record. A medical record should, according to O'Sullivan, be straightforward and flow smoothly from beginning to end. Chart records should be consistent, and inconsistencies in charting are "red flags" for further scrutiny by the attorney involved. Among noted inconsistencies are therapeutic inconsistencies between diagnoses and selected therapy or intervention and chronologic inconsistencies between objective data and resultant changes in intervention. Improper use of forms and improper reporting of information or incidents to authorities are also examples of inconsistencies. Even the smallest of inconsistencies is considered relevant, particularly to the attorney whose client alleges hospital liability or negligence on the part of the health care provider.

Progress notes should contain the recorded significant progress of the patient. Notes are expected to include changes in symptoms, complaints, objective signs, and the results of tests that contribute to the understanding of the diagnosed condition. When progress notes are complete, "there is no reason to evaluate other records" (O'Sullivan, 1975, p. 125).

Documentation serves as the interface between the physical therapist and the attorney in legal cases. Clear, objective, and accurate documentation is an essential component of quality treatment, regardless of whether it is ever evaluated by an attorney or outside party. However, in the event that records are subpoenaed, organized, clear, and objective records will serve both to protect the pediatric physical therapist from liability and to provide an accurate account of the status and progress of the patient.

When a record may be evaluated by an outside party who is not an expert in the characteristics and usual physical therapy treatment of a child, documentation such as progress notes or evaluations should be written in terms that are understandable and meaningful, even for individuals who are not physical therapists or who have not received training in a particular treatment approach or theoretic orientation.

Documentation of progress by a method that is meaningful to outsiders also poses a challenge for pediatric physical therapists. The use of norm-referenced, standardized measures may provide data concerning a child's motor performance in comparison with peers that is easily understood by others. The description of a child's motor performance on a standard measure may be useful for purposes of assessment as well as for documentation of change.

▌MEDICAL TECHNOLOGY

Another potential interface between pediatric physical therapists and the legal system involves children who are dependent on medical technology for survival. As medical technology has become more sophisticated, the ability to support children whose illnesses or injuries would, in other times, have been fatal has increased. (The reader is referred to Chapter 24 for more information.)

The point at which the continuation of technologic life support compromises the quality of a child's life is not easily determined. Because individual physicians, health care professionals, and families differ in their beliefs about issues related to quality of life and preservation of life, differences of opinion regarding the extent to which technologic life-support measures should be employed have occurred. At times, disagreements between parents and physicians and other members of the health care team, such as nurses and social workers, have been so extreme that decisions regarding the appropriateness of medical interventions have been made by the court system (National Center for State Courts, 1991).

One of the considerations in the determination of whether technologic life support should continue for a particular child may be the child's prognosis with respect to the expected future level of functioning. Although physicians have formulated prognoses for children in court cases in the past, it is not unlikely that the pediatric physical therapist may be asked to contribute a clinical opinion regarding a child's developmental outcome. The following case provides an example of a physical therapist's involvement in a health care team decision regarding the continuation of technologic life support for an infant. Although this particular case was not decided in court, it is representative of the type of situation in which pediatric physical therapists may increasingly be involved.

CASE HISTORY: KENNY

Kenny is an infant delivered at 23 to 24 weeks' gestational age at a birth weight of 770 g. Kenny's mother is a single parent who received no prenatal care. His father was involved in an emotional relationship with his mother; however, their relationship was physically abusive. One other child of Kenny's mother had been removed from the home by the Department of Family and Children's Services.

Kenny experienced multiple neonatal complications including necrotizing enterocolitis, severe bronchopulmonary dysplasia, and several unsuccessful attempts to permanently wean him from ventilator support. Kenny's other medical complications include metabolic bone disease, intrahepatic cholestasis, and multiple bouts of sepsis. He also experienced a grade III intraventricular hemorrhage. His head circumference is significantly less than would be expected for his age and other anthropometric measurements, probably as a result of cerebral atrophy.

At 10 months chronologic age, Kenny's physical therapist, Sharon, estimated Kenny's level of motor functioning to be at 1 month. At this time, he began to experience a slow deterioration of his cardiopulmonary system, including congestive heart failure. Related to the deterioration of his medical status, Sharon reported that it was difficult to follow through with physical therapy treatment plans and goals because the infant was frequently too ill to tolerate treatment. He was infrequently alert and did not demonstrate visual observation of faces or other interactional behavior. Available active movements were athetoid in quality. Just before a significant decline in his status, including the congestive heart failure, Kenny experienced a few days in which he was able to tolerate handling and treatment out of his crib on a mat.

Subsequently, Kenny experienced a decline in his status and was reintubated and ventilated. Kenny's primary physician, a pediatric intensive care specialist, and other members of Kenny's health care team began to consider the appropriateness of the repeated reintubations and ventilation and other technologic support measures. Kenny's mother frequently inquired about his prognosis and level of functioning and was willing to consider a deceleration in his care. Kenny's father, however, was not in agreement with such a plan.

Kenny's doctor approached Sharon with questions about Kenny's current level of motor functioning and his expected outcome in future years should the infant's medical condition become more stable. In light of this request, the therapist had to determine a strategy for the development of a clinical opinion regarding Kenny's present status and future level of functioning.

Response

In a situation such as Kenny's, the physical therapist, Sharon, could integrate information from a variety of sources in the formulation of her opinion. She could use her own clinical judgment, based on experience with other infants who had similar characteristic motor patterns and shared a similar medical history. Fortunately, Sharon had several years of pediatric experience with toddlers and older children in addition to her work in a neonatal intensive care unit. In this case, Kenny's lack of interactional behavior, severely delayed motor skills, and athetoid movements were considered in the formulation of Sharon's opinion.

Sharon also considered the results of outcome research studies on infants who experienced some of the same neonatal complications that Kenny experienced. In her review of outcome studies, Sharon found that grade III intracranial hemorrhage and cerebral atrophy were associated with poor neurodevelopmental outcomes. Based on assessment and observations, past experience with infants with motor performance similar to Kenny's, and a review of the literature concerning neurodevelopmental outcome, Sharon was able to formulate an opinion regarding Kenny's developmental prognosis. Sharon expected that Kenny would have significant motor impairment.

Because Kenny died before the issues related to technologic support were resolved, this case did not reach the court system. Nevertheless, Sharon's strategy for the formulation of an opinion could have been used in a legal case. Sharon's use of her past experience together with a review of the outcome literature helped her to formulate an opinion. Although not used in this instance, results of a norm-referenced standardized measure of motor development would also have been helpful.

Ethical Concerns

Although not a consideration in this case, the formulation of an opinion about Kenny might have presented an ethical dilemma for Sharon. For example, if Sharon's personal beliefs regarding the continuation or removal of technologic support for critically ill patients had not been congruent with that of the family and other members of the health care team, the formulation of an opinion might have been difficult. Health care professionals' personal beliefs regarding the sources of health improvement in their patients are as likely to contribute to the formulation of their clinical decisions as is past experience or a review of the literature.

In the development of their measurement tool the Child Health Improvement Locus of Control scales, Devellis and colleagues (1985) considered the relation between parental beliefs and behavior associated with their child's illness. The Child Improvement Locus of Control scales assess parental beliefs related to the source of control over a child's recovery and outcome. Devellis and colleagues (1985) found that factors related to the child, parents, and professionals, to chance, and to divine influence are also related to parents' beliefs regarding locus of control for health improvement in their children.

Research using the Child Health Improvement Locus

of Control scales demonstrated that parents may ascribe different amounts of responsibility for child health improvement to factors such as the child him- or herself, health care professionals, parents, chance, or divine influence as determinants of their child's recovery. For example, whereas one parent may believe that professionals are primarily responsible for their child's recovery, another may attribute recovery to divine intervention or to chance.

Health care professionals, like parents, may attribute health improvement in infants and children to various factors. Health care professionals' locus of control with respect to health improvement in children may influence their decision-making in cases such as the one previously described. For example, if Sharon had attributed health improvement to divine influence and another member of the health care team had attributed improvement to intervention by professionals, the formulation of Sharon's clinical opinion would have been influenced by factors related to her own belief system that were different from those of her colleague.

Although not often acknowledged, a pediatric physical therapist's own belief system may influence decision making or may be a source of personal stress when not congruent with that of other members of the health care team. Identification of the therapist's own beliefs with respect to locus of control for health improvement in children and of how beliefs may influence decision making increases the objectivity of clinical decision-making and the formation of opinions related to expected outcome for children.

References

California Penal Code, Section 11166 (G).

De Jong, AR, Hervada, AR, & Emmett, GA. Epidemiological variations in childhood sexual abuse. Child Abuse and Neglect, 7:155–162, 1983.

DeVellis, SR, DeVellis, SBM, Revcki, DA, Lurie, SJ, Runyan, DIC, & Bristol, M. Development and validation of the Child Health Improvement Locus of Control (CHILC) scales. Journal of Social and Clinical Psychology, 3:307–324, 1985.

Effgen, SK, Bjornson, K, Chiarello, L, Sinzer, L, & Phillips, W. Competencies for physical therapists in early intervention. Pediatric Physical Therapy 3:77–80, 1991.

Foster, M, & Phillips, W. Family systems theory as a framework for problem solving in pediatric physical therapy. Pediatric Physical Therapy, 4:70–73, 1992.

Gommes-Schwartz, B, Horowitz, JM, & Sauzier, M. Severity of emotional distress among sexually abused preschool, school aged and adolescent children. Hospital Community Psychiatry, 11:503–508, 1985.

Hampton, RH, & Newberger, EH. Child abuse incidence and reporting by hospitals: Significance of severity, class and race. American Journal of Public Health, 75:56–64, 1985.

23 Illinois Annotated Statutes. §2053, Section 4.

III Illinois Annotated Statutes. §4267-0.

Kempe, CH, Silverman, FW, Steele, BF, Droegemueller, W, & Silver, HK. The battered child syndrome. Journal of the American Medical Association, 181:17–24, 1962.

National Center for State Courts. Guidelines for state court decision making in authorizing or withholding life-sustaining medical treatment, vol. 18, No. 10. Williamsburg, VA: National Center for State Courts, 1991, pp. 253–275.

Newberger, EH, Hyde, JN, Jr, Holter, JC, & Rosenfeld, A. Child abuse and neglect. In Hoekelman, RA, Blatman, S, Friedman, SB, Nelson, NM, & Seidel, HM. (Eds.), Primary Pediatric Care. St. Louis, MO: CV Mosby, 1987, pp. 629–638.

Official Code of Georgia, Annotated. Title 19, Chapter 7. §5(2)F.

O'Sullivan, DD. Evaluation of the medical record. Medicine Trial Technique Quarterly. Chicago: Callaghan & Co., 1975.

Public Law. 93-247, Child Abuse Prevention and Treatment Act of 1974, 42 USCS §5101–5106.

Public Law 94-142, Education of All Handicapped Children Act (1975), 20 USCS §1400.

Public Law 99-457, Education of the Handicapped Act Amendments of 1986, 20 USCS §1400.

Public Law 101-336, Americans with Disabilities Act (1990), 42 USCS §12102.

Public Law 101-476, Individuals with Disabilities Education Amendments of 1990. 20 USCS §1400.

Public Law 102-119, Individuals with Disabilities Education Act Amendments of 1991, 105 Stat 587-608.

Rosenfeld, A. Sexual abuse of children: Personal and professional responses. In Newberger, E (Ed.), Child Abuse. Boston: Little, Brown & Co, 1982, pp. 57–74.

Rosenfeld, A, & Sarles, RM. Sexual misuse of children. In Hoekelman, RA, Blatman, S, Friedman, SB, Nelson, NM, & Seidel, HM. (Eds.), Primary Pediatric Care. St. Louis: CV Mosby Co, 1986, pp. 642–651.

Summit, RC. The child sexual abuse accommodation syndrome. Child Abuse and Neglect, 7:177–193, 1982.

Index

Note: Page numbers in *italics* refer to illustrations;
page numbers followed by (t) refer to tables.

Experience-expectant neural maturation, 14–15

Expiratory reserve volume (ERV), assessment of, in cystic fibrosis, 693

Extended school year (ESY), case law about, 851
eligibility for, 851

Extension, of elbow, standards for, by age, 139–140
of knees, standards for, by age, 140
of shoulders, standards for, by age, 140
of trunk, standards for, by age, 140

External load, definition of, 85

External tibial torsion, in cerebral palsy, 99–100, *100*
in myelomeningocele, 579, *580*

Extracorporeal membrane oxygenation (ECMO), after near-drowning, 567
after thoracic surgery, 747
in respiratory distress syndrome, in premature infants, 791–792

Extremity(ies), lower. See *Lower extremity(ies)*.
range of motion of, measurement of, 143, 144(t)
upper. See *Upper extremity(ies)*.

Eyes, sports injuries to, 396–397, 396(t), 397(t)

Facilitation model, 70

Fagan Test of Infant Intelligence (FTII), in mental retardation evaluation, 461

Family, contemporary, change in, *824*, 824–826, *826*
education of, about burns, 779
about cerebral palsy, 499
models of functioning, 824, 825, 826, *826*
role of, in cerebral palsy interventions, 507
in ventilator-dependent child care, 678
single-parent, 826–828, *827*
stressors on, 678, 826–832
cultural, 830–832
with dual-career parents, 828

Family Needs Survey, 838

Family Routines Inventory, 838

Family-centered intervention, 823–843, 856. See also *Parent(s)*.
caregiver competencies in, *833*, 833–834, *834*
case history of, 843
cultural considerations in, 830–832, 892, 902, 905
physical therapy competencies in, 833
prevention in, *842*, 842–843
process of, 678, 754, 834–842, *840*, 840(t), *841*
caregiver concern evaluation in, 304, 841
caretaker identification in, 835
caretaker-child involvement determination in, 835
child treatment in, 841
community assessment in, 838–839
community involvement evaluation in, 841–842

Family-centered intervention (*Continued*)
individualized family service plan development in, 839–841, *840*, *841*
initial child-caregiver observation in, 836–837
setting/timing determination in, 835–836
stressor/support assesssment in, 837–838
treatment regimen evaluation in, 841
social support in, 832–833

FAS (fetal alcohol syndrome), 798
mental retardation in, impairments with, 464(t)
myelomeningocele with, 574

Fat, body. See *Body fat*.

Feedback, extrinsic, 171–172
in cerebral palsy therapy, 503
in motor learning, 159, 171–173
precision of, 172
timing of, 172–173, *174*
in motor teaching, clinical example of, 177
intrinsic, 171–172
kinesthetic, in developmental coordination disorder, 432
visual, in developmental coordination disorder, 432

Feedback delay, 173, *174*

Feedforward, in cerebral palsy therapy, 503
in motor control, 45–46
in motor learning, 159

Feeding, in acute childhood spinal muscular atrophy, 315
in bronchopulmonary dysplasia, 668
in cerebral palsy, 497, 504–505
in congenital heart disease, 753
in premature infants, 811
with assistive technology, 631

Fees, for private practice, determination of, 883

FEF$_{25-75\%}$, assessment of, in cystic fibrosis, 694
in asthma, 720, 720(t)

Femoral anteversion, 118, *355*, 355–356, 579, *580*
treatment of, 356, *357*

Femoral head, avascular necrosis of, sports-related, 407
deformity of, factors in, 117

Femoral neck, anteversion of, in myelomeningocele, 579, *580*

Femoral retroversion, *355*, 355–356

Femur, antetorsion of, excessive, in cerebral palsy, 99, *99*

FES (functional electrical stimulation), in myelomeningocele, case history of, 616
in spinal cord injury, 538–539

FET (forced expiration technique), in cystic fibrosis management, 703

Fetal abstinence syndrome, 798–799

Fetal alcohol syndrome (FAS), 798
mental retardation in, impairments with, 464(t)
myelomeningocele with, 574

Fetters, L., 29, 56, 57

Fetus, position of, and skeletal deformities, 117

FEV$_1$, assessment of, in cystic fibrosis, 694
in asthma, 719, 720, 720(t)

FEV$_3$, assessment of, in cystic fibrosis, 694

Fibula, distal, sports injuries of, 409, *410*

Fick equation, 130
in pathologic conditions, 138, *138*

Fidgety movements, 19, 67

Field testing, in pre–sports participation examination, 389, 390(t), 391(t)

Figure-eight harness, for upper extremity prostheses, 344

Figure-ground deficit, 553

Filamentary resting tension hypothesis, 109

FIM (Functional Independence Measure), in spinal cord injury assessment, 533, 537

Financial resources, in private practice business plan, 881–883
maintenance of, 886–888, *887*

Fingers, jammed, sports-related, 406

Fitness, cardiovascular, in spinal cord injury, 539
components of, in children, 148–149, 148(t), *149*
health-related, 127–134, 128(t), 132(t), 133(t)
characteristics of, 127–128, 128(t)
components of, 130
in asthma, 722, 725–726, 729–730
in congenital heart disease, 756
in cystic fibrosis, 704, 708–709
in myelodysplasia, 610
lack of, and sports injuries, 385
level of, in juvenile rheumatoid arthritis, 219, 220(t)
motor, definition of, 127
physical. See *Physical fitness*.
program for, in disabled athletes, 412

FITNESSGRAM Program, 132–134, 133(t)
body composition standards of, 147
one-mile walk-run standards of, 137, 137(t)
sit and reach test standards of, 145
sit-up standards of, 141, 141(t)

Fitts' law, 40

Five-year-old child, functional abilities of, 26

Fixator, external, in burn management, 774, *774*

Flat foot, 361
assessment of, 361
differential diagnosis of, 361
treatment of, 361

Flexed arm hang, in muscular strength/endurance measurement, 141–142

Flexibility. See also *Contracture(s)*; *Range of motion (ROM)*
assessment of, in disabilities, 145
criterion measure of, 143
development of, physical activities in, 145